Marine Polysaccharides
Volume 3

Special Issue Editor
Paola Laurienzo

MDPI • Basel • Beijing • Wuhan • Barcelona • Belgrade

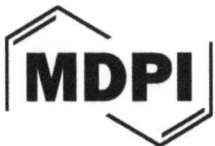

MDPI

Special Issue Editor
Paola Laurienzo
Institute for Polymers, Composites and Biomaterials, CNR
Italy

Editorial Office
MDPI AG
St. Alban-Anlage 66
Basel, Switzerland

This edition is a reprint of the Special Issue published online in the open access journal *Marine Drugs* (ISSN 1660-3397) from 2010–2017 (available at: http://www.mdpi.com/journal/marinedrugs/special_issues/polysaccharides-2010).

For citation purposes, cite each article independently as indicated on the article page online and as indicated below:

Lastname, F.M.; Lastname, F.M. Article title. *Journal Name* **Year**, *Article number, page range.*

First Edition 2018

Volume 3
ISBN 978-3-03842-901-2 (Pbk)
ISBN 978-3-03842-902-9 (PDF)

Volume 1–3
ISBN 978-3-03842-743-8 (Pbk)
ISBN 978-3-03842-744-5 (PDF)

Table of Contents

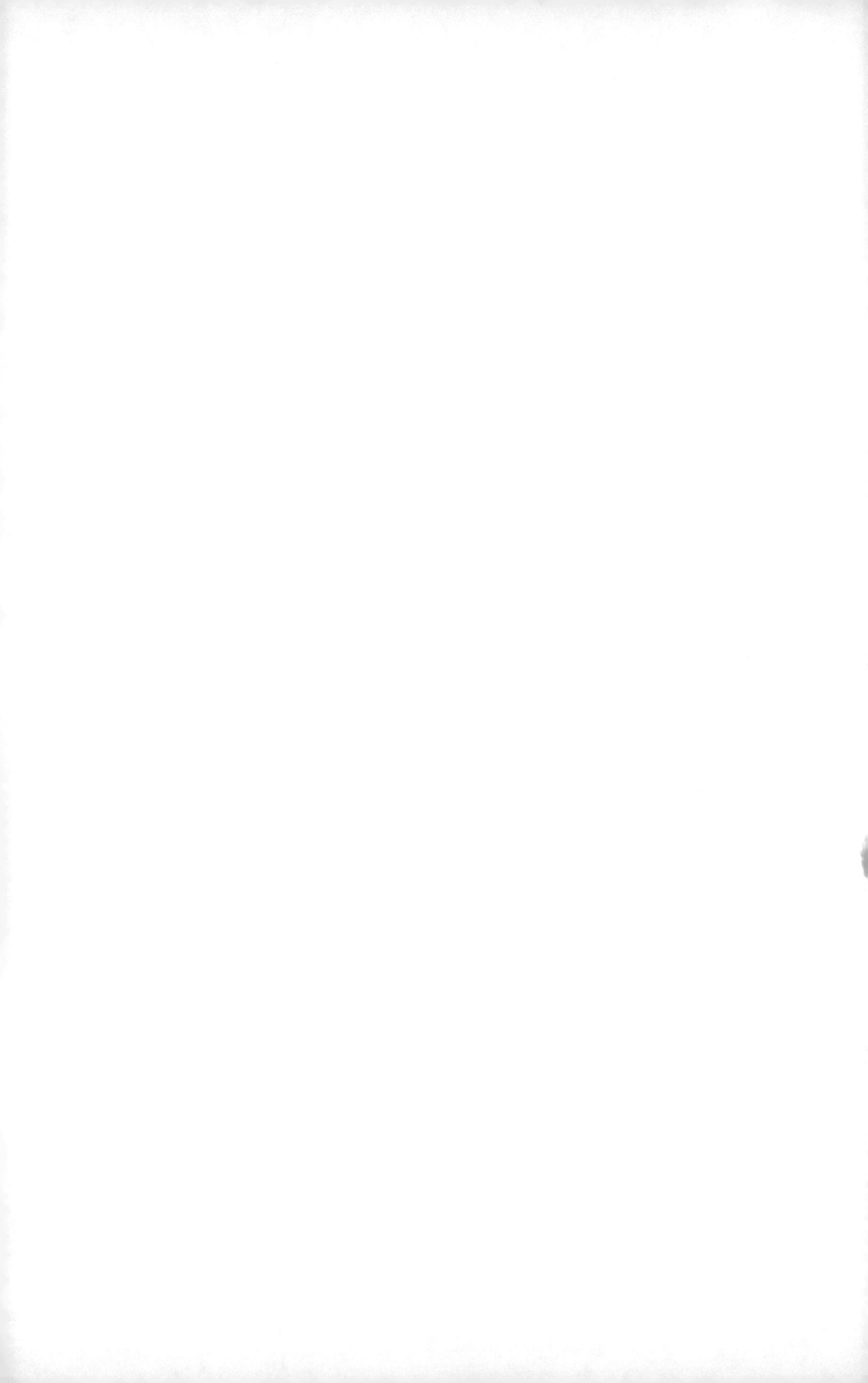

About the Special Issue Editor

Paola Laurienzo grew up in Naples, Italy. In 1983, she graduated in Chemistry at "Federico II" University of Naples. This was followed by a Post-doc position at Italian Research National Council. She was appointed as Researcher at the Institute for Polymers, Composites and Biomaterials (IPCB) of CNR in Pozzuoli (Naples, Italy) in 1986. During the first 15 years, her research activity was mainly devoted to polymer and copolymer synthesis with standard and innovative strategies; chemical modification of synthetic polymers; design and chemical–physical characterization of blends; the study of the structure–properties correlations of multiphase polymeric materials. Innovative films for food packaging, new polymers for applications as components in electro-optical devices, and recycling of plastics from waste through reactive blending were developed technologies. Two national patents were obtained in these years. From the year 2000 onwards, her interests have focused on biodegradable polyesters and natural polysaccharides for applications in tissue engineering, drug delivery, and hydrogels for wound healing. Her experience in the synthesis and chemical modification of polymers has now been extended to the realization of novel amphiphilic copolymers for the design of active targeted polymeric micelles for drug delivery, with a focus on cancer therapy.

Preface to "Marine Polysaccharides"

Volume 1: Advancements in the Discovery of Novel Marine Polysaccharides

The field of marine polysaccharides is constantly evolving, due to progress in the discovery and production of new marine polysaccharides. Seaweed remains the most abundant source of polysaccharides, but recent advances in biotechnology have allowed the production of large quantities of polysaccharides from a variety of micro-algae, by controlling growth conditions and tailoring the production of bioactive compounds in a bioreactor. Of particular interest are polysaccharides produced by micro-organisms from extreme marine environments, due to their recognized different biochemistry. Extracellular polysaccharides (EPSs) with unique properties produced by a number of micro-algae are known. The first volume is a collection of papers concerning the identification and characterization of novel marine polysaccharides. It is divided into three chapters; the first two are dedicated to polysaccharides from different marine sources (algae, micro-algae, animals), while the third one gathers information on the isolation, characterization and bioactivity of new EPSs.

Volume 2: Identification of the Methabolic Pathways Involved in the Biological Activity of Marine Polysaccharides

In the second volume, papers reporting on the elucidation of the mechanisms that underlie the biological activity of some marine polysaccharides are collected. The understanding of the underlying mechanisms is an important feature to give a rigorous scientific support to the potential use of many marine polysaccharides as natural drugs in a wide range of therapies. This volume is divided into three chapters, each of them devoted to a specific class of polysaccharides.

Volume 3: Biomedical and Pharmaceutical Applications of Marine Polysaccharides

Recently-developed technology for production of polysaccharides from marine sources makes their potential use as additives in pharmacological formulations, food supplements, and support material for biomedical implants a real possibility. Although development of low-cost and eco-friendly methods remains a challenge, many companies have developed methodologies for extraction and purification of high quantities of polysaccharides from a variety of natural sources, as confirmed by the high number of trademarks that have been registered to date. Moreover, refinements of technological approaches enable further exploitation of available resources. This volume is a collection of papers focusing on the concrete application of polysaccharides in the biomedical field. In the first chapter, review articles illustrating all the potential applications of polysaccharides are presented. The second chapter includes articles on new methodologies for extraction and purification of polysaccharides of different origins, with particular attention on the evaluation of potential toxicity strictly related to the production process. Finally, in the last chapter, papers dealing with specific examples of biomedical applications are reported. The proposals contained within this collection cover a wide range, including food supplements and services in aquaculture, among others.

Paola Laurienzo
Special Issue Editor

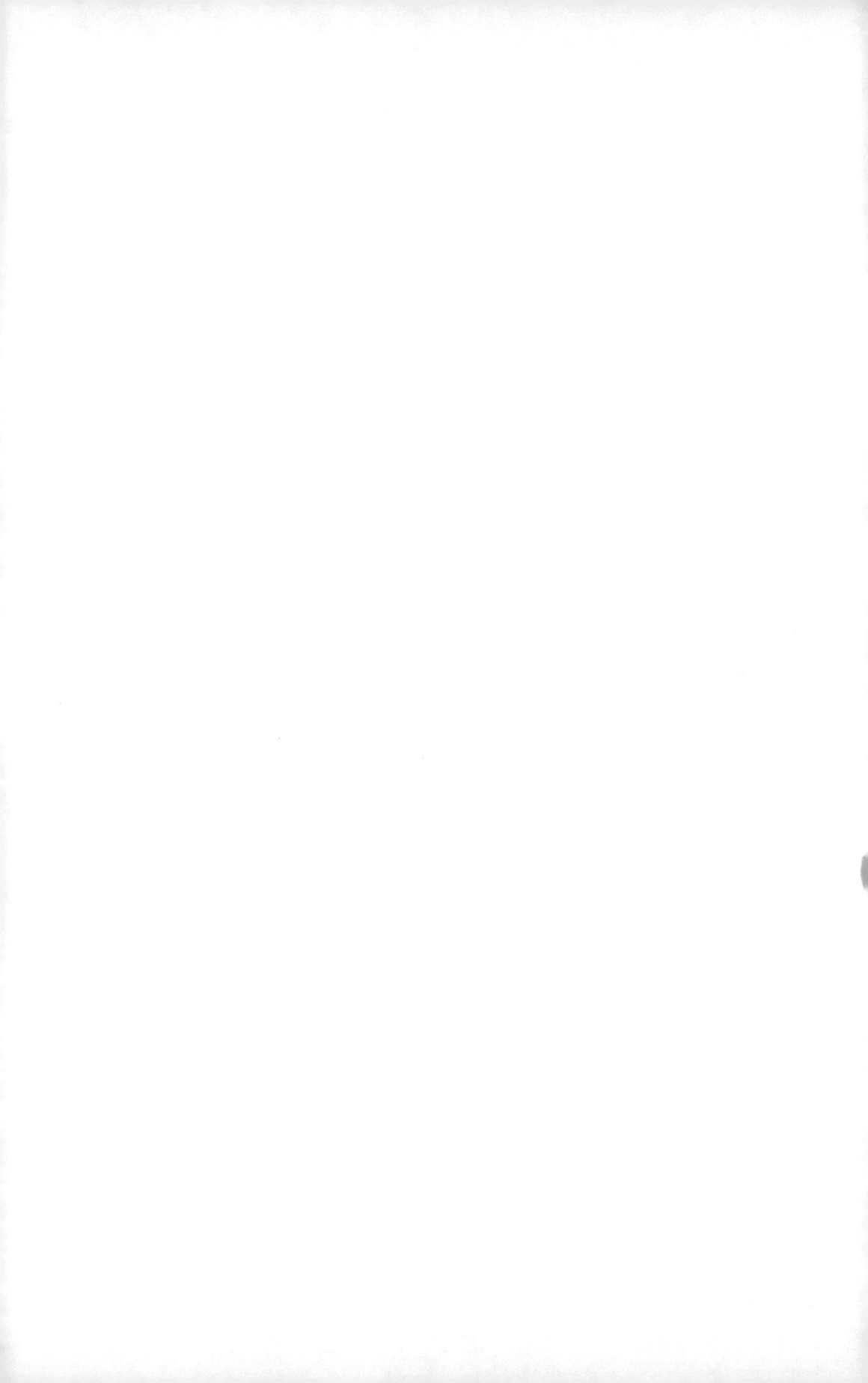

marine drugs

MDPI

Review

Marine Polysaccharides in Pharmaceutical Applications: An Overview

Paola Laurienzo

Institute of Polymers Chemistry and Technology, C.N.R.-Via Campi Flegrei, 34-80078 Pozzuoli (Naples), Italy; paola.laurienzo@ictp.cnr.it

Received: 22 July 2010; in revised form: 19 August 2010; Accepted: 20 August 2010; Published: 2 September 2010

Abstract: The enormous variety of polysaccharides that can be extracted from marine plants and animal organisms or produced by marine bacteria means that the field of marine polysaccharides is constantly evolving. Recent advances in biological techniques allow high levels of polysaccharides of interest to be produced *in vitro*. Biotechnology is a powerful tool to obtain polysaccharides from a variety of micro-organisms, by controlling the growth conditions in a bioreactor while tailoring the production of biologically active compounds. Following an overview of the current knowledge on marine polysaccharides, with special attention to potential pharmaceutical applications and to more recent progress on the discovering of new polysaccharides with biological appealing characteristics, this review will focus on possible strategies for chemical or physical modification aimed to tailor the final properties of interest.

Keywords: chitosan; alginate; agar; carrageenans; exopolysaccharides; chemical modification; drug delivery; gene delivery

1. Introduction

By the early 1950s, an impetus to learn more about marine organisms arose. The earliest biologically active substance of marine origin was a toxin named holothurin, which was extracted by Nigrelli from a marine organism, the *Actinopyga agassizi* [1]. Holothurin showed some antitumor activities in mice. Since then, the search for drugs and natural products of interest from marine organisms has continued.

The field of natural polysaccharides of marine origin is already large and expanding. Seaweeds are the most abundant source of polysaccharides, as alginates, agar and agarose as well as carrageenans. Table 1 gives an idea of the significant market of these polymers. Even cellulose and amylose have been extracted from the macroalga *ULVA*, which is present along the coasts of Mediterranean Sea and in many lagoons including that of Venice [2]. Chitin and chitosan are derived from the exoskeleton of marine crustaceans.

Table 1. Polymers from macro-algae: 2003 market data [3].

Product	Production (t y^{-1})	Algae Harvested (t y^{-1})	Comments
Carrageenan	33,000	168,400	Mainly *Eucheuma* and *Kappaphycus*
Alginate	30,000	126,500	*Laminaria, Macrocystis, Lessonia, Ascophyllum* and others
Agar	7,630	55,650	Mainly *Gelidium* and *Gracilaria*

Recently, microalgae have become particularly interesting because of the possibility to easily control the growth conditions in a bioreactor together with the demonstrated biochemical diversity of these organisms. Greater screening and selection efforts for biologically active compounds, including polysaccharides, have been developed [4]. Examples of microalgae with commercial value are the unicellular red algae *Porphyridium cruemtum* and *P. aerugineum*, because of the large quantities of extracellular polysaccharides they produce [5]. Lewis [6] screened a number of *Chlamidomonas* spp. for extracellular polysaccharide production. The most useful of these is *C. mexicana*, which yields up to 25% of its total organic production as polysaccharides. Moore and Tischer [7] have also reported high extracellular production levels for a number of green and blue-green algae. A number of patents have been issued concerning the production methods and applications for the *Porphyridium* polysaccharide [8]. The *Porphyridium* polysaccharide could also replace existing polysaccharide polymers such as carrageenan in biomedical applications.

Interest is particularly growing towards extreme marine environments. It is obvious that the various extreme marine habitats (deep-sea hydrothermal vents, cold seeps, coastal hot springs, polar regions, hypersaline ponds, *etc.*) should represent a huge source of unknown and uncultivated bacteria. Many microbial exopolysaccharides (EPSs) produced by such extreme bacteria have unique properties; the bacteria must adopt special metabolic pathways to survive in extreme conditions, and so have better capacity to produce special bioactive compounds, including EPSs, than any other microorganisms. Moreover, many thermophylic and hyperthermophylic bacteria can produce EPS under laboratory conditions.

The present review focuses on progress in discovering and producing new marine polysaccharides of interest in pharmaceuticals. The more innovative and appealing fields of application and strategies for their modification are reported. Finally, an updating of recent literature on the more common marine polysaccharides is reported.

2. Production, Applications and Modification Strategies of Marine Polysaccharides

2.1. Biotechnology of Marine Extremophylic Bacteria

The current opinion of most of the scientific community throughout the world is that knowledge of biochemical processes that adapted in extreme marine environments is the basis for discoveries in biotechnology. The fields of biotechnology that could benefit from miming the extremophiles are very broad and cover the search for new bioactive compounds for industrial, agricultural, environmental, pharmaceutical and medical uses. However, this potential remains to a large extent unexplored and, in respect of the drugs available on the market, only 30% have been developed from natural products and so far less than 10% have been isolated from marine organisms.

Also, if difficulties in culturing marine organisms in the laboratory hold still true today [9, 10], the process of industrialization of the microbial products is under recent exploitation. Marine microorganisms are now considered as efficient producers of biologically active and/or chemically novel compounds, and no "supply issue" will appear since scaled-up productions can normally be achieved through bioreactors of any capacity that can be designed nowadays [11,12]. Investigations in shake flasks are conducted with the prospect of large-scale processing in reactors.

Different bioprocess engineering approaches are used for the production of polysaccharides from microorganisms. The major modes of operation in laboratory bioreactors and pilot implants are batch, fed-batch and continuous. Batch growth refers to culturing in a vessel with an initial charge of medium that is not altered by further nutrient addition or removal. This form of cultivation is simple and widely used both in the laboratory and industrially. Growth, product formation and substrate utilization terminate after a certain time interval. Submerged processes, where the organism is grown in a liquid medium, immobilized systems, in which the producing microorganism is restricted in a fixed space, and solid-state processes cultivations, in which the bioprocess is operated at low moisture levels or water activities, are widely employed in batch mode. In a continuous process, fresh nutrient medium is continually added to a well-stirred culture and products and cells are simultaneously withdrawn. Growth and product formation can be maintained for prolonged periods, and the system usually reaches a steady state after a certain period of time. Continuous processes have been used with suspended cells as well as with immobilized cells. In fed-batch culture, nutrients are continuously or semi-continuously fed, while effluent is removed discontinuously. This type of operation is intermediate between batch and continuous processes, increasing the duration of batch cultivation and the overall reactor productivity. The fed-batch process is also applied in several bioprocesses.

2.2. Hydrogels and Superporous Hydrogels

Hydrogels based on cross-linked polysaccharides are used in key applications, such as drug delivery systems and tissue engineering. Polysaccharides may also form superabsorbent/superporous hydrogels. Superabsorbent hydrogels are hydrogels having a swelling ratio of a few hundred, and superporous hydrogels are furthermore characterized by interconnected pores with diameters on the micron to millimeter scale. Due to the presence of such big and interconnected pores, superporous hydrogels absorb a considerable amount of water in a very short period of time. These novel products may find applications in the development of drug and protein delivery systems, fast-dissolving tablets, occlusion devices for aneurysm treatment, scaffolding, cell culture, tissue engineering, hygiene products and many others [13].

Sodium alginate, chitosan, agar and carragenaan, in combination with polyacrylics such as poly(acrylic acid) and/or poly(acrylamide), form interpenetrating networks that give rise to superabsorbent and superporous hydrogels of enhanced elasticity [14,16]. Hybrid hydrogels are multi-functional, as their properties depend on cross-linking density and medium pH, and their potential for controlled release is under investigation [17]. Alternatively, polysaccharides have been cross-linked by diacrylates also leading to superabsorbent and/or superporous full-polysaccharide hydrogels [18].

2.3. Bioadhesivs and Mucoadhesives from Marine Sources

Natural bioadhesives are polymeric materials that may consist of a variety of substances, but proteins and polysaccharides feature prominently. Many actives can be released via bioadhesives, as steroids, anti-inflammatory agents, pH sensitive peptides and small proteins such as insulin, and local treatments to alleviate pain in the buccal cavity. Requirements for a successful bioadhesive device for topical administration of active agents for prolonged periods of time are:

- maintain intimate contact with the site of application for 1 to 24 hours;
- be sufficiently adhesive and cohesive;
- guarantee controlled delivery of the active ingredients in wet and moist environments;
- be non-toxic, non irritating;
- be easily removable.

Mucosal membranes are lined by epithelial or endothelial cells having "tight junctions" (physiologically connect the enterocytes apically). Membranes are located in or on the skin, ear, eye, nose, gastrointestinal tract. Mucosa have limited permeability to therapeutic agents, especially if the molecular weight is higher than 500 Daltons, thus including most peptides and proteins.

The tenacity with which marine algae cling to ships' hulls and underwater constructions suggests a remarkable water-resistant adhesive capability. Responsible for fouling growths that reduce efficiency and cause costly damage, they are highly resistant to mechanical removal and all but the most environmentally unacceptable chemical preventive agents. The responsible bioadhesives have extraordinarily high cohesive strength and binding strength to the solid surfaces, enabling the organisms to remain attached under tensional conditions that are, as a matter of fact, comparable to those found in a surgical environment. These qualities have indicated that this is a promising avenue of research in the hunt for more effective tissue adhesives for medical use, for example, surgery closures and bone glue, to replace painful traditional wound closure methods in the first case, and the use of metallic screws in the last one. Various algal bioadhesives have been isolated and characterized to find a safe and efficient candidate to be tested for use on human tissues. They are essentially based on gluing proteins; new formulations comprising polyphenolic proteins from mussels and marine origin polysaccharides are promising, especially as adhesive in ophthalmic therapies.

A bioadhesive system based exclusively on polysaccharides and potentially useful for bone glue has been recently proposed by Hoffmann *et al.* [19]. The authors developed a two-component system based on chitosan and oxidized dextran or starch. The bonding mechanism employs the reaction of aldehyde groups with amino groups in the presence of water, which covalently bind to each other in a Schiff's base reaction. Chitosan was chosen as amino carrier, and was previously partially depolymerized with acid treatment to obtain a higher ratio between amino and aminoacetyl groups. Aldehyde groups on starch or dextran are generated by oxidation with periodates. In addition, L-DOPA, an important element of mussel adhesives [20,22], was first conjugated to oxidized dextran or starch in analogy to the gluing mechanism of mussels and then oxidized to quinone. The quinone structure of L-DOPA, which is covalently bound to the aldehydes on dextran/starch, can also react with amino groups of chitosan by an imine formation or a Michael adduct formation. All of these reactions result in a strong adhesive force within the glue. With respect to fibrin glue and cyanoacrylate adhesives, which are currently used in clinical practice, biomechanical studies revealed that the new glue is superior to fibrin glue, but has less adhesive strength than cyanoacrylates. Nonetheless, cyanoacrylates, besides having toxic side effects [23], are not resorbable and thus inhibit endogenous bone repair. In conclusion, because both components are natural, biodegradable polysaccharides, without any cytotoxic effects, this bioadhesive seems to be a good candidate for bone or soft tissue gluing applications in surgery.

2.4. General Strategies of Modification of Marine Polysaccharides

Natural polysaccharides can play a relevant role in biomedical and pharmaceutical applications, particularly in the field of drug delivery, for their intrinsic biocompatibility and potential low cost. Nevertheless, the properties of such materials sometimes do not fulfill the requirements for specific applications; hence, the development of strategies aiming to chemically and/or physically modify their structure and, consequently, their physical–chemical properties is gaining increasing interest [24,25].

2.4.1. Blending

The technique of blending is particularly attractive as it allows tailoring the properties of interest of the final material in a controlled manner while using polymers already known and widely accepted in the pharmaceutical field. Properties such as biodegradation rate, adhesion to biological substrates, drug solubility inside the polymer matrix, can be modified and tailored to specific applications by simple blending. Further improvements of polymer blends are obtained through (a) addition of a third component, usually a block or graft copolymer, to impart compatibility between the two polymers; (b) chemical modification of one component aimed to create specific interactions with the other one. These strategies can solve problems arising from a bad interaction between the two polymers.

Biodegradable polymer blends usually consist in mixing natural and synthetic biodegradable polymers. Most of polysaccharides are polydispersed in terms of the molecular mass, so they are more similar to synthetic polymers than to biopolymers such as proteins and nucleic acids. Blends based on polysaccharides with natural and synthetic polymers are reported [26]. Blends of alginate with polyvinyl alcohol, a synthetic polymer that has good susceptibility to biodegradation, are proposed due to their good compatibility [27,28]. Addition of glycerol as a natural plasticizer to improve mechanical performances of alginate-based biofilms is also of interest [29].

Blends of different polysaccharides present the advantage that the components are highly compatible, and very homogeneous materials are obtained. Interesting results were obtained for alginate/chitosan blends in which chitosan was previously modified by reaction of part of the amine functionalities with succinic anhydride in order to impart solubility at neutral pH, making it possible to prepare blends of the two polymers from water solution [30,31]. Such blends show a synergistic effect of the chitosan in chelating calcium ions during the alginate gelation process, which in turn results in improved mechanical properties of the corresponding hydrogels. Materials based on such alginate/chitosan blends containing calcium sulfate as osteoinductive phase are promising for applications in bone regeneration [32].

Blends with agar are of interest due to its ability to form reversible gels simply by cooling hot aqueous solutions. This gel-forming property makes blends of agar with biocompatible polysaccharides or synthetic polymers very appealing. Blends with agar usually improve the gelation properties and water-holding capacity of the other polysaccharide component, and the obtained gels are not as strong and brittle as pure agar gels. These characteristics widen the field of potential interest of agar in biomedical applications. Blends of agar with alginate give films that are more flexible and easy to manage than pure agar, and moreover allow modulation of water permeability as a function of the blend composition, and have been proposed for dehydration of fresh fruits [33].

2.4.2. Chemical Modifications

Novel materials based on polysaccharides are being intensively sought, both through bulk and surface modifications. The chemical modification of chitin to produce chitosan represents the most fundamental process in this essay. This chemical modification is in fact particularly simple, since it just involves the hydrolysis of an amide moiety to generate the corresponding primary amino function. As in all polymer modifications, the ideal 100% conversion is very hard to achieve, and chitosans are therefore a whole family of polymers, characterized by their average molecular weight and their degree of deacetylation, *i.e.*, the percentage of amide groups converted into NH2 counterparts.

The ubiquitous hydroxyl groups in polysaccharides are the most obvious source of chemical modification that has been exploited, although all other functionalities present on polysaccharides (amino, acid, carboxylate) have been used for chemical reactions. A variety of chemical modifications (theoretically, all the reactions involving these functional groups may be performed on polysaccharides) have been realized. Hydroxyls are used for oxidation reactions with peroxide to generate the more reactive aldehyde groups, for esterification with acid or anhydrides to reduce hydrophylicity, for sulfonation reactions with a variety of sulfonating agents, for bromination or chlorination. Amino groups are more reactive than hydroxyls, so they must be protected to selectively address the reaction onto hydroxyls. Amines are specifically used for aqueous carbodiimide chemistry. Modified polysaccharides are used as such or employed for successive reactions, including copolymerization. Several examples of the more explored chemical reactions that involve hydroxyls as well as other groups on polysaccharides, widely employed to modify properties such as solubility, to impart novel characteristics to the plain polymer, or to create sites for specific binding or interactions with other molecules of biological interest, are hereafter reported.

2.4.2.1. Hydrophobic Modification

Hydrophilic polymers modified by hydrophobic moieties represent a combination of surfactant and polymer properties in one molecule. As a consequence, they self-associate in aqueous solution to form complex micellar structures. This feature can be of interest for medical diagnosis application, as micelles are used as coating of colloidal metal particles for labeling biomolecules in immunological assays [34].

Hydrophobically-modified polysaccharides are polysaccharides partially modified by cholesterol or other hydrophobic moieties. They are used as coating to stabilize liposomes for chemotherapy and immunotherapy [35]. A selective uptake by cancer cells, particularly by human colon and lung cancer cells, has been shown by liposomes coated with cholesterol derivatives of polysaccharides bearing 1-aminolactose [36]. Different cholesterol-linked celluloses of various origins, intended for applications as bile acid/cholesterol sequestrants, were prepared by reaction with monocholesteryl succinate [37]. The authors found that the introduction of a mesogenic substituent may induce a thermotropic behavior with formation of a mesophase. It has been also supposed that thermotropic cholesterol derivatives of polysaccharides would have even enhanced bile acid/cholesterol sequestration, probably through mixed mesophase formation with the free bile acids/cholesterol.

2.4.2.2. Depolymerization

Depolymerization is often used to reduce molecular weight in view of specific applications, overall as patches for controlled release of drugs, because low molecular weight polymers have an increased amount of polar end groups. The patches are adhesives based on chemically and physically modified polysaccharides, which are partially depolymerized to provide a more effective topical and transdermal drug delivery system. Such patches were really found to be highly adhesive while providing superior drug penetration.

Classical depolymerization methods include ozonolysis in aqueous solutions [38], oxidative depolymerization induced by oxygen radical generating systems [39,40], specific enzymatic degradation [41]. A recent patent reports on a method for carrying out a targeted depolymerization of polysaccharides at increased temperatures, producing simultaneously polysaccharide derivatives with a desired degree of polymerization [42]. The molecular weight of polysaccharides can be also reduced through chemical hydrolysis, ionizing radiation or electronic beam radiation [43,45].

2.4.2.3. Sulfation

Sulfated polysaccharides are polysaccharides containing high amounts of sulfate groups. They can be found in nature, but a lot of sulfated polysaccharides have been obtained by chemical modification. As sulfonating agents, sulfur trioxide-pyridin, piperidine-*N*-sulfonic acid, sodium sulfite and chlorosulfonic acid are the most used. The reaction may involve all the hydroxyls (primary and secondary) and the amines eventually present on polysaccharide, or it can be targeted to a specific site. Sulfated polysaccharides are known to have anti-retroviral [46] and/or antimalarial activity [47]. This last can further be enhanced by a combination with artemisinin or its di-hydro derivative [48]. Sulfated chitin and chitosan are found to be efficient carriers to deliver therapeutic agents across a mucosal membrane [49].

A method for inhibiting or decreasing intestinal cholesterol and fatty acids absorption in man by oral administration of synthetic sulfated polysaccharides has been the matter of an American Patent [50]. The invention is based upon the discovery that sulfated polysaccharides are potent inhibitors of human pancreatic cholesterol esterase, the enzyme responsible for promoting the intestinal absorption of cholesterol and fatty acids. A variety of polysaccharide polymers can be sulfated to produce potent inhibitors of human pancreatic cholesterol esterase. Increasing inhibitory activities are realized from increased molecular weights and sulfation at a specific position; increased efficacy is obtained by reducing absorption of the polysaccharides. Accordingly, the methodology includes non-absorbable sulfated polysaccharides having a molecular weight greater than 10 kDa; furthermore, the presence of a 3-sulfate on the sugar ring markedly enhances inhibition. Alginic acid, chitin and chitosan, agar, as well as other abundant and cheap natural polysaccharides as pectin (from vegetables and fruits), dextran and cellulose (from plants and trees), have been reacted in a controlled manner to produce sulfated derivatives. These derivatives are all water soluble, potent inhibitors of human pancreatic cholesterol esterase, whereas the parent starting polymers are either not inhibitory or poorly inhibitory. These sulfated polysaccharides can be administrated orally in pharmaceutical forms such as tablets, capsules, liquids and powders. Sulfation of polysaccharides was obtained by reaction with sulfur trioxide-pyridin. In the case of alginic acid, the reaction was performed directly on native polymer, or on the oxidized polymer, or on the product of oxidation followed by reductive amination of the native alginic acid, leading to different levels of sulfation (Figure 1). For chitin and chitosan, it is possible to target the reaction on two sites or on only one specific site, following different routes of synthesis (Figure 2).

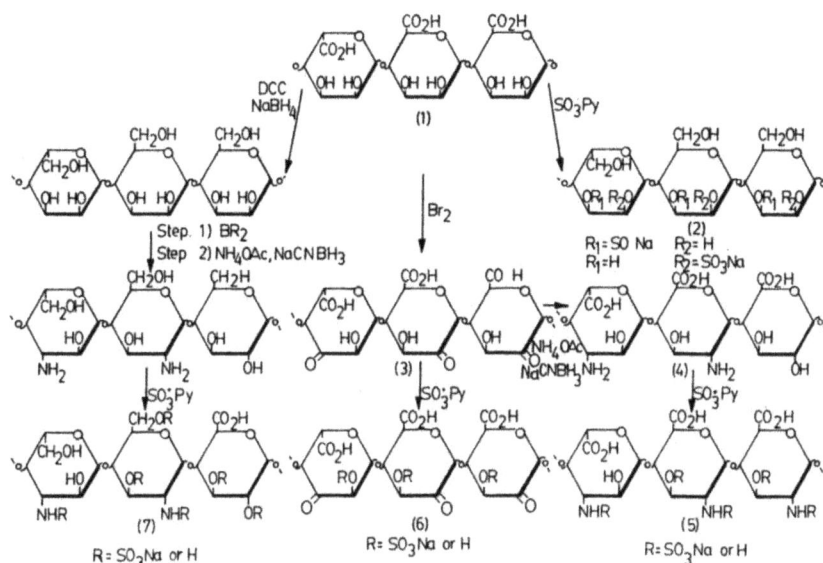

Figure 1. The synthetic strategy for preparing alginic acid sulfated derivatives.

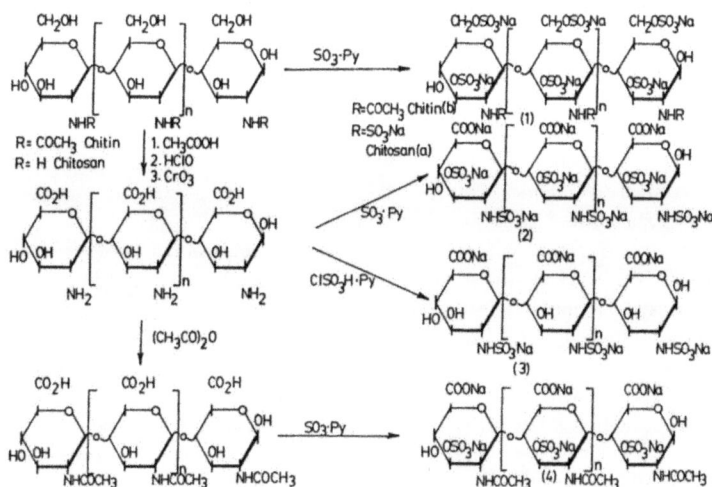

Figure 2. The synthetic strategy for preparing chitin and chitosan sulfated derivatives [50].

3. Examples of Applications of More Abundant Marine Polysaccharides in Pharmaceuticals

3.1. Alginate

Alginate is a natural occurring polysaccharide of guluronic (G) and mannuronic (M) acid, quite abundant in nature as structural component in marine brown algae (*Phaeophyceae*) and as capsular polysaccharides in soil bacteria. Brown algal biomass generally consists of mineral or inorganic components and organic components, these last mainly composed by alginates, fucans, and other carbohydrates. The isolating process of alginates from brown algal biomass is simple, including stages of pre-extraction with hydrochloric acid, followed by washing, filtration, and neutralization with alkali.

Sodium alginate is precipitated from the solution by alcohol (isopropanol or ethanol) and usually re-precipitated (to achieve higher purity) in the same way. However, the real processing scheme for alginate production is quite complicated, including 15 steps [51].

Alginate instantaneously forms gel-spheres at pH > 6 by ionotropic gelation with divalent cations such as Ca2+ [52], Ba2+, or Zn2+ and for this it is widely used for microencapsulation of drugs. On the other hand, at low pH, hydration of alginic acid leads to the formation of a high-viscosity "acid gel". The ability of alginate to form two types of gel dependent on pH, *i.e.*, an acid gel and an ionotropic gel, gives the polymer unique properties compared to neutral macromolecules, and it can be tailor-made for a number of applications.

The microencapsulation technique has been developed particularly for the oral delivery of proteins, as they are quickly denatured and degraded in the hostile environment of the stomach. The protein is encapsulated in a core material that, in turn, is coated with a biocompatible, semi permeable membrane, which controls the release rate of the protein while protecting it from biodegradation. Due to its mild gelation conditions at neutral pH, alginate gel can act as core material in this application, while poly(ethylene glycol) (PEG), which exhibits properties such as protein resistance, low toxicity and immunogenicity [53], together with the ability of preserving the biological properties of proteins [54,55], can act as a coating membrane. A chitosan/PEG-alginate microencapsulation process [56], applied to biological macromolecules such as albumin or hirudin [57], was reported to be a good candidate for oral delivery of bioactive peptides.

Several examples of alginate-encapsulated drugs, other than proteins, can also be found in literature. Qurrat-ul-Ain *et al.* [58] reported that alginate microparticles showed better drug bioavailability and reduction of systemic side effects compared with free drugs in the treatment of tuberculosis. Polyelectrolyte coating of alginate microspheres showed to be a promising tool to achieve release systems characterized by approximately zero-order release kinetics, release up to 100% of entrapped drug (dexamethasone) within 1 month, and improved biocompatibility [59].

Composites technology has been applied to alginate for drug delivery purposes. As an example, montmorillonite-alginate nanocomposites have been recently proposed as a system for sustained release of B1 and B6 vitamines [60]. The vitamins intercalated in the nanocrystals of the inorganic phase, and successively the hybrid B1/B6 montmorillonite (MMT) is further used for the synthesis of B1/B6-MMT-alginate nanocomposite.

In their simplest design, oral controlled-release dosage forms made from alginates are monolithic tablets in which the drug is homogeneously dispersed. Drug release is controlled by the formation of a hydrated viscous layer around the tablet, which acts as a diffusional barrier to drug diffusion and water penetration. Water soluble drugs are mainly released by diffusion of dissolved drug molecules across the gel layer, while poorly soluble drugs are mainly released by erosion mechanisms. Modulation of drug release rate has been achieved by incorporating pH-independent hydrocolloids gelling agents or adding polycationic hydrocolloids such as chitosan [61,62]. A number of mucoadhesive systems based on alginate have been developed [63,64]. The main shortcoming of alginates consists in their rapid erosion at neutral pH; furthermore, the adhesion to mucosal tissues is reduced when cross-linked with divalent cations. Alginates have been extensively used to modify the performances of other polysaccharides, such as chitosan, through the realization of alginate coated chitosan microspheres [65]. In the literature, it is also possible to find acrylic modified polysaccharides developed with the aim to obtain a finer control over release rate or to improve adhesive properties [66,67].

The modification of sodium alginate with amine and/or acid moieties with the aim to optimize their properties for drug delivery applications by modulating the time of erosion, the rate of release of drugs, and the adhesion to substrates has been attempted by Laurienzo *et al.* [68]. In this article, graft copolymers based on alginate and acrylic polymers were synthesized by radical polymerization of the acrylic monomers or oligomers in the presence of sodium alginate. The authors found that the modification of alginate network significantly affects water uptake and erosion rate of matrices prepared by direct compression. As a consequence, the release rate and mechanism of a highly soluble-low molecular weight drug was found to be controlled mainly by either a diffusion/erosion or erosion mechanism, depending on polymer type and medium pH. Furthermore, they found increased adhesive properties of the copolymers, and concluded that they might be good candidates in formulations for mucoadhesive systems for the treatment of heartburn and acid reflux, because of the possibility to improve the gastric protective coating action.

Hydrophobically-modified alginates can be prepared by oxidation followed by reductive amination of the 2,3-dialdehydic alginate [69]. The ability of alginate to bind cations renders these modified alginates interesting as biosurfactants environmentally friendly for the removal of organics and metal divalent cations.

Among the possible applications of alginate gel systems, one of the most promising is for tissue regeneration. The main drawback of alginate matrix gels is represented by their high density of network, which limits the cell growth [70]; moreover, cell anchorage, a strict requirement for proliferation and tissue formation, is limited on alginate gels, because of its hydrophilic nature. PEG copolymers are used to improve the biocompatibility of polysaccharides. Several PEG-alginate systems for cell entrapment have been reported [71]; recently, a new alginate-g-PEG copolymer has been described [72]. The synthesis goes via hydrophobization of alginate with alkylic amines; successively, the secondary amines grafted onto the alginate react with a low molecular weight PEG functionalized with a carboxylic acid group at one end, to produce an alginate-g-PEG copolymer. As the reactions do not involve the carboxylic acid groups of the alginate, the ability to cross-link via ionic interactions is retained. The obtained copolymers show the double function to form micelles in water above a critical concentration and to form gels with divalent cations.

Alginate for Wound Healing

Alginate dressings for wound healing have been successfully applied for many years to cleanse a wide variety of secreting lesions, and they still remain widely used in many circumstances. Alginate gels dressings are highly absorbent, and this limits wound secretions and minimizes bacterial contamination. Alginate fibers trapped in a wound are readily biodegraded [73]. Alginate dressings maintain a physiologically moist microenvironment that promotes healing and the formation of granulation tissue. Alginates can be rinsed away with saline irrigation, so removal of the dressing does not interfere with healing granulation tissue. This makes dressing changes virtually painless. Alginate dressings are very useful for moderate to heavily exudating wounds [74].

The healing of cutaneous ulcers requires the development of a vascularized granular tissue bed, the filling of large tissue defects by dermal regeneration, and the restoration of a continuous epidermal keratocyte layer. These processes were modeled *in vitro* in one study utilizing human dermal fibroblasts, microvascular endothelial cells (HMEC), and keratocyte cultures [75]. In this study, the calcium alginate was found to increase the proliferation of fibroblasts but decreased the proliferation of HMEC and keratocytes. In contrast, the calcium alginate decreased fibroblast motility but had no effect on keratinocyte motility. There was no significant effect of calcium alginate on the formation of capillary-like structures by HMEC. The effects of calcium alginate on cell proliferation and migration may have been mediated by released calcium ions. These results suggest that the calcium alginate tested may improve some cellular aspects, but not others.

Alginates have been shown to be useful also as hemostatic agents for cavity wounds [76]. A study compared the effects of calcium and zinc containing alginates and non-alginate dressings on blood coagulation and platelet activation [77]. The study showed that alginate materials activated coagulation more than non-alginate materials. The extent of coagulation activation was affected differently by the alginate M or G group concentration. Moreover, it was demonstrated that alginates containing zinc ions had the greatest potentiating effect on prothrombotic coagulation and platelet activation. However, there has been one report of a florid foreign body reaction after the use of an alginate dressing to obtain hemostasis in an apicectomy cavity. The case suggests that alginate fibers left *in situ* may elicit a long-lasting and symptomatic adverse foreign body reaction [78].

3.2. Chitosan

Chitosan is a copolymer of β-(1→4)-linked 2-acetamido-2-deoxy-D-glucopyranose and 2-amino-2-deoxy-D-glucopyranose. It is obtained by deacethylation of the natural occurring chitin. Chitin is extracted from the exoskeleton of marine organisms, mainly crabs and shrimps, as described by Burrows [79]. Briefly, the exoskeletons are crushed and washed, then treated with boiling sodium hydroxide to dissolve the proteins and sugars, thus isolating the crude chitin. The major applications of chitosan are in biomaterials, pharmaceuticals, cosmetics, metal ion sequestration, agriculture, and foodstuff treatment (flocculation, clarification, *etc.*, because of its efficient interaction with other polyelectrolytes). Development of chitosan chemistry is relevant in biomedical science, particularly in the topic of drug delivery [80,81]. Unlike its precursor chitin, which is insoluble in most common solvents, chitosan can readily be spun into fibers, cast into films, or precipitated in a variety of micromorphologies from its acidic aqueous solutions. Electrospinning from acetic acid solutions to provide nanofibers has also been reported [82]. The excellent ability to form porous structures simply by freezing and lyophilizing its solutions, or by simple techniques such as "internal bubble process" [83], makes chitosan a versatile biopolymer for tissue engineering, particularly in orthopedics for cartilage [84] and bone regeneration [85]. Possible chitosan matrix preparations for cell cultures include gels [86], sponges [87], fibers [88], or porous compositions of chitosan with ceramic [89] or other polymeric materials such as collagen or gelatin [90,91]. Chitosan has been combined with a variety of materials such as alginate, hydroxyapatite, hyaluronic acid, calcium phosphate, PMMA, poly-L-lactic acid (PLLA), and growth factors for potential application in cell-based tissue engineering [92]. Alginate is a candidate biomaterial for cartilage engineering but exhibits weak cell adherence. Iwasaki *et al.* [93] reported on alginate-based chitosan hybrid polymer fibers which showed increased cell attachment and proliferation *in vitro* compared to alginate fibers. In addition, when it is combined with alginates the system acts as a biomimetic membrane which controls the release of bioactive macromolecules such as hirudin [94]. Interpenetrated polymer networks (IPNs) of chitosan and poly(acrylic acid) (PAA) for applications as biodegradable filling systems and controlled release devices have been prepared by radical polymerization of acrylic acid in the presence of chitosan [95].

In orthopedics, chitosan is used as an adjuvant with bone cements to increase their injectability while keeping the chemical-physical properties (time setting and mechanical characteristics) suitable for surgical use [96].

Chitosan can be modified in order to improve compatibility in blends with other polymers and to impart solubility in water or in common organic solvents such as chloroform, pyridine, tetrahydrofuran. Organically soluble derivates of chitosan can be used to formulate by-designed materials for biomedical applications such as polymeric drugs and artificial organs. Acylation, alkylation and phthaloylation reactions have been widely used [97,101]. Novel formulations based on a combination of chitosan with polyol-phosphate salts have allowed neutral solutions to be obtained without any chemical modification of the chitosan [102]. These formulations possess a physiological pH and can be held liquid below room temperature for encapsulating living cells and therapeutic proteins; they form monolithic gels at body temperature. Therefore, when injected *in vivo* the liquid formulations turn into gel implants *in situ*. This system was used successfully to deliver biologically active growth factors *in vivo* as well as an encapsulating matrix for living chondrocytes for tissue engineering applications.

Due to its favorable gelling properties, chitosan can deliver morphogenic factors and pharmaceutical agents in a controlled fashion. Methodologies to produce micro and nanoparticles of chitosan and its derivates for drug delivery include spray-drying and water-in-oil emulsions techniques. Drug release from chitosan microparticles can be controlled by cross-linking the matrix. Microparticles can be cross-linked by chemicals such as glutaraldheyde, genipin, diisocyanates and ethylene glycol diglycidyl ether, or by ionic agents, or by a combination of them [103]. Among chemical agents, genipin, a naturally occurring cross-linker, significantly less cytotoxic than glutaraldehyde [104], has been largely employed for crosslinking of hydrogels and beads. Among ionic agents, tri-polyphosphate (TPP), a non toxic and multivalent polyanion, was reported to form gel by ionic interaction between positively charged amino groups of chitosan and negatively charged counterion of TPP [105,108]. By controlling the pH and the concentration of TPP solutions, cross-linked chitosan microspheres for a potentially controlled release of drugs have been obtained [109]. In alginate-chitosan mixed systems, cross-linked microcapsules are prepared either by dropping a solution of sodium alginate into an acidic solution containing chitosan, or by incubating calcium alginate beads in a chitosan solution, or by dropping a chitosan solution into a TPP solution containing sodium alginate [110].

Many applications have been proposed for chitosan-based delivery devices. Strong electrostatic interactions with mucus open the doors to possible applications as gastrointestinal or nasal delivery systems [111,112]. Additionally, the cationic character of chitosan imparts particular possibilities. pH-sensitive microspheres made of hybrid gelatine/chitosan polymer networks have been developed and showed to release drugs only in acidic medium [113]. A pH-sensitive, chitosan-based hydrogel system for controlled release of protein drugs cross-linked by genipin was developed also by Chen *et al.* [114].

Brush-like copolymers of chitosan with poly(ε-caprolactone) (PCL), polyethylene glycol (PEG) or their copolymers have been prepared following different procedures of synthesis. [115,119]. Such amphiphilic copolymers are able to self-assembly in aqueous solutions. Nanomicelles obtained from chitosan-*g*-PCL copolymers have been successfully tested as carriers of hydrophobic drugs [120].

Chitosan and its derivates or salts have been extensively investigated for alternative routes of administration of insulin, such as oral, nasal, transdermal and buccal delivery systems [121,122]. Chitosan is mucoadhesive and able to protect the insulin from enzymatic degradation, prolong the retention time of insulin, as well as open the inter-epithelial tight junction to facilitate systemic insulin transport. Targeted delivery of insulin is deemed possible in future through using chitosan with specific adhesiveness to the intended absorption mucosa. Water-soluble low molecular weight chitosan renders insulin able to be processed under mild conditions, and sulfated chitosan markedly opens the paracellular channels for insulin transport. The development of insulin carriers using chitosan base and/or its derivates involves many techniques such as nanocomplexation, mixing, solubilization, ionotropic gelation, coacervation, layer-by-layer encapsulation, water-in-oil emulsification, membrane emulsification, lyophilization, compression, capsulation, casting, adsorption and/or absorption processes.

The cationic nature of chitosan allows it to complex DNA molecules, making it an ideal candidate for gene delivery strategies. Chitosan nanoparticles appear to control the release of DNA and prolong its action both *in vitro* and *in vivo* [123,125]. Chitosan in fact provides protection against DNAase degradation [126]. Chitosan was selected also as a coating material, alone or in blends with polyvinylalcohol, for cationic surface modification of biodegradable nanoparticles for gene delivery [127]. These cationic surface modified nanospheres can readily bind DNA by electrostatic interaction, simply mixing their aqueous solutions.

Chitosan nanoparticles have been used also to transport small interfering RNAs (siRNA). The cellular RNA interference machinery is now used in cancer gene therapy to turn off, for instance, oncogene expression. Katas and Alpar [128] first studied the interaction behavior of siRNA and chitosans given that the structure and size of siRNA are quite different to that of pDNA. Studies *in vitro* demonstrated that chitosan nanoparticles are able to mediate gene silencing. Furthermore, the transfection efficiency of RNA depends on its association with chitosan. Indeed, entrapping siRNA using ionic gelation showed a better biological effect than simple complexation or siRNA adsorption onto the chitosan nanoparticles. This might be attributed to stronger interactions between the chitosan and siRNA and a better loading efficiency when using ionic gelation.

Another interesting property of chitosan is its intrinsic antibacterial activity [129]. For this reason, chitosan is a preferred carrier for drug delivery of antibiotics, combining its intrinsic antibacterial activity with that of the bound antibiotic. Studies have shown that chitosan may reduce the rate of infections induced by bacteria such as *Staphylococcus* in rabbits [130]. The mechanism involves its cationic amino groups, which associate with anions on the bacterial cell wall, suppressing biosynthesis;

moreover, chitosan disrupts the mass transport across the cell wall accelerating the death of bacteria. The antibacterial activity is retained also when it is combined with other polymers [131]. Blends of chitosan with polyvinyl alcohol (PVA) crosslinked by gamma radiation have been prepared for wound dressing [132]. Chitosan was used to prevent microbiological growth, such as fungi and bacteria, on the PVA polymer. Moreover, chitosan has antiacid and antiulcer characteristics, which prevents or weakens drug irritation in the stomach [133].

Nanostructured surface coatings based on polysaccharides have been obtained by a combination of chitosan with hyaluronic acid and heparin [134]. The engineering of the nanoscale surface features of biologically active materials is an important goal for biomaterials scientists, as it strongly influences a variety of responses of mammalian cells towards biomaterials.

3.3. Agar/Agarose and Carrageenans

Agar (or agar-agar) is a phycocolloid, which is constructed from complex saccharide molecules (mainly, β-D-galactopyranose and 3,6-anhydro-α-L-galactopyranose units) extracted from certain species of red algae (*Gelidium, Gelidiela, Pterocladia, Gracilaria, Graciliaropsis*, and *Ahfeltia*) [135]. Genetic manipulation of agarophytes in the development stages promises to minimize seasonal variations in plant growth and agar quality. Agar and its variant agarose contain also variable amounts of sulfate, piruvate and uronate substituents.

Agar is insoluble in cold water but is soluble in boiling water. Agar dissolved in hot water and permitted to cool will form thermally reversible gels (the gel will melt when heated and reformed again when cooled), without the need of acidic conditions or oxidizing agents. This characteristic gives agars the ability to perform a reversible gelling process without losing their mechanical and thermal properties. The significant thermal hysteresis of the gel is another important property for commercial applications. The gelling process in agar is due to the formation of hydrogen bonds in a continuous way [136,139]. Gelation occurs as a result of a coil-double helix transition [140,142]; helices interact among themselves and the gel is formed by linked bundles of associated right-handed double helices. The resulting three-dimensional network is capable of immobilizing water molecules in its interstices [143]. Characteristically, solutions containing 1–2% agar by weight will gel at about 35 °C and will melt at about 85 °C. The 1–2% (w/w) agar gels are strong and brittle. Typically, a force of 500–1000 g cm^{-2} is required to break these gels. The strength and brittleness of agar gels are proportional to the amount of 3-6-anhydro-α-L-galactopyranose in the agar. An alternatively way to cross-link agar is via chemical agents [144]. By crosslinking with glutaraldehyde, agar forms superabsorbent hydrogels.

The ionic nature of the agar molecules permits to complex with proteins. The presence of proteins in wine, juice and vinegar clouds these products. Agar is added during processing to bind with proteins impurities. This facilitates the removal of proteins by filtration or centrifugation.

Agar has medicinal or pharmaceutical industrial applications including use as suspending agent for radiological solutions (barium sulfate), as a bulk laxative as it gives a smooth and non-irritating hydrated bulk in the digestive tract, and as a formative ingredient for tablets and capsules to carry and release drugs. Pharmaceutical grade agar has a viscous consistency. In microbiology, agar is the medium of choice for culturing bacteria on solid substrate. Agar is also used in some molecular microbiology techniques to obtain DNA information [145]. More recently, agar was used in a newly-developed medium, *i.e.*, combined deactivators-supplemented agar medium (CDSAM), to evaluate the viability of dermatophytes in skin scales [146]. The experimental data from this clinical study indicate that CDSAM was more useful than standard media in accurately evaluating the efficacy of antifungal drugs. Agar proportion method for drug susceptibility tests has been used since 1957 [147]. Recently, the test has been replaced by more rapid tests [148].

The possibility to use agar and agarose beads for sustained release of water soluble drugs has been investigated [149]. Agarose has a significantly lower sulfate content, better optical clarity and increased gel strength with respect to agar, but it is considerably more expensive [150]. Agar beads containing phenobarbitone sodium as a water soluble and hypnotic drug were prepared [151]. The encapsulation procedure consists in dissolving the drug in a hot (around 70 °C) agar aqueous solution and then dropping the solution in a cold bath containing a non-solvent for agar (acetone or ethyl acetate). Agar beads instantaneously form by gelification. The results of dissolution and release studies indicated that agar beads could be useful for the preparation of sustained release dosage forms, although no many further studies have been developed.

Carrageenan, as well as agar and agarose, is a sulfated polysaccharide obtained by extraction with water or alkaline water of certain *Rhodophyceae* (red seaweed). It is a hydrocolloid consisting mainly of the potassium, sodium, magnesium, and calcium sulfate esters of galactose and 3,6-anhydro-galactose copolymers.

Plain carrageenans, as well as agar, are mainly used as food additive, but increasing attention is given to possible biomedical applications, in combination with synthetic polymers. The synthesis of agar-graft-polyvinylpyrrolidone (PVP) and k-carrageenan-graft-PVP blends by a microwave irradiation method has been reported [152]. The physicochemical and rheological properties of the corresponding hydrogels were studied and compared with control agar and k-carrageenan hydrogels. The novel blend hydrogels were found to be not as strong and showed better spreadability and water-holding capability, so they are potentially useful in moisturizer formulations and active carriers of drugs. The use of blended PVP with agar in hydrogel dressings has also been reported [153].

3.4. Exopolysaccharides (EPS)

Microbial polysaccharides represent a class of important products that are of growing interest for many sectors of industry. The advantages of microbial polysaccharides over plants polysaccharides are their novel functions and constant chemical and physical properties. A number of common marine bacteria widely distributed in the oceans can produce EPSs; nevertheless, most of these EPSs remain poorly understood, and only a few of them have been fully characterized. The roles of microbial EPSs in the ocean are briefly described in Table 2.

Table 2. Some roles of microbial exopolymeric material (EPSs) in the marine environment. Adapted from [151].

Role of Exopolymer	Example
Assists in attachment to surfaces	Exopolymers of marine *Vibrio* MH3 were involved in reversible attachment. Cross-linking of adjacent polysaccharide chains aided in permanent adhesion.
Facilitates biochemical interactions between cells	Exopolymer mediated bacterial attachment to the polar end of blue-green N2-fixing alga. EPS aided attachment to symbiotic host such as vent tube worm to absorb metals and detoxify microenvironment. Exopolymer buffered against sudden osmotic changes.
Provides protective barrier around the cell	Bacteria in aggregates were less preferred by grazers than freely suspended bacteria. EPS-producing deep-sea hydrothermal vent bacteria showed resistance to heavy metals. Metal binding involves cell wall components as well as polysaccharides. Exopolymer in sea-ice brine channels provided cryoprotection by interacting with water at low temperature to depress freezing point. Nutrient uptake by bacteria in aggregates was higher than for free-living cells in low nutrient systems.
Absorbs dissolved organic material	Porous and hydrated matrix acts like a sponge and sequesters and concentrates dissolved organics.

In recent years, there has been a growing interest in isolating new exopolysaccharides (EPSs)-producing bacteria from marine environments, particularly from various extreme marine environments [154]. Many new marine microbial EPSs with novel chemical compositions, properties and structures have been found to have potential applications in fields such as adhesives, textiles, pharmaceuticals and medicine for anti-cancer, food additives, oil recovery and metal removal in mining and industrial waste treatments, *etc.* General information about the EPSs produced by marine bacteria, including their chemical compositions, properties and structures, together with their potential applications in industry, are widely reported [155]. Components more commonly found in marine EPSs are listed in Table 3. Some more recent and specific examples from literature are hereafter illustrated.

Table 3. Sugar and non sugar components of bacterial exopolysaccharides [151].

Type	Component	Example	Mode of Linkage
Sugar	Pentoses	D-Arabinose	
		D-Ribose	
		D-Xylose	
	Hexoses	D-Glucose	
		D-Mannose	
		D-Galactose	
		D-Allose	
		L-Ramnose	
		L-Fucose	
	Amino sugars	D-Glucosamine	
		D-Galactosamine	
	Uronic acids	D-Glucuronic acid	
		D-Galacturonic acid	
Non sugar	Acetic acid		*O*-acyl, *N*-acyl
	Succinic acid		*O*-acyl
	Pyruvic acid		Acetal
	Phosphoric acid		Ester, Diester
	Sulfuric acid		Ester

3.5. Biological Activity of EPSs

EPS2, a polysaccharide produced by a marine filamentous fungus *Keissleriella* sp. YS 4108 exhibited profound free radical-scavenging activities [156,157]. Antioxidants are commonly used in processed foods, as they could alleviate the oxidative damage of a tissue indirectly by increasing cells' natural defenses and directly by scavenging the free radical species [158,159]. As most of antioxidants used are synthetic and have been suspected of being responsible for liver damage and carcinogenesis [160,161], it is essential to develop and utilize effective natural antioxidants. Sun, Mao *et al.* [162] isolated three different exopolysaccharides from marine fungus *Penicillium* sp. F23-2, and evaluated their antioxidant activity by assays in *in vitro* systems. The results showed that the three polysaccharides possessed good antioxidant properties, especially scavenging abilities on superoxide radicals and hydroxyl radicals.

Interesting studies concern with the roles of carbohydrates as recognition sites on the cell surfaces [163]. It has been demonstrated that micro-organisms must specifically attach to the host cell to avoid being washed away by secretions. Such attachment would permit colonization or infection, sometimes followed by membrane penetration and invasion. Bergey and Stinson [164] and Bellamy *et al.* [165] provide some evidence of the participation of the carbohydrates in the cellular recognition process of the interaction between host and pathogen. It is an attractive possibility to use carbohydrate-based drugs for blocking the early stages of an infection process. In particular, sulfated polysaccharides are involved in biological activities such as cell recognition, cell adhesion, or regulation of receptor functions [166,168]. Obtaining sulfated polysaccharides from algae has made development of biotechnology for obtaining new therapeutic products easier. The use of bioactive compounds from microalgae has been considered recently as an alternative to prevent microbial infections in animals and humans and to decrease the use of antibiotics [169]. Ascencio *et al.* [170] identified heparan sulfate glycosaminoglycan as putative host target for *Helicobacter pylori* adhesion. A number of marine and freshwater microalgal strains for the production of sulfate exopolysaccharides was screened by these authors to evaluate whether these exopolysaccharides can block adherence to human and fish cells of human gastrointestinal pathogens, such as *H. pylori* and *Aeromonas veronii*. Results indicate the sulfated polysaccharides of some species of microalgae inhibit the cytoadhesion process of *H. pylori* to animal cells. The treatment with sulfated polysaccharides could so be used to block the initial process of colonization of the host by *H. pylori*, so it may represents an alternative prophylactic therapy in microbial infections where the process of cytoadhesion of host to pathogen is likely to be blocked. Such a therapy could replace the use of antibiotics and antiparasitic drugs that are always aggressive towards the host and, moreover, can generate resistant strains to the antibiotic, making it necessary to use second generation antibiotics [171,172].

Many polysaccharides have an anticancer activity. In general, the action mechanism is via macrophage activation in the host [173,174]. More recently, Matsuda *et al.* [175] reported that a sulfated exopolysaccharide produced by *Pseudomonas* sp. shows a cytotoxic effect towards human cancer cell lines such as MT-4. These findings have resulted in further interest in this polysaccharide as a new anticancer drug suitable for clinical trials.

Several marine bacteria isolated from deep-sea hydrothermal vents have demonstrated their ability to produce, in aerobic conditions, unusual EPS. These EPS could provide biochemical entities with suitable functions for obtaining new drugs. They present original structural feature that can be modified to design compounds and improve their specificity.

Studies aimed to discover biological activity of such new EPS were performed by Colliec-Jouault *et al.* [176]. An EPS secreted by *Vibrio diabolicus*, a new species isolated from *Alvinella pompejana* of Pompei, was evaluated on the restoration of bone integrity in an experimental model and was demonstrated to be a strong bone-healing material. High molecular weight EPS produced from fermentation of *Vibrio diabolicus* stocks has been implanted in bone injuries created in the cranium of a mouse, and compared with analogous injuries not treated or treated with collagene as a reference. After 15 days, a 95% healing was found for the injuries treated with the EPS, while less than 30% healing was found for untreated or collagene treated injuries.

Another EPS produced by *Alteromonas infernos*, a new *Alteromonas* species isolated in a hydrothermal vent from the Guaymas region, was really modified in order to obtain new heparin-like compounds [177]. The native EPS was depolymerized by radical mechanism or chemical hydrolysis, and low-mass derivatives (around 24,000 Da) were sulfated to obtain an "heparin-like" or "heparin-mimetic" compound. Unlike the native EPS, the resulting sulfated EPS presented anticoagulant properties as heparin.

3.6. Exopolysaccharides from Cyanobacteria

Cyanobacteria, also known as blue-green algae or blue-green bacteria because of their color (the name comes from Greek: kyanós = blue), are a significant component of the marine nitrogen cycle and an important primary producer in many areas of the ocean. They are also found in habitats other than the marine environment; in particular, cyanobacteria are known to occur in both freshwater, hypersaline inland lakes and in arid areas where they are a major component of biological soil crusts.

Since the early 1950s, more than one hundred cyanobacteria strains of different genera have been investigated regard to the production of exocellular polysaccharides. Such polysaccharides are present as outermost investments forming sheaths, capsules and slimes that protect the bacterial cells from the environment. Moreover, most polysaccharide-producing cyanobacteria release aliquots of capsules and slimes as soluble polymers in the culture medium (RPS)[178]. In recent years the interest towards such cyanobacteria has greatly increased, in particular towards those strains that possess abundant capsules and slimes and so release large amount of soluble polysaccharides, which can be easily recovered from liquid culture.

The chemical and rheological analyses show that RPS are complex anionic hetero-polymers, in about 80% cases containing six to ten different monosaccharides, glucose being the most abundant [179]. This characteristic is unusual in EPS of industrial interest, which usually contain a lower number of monosaccharides, and is of great significance [180]. Actually, a large number of different monosaccharides in only one polymer makes many structures and architectures possible [181], thus increasing the chance of having a polymer with peculiar properties, not common to currently utilized products. The rheological properties of RPSs' aqueous solutions make them useful as thickening agents for water solutions, together with their ability to stabilize the flow properties of their own solutions under drastic changes of pH, temperature and ionic strength [182,183].

Another important feature of such RPS is their anionic nature. In fact, in about 90% cases, one or more uronic acids are present; moreover, RPS also contain sulfate groups. Both uronic and sulfate groups contribute to impart a high anionic density to the polymer. The anionic charge is an important characteristic for the affinity of these EPS towards cations, notably metal ions. Almost all RPS have significant levels of non-saccharidic components, such as ester-linked acetyl and/or pyruvyl groups and peptidic moieties which, along with other hydrophobic components as the deoxysugars fucose and rhamnose, contribute to a significant hydrophobic behavior of these otherwise hydrophilic macromolecules, conferring them emulsifying properties [184,185].

The presence of charged groups on the macromolecules may lead to several interesting industrial applications: their capability to bind water molecules can be exploited by the cosmetic and pharmaceutical industries for product formulations [186]. A promising new field of application that attracted much attention is related to antiviral activity of some RPSs isolated from the blue-green alga *Spirulina platensis* [187,188]. The presence in these polysaccharides of significantly high amounts of sulfate groups, indeed, is accounted for their antiviral activity, and an increasing amount of data is available.

4. Conclusions

A brief review of recent advances in applications of polysaccharides of marine origin in the medical and pharmaceutical fields has been reported. Many experimental results clearly indicate that novel exciting and promising marine sources of polysaccharides of applied interest, such as cyanobacteria and thermophylic or hyperthermophylic bacteria from extreme habitats, are emerging. Further investigations with a multidisciplinary approach are imperative in order to develop novel polymers useful as drugs or for healthcare in a larger sense.

References

1. Nigrelli, RF; Stempien, MF; Ruggirei, GD; Liguori, VR; Cecil, JT. Substances of potential biomedical importance from marine organisms. *Fed. Proc* **1967**, *26*, 1197–1205.
2. Immirzi, B; Laurienzo, P; Liquori, AM; Malinconico, M; Martuscelli, E; Orsello, G; Volpe, MG. Inorganic components of the macroalga ulva. *Agro Food Ind. Hi Tec* **1995**, *6*, 42–44.
3. Carlsson, AS; van Beilen, J; Möller, R; Clayton, D. Bowles, D, Ed.; Micro- and macro-algae: Utility for industrial applications. In *Outputs from the EPOBIO Project*; CPL Science: Newbury, UK, 2007.
4. De Pauw, N; Persoone, G. Borowitzka, MA, Borowitzka, LJ, Eds.; Microalgae for aquaculture. In *Microalgal Biotechnology*; Cambridge University: Cambridge, UK, 1988; pp. 197–221.
5. Ramus, JS. The production of extracellular polysaccharides by the unicellular red alga *Porphyridium eurugineum*. *J. Phycol* **1972**, *8*, 97–111.
6. Lewis, RA. Extracellular polysaccharides of green algae. *Can. J. Microbiol* **1956**, *2*, 665–672.
7. Moore, BG; Tischer, RG. Extracellular polysaccharides of algae: Effects on life-support system. *Science* **1964**, *145*, 586–587.
8. Ramus, JS. Algae biopolymer production. US Patent 4,236,349, 2 December 1980.
9. Colwell, RR. Fulfilling the promise of biothechnology. *Biotechnol. Adv* **2002**, *20*, 215–228.
10. Staley, JT; Castenholz, RW; Colwell, RR; Holt, JG; Kane, MD; Pace, NR; Salyers, AA; Tiedje, JM. The microbial world: Foundation of the biosphere. In *Report from the American Academy of Microbiology*; American Society for Microbiology: Washington, DC, USA, 1997.
11. Burgess, JG; Jordan, EM; Bregu, M; Mearns-Spragg, A; Boyd, KG. Microbial antagonism: A neglected avenue of natural products research. *J. Biotechnol* **1999**, *70*, 27–32.
12. Jensen, PR; Fenical, W. Strategies for the discovery of secondary metabolites from marine bacteria: Ecological perspectives. *Annu. Rev. Microbiol* **1994**, *48*, 559–584.
13. Omidian, H; Rocca, JG; Park, K. Advances in superporous hydrogels. *J. Control. Release* **2005**, *102*, 3–12.

14. Guilherme, MR; Reis, AV; Paulino, AT; Fajardo, AR; Muniz, EC; Tambourgi, EB. Superabsorbent hydrogel based on modified polysaccharide for removal of Pb2+ and Cu2+ from water with excellent performance. *J. Appl. Polym. Sci* **2007**, *105*, 2903–2909.

15. Omidian, H; Rocca, JG; Park, K. Elastic, superporous hydrogel hybrids of polyacrylamide and sodium alginate. *Macromol. Biosci* **2006**, *6*, 703–710.

16. Pourjavadi, A; Soleyman, R; Bardajee, GR; Ghavami, S. Novel superabsorbent hydrogel based on natural hybrid backbone: Optimized synthesis and its swelling behavior. *Bull. Korean Chem. Soc* **2009**, *30*, 2680–2686.

17. Pourjavadi, A; Farhadpour, B; Seidi, F. Synthesis and investigation of swelling behavior of new agar based superabsorbent hydrogel as a candidate for agrochemical delivery. *J. Polym. Res* **2009**, *16*, 655–665.

18. Pourjavadi, A; Barzegar, Sh; Mahdavinia, GR. MBA-crosslinked Na-Alg/CMC as a smart full-polysaccharide superabsorbent hydrogel. *Carbohydr. Polym* **2006**, *66*, 386–395.

19. Hoffmann, B; Volkmer, E; Kokott, A; Augat, P; Ohnmacht, M; Sedlmayr, N; Schieker, M; Claes, L; Mutschle, W; Ziegler, G. Characterisation of a new bioadhesives system based on polysaccharides with the potential to be used as bone glue. *J. Mater. Sci. Mater. Med* **2009**, *20*, 2001–2009.

20. Sever, MJ; Weisser, JT; Monahan, J; Srinivasan, S; Wilker, JJ. Metal-mediated cross-linking in the generation of a marine-mussel adhesive. *Angew. Chem. Int. Ed. Engl* **2004**, *43*, 448–450.

21. Yu, M; Deming, TJ. Synthetic polypeptide mimics of marine adhesives. *Macromolecules* **1998**, *31*, 4739–4745.

22. Deming, TJ. Mussel byssus and biomolecular materials. *Curr. Opin. Chem. Biol* **1999**, *3*, 100–105.

23. Montanaro, L; Arciola, CR; Cenni, E; Ciapetti, G; Ravioli, F; Filippini, F; Barsanti, LA. Cytotoxicity, blood compatibility and antimicrobial activity of two cyanoacrylate glues for surgical use. *Biomaterials* **2001**, *22*, 59–66.

24. Holte, O; Onsⵁyen, E; Myrvold, R; Karlsen, J. Sustained release of water-soluble drug from directly compressed alginate tablets. *Eur. J. Pharm. Sci* **2003**, *20*, 403–407.

25. Tonnesen, HH; Karlsen, J. Alginate in drug delivery systems. *Drug Dev. Ind. Pharm* **2002**, *28*, 621–630.

26. Rogovina, SZ; Vikhoreva, GA. Polysaccharide-based polymer blends: Methods of their production. *Glycoconj. J* **2006**, *23*, 611–618.

27. Lee, YL; Shin, DS; Kwon, OW; Park, WH; Choi, HG; Lee, YR; Han, SS; Noh, SK; Lyoo, WS. Preparation of atactic poly(vinyl alcohol)/sodium alginate blend nanowebs by electrospinning. *J. Appl. Polym. Sci* **2007**, *106*, 1337–1342.

28. Cho, SH; Oh, SH; Lee, JH. Fabrication and characterization of porous alginate/polyvinyl alcohol hybrid scaffolds for 3D cell culture. *J. Biomater. Sci. Polym. Ed* **2005**, *16*, 933–947.

29. Avella, M; Di Pace, E; Immirzi, B; Impallomeni, G; Malinconico, M; Santagata, G. Addition of glycerol plasticizer to seaweeds derived alginates: influence of microstructure on chemical-physical properties. *Carbohydr. Polym* **2007**, *69*, 503–511.

30. Daia, YN; Lia, P; Zhangc, JP; Wangc, AQ; Wei, Q. A novel pH sensitive *N*-succinyl chitosan/alginate hydrogel bead for nifedipine delivery. *Biopharm. Drug Dispos* **2008**, *29*, 173–184.

31. Nobile, MR; Pirozzi, V; Somma, E; Gomez d'Ayala, G; Laurienzo, P. Development and rheological investigation of novel alginate/*N*-succinylchitosan hydrogels. *J. Polym. Sci. B* **2008**, *46*, 1167–1182.

32. Gomez d'Ayala, G; De Rosa, A; Laurienzo, P; Malinconico, M. Development of a new calcium sulfate-based composite using alginate and chemically modified chitosan for bone regeneration. *J. Biomed. Mater. Res. A* **2007**, *81*, 811–820.

33. Laurienzo, P; Di Stasio, M; Malinconico, M; Volpe, MG. Dehydration of apples by innovative bio-films drying. *J. Food Eng* **2010**, *97*, 491–496.

34. Akiyoshi, K; Sunamoto, J. Supramolecular assembly of hydrophobized polysaccharides. *Supramol. Sci* **1996**, *3*, 157–163.

35. Sato, T. Targetability of cell-specific liposomes coated with polysaccharide-cholesterol derivatives. *Nippon Rinsho* **1989**, *47*, 1402–1407.

36. Matsukawa, S; Yamamoto, M; Ichinose, K; Ohata, N; Ishii, N; Kohji, T; Akiyoshi, K; Sunamoto, J; Kanematsu, T. Selective uptake by cancer cells of liposomes coated with polysaccharides bearing 1-aminolactose. *Anticancer Res* **2000**, *20*, 2339–2344.

37. Shaikh, VAE; Maldar, NN; Lonikar, SV; Rajan, CR; Ponrathnam, S. Thermotropic behavior of cholesterol-linked polysaccharides. *J. Appl. Polym. Sci* **1998**, *70*, 195–201.

38. Wang, Y; Hollingsworth, RI; Kasper, DL. Oxidative depolymerization of polysaccharides in aqueous solutions. *Carbohydr. Res* **1999**, *319*, 141–147.

39. Uchida, K; Kawakishi, S. Oxidative depolymerization of polysaccharides induced by the ascorbic acid-copper ion systems. *Agric. Biol. Chem* **1986**, *50*, 2579–2583.

40. Balakrishnan, B; Lesieur, S; Labarre, D; Jayakrishnan, A. Periodate oxidation of sodium alginate in water and in ethanol-water mixtures: a comparative study. *Carbohydr. Res* **2005**, *340*, 1425–1429.

41. Dutton, GGS; Savage, AV; Mignon, M. Use of a bacteriophage to depolymerize a polysaccharide to an oligosaccharide; comparison of the 1H and 13C nuclear magnetic resonance spectra of the polymer and its hexasaccharide repeating unit. *Can. J. Chem* **1980**, *58*, 2588–2591.

42. Karstens, T; Kettenbach, G; Seger, T; Stein, A; Steinmeyer, H; Mauer, G. Method for carrying out the targeted depolymerization of polysaccharides. US Patent WO/2001/007485, 1 February 2001.

43. Chrinstensen, BE; Smidsr⊘d, O; Elgsaeter, A; Stokke, BT. Depolymerization of double-stranded xanthan by acid hydrolysis: characterization of partially degraded double strands and single-stranded oligomers released from the ordered structures. *Macromolecules* **1993**, *26*, 6111–6120.

44. El-Sawy, NM; El-Rheim, HAA; Elbarbary, AM; Hegazy, ESA. Radiation induced degradation of chitosan for possible use as a growth promoter for agricultural purposes. *Carbohydr. Polym* **2010**, *79*, 555–562.

45. Pawlowski, A; Svenson, SB. Electron beam fragmentation of bacterial polysaccharides as a method of producing oligosaccharides for the preparation of conjugate vaccines. *FEMS Microbiol. Lett* **1999**, *174*, 255–263.

46. Trinchero, J; Ponce, NM; Cordoba, OL; Flores, ML; Pampuro, S; Stortz, CA; Salomon, H; Turk, G. Antiretroviral activity of fucoidans extracted from the brown seaweed Adenocystis utricularis. *Phytother. Res* **2009**, *23*, 707–712.

47. Schwartz-Albiez, R; Adams, Y; von der Lieth, CW; Mischnick, P; Andrews, KT; Kirschfink, M. Regioselectively modified sulfated cellulose as prospective drug for treatment of malaria tropica. *Glycoconj. J* **2007**, *24*, 57–65.

48. Kaneko, Y; Havlik, I. Medicinal compositions, dose and method for treating malaria. European Patent 132,945,2A1, 2003.

49. Kydonieus, A; Elson, C; Thanou, M. Drug delivery using sulfated chitinous polymers. US Patent 20,040,038,870, 26 February 2004.

50. Lange, LG, III; Spilburg, CA. Use of sulfated polysaccharides to decrease cholesterol and fatty acid absorption. US Patent 5,063,210, 5 November 1991.

51. Lewis, JG; Stanley, NF; Guist, GG. Lembi, CA, Waaland, JR, Eds.; Commercial production and applications of algal hydrocolloids. In *Algae and Human Affairs*; Cambridge University Press: Cambridge, UK, 1988; pp. 205–236.

52. Russo, R; Malinconico, M; Santagata, G. Effect on cross-linking with calcium ions on the physical properties of alginate films. *Biomacromolecules* **2007**, *8*, 3193–3197.

53. Merrill, EW; Salzman, EW. Polyethylene oxide as a biomaterial. *Am. Soc. Artif. Intern. Organs J* **1983**, *6*, 60–64.

54. Han, DK; Park, KD; Ahn, KD; Jeong, SY; Kim, YH. Preparation and surface characterization of PEO-grafted and heparin-immobolized polyurethanes. *J. Biomed. Mater. Res* **1989**, *23*, 87–104.

55. Tu, R; Lu, CL; Thyagarajan, K; Wang, E; Nguyen, H; Shen, S; Hata, C; Quijano, RC. Kinetic study of collagen fixation with polyepoxy fixatives. *J. Biomed. Mater. Res* **1993**, *27*, 3–9.

56. Chen, JP; Chu, IM; Shiao, MY; Hsu, BRS; Fu, SH. Microencapsulation of islets in PEG-amine modified alginate-poly(l-lysine)-alginate microcapsules for constructing bioartificial pancreas. *J. Ferment. Bioeng* **1998**, *86*, 185–190.

57. Chandy, T; Mooradian, DL; Rao, GHR. Chitosan/polyethylene glycol-alginate microcapsules for oral delivery of hirudin. *J. Appl. Polym. Sci* **1998**, *70*, 2143–2153.

58. Qurrat-ul-Ain; Sharma, S; Khuller, GK; Garg, SK. Alginate-based oral drug delivery system for tuberculosis: Pharmacokinetics and therapeutic effects. *J. Antimicrob. Chemother* **2003**, *51*, 931–938.

59. Jayant, RD; McShane, MJ; Srivastava, R. Polyelectrolyte-coated alginate microspheres as drug delivery carriers for dexamethasone release. *Drug Deliv* **2009**, *16*, 331–340.

60. Kevadiya, BD; Joshi, GV; Patel, HA; Ingole, PG; Mody, HM; Bajaj, HC. Montmorillonite-alginate nanocomposites as a drug delivery system: Intercalation and *in vitro* release of vitamin B1 and vitamin B6. *J. Biomater. Appl* **2010**, *25*, 161–177.

61. Miyazaki, S; Nakayama, A; Oda, M; Takada, M; Attwood, D. Chitosan and sodium alginate based bioadhesive tablets for intraoral drug delivery. *Biol. Pharm. Bull* **1994**, *17*, 745–747.

62. Tapia, C; Escobar, Z; Costa, E; Sapag-Hagar, J; Valenzuela, F; Basualto, C; Gai, MN; Yazdani-Pedram, M. Comparative studies on polyelectrolyte complexes and mixtures of chitosan-alginate and chitosan-carrageenan as prolonged diltiazem clorohydrate release systems. *Eur. J. Pharm. Biopharm* **2004**, *57*, 65–75.

63. Gavini, E; Sanna, V; Juliano, C; Bonferoni, MC; Giunchedi, P. Mucoadhesive vaginal tablets as veterinary delivery system for the controlled release of an antimicrobial drug, acriflavine. *AAPS PharmSciTech* **2002**, *3*, E20.

64. El-Kamel, A; Sokar, M; Naggar, V; Al Gamal, S. Chitosan and sodium alginate-based bioadhesive vaginal tablets. *AAPS PharmSci* **2002**, *4*, E44.

65. Strand, BL; Gaserod, O; Kulseng, B; Espevik, T; Skjak-Braek, G. Alginate-polylisine-alginate microcapsules: Effect of size reduction on capsule properties. *J. Microencapsul* **2002**, *19*, 612–630.

66. Mumper, RJ; Hoffman, AS; Puolakkainen, PA; Bouchard, LS; Gombotz, WR. Calcium-alginate beads for the oral delivery of transforming growth factor-β1 (TGF-β1): stabilization of TGF-β1 by the addition of polyacrylic acid within acid-treated beads. *J. Control. Release* **1994**, *30*, 241–251.

67. Shojaei, AH; Paulson, J; Honary, S. Evaluation of poly(acrylic acid-co-ethylhexyl acrylate) films for mucoadhesive transbuccal drug delivery: factors affecting the force of mucoadhesion. *J. Control. Release* **2000**, *67*, 223–232.

68. Laurienzo, P; Malinconico, M; Mattia, G; Russo, R; La Rotonda, MI; Quaglia, F; Capitani, D; Mannina, L. Novel alginate-acrylic polymers as a platform for drug delivery. *J. Biomed. Mater. Res. A* **2006**, *78*, 523–531.

69. Kang, HA; Shin, MS; Yang, JW. Preparation and characterization of hydrophobically modified alginate. *Polym. Bull* **2002**, *47*, 429–435.

70. Rowley, JA; Madlambayan, G; Mooney, DJ. Alginate hydrogels as synthetic extracellular matrix materials. *Biomaterials* **1999**, *20*, 45–53.

71. Seifert, DB; Phillips, JA. Porous alginate-poly(ethylene glycol) entrapment system for the cultivation of mammalian cells. *Biotechnol. Prog* **1997**, *13*, 569–576.

72. Laurienzo, P; Malinconico, M; Motta, A; Vicinanza, A. Synthesis of a novel alginate-poly(ethylene glycol) graft copolymer for cell immobilization. *Carbohydr. Polym* **2005**, *62*, 274–282.

73. Gilchrist, T; Martin, AM. Wound treatment with Sorban-an alginate fibre dressing. *Biomaterials* **1983**, *4*, 317–320.

74. Motta, GJ. Calcium alginate topical wound dressings: a new dimension in the cost-effective treatment for exudating dermal wounds and pressure sores. *Ostomy Wound Manage* **1989**, *25*, 52–56.

75. Doyle, JW; Roth, TP; Smith, RM; Li, Y-Q; Dunn, RM. Effects of calcium alginate on cellular wound healing processes modelled *in vitro*. *J. Biomed. Mater. Res* **1996**, *32*, 561–568.

76. Berry, DP; Bale, S; Harding, KG. Dressings for treating cavity wounds. *J. Wound Care* **1996**, *5*, 10–17.

77. Segan, HT; Hunt, BJ; Gilding, K. The effects of alginate and non-alginate wound dressings on blood coagulation and platelet activation. *J. Biomater. Appl* **1998**, *12*, 249–257.

78. Odell, EW; Oades, P; Lombardi, T. Symptomatic foreign body reaction to haemostatic alginate. *Br. J. Oral Maxillofac. Surg* **1994**, *32*, 178–179.

79. Burrows, F; Louime, C; Abazinge, M; Onokpise, O. Extraction and evaluation of chitin from crub exoskeleton as a seed fungicide and plant growth enhancer. *Amer.-Eurasian J. Agric. Environ. Sci* **2007**, *2*, 103–111.

80. Muzzarelli, RAA; Muzzarelli, C. Chitosan chemistry: Relevance to the biomedical sciences. *Adv. Polym. Sci* **2005**, *186*, 151–209.

81. Kumar, MNV; Muzzarelli, RAA; Muzzarelli, C; Sashiwa, H; Domb, AJ. Chitosan chemistry and pharmaceutical perspectives. *Chem. Rev* **2004**, *104*, 6017–6084.

82. Geng, X; Kwon, OH; Jang, J. Electrospinning of chitosan dissolved in concentrated acetic acid solution. *Biomaterials* **2005**, *26*, 5427–5432.

83. Chow, KS; Khor, E. Novel fabrication of open-pore chitin matrices. *Biomacromolecules* **2000**, *1*, 61–67.

84. Suh, JKF; Matthew, HWT. Application of chitosan-based polysaccharide biomaterials in cartilage tissue engineering: A review. *Biomaterials* **2000**, *21*, 2589–2598.

85. Di Martino, A; Sittinger, M; Risbud, MV. Chitosan: A versatile biopolymer for orthopaedic tissue engineering. *Biomaterials* **2005**, *26*, 5983–5990.

86. Chenite, A; Chaput, C; Wang, D; Combes, C; Buschmann, MD; Hoemann, CD; Leroux, JC; Atkinson, BL; Binette, F; Selmani, A. Novel injectable neutral solutions of chitosan form biodegradable gels *in situ*. *Biomaterials* **2000**, *21*, 2155–2161.

87. Wang, X; Yan, Y; Zhang, R. A comparison of chitosan and collagen sponges as hemostatic dressings. *J. Bioact. Compat. Polym* **2006**, *21*, 39–54.

88. Tuzlakoglu, K; Alves, CM; Mano, JF; Reis, RL. Production and characterization of chitosan fibers and 3-D fiber mesh scaffolds for tissue engineering applications. *Macromol. Biosci* **2004**, *4*, 811–819.

89. Zhang, Y; Zhang, M. Cell growth and function on calcium phosphate reinforced chitosan scaffolds. *J. Mater. Sci. Mater. Med* **2004**, *15*, 255–260.

90. Xia, W; Liu, W; Cui, L; Liu, Y; Zhong, W; Liu, D; Wu, J; Chua, K; Cao, Y. Tissue engineering of cartilage with the use of chitosan–gelatin complex scaffolds. *J. Biomed. Mater. Res* **2004**, *71B*, 373–380.

91. Risbud, M; Ringe, J; Bhonde, R; Sittinger, M. *In vitro* expression of cartilage-specific markers by chondrocytes on a biocompatible hydrogel: implications for engineering cartilage tissue. *Cell Transplant* **2001**, *10*, 755–763.

92. Hu, Q; Li, B; Wang, M; Shen, J. Preparation and characterization of biodegradable chitosan/hydroxyapatite nanocomposite rods via *in situ* hybridization: a potential material as internal fixation of bone fracture. *Biomaterials* **2004**, *25*, 779–785.

93. Iwasaki, N; Yamane, S-T; Majima, T; Kasahara, Y; Minami, A; Harada, K; Nonaka, S; Maekawa, N; Tamura, H; Tokura, S; Shiono, M; Monde, K; Nishimura, S-I. Feasibility of polysaccharide hybrid materials for scaffolds in cartilage tissue engineering: evaluation of chondrocyte adhesion to polyion complex fibers prepared from alginate and chitosan. *Biomacromolecules* **2004**, *5*, 828–833.

94. Gåser⊘d, O; Smidsr⊘d, O; Skjåsk-Bræk, G. Microcapsules of alginate-chitosan-I. A quantitative study of the interaction between alginate and chitosan. *Biomaterials* **1998**, *19*, 1815–1825.

95. Peniche, C; Arguëlles-Monal, W; Davidenko, N; Sastre, R; Gallardo, A; San Román, J. Self-curing membranes of chitosan/PAA IPNs obtained by radical polymerization: preparation, characterization and interpolymer complexation. *Biomaterials* **1999**, *20*, 1869–1878.

96. Leroux, L; Hatim, Z; Freche, M; Lacout, JL. Effects of various adjuvants (lactic acid, glycerol, and chitosan) on the injectability of a calcium phosphate cement. *Bone* **1999**, *25*, 31S–34S.

97. Zong, Z; Kimura, Y; Takahashi, M; Yamane, H. Characterization of chemical and solid state structures of acylated chitosans. *Polymer* **2000**, *41*, 899–906.

98. Hirano, S; Ohe, Y; Ono, H. Selective *N*-acylation of chitosan. *Carbohydr. Res* **1976**, *47*, 315–320.

99. Moore, GK; Roberts, GAF. Reactions of chitosan: 2. Preparation and reactivity of *N*-acyl derivatives of chitosan. *Int. J. Biol. Macromol* **1981**, *3*, 292–296.

100. Nishimura, SI; Kohgo, O; Kurita, K. Chemospecific manipulations of a rigid polysaccharide: Syntheses of novel chitosan derivatives with excellent solubility in common organic solvents by regioselective chemical modifications. *Macromolecules* **1991**, *24*, 4745–4748.

101. Yalpani, M; Hall, LD. Some chemical and analytical aspects of polysaccharide modifications. III. Formation of branched-chain, soluble chitosan derivatives. *Macromolecules* **1984**, *17*, 272–281.

102. Chenite, A; Chaput, C; Wang, D; Combes, C; Buschmann, MD; Hoemann, CD; Leroux, JC; Atkinson, BL; Binette, F; Selmani, A. Novel injectable neutral solutions of chitosan form biodegradable gels *in situ*. *Biomaterials* **2000**, *21*, 2155–2161.

103. Mi, FL; Sung, HW; Shyu, SS; Su, CC; Peng, CK. Synthesis and characterization of biodegradable TPP/genipin co-crosslinked chitosan gel beads. *Polymer* **2003**, *44*, 6521–6530.

104. Akao, T; Kobashi, K; Aburada, M. Enzymic studies on the animal and intestinal bacterial metabolism of geniposide. *Biol. Pharm. Bull* **1994**, *17*, 1573–1576.

105. Mi, FL; Shyu, SS; Lee, ST; Wong, TB. Kinetic study of chitosan-tripolyphosphate complex reaction and acid-resistive properties of the chitosan-tripolyphosphate gel beads prepared by in-liquid curing method. *J. Polym. Sci. B Polym. Phys* **1999**, *37*, 1551–1564.

106. Shu, XZ; Zhu, KJ. A novel approach to prepare tripolyphosphate/chitosan complex beads for controlled drug delivery. *Int. J. Pharm* **2000**, *201*, 51–58.

107. Shu, XZ; Zhu, KJ. Chitosan/gelatin microspheres prepared by modified emulsification and ionotropic gelation. *J. Microencapsul* **2001**, *18*, 237–245.

108. Shu, XZ; Zhu, KJ; Song, W. Novel pH-sensitive citrate cross-linked chitosan film for drug controlled release. *Int. J. Pharm* **2001**, *212*, 19–28.

109. Koa, JA; Park, HJ; Hwang, SJ; Park, JB; Lee, JS. Preparation and characterization of chitosan microparticles intended for controlled drug delivery. *Int. J. Pharm* **2002**, *249*, 165–174.

110. Aral, C; Akbuđa, J. Alternative approach to the preparation of chitosan beads. *Int. J. Pharm* **1998**, *168*, 9–15.

111. Hejazi, R; Amiji, M. Chitosan-based gastrointestinal delivery systems. *J. Control. Release* **2003**, *89*, 151–165.

112. Illum, L; Jabbal-Gill, I; Hinchcliffe, M; Fisher, AN; Davis, SS. Chitosan as a novel nasal delivery system for vaccines. *Adv. Drug Deliv. Rev* **2001**, *51*, 81–96.

113. Yao, KD; Xu, MX; Yin, YJ; Zhao, JY; Chen, XL. pH-sensitive chitosan/gelatin hybrid polymer network microspheres for delivery of cimetidine. *Polym. Int* **1996**, *39*, 333–337.

114. Chen, SC; Wu, YC; Mi, FL; Lin, YH; Yu, LC; Sung, HW. A novel pH-sensitive hydrogel composed of N,O-carboxymethyl chitosan and alginate cross-linked by genipin for protein drug delivery. *J. Control. Release* **2004**, *96*, 285–300.

115. Liu, L; Li, Y; Liu, H; Fang, Y. Synthesis and characterization of chitosan-graftpolycaprolactone copolymers. *Eur. Polym. J* **2004**, *40*, 2739–2744.

116. Yu, H; Wang, W; Chen, X; Deng, C; Jing, X. Synthesis and characterization of the biodegradable polycaprolactone-graft-chitosan amphiphilic copolymers. *Biopolymers* **2006**, *83*, 233–242.

117. Guan, X; Quan, D; Shuai, X; Liao, K; Mai, K. Chitosan-graft-poly(ε-caprolactone)s: An optimized chemical approach leading to a controllable structure and enhanced properties. *J. Polym. Sci. A Polym. Chem* **2007**, *45*, 2556–2568.

118. Bhattarai, N; Ramay, HR; Gunn, J; Matsen, FA; Zhang, M. PEG-graft-chitosan as an injectable thermosensitive hydrogel for sustained protein release. *J. Control. Release* **2005**, *103*, 609–624.

119. Lu, Y; Liu, L; Guo, S. Novel amphiphilic ternary polysaccharide derivates chitosan-g-PCL-g-mPEG: Syntesis, characterization and aggregation in aqueous solutions. *Biopolymers* **2007**, *86*, 403–408.

120. Duan, K; Zhang, X; Tang, X; Yu, J; Liu, S; Wang, D; Li, Y; Huang, J. Fabrication of cationic nanomicelle from chitosan-graft-polycaprolactone as the carrier of 7-ethyl-10-hydroxy-camptothecin. *Colloids Surf. B* **2010**, *76*, 475–482.

121. Wong, TW. Chitosan and Its Use in Design of Insulin Delivery System. *Recent Pat. Drug Deliv. Formul* **2009**, *3*, 8–25.

122. Ma, Z; Lim, LY. Uptake of chitosan and associated insulin in Caco-2 cell monolayers: A comparison between chitosan molecules and chitosan nanoparticles. *Pharm. Res* **2003**, *20*, 1812–1819.

123. Morille, M; Passirani, C; Vonarbourg, A; Clavreul, A; Benoit, JP. Progress in developing cationic vectors for non-viral systemic gene therapy against cancer. *Biomaterials* **2008**, *29*, 3477–3496.

124. Brown, MD; Schätzlein, AG; Uchegbu, IF. Gene delivery with synthetic (non viral) carriers. *Int. J. Pharm* **2001**, *229*, 1–21.

125. Erbacher, P; Zou, S; Bettinger, T; Steffan, AM; Remy, JS. Chitosan-based vector/DNA complexes for gene delivery: biophysical characteristics and transfection ability. *Pharm. Res* **1998**, *15*, 1332–1339.

126. Koping-Hoggard, M; Tubulekas, I; Guan, H; Edwards, K; Nilsson, M; Varum, KM; Artursson, P. Chitosan as a nonviral gene delivery system: structure-property relationships and characteristics compared with polyethylenimine *in vitro* and after lung administration *in vivo*. *Gene Ther* **2001**, *8*, 1108–1121.

127. Ravi Kumar, MNV; Bakowsky, U; Lehr, CM. Preparation and characterization of cationic PLGA nanospheres as DNA carriers. *Biomaterials* **2004**, *25*, 1771–1777.

128. Katas, H; Alpar, HO. Development and characterisation of chitosan nanoparticles for siRNA delivery. *J. Control. Release* **2006**, *115*, 216–225.

129. Sarasam, AR; Brown, P; Khajotia, SS; Dmytryk, JJ; Madihally, SV. Antibacterial activity of chitosan-based matrices on oral pathogens. *J. Mater. Sci. Mater. Med* **2008**, *19*, 1083–1090.

130. Aimin, C; Chunlin, H; Juliang, B; Tinyin, Z; Zhichao, D. Antibiotic loaded chitosan bar. An *in vitro, in vivo* study of a possible treatment for osteomyelitis. *Clin. Orthop* **1999**, *366*, 239–247.

131. Hu, SG; Jou, CH; Yang, MC. Protein adsorption, fibroblast activity and antibacterial properties of poly(3-hydroxybutyric acid-co-3-hydroxyvaleric acid) grafted with chitosan and chitooligosaccharide after immobilized with hyaluronic acid. *Biomaterials* **2003**, *24*, 2685–2693.

132. El, Salmawi KM. Gamma-radiation-induced crosslinked PVA/chitosan blends for wound dressing. *J. Macromol. Sci. A Pure Appl. Chem* **2007**, *44*, 541–545.

133. Gupta, KC; Ravi Kumar, MNV. Drug release behaviour of beads and microgranules of chitosan. *Biomaterials* **2000**, *21*, 1115–1119.

134. Boddohi, S; Almodóvar, J; Zhang, H; Johnson, PA; Kipper, MJ. Layer-by-layer assembly of polysaccharide-based nanostructured surfaces containing polyelectrolyte complex nanoparticles. *Colloids Surf. B* **2010**, *77*, 60–68.

135. Araki, C. Some recent studies on the polysaccharides of agarophytes. *Proc. Int. Seaweed Symp* **1966**, *5*, 3–19.

136. Stephen, AM; Phillips, GO; Williams, PA. *Food Polysaccharides and Their Applications*; Marcel Dekker: New York, NY, USA, 1995; pp. 187–203.

137. Glicksman, M. Blanshard, JMV, Mitchell, JR, Eds.; Gelling hydrocolloids in product applications. In *Polysaccharides in Foods*; Butterworths: London, UK, 1979.

138. Armisen, R; Galatas, F. Philips, GO, Williams, PA, Eds.; Agar. In *Handbook of Hydrocolloids*; CRC: New York, NY, USA, 2000.

139. Norziah, MH; Foo, SL; Karim, A. Abd. Rheological studies on mixtures of agar (Gracilaria changii) and k-carrageenan. *Food Hydrocol* **2006**, *20*, 204–217.

140. Morris, VJ. Mitchell, JA, Ledwards, DA, Eds.; Gelation of polysaccharide. In *Functional Properties of Food Macromolecules*; Elsevier: London, UK, 1986; pp. 121–170.

141. Schafer, SF; Steven, FS. A reexamination of the double-helix model for agarose gel using optical rotation. *Biopolymers* **1995**, *36*, 103–108.

142. Medina-Esquivel, R; Freile-Pelegrin, Y; Quintana-Owen, P; Yáñez-Limón, JM; Alvarado-Gil, JJ. Measurement of the Sol-Gel Transition Temperature in Agar. *Int. J. Thermophys* **2008**, *29*, 2036–2045.

143. Arnott, S; Fulner, A; Scott, WE; Dea, ICM; Morehouse, R; Rees, DA. The agarose double helix and its function in agarose gel structure. *J. Mol. Biol* **1974**, *90*, 269–284.

144. Bao, L; Yang, W; Mao, X; Mou, S; Tang, S. Agar/collagen membrane as skin dressing for wounds. *Biomed. Mater* **2008**, *3*, 044108. [CrossRef]

145. Dumitriu, S. *Polysaccharides: Structural Diversity and Functional Versatility*; Marcel Dekker: New York, NY, USA, 1988.

146. Adachi, M; Watanabe, S. Evaluation of combined deactivators-supplemented agar medium (CDSAM) for recovery of dermatophytes from patients with tinea pedis. *Med. Mycol* **2007**, *45*, 347–349.

147. Knox, R; Woodroffe, R. Semi-solid agar media for rapid drug sensitivity tests on cultures of *Mycobacterium tuberculosis*. *J. Gen. Microbiol* **1957**, *16*, 647–659.

148. Yew, WW; Tonb, SCW; Lui, KS; Leung, SKF; Chau, CH; Wang, EP. Comparison of MB/BacT system and agar proportion method in drug susceptibility testing of *Mycobacterium tuberculosis*. *Diagn. Microbiol. Infect. Dis* **2001**, *39*, 229–232.

149. Nakano, M; Nakamur, Y; Takikawa, K; Kouketsu, M; Arita, T. Sustained release of sulfamethizole from agar beads. *J. Pharm. Pharmacol* **1979**, *31*, 869–872.

150. Kojima, T; Hashida, M; Muranishi, S; Sezaki, H. Antitumor activity of timed-release derivative of mitomycin C, agarose bead conjugate. *Chem. Pharm. Bull* **1978**, *26*, 1818–1824.

151. El-Raheem El-Helw, A; El-Said, Y. Preparation and characterization of agar beads containing phenobarbitone sodium. *J. Microencapsul* **1988**, *5*, 159–163.

152. Prasad, K; Mehta, G; Meena, R; Siddhanta, AK. Hydrogel-forming Agar-graft-PVP and k-Carrageenan-graft-PVP blends: Rapid synthesis and characterization. *J. Appl. Polym. Sci* **2006**, *102*, 3654–3663.

153. Lugao, AB; Machado, LDB; Miranda, LF; Alveraz, MR; Roziak, JM. Study of wound dressing structure and hydration/dehydration properties. *Radiat. Phys. Chem* **1998**, *52*, 319–322.

154. Nichols, CA; Guezennec, J; Bowman, JP. Bacterial exopolysaccharides from extreme marine environments with special consideration of the southern ocean, sea ice and deep-sea hydrothermal vents: A review. *Mar. Biotechnol* **2005**, *7*, 253–271.

155. Weiner, R; Langille, S; Quintero, E. Structure, function an immunochemistry of bacterial exopolysaccharides. *J. Ind. Microbiol* **1995**, *15*, 339–346.

156. Sun, C; Wang, JW; Fang, L; Gao, XD; Tan, RX. Free radical scavenging and antioxidant activities of EPS2, an exopolysaccharide produced by a marine filamentous fungus *Keissleriella* sp. YS 4108. *Life Sci* **2004**, *75*, 1063–1073.

157. Sun, C; Shan, CY; Gao, XD; Tan, RX. Protection of PC12 cells from hydrogen peroxide-induced injury by EPS2, an exopolysaccharide from a marine filamentous fungus *Keissleriella* sp. YS 4108. *J. Biotechnol* **2005**, *115*, 137–144.

158. Liu, F; Ng, TB. Antioxidative and free radical scavenging activities of selected medicinal herbs. *Life Sci* **2000**, *66*, 725–735.

159. Schinella, GR; Tournier, HA; Prieto, JM; Mordujovich de Buschiazzo, P; Ríos, JL. Antioxidant activity of anti-inflammatory plant extracts. *Life Sci* **2002**, *70*, 1023–1033.

160. Grice, HC. Safety evaluation of butylated hydroxyanisole from the perspective of effects on forestomach and oesophageal squamous epithelium. *Food Chem. Toxicol* **1988**, *26*, 717–723.

161. Qi, HM; Zhang, QB; Zhao, TT; Chen, R; Zhang, H; Niu, X; Li, Z. Antioxidant activity of different sulfate content derivatives of polysaccharide extracted from Ulva pertusa (Chlorophyta) *in vitro*. *Int. J. Biol. Macromol* **2005**, *37*, 195–199.

162. Sun, H-H; Mao, W-J; Chen, Y; Guo, S-D; Li, H-Y; Qi, X-H; Chen, Y-L; Xu, J. Isolation, chemical characteristics and antioxidant properties of the polysaccharides from marine fungus *Penicillium* sp. F23-2. *Carbohydr. Polym* **2009**, *78*, 117–124.

163. Ofek, I; Beachey, EH; Sharon, N. Surface sugars of animal cells as determinants of recognition in bacterial adherence. *Trends Biochem. Sci* **1978**, *3*, 159–160.

164. Bergey, E; Stinson, M. Heparin-inhibitable basement membrane-binding protein of Streptococcus pyogenes. *Infect. Immun* **1988**, *56*, 1715–1721.

165. Bellamy, F; Horton, D; Millet, J; Picart, F; Samreth, S; Chana, JB. Glycosylated derivatives of benzophenone, benzhydrol, and benzhydril as potential venous antithrombotic agents. *J. Med. Chem* **1993**, *36*, 898–903.

166. Cassaro, CMF; Dietrich, CP. Distribution of sulfated mucopolysaccharides in invertebrates. *J. Biol. Chem* **1977**, *252*, 2254–2261.

167. Höök, M; Kjellen, L; Johansson, S; Robinson, J. Cell surface glycosaminoglycans. *Ann. Rev. Biochem* **1984**, *53*, 847–869.

168. Wight, TN; Kinsella, MG; QwarnstroÈm, E. The role of proteglycans in cell adhesion, migration and proliferation. *Curr. Opin. Cell Biol* **1992**, *4*, 793–801.

169. Guzman-Murillo, MA; Ascencio, F. Anti-adhesive activity of sulfated exopolysaccharides of microalgae on attachment of red sore disease-associated bacteria and Helicobacter pylori to tissue culture cells. *Lett. Appl. Microbiol* **2000**, *30*, 473–478.

170. Ascencio, F; Fransson, LA; Wadström, T. Affinity of the gastric pathogen Helicobacter pylori for the N-sulfated glycosaminoglycan heparan sulfate. *J. Med. Microbiol* **1993**, *38*, 240–244.

171. SjÖustrÖum, JE; Larsson, H. Factors affecting growth and antibiotic susceptibility of Helicobacter pylori: Effect of pH and urea on the survival of a wild-type strain and a urease-deficient mutant. *J. Med. Microbiol* **1996**, *44*, 425–433.

172. SjÖustrÖum, JE; Fryklund, J; KoÈhler, T; Larsson, H. *In vitro* antibacterial activity of omeprazole and its selectivity for Helicobacter spp. are dependent on incubation conditions. *Antimicrob. Agents Chemother* **1996**, *40*, 621–626.

173. Chihara, G; Hamuro, J; Maeda, Y; Araki, Y; Fukuoka, F. Fractionation and purification of the polysaccharides with marked antitumor activity, especially lentinan, from Lentinus edodes (Berk) Sing (an edible mushroom). *Cancer Res* **1970**, *30*, 2776–2781.

174. Yoshizawa, Y; Enomoto, A; Todoh, H; Ametani, A; Kaminogawa, S. Activation of murine macrophages by polysaccharide fractions from marine algae (Porphyra yezoensis). *Biosci. Biotechnol. Biochem* **1993**, *57*, 1862–1866.

175. Matsuda, M; Yamori, T; Naitoh, M; Okutani, K. Structural revision of sulfated polysaccharide B-1 isolated from a marine pseudomonas species and its cytotoxic activity against human cancer cell lines. *Mar. Biotechnol* **2003**, *5*, 13–19.

176. Colliec-Jouault, S; Zanchetta, P; Helley, D; Ratiskol, J; Sinquin, C; Fischer, AM; Guezennec, J. Les polysaccharides microbiens d'origine marine et leur potentiel en thérapeutique humaine. *Pathologie Biologie* **2004**, *52*, 127–130.

177. Guezennec, J; Pignet, P; Lijour, Y; Gentric, E; Ratiskol, J; Colliec-Jouault, S. Sulfation and depolymerization of a bacterial exopolysaccharide of hydrothermal origin. *Carbohydr. Polym* **1998**, *37*, 19–24.

178. De Philippis, R; Sili, C; Paperi, R; Vincenzini, M. Exopolysaccharide-producing cyanobacteria and their possibile exploitation: A review. *J. Appl. Phycol* **2001**, *13*, 293–299.

179. Nicolaus, B; Panico, A; Lama, L; Romano, I; Manca, MC; De Giulio, A; Gambacorta, A. Chemical composition and production of exopolysaccharides from representative members of heterocystous and non-heterocystous cyanobacteria. *Phytochemistry* **1999**, *52*, 639–647.
180. Sutherland, IW. *Biotechnology of Microbial Exopolysaccharides*; Cambridge University Press: Cambridge, UK, 1990; p. 163.
181. Atkins, EDT. Biomolecular structures of naturally occurring carbohydrate polymers. *Int. J. Biol. Macromol* **1986**, *8*, 323–329.
182. Sutherland, IW. Novel and established applications of microbial polysaccharides. *Tibtech* **1998**, *16*, 41–46.
183. De Vuyst, L; Degeest, B. Heteropolysaccharides from lactic acid bacteria. *FEMS Microbiol. Rev* **1999**, *23*, 153–177.
184. Flaibani, A; Olsen, Y; Painter, TJ. Polysaccharides in desert reclamation: Composition of exocellular proteoglycan complexes produced by filamentous blue-green and unicellular green edaphic algae. *Carbohydr. Res* **1989**, *190*, 235–248.
185. Shepherd, R; Rockey, J; Sutherland, IW; Roller, S. Novel bioemulsifiers from microorganisms for use in foods. *J. Biotechnol* **1995**, *40*, 207–217.
186. Sutherland, IW. Structure-function relationships in microbial exopolysaccharides. *Biotech. Adv* **1994**, *12*, 393–448.
187. Hayashi, K; Hayashi, T; Kojima, I. A natural sulfated polysaccharide, calcium spirulan, isolated from *Spirulina platensis*: *In vitro* and *ex vivo* evaluation of anti-herpes simplex virus and anti-human immunodeficiency virus activities. *AIDS Res. Hum. Retrovir* **1996**, *12*, 1463–1471.
188. Hayashi, T; Hayashi, K. Calcium spirulan, an inhibitor of enveloped virus replication, from a blue-green alga *Spirulina platensis*. *J. Nat. Prod. (Lloydia)* **1996**, *59*, 83–87.

Samples Availability: Available from the authors.

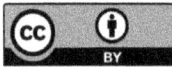

marine drugs

MDPI

Review

Marine Polysaccharides from Algae with Potential Biomedical Applications

Maria Filomena de Jesus Raposo, Alcina Maria Bernardo de Morais and
Rui Manuel Santos Costa de Morais *

CBQF—Centro de Biotecnologia e Química Fina, Laboratório Associado, Escola Superior de Biotecnologia,
Universidade Católica Portuguesa/Porto, Rua Arquiteto Lobão Vital, Apartado 2511, 4202-401 Porto, Portugal;
fraposo@porto.ucp.pt (M.F.J.R.); abmorais@porto.ucp.pt (A.M.B.M.)
* Author to whom correspondence should be addressed; rcmorais@porto.ucp.pt;
  Tel.: +351-22-5580050; Fax: +351-22-5090351.

Academic Editor: Paola Laurienzo
Received: 10 March 2015; Accepted: 4 May 2015; Published: 15 May 2015

Abstract: There is a current tendency towards bioactive natural products with applications in
various industries, such as pharmaceutical, biomedical, cosmetics and food. This has put some
emphasis in research on marine organisms, including macroalgae and microalgae, among others.
Polysaccharides with marine origin constitute one type of these biochemical compounds that have
already proved to have several important properties, such as anticoagulant and/or antithrombotic,
immunomodulatory ability, antitumor and cancer preventive, antilipidaemic and hypoglycaemic,
antibiotics and anti-inflammatory and antioxidant, making them promising bioactive products and
biomaterials with a wide range of applications. Their properties are mainly due to their structure
and physicochemical characteristics, which depend on the organism they are produced by. In the
biomedical field, the polysaccharides from algae can be used in controlled drug delivery, wound
management, and regenerative medicine. This review will focus on the biomedical applications of
marine polysaccharides from algae.

Keywords: polysaccharides; algae; bioactive; biomedical; pharmaceuticals; therapeutics;
drug delivery; regenerative medicine; wound management

---

1. Introduction

Contemporary tendency for natural products to be applied in medicine and to promote health
has put some emphasis in research on marine organisms, including macro- and microalgae, and
cyanobacteria. Extensive literature on the health benefits and uses as food or as drug carriers of
brown, red and green seaweeds, and the polysaccharides (**PS**) they produce, was published in the last
decade [1–8]. However, comparatively, there are only a handful of research papers on microalgae [9–14],
despite the richness of their composition and the ability to make them grow.

Polysaccharides already proved to have several important properties [3,8,12,15–22]. However, the
attempts to establish a relationship between the structures of the **PS** and their bioactivities/actions have
been a challenge due to the complexity of this type of polymers. In fact, aside from the homogalactan
from *Gyrodinium impudicum* (a dinoflagellate) [23], the β-glucan from *Chlorella vulgaris* (a green
microalga) [24] and the **PS** from a few species of seaweeds (Tables 1–3), most of these carbohydrates are
highly branched heteropolymers with different substituents in the various carbons of their backbone
and side-sugar components. Additionally, the monosaccharide composition and distribution within
the molecule, and the glycosidic bonds between monosaccharides can be very heterogeneous, which is
a real impairment for the study of their structures. Moreover, this heterogeneity also depends on the
species, between strains of the same species, and on the time and place of harvest.

The **PS** produced by algae are presented in Tables 1–3, according to the group of macroalga, Phaeophytes, Rhodophytes, Chlorophytes, and in Table 4, which is relative to microalgae. Nevertheless, there are always some similarities between the **PS** from each group of seaweeds: often, fucoidans are extracted from brown algal species (Table 1), agaroids and carrageenans come from red macroalgae (Table 2), and ulvans are obtained from green seaweeds (Table 3). Regarding microalgae (Table 4), and as far as we know, there are not common names for their **PS**, to the exception of spirulan from *Arthrospira platensis*. There are species that, besides producing large amounts of these useful polymers, they secrete them out into the culture medium and these polymers are easily extracted [14].

Table 1. Marine species of brown macroalgae (PHAEOPHYTES) producing polysaccharides (PS): some structural features and applications.

Type of PS	Source	Structure		Action/Application	References
		Main Mono-Sugars/Disaccharide Units	Glycosidic Bonds of Backbone		
Chromophyta Dictyotales					
Heterofucans S-fucans	Carnistrocarpus cervicornis a.k.a. Dictyota cervicornis	Fuc		Anticoagulant, antioxidant; anti-proliferative	[2,25]
S-galactofucans	D. menstrualis	Gal, fuc, xyl, glcAc		Peripheral anti-nociceptive, anti-inflammatory, antioxidant; anticoagulant, anti-proliferative	[1,2,26]
	D. mertensis			antioxidant; anticoagulant, anti-proliferative	[2]
Heterofucans	Dictyopteris delicatula	Fuc		Anticoagulant, antioxidant, antitumor, anti-proliferative	[2,27]
	D. polypodioides	Fuc		Antitumor	[28]
S-galactofucans	Lobophora variegata	Gal, fuc		Antioxidant, anticoagulant, anti-inflammatory	[29,30]
Heterofucans	Padina gymnospora	GlcAc, fuc	(1,3)- and (1,4)-β-D-glcAc	Antioxidant, anticoagulant, anti-thrombotic, antiviral	[2,31,32]
S-fucan	P. tetrastromatica	Fuc, gal, xyl, glcAc	(1,2)- and (1,3)-α-fuc		[33]
S-galactofucans; sPS; S-fucans	Spatoglossum schröederi	Gal, fuc, xyl; Fuc	(1,4)- and (1,3)-α-fuc	Anti-thrombotic; Peripheral anti-nociceptive; Anti-proliferative, anti-adhesive, antioxidant	[2,34–38]
Ectocarpales					
S-galactofucans	Adenocystis utricularis	Gal, fuc, rham, uronic acid	(1,3)-α-fuc	Antiviral	[39]
S-fucans	Cladosiphon okamuranus a.k.a. Okinawa mozuku	Fuc, glc, glcAc	(1,3)-α-L-fuc	Anti-proliferative, antiviral, anti-inflammatory, antiadhesive, antitumor, immunomodulator; angiogenic, gastroprotective, cardioprotective, restenosis preventive	[15,22,40–47]
S-fucoidan	C. novae-caledoniae	Fuc		Antitumor	[48]
Fucans	Leathesia difformis	Fuc		Antiviral	[49]
LMW-S-fucans	Nemacystus decipiens	Fuc		Anticoagulant	[50]
Fucales					
S-fucans; LMW-sPS; S-Laminaran; or otherwise modified	Ascophyllum nodosum	Fuc, xyl, gal, glcAc; Glc	(1,3)- and (1,4)-α-L-fuc (alternating); (1,3)- and (1,6)-β-glc	Immunomodulatory, anti-inflammatory, anticoagulant, anti-thrombotic, anti-metastatic, antitumor, antiadhesive, restenosis preventive; Anti-thrombotic, anticoagulant, angiogenic Antitumor; anticoagulant; serum hypocholesterolaemic, hypotensive, antibacterial, immunomodulator	[15,20,51–61]
S-fucans	Fucus spp: F. vesiculosus	Fuc, xyl, gal, glcAc	(1,3)- and (1,4)-α-L-fuc (alternating)	Immunostimulant, antiviral, antitumor, antiproliferative, antiadhesive, anticoagulant, antioxidant, anti-metastatic, anti-inflammatory; anti-angiogenic, antithrombotic (except F. vesiculosus)	[2,15,62–70]

Table 1. *Cont.*

Type of PS	Source	Structure	Action/Application	References
Laminaran; S-laminaran or otherwise modified	*Fucus* sp.	Glc	Antitumor, decreases liver triglyceride, cholesterol and phospholipid levels; serum hypocholesterolaemic, hypotensive, antibacterial, immunomodulator anticoagulant	[56,59,61]
S-fucans	*Hizikia fusiforme* a.k.a. *Sargassum fusiforme*	Fuc, gal, man, glcAc	(1,2)-α-D-man alternating with (1,4)-β-D-glcAc; some (1,4)-β-D-gal	Anticoagulant, anti-thrombotic	[71,72]
Fucans	*Pelvetia fastigiata*	Fuc		Antiviral	[73]
LMW-S-fucans	*P. canaliculata*	Fuc		Antiviral	[74]
S-fucans	*Sargassum* spp.	Fuc, gal, xyl, uronic acid		Prevent hyperlipidaemia, normalize dislipidaemia	[75–77]
S-galactofucans	*Sargassum* sp.	Gal, fuc, rham, glcAc	(1,6)-β-D-gal and/or (1,2)-β-D-man	Antitumor	[28,62,78–80]
S-heterofucans	*S. filipendula*	Fuc		Antioxidant, anti-proliferative	[2,81]
S-fucoidan	*S. henslowianum*	Fuc		Anti-proliferative, antitumor	[75]
S-fucoidan	*S. horneri*	Fuc	(1,3)-α-L-fuc, (1,3)- and (1,4)-α-L-fuc	Antitumor, antiviral	[62,80]
LMW-fucoidan	*S. patens*	Fuc		Antiviral	[32]
sPS	*Turbinaria conoides*			Antioxidant	[82]
Laminariales				
S-galactofucan	*Costaria costata*	Gal, fuc		Antitumor	[16]
S-fucans	*Ecklonia cava* or *E. kurome*	Fuc, rham, gal, glcAc	(1,3)- or (1,6)-, and (1,4)-α-L-fuc	Anti-proliferative, antitumor, anticoagulant, antioxidant, antithrombotic, anti-inflammatory	[16,83–88]
Fucoidans; laminarans	*Eisenia bicyclis*	Fuc; Glc	(1,3)- and (1,6)-β-D-glc	Anti-proliferative, antitumor, anticoagulant; Antitumor	[83,89–91]
Laminaran; S-laminaran or otherwise modified	*Laminaria* sp (or *Saccharina*)	Glc	(1,3)- and (1,6)-β-D-glc	Antitumor, anticoagulant, decreases liver triglyceride, cholesterol and phospholipid levels; serum hypocholesterolaemic, hypotensive, antibacterial, immunomodulator	[56,59,61]
S-fucoidans	*Laminaria* spp.	Fuc, xyl, man, glcAc	(1,3)-α-L-fuc	Antioxidant, anticoagulant, antithrombotic, anti-adhesive, anti-proliferative, anti-inflammatory, anti-angiogenic, anti-metastatic	[15,52,83,92–96]
S-galactofucan	*L. japonica* a.k.a. *Saccharina japonica*	Gal, fuc	(1,3)- and (1,4)-α-L-fuc (alternating)	Anti-lipidaemic, increases HDL, antiviral, antitumor, immunomodulator, antioxidant neuroprotective	[3,15,97–102]
Fucoidans	*Lessonia vadosa*	Fuc		Anticoagulant	[103]
S-fucoidan	*Saccharina cichorioides* a.k.a. *Laminaria cichorioides*	Fuc		Antitumor, anticoagulant, anti-thrombotic	[104,105]
S-galactofucans fucoidan	*Undaria pinnatifida*	Gal, fuc, xyl, uronic acid	(1,3)- and (1,4)-α-L-fuc (alternating)	Antiviral, anticoagulant, antitumor, anti-proliferative, immunomodulatory, anti-inflammatory induced osteoblastic differentiation	[3,52,69,106–111]
LMW-S-fucans			Anticoagulant	[112]
Laminaran; S-laminaran or otherwise modified		Glc	Anticoagulant, antitumor; serum hypocholesterolaemic, hypotensive, antibacterial, immunomodulator	[56,59,61]

Table 2. Marine species of red macroalgae (**RHODOPHYTES**) producing **PS**: some structural features and applications.

Type of PS	Source	Structure — Main mono-Sugars/Disaccharide Units	Structure — Glycosidic Bonds of Backbone	Action/Application	References
	Rhodophyta Bangiales				
S-galactan porphyran	*Porphyra* spp.	Gal	(1,3)-β-D-gal or (1,4)-α-L-gal	Antitumor, hypotensive, regulates blood cholesterol	[113,114]
siPS	*P. haitanensis*			Antioxidant	[115]
Porphyran	*P. yezoensis*			Antitumor, immunomodulatory, hypolipidaemic	[116-119]
	Ceramiales				
S-agarans	*Bostrychia montagnei*			Antiviral	[120]
S-agarans	*Cryptopleura ramosa*			Antiviral	[121]
	Digenea simplex			Antiviral	[122]
	Corallinales				
LMW-PS	*Corallina* sp.			Antiviral	[32]
	Cryptonemiales				
	Cryptonemia crenulata	Gal		Antiviral	[123]
S-agaran	*Gloiopeltis complanata*	Gal, Agal	[→3)-β-D-gal-(1→4)-3,6-α-L-Agal-(1→], and [→3)-β-D-gal-(1→4)-α-L-gal-(1→]		[114]
Agaroid-carrageenan	*G. furcata*	Gal	6-O-methyl-gal, 3,6Agal(1,3)-β-D-, and (1,4)-α-L-gal or (1,4)-α-L-Agal		[124]
	Gelidiales				
di-S-galactan	*Gelidium crinale*	Gal		Anticoagulant	[125]
S-agarans and hybrid DL-galactans	*Pterocladia capillacea*	Gal		Antiviral	[126]
	Gigartinales				
S-agarans S-galactans	*Aghardiella tenera*	Gal		Antiviral	[127,128]
S-λ-carrageenan	*Chondrus crispus*	Gal, Agal	(1,3)-α-D-gal, and (1,4)-β-3,6-Agal or (1,4)-β-D-gal (alternating)	Antiviral, anticoagulant, antithrombotic	[1,5,129–131]
LMW-sPS	*C. ocellatus*	Gal, Agal		Antitumor	[132]
S-galactans	*Euchema cottonii*	Gal		Antioxidant	[2]
S-κ-carrageenan	*E. spinosa*	Gal, Agal	(1,3)-α-D-gal, and (1,4)-β-3,6-Agal or (1,4)-β-D-gal (alternating)	Anticoagulant, anti-thrombotic	[5,130,131]
LMW-sPS	*Furcellaria lumbricalis*	Gal		Immunostimulant	[133]
S-galactans	*Gigartina acicularis*	Gal		Antioxidant	[2]
S-carrageenans	*G. skottsbergii*	Gal, Agal	(1,3)-α-D-gal, and (1,4)-β-3,6-Agal or (1,4)-β-D-gal (alternating)	Antiviral, anticoagulant	[130,131,134,135]
Hybrid DL-galactans	*Gymnogongrus torulosus*	Gal		Antiviral	[136]
LMW-PS	*Hymea charoides*	Gal		Antiviral	[32]
LMW-S-carrageenans	*Kappaphycus striatus*	Gal, Agal	(1,3)-α-D-gal, and (1,4)-β-3,6-Agal or (1,4)-β-D-gal (alternating)	Antitumor, immunomodulator	[1,131]
S-λ-carrageenan	*Phyllophora brodiei*	Gal, Agal	(1,3)-α-D-gal, and (1,4)-β-3,6-Agal or (1,4)-β-D-gal (alternating)	Anticoagulant, antithrombotic	[130,131,137]

Table 2. *Cont.*

Type of PS	Source	Structure	Action/ Application	References
LMW-slPS	*Soliera chordalis*		Immunostimulant	[138]
S-carrageenans	*Stenogramme interrupta*	Gal, Agal — (1,3)-α-D-gal, and (1,4)-β-3,6-Agal or (1,4)-β-D-gal (alternating)	Antiviral	[130,131,139]
Gracilariales				
slPS	*Gracilaria caudata*		Antioxidant	[2]
S-agarans S-galactans	*G. corticata*	Gal	Antiviral	[140]
slPS	*G. verrucosa*		Immunomodulator	[141]
Halymeniales				
S-galactan	*Grateloupia indica*	Gal	Anticoagulant, antithrombotic	[137]
Nemaliales				
S-mannans	*Nemalion helminthoides*	Man	Antiviral	[142]
Xylogalactans S-xylomannans	*Nothogenia fastigiata*	Xyl, gal Xyl, man	Antiviral, anticoagulant	[143–145]
Nematomatales				
S-galactans	*Schizymenia dubyi*	Gal, uronic acid	Antiviral	[146]
S-λ-carrageenan	*S. pacifica*	Gal, Agal — (1,3)-α-D-gal, and (1,4)-β-3,6-Agal or (1,4)-β-D-gal (alternating)	Antiviral	[130,131,147]
S-galactan	*S. binderi*	Gal	Anticoagulant	[148]
Rhodymeniales				
di-S-galactan; LMW-slPS	*Botryocladia occidentalis*	Gal	Anticoagulant; anti-venom	[149,150]
LMW-carrageenans	*Champia feldmannii*	Gal, Agal — (1,3)-α-D-gal, and (1,4)-β-3,6-Agal or (1,4)-β-D-gal (alternating)	Antitumor	[130,131,151]
Sebdeniales				
S-xylomannans	*Sebdenia polydactyla*	Xyl, man	Antiviral	[152]

Table 3. Marine species of green macroalgae (CHLOROPHYTES) producing **PS**: some structural features and applications.

Type of PS	Source	Structure		Action/ Application	References
		Main Mono-Sugars/Disaccharide Units	Glycosidic Bonds of Backbone		
	Chlorophyta *Bryopsidales*				
sIPS, including S-galactans	*Caulerpa* spp.			Antioxidant, anticoagulant, antithrombotic; antiviral, anti-proliferative, antitumor	[2,153,154]
sIPS and derivatives	*C. cupressoides*	Gal, man, xyl		Anti-inflammatory, antinociceptive	[8,155,156]
LMW-PS sIPS	*C. racemosa*	Gal, glc, ara, uronic acid		Antiviral; antitumor	[32,154,157]
S-arabinogalactans	*Codium* spp.	Gal, ara	(1,3)-β-D-gal	Anticoagulant, antithrombotic, antiviral	[124,153,158–161]
S-pyrulylated-galactans	*C. isthmocladum*	Gal, ara	(1,3)-β-D-gal	Antioxidant, anticoagulant, anti-proliferative	[2,162]
	Ulotrichales				
S-mannans	*Capsosiphon fulvescens*	Man, glcAc, gal		Immunomodulator	[163]
S-rhamnans and LMW-S-rhamnans	*Monostroma latissimum*	Rham	(1,3)-α-L-rham, and (1,3)-α-L-rham or (1,2)-α-L-rham or (1→2,3)-α-L-rham	Antiviral, anticoagulant	[164–168]
S-rhamnans	*M. nitidum*	Rham, glc		Anticoagulant, antithrombotic, hepatoprotective, antitumor, immunomodulator	[165,166,169–171]
	Ulvales				
Rhamnans	*Enteromorpha intestinalis*	Rham, xyl, glcAc		Antitumor, immunomodulator	[172,173]
LMW-sIPS	*E. linza*			Anticoagulant	[174]
S-ulvans and derivatives	*E. prolifera*	Rham, xyl, glc, glcAc, IduAc		Immunomodulator, antioxidant, hypolipidaemic	[124,175–177]
S-ulvans and derivatives	*Ulva* spp.	Rham, uronic acid		Anti-adhesive, antiproliferative; hepatoprotective	[178,179]
sIPS	*U. conglobata*	Rham, uronic acid		Anticoagulant	[180]
sIPS	*U. fasciata*			Antioxidant, antitumor	[181]
S-galactans sIPS	*U. lactuca*	Rham, xyl, glcAc		Antioxidant, anti-proliferative, hypocholesterolaemic, hepatoprotective, antitumor; Antiviral, anti-inflammatory, antinociceptive	[90,182–189]
S-ulvans	*U. pertusa*	Rham, xyl, glcAc, iduAc	[→4)-β-D-GlcAc-(1,4)-α-L-rham3S-(1→], and [→4)-α-L-IduAc(1,4)-α-L-rham3S-(1→]	Antioxidant, anti-proliferative, hypocholesterolaemic	[90,182–185]
LMW-S-ulvan or otherwise modified	*U. pertusa*			Antioxidant, hypotriglyceridaemic, decrease LDL- and increases HDL-cholesterol, immunostimulatory	[166,185,190,191]
S-PS	*U. rigida*	Rham, glcAc	β-D-glcAc-(1,4)-L-rham (disaccharide)	Immunostimulatory	[178,192]

31

Table 4. Marine species of microalgae/blue-green algae producing **PS**; main neutral sugars.

Type of PS	Source	Main Neutral Sugars	Action/Application	References
	MICROALGAE			
	Diatoms			
sPS	Cylindrotheca closterium	xyl, glc, man, rham		[193,194]
sPS	Navicula salinarum	glc, xyl, gal, man		[193]
s-EPS	Phaeodactylum tricornutum	glc, man, xyl, rham	Anti-adhesive	[195–197]
EPS	Haslea ostrearia			[198]
EPS	Nitzschia closterium			[199]
EPS	Skeletonema costatum			
EPS	Chaetoceros spp.	rham, fuc, gal, man		[200]
EPS	Amphora sp.			[201]
	Chlorophytes			
sPS	Chlorella stigmatophora	glc, xyl, fuc,	Anti-inflammatory, immunomodulator	[195]
sPS	C. autotrophica			[202]
PS β-(1,3)-glucan	C. vulgaris	rham, gal, arab, 2-O-methyl-rham glc	Antitumor, infection preventive agent	[24,203,204]
EPS	Dunaliella salina	gal, glc, xyl, fru		[205]
EPS	Ankistrodesmus angustus			[201]
EPS	Botryococcus braunii	gal, fuc, glc, rham		[206,207]
	Prasiophyte			
sPS	Tetraselmis sp.		Anti-adhesive	[202]
	Prymnesiophyte/haptophyte			
sPS	Isochrysis sp.			[202]
	Rhodophytes			
sPS	Porphyridium sp.	xyl, gal, glc	Anti-inflammatory, immunomodulator, prevention of tumour cell growth, anti-adhesive, antiviral, biolubricant	[208–213]
sPS	P. cruentum	xyl, gal, glc, glcAc, 3-O-methyl-xyl	Antioxidant and free radical scavenging, immunomodulator, antiviral, antibacterial, antilipidaemic, antiglycaemic	[214–222]
sPS	P. purpureum		antiviral	[223]
sPS	Rhodella reticulata	xyl, rham, 3-O-methyl-rham, 4-O-methyl-gal	Antiviral, antilipidaemic, antiglycaemic, prevention of tumour cell growth	[208,213,219],
sPS	R. maculata	xyl, gal, glc-3-O-methyl-xyl		[224,225]
	Dinoflagellates			
sPS	Cochlodinium polykrikoides	man, gal, glc	Antiviral	[226]
sPS	Gyrodinium impudicum	gal	Antiviral, anti-inflammatory, immunomodulator, anti-proliferative, prevention of tumour cell growth	[23,227–229]
	CYANOBACTERIA			
EPS	Aphanothece halophytica	glc, fuc, man, arab, glcAc		[230]
EPS s-Spirulan	Arthrospira platensis	gal, xyl, glc, fru rham, fuc, glc, 3-O-methyl-rham	Antiviral, antibacterial, prevention of tumour cell growth Anti-proliferative, anti-adhesive, anti-metastatic	[19,223,231–235]
sPS	Anabaena, Gloethece, Nostoc Aphanocapsa, Phormidium, Synechocystis, Cyanothece			[19]

Both micro- and macroalgae are excellent sources of **PS**, most of them being sulphated (**sPS**). They are associated with several biological activities and potential health benefits, making them interesting compounds for the application in pharmaceuticals, therapeutics, and regenerative medicine. Some of the beneficial bioactivities demonstrated by the crude **PS** and their derivatives, either *in vitro* or *in vivo*, upon various kinds of cell-lines and animal models, include anticoagulant and/or antithrombotic properties, immunomodulatory ability, antitumor and cancer preventive activity (as anti-proliferative agents, tumour suppressors or natural cell-killers). They are also good antidislipidaemic and hypoglycaemic agents, and can be powerful antioxidants, antibiotics and anti-inflammatory. For example, the sPS from *Enteromorpha* and *Porphyridium* have demonstrated strong antitumor and immunomodulating properties [173,211]; those from *Caulerpa cupressoides* and *Dyctiota menstrualis* are good antinociceptive agents [1,155], and the **sPS** from *Cladosiphon okaramanus* showed angiogenic, gastro- and cardioprotective bioactivities [15,46,47].

2. Some Structural Characteristics of Polysaccharides Produced by Marine Algae

The chemical structure of PS produced by macro- and microalgae may significantly determine their properties, namely physico-chemical and biochemical, and reflect their physical behavior and biological activities, as will be discussed further on in this review.

2.1. Macroalgae

Seaweeds (or marine macroalgae), whose **PS** have been studied more often, belong to the groups Chlorophyta (green seaweeds), Phaeophyceae (brown algae, Chromophyta) and Rhodophyta (red macroalgae).

Brown seaweeds usually contain fucoidans; the oligosaccharides obtained from the hydrolysis of fucoidans may often contain **gal**, **glc**, uronic acids, and/or other monosaccharides (Table 1), linked together and to the main chain by different types of glycosidic bonds. This is the case, for example, for the laminaran from *E. bicyclis* (Laminarales), or the galactofucan from *Sargassum* sp. (Fucales), and the fucan from *P. tetrastromatica* (Dictyotales) (Table 1). However, the structure complexity of these fucoidans makes difficult to establish a relationship between the **PS**-chains/composition and their biological actions, and/or some kind of protocols to design universal pharmaceuticals or other drug-like substances to prevent and/or cure specific diseases. This issue will be discussed later in this review.

The monosaccharide composition, the linkage types, the overall structure of fucoidans, and some of their di- and oligosaccharides were well explored by Ale *et al.* [75], Fedorov *et al.* [3] and Li *et al.* [103]. For example, Ale's group [75] showed the difference between **sPS** from three species of *Fucus* by focusing on the various substituents at C-2 and C-4 carbons, despite the similarities of their backbones; they also highlighted the possible structures of fucoidans from two species of *Sargassum*, already suggested by Duarte *et al.* [78] and Li *et al.* [71]. Cumashi and coworkers suggested some structures for the backbone chain of several seaweeds [15]. Among them are the schemes for the components of the main chain showing either the (1,3)-, and (1,3)- and (1,4)-linked **fuc** residues or some di- and trisaccharide repeating units for *A. nodosum*, *C. okamuranus*, *L. saccharina* (a.k.a. *Saccharina latissima*), and some species of *Fucus*. On the other hand, Fedorov *et al.* [3] focused on the structures and bioactivities of different **sPS**, such as fucoidans (e.g., galactofucan from *Laminaria* (a.k.a. *Saccharina japonica*), and laminarans (e.g., the one from *E. bicyclis*) (Table 1).

Red macroalgae contain large amounts of **sPS** (Table 2), mostly galactans (agaroids and/or carrageenans), with alternating repeating units of 1,3-α-**gal** and 1,4-β-D-**gal** [236], and/or 3,6-anhydro**gal** (3,6-**A**gal) [237]. Substituents can be other monosaccharides (**man**, **xyl**), sulphate, methoxy and/or pyruvate groups, the pattern of sulphation dividing carrageenans into different families, for example, in C-4 for κ-carrageenan, and in C-2 for λ-carrageenan. In addition, the rotation of **gal** in 1,3-linked residues divides agaroids (L-isomer) from carrageenans (D-isomer) [18]. Apart from agarans [18], found in species of *Porphyra*, *Polysiphonia*, *Acanthophora*, *Goiopeltis*,

Bostrychia or *Cryptopleura* (Table 2), red seaweeds are also good sources of κ-carrageenan (*E. spinosa*, *K. alvarezii*), λ-carrageenan (*Chondrus* sp, *G. skottsbergii* and *Phillophora*) (Table 2) [238], ι-carrageenan (*E. spinosa*) [239], and other heterogalactans with **man** and/or **xyl** bulding up their backbones. Among these, we may find xylogalactans in *N. fastigiata* [143], xylomannans in *S. polydactyla* [152] (Table 2).

Regarding green macroalgae, the information on their structures and applications is scarce. Nevertheless, Wangs's group [8] has made an excellent overview on those properties for the **sPS** from several genera of "macro-chlorophytes". These **sPS** are very diverse and complex, with various types of glycosidic bonds between monomers, and include galactans (*Caulerpa* spp.), rhamnans (*C. fulvescens* and *Enteromorpha*), arabino- and pyruvylated galactans (*Codium* spp.), and the most known ulvans from *Ulva* spp and *E. prolifera* (Table 3). Wang and coworkers [8] also included some repeating aldobiuronic di-units for the backbone of ulvans, containing **IduAc** or **glcAc** (*U. armoricana* and *U. rigida*, respectively), disaccharides (S-)**xyl-S-rham**, and a trisaccharide unit composed by 1,4-linked **glcAc**, **glcAc**, and S-rham. The backbone of rhamnans seems to be somewhat simpler (Table 3), but other types of glycosidic bonds can also appear. For example, four repeating disaccharide units were indicated for the homopolymer of *M. latissimum* [240] (Table 3). Species from *Codium* are very interesting: their **sPS** may include different percentages of arabinose (**ara**) and **gal**, giving place to arabinans (*C. adhaerens*; [153]), galactans (*C. yezoense*) [241], arabinogalactans [8]. Pyruvylated galactans were also identified in *C. yezoense* [241], *C. isthmocladium* [2] and *C. fragile* [242]. Some other species of *Codium* present other **PS**-types such as (1,4)-β-D mannans in *C. vermilara* [158], or the rare (1,3)-β-D mannans in *C. fragile* [243], with various sulphation patterns. *C. fulvescens* contains "vary branched" S-mannan as well [163].

2.2. Microalgae and Cyanobacteria

The characteristics of the various **PS** produced by microalgae, including their composition and structure, were recently discussed [14]. Some particular aspects about these polymers came to light. For example, it seems that concerning microalgae only *G. impudicum* and *C. vulgaris* contain homo-**PS** of galactose (**gal**) [23] and glucose (**glc**) [24], respectively, while the **PS** from the other species are heteropolymers of **gal**, xylose (**xyl**) and **glc** in different proportions. Rhamnose (**rham**), **fuc** and fructose can also appear, and some of the microalgal **PS** present uronic acids as well (Table 4). The glycosidic bonds are described for only a few **PS**, such as the one from *Aphanothece halophytica*, whose monosaccharides are mainly 1,3-linked, but linkages of type 1 also appear for **glc** and **glcAc** [230], which suggests that these two last molecules are terminal, and some multiple bonds, such as 1,2,4-linked and 1,3,6-linked mannose (**man**) residues [230], are present as well, suggesting some branches coming out from the backbone of the **PS**. Further, there are some special features of microalgal **PS**, as it is the case of acofriose 3-*O*-methyl-**rham** in the polymers of *Chlorella* [203], *Botryococcus braunii* and calcium-spirulan (**CaSp**) of *Arthrospira platensis* [244]. In *Porphyridium cruentum*, an aldobiuronic acid [3-*O*-(α-D-glucopyranosyluronic acid)-L-galactopyranose), or **glcAc-gal** disaccharide], and two hetero-oligosaccharides were also identified [245], and so did two other aldobiuronic acids [246], which were also found in other species of *Porphyridium* and *Rhodella* [247]. Furthermore, other repeating disaccharide-units [233,234], and some oligosaccharides were also highlighted [233]. In addition, Ford and Percival [196,197] found that the structure of the **sPS** from *Phaeodactylum tricornutum* was a ramified sulphated glucoronomannan, with a backbone composed by β-(1,3)-linked **man**; a triuronic acid, an aldobiuronic acid and a glucan made of β-(1,3)-linked **glc** were also identified as being constituents of the side chains of that polymer.

Figure 1 illustrates the structures of some **PS** from macro- and microalgae.

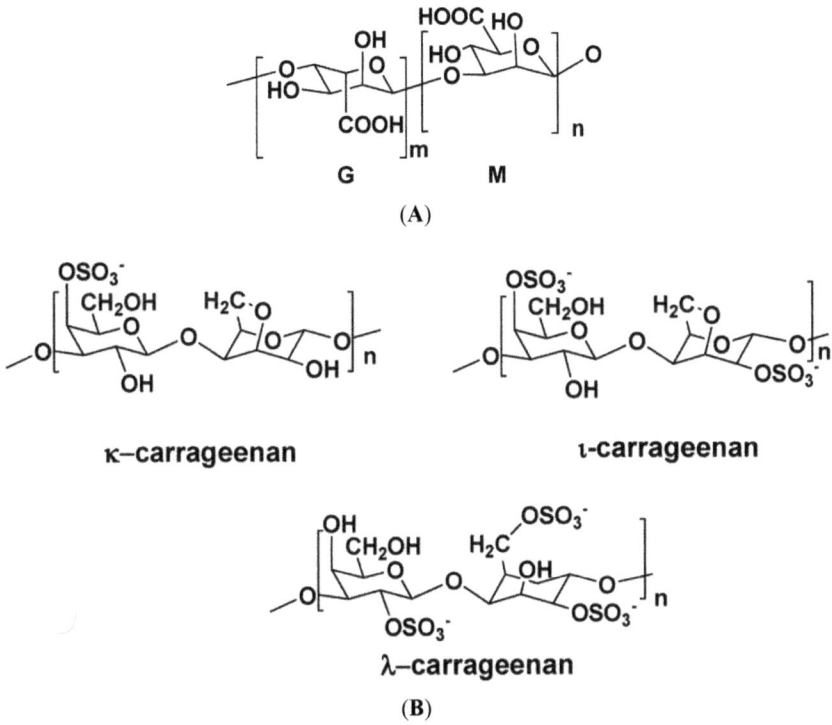

(A)

κ–carrageenan

ι-carrageenan

λ–carrageenan

(B)

Figure 1. Cont.

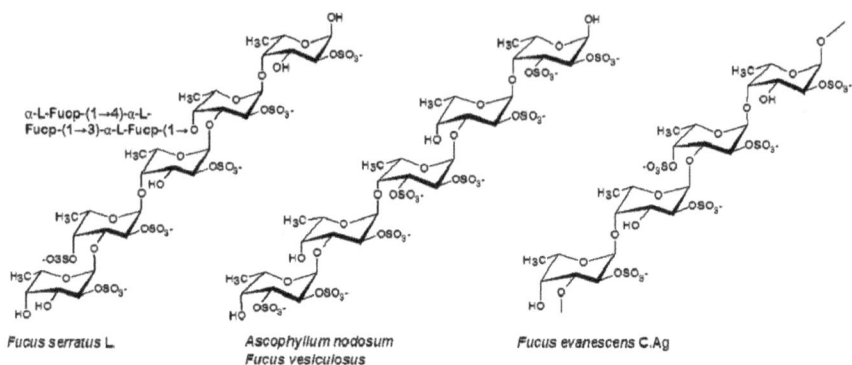

α-L-Fucp-(1→4)-α-L-
Fucp-(1→3)-α-L-Fucp-(1→

Fucus serratus L.

Ascophyllum nodosum
Fucus vesiculosus

Fucus evanescens C.Ag

(C)

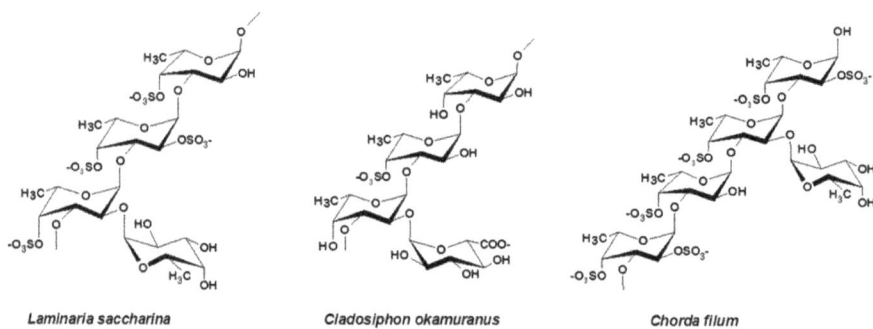

Laminaria saccharina

Cladosiphon okamuranus

Chorda filum

(D)

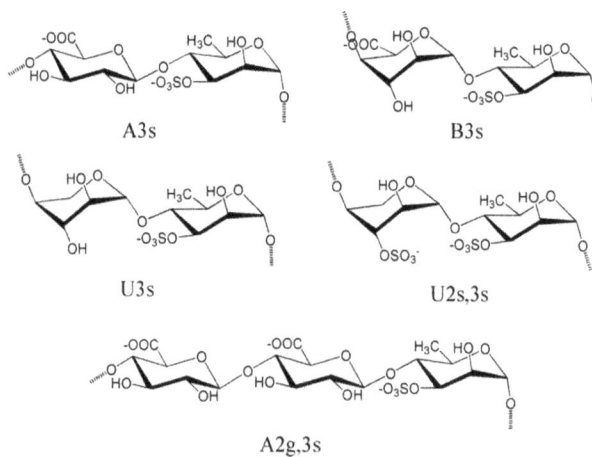

A3s

B3s

U3s

U2s,3s

A2g,3s

(E)

Figure 1. Cont.

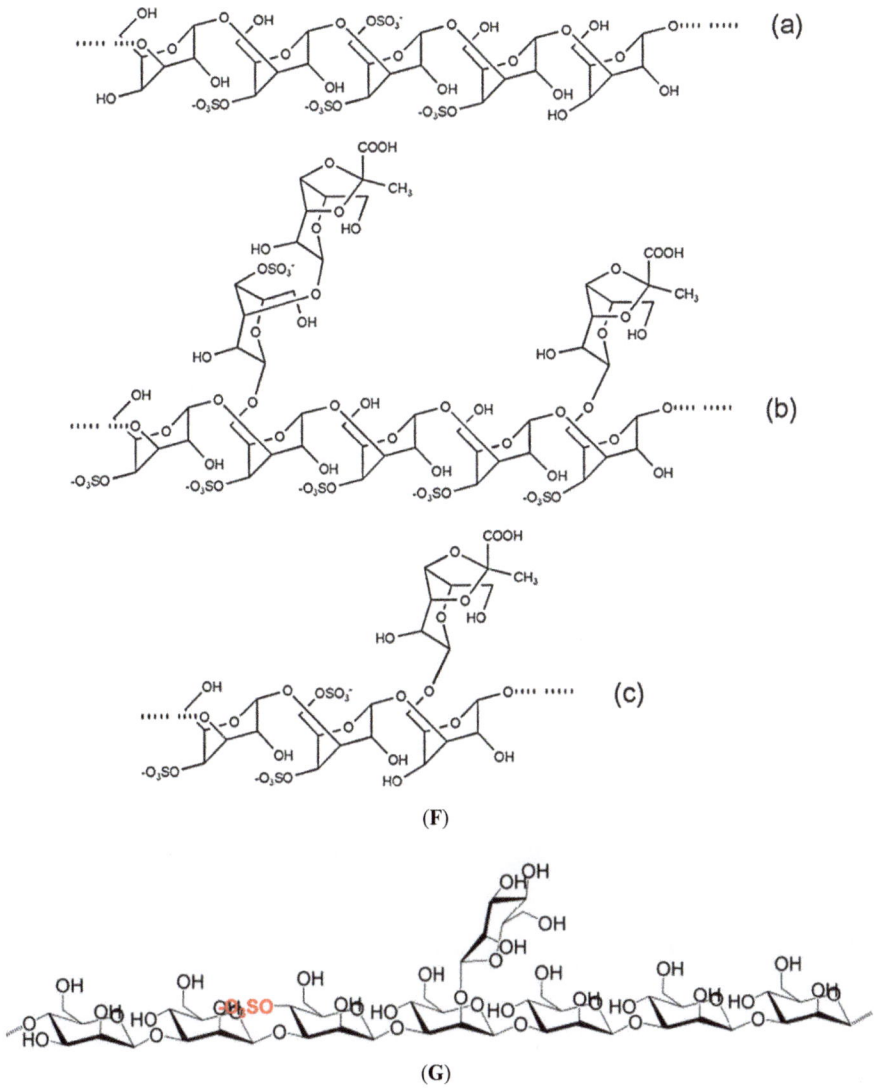

(a)

(b)

(c)

(F)

(G)

Figure 1. Cont.

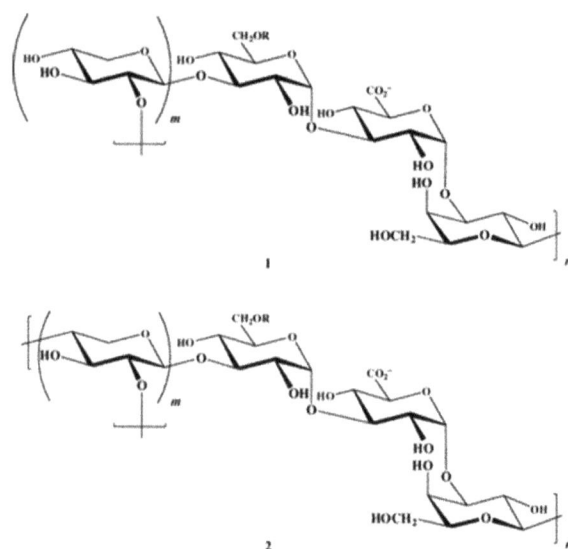

Figure 1. Examples of structures of **PS** from macro- and microalgae. (**A**) Repeating units suggested for the structure of alginates [3]; (**B**) Repeating units of some carrageenans [3]; (**C**) Fucoidan backbone of *A. nodosum* and three species of *Fucus*, showing the different distribution pattern of sulphate [75]; (**D**) Repeating units, sulphation pattern and gycosidic bounds of the backbone structures of PS of three different brown seaweeds [75]; (**E**) Alternative positions and combinations for the repeating units of ulvans. A3s and B3s are aldobiouronic repeating di-units suggested for *U. rigida* and *U. armoricana*. U3s and U2s,3s are, respectively, a xyl-(S-rham) and a (S-xyl)-(S-rham) disaccharides [8]; (**F**) Galactans of *Codium* spp. (a) linear (1,3)-β-D-galactan, (b) and (c) pyruvylated branched sulphated galactans [8]; (**G**) A rare mannan of the **PS** from *C. fragile*, with (1,3)-β-man residues and branches at C-2 [8]. Tabarsa *et al.* [243] referred that either branches or sulphates may be bound at the C-2 and/or C-4 positions along the PS backbone); (**H**) Models 1 or 2 for the possible acidic repeating unit in polysaccharide II, from *Porphyridium* sp. R = H, SO_2O, terminal **gal** or terminal **xyl**, m = 2 or 3 [14].

3. Potential Medical/Biomedical Applications of Polysaccharides from Marine Algae. Relation with Some Chemical Features of Their Structures

The **PS** are complex and heterogeneous macromolecules, coming from different genera belonging to the larger groups of algae, and species and strains of the same genus. Often, difficulties are found in identifying their chemical structure and therefore, their biological activities not being thoroughly understood. Few researchers have focused on such a challenging task as the exploitation of possible relation chemical structure–activity of **PS**. One approach to look for structure–biological activity relationships has been to make inferences based on information obtained from studies of invertebrate sulphated polysaccharides that have a regular structure and, thus, could be more easily studied [18].

The types of glycosidic linkages and the contents and positions of the sulphate groups may be significantly different in the various **sPS**, depending on species, region of the thallus, growing conditions, extraction procedures, and analytical methods [2,186]. The biological and pharmacological activities of **sPS** normally result from a complex interaction of several structural features, including the sulphation level, distribution of sulphate groups along the polysaccharide backbone, molecular weight, sugar residue composition, and stereochemistry [248,249]. For instance, the general structural features of fucans that are important in their anticoagulation activity include the sugar composition, molecular weight, sulphation level and the position of sulphate groups on the sugar backbone [84,86,250,251]. Also, it has been observed that the antiviral activity of **sPS** increases with the molecular weight [252].

Galactans, fucans and galactofucans are representative polysaccharides from brown and red seaweeds that differ in structure, sulphation level and molecular weight, and yet all were shown to inhibit HSV-1 and HSV-2 infection [253]. Recently, by using NMR, it was found that branched fucoidan oligosaccharides might present higher imuno-inflammatory activity than linear structures, because they were better at inhibiting the complement system [254]. Usov [236] compared two sulphated galactans from *Botryocladia occidentalis* and *Gelidium crinale*. He concluded that the interaction of the **sPS** with different compounds participating in the coagulation process depends on the differences in the structural features; unfortunately, data on the configuration of galactose in the galactan from G. *crinale* are not sufficient to fully understand the relationship.

3.1. Antiviral, Antibacterial and Antifungal Activities

An overview on the antiviral activity against several kinds of virus and retrovirus, enveloped or naked was well documented by Carlucci *et al.* [255] and Wijesekara *et al.* [21]. These reviews focused on the HIV type 1 and type 2, the human papilloma virus (HPV), the encephalo-myocarditis virus, the hepatitis virus type A and type B and the dengue and yellow fever virus. The inhibition of infection by most of these viruses was explained by the action of **sPS**, which might block the attachment of virions to the host cell surfaces [140,256]. Another way of exerting their activity is by inhibiting the replication of the enveloped virus, such as the HIV, the human cytomegalovirus (HCMV) and the respiratory syncytial virus (RSV) [18,147,153], either by inhibiting the virus adsorption or the entry into the host cells. Some of the **sPS** are effective only if applied simultaneously with the virus or immediately after infection [18]. Another mechanism of action of fucoidans and other **sPS** is through the inhibition of the syncytium formation induced by viruses [21,257].

Some S-xylomannans were reported to present antiviral sulphate-dependent activity, as it was the case of **PS** from *S. polydactyla* and *S. latifolium*, which inhibited the multiplication of HSV-1 in Vero-cells [152,258]. In addition, the molecular weight (MW) seems to play an important role in the antiviral properties of the **sPS**, the effect increasing with the MW [18]. However, other structural features can be co-responsible for the reinforcement of the antiviral effectiveness, like sulphation patterns, composition and distribution of sugar residues along the backbone, and the complexity of the polymers [18,152,248,253]. Further, the fucoidans from *L. japonica* already proved their effectiveness in fighting both RNA and DNA viruses [103], such as poliovirus III, adenovirus III, ECHO6 virus, coxsackie B3 and A16 viruses. Moreover, these **sPS** can protect host cells by inhibiting the cytopathic activity of those viruses [99].

In addition to their virucidal activity against HIV and other viruses associated to sexually transmitted diseases (STD) [5], including HPV, some carrageenans might find application as vaginal lubricant gels and coatings of condoms, with microbicidal activity, for they do not present any significant anticoagulant properties or cytotoxicity [259,260]. Furthermore, some fucoidans, apart from inhibiting attachment of virus particles to host cells, were able to inhibit the attachment of human spermatozoids to the *zona pellucida* of oocytes [261]; this property could be used for the development of a contraceptive gel with microbicidal characteristics [20].

The polysaccharides produced by some marine microalgae, and which may be released into the culture medium, showed antiviral activity against different kinds of viruses, such as the HIV-1, HSV-1 and HSV-2, VACV and Flu-A (Table 4), as described by Raposo *et al.* [14]. Sulphated **PS**, in particular, proved to increase the antiviral capacity [231]. In fact, the antiviral activity of the **PS** may depend on the culture medium, algal strain and cell line used for testing, but also on the methodology, and the degree of sulphation, as is the case of **EPS** from *P. cruentum* [216,262]. Despite the slight toxicity that some **PS** may present, they could be safely applied in *in vivo* experiments, decreasing the replication of the virus VACV, for instance [223].

The mechanisms involved in the antiviral activity of **sPS** may be understood analyzing what happens when cells are infected by a virus. Just before infection, viruses have to interact with some glycosaminoglycan receptors (GAG), such as heparin sulphate (HS) [263]. The GAG to which a protein can be covalently bound are part of the target cell surface and can also be found in the intracellular matrix of various connective and muscle tissues. **SPS** may impair the attachment of the virus particles by competing for those GAG-receptors, as they are chemically similar to HS [130,255], most of them having a covalently linked core protein [264,265]. Besides, as it happens with GAG, **sPS** are negatively charged and highly sulphated polymers [40,255,266], whose monosaccharide distribution pattern might influence the specificity of the bound protein, determining several biological functions [263]. For viruses to attach to the host cell surface, the linkage between the basic groups of the glycoproteins of the virus and the anionic components of the **PS** (sulphate, for example) at the cell surface must be established [248]. In fact, whichever the algal **PS** is, either from seaweeds or microalgae, by mimicking these GAG, they may induce the formation of a virus-algal **PS** complex, thus, impairing the cell infection by blocking the interaction virus-host cell receptor. Hidari and coworkers [40], for instance, showed that dengue virus (DENV) establishes an exclusive complex with fucoidan, and viral infection is, therefore, inhibited. They suggested that arginine-323 had a high influence on the interaction between the DENV-2 virus and the fucoidan, in an *in vitro* experiment with BHK-21 cells. These researchers also found that glucuronic acid seems to be crucial since no antiviral activity was observed when this compound was reduced to glucose.

Sulphated polysaccharides from seaweeds, such as alginates, fucoidans and laminaran appear to have antibacterial activity against *E. coli* and species from *Staphylococcus*. A fucoidan from *L. japonica* and sodium alginate were found to inhibit *E. coli* [267], for example, by adhering to bacteria and killing those microorganisms [5], thus showing bactericidal properties. This type of **PS** is also a good antibacterial agent against *Helicobacter pylori*, eradicating their colonies, restoring the stomach mucosa, in clinical trial studies, and regenerating biocenosis in the intestines [268]. Laminaran from *Fucus*, *Laminaria*, *A. nodosum* and *U. pinnatifida* demonstrated to have an effect on pathogenic bacteria [56] as well, with the advantage of being unable to promote blood coagulation [269]. An S-galactan from *Chaetomorpha aerea* inhibited the growth of *Staphylococcus aureus* (50 mg/mL of extract) but not that of *Salmonella enteritidis* [270]. In contrast, the carrageenans from some seaweeds [271] and the sulphated exopolysaccharide (**sEPS**) from the red microalga *Porphyridium cruentum*, despite the higher concentration used [216], showed a significant inhibitory activity against *S. enteritidis*. In fact, some **PS** from microalgae, such as *A. platensis* (Table 4), may present antibacterial properties against some specific bacteria, the activity depending on the solvent used to extract the polymer, as referred to by Raposo *et al.* [14].

By stimulating the production and/or expression of ILs, dectin-1 and toll-like receptors-2 on macrophages and dendritic cells, respectively, (1,3)-β-glucans from, e.g., *C. vulgaris*, and laminarans, also induced antifungal and antibacterial responses in rats [272], and some resistance to mammal organisms towards infections by *E. coli* [273]. Therefore, these types of **PS** promise to be good antimicrobial agents.

3.2. Anti-Inflammatory and Immunomodulatory Activities

Polysaccharides from macro- and microalgae have long demonstrated to have biological and pharmaceutical properties, such as anti-inflammatory and immunomodulation (Tables 1–4) [14]. Neverthless, the anti-inflammatory properties may be shown in several ways, depending on the **PS**, its source and type/site of inflammation. There is growing evidence that **sPS** are able to interefere with the migration of leukocytes to the sites of inflammation. For example, the heterofucan from *D. menstrualis* decreases inflammation by directly binding to the cell surface of leukocytes, especially polymorphonuclear cells (PMNs). It completely inhibits the migration of the leukocytes into the peritoneal cavity of mice where the injured tissue was after being submitted to simulated pain and inflammation, without the production of pro-inflammatory cytokines [1]. Sometimes, the recruitment of these PMNs shows to be dependent on P- and/or L-selectins, as it was demonstrated for fucoidans of some brown seaweeds [15,112].

Some other studies refer the association of the anti-inflammatory activity with the immunomodulatory ability. This seems to be the case in the work by Kang *et al.* [88], who simulated an inflammation process in RAW 264.7 cells (peritoneal macrophage primary cells) induced by lipopolysaccharides (LPS). They found that the fucoidan from *E. cava* inhibited, in a dose-dependent manner, the enzyme nitric oxide synthase induced by LPS (iNOS) and the gene expression for the enzyme cyclooxygenase-2 (COX-2) and, as a consequence, the production of nitric oxide (NO) and prostaglandin E2 (PGL2). Li *et al.* [274] confirmed the anti-inflammation mechanism *in vivo* via the immunomodulatory system *in vivo*, since the fucoidan from *L. japonica* reduced the inflammation of rats' myocardium damaged cells, by inactivating the cytokines HMG B1 and NF-κB, two groups of proteins secreted by the immune cells during inflammatory diseases. These protective and regenerative effects of fucoidans (from *A. nodosum*), via the immunomodulatory system, were also verified in the destruction/proteolysis of connective tissue by Senni *et al.* [275]. These researchers referred to the fact that severe inflammation and the subsequent excessive release of cytokines and matrix proteinases could result in rheumatoid arthritis or chronic wounds and leg ulcers, which could be treated with fucoidans [275].

In addition to the polysaccharide from *Ulva rigida*, a green seaweed [192], the **sPS** p-KG03 from the marine dinoflagellate *G. impudicum*, also activates the production of nitric oxide and immunostimulates the production of cytokines in macrophages [227].

The enhancement of the immunomodulatory system by some **sPS** from marine algae is also a way for **sPS** to suppress tumour cell's growth and their proliferation, and to be natural neoplastic-cell killers (apoptotic effect).

Studies with arabinogalactan and other fucoidans revealed them to be immunostimulators by activating macrophages and lymphocytes, which suggests their effectiveness in the immuno-prevention of cancer [22,276]. The **PS** from *U. pinnatifida* was also suggested to treat/relieve the symptoms of pulmonary allergic inflammation as it supresses the activity of Th2 immune responses [111]. On the other hand, fucoidan activated macrophages and splenocytes to produce cytokines and chemokines [277].

Polysaccharides from marine microalgae, such as *Porphyridium*, *Phaeodactylum*, and *C. stigmatophora* (Table 4), showed pharmacological properties, such as anti-inflammatory activity and as immunomodulatory agents, as reported by Raposo *et al.* [14]. Some of these **sPS**, for example, the ones from *C. stigmatophora* and *P. tricornutum* (Table 4), have revealed anti-inflammatory efficacy *in vivo* and *in vitro* [195]. The mechanisms underlying the anti-inflammatory and immunomodulatory activities may be unsderstood by making some considerations at the molecular level. On one side, the protein moiety that is covalently bound to most **PS** seems to play a critical role in the activation of NF-κB and MAPK pathways involved in the macrophage stimulation [265,278]. This was evidenced in an *in vitro* experiment performed by Tabarsa and colleagues [265]. They showed that the **PS** from *C. fragile* was not able to stimulate RAW264.7 cells to produce NO and the protein alone was also unable to induce NO release, but the complex **sPS**-protein did inhibit the inflammatory process. On the other side, several other researchers found that proteins were not essential or responsible for the immunostimulatory responses of the cells [192,279]. In addition, Tabarsa and coworkers [265] demonstrated that the sulphate content and the MW were not crucial for the stimulation of murine macrophage cells. In fact, both desulphated and LMW-PS derivatives of *C. fragile* produced immunomodulatory responses similar to the ones of the original **PS**. In contrast, the **sPS** from *U. rigida* induced a strong sulphate-dependent release of NO [192], thus, the sulphate content showing to be essential for the stimulation of macrophages. These researchers mentioned the possibility of the sulphate interfering in the interaction **PS**-cell surface receptors.

The interaction of algal **sPS** with the complement system suggests that they might influence the innate immunity to reduce the pro-inflammatory state [254]. In addition, algal polysaccharides have been shown to regulate the innate immune response directly by binding to pattern recognition receptors (PRRs) [280]. For example, λ-carrageenan stimulated mouse T cell cultures in a toll-like receptor-4 (TLR4) [281].

Different effects were observed in other types of **sPS**: Zhou *et al.* [282] proved that carrageenans from *Chondrus* with lower molecular weights better stimulated the immune system. The same trend was verified for the **sEPS** from the red microalga *Porphyridium* [221], a 6.53 kDa LMW-fragment at 100 μg/mL presenting the strongest immunostimulating activity.

It is worth remarking that carrageenans from red seaweeds are recognized for triggering potent inflammatory and carcinogenic effects either in rats and mice cells [130]. However, while some carrageenans stimulate the activity of macrophages, others inhibit macrophage activities [21].

Although **PS** from various macro- and microalgae do not show anticoagulant and/or antithrombotic activities, attention should be paid to the anticoagulant properties of some **PS**, since their use could cause severe bleeding complications. This issue will be discussed further on in this review.

3.3. Anti-Proliferative, Tumour Suppressor, Apoptotic and Cytotoxicity Activities

Because of the growing number of individuals suffering from different types of cancer and the secondary effects of synthetic chemicals and other types of treatment used against tumour damages, research was driven towards demand for natural therapeutics with bioactive compounds. In this context, **sPS** from both macro- and microalgae already proved to have antitumor biological activities.

An S-fucoidan from *C. okamuranus* exhibited anti-proliferative activity in U937 cells (myeloid cancer cell-line) by inducing cell apoptosis following a pathway dependent of Caspases-3 and -7 [43]. In another study, conducted by Heneji's group [283], a similar fucoidan induced apoptosis in two different leukaemia cell lines. These results indicate that fucoidans might be good candidates for alternative therapeutics in treating adult T-cell leukaemia [22]. S-fucoidans from *E. cava* also seem to be promising to treat other types of human leukaemia (monocyte- and promyelocytic-origin) cell-lines [284]. There was some evidence that the fucoidan from *L. guryanovae* inactivated the epidermal growth factor (tyrosine kinase) receptor (EGFR), which is greatly involved in cell transformation, differentiation and proliferation [285,286]. Therefore, this kind of **sPS** could be used as antitumor and anti-metastatic therapeutical/preventing agent, which might act either on tumour cells or by stimulating the immune response [287].

Further, the **sPS** from *E. bicyclis* and several other seaweeds (Tables 1–3) have demonstrated their potent bioactivity against different kinds of tumours, including lung and skin, both *in vitro* and *in vivo* [62,83,288,289] causing apoptosis in various tumour cell-lines [62,290–292]. The mechanisms involved in this antitumor activity might be associated again with the production of pro-inflammatory interleukins IL-2 and IL-12 and cytokine interferon-gamma (INF-γ) by the immune-stimulated macrophages, together with the increase of the activity of the natural killer cells (NK cells) and the induction of apoptosis [62,293]. NK cells can also upregulate the secretion of IFN-γ, which can activate either the T-cells for the production of IL-2 or the macrophages, which, after being activated, keep on producing IL-12 and activating NK cells [293,294]. The enhancement of the cytotoxicity of these NK cells (lymphocytes and macrophages) can be stimulated by other **sPS** such as fucoidans and carrageenans from other seaweeds [276,282]. Polysaccharides can also activate some signalling receptors in the membranes of macrophages, such as Toll-like receptor-4 (TLR-4), cluster of differentiation 14 (CD14), competent receptor-3 (CR-3) and scavenging receptor (SR) [295]; these are also activated by other intracellular pathways, involving several other protein-kinases, that enhance the production of NO, which, in turn, plays an important role in causing tumour apoptosis [295]. These immunomodulation properties of S-fucoidans could be used for the protection of the damaged gastric mucosa as it was already demonstrated by using rat-models [296]. More information on the pathways and mechanisms responsible for the immune-inflammatory activities, including the involvement of the complementary system, may be found in Jiao and colleagues' work [18].

The anti-adhesive properties of some **sPS**, especially fucoidans might also explain their anti-metastatic activity (Tables 1–3), both *in vitro* and *in vivo*, in various animal-models [15,297], as they can inhibit the adhesion of tumour cells to platelets, thus decreasing the possibilities of proliferation of neoplastic cells. The mechanisms by which fucoidans and other **sPS** exert their anti-adhesive ability were well documented by Li's group [103]. Some researchers also highlighted the mitogenic properties and the cytotoxicity and tumoricidal activity of some arabinogalactans and fucoidans as well [42,276], either in different cell-lines or various animal-models.

The anti-adhesive properties of algal **sPS** may also be relevant as these polymers can block the adhesion of tumour cells to the basal membrane, thus demonstrating to impair implantation of tumour cells and metastatic activity by binding to the extracellular matrix [37]. For example, the **sPS** from *Cladosiphon* was shown to prevent gastric cancer *in vivo*, since it inhibited the adhesion of *H. pylori* to the stomach mucosa (mucin) of gerbils [45]. Metastasis appearance could also be reduced *in vivo* by S-laminaran, a 1,3:1,6-β-D-glucan, because this compound inhibited the activity of heparanase, an endo-β-D-glucuronidase involved in the degradation of the main **PS** component in the basal membrane and the extracellular matrix. The expression of this enzyme is known to be associated with tumour metastasis [59].

These antitumor properties may also be found in some **PS** from microalgae, such as *A. platensis*, which are inhibitors of cell proliferation [234]. Other **sPS**, such as **sPS** p-KG03 from *G. impudicum*, have also anti-proliferative activity in cancer cell lines (*in vitro*) and inhibitory activity against tumour growth (*in vivo*) [227,228,298]. Other **PS** from microalgae, such as *C. vulgaris* (Table 4), and **sPS** or LMW-derivatives of **sPS** from *P. cruentum* (Table 4), for example, are described as having similar properties in the review performed by Raposo *et al.* [14].

In some research work, the immunomodulatory activity was associated to the ability of inhibiting carcinogenesis. For example, Jiao's group [172] found that a sulphated rhamnan and some derivatives from the green seaweed *E. intestinalis* suppressed tumour cell growth *in vivo* (mice), but they did not show any toxicity against tumour cells *in vitro*. The oral administration of the **sPS** to mice enhanced the spleen and thymus indexes, and also induced the production of TNF-α and NO in macrophages, increased lymphocyte proliferation, and enhanced TNF-α release into serum.

The degree of sulphation may play some role in the carcinogenesis process, although the action of the **sPS** may also depend on the type of tumour. In fact, an oversulphated **PS** demonstrated the capacity of inhibiting the growth of L-1210 leukaemia tumour in mice, but, on the other hand, it was unable to inhibit the growth of Sarcoma-180 tumour in mice [83]. In addition to the sulphation level, MW may also influence the anticancer activity. For instance, LMW-PS derivatives showed to enhance antitumor activity [91,299]. However, the increment in the anticancer activity greatly depends on the conditions of the **PS** depolymerisation [299]. Kaeffer *et al.* [186] suggested that the *in vitro* antitumor activity of LMW-PS, sulphated or not, against cancerous colonic epithelial cells (Caco cells) might be associated with the inhibition of tumour cells proliferation and/or differentiation.

3.4. Anticoagulant and Antithrombotic Activities

There are several studies on the anticoagulant properties of **PS** isolated from seaweeds, presented in a recent review [14] by different groups of researchers: Wang *et al.* [8], Costa and colleagues [2], Cumashi *et al.* [15], Athukorala *et al.* [300] and Wijesekara and coworkers [21].

The main sources of the **sPS** from green seaweeds with anticoagulant properties are *Codium* and *Monostroma* [167,301]. Some of the **PS**, such as S-rhamnans, showed their action by extending the clotting time via the intrinsic and extrinsic pathways [167]. In fact, *Codium* spp present strong anticoagulant effects [159,160], but other species from Division/Phyllum Chlorophyta also contain **sPS** (native, low-molecular or otherwise modified) with anticoagulant properties (Table 3). The mechanism of action of the referred **PS** is mostly attributed to either a direct inhibition of thrombin or by enhancing the power of antithrombin III [302,303].

Some other **PS** from green seaweeds also showed potent anticoagulant properties but their mechanisms of action are associated not only to a direct increase in the clotting time (APTT assays) by inhibiting the contact activation pathway (intrinsic pathway), but also by inhibiting the heparin cofactor II-mediated action of thrombin [180,304] thus showing a potent antithrombotic bioactivity.

In addition to their anticoagulant properties demonstrated *in vitro* by APTT and TT tests, several **sPS** from algae of different groups (Tables 1–3) present antithrombotic qualities *in vivo* [305,306] by increasing the time of clot formation. In fact, Wang and colleagues [8] published an exhaustive work on this issue by including a summary table with 24 references about both the anticoagulant, and anti- and prothrombotic activities of several **sPS** from various green seaweeds. In two other studies, Wijesekara *et al.* [21] and Costa and coworkers [2] also included the **sPS** from brown and red macroalgae that present effects on the blood clotting time. Wijesekara and colleagues [21] referred to the fact that there are few reports on the interference of **PS** from algae on the PT (prothrombin) pathway, meaning that most of the marine **sPS** may not affect the extrinsic pathway of coagulation [21]. As a matter of fact, Costa *et al.* [2] did not detect any inhibition in the extrinsic coagulation pathway (PT test), for the concentrations used; only *C. cupressoides* increased the clotting time. In addition, they found no anticoagulant properties (APTT and PT assays) in the **sPS** from a brown seaweed (*S. filipendula*) and a red macroalga (*G. caudate*). Further, in our laboratory we found no anticoagulant properties in the **sEPS** from different strains of the red microalga *P. cruentum*, despite the high content in sulphate and molecular weight. As Costa *et al.* [2] observed, this could be due to the absence of sulphate groups in the monosaccharides at the non-reducing ends of the branches, which impaired the interaction between target proteases and coagulation factors. Nishino *et al.* [84] and Dobashi *et al.* [72] defended that there might be no effect above an upper limit for the content in sulphate, since the difference in the anticoagulant and antithrombotic activities decreased with the increase of the sulphate content.

It seems that some of the chemical and structural features of the **sPS** may have some influence on their anticoagulant and/or antithrombotic activities. The degree and distribution pattern of sulphate, the nature and distribution of monosaccharides and their glycosidic bonds, and also the molecular weight showed to play some role on the coagulation and platelet aggregation processes induced by S-galactans and S-fucoidans [2,307,308]. In fact, at least for some fucoidans, the anticoagulant properties are related to the content in C-2 and C-2,3 (di)sulphate, this last feature being usually common in these **PS** [52,53,105]. Several other studies documented the anticoagulant activity and inhibition of platelet aggregation [22,103,130], supplying more information on the mechanisms of different **sPS** for these biological activities. Higher MW-**PS** usually present stronger anticoagulant activity [309] and if a **PS** has a more linear backbone, a longer polymer is required to accomplish the same anticoagulant effects [251]. However, both the native **PS** and LMW-derivatives of the green seaweed *M. latissimum* presented strong anticoagulant activities [168]. Nishino and colleagues also observed that high molecular weight fucans (e.g., 27 and 58 kDa) showed greater anticoagulant activity than the ones with lower molecular weight (~10 kDa) [85]. They found that a higher content of fucose and sulphate groups coincided with higher anticoagulant activities of sulphated polysaccharide fractions from *E. kurome* [84]. However, despite its high sulphation level, the galactofucan from *U. pinnatifida* lacks significant anticoagulation activity [38]. Moreover, an S-galactofucan from the brown seaweed *S. schröederi* did not present any anticoagulant properties *in vitro*, but demonstrated a strong antithrombotic activity when administered to an animal-model during an experimental induced venous thrombosis, this effect disappearing with the desulphation of the polymer [38].

As for other **PS**, the anticoagulant properties of the **PS** from marine microalgae may not only depend on the percentage of sulphate residues, but rather on the distribution/position of sulphate groups and, probably, on the configuration of the polymer chains [14]. Spirulan from *A. platensis* (Table 4) is one of the **PS** from marine microalgae that strongly interferes with the blood coagulation-fibrinolytic system and exhibits antithrombogenic properties [159,310], therefore, promising to be an anti-thrombotic agent in clots' breakdown, although care should be taken regarding hemorrhagic strokes [14].

It seems that the anticoagulant mechanisms of action of **PS** may be attributed to: (i) the inhibition of thrombin directly or via antithrombin III (AT-III) [66,302,303,311,312]; (ii) the increment in the activity of thrombin inhibitors, such as AT-III and/or heparin cofactor II (HC-II) [130,304,313], in both the intrinsic (contact activation or normal, measured by APPT test) and extrinsic (Tissue factor, TF, measured by PT test) pathways [314], the activation of HC-II seeming to be sulphate-dependent [315].

One explanation for the **sPS** to act directly on thrombin may be associated with the ability of those polymers to bind to thrombin, thus, hindering its catalytic activity [15,316]. In addition, some **sPS** may also inhibit thrombin from linking to their receptors in human platelets (protease activated receptor-1 and GP-1b) [317]. However, a high content of glucuronic acid might render a **sPS** unable to interfere in the coagulation process [15].

3.5. Antilipidaemic (Hypocholesterolaemic and Hypotriglyreridaemic), Hypoglycaemic and Hypotensive Activities

Sulphated **PS** from seaweeds are potent inhibitors of human pancreatic cholesterol esterase, an enzyme that promotes its absorption at the intestinal level; this inhibitory effect is enhanced by higher molecular weights and degree of sulphation [6].

An S-ulvan from *U. pertusa* in an *in vivo* study using mice-models regulated the ratio HDL/LDL-cholesterol and reduced the levels of triglycerides (TG) in serum [185]. However, in another experiment with rats and mice, using native ulvans from the same species, the animals experienced a hypocholesterolaemic effect but no reduction in the TG profile [318]. An opposite reaction was observed when the **PS** was acetylated and oversulphated, as TG levels were normalized. It seems that the ability to sequester bile extracts may be involved [185]. The contents in sulphate and acetylate groups play important roles during the dislipidaemia process [191,319]. Ulvans from *Ulva* spp also showed antiperoxidative properties, preventing liver tissues from hyperlipidaemia, including that induced by toxic chemicals and protecting the injured tissue from the oxidative stress [189], and improving antioxidant performance of the animal models. In fact, these **sPS** regulated superoxide dismutase (SOD) and catalase, increased vitamins E and C, and reduced-glutathione, and had some role in reducing the levels of aspartate and alanine transaminases in the rats' liver [179,185]. Further, the **sPS** from *M. nitidum* also demonstrated hepatoprotective activity by increasing the expression of liver detoxifying enzymes, and, therefore, showed to be good agents for chemoprevention medicine [171]. The activity of these **PS** may be related to their uronic acid and sulphate content, which are able to sequester and bind to bile acids [320], reducing their levels. Other **sPS** from green seaweeds also revealed hypolipidaemic properties, such as that from *E. prolifera*. This **PS** regulated the lipidic profile both in plasma and liver, increasing HDL-cholesterol, in rats [177]. Fucoidans from *L. japonica*, the native or LMW-derivate, have hypolipidaemic effects, decreasing total and LDL-cholesterol in the serum and TG in rats [321], and they prevented hypercholesterolaemia in mice [322]. Another mechanism to reduce blood cholesterol in humans by **sPS** is associated to their high capacity to inhibit pancreatic cholesterol esterase, which is responsible for the absorption of cholesterol and fatty acids at the intestine [6]. It seems that the presence of sulphate at the C-3 position of the sugar residues greatly enhances that inhibition [6]. Porphyran from *P. yezoensis* has anti-hyperlipidaemic properties [119,323] by reducing the release of apolipoprotein-B100 (apoB100) and decreasing the synthesis of lipids in human liver cultured cells [324]. By reducing the secretion of apoB100, porphyran has the potential to be used as a therapeutic agent to treat CVD. In addition, some types of carrageenans have already proved to decrease blood cholesterol in humans [325] and in rats fed on a diet enriched with a mixture of κ/λ-carrageenans from *G. radula* [326].

Most of the **PS** from marine microalgae are naturally highly sulphated, with high molecular weights, making them not-easily absorbable and thus enabling them to be used as anticholesterolaemic agents. Few studies were carried out in this area, namely focusing on *Porphyridium*, *P. cruentum*, *R. reticulata* (Table 4) [327–330], but these suggest a strong potential of sulphated polysaccharides from unicellular algae to be used as hypolipidaemic and hypoglycaemic agents, and as promising agents for reducing coronary heart disease, due to their hypocholesterolaemic effects [14].

As far as we know, scarce research was performed on the mechanisms underlying the antihyperlipidaemic activity. However, the sequestration and disruption of the enterophatic circulation of the bile acids may be involved [185,331,332]. For example, ulvans and their LMW-derivatives, and also the **sEPS** from *Porphyridium* showed to increase the excretion of bile [185,333]. Another explanation for the antihyperlipidaemic activity of **sPS** may be associated to the fact that they can effectively increase the anionic charges on the cell surface, which improve the removal of cholesterol excess from the blood, thus, resulting in a decrease of serum cholesterol [103]. In addition, most **PS** have ion exchange capacity, such as those from *Porphyridium* and *Rhodella* [334], and they can function as dietary fibres. This could also explain the ability to lower down cholesterol [335]. **PS** may act as dietary fibres, immunostimulating the goblet cells in the intestine to increase the release and effects of mucin [336]. Moreover, the administration of **PS** may increase the viscosity of the intestinal contents, interfering with the formation of micelles and nutrient absorption, thus, lowering lipid absorption, and reducing gastrointestinal transit time (GTT) [333,337].

Other **PS** have the ability to inhibit the enzyme α-glucosidase, thus improving the postprandial hyperglycaemia [338], and another can also reduce the blood pressure by inhibiting the release of plasma angiotensin II [339].

3.6. Antiaging (Antioxidant) Activity

The main mechanism by which **sPS** from green seaweeds exert their primary antioxidant action is by scavenging free-radicals (superoxide, hydroxyl, 1,1-diphenyl-2-picrylhydrazyl (DPPH)-radicals) or by inhibiting their appearance [8]. They also demonstrated to have total antioxidant capacity, and a strong ability as reducing agents and as ferrous chelators [8]. However, some other **sPS**, such as S-heterogalactan (*C. cupressoides*) do not show a good scavenging power, but they are rather powerful against reactive oxygen species (ROS) [340]. It is interesting to note that fucoidans from brown seaweeds seem to exert a reducing power bigger than the **sPS** from other groups [2]; the **PS** from *S. filipendula* has an effect even stronger than vitamin C. Moreover, the fucoidan from *L. japonica* has a great potential to be used in medicine in order to prevent free-radical-mediated diseases, as it successfully prevented peroxidation of lipids in plasma, liver and spleen *in vivo* (mice), despite showing no effects *in vitro* [100]. The **sPS** from another species of *Sargassum* (*S. fulvellum*) has shown a NO scavenging activity higher than some commercial antioxidants [341]. In addition, the **sPS** from the red macroalga *P. haitanensis* demonstrated to decrease antioxidant damages in aging mice [115].

It seems that LMW-**sPS** may present higher antioxidant activity than the native polymers, as it was verified with the **PS** from *U. pertusa* and *E. prolifera* [166,342]. It is probably related with the ability of **PS** to be incorporated in the cells and to donate protons [21].

As noted by Raposo *et al.* [14], sulphated **PS** produced and secreted out by marine microalgae have shown the capacity to prevent the accumulation and the activity of free radicals and reactive chemical species. Therefore, **sPS** might act as protecting systems against these oxidative and radical stress agents. The **sPS** from *Porphyridium* and *Rhodella reticulata* (Table 4) exhibited antioxidant activity [343,344], although some research revealed no scavenging activity and no ability to inhibit the oxidative damage in cells and tissues for the crude **sPS** with high molecular weight from *Porphyridium cruentum*, while the **EPS**-derived products after microwave treatment showed antioxidant activity [220]. In all cases, the antioxidant activity was dose-dependent. Methanolic extracts of **EPS** from *A. platensis* also exhibit a very high antioxidant capacity [235].

Due to their strong antioxidant properties, most of the **sPS** from marine macro- and microalgae are promising since they may protect human health from injuries induced by ROS, which can result in cancer, diabetes, some inflammatory and neurodegenerative diseases, and some other aging-related disorders, such as Alzheimer and CVD.

The influence of sulphate content on the antioxidant activity depends rather on the origin of the **PS**. For example, the **PS** from *U. fasciata* and other macro- and microalgae with lower sulphate content demonstrated a strong antioxidative power [165,181,220,343], while the antioxidant activity observed in **PS** from *E. linza* and other seaweeds showed to be sulphate-dependent [174,345]. Furthermore, high sulphated **PS** was shown to have an enhanced scavenging power [97,182], this property being also dependent on the sulphate distribution pattern [2]. It seems, in addition, that the protein moiety of **PS** may play some role on the antioxidative power. For example, Tannin-Spitz *et al.* [343] reported a stronger antioxidant activity for the crude **PS** of *Porphyridium* than for the denatured **PS**.

Zhao *et al.* [346] found that the antioxidant activity of **sPS** was apparently related, not only to molecular weight and sulphated ester content, but also to glucuronic acid and fructose content. This antioxidant activity seems to be attributable to metal chelating, free radical and hydroxyl radical scavenging activities of the **sPS**.

3.7. Nutritional Applications: Fibres (Dietary), Prebiotic and Probiotic

As already mentioned by Raposo *et al.* [14], **PS** can find applications in the food industry as emulsifying and gelling agents, as flocculant and hydrating agents, emulsifiers, stabilizers, thickening agents, *i.e.*, food additives [347], like agar E406, alginates E400-404, carrageenan E407. The **sPS** from marine microalgae could be used as nutraceuticals due to their content in fibres, the ability of acid binding and for cation exchange, and the properties of faecal bulking as well, being also good candidates as prebiotics [348]. The **PS** alone or in combination with other compounds have a great potential to be used in edible films and coatings of foods, while carriers of flavors, colorants, spices and nutraceuticals [349]. In our laboratory, experiments have already been carried out with based **EPS** from *P. cruentum*-coatings applied to fresh-cut apple. These polymers also have the potential to be used in low-fat or fat-free food products, as fat substitutes in mayonnaises [350,351], salad dressings and other food emulsions [352].

3.8. Other Biological Activities

As it happens in relation to the fucoidan from *S. schröederi* (Dictyotales) [36], a heterofucan-derivative from *D. menstrualis*, another member of Dictyotales, also presented antinociceptive activity. It acted as a peripheral analgesic agent, reaching 61.2% of pain reduction (4 mg/kg) in mice, this effect being as potent as dipyrone's, and it was dose-dependent [1]. This suggests that this kind of S-fucans and some S-galactans can act as analgesic agents but not as anaesthetic ones, as they do not decrease pain when it involves the CNS. S-galactan from *G. cornea* is another **sPS** with analgesic characteristics, but at a higher concentration (9 mg/kg) [353]. A S-galactan from *C. feldmannii* is a more potent antinociceptive agent (80% reduction in contractions), but it also presents good anticoagulant properties [354]. Sulphated **PS** from *C. cupressoides* [155,156], at a dose of 27 mg/kg/day, reduced by 90% the writhes induced in mice by acetic acid, but they also showed analgesic effects only via peripheral mechanisms [156]. It seems that these **sPS** act by binding to the surface of the leukocytes, hindering their migration to the focus of tissue injury [1,355], therefore, demonstrating anti-inflammatory properties as well. Thus, all these **sPS** promise to be good peripheral antinociceptive agents, with some special care in relation to the galactan from *Champia feldmannii* due to its anticoagulant properties.

The angiogenic (neovascularization) properties of **PS** can be considered according to two angles. When dealing with treatment/prevention of neoplasias it is very important that the **PS** in question does not show that ability, so that the tumour will be reduced, and cells might die if not irrigated. Therefore, **sPS**, such as fucoidans may function as tumour supressors by inhibiting angiogenesis induced by tumour cells [3]. However, if the disorder we are dealing with is the result of an ischaemic issue, a **PS** with angiogenic activity should be used in order to re-establish the blood flow of the injured tissues, thus, acting as cardioprotective after ischaemia. The angiogenic mechanisms of fucoidans and glucans were well explained by Fedorov *et al.* [3] and Cumashi *et al.* [15].

Angiogenesis involves the differentiation of mature endothelial cells, their proliferation and migration. In fact, some **sPS** demonstrated the capacity to promote therapeutic revascularization in animal models, increasing the vessel formation when administered by injection in rats with ischaemic hind limb [57]. The mechanisms involved in the angiogenic properties of modified fucoidans are associated with the ability of these polymers to interact with endothelial cells, modulating the activity of proangiogenic growth factors, such as fibroblast growth factor-2 (FGF-2). The latter is mitogenic for that type of cells, fibroblasts and smooth muscle cells [103], and extracellular matrix components [58,356,357]. In fact, there is a correlation of the reduction of plasminogen-activator inhibitor (PAI-1) secretion with the upregulation of cell-surface α-6 integrin sub-unit. This could be an explanation for the proangiogenic ability, including the induction *in vitro* of tube formation by human endothelial cells. The fucoidans of *C. okamuranus* and *F. vesiculosus* are promising in treatment of ischaemic disorders, including infarcted myocardium, as they did not show to inhibit tubulogenesis in HUVEC cells. This cardioprotective activity was confirmed in animal models by enhancing creatinine phosphokinase, lactate dehydrogenase, and alanine and aspartate transaminases [47].

Fucoidans from two species of *Laminaria* and three species of *Fucus* revealed antiangiogenic properties, through the inhibition of the *in vitro* neogenesis of tubules in human umbilical vein endothelial cells (HUVEC), while a decrease in PAI-1 in HUVEC supernatants was also observed [15]. It is worth noting that these **sPS** revealed anticoagulant and antithrombotic activities, and some of these fucoidans inhibited the adhesion of breast cancer cells to platelets, as well, thus showing anti-adhesive and anti-metastatic properties. These features suggest that this type of polymers could be used as complementary agents in the therapeutical treatment of cancer.

In addition to the cardioprotective effects, the fucoidan from *C. okamuranus* Tokida demonstrated a great potential to be used as a gastroprotective agent [46]. It was used as a component of a new drug to treat/prevent gastric ulcers, and to inhibit *Helicobacter pylori* from adhering to the mucosa of the stomach [358], and also inhibited stomach cancer [44].

The fucoidans from other seaweeds are promising as well, not only as hepatoprotective agents against chemical damages, stimulating the release of IL-10 and inhibiting proinflammatory cytokines [359,360], but also against hepatic fibrosis, protecting hepatocytes and inhibiting the proliferation of hepatic stellate cells, which are co-responsible in the process [361].

Being an antioxidant against free radicals, fucoidan from *F. vesiculosus* might be an alternative or complementary therapeutic in uropathy and renalpathy, since it could prevent from the injuries caused by oxalate-induced free radicals [362] and from the mitochondrial damages associated to the process [363]. Several other disorders of the urinary system, including Heymann nephritis, are also liable to treatment or complementary therapeutics through the use of fucoidans [293,364–367].

The **PS** from other seaweeds demonstrated either stimulatory or inhibitory effects on some enzymes as was reported in the review by Smit [20], and inhibited cytotoxic and myotoxic effects against snake venoms as well, thus protecting the muscle from necrosis [368].

3.9. Biomedical Applications

Biomedical field is constantly demanding for new biomaterials with innovative properties. Natural polymers appear as materials of election for this objective due to their biocompatibility and biodegradability [369].

Alongside their biological activity and potential pharmaceutical use, as has already been addressed in this review, **PS** may be used as biomaterials, as such, or in combination with other synthetic or natural substances. There are several potential biomedical applications for **PS** in: regenerative medicine, such as wound management products, drug delivery systems (DDSs), tissue engineering, and medical fibres and biotextiles [369,370] (Table 5).

Table 5. Some applications of algal **PS** in biomedicine.

Groups of PSs	Possible Sources	Applications	References
Alginates	*Laminaria* spp, *A. nodosum*, *Ecklonia* sp., *M. pyrifera*, *Durvillaea*, *Lessonia*	Drugs carriers Encapsulation	[371]
		Scaffolds for ligaments and tissue engineering Regeneration of tissues Moulding in dentistry	[372–374]
		Wound healing and dressings	[375–377]
Agaroids	*B. montaignei*, *Goiopeltis* spp., *A. tenera*, *P. capillacea*	Cell encapsulation	
		Scaffolds for tissue engineering	[378]
		Wound healing and dressings	[379]
		Revascularization	[380]
Ulvans	*Ulva rigida*, *Ulva* spp.	Drug carriers	[381]
		Wound dressings	[382,383]
		Tissue engineering	[384]
β-glucans	*A. nodosum*, *E. bicyclis*, *Fucus* sp., *Laminaria* sp., *U. pinnatifida* (laminaran); *C. vulgaris*	Wound healing	[385–387]
		Burn-wound dressings	
		Tissue regeneration	[388–390]
fucoidans	*U. pinnatifida*	Vaccines for immunotherapy	[299]
PSs from microalgae	*A. platensis*	Production of nanofibers	[391]
		Gluing and soft tissue closure after surgery	[6]
	Porphyridium	Lubricants for bone joints	[212,392]

Alginates from macroalgae have been most used in several applications: controlled drug release [371], cell encapsulation, scafold in ligament, tissue engineering and regeneration of almost all tissues in the human organism, or even preparation of moulds in dentistry [372–374]. A review recently made available was devoted to the processing of alginate fibres for use as wound management materials [375,376]. **PS** have been widely applied as hydrogels, eventually combined with other substances, for: the encapsulation and delivery of Langerhans islets [393], ovarian follicles [394] and stem cells in neural tissue engineering [395], skin tissue engineering [396], bone tissue engineering [397] and skeletal muscle regeneration [398]; regenerating the osteochondral interface [399]; capturing of endothelial progenitor cells from the human blood [400]. Kaltostat® is a commercially available alginate dressing that promotes haemostasis and manages exudate in low to moderately exuding wounds. In the form of porous scaffolds, alginate has been used for creating a capillary bed in newly reconstructed tissues [401], and in the form of electrospin nanofibrous scaffolds, for constructing vascular replacements containing endothelial cells and smooth muscle cells (SMC) [402]. Alginate may also be used as a component of scaffolds for heart valve engineering [403], and for cardiac tissue engineering [404].

Similarly to alginate, agar can be used for cell encapsulation in tissue engineering applications. Due to its chondrogenic potential, agar was selected to entrap chondrocytes within poly-L-lactide scaffolds [378]. Composite membranes with agar proved to be promising wound dressings for healing burns or ulcers [379]. Agar gel supported the formation of *in vivo* autologous vascular prosthetic tissues, called "biotubes" [380].

However, not all polysaccharides are suitable for tissue engineering, mainly due to their jelly-like consistency and insufficient mechanical properties. As referred above, even **PS** used in tissue engineering usually need to be combined with other natural or synthetic polymers, or reinforced with inorganic substances [405].

A new generation of medical textiles incorporated with **PS**, such as alginate, is growing with respect to, in wound management products [406]. The main qualities of fibres and wound dressing products include antiviral, fungistatic, non-toxic, highly absorbent, non-allergic, breathable, haemostatic, and biocompatible. Such products with good mechanical properties may incorporate medication [377].

sPS are capable of binding to protein and may be involved in the cell development, cell differentiation, cell adhesion, cell signaling and cell matrix interactions. These bioactive molecules present a great potential for medical, pharmaceutical and biotechnological applications, such as wound dressings, biomaterials, tissue regeneration and 3D culture scaffolds, and even drugs [19]. Their biological activities and their resemblance to glycosaminoglycans (GAGs), which have been most studied, might position these **PS** in advantage. For example, ulvans from green algae, may be processed into porous structures, including nanofibres [381], particles [382], membranes [383] and hydrogels [384], which make them good candidates for medical applications, such as drug delivery, wound dressing and bone tissue engineering [381–384]. Carrageenans, besides being hydrogels, may also be processed into fibres, membranes or porous structures for several biomedical applications [407].

Fucoidans from brown algae besides having application in the biopharmaceutical industry (immunomodulatory, antiviral and anticoagulant agents), have found new applications in biomedicine, for instance, as nanoparticles of fucoidan and chitosan [408], and more recently in the synthesis of biohybrid glycopolymers [409].

The (1,3)-β-glucans have been used to help healing wounds, by inducing the migration of macrophages to the wound site [385], to accelerate the healing process as a constituent in composites [386,410], and in burn-wound dressings, therefore, reducing the need for analgesics [387]. Fucoidan-chitosan films and/or gels may be used to treat dermal burns and regenerate epithelial tissue [388]. The mechanism of action of hydrocolloids may be associated to the fact that wound dressings with **sPS** decrease wound secretions and scars, reducing the bacterial inflammation [389,390], with the advantage of being free from prions or other animal contaminants.

Native **sPS**, LMW- or otherwise modified derivatives, are also promising in the prevention of arteriosclerosis after cardiac transplantation [411,412], in coating encapsulates for controlled drug delivering, as new materials for cell immobilization and tissue engineering [7,413], and as carrier-materials for transplantation of chondrocytes and osteoblasts, improving neo-cartilage and neo-bone formation [414].

The use of fucoidans in dendritic cell-based vaccines for cancer immunotherapy has been also suggested [299].

Another promising and emerging application of the **PS** from microalgae might be associated to the production of nanofibres from the biomass of *A. platensis* (Table 4), to be used as extracellular matrices for the culture of stem cells in order to treat spinal cord injuries [391].

Their gluing and adhesive capacities, as well as their strong cohesive and binding strength, allied to their non-toxic and non-irritating properties, make the bioadhesive **PS** produced by marine microalgae good candidates as mucobioadhesives or glues for bone gluing and soft tissue closure after surgery. They might also replace the metallic screws and traditional wound closure methods, respectively [6].

The **sEPS** from *Porphyridium* (Table 4) has already shown a good lubrication capacity [355], being an excellent candidate to substitute for hyaluronic acid as a biolubricant. Another promising application could be as a component of a joint-lubricating solution, as it was demonstrated by injecting the **EPS** from *Porphyridium* into the joints of rabbits' knees [212], thus mitigating degenerative joint disorders caused by arthritis.

4. Conclusions

Polysaccharides may be regarded as key ingredients for the production of bio-based materials in life sciences (e.g., medical devices, pharmaceutics, food, cosmetics). There are an enormous variety of polysaccharides that can be synthetized and/or released by marine macro- and microalgae. Both these marine organisms are excellent sources of **PS**, most of them sulphated (**sPS**). Although some similarities may be found between the **PS** from each group of organisms, they can be very heterogeneous and structurally different. The biological source and biodegradability of these biopolymers, coupled to the large variety of functionalities they encompass, make them promising compounds for the application in pharmaceuticals, therapeutics, and regenerative medicine. Some of the beneficial bioactivities demonstrated by the crude **PS** and their derivatives, either *in vitro* or *in vivo*, include anticoagulant and/or antithrombotic properties, immunomodulatory ability, antitumor and cancer preventive activity. They are also good antilipidaemic and hypoglycaemic agents, and can be powerful antioxidants, antibiotics and anti-inflammatory. Other biomedical properties of **PS** have been discussed, such as antinociceptive, angiogenic, cardioprotective, gastroprotective and hepatoprotective activities. The biomedical applications and potentialities of **PS** in this area were listed, such as healing wound agents, mucobioadhesives for bone and soft tissue closure, biolubricants to mitigate joint disorders caused by arthritis, vaccines for cancer immunotherapy, or in a new generation of biotextiles and medical fibres, in drug delivery systems, and scaffolds in regenerative medicine.

From the extensive list above, the importance of this type of compounds—**PS** from macro- and microalgae—for medical use is quite obvious. However, despite all the interesting properties and potentialities for human health, the use of these **PS**, especially those from microalgae need to be further explored. In particular, the toxicity and bioavailability of some of these polymers are yet to be studied on humans.

Acknowledgments: This work was supported by Fundação para a Ciência e Tecnologia (FCT) of Portuguese Republic Government, in the frame of the project PEst-OE/EQB/LA0016/2013.

Conflicts of Interest: The authors declare no conflict of interest.

References

1. Albuquerque, I.R.L.; Cordeiro, S.L.; Gomes, D.L.; Dreyfuss, J.L.; Filgueira, L.G.A.; Leite, E.L.; Nader, H.B.; Rocha, H.A.O. Evaluation of anti-nociceptive and anti-inflammatory activities of a heterofucan from *Dictyota menstrualis*. *Mar. Drugs* **2013**, *11*, 2722–2740.
2. Costa, L.S.; Fidelis, G.P.; Cordeiro, S.L.; Oliveira, R.M.; Sabry, D.A.; Câmara, R.B.G.; Nobre, L.T.D.B.; Costa, M.S.S.P.; Almeida-Lima, J.; Farias, E.H.C.; *et al.* Biological activities of sulfated polysaccharides from tropical seaweeds. *Biomed. Pharmacother.* **2010**, *64*, 21–28. [CrossRef] [PubMed]
3. Fedorov, S.N.; Ermakova, S.P.; Zvyagintseva, T.N.; Stonik, V.A. Anticancer and cancer preventive properties of marine polysaccharides: Some results and prospects. *Mar. Drugs* **2013**, *11*, 4876–4901. [CrossRef] [PubMed]
4. Jiménez-Escrig, A.; Gómez-Ordóñez, E.; Rupérez, P. Seaweed as a source of novel nutraceuticals: Sulfated polysaccharides and peptides. *Adv. Food Nutr. Res.* **2011**, *64*, 325–337. [PubMed]
5. Kraan, S. Algal polysaccharides, novel applications and outlook. In *Carbohydrates-Comprehensive Studies on Glycobiology and Glycotechnology*; InTech: Rijeka, Croatia, 2012; Chapter 22; pp. 489–524.
6. Laurienzo, P. Marine polysaccharides in pharmaceutical applications: An overview. *Mar. Drugs* **2010**, *8*, 2435–2465. [CrossRef] [PubMed]
7. Gomez d'Ayala, G.; Malinconico, M.; Laurienzo, P. Marine derived polysaccharides for biomedical applications: Chemical modification approaches. *Molecules* **2008**, *13*, 2069–2106.
8. Wang, L.; Wang, X.; Wu, H.; Liu, R. Overview on biological activities and molecular characteristics of sulfated polysaccharides from marine green algae in recent years. *Mar. Drugs* **2014**, *12*, 4984–5020. [CrossRef] [PubMed]
9. Burja, A.M.; Banaigs, B.; Abou-Mansor, E.; Burgess, J.G.; Wright, P.C. Marine cyanobacteria—A prolific source of natural products. *Tetrahedron* **2001**, *57*, 9347–9377. [CrossRef]
10. Pulz, O.; Gross, W. Valuable products from biotechnology of microalgae. *Appl. Microbiol. Biotechnol.* **2004**, *65*, 635–648. [CrossRef] [PubMed]
11. De Jesus Raposo, M.F.; de Morais, A.M.M.B. Microalgae for the prevention of cardiovascular disease and stroke. *Life Sci.* **2015**, *125*, 32–41. [CrossRef] [PubMed]
12. De Jesus Raposo, M.F.; de Morais, R.M.S.C.; de Morais, A.M.M.B. Bioactivity and applications of sulphated polysaccharides from marine microalgae. *Mar. Drugs* **2013**, *11*, 233–252. [CrossRef] [PubMed]
13. De Jesus Raposo, M.F.; de Morais, R.M.S.C.; de Morais, A.M.M.B. Health applications of bioactive compounds from marine microalgae. *Life Sci.* **2013**, *93*, 479–486. [CrossRef] [PubMed]
14. De Jesus Raposo, M.F.; de Morais, A.M.M.B.; de Morais, R.M.S.C. Bioactivity and Applications of polysaccharides from marine microalgae. In *Polysaccharides: Bioactivity and Biotechnology*; Merillon, J.-M., Ramawat, K.G., Eds.; Springer: Cham, Switzerland, 2014. [CrossRef]
15. Cumashi, A.; Ushakova, N.A.; Preobrazhenskaya, M.E.; D'Incecco, A.; Piccoli, A.; Totani, L.; Tinari, N.; Morozevich, G.E.; Berman, A.E.; Bilan, M.I.; *et al.* A comparative study of the anti-inflammatory, anticoagulant, antiangiogenic, and antiadhesive activities of nine different fucoidans from brown seaweeds. *Glycobiology* **2007**, *5*, 541–552.

16. Ermakova, S.; Sokolova, R.; Kim, S.-M.; Um, B.-H.; Isakov, V.; Zvyagintseva, T. Fucoidans from Brown seaweeds *Sargassum hornery, Ecklonia cava, Costaria costata*: Structural characteristics and anticancer activity. *Appl. Biochem. Biotechnol.* **2011**, *164*, 841–850. [CrossRef] [PubMed]

17. Fujitani, N.; Sakari, S.; Yamagushi, Y.; Takenaka, H. Inhibitory effects of microalgae on activation of hyaluronidase. *J. Appl. Phycol.* **2001**, *13*, 489–492. [CrossRef]

18. Jiao, G.; Yu, G.; Zhang, J.; Ewart, H.S. Chemical structures and bioactivities of sulphated polysaccharides from marine algae. *Mar. Drugs* **2011**, *9*, 196–223. [CrossRef] [PubMed]

19. Senni, K.; Pereira, J.; Gueniche, F.; Delbarre-Ladrat, C.; Sinquin, C.; Ratiskol, J.; Godeau, G.; Fisher, A.M.; Helley, D.; Colliec-Jouault, S. Marine polysaccharides: A source of bioactive molecules for cell therapy and tissue engineering. *Mar. Drugs* **2011**, *9*, 1664–1681. [CrossRef] [PubMed]

20. Smitt, A.J. Medicinal and pharmaceutical uses of seaweed natural products: A review. *J. Appl. Phycol.* **2004**, *16*, 245–262. [CrossRef]

21. Wijesekara, I.; Pangestuti, R.; Kim, S.-K. Biological activities and potential health benefits of sulfated polysaccharides derived from marine algae. *Carbohydr. Polym.* **2011**, *84*, 14–21. [CrossRef]

22. Wijesinghe, W.A.J.P.; Jeon, Y.-J. Biological activities and potential industrial applications of fucose rich sulphated polysaccharides and fucoidans from brown seaweeds: A review. *Carbohydr. Polym.* **2012**, *88*, 13–20. [CrossRef]

23. Yim, J.H.; Kim, S.J.; Ahn, S.H.; Lee, H.K. Characterization of a novel bioflocculant, p-KG03, from a marine dinoflagellate, *Gyrodinium impudicum* KG03. *Bioresour. Technol.* **2007**, *98*, 361–367. [CrossRef] [PubMed]

24. Nomoto, K.; Yokokura, T.; Satoh, H.; Mutai, M. Anti-tumor effect by oral administration of *Chlorella* extract, PCM-4 by oral admission. *Gan To Kagaku Zasshi* **1983**, *10*, 781–785. (In Japanese)

25. Camara, R.B.G.; Costa, L.S.; Fidelis, G.P.; Nobre, L.T.D.B.; Dantas-Santos, N.; Cordeiro, S.L.; Costa, M.S.S.P.; Alves, L.G.; Rocha, H.A.O. Heterofucans from the brown seaweed *Canistrocarpus cervicornis* with anticoagulant and antioxidant activities. *Mar. Drugs* **2011**, *9*, 124–138. [CrossRef] [PubMed]

26. Albuquerque, I.R.L.; Queiroz, K.C.S.; Alves, L.G.; Santos, E.A.; Leite, E.L.; Rocha, H.A.O. Heterofucans from *Dictyota menstrualis* have anticoagulant activity. *Braz. J. Med. Biol. Res.* **2004**, *37*, 167–171. [CrossRef] [PubMed]

27. Bilan, M.I.; Usov, A.I. Structural analysis of fucoidans. *Nat. Prod. Commun.* **2008**, *3*, 1639–1648.

28. Sokolova, R.V.; Ermakova, S.P.; Awada, S.M.; Zvyagintseva, T.N.; Kanaan, H.M. Composition, structural characteristics, and antitumor properties of polysaccharides from the brown algae *Dictyopteris polypodioides* and *Sargassum* sp. *Chem. Nat. Comp.* **2011**, *47*, 329–334. [CrossRef]

29. Medeiros, V.P.; Queiroz, K.C.; Cardoso, M.L.; Monteiro, G.R.; Oliveira, F.W.; Chavante, S.F.; Guimarães, L.A.; Rocha, H.A.; Leite, E.L. Sulfated galactofucan from *Lobophora variegata*: Anticoagulant and anti-inflammatory properties. *Biochemistry (Mosc.)* **2008**, *73*, 1018–1024. [CrossRef]

30. Paiva, A.A.; Castro, A.J.; Nascimento, M.S.; Will, L.S.; Santos, N.D.; Araújo, R.M.; Xavier, C.A.; Rocha, F.A.; Leite, E.L. Antioxidant and anti-inflammatory effect of polysaccharides from *Lobophora variegata* on zymosan-induced arthritis in rats. *Int. Immunopharmacol.* **2011**, *11*, 1241–1250. [CrossRef] [PubMed]

31. Silva, T.M.; Alves, L.G.; de Queiroz, K.C.; Santos, M.G.; Marques, C.T.; Chavante, S.F.; Rocha, H.A.O.; Leite, E.L. Partial characterization and anticoagulant activity of a heterofucan from the brown seaweed *Padina gymnospora*. *Braz. J. Med. Biol. Res.* **2005**, *38*, 523–533. [PubMed]

32. Zhu, W.; Ooi, V.E.C.; Chan, P.K.S.; Ang, P.O., Jr. Inhibitory effect of extracts of marine algae from Hong Kong against *Herpes simplex* viruses. In Proceedings of the 17th International Seaweed Symposium; Chapman, A.R.O., Anderson, R.J., Vreeland, V.J., Davison, I.R., Eds.; Oxford University Press: Oxford, UK, 2003; pp. 159–164.

33. Karmakar, P.; Ghosh, T.; Sinha, S.; Saha, S.; Mandal, P.; Ghosal, P.K.; Ray, B. Polysaccharides from the brown seaweed *Padina tetrastromatica*: Characterization of a sulfated fucan. *Carbohyd. Polym.* **2009**, *78*, 416–421. [CrossRef]

34. Almeida-Lima, J.; Dantas-Santos, N.; Gomes, D.L.; Cordeiro, S.L.; Sabry, D.A.; Costa, L.S.; Freitas, M.L.; Silva, N.B.; Moura, C.E.B.; Lemos, T.M.A.M.; *et al.* Evaluation of acute and subchronic toxicity of a non-anticoagulant, but antithrombotic algal heterofucan from the *Spatoglossum schröederi* in wistar rats. *Rev. Bras. Farmacogn.* **2011**, *21*, 674–679. [CrossRef]

35. Almeida-Lima, J.; Costa, L.S.; Silva, N.B.; Melo-Silveira, R.F.; Silva, F.V.; Felipe, M.B.M.C.; Medeiros, S.R.B.M.; Leite, E.L.; Rocha, H.A.O. Evaluating the possible genotoxic, mutagenic and tumor cell proliferation-inhibition effects of a non-anticoagulant, but antithrombotic algal heterofucan. *J. Appl. Toxicol.* **2010**, *30*, 708–715. [CrossRef] [PubMed]

36. Farias, W.R.; Lima, P.C.; Rodrigues, N.V.; Siqueira, R.C.; Amorim, R.M.; Pereira, M.G.; Assreuy, A.M. A novel antinociceptive sulphated polysaccharide of the brown marine alga *Spatoglossum schröederi*. *Nat. Prod. Commun.* **2011**, *6*, 863–866. [PubMed]

37. Rocha, H.A.O.; Franco, C.R.C.; Trindade, E.S.; Veiga, S.S.; Leite, E.L.; Dietrich, C.P.; Nader, H.B. Fucan inhibits Chinese hamster ovary cell (CHO) adhesion to fibronectin by binding to the extracellular matrix. *Planta Med.* **2005**, *71*, 628–633. [CrossRef] [PubMed]

38. Rocha, H.A.O.; Moraes, F.A.; Trindade, E.S.; Franco, C.R.C.; Torquato, R.J.S.; Veiga, S.S.; Valente, A.P.; Mourão, P.A.; Leite, E.L.; Nader, H.B.; *et al.* Structural and haemostatic activities of a sulfated galactofucan from the brown alga *Spatoglossum schröederi*. An ideal antithrombotic agent? *J. Biol. Chem.* **2005**, *280*, 41278–41288. [CrossRef] [PubMed]

39. Ponce, N.M.A.; Pujol, C.A.; Damonte, E.B.; Flores, M.L.; Stortz, C.A. Fucoidans from the brown seaweed *Adenocystis utricularis*: Extraction methods, antiviral activity and structural studies. *Carbohydr. Res.* **2003**, *338*, 153–165. [CrossRef] [PubMed]

40. Hidari, K.I.P.J.; Takahashi, N.; Arihara, M.; Nagaoka, M.; Morita, K.; Suzuki, T. Structure and anti-dengue virus activity of sulfated polysaccharide from a marine alga. *Biochem. Biophys. Res. Commun.* **2008**, *376*, 91–95. [CrossRef] [PubMed]

41. Nagaoka, M.; Shibata, H.; Kimura-Takagi, I.; Hashimoto, S.; Kimura, K.; Makino, T.; Aiyama, R.; Ueyama, S.; Yokokura, T. Structural study of fucoidan from *Cladosiphon okamuranus* Tokida. *Glycoconj. J.* **1999**, *16*, 19–26. [CrossRef] [PubMed]

42. Shimizu, J.; Wada-Funada, U.; Mano, H.; Matahira, Y.; Kawaguchi, M.; Wada, M. Proportion of murine cytotoxic T cells is increased by high molecular-weight fucoidan extracted from *Okinawa mozuku* (*Cladosiphon okamuranus*). *J. Health Sci.* **2005**, *51*, 394–397. [CrossRef]

43. Teruya, T.; Konishi, T.; Uechi, S.; Tamaki, H.; Tako, M. Anti-proliferative activity of oversulfated fucoidan from commercially cultured *Cladosiphon okamuranus* Tokida in U937 cells. *Int. J. Biol. Macromol.* **2007**, *41*, 221–226. [CrossRef] [PubMed]

44. Kawamoto, H.; Miki, Y.; Kimura, T.; Tanaka, K.; Nakagawa, T.; Kawamukai, M.; Matsuda, H. Effects of fucoidan from Mozuku on human stomach cell lines. *Food Sci. Technol. Res.* **2006**, *12*, 218–222. [CrossRef]

45. Shibata, H.; Iimuro, M.; Uchiya, N.; Kawamori, T.; Nagaoka, M.; Ueyama, S.; Hashimoto, S.; Yokokura, T.; Sugimura, T.; Wakabayashi, K. Preventive effects of *Cladosiphon* fucoidan against *Helicobacter pylori* infection in Mongolian gerbils. *Helicobacter* **2003**, *8*, 59–65. [CrossRef] [PubMed]

46. Shibata, H.; Kimura-Takagi, I.; Nagaoka, M.; Hashimoto, S.; Aiyama, R.; Iha, M.; Ueyama, S.; Yokokura, T. Properties of fucoidan from *Cladosiphon okamuranus* Tokida in gastric mucosal protection. *Biofactors* **2000**, *11*, 235–245. [CrossRef] [PubMed]

47. Thomes, P.; Rajendran, M.; Pasanban, B.; Rengasamy, R. Cardioprotective activity of *Cladosiphon okamuranus* against isoproterenol induced myocardial infraction in rats. *Phytomedicine* **2010**, *18*, 52–57. [CrossRef] [PubMed]

48. Zhang, Z.; Teruya, K.; Eto, H.; Shirahata, S. Fucoidan extract induces apoptosis in MCF-7 cells via a mechanism involving the ROS-dependent JNK activation and mitochondria-mediated pathways. *PLoS ONE* **2011**, *6*, e27441. [CrossRef] [PubMed]

49. Feldman, S.C.; Reynaldi, S.; Stortz, C.A.; Cerezo, A.S.; Damonte, E.B. Antiviral properties of fucoidan fractions from *Leathesia difformis*. *Phytomedicine* **1999**, *6*, 335–340. [CrossRef] [PubMed]

50. Kim, K.J.; Lee, O.H.; Lee, H.H.; Lee, B.Y. A 4-week repeated oral dose toxicity study of fucoidan from the sporophyll of *Undaria pinnatifida* in Sprague-Dawley rats. *Toxicology* **2010**, *267*, 154–158. [CrossRef] [PubMed]

51. Anastase-Ravion, S.; Carreno, M.P.; Blondin, C.; Ravion, O.; Champion, J.; Chaubet, F.; Haeffner-Cavaillon, N.; Letourneur, D. Heparin-like polymers modulate proinflammtory cytokine production by lipopolysaccharide-stimulated human monocytes. *J. Biomed. Mat. Res.* **2002**, *60*, 375–383. [CrossRef]

52. Chevolot, L.; Foucault, A.; Chaubet, F.; Kervarec, N.; Sinquin, C.; Fisher, A.M.; Boisson-Vidal, C. Further data on the structure of brown seaweed fucans: Relationships with anticoagulant activity. *Carbohydr. Res* **1999**, *319*, 154–165. [CrossRef] [PubMed]

53. Chevolot, L.; Mulloy, B.; Racqueline, J. A disaccharide repeat unit is the structure structure in fucoidans from two species of brown algae. *Carbohydr. Res.* **2001**, *330*, 529–535. [CrossRef] [PubMed]

54. Colliec-Jouault, S.; Millet, J.; Helley, D.; Sinquin, C.; Fischer, A.M. Effect of low-molecular-weight fucoidan on experimental arterial thrombosis in the rabbit and rat. *J. Thromb. Haemost.* **2003**, *1*, 1114–1115. [CrossRef] [PubMed]

55. Foley, S.A.; Szegezdi, E.; Mulloy, B.; Samali, A.; Tuohy, M.G. An unfractionated fucoidan from *Ascophyllum nodosum*: Extraction, characterization, and apoptotic effects *in vitro*. *J. Nat. Prod.* **2011**, *74*, 1851–1861. [CrossRef] [PubMed]

56. Hoffman, R.; Paper, D.H.; Donaldson, J.; Alban, S.; Franz, G. Characterization of a laminarin sulfate which inhibits basic fibroblast growth-factor binding and endothelial-cell proliferation. *J. Cell Sci.* **1995**, *108*, 3591–3598. [PubMed]

57. Luyt, C.E.; Meddahi-Pellé, A.; Ho-Tin-Noe, B.; Colliec-Jouault, S.; Guezennec, J.; Louedec, L.; Prats, H.; Jacob, M.P.; Osborne-Pellegrin, M.; Letourneur, D.; *et al.* Low-molecular-weight fucoidan promotes therapeutic revascularization in a rat model of critical hindlimb ischemia. *J. Pharmacol. Exp. Therapeut.* **2003**, *305*, 24–30. [CrossRef]

58. Matou, S.; Helley, D.; Chabut, D.; Bros, A.; Fischer, A.M. Effect of fucoidan on fibroblast growth factor-2-induced angiogenesis *in vitro*. *Thromb. Res.* **2002**, *106*, 213–221. [CrossRef] [PubMed]

59. Miao, H.Q.; Elkin, M.; Aingorn, E.; Ishai-Michaeli, R.; Stein, C.A.; Vlodavsky, I. Inhibition of heparanase activity and tumor metastasis by laminarin sulfate and synthetic phosphorothioate oligodeoxynucleotides. *Int. J. Cancer* **1999**, *83*, 424–431. [CrossRef] [PubMed]

60. Percival, E. Glucuronoxylofucan, a cell-wall component of *Ascophyllum nodosum*. *Carbohydr. Res.* **1968**, *7*, 272–277. [CrossRef]

61. Renn, D.W.; Noda, H.; Amano, H.; Nishino, T.; Nishizana, K. Antihypertensive and antihyperlipidemic effects of funoran. *Fisch. Sci.* **1994**, *60*, 423–427.

62. Ale, M.T.; Maruyama, H.; Tamauchi, H.; Mikkelsen, J.D.; Meyer, A.S. Fucoidan from *Sargassum* sp. and *Fucus vesiculosus* reduces cell viability of lung carcinoma and melanoma cells *in vitro* and activates natural killer cells in mice *in vivo*. *Int. J. Biol. Macromol.* **2011**, *49*, 331–336. [CrossRef] [PubMed]

63. Beress, A.; Wassermann, O.; Tahhan, S.; Bruhn, T.; Beress, L.; Kraiselburd, E.N.; Gonzalez, L.V.; de Motta, G.E.; Chavez, P.I. A new procedure for the isolation of anti-HIV compounds (polysaccharides and polyphenols) from the marine alga *Fucus vesiculosus*. *J. Nat. Prod.* **1993**, *56*, 478–488. [CrossRef] [PubMed]

64. Bilan, M.I.; Grachev, A.A.; Ustuzhanina, N.E.; Shashkov, A.S.; Nifantiev, N.E.; Usov, A.I. Structure of a fucoidan from brown seaweed *Fucus evanescens*. *Carbohydr. Res.* **2002**, *337*, 719–730. [CrossRef] [PubMed]

65. Mourão, P.A.; Pereira, M.S. Searching for alternatives to heparin: Sulfated fucans from marine invertebrates. *Trends Cardiovasc. Med.* **1999**, *9*, 225–232. [CrossRef] [PubMed]

66. Pereira, M.S.; Mulloy, B.; Mourão, P.A. Structure and anticoagulant activity of sulfated fucans. Comparison between the regular, repetitive, and linear fucans from echinoderms with the more heterogeneous and branched polymers from brown algae. *J. Biol. Chem.* **1999**, *274*, 7656–7667. [CrossRef] [PubMed]

67. Nakamura, T.; Suzuki, H.; Wada, Y.; Kodama, T.; Doi, T. Fucoidan induces nitric oxide production via p38 mitogen-activated protein kinase and NF-κB-dependent signaling pathways through macrophage scavenger receptors. *Biochem. Biophys. Res. Commun.* **2006**, *343*, 286–294. [CrossRef] [PubMed]

68. Park, H.S.; Kim, G.Y.; Nam, T.J.; Deuk Kim, N.; Hyun Choi, Y. Antiproliferative activity of fucoidan was associated with the induction of apoptosis and autophagy in AGS human gastric cancer cells. *J. Food Sci.* **2011**, *76*, T77–T83. [CrossRef] [PubMed]

69. Synytsya, A.; Kim, W.J.; Kim, S.M.; Pohl, R.; Synytsya, A.; Kvasnicka, F.; Copikova, J.; Park, Y.I. Structure and antitumor activity of fucoidan isolated from sporophyll of Korean brown seaweed *Undaria pinnatifida*. *Carbohydr. Polym.* **2010**, *81*, 41–48. [CrossRef]

70. Yang, J.W.; Yoon, S.Y.; Oh, S.J.; Kim, S.K.; Kang, K.W. Bifunctional effects of fucoidan on the expression of inducible nitric oxide synthase. *Biochem. Biophys. Res. Commun.* **2006**, *346*, 345–350. [CrossRef] [PubMed]

71. Li, B.; Wei, X.J.; Sun, J.L.; Xu, S.Y. Structural investigation of a fucoidan containing a fucose-free core from the brown seaweed, *Hizikia fusiforme*. *Carbohydr. Res.* **2006**, *341*, 1135–1146. [CrossRef] [PubMed]

72. Dobashi, K.; Nishino, T.; Fujihara, M. Isolation and preliminary characterization of fucose-containing sulfated polysaccharides with blood-anticoagulant activity from seaweed *Hizikia fusiforme. Carbohydr. Res.* **1989**, *194*, 315–320. [CrossRef] [PubMed]

73. Venkateswaran, P.S.; Millman, I.; Blumberg, B.S. Interaction of fucoidan from *Pelvetia fastigiata* with surface antigens of hepatitis B and woodchuck hepatitis viruses. *Planta Med.* **1989**, *55*, 265–270. [CrossRef] [PubMed]

74. Klarzynski, O.; Descamps, V.; Plesse, B.; Yvin, J.C.; Kloareg, B.; Fritig, B. Sulfated fucan oligosaccharides elicit defense responses in tobacco and local and systemic resistance against tobacco mosaic virus. *Mol. Plant Microbe Interact.* **2003**, *16*, 115–122. [CrossRef] [PubMed]

75. Ale, M.T.; Mikkelsen, J.D.; Meyer, A.S. Important determinants for fucoidan bioactivity: A critical review of structure-function relations and extraction methods for fucose-containing sulfated polysaccharides from brown seaweeds. *Mar. Drugs* **2011**, *9*, 2106–2130. [CrossRef] [PubMed]

76. Raghavendran, H.R.; Sathivel, A.; Devaki, T. Effect of *Sargassum polycystum* (Phaeophyceae)-sulphated polysaccharide extract against acetaminophen-induced hyperlipidemia during toxic hepatitis in experimental rats. *Mol. Cell. Biochem.* **2005**, *276*, 89–96. [CrossRef] [PubMed]

77. Josephine, A.; Veena, C.K.; Amudha, G.; Preetha, S.P.; Varalakshmi, P. Protective role of sulphated polysaccharides in abating the hyperlipidemic nephropathy provoked by cyclosporine A. *Arch. Toxicol.* **2007**, *81*, 371–379. [CrossRef] [PubMed]

78. Duarte, M.E.; Cardoso, M.A.; Noseda, M.D.; Cerezo, A.S. Structural studies on fucoidans from the brown seaweed *Sargassum stenophyllum. Carbohydr. Res.* **2001**, *333*, 281–293. [CrossRef] [PubMed]

79. Ale, M.T.; Mikkelsen, J.D.; Meyer, A.S. Designed optimization of a single-step extraction of fucose-containing sulfated polysaccharides from *Sargassum* sp. *J. Appl. Phycol.* **2011**, *24*, 715–723. [CrossRef]

80. Hoshino, T.; Hayashi, T.; Hayashi, K.; Hamada, J.; Lee, J.B.; Sankawa, U. An antivirally active sulfated polysaccharide from *Sargassum horneri* (Turner) C. Agardh. *Biol. Pharm. Bull.* **1998**, *21*, 730–734. [CrossRef] [PubMed]

81. Costa, L.S.; Fidelis, G.P.; Telles, C.B.S.; Dantas-Santos, N.; Camara, R.B.G.; Cordeiro, S.L.; Costa, M.S.S.P.; Almeida-Lima, J.; Melo-Silveira, R.F.; Albuquerque, I.R.L.; *et al.* Antioxidant and antiproliferative activities of heterofucans from the seaweed *Sargassum filipendula. Mar. Drugs* **2011**, *9*, 952–966.

82. Chattopadhyay, N.; Ghosh, T.; Sinha, S.; Chattopadhyay, K.; Karmakar, P.; Ray, B. Polysaccharides from *Turbinaria conoides*: Structural features and antioxidant capacity. *Food Chem.* **2010**, *11*, 823–829. [CrossRef]

83. Yamamoto, I.; Takahashi, M.; Tamura, E.; Maruyama, H.; Mori, H. Antitumor activity of edible marine algae: Effect of crude fucoidan fractions prepared from edible brown seaweed against L-1210 leukemia. *Hydrobiology* **1984**, *116/117*, 145–148. [CrossRef]

84. Nishino, T.; Yokoyama, G.; Dobahi, K. Isolation, purification and characterization of fucose-containing sulfated polysaccharides from the brown seaweed *Ecklonia kurome* and their blood-anticoagulant activities. *Carbohydr. Res.* **1989**, *186*, 119–129. [CrossRef] [PubMed]

85. Nishino, T.; Aizu, Y.; Nagumo, T. The influence of sulfate content and molecular weight of a fucan sulfate from the brown seaweed *Ecklonia kurome* on its antithrombin activity. *Thromb. Res.* **1991**, *64*, 723–731. [CrossRef] [PubMed]

86. Nishino, T.; Kiyohara, H.; Yamada, H.; Nagumo, T. An anticoagulant fucoidan from the brown seaweed *Ecklonia kurome. Phytochemistry* **1991**, *30*, 535–539. [CrossRef] [PubMed]

87. Hu, J.F.; Geng, M.Y.; Zhang, J.T.; Jiang, H.D. An *in vitro* study of the structure-activity relationships of sulfated polysaccharide from brown algae to its antioxidant effect. *J. Asian Nat. Prod. Res.* **2001**, *3*, 353–358. [CrossRef] [PubMed]

88. Kang, S.M.; Kim, K.N.; Lee, S.H.; Ahn, G.; Cha, S.H.; Kim, A.D.; Yang, X.-D.; Kang, M.-C.; Jeon, Y.-J. Anti-inflammatory activity of polysaccharide purified from AMG-assistant extract of *Ecklonia cava* in LPS-stimulated RAW264.7 macrophages. *Carbohydr. Polym.* **2011**, *85*, 80–85. [CrossRef]

89. Takahashi, M. Studies on the mechanism of host mediated antitumor action of fucoidan from a brown alga *Eisenia bicyclis. J. Jpn. Soc. Reticuloendothel. Syst.* **1983**, *22*, 269–283.

90. Usui, T.; Asari, K.; Mizuno, T. Isolation of highly purified fucoidan from *Eisenia bicyclis* and its anticoagulant and antitumor activities. *Agric. Biol. Chem.* **1980**, *44*, 2. [CrossRef]

91. Rioux, L.E.; Turgeon, S.L.; Beaulieu, M. Structural characterization of laminaran and galactofucan extracted from the brown seaweed *Saccharina longicruris. Phytochemistry* **2010**, *71*, 1586–1595. [CrossRef] [PubMed]

92. Usov, A.I.; Smirnova, G.P.; Bilan, M.I.; Shashkov, A.S. Polysaccharides of algae: 53. Brown alga *Laminaria saccharina* (L.) Lam. as a source of fucoidan. *Bioorg. Khim* **1998**, *24*, 382–389.

93. Maruyama, H.; Yamamoto, I. An antitumor fraction from an edible brown seaweed *Laminaria religiosa*. *Hydrobiologia* **1984**, *116/177*, 534–536. [CrossRef]

94. Kitamura, K.; Matsuo, M.; Yasui, T. Enzymic degradation of fucoidan by fucoidanase from the hepatopancreas of *Patinopecten yessoensis*. *Biosci. Biotechnol. Biochem.* **1992**, *56*, 490–494. [CrossRef]

95. Huang, L.; Wen, K.; Gao, X.; Liu, Y. Hypolipidemic effect of fucoidan from *Laminaria japonica* in hyperlipidemic rats. *Pharm. Biol.* **2010**, *48*, 422–426. [CrossRef] [PubMed]

96. Xue, C.H.; Chen, L.; Li, Z.J.; Cai, Y.P.; Lin, H.; Fang, Y. Antioxidative activities of low molecular fucoidans from kelp *Laminaria japonica*. *Dev. Food Sci.* **2004**, *42*, 139–145.

97. Wang, J.; Zhang, Q.; Zhang, Z.; Li, Z. Antioxidant activity of sulfated polysaccharide fractions extracted from *Laminaria japonica*. *Int. J. Biol. Macromol.* **2008**, *42*, 127–132. [CrossRef] [PubMed]

98. Vishchuk, O.S.; Ermakova, S.P.; Zvyagintseva, T.N. Sulfated polysaccharides from brown seaweeds *Saccharina japonica* and *Undaria pinnatifida*: Isolation, structural characteristics, and antitumor activity. *Carbohydr. Res.* **2011**, *346*, 2769–2776. [CrossRef] [PubMed]

99. Li, F.; Tian, T.C.; Shi, Y.C. Study on antivirus effect of fucoidan *in vitro*. *J. N. Bethune Univ. Med. Sci.* **1995**, *21*, 255–257.

100. Li, D.Y.; Xu, R.Y.; Zhou, W.Z.; Sheng, X.B.; Yang, A.Y.; Cheng, J.L. Effects of fucoidan extracted from brown seaweed on lipid peroxidation in mice. *Acta Nutrim. Sin.* **2002**, *24*, 389–392.

101. Wang, W.T.; Zhou, J.H.; Xing, S.T.; Guan, H.S. Immunomodulating action of marine algae sulfated polysaccharides on normal and immunosuppressed mice. *Chin. J. Pharm Toxicol.* **1994**, *8*, 199–202.

102. Luo, D.; Zhan, Q.; Wang, H.; Cui, Y.; Sun, Z.; Yang, J.; Zheng, Y.; Jia, J.; Yu, F.; Wang, X. Fucoidan protects against dopaminergic neuron death *in vivo* and *in vitro*. *Eur. J. Pharmacol.* **2009**, *617*, 33–40. [CrossRef] [PubMed]

103. Li, B.; Lu, F.; Wei, X.; Zhao, R. Fucoidan: Structure and bioactivity. *Molecules* **2008**, *13*, 1671–1695. [CrossRef] [PubMed]

104. Lee, S.H.; Athukorala, Y.; Lee, J.S.; Jeon, Y.J. Simple separation of anticoagulant sulfated galactan from red algae. *J. Appl. Phycol.* **2008**, *20*, 1053–1059. [CrossRef]

105. Yoon, S.J.; Pyun, Y.R.; Hwang, J.K.; Mourão, P.A.S. A sulfated fucan from the brown alga *Laminaria cichorioides* has mainly heparin cofactor II-dependent anticoagulant activity. *Carbohydr. Res.* **2007**, *342*, 2326–2330. [CrossRef] [PubMed]

106. Thompson, K.D.; Dragar, C. Antiviral activity of *Undaria pinnatifida* against herpes simplex virus. *Phytother. Res.* **2004**, *18*, 551–555. [CrossRef] [PubMed]

107. Hemmingson, J.A.; Falshow, R.; Furneaux, R.H.; Thompsom, K. Structure and antiviral activity of the galactofucans sulfates extracted from *Undaria pinnatifida* (Phaeophyta). *J. Appl. Phycol.* **2006**, *18*, 185–193. [CrossRef]

108. Maruyama, H.; Tamauchi, H.; Hashimoto, M.; Nakano, T. Antitumor activity and immune response of Mekabu fucoidan extracted from Sporophyll of *Undaria pinnatifida*. *Vivo* **2003**, *17*, 245–249.

109. Cho, Y.S.; Jung, W.K.; Kim, J.A.; Choi, I.W.; Kim, S.K. Beneficial effects of fucoidan on osteoblastic MG-63 cell differentiation. *Food Chem.* **2009**, *116*, 990–994. [CrossRef]

110. Cho, M.L.; Lee, B.Y.; You, S.G. Relationship between oversulfation and conformation of low and high molecular weight fucoidans and evaluation of their *in vitro* anticancer activity. *Molecules* **2011**, *16*, 291–297. [CrossRef]

111. Maruyamaa, H.; Tamauchib, H.; Hashimotoc, M.; Nakano, T. Suppression of Th2 immune responses by Mekabu fucoidan from *Undaria pinnatifida* sporophylls. *Int. Arch. Allergy Immunol.* **2005**, *137*, 289–294. [CrossRef] [PubMed]

112. Preobrazhenskaya, M.E.; Berman, A.E.; Mikhailov, V.I.; Ushakova, N.A.; Mazurov, A.V.; Semenov, A.V.; Usov, A.I.; Nifant'ev, N.E.; Bovin, N.V. Fucoidan inhibits leukocyte recruitment in a model peritoneal inflammation in rat and blocks interaction of P-selectin with its carbohydrate ligand. *Biochem. Mol. Biol. Int.* **1997**, *43*, 443–451. [PubMed]

113. Noda, H. Health benefits and nutritional properties of nori. *J. Appl. Phycol.* **1993**, *5*, 255–258. [CrossRef]

114. Takano, R.; Hayashi, K.; Hara, S.; Hirase, S. Funoran from the red seaweed *Gloiopeltis complanata*: Polysaccharides with sulphated agarose structure and their precursor structure. *Carbohydr. Polym.* **1995**, *27*, 305–311. [CrossRef]

115. Zhang, Q.B.; Li, N.; Zhou, G.F.; Lu, X.L.; Xu, Z.H.; Li, Z. *In vivo* antioxidant activity of polysaccharide fraction from *Porphyra haitanensis* (Rhodophyta) in aging mice. *Pharmacol. Res.* **2003**, *48*, 151–155. [CrossRef] [PubMed]

116. Kwon, M.J.; Nam, T.J. Porphyran induces apoptosis related signal pathway in AGS gastric cancer cell lines. *Life Sci.* **2006**, *79*, 1956–1962. [CrossRef] [PubMed]

117. Yoshizawa, Y.; Enomoto, A.; Todoh, H.; Ametani, A.; Kaminogawa, S. Activation of murine macrophages by polysaccharide fractions from marine algae (*Porphyra yezoensis*). *Biosci. Biotechnol. Biochem.* **1993**, *57*, 1862–1866. [CrossRef] [PubMed]

118. Yoshizawa, Y.; Ametani, A.; Tsunehiro, J.; Nomura, K.; Itoh, M.; Fukui, F.; Kaminogawa, S. Macrophage stimulation activity of the polysaccharide fraction from a marine alga (*Porphyra yezoensis*): Structure-function relationships and improved solubility. *Biosci. Biotechnol. Biochem.* **1995**, *59*, 1933–1937. [CrossRef] [PubMed]

119. Tsuge, K.; Okabe, M.; Yoshimura, T.; Sumi, T.; Tachibana, H.; Yamada, K. Dietary effect of porphyran from *Porphyra yezoensis* on growth and lipid metabolism of Sprague-Dawley rats. *Food Sci. Technol. Res.* **2004**, *10*, 147–151. [CrossRef]

120. Duarte, M.E.; Noseda, D.G.; Noseda, M.D.; Tulio, S.; Pujol, C.A.; Damonte, E.B. Inhibitory effect of sulfated galactans from the marine alga *Bostrychia montagnei* on herpes simplex virus replication *in vitro*. *Phytomedicine* **2001**, *8*, 53–58. [CrossRef] [PubMed]

121. Carlucci, M.J.; Scolaro, L.A.; Matulewicz, M.C.; Damonte, E.B. Antiviral activity of natural sulphated galactans on herpes virus multiplication in cell culture. *Planta Med.* **1997**, *63*, 429–432. [CrossRef] [PubMed]

122. Sekine, H.; Ohonuki, N.; Sadamasu, K.; Monma, K.; Kudoh, Y.; Nakamura, H.; Okada, Y.; Okuyama, T. The inhibitory effect of the crude extract from the seaweed *Dygenea simplex* C. Agardh on the *in vitro* cytopathic activity of HIV-1 and its antigen production. *Chem. Pharm. Bull. (Tokyo)* **1995**, *43*, 1580–1584. [CrossRef]

123. Talarico, L.B.; Zibetti, R.G.M.; Faria, P.C.S.; Scolaro, L.A.; Duarte, M.E.R.; Noseda, M.D.; Pujol, C.A.; Damonte, E.B. Anti-herpes simplex virus activity of sulfated galactans from the red seaweed *Gymnogongrus griffithsiae* and *Cryptonemia crenulata*. *Int. J. Biol. Macromol.* **2004**, *34*, 63–71. [CrossRef] [PubMed]

124. Takano, R.; Iwane-Sakata, H.; Hayashi, K.; Hara, S.; Hirase, S. Concurrence of agaroid and carrageenan chains in funoran from the red seaweed *Gloiopeltis furcata* Post. Et Ruprecht (Cryptonemiales, Rhodophyta). *Carbohydr. Polym.* **1998**, *35*, 81–87. [CrossRef]

125. Pereira, M.G.; Benevides, N.M.B.; Melo, M.R.S.; Valente, A.P.; Melo, F.R.; Mourão, P.A.S. Structure and anticoagulant activity of a sulfated galactan from the red alga, *Gelidium crinale*. Is there a specific structural requirement for the anticoagulant action? *Carbohydr. Res.* **2005**, *340*, 2015–2023. [CrossRef] [PubMed]

126. Pujol, C.A.; Errea, M.I.; Matulewicz, M.C.; Damonte, E.B. Antiherpetic activity of S1, an algal derived sulphated galactan. *Phytother Res.* **1996**, *10*, 410–413. [CrossRef]

127. De Clercq, E. Current lead natural products for the chemotherapy of human immunodeficiency virus (HIV) infection. *Med. Res. Rev.* **2000**, *20*, 323–349. [CrossRef] [PubMed]

128. Witvrouw, M.; Este, J.A.; Mateu, M.Q.; Reymen, D.; Andrei, G.; Snoeck, R.; Ikeda, S.; Pauwels, R.; Bianchini, N.V.; Desmyter, J.; de Clercq, E. Activity of a sulfated polysaccharide extracted from the red seaweed *Aghardhiella tenera* against human immunodeficiency virus and other enveloped viruses. *Antivir. Chem. Chemother.* **1994**, *5*, 297–303. [CrossRef]

129. Luescher-Mattli, M. Algae, a possible source for new drugs in the treatment of HIV and other viral diseases. *Curr. Med. Chem.* **2003**, *2*, 219–225.

130. Prajapati, V.D.; Maherereriya, P.M.; Jani, G.K.; Soalnki, H.K. Carrageenan: A natural seaweed polysaccharide and its applications. *Carbohydr. Polym.* **2014**, *105*, 97–112. [CrossRef] [PubMed]

131. Campo, V.L.; Kawano, D.F.; da Silva, D.B.; Carvalho, I. Carrageenans: Biological properties, chemical modifications and structural analysis. *Carbohydr. Polym.* **2009**, *77*, 167–180. [CrossRef]

132. Mou, H.; Xiaolu, J.; Huashi, G. A kappa-carrageenan derived oligosaccharide prepared by enzymatic degradation containing anti-tumor activity. *J. Appl. Phycol.* **2003**, *15*, 297–303. [CrossRef]

133. Yang, B.; Yu, G.; Zhao, X.; Ren, W.; Jiao, G.; Fang, L.; Wang, Y.; Du, G.; Tiller, C.; Girouard, G.; *et al.* Structural characterisation and bioactivities of hybrid carrageenan-like sulphated galactan from red alga *Furcellaria lumbricalis*. *Food Chem.* **2011**, *124*, 50–57. [CrossRef]

134. Carlucci, M.J.; Pujol, C.A.; Ciancia, M.; Noseda, M.D.; Matulewicz, M.C.; Damonte, E.B.; Cerezo, A.S. Antiherpetic and anticoagulant properties of carrageenans from the red seaweed *Gigartina skottsbergii* and their cyclized derivatives: Correlation between structure and biological activity. *Int. J. Biol. Macromol.* **1997**, *20*, 97–105. [CrossRef] [PubMed]

135. Carlucci, M.J.; Ciancia, M.; Matulewicz, M.C.; Cerezo, A.S.; Damonte, E.B. Antiherpetic activity and mode of action of natural carrageenans of diverse structural types. *Antivir. Res.* **1999**, *43*, 93–102. [CrossRef] [PubMed]

136. Pujol, C.A.; Estevez, J.M.; Carlucci, M.J.; Ciancia, M.; Cerezo, A.S.; Damonte, E.B. Novel DL-galactan hybrids from the red seaweed *Gymnogongrus torulosus* are potent inhibitors of herpes simplex virus and dengue virus. *Antivir. Chem. Chemother.* **2002**, *13*, 83–89. [CrossRef] [PubMed]

137. Sen, A.K.; Das, A.K.; Banerji, N.; Siddhanta, A.K.; Mody, K.H.; Ramavat, B.K.; Chauhan, V.D.; Vedasiromoni, J.R.; Ganguly, D.K. A new sulfated polysaccharide with potent blood anti-coagulant activity from the red seaweed *Grateloupia indica*. *Int. J. Biol. Macromol.* **1994**, *16*, 279–280. [CrossRef] [PubMed]

138. Bondu, S.; Deslandes, E.; Fabre, M.S.; Berthou, C.; Yu, G. Carrageenan from *Solieria chordalis* (Gigartinales): Structural analysis and immunological activities of the low molecular weight fractions. *Carbohydr. Polym.* **2010**, *81*, 448–460. [CrossRef]

139. Caceres, P.J.; Carlucci, M.J.; Damonte, E.B.; Matsuhiro, B.; Zuniga, E.A. Carrageenans from chilean samples of *Stenogramme interrupta* (Phyllophoraceae): Structural analysis and biological activity. *Phytochemistry* **2000**, *53*, 81–86. [CrossRef]

140. Mazumder, S.; Ghosal, P.K.; Pujol, C.A.; Carlucci, M.J.; Damonte, E.B.; Ray, B. Isolation, chemical investigation and antiviral activity of polysaccharides from *Gracilaria corticata* (Gracilariaceae, Rhodophyta). *Int. J. Biol. Macromol.* **2002**, *31*, 87–95. [CrossRef] [PubMed]

141. Yoshizawa, Y.; Tsunehiro, J.; Nomura, K.; Itoh, M.; Fukui, F.; Ametani, A.; Kaminogawa, S. *In vivo* macrophage-stimulation activity of the enzyme-degraded water-soluble polysaccharide fraction from a marine alga (*Gracilaria verrucosa*). *Biosci. Biotechnol. Biochem.* **1996**, *60*, 1667–1671. [CrossRef] [PubMed]

142. Recalde, M.P.; Noseda, M.D.; Pujol, C.A.; Carlucci, M.J.; Matulewicz, M.C. Sulfated mannans from the red seaweed *Nemalion helminthoides* of the South Atlantic. *Phytochemistry* **2009**, *70*, 1062–1068. [CrossRef] [PubMed]

143. Damonte, E.; Neyts, J.; Pujol, C.A.; Snoeck, R.; Andrei, G.; Ikeda, S.; Witvrouw, M.; Reymen, D.; Haines, H.; Matulewicz, M.C.; *et al.* Antiviral activity of a sulphated polysaccharide from the red seaweed *Nothogenia fastigiata*. *Biochem Pharmacol.* **1994**, *47*, 2187–2192. [CrossRef] [PubMed]

144. Damonte, E.B.; Matulewicz, M.C.; Cerezo, A.S.; Coto, C.E. Herpes simplex virus-inhibitory sulfated xylogalactans from the red seaweed *Nothogenia fastigiata*. *Chemotherapy* **1996**, *42*, 57–64. [CrossRef] [PubMed]

145. Kolender, A.A.; Pujol, C.A.; Damonte, E.B.; Matulewicz, M.C.; Cerezo, A.S. The system of sulfated alpha-(1→3)-linked D-mannans from the red seaweed *Nothogenia fastigiata*: Structures, antiherpetic and anticoagulant properties. *Carbohydr. Res.* **1997**, *304*, 53–60. [CrossRef] [PubMed]

146. Bourgougnon, N.; Roussakis, C.; Kornprobst, J.M.; Lahaye, M. Effects *in vitro* of sulfated polysaccharide from *Schizymenia dubyi* (Rhodophyta, Gigartinales) on a non-small-cell bronchopulmonary carcinoma line (NSCLC-N6). *Cancer Lett.* **1994**, *85*, 87–92. [CrossRef] [PubMed]

147. Nakashima, H.; Kido, Y.; Kobayashi, N.; Motoki, Y.; Neushul, M.; Yamamoto, N. Purification and characterization of an avian myeloblastosis and human immunodeficiency virus reverse transcriptase inhibitor, sulfated polysaccharides extracted from sea algae. *Antimicrob. Agents Chemother.* **1987**, *31*, 1524–1528. [CrossRef] [PubMed]

148. Zuniga, E.A.; Matsuhiro, B.; Mejias, E. Preparation of a low-molecular weight fraction by free radical depolymerization of the sulfated galactan from *Schizymenia binderi* (Gigartinales, Rhodophyta) and its anticoagulant activity. *Carbohydr. Polym.* **2006**, *66*, 208–215. [CrossRef]

149. Farias, W.R.L.; Valente, A.P.; Pereira, M.S.; Mourão, P.A.S. Structure and anticoagulant activity of sulfated galactans. Isolation of a unique sulfated galactan from the red alga *Botryocladia occidentalis* and comparison of its anticoagulant action with that of sulfated galactans from invertebrates. *J. Biol. Chem.* **2000**, *275*, 29299–29307. [CrossRef] [PubMed]

150. Toyama, M.H.; Toyama, D.O.; Torres, V.M.; Pontes, G.C.; Farias, W.R.L.; Melo, F.R.; Oliveira, S.C.B.; Fagundes, F.H.R.; Diz Filho, E.B.S.; Cavada, B.S. Effects of Low Molecular Weight Sulfated Galactan Fragments From *Botryocladia occidentalis* on the Pharmacological and Enzymatic Activity of Spla2 from *Crotalus durissus cascavella*. *Protein J.* **2010**, *29*, 567–571. [CrossRef] [PubMed]

151. Lins, K.O.; Bezerra, D.P.; Alves, A.P.; Alencar, N.M.; Lima, M.W.; Torres, V.M.; Farias, W.R.; Pessoa, C.; de Moraes, M.O.; Costa-Lotufo, L.V. Antitumor properties of a sulfated polysaccharide from the red seaweed *Champia feldmannii* (Diaz-Pifferer). *J. Appl. Toxicol.* **2009**, *29*, 20–26. [CrossRef] [PubMed]

152. Ghosh, T.; Pujol, C.A.; Damonte, E.B.; Sinha, S.; Ray, B. Sulfated xylomannans from the red seaweed *Sebdenia polydactyla*: Structural features, chemical modification and antiviral activity. *Antivir. Chem. Chemother.* **2009**, *19*, 235–242. [CrossRef] [PubMed]

153. Lee, J.B.; Hayashi, K.; Maeda, M.; Hayashi, T. Antiherpetic activities of sulfated polysaccharides from green algae. *Planta Med.* **2004**, *70*, 813–817. [CrossRef] [PubMed]

154. Ji, H.; Shao, H.; Zhang, C.; Hong, P.; Xiong, H. Separation of the polysaccharides in *Caulerpa racemosa* and their chemical composition and antitumor activity. *J. Appl. Polym. Sci.* **2008**, *110*, 1435–1440. [CrossRef]

155. Rodrigues, J.A.G.; Oliveira Vanderlei, E.D.S.; Silva, L.M.; de Araujo, I.W.; de Queiroz, I.N.; de Paula, G.A.; Abreu, T.M.; Ribeiro, N.A.; Bezerra, M.M.; Chaves, H.V.; *et al.* Antinociceptive and anti-inflammatory activities of a sulfated polysaccharide isolated from the green seaweed *Caulerpa cupressoides*. *Pharmacol. Rep.* **2012**, *64*, 282–292. [CrossRef] [PubMed]

156. Rodrigues, J.A.G.; Oliveira Vanderlei, E.D.S.; Gomes Quindere, A.L.; Monteiro, V.S.; Mendes de Vasconcelos, S.M.; Barros Benevides, N.M. Antinociceptive activity and acute toxicological study of a novel sulfated polysaccharide from *Caulerpa cupressoides* var. *lycopodium* (Chlorophyta) in Swiss mice. *Acta Sci. Technol.* **2013**, *35*, 417–425.

157. Chattopadhyay, K.; Adhikari, U.; Lerouge, P.; Ray, B. Polysaccharides from *Caulerpa racemosa*: Purification and structural features. *Carbohydr. Polym.* **2007**, *68*, 407–415. [CrossRef]

158. Fernández, P.V.; Ciancia, M.; Miravalles, A.B.; Estevez, J.M. Cell wall polymer mapping in the coenocytic macroalga *Codium vermilara*. *J. Phycol.* **2010**, *46*, 456–465. [CrossRef]

159. Hayakawa, Y.; Hayashi, T.; Hayashi, K.; Osawa, T.; Niiya, K.; Sakuragawa, N. Activation of heparin cofactor II by calcium spirulan. *J. Biol. Chem.* **2000**, *275*, 11379–11382. [CrossRef] [PubMed]

160. Shanmugam, M.; Mody, K.H.; Ramavat, B.K.; Murthy, A.S.K.; Siddhanta, A.K. Screening of Codiacean algae (Chlorophyta) of the Indian coasts for blood anticoagulant activity. *Indian J. Mar. Sci.* **2002**, *31*, 33–38.

161. Ciancia, M.; Quintana, I.; Vizcarguenaga, M.I.; Kasulin, L.; de Dios, A.; Estevez, J.M.; Cerezo, A.S. Polysaccharides from the green seaweeds *Codium fragile* and *C. vermilara* with controversial effects on hemostasis. *Int. J. Biol. Macromol.* **2007**, *41*, 641–649. [CrossRef] [PubMed]

162. Farias, E.H.; Pomin, V.H.; Valente, A.P.; Nader, H.B.; Rocha, H.A.; Mourão, P.A. A preponderantly 4-sulfated, 3-linked galactan from the green alga *Codium isthmocladum*. *Glycobiology* **2008**, *18*, 250–259. [CrossRef] [PubMed]

163. Na, Y.S.; Kim, W.J.; Kim, S.M.; Park, J.K.; Lee, S.M.; Kim, S.O.; Synytsya, A.; Park, Y.I. Purification, characterization and immunostimulating activity of water-soluble polysaccharide isolated from *Capsosiphon fulvescens*. *Int. Immunopharmacol.* **2010**, *10*, 364–370. [CrossRef] [PubMed]

164. Lee, J.B.; Hayashi, K.; Hayashi, T.; Sankawa, U.; Maeda, M. Antiviral activities against HSV-1, HCMV, and HIV-1 of rhamnan sulfate from *Monostroma latissimum*. *Planta Med.* **1999**, *65*, 439–441. [CrossRef] [PubMed]

165. Qi, H.M.; Zhang, Q.B.; Zhao, T.T.; Chen, R.; Zhang, H.; Niu, X.Z.; Li, Z. Antioxidant activity of different sulfate content derivatives of polysaccharide extracted from *Ulva pertusa* (Chlorophyta) *in vitro*. *Int. J. Biol. Macromol.* **2005**, *37*, 195–199. [CrossRef] [PubMed]

166. Qi, H.M.; Zhao, T.T.; Zhang, Q.B.; Li, Z.; Zhao, Z.Q.; Xing, R. Antioxidant activity of different molecular weight sulfated polysaccharides from *Ulva pertusa* Kjellm (Chlorophyta). *J. Appl. Phycol.* **2005**, *17*, 527–534. [CrossRef]

167. Mao, W.; Li, H.; Li, Y.; Zhang, H.; Qi, X.; Sun, H.; Chen, Y.; Guo, S. Chemical characteristic and anticoagulant activity of the sulfated polysaccharide isolated from *Monostroma latissimum* (Chlorophyta). *Int. J. Biol. Macromol.* **2009**, *44*, 70–74. [CrossRef] [PubMed]

168. Zhang, H.J.; Mao, W.J.; Fang, F.; Li, H.Y.; Sun, H.H.; Chen, Y.; Qi, X.H. Chemical characteristics and anticoagulant activities of a sulfated polysaccharide and its fragments from *Monostroma latissimum*. *Carbohydr. Polym.* **2008**, *71*, 428–434. [CrossRef]

169. Hayakawa, Y.; Hayashi, T.; Lee, J.B.; Srisomporn, P.; Maeda, M.; Ozawa, T.; Sakuragawa, N. Inhibition of thrombin by sulfated polysaccharides isolated from green algae. *Biochim. Biophys. Acta Protein Struct. Mol. Enzymol.* **2000**, *1543*, 86–94. [CrossRef]

170. Karnjanapratum, S.; You, S. Molecular characteristics of sulfated polysaccharides from *Monostroma nitidum* and their *in vitro* anticancer and immunomodulatory activities. *Int. J. Biol. Macromol.* **2011**, *48*, 311–318. [CrossRef] [PubMed]

171. Charles, A.L.; Chang, C.K.; Wu, M.L.; Huang, T.C. Studies on the expression of liver detoxifying enzymes in rats fed seaweed (*Monostroma nitidum*). *Food Chem. Toxicol.* **2007**, *45*, 2390–2396. [CrossRef] [PubMed]

172. Jiao, L.; Li, X.; Li, T.; Jiang, P.; Zhang, L.; Wu, M.; Zhang, L. Characterization and anti-tumor activity of alkali-extracted polysaccharide from *Enteromorpha intestinalis*. *Int. Immunopharmacol.* **2009**, *9*, 324–329. [CrossRef] [PubMed]

173. Jiao, L.; Jiang, P.; Zhang, L.; Wu, M. Antitumor and immunomodulating activity of polysaccharides from *Enteromorpha intestinalis*. *Biotechnol. Biopro. Eng.* **2010**, *15*, 421–428. [CrossRef]

174. Wang, X.; Zhang, Z.; Yao, Z.; Zhao, M.; Qi, H. Sulfation, anticoagulant and antioxidant activities of polysaccharide from green algae *Enteromorpha linza*. *Int. J. Biol. Macromol.* **2013**, *58*, 225–230. [CrossRef] [PubMed]

175. Kim, J.K.; Cho, M.L.; Karnjanapratum, S.; Shin, I.S.; You, S.G. *In vitro* and *in vivo* immunomodulatory activity of sulfated polysaccharides from *Enteromorpha prolifera*. *Int. J. Biol. Macromol.* **2011**, *49*, 1051–1058. [CrossRef] [PubMed]

176. Li, B.; Liu, S.; Xing, R.; Li, K.; Li, R.; Qin, Y.; Wang, X.; Wei, Z.; Li, P. Degradation of sulfated polysaccharides from *Enteromorpha prolifera* and their antioxidant activities. *Carbohydr. Polym.* **2013**, *92*, 1991–1996. [CrossRef] [PubMed]

177. Teng, Z.; Qian, L.; Zhou, Y. Hypolipidemic activity of the polysaccharides from *Enteromorpha prolifera*. *Int. J. Biol. Macromol.* **2013**, *62*, 254–256. [CrossRef] [PubMed]

178. Lahaye, M.; Robic, A. Structure and functional properties of ulvan, a polysaccharide from green seaweeds. *Biomacromolecules* **2007**, *8*, 1765–1774. [CrossRef] [PubMed]

179. Rao, H.B.R.; Sathivel, A.; Devaki, T. Antihepatotoxic nature of *Ulva reticulata* (Chlorophyceae) on acetaminophen-induced hepatoxicity in experimental rats. *J. Med. Food* **2004**, *7*, 495–497. [CrossRef] [PubMed]

180. Mao, W.; Zang, X.; Li, Y.; Zhang, H. Sulfated polysaccharides from marine green algae *Ulva conglobata* and their anticoagulant activity. *J. Appl. Phycol.* **2006**, *18*, 9–14. [CrossRef]

181. Shao, P.; Chen, X.; Sun, P. *In vitro* antioxidant and antitumor activities of different sulfated polysaccharides isolated from three algae. *Int. J. Biol. Macromol.* **2013**, *62*, 155–161. [CrossRef] [PubMed]

182. Xing, R.G.; Liu, S.; Yu, H.H.; Guo, Z.Y.; Li, Z.; Li, P.C. Preparation of high-molecular weight and high-sulfate content chitosans and their potential antioxidant activity *in vitro*. *Carbohydr. Polym.* **2005**, *61*, 148–154. [CrossRef]

183. Lahaye, M.; Ray, B. Cell-wall polysaccharides from the marine green alga *Ulva rigida* (Ulvales, Chlorophyta)-NMR analysis of ulvan oligosaccharides. *Carbohydr. Res.* **1996**, *283*, 161–173. [CrossRef] [PubMed]

184. Lahaye, M.; Brunel, M.; Bonnin, E. Fine chemical structure analysis of oligosaccharides produced by an ulvan-lyase degradation of the water-soluble cell-wall polysaccharides from *Ulva* sp. (Ulvales, Chlorophyta). *Carbohydr. Res.* **1997**, *304*, 325–333. [CrossRef] [PubMed]

185. Yu, P.Z.; Li, N.; Liu, X.G.; Zhou, G.F.; Zhang, Q.B.; Li, P.C. Antihyperlipidemic effects of different molecular weight sulfated polysaccharides from *Ulva pertusa* (Chlorophyta). *Pharmacol. Res.* **2003**, *48*, 543–549. [CrossRef] [PubMed]

186. Kaeffer, B.; Benard, C.; Lahaye, M.; Blottiere, H.M.; Cherbut, C. Biological properties of ulvan, a new source of green seaweed sulfated polysaccharides, on cultured normal and cancerous colonic epithelial tells. *Planta Med.* **1999**, *65*, 527–531. [CrossRef] [PubMed]

187. Margret, R.J.; Kumaresan, S.; Ravikumar, S. A preliminary study on the anti-inflammatory activity of methanol extract of *Ulva lactuca* in rat. *J. Environ. Biol.* **2009**, *30*, 899–902. [PubMed]

188. Chiu, Y.H.; Chan, Y.L.; Li, T.L.; Wu, C.J. Inhibition of Japanese encephalitis virus infection by the sulfated polysaccharide extracts from *Ulva lactuca*. *Mar. Biotechnol.* **2012**, *14*, 468–478. [CrossRef] [PubMed]

189. Sathivel, A.; Raghavendran, H.R.B.; Srinivasan, P.; Devaki, T. Anti-peroxidative and anti-hyperlipidemic nature of *Ulva lactuca* crude polysaccharide on D-Galactosamine induced hepatitis in rats. *Food Chem. Toxicol.* **2008**, *46*, 3262–3267. [CrossRef] [PubMed]

190. Tabarsa, M.; Han, J.H.; Kim, C.Y.; You, S.G. Molecular characteristics and immunomodulatory activities of water-soluble sulfated polysaccharides from *Ulva pertusa*. *J. Med. Food* **2012**, *15*, 135–144. [CrossRef] [PubMed]

191. Qi, H.; Liu, X.; Zhang, J.; Duan, Y.; Wang, X.; Zhang, Q. Synthesis and antihyperlipidemic activity of acetylated derivative of ulvan from *Ulva pertusa*. *Int. J. Biol. Macromol.* **2012**, *50*, 270–272. [CrossRef] [PubMed]

192. Leiro, J.M.; Castro, R.; Arranz, J.A.; Lamas, J. Immunomodulating activities of acidic sulphated polysaccharides obtained from the seaweed *Ulva rigida* C. Agardh. *Int. Immunopharmacol.* **2007**, *7*, 879–888. [CrossRef] [PubMed]

193. Staats, N.; de Winder, B.; Stal, L.J.; Mur, L.R. Isolation and characterization of extracellular polysaccharides from the epipelic diatoms *Cylindrotheca closterium* and *Navicula salinarum*. *Eur. J. Phycol.* **1999**, *34*, 161–169. [CrossRef]

194. Pletikapic, G.; Radic, T.M.; Zimmermann, A.H.; Svetlicic, V.; Pfannkuchen, M.; Maric, D.; Godrjan, J.; Zutic, V. AFM imaging of extracellular polymer release by marine diatom *Cylindrotheca closterium* (Ehrenberg) Reiman & JC Lewin. *J. Mol. Recogn.* **2011**, *24*, 436–445. [CrossRef]

195. Guzman, S.; Gato, A.; Lamela, M.; Freire-Garabal, M.; Calleja, J.M. Anti-Inflammatory and immunomodulatory activities of polysaccharide from *Chlorella stigmatophora* and *Phaeodactylum tricornutum*. *Phytother. Res.* **2003**, *17*, 665–670. [CrossRef] [PubMed]

196. Ford, C.W.; Percival, E. The carbohydrates of *Phaeodactylum tricornutum*. Part I. Preliminary examination of the organism and characterization of low molecular weight material and of a glucan. *J. Chem. Soc.* **1965**, *1298*, 7035–7041. [CrossRef]

197. Ford, C.W.; Percival, E. The carbohydrates of *Phaeodactylum tricornutum*. Part II. A sulphated glucuronomannan. *J. Chem. Soc.* **1965**, *1299*, 7042–7046. [CrossRef]

198. Rincé, Y.; Lebeau, T.; Robert, J.M. Artificial cell-immobilization: A model simulating immobilization in natural environments? *J. Appl. Phycol.* **1999**, *11*, 263–272. [CrossRef]

199. Penna, A.; Berluti, S.; Penna, N.; Magnani, M. Influence of nutrient ratios on the *in vitro* extracellular polysaccharide production by marine diatoms from Adriatic Sea. *J. Plankton Res.* **1999**, *21*, 1681–1690. [CrossRef]

200. Urbani, R.; Sist, P.; Pletikapić, G.; Radić, T.M.; Svetličić, V.; Žutic, V. Diatom Polysaccharides: Extracellular Production, Isolation and Molecular Characterization. In *The Complex World of Polysaccharides*; Karunaratne, D.N., Ed.; InTech: Rijeka, Croatia, 2012; Chapter 12. [CrossRef]

201. Chen, C.-S.; Anaya, J.M.; Zhang, S.; Spurgin, J.; Chuang, C.-Y.; Xu, C.; Miao, A.-J.; Chen, E.Y.-T.; Schwehr, K.A.; Jiang, Y.; *et al.* Effects of engineered nanoparticles on the assembly of exopolymeric substances from phytoplankton. *PLoS ONE* **2011**, *6*, e21865. [CrossRef] [PubMed]

202. Guzmán-Murillo, M.A.; Ascencio, F. Anti-adhesive activity of sulphated exopolysaccharides of microalgae on attachment of the red sore disease-associated bacteria and *Helicobacter pylori* to tissue culture cells. *Lett. Appl. Microbiol.* **2000**, *30*, 473–478. [CrossRef] [PubMed]

203. Ogawa, K.; Yamaura, M.; Maruyama, I. Isolation and identification of 2-O-methyl-L-rhamnose and 3-O-methyl-L-rhamnose as constituents of an acidic polysaccharide of *Chlorella vulgaris*. *Biosci. Biotechnol. Biochem.* **1997**, *61*, 539–540. [CrossRef]

204. Ogawa, K.; Ikeda, Y.; Kondo, S. A new trisaccharide, α-D-glucopyranuronosyl-(1→3)-α-L-rhamnopyranosyl-(1→2)-α-L-rhamnopyranose from *Chlorella vulgaris*. *Carbohydr. Res.* **1999**, *321*, 128–131. [CrossRef]

205. Mishra, A.; Kavita, K.; Jha, B. Characterization of extracellular polymeric substances produced by micro-algae *Dunaliella salina*. *Carbohydr. Polym.* **2011**, *83*, 852–857. [CrossRef]

206. Allard, B.; Guillot, J.P. The production of extracellular polysaccharides by fresh-water microalgae. Investigation of the polysaccharide components. In *Biomass for Energy and Industry*; Grassi, G., Delmon, B., Molle, J.F., Zibetta, H., Eds.; Elsevier Applied Science: London, UK, 1987; pp. 603–607.

207. Allard, B.; Casadeval, E. Carbohydrate composition and characterization of sugars from the green alga *Botryococcus braunii*. *Phytochemistry* **1990**, *29*, 1875–1878. [CrossRef]

208. Geresh, S.; Arad, S.M. The extracellular polysaccharides of the red microalgae: Chemistry and rheology. *Bioresour. Technol.* **1991**, *38*, 195–201. [CrossRef]

209. Dubinsky, O.; Barak, Z.; Geresh, S.; Arad, S.M. Composition of the cell-wall polysaccharide of the unicellular red alga *Rhodella reticulata* at two phases of growth. In Recent Advances in Algal Biotechnology, Proceedings of the 5th International Conference of the Society of Applied Algology, Tiberias, Israel, 28 January–2 February 1990; US Office of Naval Research: London, UK, 1990; p. 17.

210. Arad, S.M. Production of sulphated polysaccharides from red unicellular algae. In *Algal Biotechnology*; Stadler, T., Mollion, J., Verdus, M.C., Karamanos, Y., Morvan, H., Christiaen, D., Eds.; Elsevier Applied Science: London, UK, 1988; pp. 65–87.

211. Matsui, S.M.; Muizzudin, N.; Arad, S.M.; Marenus, K. Sulfated polysaccharides from red microalgae anti-inflammatory properties *in vitro* and *in vivo*. *Appl. Biochem. Biotechnol.* **2003**, *104*, 13–22. [CrossRef] [PubMed]

212. Arad, S.M.; Atar, D. Viscosupplementation with Algal Polysaccharides in the Treatment of Arthritis. Patent WO/2007/066340, 2007.

213. Talyshinsky, M.M.; Souprun, Y.Y.; Huleihel, M.M. Antiviral activity of red microalgal polysaccharides against retroviruses. *Cancer Cell Int.* **2002**, *2*, 8–14. [CrossRef] [PubMed]

214. Garcia, D.; Morales, E.; Dominguez, A.; Fábregas, J. Productividad mixotrófica del exopolisacárido sulfatado com la microalga marina *Porphyridium cruentum*. In *Communicaciones del III Congreso Ibérico de Biotecnología—Biotec'96*; Universidad de Valladolid: Valladolid, Spain, 1996; pp. 591–592.

215. Heaney-Kieras, J.H. Study of the Extracellular Polysaccharide of *Porphyridium cruentum*. Ph.D. Thesis, University of Chicago, Chicago, IL, USA, 1972.

216. Raposo, M.F.J.; Morais, A.M.M.B.; Morais, R.M.S.C. Influence of sulphate on the composition and antibacterial and antiviral properties of the exopolysaccharide from *Porphyridium cruentum*. *Life Sci.* **2014**, *101*, 56–63. [CrossRef]

217. Gloaguen, V.; Ruiz, G.; Morvan, H.; Mouradi-Givernaud, A.; Maes, E.; Krausz, P.; Srecker, G. The extracelular polysaccharide of *Porphtyridium* sp.: An NMR study of lithium-resistant oligosaccharidic fragments. *Carbohydr. Res.* **2004**, *339*, 97–103. [CrossRef] [PubMed]

218. Geresh, S.; Adin, I.; Yarmolinsky, E.; Karpasas, M. Characterization of the extracellular polysaccharide of *Porphyridium* sp.: Molecular weight determination and rheological properties. *Carbohydr. Polym.* **2002**, *50*, 183–189. [CrossRef]

219. Dubinsky, O.; Simon, B.; Karamanos, Y.; Geresh, S.; Barak, Z.; Arad, S.M. Composition of the cell wall polysaccharide produced by the unicellular red alga *Rhodella reticulata*. *Plant Physiol. Biochem.* **1992**, *30*, 409–414.

220. Sun, L.; Wang, C.; Shi, Q.; Ma, C. Preparation of different molecular weight polysaccharides from *Porphyridium cruentum* and their antioxidant activities. *Int. J. Biol. Macromol.* **2009**, *45*, 42–47. [CrossRef] [PubMed]

221. Sun, L.; Wang, L.; Zhou, Y. Immunomodulation and antitumor activities of different molecular weight polysaccharides from *Porphyridium cruentum*. *Carbohydr. Polym.* **2012**, *87*, 1206–1210. [CrossRef]

222. Huang, J.; Chen, B.; You, W. Studies on separation of extracellular polysaccharide from Porphyridium cruentum and its anti-HBV activity *in vitro*. *Chin. J. Mar. Drugs (Chin.)* **2005**, *24*, 18–21.

223. Radonic, A.; Thulke, S.; Achenbach, J.; Kurth, A.; Vreemann, A.; König, T.; Walter, C.; Possinger, K.; Nitsche, A. Anionic polysaccharides from phototrophic microorganisms exhibit antiviral activities to *Vaccinia* virus. *J. Antivir. Antiretrovir.* **2010**, *2*, 51–55.

224. Evans, L.V.; Callow, M.E.; Percival, E.; Fareed, V.S. Studies on the synthesis and composition of extracellular mucilage in the unicellular red alga *Rhodella*. *J. Cell Sci.* **1974**, *16*, 1–21. [PubMed]

225. Fareed, V.S.; Percival, E. The presence of rhamnose and 3-O-methylxylose in the extracellular mucilage from the red alga *Rhodella maculata*. *Carbohydr. Res.* **1977**, *53*, 276–277. [CrossRef]

226. Hasui, M.; Matsuda, M.; Okutani, K.; Shigeta, S. *In vitro* antiviral activities of sulphated polysaccharides from a marine microalga (*Cochlodinium polykrikoides*) against human immunodeficiency virus and other enveloped virus. *Int. J. Biol. Macromol.* **1995**, *17*, 293–297. [CrossRef] [PubMed]

227. Bae, S.Y.; Yim, J.H.; Lee, H.K.; Pyo, S. Activation of murine peritoneal macrophages by sulphated exopolysaccharide from marine microalga *Gyrodinium impudicum* (strain KG03): Involvement of the NF-kappa B and JNK pathway. *Int. Immunopharmacol.* **2006**, *6*, 473–484. [CrossRef] [PubMed]

228. Yim, J.H.; Son, E.; Pyo, S.; Lee, H.K. Novel sulfated polysaccharide derived from red-tide microalga *Gyrodinium impudicum* strain KG03 with immunostimulating activity *in vivo*. *Mar. Biotechnol.* **2005**, *7*, 331–338. [CrossRef] [PubMed]

229. Yim, J.H.; Kim, S.J.; Ahn, S.H.; Lee, C.K.; Rhie, K.T.; Lee, H.K. Antiviral effects of sulphated polysaccharide from the marine microalga *Gyrodinium impudicum* strain KG03. *Mar. Biotech.* **2004**, *6*, 17–25. [CrossRef]

230. Li, P.; Liu, Z.; Xu, R. Chemical characterization of the released polysaccharides from the cyanobacterium *Aphanothece halophytica* GR02. *J. Appl. Phycol.* **2001**, *13*, 71–77. [CrossRef]

231. Hayashi, T.; Hayashi, K.; Maeda, M.; Kojima, I. Calcium spirulan, an inhibitor of enveloped virus replication, from a blue-green alga *Spirulina platensis*. *J. Nat. Prod.* **1996**, *59*, 83–87. [CrossRef] [PubMed]

232. Martinez, M.J.A.; del Olmo, L.M.B.; Benito, P.B. Antiviral activities of polysaccharides from natural sources. *Stud. Nat. Prod. Chem.* **2005**, *30*, 393–418.

233. Lee, J.-B.; Hayashi, T.; Hayashi, K.; Sankawa, U. Structural analysis of calcium spirulan (Ca-SP)-derived oligosaccharides using electrospray ionization mass spectrometry. *J. Nat. Prod.* **2000**, *63*, 136–138. [CrossRef] [PubMed]

234. Kaji, T.; Okabe, M.; Shimada, S.; Yamamoto, C.; Fujiwara, Y.; Lee, J.-B.; Hayashi, T. Sodium spirulan as a potent inhibitor of arterial smooth muscle cell proliferation *in vitro*. *Life Sci.* **2004**, *74*, 1–9. [CrossRef]

235. Challouf, R.; Trabelsi, L.; Dhieb, R.B.; El Abed, O.; Yahia, A.; Ghozzi, K.; Ammar, J.B.; Omran, H.; Ouada, H.B. Evaluation of cytotoxicity and biological activities in extracellular polysaccharides released by cyanobacterium *Arthrospira platensis*. *Braz. Arch. Biol. Technol.* **2011**, *54*, 831–838. [CrossRef]

236. Usov, A.I. Polysaccharides of the red algae. *Adv. Carbohydr. Chem. Biochem.* **2011**, *65*, 115–217.

237. Pomin, V.H. Fucanomics and Galactanomics: Marine Distribution, Medicinal Impact, Conceptions, and Challenges. *Mar. Drugs* **2012**, *10*, 793–811. [CrossRef]

238. Anderson, N.S.; Dolan, T.C.S.; Rees, D.A. Carrageenans. Part VII. Polysaccharides from *Eucheuma spinosum* and *Eucheuma cottonii*. The covalent structure of λ-carrageenan. *J. Chem. Soc. Perkin. Trans. I* **1973**, *19*, 2173–2176. [CrossRef] [PubMed]

239. Funami, T.; Hiroe, M.; Noda, S.; Asai, I.; Ikeda, S.; Nishinari, K. Influence of molecular structure imaged with atomic force microscopy on the rheological behavior of carrageenan aqueous systems in the presence or absence of cations. *Food Hydrocolloid* **2007**, *21*, 617–629. [CrossRef]

240. Li, H.; Mao, W.; Zhang, X.; Qi, X.; Chen, Y.; Chen, Y.; Chena, Y.; Xua, J.; Zhaoa, C.; Houa, Y.; *et al.* Structural characterization of an anticoagulant-active sulfated polysaccharide isolated from green alga *Monostroma latissimum*. *Carbohydr. Polym.* **2011**, *85*, 394–400. [CrossRef]

241. Bilan, M.I.; Vinogradova, E.V.; Shashkov, A.S.; Usov, A.I. Structure of a highly pyruvylated galactan sulfate from the Pacific green alga *Codium yezoense* (Bryopsidales, Chlorophyta). *Carbohydr. Res.* **2007**, *342*, 586–596. [CrossRef] [PubMed]

242. Ohta, Y.; Lee, J.B.; Hayashi, K.; Hayashi, T. Isolation of sulfated galactan from *Codium fragile* and its antiviral effect. *Biol. Pharm. Bull.* **2009**, *32*, 892–898. [CrossRef] [PubMed]

243. Tabarsa, M.; Karnjanapratum, S.; Cho, M.; Kim, J.K.; You, S. Molecular characteristics and biological activities of anionic macromolecules from *Codium fragile*. *Int. J. Biol. Macromol.* **2013**, *59*, 1–12. [CrossRef] [PubMed]

244. Lee, J.-B.; Hayashi, T.; Hayashi, K.; Sankawa, U.; Maeda, M.; Nemoto, T.; Nakanishi, H. Further purification and structural analysis of calcium spirulan from *Spirulina platensis*. *J. Nat. Prod.* **1998**, *61*, 1101–1104. [CrossRef] [PubMed]

245. Pignolet, O.; Jubeau, S.; Vaca-Garcia, C.; Michaud, P. Highly valuable microalgae: Biochemical and topological aspects. *J. Ind. Microbiol. Biotechnol.* **2013**, *40*, 781–796. [CrossRef] [PubMed]

246. Heaney-Kieras, J.H.; Chapman, D. Structural studies on the extracellular polysaccharide of the red alga *Porphyridium cruentum*. *Carbohydr. Res.* **1976**, *52*, 169–177. [CrossRef] [PubMed]

247. Geresh, S.; Dubinsky, O.; Arad, S.M.; Christian, D.; Glaser, R. Structure of 3-*O*-(α-D-glucopyranosyluronic acid)-L-galactopyranose, an aldobiuronic acid isolated from the polysaccharides of various unicellular red algae. *Carbohydr. Res.* **1990**, *208*, 301–305. [CrossRef] [PubMed]

248. Damonte, E.B.; Matulewicz, M.C.; Cerezo, A.S. Sulfated seaweed polysaccharides as antiviral agents. *Curr. Med. Chem.* **2004**, *11*, 2399–2419. [CrossRef] [PubMed]

249. Ghosh, T.; Chattopadhyay, K.; Marschall, M.; Karmakar, P.; Mandal, P.; Ray, B. Focus on antivirally active sulfated polysaccharides: From structure-activity analysis to clinical evaluation. *Glycobiology* **2009**, *19*, 2–15. [CrossRef] [PubMed]

250. Nishino, T.; Nagumo, T. The sulfate-content dependence of the anticoagulant activity of a fucan sulfate from the brown seaweed *Ecklonia kurome*. *Carbohydr. Res.* **1991**, *214*, 193–197. [CrossRef] [PubMed]

251. Pomin, V.H.; Pereira, M.S.; Valente, A.P.; Tollefsen, D.M.; Pavao, M.S.G.; Mourao, P.A.S. Selective cleavage and anticoagulant activity of a sulfated fucan: Stereospecific removal of a 2-sulfate ester from the polysaccharide by mild acid hydrolysis, preparation of oligosaccharides, and heparin cofactor II-dependent anticoagulant activity. *Glycobiology* **2005**, *15*, 369–381. [CrossRef] [PubMed]

252. Witvrouw, M.; de Clercq, E. Sulfated polysaccharides extracted from sea algae as potential antiviral drugs. *Gen. Pharmacol.* **1997**, *29*, 497–511. [CrossRef] [PubMed]

253. Harden, E.A.; Falshaw, R.; Carnachan, S.M.; Kern, E.R.; Prichard, M.N. Virucidal activity of polysaccharide extracts from four algal species against herpes simplex virus. *Antivir. Res.* **2009**, *83*, 282–289. [CrossRef] [PubMed]

254. Clement, M.J.; Tissot, B.; Chevolot, L.; Adjadj, E.; Du, Y.; Curmi, P.A.; Daniel, R. NMR characterization and molecular modeling of fucoidan showing the importance of oligosaccharide branching in its anticomplementary activity. *Glycobiology* **2010**, *20*, 883–894. [CrossRef] [PubMed]

255. Carlucci, M.J.; Mateu, C.G.; Artuso, M.C.; Scolaro, L.A. Polysaccharides from red algae: Genesis of a renaissance. In *The Complex World of Polysaccharides*; Karunaratne, D.N., Ed.; InTech: Rijeka, Croatia, 2012; Chapter 20; pp. 535–554. Available online: http://www.intechopen.com/books/the-complex-world-of-polysaccharides/polysaccharides-from-red-algae-genesis-of-a-renaissance (accessed on 2 February 2015). [CrossRef]

256. Baba, M.; Snoeck, R.; Pauwels, R.; de Clercq, E. Sulfated polysaccharides are potent and selective inhibitors of various enveloped viruses, including herpes simplex virus, cytomegalovirus, vesicular stomatitis virus, and human immunodeficiency virus. *Antimicrob. Agents Chemother.* **1988**, *32*, 1742–1745. [CrossRef] [PubMed]

257. Mandal, P.; Mateu, C.G.; Chattopadhyay, K.; Pujol, C.A.; Damonte, E.B.; Ray, B. Structural features and antiviral activity of sulphated fucans from the brown seaweed *Cystoseira indica*. *Antivir. Chem. Chemother.* **2007**, *18*, 153–162. [CrossRef] [PubMed]

258. Mohsen, M.S.A.; Mohamed, S.F.; Ali, F.M.; El-Sayed, O.H. Chemical Structure and Antiviral Activity of Water-soluble Sulfated Polysaccharides from Sargassum latifolium. *J. Appl. Sci. Res.* **2007**, *3*, 1178–1185.

259. Buck, C.B.; Thompson, C.D.; Roberts, J.N.; Muller, M.; Lowy, D.R.; Schiller, J.T. Carrageenan is a potent inhibitor of papillomavirus infection. *PLoS Pathog.* **2006**, *2*, 671–680. [CrossRef]

260. Zeitlin, L.; Whaley, K.J.; Hegarty, T.A.; Moench, T.R.; Cone, R.A. Tests of vaginal microbicides in the mouse genital herpes model. *Contraception* **1997**, *56*, 329–335. [CrossRef] [PubMed]

261. Oehninger, S.; Clark, G.F.; Acosta, A.A.; Hodgen, G.D. Nature of the inhibitory effect of complex saccharide moieties on the tight binding of human spermatozoa to the human *zona pellucida*. *Fertil. Steril.* **1991**, *55*, 165–169. [PubMed]

262. Huleihel, M.; Ishanu, V.; Tal, J.; Arad, S.M. Antiviral effect of the red microalgal polysaccharides on *Herpes simplex* and *Varicella zoster* viruses. *J. Appl. Phycol.* **2001**, *13*, 127–134. [CrossRef]

263. Esko, J.D.; Selleck, S.B. Order out of chaos: Assembly of ligand binding sites in heparin sulfate. *Annu. Rev. Biochem.* **2002**, *71*, 435–471. [CrossRef] [PubMed]

264. Heaney-Kieras, J.; Roden, L.; Chapman, D.J. The covalent linkage of protein to carbohydrate in the extracellular protein-polysaccharide from the red alga *Porphyridium cruentum*. *Biochemistry* **1977**, *165*, 1–9.

265. Tabarsa, M.; Park, G.M.; Shin, I.S.; Lee, E.; Kim, J.K.; You, S. Structure-activity relationships of sulphated glycoproteins from *Codium fragile* on nitric oxide releasing capacity from RAW264.7 cells. *Mar. Biotechnol.* **2015**, *17*, 266–276. [CrossRef] [PubMed]

266. Huleihel, M.; Ishanu, V.; Tal, J.; Arad, S.M. Activity of *Porphyridium* sp. polysaccharide against *Herpes simplex* viruses *in vitro* and *in vivo*. *J. Biochem. Biophys. Met.* **2002**, *50*, 189–200. [CrossRef]

267. Li, L.-Y.; Li, L.-Q.; Guo, C.-H. Evaluation of *in vitro* antioxidant and antibacterial activities of *Laminaria japonica* polysaccharides. *J. Med. Plants Res.* **2010**, *4*, 2194–2198.

268. Miroshnichenko, V.A.; Yansons, T.Y.; Polushin, O.G. Differentiated approach to the treatment of gastroduodenal pathology with the use of bioactive substances of marine hydrocele. In *New Biomedical Technologies to Use of Dietary Supplements*; Ivanov, E.M., Ed.; IMKVL Siberian Branch, Ross. Akad. Med. Nank.: Vladivostok, Russia, 1998; pp. 146–150.

269. Shanmugam, M.; Mody, K.H. Heparinoid-active sulfated polysaccharides from marine algae as potential blood anticoagulant agents. *Curr. Sci.* **2000**, *79*, 1672–1683.

270. Pierre, G.; Sopena, V.; Juin, C.; Mastouri, A.; Graber, M.; Mangard, T. Antibacterial activity of a sulphated galactan extracted from the marine alga *Chaetomorpha aerea* against *Staphylococcus aureus*. *Biotechnol. Bioproc. Eng.* **2011**, *16*, 937–945. [CrossRef]

271. Yamashita, S.; Sugita-Konishi, Y.; Shimizu, M. *In vitro* bacteriostatic effects of dietary polysaccharides. *Food Sci. Technol. Res.* **2001**, *7*, 262–264. [CrossRef]

272. Rice, P.J.; Adams, E.L.; Ozment-Skelton, T.; Gonzalez, A.J.; Goldman, M.P.; Lockhart, B.E.; Barker, L.A.; Breuel, K.F.; Deponti, W.K.; Kalbfleisch, J.H.; *et al.* Oral delivery and gastrointestinal absorption of soluble glucans stimulate increased resistance to infectious challenge. *J. Pharmacol. Exper. Ther.* **2005**, *314*, 1079–1086. [CrossRef]

273. Verma, M.S.; Gu, F.X. 1,3-β-Glucans: Drug delivery and pharmacology. In *The Complex World of Polysaccharides*; Karunaratne, D.N., Ed.; InTech: Rijeka, Croatia, 2012; Chapter 21; pp. 555–572. [CrossRef]

274. Li, C.; Gao, Y.; Xing, Y.; Zhu, H.; Shen, J.; Tian, J. Fucoidan, a sulfated polysaccharide from brown algae, against myocardial ischemia–reperfusion injury in rats via regulating the inflammation response. *Food Chem. Toxicol.* **2011**, *49*, 2090–2095. [CrossRef] [PubMed]

275. Senni, K.; Gueniche, F.; Bertaud, A.F.; Tchen, S.I.; Fioretti, F.; Jouault, S.C.; Durand, P.; Guezennec, J.; Godeau, G.; Letourneur, D. Fucoidan a sulfated polysaccharide from brown algae is a potent modulator of connective tissue proteolysis. *Arch. Biochem. Biophys.* **2006**, *445*, 56–64. [CrossRef] [PubMed]

276. Choi, E.M.; Kim, A.J.; Kim, Y.O.; Hwang, J.K. Immunomodulating activity of arabinogalactan and fucoidan *in vitro. J. Med. Food* **2005**, *8*, 446–453. [CrossRef] [PubMed]

277. Yoo, Y.C.; Kim, W.J.; Kim, S.Y.; Kim, S.M.; Chung, M.K.; Park, J.W.; Suh, H.H.; Lee, K.B.; Park, Y.I. Immunomodulating activity of a fucoidan isolated from Korean *Undaria pinnatifida* sporophyll. *Algae* **2007**, *22*, 333–338. [CrossRef]

278. Chen, Z.; Soo, M.Y.; Srinivasan, N.; Tan, B.K.H.; Chan, S.H. Activation of macrophages by polysaccharide-protein complex from *Licium barbarum. Phytother. Res.* **2009**, *23*, 1116–1122. [CrossRef] [PubMed]

279. Karnjanapratum, S.; Tabarsa, M.; Cho, M.; You, S.G. Characterization and immunomodulatory activities of sulfated polysaccharides from *Capsosiphon fulvescens. Int. J. Biol. Macromol.* **2012**, *51*, 720–729. [CrossRef] [PubMed]

280. Chen, D.; Wu, X.Z.; Wen, Z.Y. Sulfated polysaccharides and immune response: Promoter or inhibitor? *Panminerva Med.* **2008**, *50*, 177–183. [PubMed]

281. Tsuji, R.F.; Hoshino, K.; Noro, Y.; Tsuji, N.M.; Kurokawa, T.; Masuda, T.; Akira, S.; Nowak, B. Suppression of allergic reaction by lambda-carrageenan: Toll-like receptor 4/MyD88-dependent and -independent modulation of immunity. *Clin. Exp. Allergy* **2003**, *33*, 249–258. [CrossRef] [PubMed]

282. Zhou, G.; Sun, Y.; Xin, H.; Zhang, Y.; Li, Z.; Xu, Z. *In vivo* antitumor and immunomodulation activities of different molecular weight lambda-carrageenans from *Chondrus ocellatus. Pharmacol. Res.* **2004**, *50*, 47–53. [CrossRef] [PubMed]

283. Heneji, K.; Matsuda, T.; Tomita, M.; Kawakami, H.; Ohshiro, K.; Masuda, M.; Takasu, N.; Tanaka, Y.; Ohta, T.; *et al.* Fucoidan extracted from *Cladosiphon okamuranus* Tokida induces apoptosis of human T-cell leukemia virus type 1-infected T-cell lines and primary adult T-cell leukemia cells. *Nutr. Cancer* **2005**, *52*, 189–201. [CrossRef] [PubMed]

284. Athukorala, Y.; Ahn, G.N.; Jee, Y.H.; Kim, G.Y.; Kim, S.H.; Ha, J.H.; Kang, J.-S.; Lee, K.-W.; Jeon, Y.-J. Antiproliferative activity of sulfated polysaccharide isolated from an enzymatic digest of *Ecklonia cava* on the U-937 cell line. *J. Appl. Phycol.* **2009**, *21*, 307–314. [CrossRef]

285. Chen, W.S.; Lazar, C.S.; Poenie, M.; Tsien, R.Y.; Gill, G.N.; Rosenfeld, M.G. Requirement for intrinsic protein tyrosine kinase in the immediate and late actions of the EGF receptor. *Nature* **1987**, *328*, 820–823. [CrossRef] [PubMed]

286. Lee, N.Y.; Ermakova, S.P.; Choi, H.K.; Kusaykin, M.I.; Shevchenko, N.M.; Zvyagintseva, T.N.; Choi, H.S. Fucoidan from *Laminaria cichorioides* inhibits AP-1 transactivation and cell transformation in the mouse epidermal JB6 cells. *Mol. Carcinog.* **2008**, *47*, 629–637. [CrossRef] [PubMed]

287. Khotimchenko, Y.S. Antitumor properties of non-starch polysaccharides: Fucoidans and Chitosans. *Rus. J. Mar. Biol.* **2010**, *36*, 321–330. [CrossRef]

288. Yamamoto, I.; Nagumo, T.; Yagi, K.; Tominaga, H.; Aoki, M. Antitumor effect of seaweeds, 1. Antitumor effect of extract from *Sargassum* and *Laminaria. Jpn. J. Exp. Med.* **1974**, *44*, 543–546. [PubMed]

289. Yamamoto, I.; Nagumo, T.; Takahashi, M.; Fujihara, M.; Suzuki, Y.; Iizima, N. Antitumor effect of seaweeds, 3. Antitumor effect of an extract from *Sargassum kjellmanianum*. *Jpn. J. Exp. Med.* **1981**, *51*, 187–189.

290. Aisa, Y.; Miyakawa, Y.; Nakazato, T.; Shibata, H.; Saito, K.; Ikeda, Y.; Kizaki, M. Fucoidan induces apoptosis of human HS-sultan cells accompanied by activation of caspase-3 and down-regulation of ERK pathways. *Am. J. Hematol.* **2005**, *78*, 7–14. [CrossRef] [PubMed]

291. Kim, E.J.; Park, S.Y.; Lee, J.Y.; Park, J.H. Fucoidan present in brown algae induces apoptosis of human colon cancer cells. *BMC Gastroenterol.* **2010**, *10*, 96–106. [CrossRef] [PubMed]

292. Yamasaki-Miyamoto, Y.; Yamasaki, M.; Tachibana, H.; Yamada, K. Fucoidan induces apoptosis through activation of caspase-8 on human breast cancer MCF-7 cells. *J. Agric. Food Chem.* **2009**, *57*, 8677–8682. [CrossRef] [PubMed]

293. Zhang, Q.; Li, N.; Zhao, T.; Qi, H.; Xu, Z.; Li, Z. Fucoidan inhibits the development of proteinuria in active Heymann nephritis. *Phytother. Res.* **2005**, *19*, 50–53. [CrossRef] [PubMed]

294. Maruyama, H.; Tamauchi, H.; Iizuka, M.; Nakano, T. The role of NK cells in antitumor activity of dietary fucoidan from *Undaria pinnatifida* sporophylls (Mekabu). *Planta Med.* **2006**, *72*, 1415–1417. [CrossRef] [PubMed]

295. Teruya, T.; Tatemoto, H.; Konishi, T.; Tako, M. Structural characteristics and *in vitro* macrophage activation of acetyl fucoidan from *Cladosiphon okamuranus*. *Glycoconj. J.* **2009**, *26*, 1019–1028. [CrossRef] [PubMed]

296. Raghavendran, H.R.; Srinivasan, P.; Rekha, S. Immunomodulatory activity of fucoidan against aspirin-induced gastric mucosal damage in rats. *Int. Immunopharmacol.* **2011**, *11*, 157–163. [CrossRef] [PubMed]

297. Alekseyenko, T.V.; Zhanayeva, S.Y.; Venediktova, A.A.; Zvyagintseva, T.N.; Kuznetsova, T.A.; Besednova, N.N.; Korolenko, T.A. Antitumor and antimetastatic activity of fucoidan, a sulfated polysaccharide isolated from the Okhotsk sea *Fucus evanescens* brown alga. *Bull. Exper. Biol. Med.* **2007**, *143*, 730–732. [CrossRef]

298. Namikoshi, M. Bioactive compounds produced by cyanobacteria. *J. Int. Microbiol. Biotechnol.* **1996**, *17*, 373–384. [CrossRef]

299. Yang, C.; Chung, D.; Shin, I.S.; Lee, H.Y.; Kim, J.C.; Lee, Y.J.; You, S.G. Effects of molecular weight and hydrolysis conditions on anticancer activity of fucoidans from sporophyll of *Undaria pinnatifida*. *Int. J. Biol. Macromol.* **2008**, *43*, 433–437. [CrossRef] [PubMed]

300. Athukorala, Y.; Lee, K.W.; Kim, S.K.; Jeon, Y.J. Anticoagulant activity of marine green and brown algae collected from Jeju Island in Korea. *Bioresour. Technol.* **2007**, *98*, 1711–1716. [CrossRef] [PubMed]

301. Maeda, M.; Uehara, T.; Harada, N.; Sekiguchi, M.; Hiraoka, A. Heparinoid-active sulfated polysaccharide from *Monostroma-nitidum* and their distribution in the Chlorophyta. *Phytochemistry* **1991**, *30*, 3611–3614. [CrossRef]

302. Matsubara, K.; Matsuura, Y.; Hori, K.; Miyazawa, K. An anticoagulant proteoglycan from the marine green alga, *Codium pugniformis*. *J. Appl. Phycol.* **2000**, *12*, 9–14. [CrossRef]

303. Matsubara, K.; Matsuura, Y.; Bacic, A.; Liao, M.L.; Hori, K.; Miyazawa, K. Anticoagulant properties of a sulfated galactan preparation from a marine green alga, *Codium cylindricum*. *Int. J. Biol. Macromol.* **2001**, *28*, 395–399. [CrossRef] [PubMed]

304. Li, H.; Mao, W.; Hou, Y.; Gao, Y.; Qi, X.; Zhao, C.; Chen, Y.; Chen, Y.; Li, N.; Wang, C. Preparation, structure and anticoagulant activity of a low molecular weight fraction produced by mild acid hydrolysis of sulfated rhamnan from *Monostroma latissimum*. *Bioresour. Technol.* **2012**, *114*, 414–418. [CrossRef] [PubMed]

305. Rodrigues, J.A.G.; Oliveira Vanderlei, E.D.S.; Bessa, E.F.; Magalhaes, F.D.A.; Monteiro de Paula, R.C.; Lima, V.; Barros Benevides, N.M. Anticoagulant activity of a sulfated polysaccharide isolated from the green seaweed *Caulerpa cupressoides*. *Braz. Arch. Biol. Technol.* **2011**, *54*, 691–700. [CrossRef]

306. Rodrigues, J.A.G.; Lino de Queiroz, I.N.; Gomes Quindere, A.L.; Vairo, B.C.; de Souza Mourao, P.A.; Barros Benevides, N.M. An antithrombin-dependent sulfated polysaccharide isolated from the green alga *Caulerpa cupressoides* has *in vivo* anti- and prothrombotic effects. *Cienc. Rural* **2011**, *41*, 634–639. [CrossRef]

307. Melo, F.R.; Pereira, M.S.; Foguel, D.; Mourão, P.A.S. Antithrombin-mediated anticoagulant activity of sulfated polysaccharides. *J. Biol. Chem.* **2004**, *279*, 20824–20835. [CrossRef] [PubMed]

308. Silva, F.R.F.; Dore, C.M.P.G.; Marques, C.T.; Nascimento, M.S.; Benevides, N.M.B.; Rocha, H.A.O.; Chavante, S.F.; Leite, E.L. Anticoagulant activity, paw edema and pleurisy induced carrageenan: Action of major types of commercial carrageenans. *Carbohydr. Polym.* **2010**, *79*, 26–33. [CrossRef]

309. Chandía, N.P.; Matsuhiro, B. Characterization of a fucoidan from *Lessonia vadosa* (Phaeophyta) and its anticoagulant and elicitor properties. *Int. J. Biol. Macromol.* **2008**, *42*, 235–240. [CrossRef] [PubMed]

310. Hayakawa, Y.; Hayashi, T.; Hayashi, K.; Osawa, T.; Niiya, K.; Sakuragawa, N. Heparin cofactor II-dependent antithrombin activity of calcium spirulan. *Blood Coagul. Fibrinol.* **1996**, *7*, 554–560. [CrossRef]

311. Grauffel, V.; Koareg, B.; Mabeau, S.; Duran, P.; Jozefonvicz, J. New natural polysaccharides with potent antithrombotic activity: Fucans from brown algae. *Biomaterials* **1989**, *10*, 363–368. [CrossRef] [PubMed]

312. Kindness, G.; Williamson, F.B.; Long, W.F. Effect of polyanetholesulfonic acid and xylan sulphate on antithrombin III activity. *Biochem. Biophys. Res. Com.* **1979**, *13*, 1062–1068. [CrossRef]

313. Qiu, X.; Amarasekara, A.; Doctor, V. Effect of oversulfation on the chemical and biological properties of fucoidan. *Carbohydr. Polym.* **2006**, *63*, 224–228. [CrossRef]

314. Jung, W.K.; Athukorala, Y.; Lee, Y.J.; Cha, S.H.; Lee, C.H.; Vasanthan, T.; Choi, K.-S.; Yoo, S.-H.; Kim, S.-K.; Jeon, Y.J. Sulfated polysaccharide purified from *Ecklonia cava* accelerates antithrombin III-mediated plasma proteinase inhibition. *J. Appl. Phycol.* **2007**, *19*, 425–430. [CrossRef]

315. Nishino, T.; Nagumo, T. Anticoagulant and antithrombotic activities of oversulfated fucans. *Carbohydr. Res.* **1992**, *229*, 355–362. [CrossRef] [PubMed]

316. Minix, R.; Doctor, V.M. Interaction of fucoidan with proteases and inhibitors of coagulation and fibrinolysis. *Thromb. Res.* **1997**, *87*, 419–429. [CrossRef] [PubMed]

317. De Candia, E.; de Cristofaro, R.; Landolfi, R. Thrombin-induced platelet activation is inhibited by high- and low-molecular-weight heparin. *Circulation* **1999**, *99*, 3308–3314. [CrossRef] [PubMed]

318. Yu, P.Z.; Zhang, Q.B.; Li, N.; Xu, Z.H.; Wang, Y.M.; Li, Z.E. Polysaccharides from *Ulva pertusa* (Chlorophyta) and preliminary studies on their antihyperlipidemia activity. *J. Appl. Phycol.* **2003**, *15*, 21–27. [CrossRef]

319. Qi, H.; Huang, L.; Liu, X.; Liu, D.; Zhang, Q.; Liu, S. Antihyperlipidemic activity of high sulfate content derivative of polysaccharide extracted from *Ulva pertusa* (Chlorophyta). *Carbohydr. Polym.* **2012**, *87*, 1637–1640. [CrossRef]

320. Lahaye, M. Marine algae as sources of fibres: Determination of soluble and insoluble dietary fibre contents in some "sea vegetables". *J. Sci. Food Agric.* **1991**, *54*, 587–594. [CrossRef]

321. Li, Z.J.; Xue, C.H.; Lin, H. The hypolipidemic effects and antioxidative activity of sulfated fucan on the experimental hyperlipidemia in rats. *Acta Nutrim. Sin.* **1999**, *21*, 280–283.

322. Li, D.Y.; Xu, Z.; Zhang, S.H. Prevention and cure of fucoidan of *L. japonica* on mice with hypercholesterolemia. *Food Sci.* **1999**, *20*, 45–46.

323. Ren, D.; Noda, H.; Amano, H.; Nishino, T.; Nishizawa, K. Study on antihypertensive and antihyperlipidemic effects of marine algae. *Fish. Sci.* **1994**, *60*, 33–40.

324. Inoue, N.; Yamano, N.; Sakata, K.; Nagao, K.; Hama, Y.; Yanagita, T. The sulfated polysaccharide porphyran reduces apolipoprotein B100 secretion and lipid synthesis in HepG2 cells. *Biosci. Biotechnol. Biochem.* **2009**, *73*, 447–449. [CrossRef] [PubMed]

325. Panlasigui, L.N.; Baello, O.Q.; Dimatangal, J.M.; Dumelod, D.B. Blood cholesterol and lipid-lowering effects of carrageenan on human volunteers. *Asia Pac. J. Clin. Nutr.* **2003**, *12*, 209–214. [PubMed]

326. Reddy, B.S.; Watanabe, K.; Sheinfil, A. Effect of dietary wheat bran, alfalfa, pectin and carrageenan on plasma cholesterol and fecal bile acid and neutral sterol excretion in rats. *J. Nutr.* **1980**, *110*, 1247–1254. [PubMed]

327. Ginzberg, A.; Cohen, M.; Sod-Moriah, U.A.; Shany, S.; Rosenshtrauch, A.; Arad, S.M. Chickens fed with biomass of the red microalga *Porphyridium* sp. have reduced blood cholesterol levels and modified fatty acids composition in egg yolk. *J. Appl. Phycol.* **2000**, *12*, 325–330. [CrossRef]

328. Dvir, I.; Maislos, M.; Arad, S.M. Feeding rodents with red microalgae. In *Dietary Fiber, Mechanisms of Action in Human Physiology and Metabolism*; Cherbut, C., Barry, J.L., Lairon, D., Durand, M., Eds.; John Libbey Eurotext: Paris, France, 1995; pp. 86–91.

329. Dvir, I.; Stark, A.H.; Chayoth, R.; Madar, Z.; Arad, S.M. Hycholesterolemic effects of nutraceuticals produced from the red microalga *Porphyridium* sp. in rats. *Nutrients* **2009**, *1*, 156–167. [CrossRef] [PubMed]

330. Huang, J.; Liu, L.; Yu, Y.; Lin, W.; Chen, B.; Li, M. Reduction in the blood glucose level of exopolysaccharide of *Porphyridium cruentum* in alloxan-induced diabetic mice. *J. Fujian Norm. Univ.* **2006**, *22*, 77–80. (In Chinese)

331. Glore, S.R.; van Treeck, D.; Knehans, A.W.; Guild, M. Soluble fiber in serum lipids: A literature review. *J. Am. Diet. Assoc.* **1994**, *94*, 425–436. [CrossRef] [PubMed]

332. Marlett, J. Dietary fibre and cardiovascular disease. In *Handbook of Dietary Fibers*; Cho, S.S., Dreher, M.D., Eds.; Marcel Dekker: New York, NY, USA, 2001; pp. 17–30.

333. Dvir, I.; Chayoth, R.; Sod-Moriah, U.; Shany, S.; Nyska, A.; Stark, A.H.; Madar, Z.; Arad, S.M. Soluble polysaccharide of red microalga *Porphyridium* sp. alters intestinal morphology and reduces serum cholesterol in rats. *Br. J. Nutr.* **2000**, *84*, 469–476. [PubMed]

334. Lupescu, N.; Geresh, S.; Arad, S.M.; Bernstein, M.; Glaser, R. Structure of some sulfated sugars isolated after acid hydrolysis of the extracellular polysaccharide of *Porphyridium* sp. unicellular red alga. *Carbohydr. Res.* **1991**, *210*, 349–352. [CrossRef]

335. Guillon, F.; Champ, M. Structural and physical properties of dietary fibres, and consequences of processing on human physiology. *Food Res. Int.* **2000**, *33*, 233–245. [CrossRef]

336. Barcelo, A.; Claustre, J.; Moro, F.; Chayvaille, J.A.; Cuber, J.C.; Plaisancie, P. Mucin secretion is modulated by luminal factors in the isolated vascularly perfused rat colon. *Gut* **2000**, *46*, 218–224. [CrossRef] [PubMed]

337. Oakenfull, D. Physicochemical properties of dietary fiber: Overview. In *Handbook of Dietary Fibers*; Cho, S.S., Dreher, M.D., Eds.; Marcel Dekker: New York, NY, USA, 2001; pp. 195–206.

338. Ohta, T.; Sasaki, S.; Oohori, T.; Yoshikawa, S.; Kurihara, H. β-Glucosidase inhibitory activity of a 70% methanol extract from ezoishe (*Pelvetia babingtonii* de Toni) and its effect on the elevation of blood glucose level in rats. *Biosci. Biotechnol. Biochem.* **2002**, *66*, 1552–1554. [CrossRef] [PubMed]

339. Fu, X.Y.; Xue, C.H.; Ning, Y.; Li, Z.J.; Xu, J.C. Acute antihypertensive effects of fucoidan oligosaccharides prepared from *Laminaria japonica* on renovascular hypertensive rat. *J. Ocean Univ. Qingdao* **2004**, *34*, 560–564.

340. Costa, M.S.S.P.; Costa, L.S.; Cordeiro, S.L.; Almeida-Lima, J.; Dantas-Santos, N.; Magalhaes, K.D.; Sabry, D.A.; Lopes Albuquerque, I.R.; Pereira, M.R.; Leite, E.L. Evaluating the possible anticoagulant and antioxidant effects of sulfated polysaccharides from the tropical green alga *Caulerpa cupressoides* var. *flabellata*. *J. Appl. Phycol.* **2012**, *24*, 1159–1167. [CrossRef]

341. Kim, S.H.; Choi, D.S.; Athukorala, Y.; Jeon, Y.J.; Senevirathne, M.; Rha, C.K. Antioxidant activity of sulfated polysaccharides isolated from *Sargassum fulvellum*. *J. Food Sci. Nutr.* **2007**, *12*, 65–73. [CrossRef]

342. Cho, M.L.; Lee, H.-S.; Kang, I.-J.; Won, M.-H.; You, S.G. Antioxidant properties of extract and fractions from *Enteromorpha prolifera*, a type of green seaweed. *Food Chem.* **2011**, *127*, 999–1006. [CrossRef] [PubMed]

343. Tannin-Spitz, T.; Bergman, M.; van Moppes, D.; Grossman, S.; Arad, S.M. Antioxidant activity of the polysaccharide of the red microalga *Porphyridium* sp. *J. Appl. Phycol.* **2005**, *17*, 215–222. [CrossRef]

344. Chen, B.; You, B.; Huang, J.; Yu, Y.; Chen, W. Isolation and antioxidant property of the extracellular polysaccharide from *Rhodella reticulata*. *World J. Microbiol. Biotechnol.* **2010**, *26*, 833–840. [CrossRef]

345. Zhang, Z.; Wang, X.; Yu, S.; Yin, L.; Zhao, M.; Han, Z. Synthesized oversulfated and acetylated derivatives of polysaccharide extracted from *Enteromorpha linza* and their potential antioxidant activity. *Int. J. Biol. Macromol.* **2011**, *49*, 1012–1015. [CrossRef] [PubMed]

346. Zhao, X.; Xue, C.H.; Li, B.F. Study of antioxidant activities of sulfated polysaccharides from *Laminaria japonica*. *J. Appl. Phycol.* **2008**, *20*, 431–436. [CrossRef]

347. Bernal, P.; Llamas, M.A. Promising biotechnological applications of antibiofilm exopolysaccharides. *Microb. Biotechnol.* **2012**, *5*, 670–673. [CrossRef] [PubMed]

348. Ciferri, O. *Spirulina*, the edible microorganism (algae, single-cell protein). *Microbiol. Rev.* **1983**, *47*, 551–578. [PubMed]

349. Marceliano, M.B. Structure and Function of Polysaccharide Gum-Based Edible Films and Coatings. In *Edible Films and Coatings for Food Applications*; Embuscado, M.E., Huber, K.C., Eds.; Springer: London, UK, 2009.

350. Franco, J.M.; Raymundo, A.; Sousa, I.; Gallegos, C. Influence of Processing Variables on the Rheological and Textural Properties of Lupin Protein-Stabilized Emulsions. *J. Agric. Food Chem.* **1998**, *46*, 3109–3115. [CrossRef]

351. Raymundo, A.; Franco, J.; Gallegos, C.; Empis, J.; Sousa, I. Effect of thermal denaturation of lupin protein on its emulsifying properties. *Nahrung* **1998**, *42*, 220–224. [CrossRef]

352. Raymundo, A.; Gouveia, L.; Batista, A.P.; Empis, J.; Sousa, I. Fat mimetic capacity of *Chlorella vulgaris* biomass in oil-in-water food emulsions stabilized by pea protein. *Food Res. Int.* **2005**, *38*, 961–965. [CrossRef]

353. Coura, C.O.; de Araújo, I.W.; Vanderlei, E.S.; Rodrigues, J.A.; Quinderé, A.L.; Fontes, B.P.; de Queiroz, I.N.; de Menezes, D.B.; Bezerra, M.M.; e Silva, A.A.; *et al.* Antinociceptive and anti-inflammatory activities of sulphated polysaccharides from the red seaweed *Gracilaria cornea*. *Basic Clin. Pharmacol. Toxicol.* **2012**, *110*, 335–341. [CrossRef] [PubMed]

354. Assreuy, A.M.S.; Gomes, D.M.; Silva, M.S.J.; Torres, V.M.; Siqueira, R.C.L.; Pires, A.F.; Criddle, D.N.; Alencar, N.M.N.; Cavada, B.S.; Sampaio, A.H.; *et al.* Biological effects of a sulfated-polysaccharide isolated from the marine red algae *Champia feldmannii. Biol. Pharm. Bull.* **2008**, *31*, 691–695.

355. Ribeiro, R.A.; Vale, M.L.; Thomazzi, S.M.; Paschoalato, A.B.; Poole, S.; Ferreira, S.H.; Cunha, F.Q. Involvement of resident macrophages and mast cells in the writhing nociceptive response induced by zymosan and acetic acid in mice. *Eur. J. Pharmacol.* **2000**, *387*, 111–118. [CrossRef] [PubMed]

356. Chabut, D.; Fischer, A.M.; Colliec-Jouault, S.; Laurendeau, I.; Matou, S.; Le Bonniec, B.; Helley, D. Low molecular weight fucoidan and heparin enhance the basic fibroblast growth factor-induced tube formation of endothelial cells through heparan sulfate-dependent alpha 6 overexpression. *Mol. Pharmacol.* **2003**, *64*, 696–702. [CrossRef] [PubMed]

357. Carmeliet, P. Angiogenesis in health and disease. *Nat. Med.* **2003**, *9*, 653–660. [CrossRef] [PubMed]

358. Itsuko, K.; Hideyuki, S.; Masato, N.; Shusuke, H.; Haruji, S.; Teruo, Y. Antiulcer agent and adhesion inhibitor for *Helicobacter pylori*. Patent EP0645143 B1, 21 September 1994.

359. Saito, A.; Yoneda, M.; Yokohama, S.; Okada, M.; Haneda, M.; Nakamura, K. Fucoidan prevents concanavalin A-induced liver injury through induction of endogenous IL-10 in mice. *Hepatol. Res.* **2006**, *35*, 190–198. [PubMed]

360. Kawano, N.; Egashira, Y.; Sanada, H. Effect of dietary fiber in edible seaweeds on the development of D-galactosamine-induced hepatopathy in rats. *J. Nutr. Sci. Vitaminol. (Tokyo)* **2007**, *53*, 446–450. [CrossRef]

361. Hayashi, K.; Nakano, T.; Hashimoto, M.; Kanekiyo, K.; Hayashi, T. Defensive effects of a fucoidan from brown alga *Undaria pinnatifida* against herpes simplex virus infection. *Int. Immunopharmacol.* **2008**, *8*, 109–116. [CrossRef]

362. Veena, C.K.; Josephine, A.; Preetha, S.P.; Varalakshmi, P.; Sundarapandiyan, R. Renal peroxidative changes mediated by oxalate: The protective role of fucoidan. *Life Sci.* **2006**, *79*, 1789–1795. [CrossRef] [PubMed]

363. Veena, C.K.; Josephine, A.; Preetha, S.P.; Rajesh, N.G.; Varalakshmi, P. Mitochondrial dysfunction in an animal model of hyperoxaluria: A prophylactic approach with fucoidan. *Eur. J. Pharmacol.* **2008**, *579*, 330–336. [CrossRef] [PubMed]

364. Veena, C.K.; Josephine, A.; Preetha, S.P.; Varalakshmi, P. Effect of sulphated polysaccharides on erythrocyte changes due to oxidative and nitrosative stress in experimental hyperoxaluria. *Hum. Exp. Toxicol.* **2007**, *26*, 923–932. [CrossRef] [PubMed]

365. Veena, C.K.; Josephine, A.; Preetha, S.P.; Varalakshmi, P. Physico-chemical alterations of urine in experimental hyperoxaluria: A biochemical approach with fucoidan. *J. Pharm. Pharmacol.* **2007**, *59*, 419–527. [CrossRef] [PubMed]

366. Veena, C.K.; Josephine, A.; Preetha, S.P.; Varalakshmi, P. Beneficial role of sulfated polysaccharides from edible seaweed *Fucus vesiculosus* in experimental hyperoxaluria. *Food Chem.* **2007**, *100*, 1552–1559. [CrossRef]

367. Liu, J.C.; Zheng, F.L.; Liu, Y.P. Effect of fucoidan on renal interstitial fibrosis in adenine-induced chronic renal failure in rats. *Nephrology* **2008**, *13*, 158. [CrossRef]

368. Angulo, Y.; Lomonte, B. Inhibitory effect of fucoidan on the activities of crotaline snake venom myotoxic phospholipases A(2). *Biochem. Pharmacol.* **2003**, *66*, 1993–2000. [CrossRef] [PubMed]

369. Silva, T.H.; Alves, A.; Popa, E.G.; Reys, L.L.; Gomes, M.E.; Sousa, R.A.; Silva, S.S.; Mano, J.F.; Reis, R.L. Marine algae sulfated polysaccharides for tissue engineering and drug delivery approaches. *Biomatter* **2012**, *2*, 278–289. [CrossRef] [PubMed]

370. Ige, O.O.; Umoru, L.E.; Aribo, S. Natural Products: A Minefield of Biomaterials. *ISRN Mater. Sci.* **2012**, *2012*. [CrossRef]

371. Fundueanu, G.; Esposito, E.; Mihai, D.; Carpov, A.; Desbrieres, J.; Rinaudo, M.; Nastruzzi, C. Preparation and characterization of Ca-alginate microspheres by a new emulsification. *Int. J. Pharm.* **1998**, *170*, 11–21. [CrossRef]

372. Lee, K.Y.; Mooney, D.J. Alginate: Properties and biomedical applications. *Prog. Polym. Sci.* **2012**, *7*, 106–126. [CrossRef]

373. Draget, K.I.; Taylor, C. Chemical, physical and biological properties of alginates and their biomedical implications. *Food Hydrocolloid* **2011**, *25*, 251–256. [CrossRef]

374. Kong, H.; Mooney, D. Polysaccharide-based hydrogels in tissue engineering. In *Polysacharides. Structural Diversity and Functional Versatility*, 2nd ed.; Dumitriu, S., Ed.; Marcel Dekker: New York, NY, USA, 2005; pp. 817–837.

375. Qin, Y. The characterization of alginate wound dressing with different fiber and textile structures. *J. Appl. Polym. Sci.* **2006**, *100*, 2516–2520. [CrossRef]

376. Qin, Y. Alginate fibbers: An overview of the production processes and applications in wound management. *Polym. Int.* **2008**, *57*, 171–108. [CrossRef]

377. Rinaudo, M. Biomaterials based on a natural polysaccharide: Alginate. *TIP. Revista Especializada en Ciencias Químico-Biológicas* **2014**, *17*, 92–96.

378. Gong, Y.; He, L.; Li, J.; Zhou, Q.; Ma, Z.; Gao, C.; Shen, J. Hydrogel-filled polylactide porous scaffolds for cartilage tissue engineering. *J. Biomed. Mater. Res. B Appl. Biomater.* **2007**, *82*, 192–204. [CrossRef] [PubMed]

379. Bao, L.; Yang, W.; Mao, X.; Mou, S.; Tang, S. Agar/collagen membrane as skin dressing for wounds. *Biomed. Mater.* **2008**, *3*, 1–7. [CrossRef]

380. Nakayama, Y.; Tsujinaka, T. Acceleration of robust "biotube" vascular graft fabrication by in-body tissue architecture technology using a novel eosin Y-releasing mold. *J. Biomed. Mater. Res. B Appl. Biomater.* **2014**, *102*, 231–238. [CrossRef] [PubMed]

381. Toskas, G.; Hund, R.-D.; Laourine, E.; Cherif, C.; Smyrniotopoulos, V.; Roussis, V. Nanofibers based on polysaccharides from the green seaweed *Ulva rigida*. *Carbohydr. Polym.* **2011**, *84*, 1093–1102. [CrossRef]

382. Alves, A.; Duarte, A.R.C.; Mano, J.F.; Sousa, R.A.; Reis, R.L. PDLLA enriched with ulvan particles as a novel 3D porous scaffold targeted for bone engineering. *J. Supercrit. Fluids* **2012**, *65*, 32–38. [CrossRef]

383. Alves, A.; Sousa, R.A.; Reis, R.L. Processing of degradable ulvan 3D porous structures for biomedical applications. *J. Biomed. Mater. Res. A* **2013**, *101*, 998–1006. [CrossRef] [PubMed]

384. Morelli, A.; Chiellini, F. Ulvan as a New Type of Biomaterial from Renewable Resources: Functionalization and Hydrogel Preparation. *Macromol. Chem. Phys.* **2010**, *211*, 821–832. [CrossRef]

385. Browder, W.; Williams, D.; Lucore, P.; Pretus, H.; Jones, E.; Mcnamee, R. Effect of Enhanced Macrophage Function on Early Wound-Healing. *Surgery* **1988**, *104*, 224–230. [PubMed]

386. Kofuji, K.; Huang, Y.; Tsubaki, K.; Kokido, F.; Nishikawa, K.; Isobe, T.; Murata, Y. Preparation and evaluation of a novel wound dressing sheet comprised of beta-glucan-chitosan complex. *React. Funct. Polym.* **2010**, *70*, 784–789. [CrossRef]

387. Delatte, S.J.; Evans, J.; Hebra, A.; Adamson, W.; Othersen, H.B.; Tagge, E.P. Effectiveness of beta-glucan collagen for treatment of partial-thickness burns in children. *J. Ped. Sur.* **2001**, *36*, 113–118. [CrossRef]

388. Sezer, A.D.; Hatipoğlu, F.; Cevher, E.; Oğurtan, Z.; Baş, A.L.; Akbuğa, J. Chitosan films containing fucoidan as a wound dressing for dermal burn healing: Preparation and *in vitro/in vivo* evaluation. *AAPS PharmSciTech* **2007**, *8*, E94–E101. [CrossRef] [PubMed]

389. Gilchrist, T.; Martin, A.M. Wound treatment with Sorban-an alginate fibre dressing. *Biomaterials* **1983**, *4*, 317–320. [CrossRef] [PubMed]

390. Motta, G.J. Calcium alginate topical wound dressings: A new dimension in the cost-effective treatment for exudating dermal wounds and pressure sores. *Ostomy Wound Manag.* **1989**, *25*, 52–56.

391. De Morais, M.G.; Stillings, C.; Dersch, R.; Rudisile, M.; Pranke, P.; Costa, J.A.V.; Wendorff, J. Preparation of nanofibers containing the microalga *Spirulina* (*Arthrospira*). *Bioresour. Technol.* **2010**, *101*, 2872–2876. [CrossRef] [PubMed]

392. Arad, S.M.; Rapoport, L.; Moshkovich, A.; van Moppes, D.; Karpasan, M.; Golan, R.; Golan, Y. Superior biolubricant from a species of red microalga. *Langmuir* **2006**, *2*, 7313–7317. [CrossRef]

393. Johnson, A.S.; O'Sullivan, E.; D'Aoust, L.N.; Omer, A.; Bonner-Weir, S.; Fisher, R.J.; Weir, G.C.; Colton, C.K. Quantitative assessment of islets of langerhans encapsulated in alginate. *Tissue Eng. Part C Methords* **2011**, *17*, 435–449. [CrossRef]

394. Tagler, D.; Tu, T.; Smith, R.M.; Anderson, N.R.; Tingen, C.M.; Woodruff, T.K.; Shea, L.D. Embryonic fibroblasts enable the culture of primary ovarian follicles within alginate hydrogels. *Tissue Eng. Part A* **2012**, *18*, 1229–1238. [CrossRef] [PubMed]

395. Banerjee, A.; Arha, M.; Choudhary, S.; Ashton, R.S.; Bhatia, S.R.; Schaffer, D.V.; Kane, R.S. The Influence of Hydrogel Modulus on the Proliferation and Differentiation of Encapsulated Neural Stem Cells. *Biomaterials* **2009**, *30*, 4695–4699. [CrossRef] [PubMed]

396. Jeong, S.I.; Jeon, O.; Krebs, M.D.; Hill, M.C.; Alsberg, E. Biodegradable photo-crosslinked alginate nanofibre scaffolds with tuneable physical properties, cell adhesivity and growth factor release. *Eur. Cells Mater.* **2012**, *24*, 331–343.

397. Zhou, H.; Xu, H.H.K. The fast release of stem cells from alginate-fibrin microbeads in injectable scaffolds for bone tissue engineering. *Biomaterials* **2011**, *32*, 7503–7513. [CrossRef] [PubMed]

398. Liu, J.; Xu, H.H.K.; Zhou, H.; Weir, M.D.; Chen, Q.; Trotman, C.A. Human umbilical cord stem cell encapsulation in novel macroporous and injectable fibrin for muscle tissue engineering. *Acta Biomater.* **2013**, *9*, 4688–4697. [CrossRef] [PubMed]

399. Khanarian, N.T.; Jiang, J.; Wan, L.Q.; Mow, V.C.; Lu, H.H. A hydrogel-mineral composite scaffold for osteochondral interface tissue engineering. *Tissue Eng. Part A* **2012**, *18*, 533–545. [CrossRef] [PubMed]

400. Hatch, A.; Hansmann, G.; Murthy, S.K. Engineered alginate hydrogels for effective microfluidic capture and release of endothelial progenitor cells from whole blood. *Langmuir* **2011**, *27*, 4257–4264. [CrossRef] [PubMed]

401. Yamamoto, M.; James, D.; Li, H.; Butler, J.; Rafii, S.; Rabbany, S. Generation of stable co-cultures of vascular cells in a honeycomb alginate scaffold. *Tissue Eng. Part A* **2010**, *16*, 299–308. [CrossRef] [PubMed]

402. Hajiali, H.; Shahgasempour, S.; Naimi-Jamal, M.R.; Petrovi, H. Electrospun PGA/gelatin nanofibrous scaffolds and their potential application in vascular tissue engineering. *Int. J. Nanomed.* **2011**, *6*, 2133–2141. [CrossRef]

403. Hockaday, L.A.; Kang, K.H.; Colangelo, N.W.; Cheung, P.Y.; Duan, B.; Malone, E.; Wu, J.; Girardi, L.N.; Bonassar, L.J.; Lipson, H.; *et al.* Rapid 3D printing of anatomically accurate and mechanically heterogeneous aortic valve hydrogel scaffolds. *Biofabrication* **2012**, *4*. [CrossRef]

404. Dvir, T.; Timko, B.P.; Brigham, M.D.; Naik, S.R.; Karajanagi, S.S.; Levy, O.; Jin, H.; Parker, K.K.; Langer, R.; Kohane, D.S. Nanowired three dimensional cardiac patches. *Nat. Nanotechnol.* **2011**, *6*, 720–725. [CrossRef] [PubMed]

405. Bacakova, L.; Novotna, K.; Parizek, M. Polysaccharides as Cell Carriers for Tissue Engineering: The Use of Cellulose in Vascular Wall Reconstruction. *Physiol. Res.* **2014**, *63*, 29–47.

406. Petrulyte, S. Advanced textile materials and biopolymers in wound management. *Dan. Med. Bull.* **2008**, *55*, 72–77. [PubMed]

407. Popa, E.G.; Gomes, M.E.; Reis, R.L. Cell delivery systems using alginate-carrageenan hydrogel beads and fibers for regenerative medicine applications. *Biomacromolecules* **2011**, *12*, 3952–3961. [CrossRef]

408. Yoon, H.Y.; Son, S.; Lee, S.J.; You, D.G.; Yhee, J.Y.; Park, J.H.; MSwierczewska, M.; Lee, S.; Kwon, I.C.; Kim, S.H.; *et al.* Glycol chitosan nanoparticles as specialized cancer therapeutic vehicles: Sequential delivery of doxorubicin and Bcl-2 siRNA. *Sci. Rep.* **2014**, *4*. [CrossRef] [PubMed]

409. Ghadban, A.1.; Albertin, L.; Rinaudo, M.; Heyraud, A. Biohybrid glycopolymer capable of ionotropic gelation. *Biomacromolecules* **2012**, *13*, 3108–3119. [CrossRef] [PubMed]

410. Huang, M.; Yang, M. Evaluation of glucan/poly(vinyl alcohol) blend wound dressing using rat models. *Int. J. Pharm.* **2008**, *346*, 38–46. [CrossRef] [PubMed]

411. Alkhatib, B.; Freguin-Bouilland, C.; Lallemand, F.; Henry, J.P.; Litzler, P.Y.; Marie, J.P.; Richard, V.; Thuillez, C.; Plissonnier, D. Low molecular weight fucan prevents transplant coronaropathy in rat cardiac allograft model. *Transpl. Immunol.* **2006**, *16*, 14–19. [CrossRef] [PubMed]

412. Fréguin-Bouilland, C.; Alkhatib, B.; David, N.; Lallemand, F.; Henry, J.P.; Godin, M.; Thuillez, C.; Plissonnier, D. Low molecular weight fucoidan prevents neointimal hyperplasia after aortic allografting. *Transplantation* **2007**, *83*, 1234–1241. [CrossRef] [PubMed]

413. Yang, J.-S.; Xie, Y.-J.; He, W. Research progress on chemical modification of alginate: A review. *Carbohydr. Polym.* **2011**, *84*, 33–39. [CrossRef]

414. Augst, A.D.; Kong, H.J.; Mooney, D.J. Alginate Hydrogels as Biomaterials. *Macromol. Biosci.* **2006**, *6*, 623–633. [CrossRef] [PubMed]

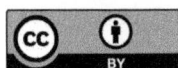

marine drugs

MDPI

Review

Marine Origin Polysaccharides in Drug Delivery Systems

Matias J. Cardoso [1,2], Rui R. Costa [1,2,*] and João F. Mano [1,2,*]

[1] 3B's Research Group—Biomaterials, Biodegradables and Biomimetics, University of Minho, Headquarters of the European Institute of Excellence of Tissue Engineering and Regenerative Medicine, Avepark—Parque de Ciência e Tecnologia, Zona Industrial da Gandra, 4805-017 Barco GMR, Portugal; matjcardoso@gmail.com

[2] ICVS/3B's, PT Government Associated Laboratory, Braga/Guimarães, Portugal

* Correspondence: rui.costa@dep.uminho.pt (R.R.C.); jmano@dep.uminho.pt (J.F.M.); Tel.: +351-253-510-900 (R.R.C. & J.F.M.)

Academic Editor: Paola Laurienzo
Received: 14 December 2015; Accepted: 25 January 2016; Published: 5 February 2016

Abstract: Oceans are a vast source of natural substances. In them, we find various compounds with wide biotechnological and biomedical applicabilities. The exploitation of the sea as a renewable source of biocompounds can have a positive impact on the development of new systems and devices for biomedical applications. Marine polysaccharides are among the most abundant materials in the seas, which contributes to a decrease of the extraction costs, besides their solubility behavior in aqueous solvents and extraction media, and their interaction with other biocompounds. Polysaccharides such as alginate, carrageenan and fucoidan can be extracted from algae, whereas chitosan and hyaluronan can be obtained from animal sources. Most marine polysaccharides have important biological properties such as biocompatibility, biodegradability, and anti-inflammatory activity, as well as adhesive and antimicrobial actions. Moreover, they can be modified in order to allow processing them into various shapes and sizes and may exhibit response dependence to external stimuli, such as pH and temperature. Due to these properties, these biomaterials have been studied as raw material for the construction of carrier devices for drugs, including particles, capsules and hydrogels. The devices are designed to achieve a controlled release of therapeutic agents in an attempt to fight against serious diseases, and to be used in advanced therapies, such as gene delivery or regenerative medicine.

Keywords: drug delivery; polysaccharides; marine excipients; biomaterials; polysaccharide/drug conjugates

1. Introduction

Marine organisms are a vast source of different compounds with diverse biological properties and bioactivity. Recently, a growing interest in many scientific areas that study the diverse applications of marine compounds has been found, justified by their large biodiversity and simplicity of the extraction and purification processes [1,2]. Marine biomaterials have wide applicability in biomedicine because of their noncytotoxic characteristics, biodegradability and biocompatibility. These biological properties have allowed the discovery of a broad range of novel bioactive compounds with pharmacological properties and constitute a fundamental cornerstone of the pharmaceutical industry [2–4]. Some of these compounds have been studied for cancer treatment due to their antitumoral properties [5–7], among which are polypeptides extracted from tunicates [8] and sponges [9]. Many of these compounds are already used clinical trials, such as Aplidin [10] and Ecteinascidin 743 [11].

Marine polysaccharides are mostly used in food and cosmetic industries, but are also widely present in pharmaceutical sciences, with an increasing interest in integrating them as materials for the incorporation of bioactive agents [12]. Marine algae are the main source of marine polysaccharides, but they can also be obtained from animal sources, such as the skeletons of crustaceans and cartilaginous fish tissue. There are also some polysaccharides that can be extracted from marine microorganism, like some prokaryotes [13]. Marine polysaccharides can be described as a large complex group consisting of different macromolecules with different biological properties [14,15]. Polysaccharides may exhibit different chemical structures and different biological properties such as biocompatibility, biodegradability, adhesive properties and the ability to form hydrogels. Among the many marine polysaccharides there is one group that stands out: sulfated polysaccharides [16]. In comparison with other marine polysaccharides, they exhibit bioactivities that include antioxidant [17], anticoagulant [18], anticancer [19], antiviral [20], anti-allergic [21], anti-adhesive, anti-angiogenic and anti-inflammatory actions [22]. The systematic study of some of these materials for drug delivery systems (DDSs) allowed discovering new chemical modification methods aiming to harness such biological activities and change their affinity to specific drugs. Considering the latter, it has been possible to increase the ability to incorporate drugs and increase the efficacy of their release, either by chemical reactions or by interactions with other natural or synthetic polymers [23].

The interest in the study of marine polysaccharides for DDSs with therapeutic purposes relies in the possibility of developing novel approaches of less invasive and more personalized treatments. Several experiments have already shown that many of these biomaterials allow loading lower drug dosages, which may lead to a drastic reduction of the side effects caused by the drugs. These materials can be used as a signaling marker that could lead the delivery of a carrier to a specific location and widening the function of DDSs as diagnostic instruments [24,25]. These systems also have a wide applicability in gene therapy, which is usually limited by the health risk of associated with viral vectors [26]. In contrast, biomaterials have been shown to offer numerous advantages for the encapsulation of genetic material and others therapeutic agents, by ensuring stabilization and protection, also increasing its solubility and promoting a sustained release as well their biocompatibility and in some cases biodegradability [27,28]. In this review, we focus on the use of marine polysaccharides as raw materials for the construction of DDSs (Figure 1).

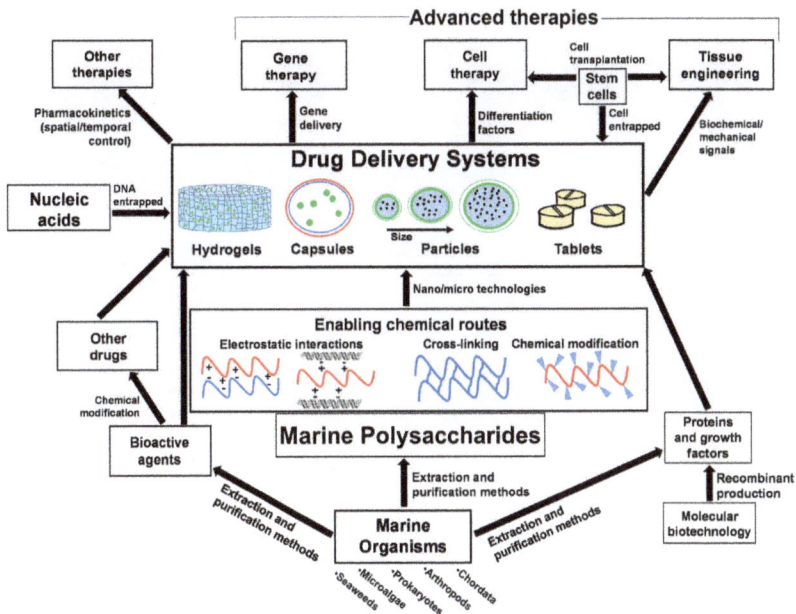

Figure 1. Interrelations of marine origin polysaccharides in drug delivery systems for advances therapies and applications.

We identified alginate, chitosan, carrageenan, hyaluronan (also known as hyaluronic acid) and chondroitin sulfate as the major marine polysaccharides used currently in—or being considered for—the pharmaceutical industry. The various means to modify and adapt these biopolymers to achieve drug protection and delivery, stimuli-responsiveness and targeting capability will be discussed.

2. Polysaccharides from Marine Algae

Among the vast marine organism diversity, algae are the main source of marine polysaccharides. There are some polysaccharides that can be extracted from marine prokaryotes like microalgae, which can also be grown in bioreactors under controlled conditions. Red macroalgae are the most used sources of polysaccharides but it is possible to obtain polysaccharides from green or brown macroalgae. Seaweeds are a different type of multicellular marine algae and are also a major source of polysaccharides. The latter are also divided in groups: red, green and brown. Nowadays, the large quantity of marine algae that reach and deposit in coast regions has led to a widespread use of marine compounds to produce cosmetics, and food supplements and emulsifiers, among others. Despite their large bioavailability, polysaccharides remain relatively unexploited in the medical industry. Figure 2 represents the main polysaccharides that will be discussed herein.

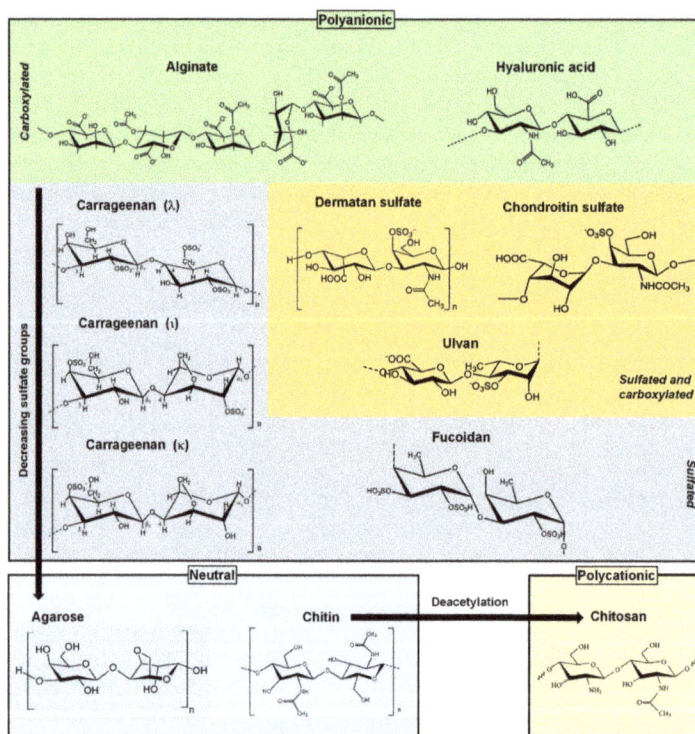

Figure 2. Marine origin polysaccharides categorized by electrostatic nature and carboxylated/sulfated structure.

2.1. Alginates

Alginate is a polysaccharide extracted from brown seaweeds, including *Laminaria hyperborea*, *Laminaria digitata*, *Laminaria japonica*, *Ascophyllum nodosum*, and *Macrocystis pyrifera* [29]. It is composed by a sequence of two (1→4)-linked α-L-guluronate (G) and β-D-mannuronate (M) monomers (Figure 2). The proportion of M and G blocks may vary with the type of seaweed that it is extracted from.

For example, alginate extracted from *Laminaria digitata* and *Ascophyllum nodosum* have been shown to have M/G ratios of 1.16 and 1.82, respectively [30]. Alginate is biocompatible, has low toxicity and high bioavailability as well. These are the main advantages that make alginate one of the biopolymers with the widest biomedical applicability. One of the most common applications of alginate is their use as an excipient in DDSs, namely acting as a stabilizer agent in pharmaceutical formulations [31]. Alginate has carboxyl groups which are charged at pH values higher than 3–4, making alginate soluble at neutral and alkaline conditions [32]. Such pH sensitivity promotes greater protection for drugs with preferential absorption in the intestinal tract: the acidic environment of the stomach does not disturb the stability of the alginate carrier, whereas in the intestine (where the pH is alkaline) the solubility of this biopolymer—as well as the drug release—is promoted [33]. Thus, solubility and pH sensitivity make alginate a good biomaterial for the construction of DDSs [34].

Alginate is widely used for its biocompatibility, low toxicity, high bioavailability, lower extraction and purification costs as compared with other biopolymers, and for the capability to be processed in the form of hydrogel matrices, beads and particles [12,35–37]. Alginate is also used as an excipient in pharmaceutical tablets to promote greater protection and stabilization of the drug. Sodium alginate is the type of alginate mainly used in the pharmaceutical industry in the manufacture of tablets, especially when the drug is not soluble in water. Sodium alginate may be used for the purpose of extending the drug release [31]. Studies using tablets containing ibuprofen demonstrated that it is possible to control the absorption ratio of the tablets. By using sodium alginate with different chemical structure and degree of viscosity, Sirkia *et al.* obtained carriers that triggered either an immediate ibuprofen release or prolonged it, proving that the chemical structure of alginate may influence the release rate of the bioactive agent [38].

In acidic environments, alginate carboxyl groups are protonated, *i.e.*, in the –COOH form, being thus uncharged and exhibiting higher viscosity [32]. This may interfere with the elution of the bioactive agent from the device, thereby limiting drug release when the pH is low [39–41]. However, gelling sodium alginate with Ca^{2+} ions can solve pH dependent limitations related to the hydration, dilation and erosion of the carrier. Alginate has the ability of cross-linking with Ca^{2+} ions through an ionotropic gelation process, usually above pH 6 [42]. Ca^{2+} is not the only ion capable of promoting ionotropic gelation of alginate: Ba^{2+} or Zn^{2+} ions may also be used for that propose [43]. Virtually any drug may be entrapped during such mild cross-linking process, and its subsequent release may be dependent on several factors, such as cross-linking extension [44]. Giunchedi *et al.* reported that using sodium alginate, hydroxypropyl methylcellulose (HPMC), calcium gluconate, and ketoprofen as a model drug in the preparation of tablets by direct compression in different combination and ratios may prolong drug release, in particular in tablets with 20% of HPMC [45]. Alginate hydrogels also have applications in wound healing treatments through the construction of structures used for wound dressings. Several studies show that the bioavailability of drugs encapsulated in alginate hydrogels is greater than if free drug was applied directly at the lesion site, thus increasing the efficacy of healing [46]. Alginate hydrogels are also used widely in tissue regeneration treatments and cell encapsulation [47,48]. Hydrogels obtained from alginate, in particular, present some similar features of the extracellular matrix, thus being appropriate materials to be used in tissue engineering and regenerative medicine applications [46]. However, it should be noted that the gelling capability of alginate varies with the proportion of G and M groups, with alginates rich in G content yielding higher strength when compared to alginates rich in M groups [49].

Alginate is also used in the construction of microparticles with the ability to incorporate different bioactive agents, particularly proteins. Alginate microparticles have the capability of retaining large amounts of drug and also promoting protection of the cargo from any proteolytic attack. There are different mechanisms of release of a bioactive agent from the carrier, such as through variations of temperature and pH, and the use of biodegradable materials or enzymatic degradation, among other chemical and physical stimuli-responsive methods [32,33,35,50]. These parameters are difficult to control and program, since they can vary significantly. However, new release mechanisms from microparticles have been developed, that depended on fully controlled external stimuli, such as ultrasound-triggering. Duarte *et al.* developed a type of alginate microparticles which were shown to have perfluorocarbon breakthrough capacity when subjected to vibration by ultrasound waves [51]. Results showed a disruption of these microparticles after 15 min of exposure, suggesting that such structures are promising DDSs controlled externally by acoustic stimuli (Figure 3).

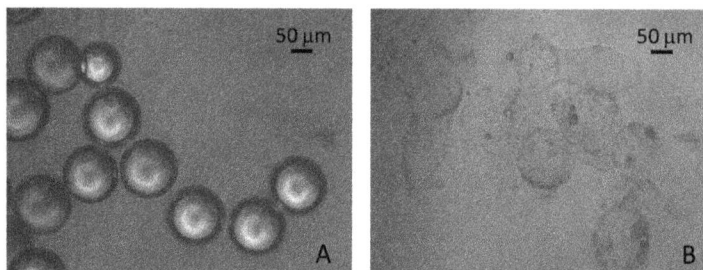

Figure 3. Optical microscope images of alginate microspheres before (**A**) and after (**B**) ultrasound exposure. Reprinted with permission from [51], Copyright © 2014 American Chemical Society.

Over the years, other methods have been developed to fabricate drug delivery particles that promote a better loading efficacy of bioactive substances. Using superhydrophobic surfaces it is possible to produce polymer particles suitable as DDSs. This method allows loading drugs into spherical structures with an encapsulation efficiency close to 100% [52–54]. Another strategy to synthesize particles relies on complexation, based on the electrostatic interactions between alginate at neutral and alkaline pH values, bioactive agents and other kinds of naturally occurring polymers, such as the polycation chitosan [23,31,33,47]. In this matter, alginate complexes have been used to construct DDSs (especially nanoparticles) for gene therapy treatments. The very first systems for the gene delivery were based on genetic material encapsulated within viral vectors. These have several limitations such as the possibility to trigger an immune and inflammatory reactions, infections and mutations. These systems also have high costs of production due to complexity in the processing of viral vectors [26]. Taking advantage of the capability of natural polymers to form complexes with DNA, safer DDSs could be synthesized to deliver genetic material. The most commonly used polymers in the construction of DNA load vehicles are usually of synthetic origin, for example polyethylenimine (PEI), poly-L-lysine (PLL), poly(L-ornithine) and poly(4-hydroxy-L-proline ester) [55]. The use of these synthetic materials has allowed the synthesis of complexes via electrostatic interactions between the polymer and the DNA, allowing the creation of a stable complex and the possibility of size adjustment. One of the major limitations of using synthetic materials is their often adverse biological effect in the body. PEI, for example, exhibits elevated levels of cytotoxicity [56]. In contrast, most natural materials are biocompatibile, biodegradable (in some cases) and show similar capacity to form ionic bonds, therefore providing ensuring good protection for genetic material [57–59]. Krebs *et al.* developed a calcium phosphate-DNA nanoparticle system incorporated in alginate-based hydrogel for gene delivery to promote bone formation. Results showed a DNA sustained release from the alginate hydrogel around 45% of DNA released after approximately 75 days. *In vivo* studies, through the injection of alginate hydrogels containing calcium phosphate nanoparticles and osteoblast-like cells in mice, showed evidence of bone formation [60].

Taking its anionic nature, alginate can be assembled with polycations as structures other than particles using layer-by-layer (LbL). LbL is used to fabricate ultrathin nanostructured films in a multilayer fashion based on complementary interactions between building blocks, such as polyelectrolytes [61–63]. This technique may be useful as a biomimetic approach applied in deconstructing and reconstructing the physiological conditions found in native biological environments, such as the human body [64]. Polyelectrolyte freestanding films (*i.e.*, films with a few micrometers in thickness) have been shown to be suitable drug reservoirs of biomolecules, such as growth factors and antibiotics [65]. This type of films exhibit a good cell adhesion, possibility of cargo entrapment and fast release by variations of electrostatic interactions strength, and also promote a sustained release due to the slow film degradation [66–70]. Such multilayer systems can be also used as barriers with controlled mass transporter properties [71]. The versatility of LbL allows it to be extrapolated to the third dimension to conceive more complex DDSs, such as spherical capsules and tubular structures [72].

Microcapsules are also typical shapes of alginate processing following different techniques, including emulsion [73–75], multiple-phase emulsion [31,76] and calcium cross-linked encapsulation [77]. The ability of alginate to create complexes with other biomaterials by electrostatic interactions, chemical modification or cross-linking can be exploited for building hybrid and more versatile DDSs. Capsules constructed from chitosan/alginate-PEG complexes are reliable models for encapsulating proteins, such as albumin, one of the most common model proteins used in controlled release studies [78]. The construction of alginate spherical structures with other types of synthetic materials can be a good strategy to extend the versatility of these systems. Using poly(N-isopropylacrylamide) (PNIPAAm) to take advantage of its thermosensitive properties [79] in combination with alginate can lead to devices capable of delivering biomolecules with a dual stimuli-responsive dependence (both pH and temperature) [80]. Studies using indomethacin as a model drug reported that chitosan-alginate-PNIPAAm beads showed lower release rates with decreasing temperatures [81]. The same occurs when there is a decrease in pH, indicating that it is possible to control the permeability of the particles by controlling both pH and temperature. This approach can lead to the development of DDSs capable of promoting higher control over the release of drugs, proteins and others biomolecules with pharmaceutical interest. Following a similar concept of polymer conjugation, alginate can also undergo complexation with natural polymers, like chitosan, to enhance the absorption and cargo protection in oral delivery, for example, for the administration of insulin [73,82].

Alginate may be used in the construction of capsules for cell encapsulation often associated with cytotherapy treatments or simply the creation of cellular microcultures in more complex systems where the use of a conventional bioreactor is not possible. In this context, a new approach to the construction of alginate-based capsules for the incorporation of different types of cells has been presented [83,84]. Cells were encapsulated in alginate liquefied particles, coated with multilayer of alternating chitosan and alginate. Along with the cells, poly (lactic acid) microparticles were co-encapsulated to provide anchorage points so that cell survival is promoted. Results demonstrated a high viability of the encapsulated cells and usefulness of these capsules as culture systems. This type of system has wide applicability not only for the cell culture but also in other biomedical applications, since it will allow the encapsulation of different types of cells in combination with other biomolecules such as, for example, growth factors and other cytokines.

2.2. Carrageenans

Carrageenan is a sulfated polysaccharide present in red algae, which structure consists in a linear sequence of alternate residues forming $(AB)_n$ sequence, where A and B are units of galactose residues. These residues may or may not be sulfated. They are linked by alternating α-(1→3) (unit A) and β-(1→4) (unit B) glycosidic bonds (Figure 2). Unit A is always in D- conformation, while unit B can be found either in D- or L-configuration. The sulfated groups give it a negative charge, which categorizes carrageenans as polyanions [85]. Carrageenans are classified according to their degree of sulfation: they can be kappa (κ), iota (ι), and lambda (λ), if they have one, two or three sulfate groups respectively. The extraction process is straightforward, consisting in the immersion of the raw material in alkaline solution so that a gel forms. Then follows an extraction step, where the gel is immersed in water heated at 74 °C. Depending on the type of carrageenan and desired degree of purification, it is possible to execute additional purification steps, such as dialysis. The process finishes with filtration, precipitation and drying [85]. κ and ι types are most frequently extracted from algae of the *Kappaphycus* and *Eucheuma* genera, while λ type is often extracted from algae belonging to the family Gigantinaceae. The number of sulfated groups influences the gelation capability. Carrageenans κ and ι

can form gels in the presence of cations, while the high sulfation degree of λ carrageenan prevent its gelation. Gelation capability has been used in many areas, such as food industries (using carrageenan as an emulsifier and stabilizer), as well as in the cosmetic and pharmaceutical industries [86].

Contrary to what happens with other biomaterials of marine origin, the use of carrageenan as an excipient in the pharmaceutical industry is not common, thus reports about their applications, characteristics and functions are infrequent. As an example, a study was conducted where two types of carrageenan (κ and ι) were analyzed in terms of compression behavior and their capability of tablet formation [87]. Results showed that both carrageenans are suitable excipients for controlled release. Carrageenans are also present in various biomedical applications due to their anticoagulant properties [88], antitumor, immunomodulatory [89], anti-hyperlipidemic [90] and antioxidant activities [91]. They also have a protective activity against bacteria, fungi and some viruses [92,93]. Due to the latter, carrageenans have been suggested for possible treatments of respiratory diseases, such as the famous bird flu, and is also being tested for killing other viruses, such as the dengue fever, hepatitis A, HIV [94] and herpes viruses [95]. Studies showed that carrageenan, and derivatives of degradation have different levels of toxicity, but do not endanger the health of the patients [93,96]. These properties make carrageenan a promising biomaterial for biomedical applications.

The use of carrageenan as an excipient in the manufacture of devices for oral delivery depends mostly on their physicochemical properties, such as water solubility and jellification capability. Carrageenan load capacity depends largely on the sulfation extent, which affects its mechanical properties and its dissolution rate. These factors may affect the release of the cargo, prolonging or accelerating its release [97]. A greater control over the drug release profile—regardless of other conditions, such as carrageenan type and pH—is possible by association or conjugation with other polymers. The addition of polymers such as hydroxypropyl methylcellulose (HPMC), a temperature sensitive semi-synthetic polymer, can solve problems related to pH erosion and provide higher protection to the drug, thus promoting a sustained release that does not depend on pH [98]. However, the opposite response may be desired (*i.e.*, pH-triggered degradation) and, for that, pH responsive polymers may be conjugated. By varying the pH, it is possible to control not only the loading but also the release mechanisms of carrageenan/alginate interpenetrated networks [99]. The use of stimuli-responsive materials offers another perspective for drug and gene delivery where the carrier may be an active trigger and function as a therapy optimizer. Using temperature-sensitive materials for nanocarriers construction can promote a controlled release at temperatures above 37 °C. Such a system could be helpful in situations as common as a fever. However, it is possible to use other nanocarriers in situations of hyperthermia, where the drug would be available in a localized region [100,101].

Carrageenan in the pharmaceutical industry is generally used as a raw material for the construction of DDSs, cell capsules for cell therapies and cartilage regeneration applications [27,102]. The use of carrageenan-based hydrogels as a vehicle for the controlled delivery of biomolecules can be a good strategy especially for cargo stabilization Popa *et al.* showed that κ-carrageenan hydrogels are adequate environments to encapsulate different types of human cells achieving chondrogenic differentiation [103]. This system proved to have potential for cartilage regeneration strategies, not only due to the referred differentiation but also because these hydrogels can be easily injectable *in situ* and may be used as reservoirs for growth factors [104]. Carrageenan-based hydrogels, along with other materials of marine origin, have also proved to be suitable good devices for cell encapsulation [105,106]. New methods on the production of spherical beads and fibrillar carrageenan/alginate based hydrogel have been developed. Fibrillar hydrogels obtained by wet spinning showed great potential for applications as a cell carrier for cell delivery systems [107]. Knowing the biological properties of carrageenan, it is hypothesized that carrageenan-based devices are suitable DDSs for the delivery of not only bioactive agents but also of cells for cytotherapies.

Taking advantage of the polyanionic nature of carragenans, they can be combined with polycations via electrostatic interactions. Grenha *et al.* developed carrageenan/chitosan nanoparticles through a simple construction method by ionic interactions between polycationic groups of chitosan and polyanionic ones of carrageenan (Figure 4A) [108]. This method has the advantage of avoiding the use of organic solvents and harmful cross-linkers. These nanoparticles had a diameter size between 350 and 650 nm. Using albumin as a model protein, *in vitro* release tests demonstrated a prolonged release over time, with a 100% of albumin release after three weeks (Figure 4B). Having a slow release rate is important since it enables the reduction of the encapsulated dose and also provides continuous long-term release without the need for repeated administrations. Cytotoxicity tests demonstrated that these devices present low toxicity. These results are a good indicator that these structures may be feasible for the encapsulation of agents with therapeutic purposes. Carrageenan has also been used in the construction of multilayer structures [109], microcapsules [110] and micro/nanoparticles [111].

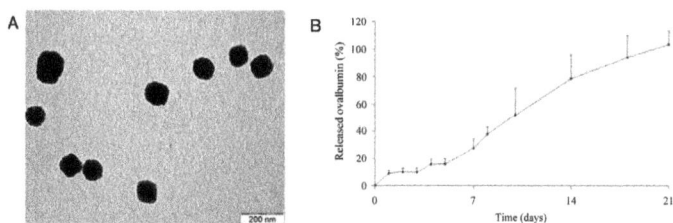

Figure 4. Transmission electron microscopy (TEM) micrograph of chitosan/carrageenan nanoparticles (**A**). Ovalbumin release profile from chitosan-carrageenan nanoparticles (**B**). Adapted with permission from [108], Copyright © 2009 Wiley Periodicals, Inc.

2.3. Fucoidans

Fucoidan is a sulfated polysaccharide found in many species of brown algae. It is a polymer chain of (1→3)-linked α-L-fucopyranosyl residues (Figure 2), although it is possible to find alternating (1→3) and (1→4)-linked α-L-fucopyranosyl residues. The structure of fucoidan and its composition depend largely on the extraction source, especially the type of algae. For example, fucoidan extracted from *Fucus vesiculosus* is rich in fucose and sulfate, whereas that obtained from *Sargassum stenophyllum* contains many more types of residues besides fucose and sulfate, such as galactose, mannose, glucuronic acid, glucose and xylose. A more detailed comparison between several fucoidans and their extraction sources can be found elsewhere [112]. The extraction can be processed by precipitation using salts or organic solvents, followed by a purification step by chromatography. Recently it was reported that fucoidan has antitumor activity dependent on the degree of sulfation and can inhibit tumor cell proliferation and growth [113,114]. However, fucoidan may have inhibitory effects over some cellular functions. Cumashi *et al.* demonstrated that fucoidans may exhibit strong antithrombin properties and suppresses tubulogenesis on HUVECs [22]. Fucoidan has also shown anticoagulant and anti-inflammatory properties, as well as anti-adhesive and antiviral properties [115,116].

Like other marine polysaccharides, fucoidan can also be used as a raw material for the construction of DDSs. A typical way of processing fucoidan DDSs is by electrostatic interactions with chitosan, to make microspheres, so-called fucospheres [117], which have been suggested for burn treatments. Particles with sizes ranging between 367 and 1017 nm were shown to trigger both *in vitro* and *in vivo* a decrease of the normal burn treatment time due to the increase of regeneration and healing of epithelial tissue [118]. Taking advantage of the great bioactivity of fucoidan, and the ability to complex with other materials like chitosan, other approaches can be pursued. Huang and Li developed novel chitosan/fucoidan nanoparticles with antioxidant properties for antibiotics delivery (Figure 5A) [119]. These nanoparticles presented a spherical morphology and diameter of 200–250 nm. Results showed a highly anti-oxidant effect by reducing concentration of reactive oxygen spices (ROS), using gentamicin as a model drug, release studies showed a controlled release around 99% of gentamicin in 72 h (Figure 5B). The antioxidant chitosan/fucoidan nanoparticles could thus be effective in delivering antibiotics to airway inflammatory diseases, where the amount of ROS it significantly high. Another approach to take advantage of chitosan/fucoidan interactions as DDSs is to synthesize hydrogels, as described by Nakamura *et al.* The authors developed a chitosan/fucoidan microcomplex hydrogel for the delivery of heparin binding growth factors, which showed high affinity with growth factors and were able to promote growth factor activity and also a controlled release [120]. *In vivo* studies showed a neovascularization promoted by the growth factors released from the chitosan/fucoidan hydrogel.

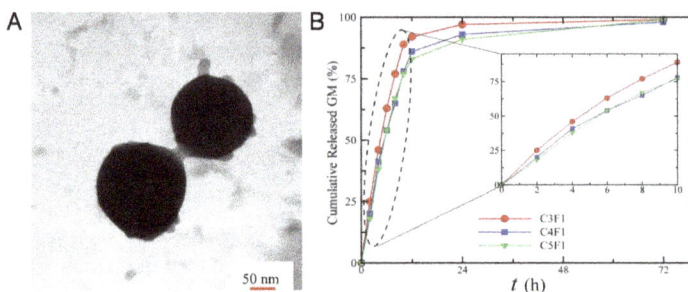

Figure 5. TEM image of chitosan/fucoidan nanoparticles (**A**). Gentamicin release kinetics from chitosan/fucoidan particles (**B**). Adapted with permission from [119], Copyright © 2014 distributed under a Creative Commons Attribution License.

Another shape that can be obtained resorting to the polyanionic character of fucoidan are capsules, processed by LbL, particularly fucoidan-chitosan pH sensitive capsules for insulin controlled release [121]. Pinheiro *et al.* used polystyrene nanoparticles with a diameter approximately 100 nm as a template for the deposition of a fucoidan-chitosan multilayered coating [122]. After construction of the coating, the polystyrene core was removed, being thus possible to incorporate into the capsule numerous bioactive agents. Using PLL as a model molecule, results showed that the release profile was pH dependent and also that the release occurred by diffusion. These results indicate the sensitivity of these particles to pH variations found along the gastro-intestinal tract and the possibility of using these particles as DDSs for oral administration.

2.4. Ulvans

Ulvan is a sulfated polysaccharide extracted from the green algae of the *Ulva* and *Enteromorpha* genera. Ulvan consists in a polymer chain of different sugar residues like glucose, rhamnose, xylose, glucuronic and iduronic acid with α- and β-(1→4) linkages (Figure 2). Because of the large number of sugars in its composition, ulvan may exhibit variations in the electronic density and charge distribution, as well as variations of molecular weight. Since it contains rare sugars, ulvan is a natural source for obtaining them upon depolymerization, instead of resorting to chemical synthesis. The extraction process is simple, consisting in adding an organic solvent over the feedstock followed by successive washing steps with hot water, filtration and centrifugation [123]. Ulvan has several properties of biological interest, such as exhibiting antiviral, antioxidant, antitumor, anticoagulant, anti-hyperlipidemic and immune system enhancing activities. Ulvan also presents low cytotoxicity levels in a wide range of concentrations [124]. Ulvan is typically used in the food and cosmetic industries, but because of their biological properties, it has a great potential for the development of new DDSs, such as being used as an active principle in pharmacological formulations [125]. Because of their ability for complexing with metal ions, ulvan can also be used as a chelating agent in the treatment against heavy metal poisoning [126]. Furthermore, the capacity to process ulvan as nanofibers and membranes has been useful for tissue engineering and regenerative medicine, for example in wound healing treatments [127].

Ulvan has been used in construction of nanocarriers for biomolecules. Alves *et al.* constructed a two-dimensional ulvan-based structure for drug delivery by chemical cross-linking for wound healing [128]. Using dexamethasone as a model drug, there was a rapid release in the first hour (around 49%), followed by a slower and sustained release, around 75% up to 14 days. Additionally, it is also possible to obtain three-dimensional ulvan-based structures. In this context, ulvan/chitosan particles were produced for the encapsulation and release of dexamethasone [129]. These particles were incorporated in three-dimensional poly (D,L-lactic acid) porous scaffolds for bone tissue regeneration. *In vitro* release assays demonstrated a fast release in the first three hours (around 52%), followed by a sustained cumulative release up to 60% in the next 21 days.

Like other marine polysaccharides, ulvan may undergo chemical modifications to synthesize thermostable hydrogels. The addition of other functional groups is also possible so that temperature and light responsive hydrogels are conceived. In this case, ulvan was modified with methacrylate groups to allow jellification by photopolymerization through the irradiation with ultraviolet light [130]. This is a useful approach to develop cell encapsulation strategies for cytotherapy applications. Ulvan is also used in the construction of membranes, due to electrostatic interactions with other cationic polymers [131]. Through chemical modification, ulvan and chitosan can also be used as a polymeric component of bone cement, especially due to their mechanical properties [132].

3. Polysaccharides from Marine Animals

There are other marine sources beside algae and microorganisms: marine animals are also an excellent source for polysaccharides. In this section, the most important animal origin polymers used in DDSs will be presented. There are two main categories of polymers: chitin-derived polymers and glycosaminoglycans (GAGs).

3.1. Chitosans

Chitosan is a linear polysaccharide derived from chitin, one of the most abundant natural polymers of our ecosystem [133]. Chitosan is obtained by the deacetylation of chitin, resulting in a compound with randomly distributed D-glucosamine residues (deacetylated unit) and N-acetyl-D-glucosamine (acetylated unit) (Figure 2) [134,135]. Chitosan, as well as chitin, can be degraded by enzymes such as chitinase and lysozyme [136]. Chitin is the main component of the exoskeleton of arthropods and crustaceans such as crabs, shrimps and lobsters, and can also be extracted from some fungi and nematodes. Chitin is not water soluble, and thus it is usually converted into soluble derivatives including chitosan (soluble in acidic conditions) and carboxymethyl chitosan (soluble in a wide range of acidic and alkaline solutions). Chitosan has amine groups sensitive to pH variations, being positively charged in acidic environments and neutral in alkaline pH values (pK_a close to 6) [32]. Chitosan is one of the marine polysaccharides most widely used and studied for biomedical applications, in particular in the construction of nanoparticles, beads and capsules for controlled drug delivery systems, and also membranes, films and scaffolds for tissue engineering and regenerative medicine [137–140].

Chitosan has antimicrobial activity, a useful property to build films that prevent wound infection [141,142]. It also shows antitumor and anti-inflammatory activity [143,144]. All of these biological properties make chitosan an excellent candidate for constructing devices that require the contact with biological environments, and as excipients for DDSs [145,146]. For chitosan-based DDSs, electrostatic interactions between the polysaccharide and a bioactive agent are a key to drug stabilization, protection and acceleration (or deceleration) of its release. This means that, if a drug is anionic, positively-charged polymers (like chitosan) are used as excipient, and *vice-versa*. The release profile and rate of biomolecules from within chitosan-based carriers may depend on the morphology, size, density, cross-linking degree, as well as the deacetylation degree of chitosan and physicochemical properties of the bioactive agent. The release will also be affected by the pH and by the presence or absence of enzymes. The release may occur in different ways: (i) release from the surface of DDSs; (ii) passive diffusion; and (iii) erosion of the DDS. Deacetylation degree of chitosan can be also used as a degradation control parameter [137,147]. Another mechanism of release exploited for chitosan-based carriers is triggered by enzymatic degradation [148].

It is also possible to increase the binding capacity of poorly water-soluble drugs by introducing different chemical modifications onto chitosan. Chitosan chemical modification can be a good strategy to increase the effectiveness of release and attribute other properties such as drug protection and stabilization [135]. Hydroxypropyl chitosan (HPCH), obtained from the reaction between chitosan and propylene epoxide under alkali condition, can be grafted with carboxymethyl β-cyclodextrin mediated via a water-soluble 1-ethyl-3-(3-dimethylaminopropyl) carbodiimide (EDC) [80]. Hydrophobic drugs can be encapsulated due the presence of hydrophobic groups present in HPCH. In addition, due to the free amine groups that can be protonated at lower pH values such DDSs can be pH-responsive. Using ketoprofen as a hydrophobic drug model, *in vitro* release results showed that this chitosan derivate has a great potential as a biodegradable delivery system for hydrophobic drugs in a pH-sensitive controlled release [149,150]. The introduction of thiol groups has also been shown to increase the solubility of chitosan in water, maintaining the pH dependence of chitosan particles [151]. *N,O*-carboxymethyl chitosan (NOCC, also known as carboxymethylated chitosan) is a water soluble derivative that retains a fraction of the amine residues and its polycationic properties under acidic conditions [34]. Ketoprofen-loaded beads of NOCC and a PNIPAAm with a telechelic amine group (PNIPAAm-NH$_2$) were developed for the study of controlled release system. Release studies taking in acidic and physiological conditions at 21 and 37 °C showed that these particular beads are sensitive to temperature and pH variations [152]. Acetylated chitosan grafted with fatty acid like palmitoyl is another strategy to develop chitosan-based excipients to entrap and release hydrophobic drugs [153–155]. Photo-sensitive products can also be synthesized. Methacrylamide chitosan, a water-soluble modified chitosan, is suitable for photo-cross-linking and has been used for the construction of delivery carriers. Wijekoon *et al.* developed a fluorinated methacrylamide chitosan hydrogel for oxygen delivery in wound healing [156]. During the methacrylation process, different fluorinated ligands were added to chitosan to obtain different fluorinated methacrylamide chitosans. Hydrogels were constructed by photo-cross-linking. This new biocompatible, injectable moldable photo-cross-linked chitosan-based hydrogel allowed controlling both the capacity and rate of oxygen delivery, maintaining beneficial oxygen level up to five days.

The reactivity of chitosan with other materials may also promote sustained release, as well as cargo stabilization and protection. This can be achieved using different methods, such as graft copolymerization with synthetic polymers like poly(ethylene glycol) (PEG) and PEI [148,157]. Several studies showed the ability of chitosan to enhance and prolong the absorption of hydrophilic drugs taken by oral [158] and pulmonary [159] administration routes. Chemical modification of chitosan with PEG is a way of improving the biocompatibility of chitosan, especially to reduce chitosan toxicity, as well as to enhance protein adsorption, cell adhesion, growth and proliferation [160,161]. Prego *et al.* showed that chitosan-PEG nanocapsules for oral delivery of peptides exhibited low cytotoxicity and enhanced intestinal absorption capability [162]. Other studies showed that this approach can also be applied to deliver other drugs such as insulin [163–166]. Taking advantage of the jellification capability of some copolymers containing chitosan, Bhattarai and coworkers presented an injectable PEG-grafted chitosan hydrogel for controlled release [167]. These hydrogels were liquid at room temperature and a gel at physiological temperature. Using albumin as a protein model, *in vitro* release studies at 37 °C showed a high release in the first 5 h, up to 50%–60% followed by a sustained release for the next days with a cumulative release up to 80%.

Hydrogels based on cross-linked chitosan may have the ability to promote a sustained release upon nasal administration. Hydrogels were constructed by joining *N*-[(2-hydroxy-3-trimethylammonium) propyl] chitosan chloride (HTCC) and PEG with the addition of a small quantity of α-β-glycerophosphate (α-β-GP) as a gelling agent [168]. These hydrogels are pH sensitive and have the particularity of being liquid at room temperature and exhibit higher rigidity at 37 °C. Wu and coworkers developed these hydrogels as smart devices for the controlled release of biomolecules through nasal administration as drops or spray. Once applied, the solution is exposed to physiological temperature, becoming a viscous hydrogel which can be absorbed by mucosa. Because of their ease of production and administration, this new formulation was tested as a loading device for the controlled release of insulin. Assays in rats showed an increased absorption in the nasal cavities and a decrease in blood glucose, without any evidence of cytotoxicity. These results demonstrated the great potential of these hydrogels as carriers for the controlled release of bioactive agents, especially hydrophilic biomolecules [169]. Nasal administration is less compliant for the patient, causing no discomfort and pain, leading to a reliable management and patient satisfaction [170]. Furthermore, the fact that this type of hydrogels are liquid at room temperature also enhances their ease of application as a DDS for parenteral administration [171].

Chitosan can form stable and highly dense electrostatic complexes capable of providing stability and protection to drugs. Being a polycationic polysaccharide, chitosan can form particle complexes with nucleic acids for gene therapy [172–175]. The formation of particle complexes between the polymer and the nucleic acids depends on many intrinsic factors, such as the deacetylation degree, the molecular weight, as well external factors like temperature and pH, and represent crucial factors on the efficiency of transfection [176]. The positive charge of chitosan allows interacting with the negatively charged peptidoglycans present in the cell membrane, facilitating the entry of a chitosan/DNA complex into the cell by pre-established endocytic pathways [177,178]. The amount of genetic material available to react with chitosan is also very important: an improper ratio can lead to the dissociation of the complex or to a lack of synthesized complexed particles, resulting in low transfection rate [176]. It has been reported that using chitosan overcomes some of these limitations: chemically modifying chitosan can increase the affinity with the DNA to yield a more stable complex, which can lead to an increase in the transfection efficacy [179]. The modifications can also increase chitosan solubility and thus offer greater protection to the cargo from the degradative action of DNases on DNA [176]. Chemical derivatives opened a new range of possibilities to construct DDSs for the intracellular release of the genetic material, with wide applicability in the treatment of various genetic diseases. Following this line, Forrest and coworkers presented a PEI-PEG-chitosan-copolymer for gene delivery with good loading capacity and high transfection efficacy, as well as low toxicity that makes these particles good candidates for *in vivo* gene delivery [180].

Chitosan-based capsules can also be synthesized resorting to electrostatic complexation, and, in some cases, are able to respond to external stimuli other than pH. One such example is the conception of LbL microcapsules made by complexation of chitosan with negatively charged elastin-like recombinamers (ELRs), recombinant polypeptides with intrinsic response towards temperature [181]. Novel thermoresponsive ELR/chitosan microcapsules were developed for the delivery of active molecules [182]. Using bovine serum albumin (BSA) as a model molecule, the results showed a greater BSA retention at physiological temperature (37 °C), when compared to room temperature (25 °C). Studies with cells also showed a low cytotoxicity for such structures. The pH response of these microcapsules was not studied, but the results are a good indicator that chitosan can bond with other sources of stimuli-responsive biomaterials, including unconventional ones such as genetically engineered polypeptides. While thermal responses are perhaps the most exploited mechanism integrated in smart DDSs, it is debatable whether their sensitivity would be enough to treat, for example, a common fever, where the body temperature varies just 1–2 °C. Besides, not all people have exactly the same body temperature. Therefore, conjugating two or more physiological parameters could be a solution for diseases that require administration based on triggers operating within tight ranges.

3.2. Hyaluronans

Hyaluronan belongs to the family of glycosaminoglycans. GAGs are linear, negatively charged heteropolysaccharides composed of repeating disaccharide units of N-acetylated hexosamine and uronic acid (with the exception of keratan sulfate) [183]. It is a linear polysaccharide consisting of an alternating chain disaccharide units of N-acetyl-D-glucosamine and D-glucuronic linked by β-(1→3) and β-(1→4) glycosidic bonds (Figure 2) [184]. Hyaluronan is a major component of extracellular matrix and is present in the synovial fluid, vitreous humor and cartilage tissue. Due to its high viscoelasticity, hyaluronan has an important role in several biological functions and also as an excellent material for different biomedical applications. Namely, it is involved in tissue regeneration, cell proliferation, differentiation and migration [185]. Because of its presence in the synovial fluid in joints, hyaluronan can be used as a biological marker to diagnose diseases associated with rheumatoid arthritis [186]. Due to its biocompatibility and biodegradability, hyaluronan has also been proposed for tissue engineering applications for manufacturing wound healing structures [187] and as a supplement for patients with arthritis [185]. Nowadays, hyaluronan production is done on a large scale using different methods and sources, such as bacterial fermentation [188–190]. hyaluronan may also be extracted directly from marine animal sources, such as cartilage and also from the vitreous humor of several fish species [191]. His biodegradability is mediated by the action of hydrolases, such as hyaluronidase, which breaks the glycosidic bond between two residues [192]. In the human body, hyaluronan is present in various biological fluids, allowing its use as a biomarker to monitoring its movement in biological fluids [193,194].

Hyaluronan hydrogels with dual stimuli-responsiveness can be made, namely towards pH and temperature variations. Hydrogels were obtained from hyaluronan and PNIPAAm with TEMED as a cross-linker [195]. Using gentamicin as a model drug, *in vitro* release assays at 37 °C and pH 7.4 showed an initial release of around 25% in the first 60 min, followed by a sustainable release up to 30% over the following 20 h. These results also showed that the release rate increases with increasing hyaluronan ratio in the hydrogel composition. These structures showed sensitivity to variations in temperature, showing potential as a device for biomolecules loading with smart controlled release system. There are other interesting types of hyaluronan conjugate-based hydrogels. Hyaluronan-tyramine (HA-Tyr) conjugates can be obtained by the enzymatic oxidative reaction of tyramine moieties using H_2O_2 and horseradish peroxidase (HRP). These hydrogels are highly biodegradable, which can be controlled by the cross-linking degree [196], and can encapsulate drugs. It was reported that the concentration of H_2O_2 has an influence in the mechanical strength of the hydrogel and on the release rate of drugs [197]. It was also reported that, in contact with hyaluronidase, the entrapped protein can be released continuously and completely from a hydrogel due to the polymer network degradation. On the same line of work, a new hyaluronidase incorporated-hyaluronan-tyramine hydrogel was developed for the delivery of trastuzumab, an antibody drug against breast cancer. *In vitro* release studies showed an antibody tunable release accompanied by the hydrogel degradation controlled by the concentration of hyaluronidase, as well as trastuzumab-dependent inhibition on the proliferation on cells [198].

Like other polyanions, hyaluronan can be complexed with polycations such as chitosan to form nanoparticles [199] and microspheres [200]. Recent studies presented these systems as a new approach for the treatment of ocular disorders. Hyaluronan/chitosan nanoparticles have been synthesized by means of electrostatic interactions to develop nanoparticles for the delivery of genes to the cornea and conjunctiva [201,202]. Results indicated an appropriate size distribution (100–230 nm) and internalization of these particles by endocytic processes mediated by membrane receptors. This result reveals the great biomedical applications potential of these nanoparticles as gene delivery device for treating diseases at the level of the human conjunctiva and other ocular diseases.

Hyaluronan has also been used as a coating material for spherical structures. Cross-linked chitosan spheres can serve as templates for the alternating adsorption of hyaluronan and chitosan multilayers [203]. *In vitro* release using gentamycin sulfate as a model drug indicated a sustained release from the microspheres, compared to the release from uncoated cores. These results show that a LbL coating can promote stabilization to the cargo and for that reason allows an enhanced sustained release. Liposomes are also viable spherical templates for hyaluronan coatings. Liposomes are pH sensitive lipid-based structures, and have been used as carriers for the controlled release of bioactive agents for cancer treatments [204]. One useful application of such pH sensitiveness is for the intracellular delivery of peptides. Jiang *et al.* presented a new liposome coated with hyaluronan for anticancer drug delivery [205]. In this case, the coating protected the liposome and the cargo against attacks by proteins present in the bloodstream. Entering the tumor extracellular matrix, where the hyaluronidase degrades the outer layer of hyaluronan, exposes the liposome to pH changes existing in the cytoplasm, enabling the intracellular drug release. A high antitumor activity was also detected during *in vivo* tests.

One interesting feature of hyaluronan is the ability to interact with several proteins. Such capability can be useful as a diagnostic tool, in particular due to existence of membrane receptors specific for hyaluronan. It is the case of CD44, a receptor that is highly expressed when there is an increase in cell proliferation. Determining an increased expression level of CD44 by means of hyaluronan devices can be an excellent marker for the early diagnosis of cancer [206]. Hyaluronan hydrogels can be used as reservoirs of bioactive agents obtained via various methods of constructions [207]. Nanoparticles based on the interaction of hyaluronan with metals, such as gold, have been widely used as markers for diagnosing diseases such as rheumatoid arthritis and cancer due to the ability of some of these devices to emit fluorescence [194,208–210].

3.3. Chondroitin Sulfates

Chondroitin sulfate is a sulfated glycosaminoglycan composed of a single chain of repeating disaccharide units of glucuronic acid (GlcA) and N-acetylgalactosamine (GalNAc) linked by β-(1→3) and can be sulfated in different carbon positions (Figure 2). It is usually extracted from the cartilage of bovine and porcine cattle but can also be extracted from some marine animals, like the whale and shark. However, due to ecological reasons, the extraction of protected species is currently quite limited. There are nonetheless other non-mammalian marine animal sources, such as the ray, the salmon fish, the sea cucumber, some cnidarians and mollusks [27]. Chondroitin sulfate has anticoagulant properties and has been suggested as a natural substitute for heparin, one of the most widely used anticoagulants [211,212]. In the pharmaceutical industry, this polysaccharide has been used as an active principle in drugs with anticoagulant properties, as a supplement to prevent arthritis [213], and as hydrogels for cartilage tissue regeneration [214]. Therefore, chondroitin sulfate is a suitable material to build DDSs. Studies with chondroitin sulfate/chitosan nanoparticles have indicated a large retention capacity of proteins and polypeptides, like growth factors [215]. Release assays showed a sustained release of the cargo in the order of 65% in the first 30 days. Studies *in vitro* performed on human adipose derived stem cells stem showed the ability of these nanoparticles to enter the cells promoting osteogenic differentiation. Cell internalization proved to be dependent on the particles concentration in the culture media, as well as on the incubation time.

Electrostatic interactions between different materials can be used for the construction of DDSs with the ability to incorporate different bioactive agents, as well as to enhance the cargo loading and to promote a sustained controlled release [216]. Despite the numerous advantages of using natural materials, synthetic polymers are still commonly used in the pharmaceutical industry, though they can be conjugated with natural ones. For example, chondroitin sulfate/PEG hydrogels was developed and proposed for a variety of biomedical applications, such as in wound healing and regenerative medicine [217]. This type of hydrogels proved to be biocompatible, since no inflammatory response when implanted has been observed, and is also biodegradable by enzymatic activity.

While 3D hydrogels and spherical objects are common designs for DDSs, a recent study showed that porous tubular structures can be constructed from hydroxyapatite and chondroitin sulfate for the delivery of chemotherapeutics [218]. Results for doxorubicin hydrochloride release showed a high encapsulation capacity around of 91% of efficacy due to the tubes geometry and porosity. *In vitro* release assays at different pH values (5, 6, and 7.4) revealed a pH dependent controlled release. These results revealed the potential use of these structures as controlled drug delivery devices for chemotherapy treatments, not only because of their pH dependent release, but also due to the long-term sustained release that eliminates the need for regular administration.

4. Emerging Glycosaminoglycan-Like Polysaccharides from Marine Origin

There are several types of glycosaminoglycans with different biological properties but, unlike hyaluronan and chondroitin sulfate, their bioavailability is low, they are difficult to extract and to produce, therefore they are not widely used in pharmaceutical sciences. However, due to their biological properties, they can be used as active agents in supplements. Examples include the sulfated glycosaminoglycans dermatan sulfate, heparan sulfate and keratan sulfate, and the nonsulfated agarose.

4.1. Dermatan Sulfates

Dermatan sulfate is a glycosaminoglycan with a linear disaccharide chain containing units of hexosamine, N-acetyl-galactosamine or glucuronic acid linked by β-(1→4) or (1→3). In some cases, this compound may present residues of L-iduronic acid, being the main structural difference between dermatan sulfate and chondroitin sulfate. Dermatan sulfate is extracted mainly from ray skin and can be used as a stabilizer for growth factors and cytokines. Recent studies have shown anticoagulant activity for dermatan sulfate without causing the possible complications present in the treatments made with heparin [219–221]. Dermatan sulfate anticoagulant character inhibits thrombin, showing no effect on factor X of the clotting cascade. It also has no interaction in platelet function. Thus, dermatan sulfate is a good alternative for heparin [222]. Thanks to its anticoagulant and antithrombotic activities, dermatan sulfate is seen as a potential substitute for heparin [211].

4.2. Heparan Sulfates

Heparan sulfate is another glycosaminoglycan which structure is very similar to heparin. It consists in a linear chain of alternating D-glucuronic acid or iduronic acid and D-glucosamine residues, which can be sulfated or acetylated. The distribution of sulfated residues can set some of the biological properties of heparan sulfate. The number of sulfated groups can influence the affinity with other proteins and so may influence their biological properties [223]. For example, heparan sulfate can block DNA topoisomerase activity in cell nucleus [224], and also has a role in the control of cell cycle and proliferation. Regarding the latter, heparin sulfate/cell complexes are often associated with increased cell proliferation which can lead to processes of oncogenesis. Thus, heparan sulfate has a significant role in the development of cancer, which is being associated with the increase of cell proliferation, angiogenesis in tumors, cancer cells differentiation and metastasis formation [225]. However, the effect of heparan sulfate on tumor cells may depend on the glycosaminoglycan structure, the type of tumor cell and/or the tumor microenvironment [226].

Independently of its role in cancer, this sulfated polysaccharide is also biodegradable, particularly by enzymatic action of heparanase [227]. Due to the presence of sulfated groups, it may bind to a number of different proteins and regulate biological processes such as coagulation and regulation. Heparan sulfate has the ability to bind to various polypeptides, such as the complex formed by the cellular receptor and growth factors [228]. Chemical modification of heparan sulfate can interfere with its anticoagulant activity and can have therapeutic effects in tumors. Regardless of the heavy involvement of heparan sulfate in different stages of tumor formation, it is possible that this polymer could be helpful as a new diagnostic method in the discovery and in the development of new drugs for cancer treatments, as well as in the development of DDSs with sensing capability. [229]. Due to the biological properties of heparan sulfate, it is not unreasonable to state that the production of heparan sulfate-based DDSs based could be a strategic approach to develop new chemotherapeutic strategies.

4.3. Keratan Sulfates

Keratan sulfate is a glycosaminoglycan that lacks the uronic acid unit. The disaccharide unit normally consists in galactose residues and N-acetylglucosamine bonded by β-(1→4) linkages. The extremities of keratan sulfate have a protein binding region at the extremities. There are three different classes of keratan sulfate which differ in the nature of the protein binding region. Class I is known for its presence in the cornea and in small cartilage. The protein binding occurs between the N- of a N-acetylglucosamine and an asparagine. In Class II, also present in small cartilage, the protein binding is made between the O- of N-acetylglucosamine with either a serine or a threonine. Finally, in Class III (first isolated from nervous tissue), the protein binding occurs in the O- of the mannose residue to a serine or threonine [230]. The presence of keratan sulfate in corneal tissue is related to the maintenance of the moisture level of the corneal tissue, which may influence its levels of transparency. Studies at the cellular level have shown that keratan sulfate has anti-adhesive properties. In nervous tissues, keratan sulfate can prevent the growth of axons, and in cartilage it may decrease the immune response in diseases such as osteoarthritis [231]. However, keratan sulfate presents an inhibitory action in nerve regeneration after nerve injury [232,233].

4.4. Agarose

Agarose is a marine biomaterial with a structure similar to carrageenan, present in the cell wall of red algae. Its structure comprises monosaccharide residues connected alternately in the conformation $(AB)_n$. The units consist of galactose residues linked by α-(1→3) (unit A) and β-(1→4) (unit B) linkages. The main difference between carrageenan and agar is that the carrageenan unit A is always in the D- conformation, while in the agar unit A can only be in the L- conformation [234]. Unlike carrageenan, agarose is not classified according to the sulfation degree, since the best known type of agarose is a neutral type without any sulfated group. Agarose is widely used in food industry and also in microbiology in the form of gel to be used as culture medium in the form of agar. Agarose is associated with several biomedical applications especially as hydrogels for the release of bioactive agents, taking advantage of its ability to jellify, biocompatibility and native biodegradability [235,236].

5. Conclusions

Marine polysaccharides have been widely used to synthesize DDSs. The fact that they are biocompatible, nontoxic and often biodegradable and stimuli-responsive makes these polymers suitable raw materials for the construction of increasingly complex loading devices with a release that can be potentially controlled. We showed that such devices can be constructed using different methods and can be synthesized in various shapes, such as hydrogels, particles and capsules, capable of protecting different bioactive agents like proteins and nuclei acids. Each and every polymer exhibits several chemical and biological properties, making marine biomaterials and their derivatives excellent materials not only for the construction of load devices but also for other pharmaceutical formulations as excipients or even active compounds in some food supplements. Natural-origin biomaterials allow incorporating a wide variety of proteins, drugs and nucleic acids, which for many new drugs would not be possible with many synthetic materials, which may be even toxic for the body. The release of bioactive agents may occur through various mechanisms, which may be controlled by using stimuli-responsive polymers to promote a fast or a sustained release. Because these materials are often biocompatible and biodegradable, their use may augment the efficiency of encapsulation and promote the protection of a bioactive agent.

Nowadays, it is already possible to find systems able to control the release of therapeutic molecules for the treatment of genetic diseases. Despite the great knowledge and wide use of marine polysaccharides in the pharmaceutical industry, some challenges remain unsolved, such as the efficient targeted delivery, the perfect control over the release rate to fit within a therapeutic window, and the adaptability to administration routes that are more patient compliant (e.g., oral instead of intravenous). Therefore, further investigation will be required to improve the isolation and purification of marine biopolymers, as well as the synthesis of their chemical modification and processing into the various possible matrices shapes. It is expected that in the short-term such control will lead to more efficient loading, higher degrees of control over the release and improved DDS designs, that could be used in advanced therapies. This could be possible by looking into the interactions between polymer, drugs and native biological tissues, as well the intelligent response of the polysaccharides and targeting capability. Future strategies should also combine the possibility of controlled release from this type of devices with diagnostic capability (theranostics approaches) where platforms involving nanotechnologies and image should be taken into consideration.

Acknowledgments: This work was supported by Fundação para a Ciência e Tecnologia (FCT, Grant SFRH/BPD/95446/2013), "Fundo Social Europeu" (FSE), "Programa Operacional de Potencial Humano" (POPH), and by European Research Council grant agreement ERC-ADG-2014-669858 for project ATLAS.

Conflicts of Interest: The authors declare no conflict of interest.

References

1. Pomponi, S.A. The bioprocess-technological potential of the sea. *J. Biotechnol.* **1999**, *70*, 5–13. [CrossRef]
2. Silva, T.H.; Duarte, A.R.; Moreira-Silva, J.; Mano, J.F.; Reis, R.L. Biomaterials from marine-origin biopolymers. In *Biomimetic Approaches for Biomaterials Development*; Mano, J.F., Ed.; Wiley-VCH Verlag: Weinheim, Germany, 2012; pp. 1–23.
3. Munro, M.H.; Blunt, J.W.; Dumdei, E.J.; Hickford, S.J.; Lill, R.E.; Li, S.; Battershill, C.N.; Duckworth, A.R. The discovery and development of marine compounds with pharmaceutical potential. *J. Biotechnol.* **1999**, *70*, 15–25. [CrossRef]
4. Molinski, T.F.; Dalisay, D.S.; Lievens, S.L.; Saludes, J.P. Drug development from marine natural products. *Nat. Rev. Drug Discov.* **2009**, *8*, 69–85. [CrossRef] [PubMed]
5. Schwartsmann, G.; da Rocha, A.B.; Berlinck, R.G.S.; Jimeno, J. Marine organisms as a source of new anticancer agents. *Lancet Oncol.* **2001**, *2*, 221–225. [CrossRef]
6. Jimeno, J.; Lopez-Martin, J.A.; Ruiz-Casado, A.; Izquierdo, M.A.; Scheuer, P.J.; Rinehart, K. Progress in the clinical development of new marine-derived anticancer compounds. *Anticancer Drugs* **2004**, *15*, 321–329. [CrossRef] [PubMed]
7. Newman, D.J.; Cragg, G.M. Marine-sourced anti-cancer and cancer pain control agents in clinical and late preclinical development. *Mar. Drugs* **2014**, *12*, 255–278. [CrossRef] [PubMed]
8. Rinehart, K.L. Antitumor compounds from tunicates. *Med. Res. Rev.* **2000**, *20*, 1–27. [CrossRef]
9. Suarez-Jimenez, G.M.; Burgos-Hernandez, A.; Ezquerra-Brauer, J.M. Bioactive peptides and depsipeptides with anticancer potential: Sources from Marine Animals. *Mar. Drugs* **2012**, *10*, 963–986. [CrossRef] [PubMed]
10. Jimeno, J.M. A clinical armamentarium of marine-derived anti-cancer compounds. *Anticancer Drugs* **2002**, *13*, S15–S19. [PubMed]
11. Valoti, G.; Nicoletti, M.I.; Pellegrino, A.; Jimeno, J.; Hendriks, H.; D'Incalci, M.; Faircloth, G.; Giavazzi, R. Ecteinascidin-743, a new marine natural product with potent antitumor activity on human ovarian carcinoma xenografts. *Clin. Cancer Res.* **1998**, *4*, 1977–1983. [PubMed]
12. Laurienzo, P. Marine polysaccharides in pharmaceutical applications: An Overview. *Mar. Drugs* **2010**, *8*, 2435–2465. [CrossRef] [PubMed]
13. Senni, K.; Pereira, J.; Gueniche, F.; Delbarre-Ladrat, C.; Sinquin, C.; Ratiskol, J.; Godeau, G.; Fischer, A.M.; Helley, D.; Colliec-Jouault, S. Marine polysaccharides: A source of bioactive molecules for cell therapy and tissue engineering. *Mar. Drugs* **2011**, *9*, 1664–1681. [CrossRef] [PubMed]
14. Ngo, D.H.; Kim, S.K. Sulfated polysaccharides as bioactive agents from marine algae. *Int. J. Biol. Macromol.* **2013**, *62*, 70–75. [CrossRef] [PubMed]
15. Costa, L.S.; Fidelis, G.P.; Cordeiro, S.L.; Oliveira, R.M.; Sabry, D.A.; Camara, R.B.; Nobre, L.T.; Costa, M.S.; Almeida-Lima, J.; Farias, E.H.; *et al.* Biological activities of sulfated polysaccharides from tropical seaweeds. *Biomed. Pharmacother.* **2010**, *64*, 21–28. [CrossRef] [PubMed]
16. Wijesekara, I.; Pangestuti, R.; Kim, S.K. Biological activities and potential health benefits of sulfated polysaccharides derived from marine algae. *Carbohydr. Polym.* **2011**, *84*, 14–21. [CrossRef]
17. Barahona, T.; Chandia, N.P.; Encinas, M.V.; Matsuhiro, B.; Zuniga, E.A. Antioxidant capacity of sulfated polysaccharides from seaweeds. A kinetic approach. *Food Hydrocoll.* **2011**, *25*, 529–535. [CrossRef]
18. Ciancia, M.; Quintana, I.; Cerezo, A.S. Overview of anticoagulant activity of sulfated polysaccharides from seaweeds in relation to their structures, focusing on those of green seaweeds. *Curr. Med. Chem.* **2010**, *17*, 2503–2529. [CrossRef] [PubMed]
19. Sithranga Boopathy, N.; Kathiresan, K. Anticancer drugs from marine flora: An Overview. *J. Oncol.* **2010**, *2010*, 1–18. [CrossRef] [PubMed]
20. Bouhlal, R.; Haslin, C.; Chermann, J.C.; Colliec-Jouault, S.; Sinquin, C.; Simon, G.; Cerantola, S.; Riadi, H.; Bourgougnon, N. Antiviral activities of sulfated polysaccharides isolated from *sphaerococcus coronopifolius* (*rhodophyta, gigartinales*) and *boergeseniella thuyoides* (*rhodophyta, ceramiales*). *Mar. Drugs* **2011**, *9*, 1187–1209. [CrossRef] [PubMed]
21. Vo, T.S.; Ngo, D.H.; Kim, S.K. Potential targets for anti-inflammatory and anti-allergic activities of marine algae: An Overview. *Inflamm. Allergy Drug Targets* **2012**, *11*, 90–101. [CrossRef] [PubMed]

22. Cumashi, A.; Ushakova, N.A.; Preobrazhenskaya, M.E.; D'Incecco, A.; Piccoli, A.; Totani, L.; Tinari, N.; Morozevich, G.E.; Berman, A.E.; Bilan, M.I.; *et al.* A comparative study of the anti-inflammatory, anticoagulant, antiangiogenic, and antiadhesive activities of nine different fucoidans from brown seaweeds. *Glycobiology* **2007**, *17*, 541–552. [CrossRef] [PubMed]

23. D'Ayala, G.G.; Malinconico, M.; Laurienzo, P. Marine derived polysaccharides for biomedical applications: Chemical modification approaches. *Molecules* **2008**, *13*, 2069–2106. [CrossRef] [PubMed]

24. Allen, T.M.; Cullis, P.R. Drug delivery systems: Entering the mainstream. *Science* **2004**, *303*, 1818–1822. [CrossRef] [PubMed]

25. Brannon-Peppas, L.; Blanchette, J.O. Nanoparticle and targeted systems for cancer therapy. *Adv. Drug Deliv. Rev.* **2012**, *64*, 206–212. [CrossRef]

26. Thomas, C.E.; Ehrhardt, A.; Kay, M.A. Progress and problems with the use of viral vectors for gene therapy. *Nat. Rev. Genet.* **2003**, *4*, 346–358. [CrossRef] [PubMed]

27. Silva, T.H.; Alves, A.; Popa, E.G.; Reys, L.L.; Gomes, M.E.; Sousa, R.A.; Silva, S.S.; Mano, J.F.; Reis, R.L. Marine algae sulfated polysaccharides for tissue engineering and drug delivery approaches. *Biomatter* **2012**, *2*, 278–289. [CrossRef] [PubMed]

28. Nitta, S.K.; Numata, K. Biopolymer-based nanoparticles for drug/gene delivery and tissue engineering. *Int. J. Mol. Sci.* **2013**, *14*, 1629–1654. [CrossRef] [PubMed]

29. Lee, K.Y.; Mooney, D.J. Alginate: Properties and biomedical applications. *Prog. Polym. Sci.* **2012**, *37*, 106–126. [CrossRef] [PubMed]

30. Haug, A.; Larsen, B. Quantitative determination of uronic acid compositions of alginates. *Acta Chem. Scand.* **1962**, *16*, 1908–1918. [CrossRef]

31. Tonnesen, H.H.; Karlsen, J. Alginate in drug delivery systems. *Drug Dev. Ind. Pharm.* **2002**, *28*, 621–630. [CrossRef] [PubMed]

32. Mano, J.F. Stimuli-responsive polymeric systems for biomedical applications. *Adv. Eng. Mater.* **2008**, *10*, 515–527. [CrossRef]

33. George, M.; Abraham, T.E. Polyionic hydrocolloids for the intestinal delivery of protein drugs: Alginate and chitosan—A review. *J. Control. Release* **2006**, *114*, 1–14. [CrossRef] [PubMed]

34. Chen, S.C.; Wu, Y.C.; Mi, F.L.; Lin, Y.H.; Yu, L.C.; Sung, H.W. A novel pH-sensitive hydrogel composed of *N,O*-carboxymethyl chitosan and alginate cross-linked by genipin for protein drug delivery. *J. Control. Release* **2004**, *96*, 285–300. [CrossRef] [PubMed]

35. Gombotz, W.R.; Wee, S.F. Protein release from alginate matrices. *Adv. Drug Deliv. Rev.* **2012**, *64*, 194–205. [CrossRef]

36. Beneke, C.E.; Viljoen, A.M.; Hamman, J.H. Polymeric plant-derived excipients in drug delivery. *Molecules* **2009**, *14*, 2602–2620. [CrossRef] [PubMed]

37. Sudhakar, Y.; Kuotsu, K.; Bandyopadhyay, A.K. Buccal bioadhesive drug delivery—A promising option for orally less efficient drugs. *J. Control. Release* **2006**, *114*, 15–40. [CrossRef] [PubMed]

38. Sirkia, T.; Salonen, H.; Veski, P.; Jurjenson, H.; Marvola, M. Biopharmaceutical evaluation of new prolonged-release press-coated ibuprofen tablets containing sodium alginate to adjust drug-release. *Int. J. Pharm.* **1994**, *107*, 179–187. [CrossRef]

39. Xu, Y.; Zhan, C.; Fan, L.; Wang, L.; Zheng, H. Preparation of dual crosslinked alginate-chitosan blend gel beads and *in vitro* controlled release in oral site-specific drug delivery system. *Int. J. Pharm.* **2007**, *336*, 329–337. [CrossRef] [PubMed]

40. Pillay, V.; Fassihi, R. *In vitro* release modulation from crosslinked pellets for site-specific drug delivery to the gastrointestinal tract: I. Comparison of pH-responsive drug release and associated kinetics. *J. Control. Release* **1999**, *59*, 229–242. [CrossRef]

41. Pillay, V.; Fassihi, R. *In vitro* release modulation from crosslinked pellets for site-specific drug delivery to the gastrointestinal tract: II. Physicochemical characterization of calcium-alginate, calcium-pectinate and calcium-alginate-pectinate pellets. *J. Control. Release* **1999**, *59*, 243–256. [CrossRef]

42. Mandal, S.; Basu, S.K.; Sa, B. Ca^{2+} ion cross-linked interpenetrating network matrix tablets of polyacrylamide-grafted-sodium alginate and sodium alginate for sustained release of diltiazem hydrochloride. *Carbohydr. Polym.* **2010**, *82*, 867–873. [CrossRef]

43. Russo, R.; Malinconico, M.; Santagata, G. Effect of cross-linking with calcium ions on the physical properties of alginate films. *Biomacromolecules* **2007**, *8*, 3193–3197. [CrossRef] [PubMed]

44. Oliveira, M.B.; Mano, J.F. On-chip assessment of the protein-release profile from 3D hydrogel arrays. *Anal. Chem.* **2013**, *85*, 2391–2396. [CrossRef] [PubMed]

45. Giunchedi, P.; Gavini, E.; Moretti, M.D.; Pirisino, G. Evaluation of alginate compressed matrices as prolonged drug delivery systems. *AAPS PharmSciTech* **2000**, *1*, 31–36. [CrossRef] [PubMed]

46. Hamidi, M.; Azadi, A.; Rafiei, P. Hydrogel nanoparticles in drug delivery. *Adv. Drug Deliv. Rev.* **2008**, *60*, 1638–1649. [CrossRef] [PubMed]

47. Augst, A.D.; Kong, H.J.; Mooney, D.J. Alginate hydrogels as biomaterials. *Macromol. Biosci.* **2006**, *6*, 623–633. [CrossRef] [PubMed]

48. Lee, K.Y.; Mooney, D.J. Hydrogels for tissue engineering. *Chem. Rev.* **2001**, *101*, 1869–1880. [CrossRef] [PubMed]

49. Draget, K.I.; Skjåk Bræk, G.; Smidsrød, O. Alginic acid gels: The effect of alginate chemical composition and molecular weight. *Carbohydr. Polym.* **1994**, *25*, 31–38. [CrossRef]

50. Mura, S.; Nicolas, J.; Couvreur, P. Stimuli-responsive nanocarriers for drug delivery. *Nat. Mater.* **2013**, *12*, 991–1003. [CrossRef] [PubMed]

51. Duarte, A.R.; Unal, B.; Mano, J.F.; Reis, R.L.; Jensen, K.F. Microfluidic production of perfluorocarbon-alginate core-shell microparticles for ultrasound therapeutic applications. *Langmuir* **2014**, *30*, 12391–12399. [CrossRef] [PubMed]

52. Song, W.L.; Lima, A.C.; Mano, J.F. Bioinspired methodology to fabricate hydrogel spheres for multi-applications using superhydrophobic substrates. *Soft Matter* **2010**, *6*, 5868–5871. [CrossRef]

53. Costa, A.M.; Alatorre-Meda, M.; Alvarez-Lorenzo, C.; Mano, J.F. Superhydrophobic surfaces as a tool for the fabrication of hierarchical spherical polymeric carriers. *Small* **2015**, *11*, 3648–3652. [CrossRef] [PubMed]

54. Costa, A.M.; Alatorre-Meda, M.; Oliveira, N.M.; Mano, J.F. Biocompatible polymeric microparticles produced by a simple biomimetic approach. *Langmuir* **2014**, *30*, 4535–4539. [CrossRef] [PubMed]

55. Thomas, M.; Klibanov, A.M. Non-viral gene therapy: Polycation-mediated DNA delivery. *Appl. Microbiol. Biotechnol.* **2003**, *62*, 27–34. [CrossRef] [PubMed]

56. Pack, D.W.; Hoffman, A.S.; Pun, S.; Stayton, P.S. Design and development of polymers for gene delivery. *Nat. Rev. Drug Discov.* **2005**, *4*, 581–593. [CrossRef] [PubMed]

57. Liu, Z.; Jiao, Y.; Wang, Y.; Zhou, C.; Zhang, Z. Polysaccharides-based nanoparticles as drug delivery systems. *Adv. Drug Deliv. Rev.* **2008**, *60*, 1650–1662. [CrossRef] [PubMed]

58. Panyam, J.; Labhasetwar, V. Biodegradable nanoparticles for drug and gene delivery to cells and tissue. *Adv. Drug Deliv. Rev.* **2003**, *55*, 329–347. [CrossRef]

59. Quick, D.J.; Macdonald, K.K.; Anseth, K.S. Delivering DNA from photocrosslinked, surface eroding polyanhydrides. *J. Control. Release* **2004**, *97*, 333–343. [CrossRef] [PubMed]

60. Krebs, M.D.; Salter, E.; Chen, E.; Sutter, K.A.; Alsberg, E. Calcium phosphate-DNA nanoparticle gene delivery from alginate hydrogels induces *in vivo* osteogenesis. *J. Biomed. Mater. Res. A* **2010**, *92*, 1131–1138. [PubMed]

61. Becker, A.L.; Johnston, A.P.; Caruso, F. Layer-by-layer-assembled capsules and films for therapeutic delivery. *Small* **2010**, *6*, 1836–1852. [CrossRef] [PubMed]

62. Zhao, Q.; Han, B.; Wang, Z.; Gao, C.; Peng, C.; Shen, J. Hollow chitosan-alginate multilayer microcapsules as drug delivery vehicle: Doxorubicin loading and *in vitro* and *in vivo* studies. *Nanomed. NBM* **2007**, *3*, 63–74. [CrossRef] [PubMed]

63. Costa, N.L.; Sher, P.; Mano, J.F. Liquefied capsules coated with multilayered polyelectrolyte films for cell immobilization. *Adv. Eng. Mater.* **2011**, *13*, B218–B224. [CrossRef]

64. Mano, J.F. Designing biomaterials for tissue engineering based on the deconstruction of the native cellular environment. *Mater. Lett.* **2015**, *141*, 198–202. [CrossRef]

65. Chen, D.; Wu, M.; Chen, J.; Zhang, C.; Pan, T.; Zhang, B.; Tian, H.; Chen, X.; Sun, J. Robust, flexible, and bioadhesive free-standing films for the co-delivery of antibiotics and growth factors. *Langmuir* **2014**, *30*, 13898–13906. [CrossRef] [PubMed]

66. Caridade, S.G.; Monge, C.; Gilde, F.; Boudou, T.; Mano, J.F.; Picart, C. Free-standing polyelectrolyte membranes made of chitosan and alginate. *Biomacromolecules* **2013**, *14*, 1653–1660. [CrossRef] [PubMed]

67. Jiang, C.; Tsukruk, V.V. Freestanding nanostructures via layer-by-layer assembly. *Adv. Mater.* **2006**, *18*, 829–840. [CrossRef]

68. Okamura, Y.; Kabata, K.; Kinoshita, M.; Saitoh, D.; Takeoka, S. Free-standing biodegradable poly(lactic acid) nanosheet for sealing operations in surgery. *Adv. Mater.* **2009**, *21*, 4388–4392. [CrossRef] [PubMed]

69. Fujie, T.; Matsutani, N.; Kinoshita, M.; Okamura, Y.; Saito, A.; Takeoka, S. Adhesive, flexible, and robust polysaccharide nanosheets integrated for tissue-defect repair. *Adv. Funct. Mater.* **2009**, *19*, 2560–2568. [CrossRef]
70. Fujie, T.; Okamura, Y.; Takeoka, S. Ubiquitous transference of a free-standing polysaccharide nanosheet with the development of a nano-adhesive plaster. *Adv. Mater.* **2007**, *19*, 3549–3553. [CrossRef]
71. Silva, J.M.; Duarte, A.R.; Caridade, S.G.; Picart, C.; Reis, R.L.; Mano, J.F. Tailored freestanding multilayered membranes based on chitosan and alginate. *Biomacromolecules* **2014**, *15*, 3817–3826. [CrossRef] [PubMed]
72. Costa, R.R.; Mano, J.F. Polyelectrolyte multilayered assemblies in biomedical technologies. *Chem. Soc. Rev.* **2014**, *43*, 3453–3479. [CrossRef] [PubMed]
73. Zhang, Y.; Wei, W.; Lv, P.; Wang, L.; Ma, G. Preparation and evaluation of alginate-chitosan microspheres for oral delivery of insulin. *Eur. J. Pharm. Biopharm.* **2011**, *77*, 11–19. [CrossRef] [PubMed]
74. Lima, A.C.; Sher, P.; Mano, J.F. Production methodologies of polymeric and hydrogel particles for drug delivery applications. *Expert Opin. Drug Deliv.* **2012**, *9*, 231–248. [CrossRef] [PubMed]
75. Soppimath, K.S.; Aminabhavi, T.M.; Kulkarni, A.R.; Rudzinski, W.E. Biodegradable polymeric nanoparticles as drug delivery devices. *J. Control. Release* **2001**, *70*, 1–20. [CrossRef]
76. Ribeiro, A.J.; Neufeld, R.J.; Arnaud, P.; Chaumeil, J.C. Microencapsulation of lipophilic drugs in chitosan-coated alginate microspheres. *Int. J. Pharm.* **1999**, *187*, 115–123. [CrossRef]
77. Lin, Y.H.; Liang, H.F.; Chung, C.K.; Chen, M.C.; Sung, H.W. Physically crosslinked alginate/*N,O*-carboxymethyl chitosan hydrogels with calcium for oral delivery of protein drugs. *Biomaterials* **2005**, *26*, 2105–2113. [CrossRef] [PubMed]
78. Chandy, T.; Mooradian, D.L.; Rao, G.H.R. Chitosan polyethylene glycol alginate microcapsules for oral delivery of hirudin. *J. Appl. Polym. Sci.* **1998**, *70*, 2143–2153. [CrossRef]
79. Schmaljohann, D. Thermo- and pH-responsive polymers in drug delivery. *Adv. Drug Deliv. Rev.* **2006**, *58*, 1655–1670. [CrossRef] [PubMed]
80. Prabaharan, M.; Mano, J.F. Stimuli-responsive hydrogels based on polysaccharides incorporated with thermo-responsive polymers as novel biomaterials. *Macromol. Biosci.* **2006**, *6*, 991–1008. [CrossRef] [PubMed]
81. Shi, J.; Alves, N.M.; Mano, J.F. Chitosan coated alginate beads containing poly(*N*-isopropylacrylamide) for dual-stimuli-responsive drug release. *J. Biomed. Mater. Res. B Appl. Biomater.* **2008**, *84*, 595–603. [CrossRef] [PubMed]
82. Sarmento, B.; Ribeiro, A.; Veiga, F.; Sampaio, P.; Neufeld, R.; Ferreira, D. Alginate/chitosan nanoparticles are effective for oral insulin delivery. *Pharm. Res.* **2007**, *24*, 2198–2206. [CrossRef] [PubMed]
83. Correia, C.R.; Reis, R.L.; Mano, J.F. Multilayered hierarchical capsules providing cell adhesion sites. *Biomacromolecules* **2013**, *14*, 743–751. [CrossRef] [PubMed]
84. Correia, C.R.; Sher, P.; Reis, R.L.; Mano, J.F. Liquified chitosan-alginate multilayer capsules incorporating poly(L-lactic acid) microparticles as cell carriers. *Soft Matter* **2013**, *9*, 2125–2130. [CrossRef]
85. Rinaudo, M. Main properties and current applications of some polysaccharides as biomaterials. *Polym. Int.* **2008**, *57*, 397–430. [CrossRef]
86. Li, L.; Ni, R.; Shao, Y.; Mao, S. Carrageenan and its applications in drug delivery. *Carbohydr. Polym.* **2014**, *103*, 1–11. [CrossRef] [PubMed]
87. Picker, K.M. Matrix tablets of carrageenans. I. A compaction study. *Drug Dev. Ind. Pharm.* **1999**, *25*, 329–337. [CrossRef] [PubMed]
88. Silva, F.R.F.; Dore, C.M.P.G.; Marques, C.T.; Nascimento, M.S.; Benevides, N.M.B.; Rocha, H.A.O.; Chavante, S.F.; Leite, E.L. Anticoagulant activity, paw edema and pleurisy induced carrageenan: Action of major types of commercial carrageenans. *Carbohydr. Polym.* **2010**, *79*, 26–33. [CrossRef]
89. Zhou, G.; Sun, Y.; Xin, H.; Zhang, Y.; Li, Z.; Xu, Z. *In vivo* antitumor and immunomodulation activities of different molecular weight lambda-carrageenans from *Chondrus ocellatus*. *Pharmacol. Res.* **2004**, *50*, 47–53. [CrossRef] [PubMed]
90. Panlasigui, L.N.; Baello, O.Q.; DimatangalBSc, J.M.; DumelodMSc, B.D. Blood cholesterol and lipid-lowering effects of carrageenan on human volunteers. *Asia Pac. J. Clin. Nutr.* **2003**, *12*, 209–214. [PubMed]
91. De Souza, M.C.R.; Marques, C.T.; Dore, C.M.G.; da Silva, F.R.F.; Rocha, H.A.O.; Leite, E.L. Antioxidant activities of sulfated polysaccharides from brown and red seaweeds. *J. Appl. Phycol.* **2007**, *19*, 153–160. [CrossRef] [PubMed]
92. Carlucci, M.J.; Ciancia, M.; Matulewicz, M.C.; Cerezo, A.S.; Damonte, E.B. Antiherpetic activity and mode of action of natural carrageenans of diverse structural types. *Antiviral Res.* **1999**, *43*, 93–102. [CrossRef]

93. Campo, V.L.; Kawano, D.F.; da Silva, D.B.; Carvalho, I. Carrageenans: Biological properties, chemical modifications and structural analysis—A review. *Carbohydr. Polym.* **2009**, *77*, 167–180. [CrossRef]

94. Schaeffer, D.J.; Krylov, V.S. Anti-HIV activity of extracts and compounds from algae and cyanobacteria. *Ecotoxicol. Environ. Saf.* **2000**, *45*, 208–227. [CrossRef] [PubMed]

95. Carlucci, M.J.; Scolaro, L.A.; Noseda, M.D.; Cerezo, A.S.; Damonte, E.B. Protective effect of a natural carrageenan on genital herpes simplex virus infection in mice. *Antiviral Res.* **2004**, *64*, 137–141. [CrossRef]

96. Prajapati, V.D.; Maheriya, P.M.; Jani, G.K.; Solanki, H.K. Carrageenan: A natural seaweed polysaccharide and its applications. *Carbohydr. Polym.* **2014**, *105*, 97–112. [CrossRef] [PubMed]

97. Bornhöft, M.; Thommes, M.; Kleinebudde, P. Preliminary assessment of carrageenan as excipient for extrusion/spheronisation. *Eur. J. Pharm. Biopharm.* **2005**, *59*, 127–131. [CrossRef] [PubMed]

98. Bonferoni, M.C.; Rossi, S.; Ferrari, F.; Bertoni, M.; Bolhuis, G.K.; Caramella, C. On the employment of *lambda carrageenan* in a matrix system. III. Optimization of a lambda carrageenan-HPMC hydrophilic matrix. *J. Control. Release* **1998**, *51*, 231–239. [CrossRef]

99. Mohamadnia, Z.; Zohuriaan-Mehr, A.J.; Kabiri, K.; Jamshidi, A.; Mobedi, H. pH-sensitive IPN hydrogel beads of carrageenan-alginate for controlled drug delivery. *J. Bioact. Compat. Polym.* **2007**, *22*, 342–356. [CrossRef]

100. Ganta, S.; Devalapally, H.; Shahiwala, A.; Amiji, M. A review of stimuli-responsive nanocarriers for drug and gene delivery. *J. Control. Release* **2008**, *126*, 187–204. [CrossRef] [PubMed]

101. Meyer, D.E.; Shin, B.C.; Kong, G.A.; Dewhirst, M.W.; Chilkoti, A. Drug targeting using thermally responsive polymers and local hyperthermia. *J. Control. Release* **2001**, *74*, 213–224. [CrossRef]

102. Popa, E.G.; Rodrigues, M.T.; Coutinho, D.F.; Oliveira, M.B.; Mano, J.F.; Reis, R.L.; Gomes, M.E. Cryopreservation of cell laden natural origin hydrogels for cartilage regeneration strategies. *Soft Matter* **2013**, *9*, 875–885. [CrossRef]

103. Popa, E.G.; Caridade, S.G.; Mano, J.F.; Reis, R.L.; Gomes, M.E. Chondrogenic potential of injectable kappa-carrageenan hydrogel with encapsulated adipose stem cells for cartilage tissue-engineering applications. *J. Tissue Eng. Regen. Med.* **2015**, *9*, 550–563. [CrossRef] [PubMed]

104. Rocha, P.M.; Santo, V.E.; Gomes, M.E.; Reis, R.L.; Mano, J.F. Encapsulation of adipose-derived stem cells and transforming growth factor-β1 in carrageenan-based hydrogels for cartilage tissue engineering. *J. Bioact. Compat. Polym.* **2011**, *26*, 493–507. [CrossRef]

105. Luna, S.M.; Gomes, M.E.; Mano, J.F.; Reis, R.L. Development of a novel cell encapsulation system based on natural origin polymers for tissue engineering applications. *J. Bioact. Compat. Polym.* **2010**, *25*, 341–359. [CrossRef]

106. Gasperini, L.; Mano, J.F.; Reis, R.L. Natural polymers for the microencapsulation of cells. *J. R. Soc. Interface* **2014**, *11*, 1–19. [CrossRef] [PubMed]

107. Popa, E.G.; Gomes, M.E.; Reis, R.L. Cell delivery systems using alginate—Carrageenan hydrogel beads and fibers for regenerative medicine applications. *Biomacromolecules* **2011**, *12*, 3952–3961. [CrossRef] [PubMed]

108. Grenha, A.; Gomes, M.E.; Rodrigues, M.; Santo, V.E.; Mano, J.F.; Neves, N.M.; Reis, R.L. Development of new chitosan/carrageenan nanoparticles for drug delivery applications. *J. Biomed. Mater. Res. A* **2010**, *92*, 1265–1272. [CrossRef] [PubMed]

109. Oliveira, S.M.; Silva, T.H.; Reis, R.L.; Mano, J.F. Nanocoatings containing sulfated polysaccharides prepared by layer-by-layer assembly as models to study cell-material interactions. *J. Mater. Chem. B* **2013**, *1*, 4406–4418. [CrossRef]

110. Yeo, Y.; Baek, N.; Park, K. Microencapsulation methods for delivery of protein drugs. *Biotechnol. Bioprocess. Eng.* **2001**, *6*, 213–230. [CrossRef]

111. Rodrigues, S.; da Costa, A.M.; Grenha, A. Chitosan/carrageenan nanoparticles: Effect of cross-linking with tripolyphosphate and charge ratios. *Carbohydr. Polym.* **2012**, *89*, 282–289. [CrossRef] [PubMed]

112. Li, B.; Lu, F.; Wei, X.; Zhao, R. Fucoidan: Structure and bioactivity. *Molecules* **2008**, *13*, 1671–1695. [CrossRef] [PubMed]

113. Ermakova, S.; Sokolova, R.; Kim, S.M.; Um, B.H.; Isakov, V.; Zvyagintseva, T. Fucoidans from brown seaweeds *sargassum hornery, eclonia cava, costaria costata*: Structural characteristics and anticancer activity. *Appl. Biochem. Biotechnol.* **2011**, *164*, 841–850. [CrossRef] [PubMed]

114. Anastyuk, S.D.; Shevchenko, N.M.; Ermakova, S.P.; Vishchuk, O.S.; Nazarenko, E.L.; Dmitrenok, P.S.; Zvyagintseva, T.N. Anticancer activity *in vitro* of a fucoidan from the brown alga *fucus evanescens* and its low-molecular fragments, structurally characterized by tandem mass-spectrometry. *Carbohydr. Polym.* **2012**, *87*, 186–194. [CrossRef]

115. Kim, S.K.; Ravichandran, Y.D.; Khan, S.B.; Kim, Y.T. Prospective of the cosmeceuticals derived from marine organisms. *Biotechnol. Bioprocess. Eng.* **2008**, *13*, 511–523. [CrossRef]

116. Sezer, A.; Cevher, E. Fucoidan: A versatile biopolymer for biomedical applications. In *Active Implants and Scaffolds for Tissue Regeneration*; Zilberman, M., Ed.; Springer: Berlin/Heidelberg, Germany, 2011; Volume 8, pp. 377–406.

117. Sezer, A.D.; Akbuga, J. Fucosphere—New microsphere carriers for peptide and protein delivery: Preparation and *in vitro* characterization. *J. Microencapsul.* **2006**, *23*, 513–522. [CrossRef] [PubMed]

118. Sezer, A.D.; Cevher, E.; Hatipoglu, F.; Ogurtan, Z.; Bas, A.L.; Akbuga, J. The use of fucosphere in the treatment of dermal burns in rabbits. *Eur. J. Pharm. Biopharm.* **2008**, *69*, 189–198. [CrossRef] [PubMed]

119. Huang, Y.C.; Li, R.Y. Preparation and characterization of antioxidant nanoparticles composed of chitosan and fucoidan for antibiotics delivery. *Mar. Drugs* **2014**, *12*, 4379–4398. [CrossRef] [PubMed]

120. Nakamura, S.; Nambu, M.; Ishizuka, T.; Hattori, H.; Kanatani, Y.; Takase, B.; Kishimoto, S.; Amano, Y.; Aoki, H.; Kiyosawa, T.; *et al.* Effect of controlled release of fibroblast growth factor-2 from chitosan/fucoidan micro complex-hydrogel on *in vitro* and *in vivo* vascularization. *J. Biomed. Mater. Res. A* **2008**, *85*, 619–627. [CrossRef] [PubMed]

121. Sato, K.; Takahashi, S.; Anzai, J. Layer-by-layer thin films and microcapsules for biosensors and controlled release. *Anal. Sci.* **2012**, *28*, 929–938. [CrossRef] [PubMed]

122. Pinheiro, A.C.; Bourbon, A.I.; Cerqueira, M.A.; Maricato, E.; Nunes, C.; Coimbra, M.A.; Vicente, A.A. Chitosan/fucoidan multilayer nanocapsules as a vehicle for controlled release of bioactive compounds. *Carbohydr. Polym.* **2015**, *115*, 1–9. [CrossRef] [PubMed]

123. Lahaye, M.; Robic, A. Structure and functional properties of ulvan, a polysaccharide from green seaweeds. *Biomacromolecules* **2007**, *8*, 1765–1774. [CrossRef] [PubMed]

124. Alves, A.; Sousa, R.A.; Reis, R.L. *In vitro* cytotoxicity assessment of ulvan, a polysaccharide extracted from green algae. *Phytother. Res.* **2013**, *27*, 1143–1148. [CrossRef] [PubMed]

125. Ahmed, O.M.; Ahmed, R.R. Anti-proliferative and apoptotic efficacies of ulvan polysaccharides against different types of carcinoma cells *in vitro* and *in vivo*. *J. Cancer Sci. Ther.* **2014**, *6*, 202–208. [CrossRef]

126. Alves, A.; Sousa, R.A.; Reis, R.L. A practical perspective on ulvan extracted from green algae. *J. Appl. Phycol.* **2013**, *25*, 407–424. [CrossRef]

127. Dash, M.; Samal, S.K.; Bartoli, C.; Morelli, A.; Smet, P.F.; Dubruel, P.; Chiellini, F. Biofunctionalization of ulvan scaffolds for bone tissue engineering. *ACS Appl. Mater. Interfaces* **2014**, *6*, 3211–3218. [CrossRef] [PubMed]

128. Alves, A.; Pinho, E.D.; Neves, N.M.; Sousa, R.A.; Reis, R.L. Processing ulvan into 2D structures: Cross-linked ulvan membranes as new biomaterials for drug delivery applications. *Int. J. Pharm.* **2012**, *426*, 76–81. [CrossRef] [PubMed]

129. Alves, A.; Duarte, A.R.C.; Mano, J.F.; Sousa, R.A.; Reis, R.L. PDLLA enriched with ulvan particles as a novel 3D porous scaffold targeted for bone engineering. *J. Supercrit. Fluids* **2012**, *65*, 32–38. [CrossRef]

130. Morelli, A.; Chiellini, F. Ulvan as a new type of biomaterial from renewable resources: Functionalization and hydrogel preparation. *Macromol. Chem. Phys.* **2010**, *211*, 821–832. [CrossRef]

131. Toskas, G.; Heinemann, S.; Heinemann, C.; Cherif, C.; Hund, R.D.; Roussis, V.; Hanke, T. Ulvan and ulvan/chitosan polyelectrolyte nanofibrous membranes as a potential substrate material for the cultivation of osteoblasts. *Carbohydr. Polym.* **2012**, *89*, 997–1002. [CrossRef] [PubMed]

132. Barros, A.A.; Alves, A.; Nunes, C.; Coimbra, M.A.; Pires, R.A.; Reis, R.L. Carboxymethylation of ulvan and chitosan and their use as polymeric components of bone cements. *Acta Biomater.* **2013**, *9*, 9086–9097. [CrossRef] [PubMed]

133. Bansal, V.; Sharma, P.K.; Sharma, N.; Pal, O.P.; Malviya, R. Applications of chitosan and chitosan derivatives in drug delivery. *Adv. Biol. Res.* **2011**, *5*, 28–37.

134. Rinaudo, M. Chitin and chitosan: Properties and applications. *Prog. Polym. Sci.* **2006**, *31*, 603–632. [CrossRef]

135. Alves, N.M.; Mano, J.F. Chitosan derivatives obtained by chemical modifications for biomedical and environmental applications. *Int. J. Biol. Macromol.* **2008**, *43*, 401–414. [CrossRef] [PubMed]

136. Varum, K.M.; Myhr, M.M.; Hjerde, R.J.; Smidsrod, O. *In vitro* degradation rates of partially N-acetylated chitosans in human serum. *Carbohydr. Res.* **1997**, *299*, 99–101. [CrossRef]

137. Agnihotri, S.A.; Mallikarjuna, N.N.; Aminabhavi, T.M. Recent advances on chitosan-based micro- and nanoparticles in drug delivery. *J. Control. Release* **2004**, *100*, 5–28. [CrossRef] [PubMed]

138. Sinha, V.R.; Singla, A.K.; Wadhawan, S.; Kaushik, R.; Kumria, R.; Bansal, K.; Dhawan, S. Chitosan microspheres as a potential carrier for drugs. *Int. J. Pharm.* **2004**, *274*, 1–33. [CrossRef] [PubMed]
139. Prabaharan, M.; Mano, J.F. Chitosan-based particles as controlled drug delivery systems. *Drug Deliv.* **2005**, *12*, 41–57. [CrossRef] [PubMed]
140. Couto, D.S.; Hong, Z.; Mano, J.F. Development of bioactive and biodegradable chitosan-based injectable systems containing bioactive glass nanoparticles. *Acta Biomater.* **2009**, *5*, 115–123. [CrossRef] [PubMed]
141. Rabea, E.I.; Badawy, M.E.; Stevens, C.V.; Smagghe, G.; Steurbaut, W. Chitosan as antimicrobial agent: Applications and mode of action. *Biomacromolecules* **2003**, *4*, 1457–1465. [CrossRef] [PubMed]
142. Kim, I.Y.; Seo, S.J.; Moon, H.S.; Yoo, M.K.; Park, I.Y.; Kim, B.C.; Cho, C.S. Chitosan and its derivatives for tissue engineering applications. *Biotechnol. Adv.* **2008**, *26*, 1–21. [CrossRef] [PubMed]
143. Qin, C.Q.; Du, Y.M.; Xiao, L.; Li, Z.; Gao, X.H. Enzymic preparation of water-soluble chitosan and their antitumor activity. *Int. J. Biol. Macromol.* **2002**, *31*, 111–117. [CrossRef]
144. Chung, M.J.; Park, J.K.; Park, Y.I. Anti-inflammatory effects of low-molecular weight chitosan oligosaccharides in IgE-antigen complex-stimulated RBL-2H3 cells and asthma model mice. *Int. Immunopharmacol.* **2012**, *12*, 453–459. [CrossRef] [PubMed]
145. Ilium, L. Chitosan and its use as a pharmaceutical excipient. *Pharm. Res.* **1998**, *15*, 1326–1331. [CrossRef]
146. Singla, A.; Chawla, M. Chitosan: Some pharmaceutical and biological aspects—An update. *J. Pharm. Pharmacol.* **2001**, *53*, 1047–1067. [CrossRef] [PubMed]
147. Bhise, K.S.; Dhumal, R.S.; Paradkar, A.R.; Kadam, S.S. Effect of drying methods on swelling, erosion and drug release from chitosan-naproxen sodium complexes. *AAPS PharmSciTech* **2008**, *9*, 1–12. [CrossRef] [PubMed]
148. Felt, O.; Buri, P.; Gurny, R. Chitosan: A unique polysaccharide for drug delivery. *Drug Dev. Ind. Pharm.* **1998**, *24*, 979–993. [CrossRef] [PubMed]
149. Prabaharan, M.; Reis, R.L.; Mano, J.F. Carboxymethyl chitosan-graft-phosphatidylethanolamine: Amphiphilic matrices for controlled drug delivery. *React. Funct. Polym.* **2007**, *67*, 43–52. [CrossRef]
150. Prabaharan, M.; Mano, J.F. Hydroxypropyl chitosan bearing beta-cyclodextrin cavities: Synthesis and slow release of its inclusion complex with a model hydrophobic drug. *Macromol. Biosci.* **2005**, *5*, 965–973. [CrossRef] [PubMed]
151. Jayakumar, R.; Reis, R.L.; Mano, J.F. Synthesis and characterization of pH-sensitive thiol-containing chitosan beads for controlled drug delivery applications. *Drug Deliv.* **2007**, *14*, 9–17. [CrossRef] [PubMed]
152. Prabaharan, M.; Mano, J.F. A novel pH and thermo-sensitive *N,O*-carboxymethyl chitosan-graft-poly(*N*-isopropylacrylamide) hydrogel for controlled drug delivery. *E-Polymers* **2007**, *7*, 503–516. [CrossRef]
153. Le Tien, C.; Lacroix, M.; Ispas-Szabo, P.; Mateescu, M.A. *N*-acylated chitosan: Hydrophobic matrices for controlled drug release. *J. Control. Release* **2003**, *93*, 1–13. [CrossRef]
154. Martin, L.; Wilson, C.G.; Koosha, F.; Uchegbu, I.F. Sustained buccal delivery of the hydrophobic drug denbufylline using physically cross-linked palmitoyl glycol chitosan hydrogels. *Eur. J. Pharm. Biopharm.* **2003**, *55*, 35–45. [CrossRef]
155. Jiang, G.B.; Quan, D.; Liao, K.; Wang, H. Novel polymer micelles prepared from chitosan grafted hydrophobic palmitoyl groups for drug delivery. *Mol. Pharm.* **2006**, *3*, 152–160. [CrossRef] [PubMed]
156. Wijekoon, A.; Fountas-Davis, N.; Leipzig, N.D. Fluorinated methacrylamide chitosan hydrogel systems as adaptable oxygen carriers for wound healing. *Acta Biomater.* **2013**, *9*, 5653–5664. [CrossRef] [PubMed]
157. Prashanth, K.V.H.; Tharanathan, R.N. Chitin/chitosan: Modifications and their unlimited application potential—An overview. *Trends Food Sci. Technol.* **2007**, *18*, 117–131. [CrossRef]
158. Thanou, M.; Verhoef, J.C.; Junginger, H.E. Oral drug absorption enhancement by chitosan and its derivatives. *Adv. Drug Deliv. Rev.* **2001**, *52*, 117–126. [CrossRef]
159. Andrade, F.; Goycoolea, F.; Chiappetta, D.A.; das Neves, J.; Sosnik, A.; Sarmento, B. Chitosan-grafted copolymers and chitosan-ligand conjugates as matrices for pulmonary drug delivery. *Int. J. Carbohydr. Chem.* **2011**, *2011*, 1–14. [CrossRef]
160. Zhang, M.; Li, X.H.; Gong, Y.D.; Zhao, N.M.; Zhang, X.F. Properties and biocompatibility of chitosan films modified by blending with PEG. *Biomaterials* **2002**, *23*, 2641–2648. [CrossRef]
161. Casettari, L.; Vllasaliu, D.; Castagnino, E.; Stolnik, S.; Howdle, S.; Illum, L. PEGylated chitosan derivatives: Synthesis, characterizations and pharmaceutical applications. *Prog. Polym. Sci.* **2012**, *37*, 659–685. [CrossRef]

162. Prego, C.; Fabre, M.; Torres, D.; Alonso, M.J. Efficacy and mechanism of action of chitosan nanocapsules for oral peptide delivery. *Pharm. Res.* **2006**, *23*, 549–556. [CrossRef] [PubMed]

163. Mao, S.; Germershaus, O.; Fischer, D.; Linn, T.; Schnepf, R.; Kissel, T. Uptake and transport of PEG-graft-trimethyl-chitosan copolymer-insulin nanocomplexes by epithelial cells. *Pharm. Res.* **2005**, *22*, 2058–2068. [CrossRef] [PubMed]

164. Mao, S.; Shuai, X.; Unger, F.; Wittmar, M.; Xie, X.; Kissel, T. Synthesis, characterization and cytotoxicity of poly(ethylene glycol)-graft-trimethyl chitosan block copolymers. *Biomaterials* **2005**, *26*, 6343–6356. [CrossRef] [PubMed]

165. Zhang, X.; Zhang, H.; Wu, Z.; Wang, Z.; Niu, H.; Li, C. Nasal absorption enhancement of insulin using PEG-grafted chitosan nanoparticles. *Eur. J. Pharm. Biopharm.* **2008**, *68*, 526–534. [CrossRef] [PubMed]

166. Jintapattanakit, A.; Junyaprasert, V.B.; Mao, S.; Sitterberg, J.; Bakowsky, U.; Kissel, T. Peroral delivery of insulin using chitosan derivatives: A comparative study of polyelectrolyte nanocomplexes and nanoparticles. *Int. J. Pharm.* **2007**, *342*, 240–249. [CrossRef] [PubMed]

167. Bhattarai, N.; Ramay, H.R.; Gunn, J.; Matsen, F.A.; Zhang, M. PEG-grafted chitosan as an injectable thermosensitive hydrogel for sustained protein release. *J. Control. Release* **2005**, *103*, 609–624. [CrossRef] [PubMed]

168. Wu, J.; Su, Z.G.; Ma, G.H. A thermo- and pH-sensitive hydrogel composed of quaternized chitosan/glycerophosphate. *Int. J. Pharm.* **2006**, *315*, 1–11. [CrossRef] [PubMed]

169. Wu, J.; Wei, W.; Wang, L.Y.; Su, Z.G.; Ma, G.H. A thermosensitive hydrogel based on quaternized chitosan and poly(ethylene glycol) for nasal drug delivery system. *Biomaterials* **2007**, *28*, 2220–2232. [CrossRef] [PubMed]

170. Nazar, H.; Fatouros, D.G.; van der Merwe, S.M.; Bouropoulos, N.; Avgouropoulos, G.; Tsibouklis, J.; Roldo, M. Thermosensitive hydrogels for nasal drug delivery: The formulation and characterisation of systems based on N-trimethyl chitosan chloride. *Eur. J. Pharm. Biopharm.* **2011**, *77*, 225–232. [CrossRef] [PubMed]

171. Tahrir, F.G.; Ganji, F.; Ahooyi, T.M. Injectable thermosensitive chitosan/glycerophosphate-based hydrogels for tissue engineering and drug delivery applications: A review. *Recent Pat. Drug Deliv. Formul.* **2015**, *9*, 107–120. [CrossRef] [PubMed]

172. Roy, K.; Mao, H.Q.; Huang, S.K.; Leong, K.W. Oral gene delivery with chitosan—DNA nanoparticles generates immunologic protection in a murine model of peanut allergy. *Nat. Med.* **1999**, *5*, 387–391. [PubMed]

173. Borchard, G. Chitosans for gene delivery. *Adv. Drug Deliv. Rev.* **2001**, *52*, 145–150. [CrossRef]

174. Sato, T.; Ishii, T.; Okahata, Y. *In vitro* gene delivery mediated by chitosan. Effect of pH, serum, and molecular mass of chitosan on the transfection efficiency. *Biomaterials* **2001**, *22*, 2075–2080. [CrossRef]

175. Leong, K.W.; Mao, H.Q.; Truong-Le, V.L.; Roy, K.; Walsh, S.M.; August, J.T. DNA-polycation nanospheres as non-viral gene delivery vehicles. *J. Control. Release* **1998**, *53*, 183–193. [CrossRef]

176. Saranya, N.; Moorthi, A.; Saravanan, S.; Devi, M.P.; Selvamurugan, N. Chitosan and its derivatives for gene delivery. *Int. J. Biol. Macromol.* **2011**, *48*, 234–238. [CrossRef] [PubMed]

177. De Smedt, S.C.; Demeester, J.; Hennink, W.E. Cationic polymer based gene delivery systems. *Pharm. Res.* **2000**, *17*, 113–126. [CrossRef] [PubMed]

178. Cho, Y.W.; Kim, J.D.; Park, K. Polycation gene delivery systems: Escape from endosomes to cytosol. *J. Pharm. Pharmacol.* **2003**, *55*, 721–734. [CrossRef] [PubMed]

179. Kean, T.; Roth, S.; Thanou, M. Trimethylated chitosans as non-viral gene delivery vectors: Cytotoxicity and transfection efficiency. *J. Control. Release* **2005**, *103*, 643–653. [CrossRef] [PubMed]

180. Kievit, F.M.; Veiseh, O.; Bhattarai, N.; Fang, C.; Gunn, J.W.; Lee, D.; Ellenbogen, R.G.; Olson, J.M.; Zhang, M. PEI–PEG–chitosan-copolymer-coated iron oxide nanoparticles for safe gene delivery: Synthesis, complexation, and transfection. *Adv. Funct. Mater.* **2009**, *19*, 2244–2251. [CrossRef] [PubMed]

181. Costa, R.R.; Martín, L.; Mano, J.F.; Rodríguez-Cabello, J.C. Elastin-like macromolecules. In *Biomimetic Approaches for Biomaterials Development*; Mano, J.F., Ed.; Wiley-VCH Verlag: Weinheim, Germany, 2012; pp. 93–116.

182. Costa, R.R.; Custodio, C.A.; Arias, F.J.; Rodriguez-Cabello, J.C.; Mano, J.F. Nanostructured and thermoresponsive recombinant biopolymer-based microcapsules for the delivery of active molecules. *Nanomed. NBM* **2013**, *9*, 895–902. [CrossRef] [PubMed]

183. Afratis, N.; Gialeli, C.; Nikitovic, D.; Tsegenidis, T.; Karousou, E.; Theocharis, A.D.; Pavão, M.S.; Tzanakakis, G.N.; Karamanos, N.K. Glycosaminoglycans: Key players in cancer cell biology and treatment. *FEBS J.* **2012**, *279*, 1177–1197. [CrossRef] [PubMed]

184. Burdick, J.A.; Prestwich, G.D. Hyaluronic acid hydrogels for biomedical applications. *Adv. Mater.* **2011**, *23*, H41–H56. [CrossRef] [PubMed]

185. Kogan, G.; Soltes, L.; Stern, R.; Gemeiner, P. Hyaluronic acid: A natural biopolymer with a broad range of biomedical and industrial applications. *Biotechnol. Lett.* **2007**, *29*, 17–25. [CrossRef] [PubMed]

186. Lee, H.; Lee, K.; Kim, I.K.; Park, T.G. Synthesis, characterization, and *in vivo* diagnostic applications of hyaluronic acid immobilized gold nanoprobes. *Biomaterials* **2008**, *29*, 4709–4718. [CrossRef] [PubMed]

187. Chen, W.Y.; Abatangelo, G. Functions of hyaluronan in wound repair. *Wound Repair Regen.* **1999**, *7*, 79–89. [CrossRef] [PubMed]

188. Kim, S.J.; Park, S.Y.; Kim, C.W. A novel approach to the production of hyaluronic acid by streptococcus zooepidemicus. *J. Microbiol. Biotechnol.* **2006**, *16*, 1849–1855.

189. Vazquez, J.A.; Montemayor, M.I.; Fraguas, J.; Murado, M.A. High production of hyaluronic and lactic acids by *Streptococcus zooepidemicus* in fed-batch culture using commercial and marine peptones from fishing by-products. *Biochem. Eng. J.* **2009**, *44*, 125–130. [CrossRef]

190. Rangaswamy, V.; Jain, D. An efficient process for production and purification of hyaluronic acid from *Streptococcus equi* subsp. *Zooepidemicus. Biotechnol. Lett.* **2008**, *30*, 493–496. [CrossRef] [PubMed]

191. Murado, M.A.; Montemayor, M.I.; Cabo, M.L.; Vazquez, J.A.; Gonzalez, M.P. Optimization of extraction and purification process of hyaluronic acid from fish eyeball. *Food Bioprod. Process.* **2012**, *90*, 491–498. [CrossRef]

192. Zhong, S.P.; Campoccia, D.; Doherty, P.J.; Williams, R.L.; Benedetti, L.; Williams, D.F. Biodegradation of hyaluronic acid derivatives by hyaluronidase. *Biomaterials* **1994**, *15*, 359–365. [CrossRef]

193. Lokeshwar, V.B.; Rubinowicz, D.; Schroeder, G.L.; Forgacs, E.; Minna, J.D.; Block, N.L.; Nadji, M.; Lokeshwar, B.L. Stromal and epithelial expression of tumor markers hyaluronic acid and HYAL1 hyaluronidase in prostate cancer. *J. Biol. Chem.* **2001**, *276*, 11922–11932. [CrossRef] [PubMed]

194. Rousseau, J.C.; Delmas, P.D. Biological markers in osteoarthritis. *Nat. Clin. Pract. Rheumatol.* **2007**, *3*, 346–356. [CrossRef] [PubMed]

195. Santos, J.R.; Alves, N.M.; Mano, J.F. New thermo-responsive hydrogels based on poly (*N*-isopropylacrylamide)/hyaluronic acid semi-interpenetrated polymer networks: Swelling properties and drug release studies. *J. Bioact. Compat. Polym.* **2010**, *25*, 169–184. [CrossRef]

196. Kurisawa, M.; Chung, J.E.; Yang, Y.Y.; Gao, S.J.; Uyama, H. Injectable biodegradable hydrogels composed of hyaluronic acid-tyramine conjugates for drug delivery and tissue engineering. *Chem. Commun.* **2005**, 4312–4314. [CrossRef] [PubMed]

197. Lee, F.; Chung, J.E.; Kurisawa, M. An injectable hyaluronic acid-tyramine hydrogel system for protein delivery. *J. Control. Release* **2009**, *134*, 186–193. [CrossRef] [PubMed]

198. Xu, K.; Lee, F.; Gao, S.; Tan, M.H.; Kurisawa, M. Hyaluronidase-incorporated hyaluronic acid-tyramine hydrogels for the sustained release of trastuzumab. *J. Control. Release* **2015**, *216*, 47–55. [CrossRef] [PubMed]

199. Oyarzun-Ampuero, F.A.; Brea, J.; Loza, M.I.; Torres, D.; Alonso, M.J. Chitosan-hyaluronic acid nanoparticles loaded with heparin for the treatment of asthma. *Int. J. Pharm.* **2009**, *381*, 122–129. [CrossRef] [PubMed]

200. Lim, S.T.; Martin, G.P.; Berry, D.J.; Brown, M.B. Preparation and evaluation of the *in vitro* drug release properties and mucoadhesion of novel microspheres of hyaluronic acid and chitosan. *J. Control. Release* **2000**, *66*, 281–292. [CrossRef]

201. de la Fuente, M.; Seijo, B.; Alonso, M.J. Novel hyaluronic acid-chitosan nanoparticles for ocular gene therapy. *Invest. Ophthalmol. Vis. Sci.* **2008**, *49*, 2016–2024. [CrossRef] [PubMed]

202. Contreras-Ruiz, L.; de la Fuente, M.; Parraga, J.E.; Lopez-Garcia, A.; Fernandez, I.; Seijo, B.; Sanchez, A.; Calonge, M.; Diebold, Y. Intracellular trafficking of hyaluronic acid-chitosan oligomer-based nanoparticles in cultured human ocular surface cells. *Mol. Vis.* **2011**, *17*, 279–290. [PubMed]

203. Grech, J.M.R.; Mano, J.F.; Reis, R.L. Chitosan beads as templates for layer-by-layer assembly and their application in the sustained release of bioactive agents. *J. Bioact. Compat. Polym.* **2008**, *23*, 367–380. [CrossRef]

204. Simoes, S.; Moreira, J.N.; Fonseca, C.; Duzgunes, N.; de Lima, M.C. On the formulation of pH-sensitive liposomes with long circulation times. *Adv. Drug Deliv. Rev.* **2004**, *56*, 947–965. [CrossRef] [PubMed]

205. Jiang, T.; Zhang, Z.; Zhang, Y.; Lv, H.; Zhou, J.; Li, C.; Hou, L.; Zhang, Q. Dual-functional liposomes based on pH-responsive cell-penetrating peptide and hyaluronic acid for tumor-targeted anticancer drug delivery. *Biomaterials* **2012**, *33*, 9246–9258. [CrossRef] [PubMed]

206. Kramer, M.W.; Escudero, D.O.; Lokeshwar, S.D.; Golshani, R.; Ekwenna, O.O.; Acosta, K.; Merseburger, A.S.; Soloway, M.; Lokeshwar, V.B. Association of hyaluronic acid family members (HAS1, HAS2, and HYAL-1) with bladder cancer diagnosis and prognosis. *Cancer* **2011**, *117*, 1197–1209. [CrossRef] [PubMed]

207. Luo, Y.; Kirker, K.R.; Prestwich, G.D. Cross-linked hyaluronic acid hydrogel films: New biomaterials for drug delivery. *J. Control. Release* **2000**, *69*, 169–184. [CrossRef]

208. Mohammad, E.-D.; Xuefei, H. Biological applications of hyaluronic acid functionalized nanomaterials. In *Petite and Sweet: Glyco-Nanotechnology as a Bridge to New Medicines*; Xuefei, H., Barchi, J., Jr., Eds.; American Chemical Society: Washington, DC, USA, 2011; Volume 1091, pp. 181–213.

209. Lokeshwar, V.B.; Obek, C.; Pham, H.T.; Wei, D.; Young, M.J.; Duncan, R.C.; Soloway, M.S.; Block, N.L. Urinary hyaluronic acid and hyaluronidase: Markers for bladder cancer detection and evaluation of grade. *J. Urol.* **2000**, *163*, 348–356. [CrossRef]

210. Leroy, V.; Monier, F.; Bottari, S.; Trocme, C.; Sturm, N.; Hilleret, M.N.; Morel, F.; Zarski, J.P. Circulating matrix metalloproteinases 1, 2, 9 and their inhibitors TIMP-1 and TIMP-2 as serum markers of liver fibrosis in patients with chronic hepatitis C: Comparison with PIIINP and hyaluronic acid. *Am. J. Gastroenterol.* **2004**, *99*, 271–279. [CrossRef] [PubMed]

211. Teien, A.N.; Abildgaard, U.; Hook, M. The anticoagulant effect of heparan sulfate and dermatan sulfate. *Thromb. Res.* **1976**, *8*, 859–867. [CrossRef]

212. Lindahl, U.; Lidholt, K.; Spillmann, D.; Kjellen, L. More to heparin than anticoagulation. *Thromb. Res.* **1994**, *75*, 1–32. [CrossRef]

213. Clegg, D.O.; Reda, D.J.; Harris, C.L.; Klein, M.A.; O'Dell, J.R.; Hooper, M.M.; Bradley, J.D.; Bingham III, C.O.; Weisman, M.H.; Jackson, C.G.; *et al.* Glucosamine, chondroitin sulfate, and the two in combination for painful knee osteoarthritis. *N. Engl. J. Med.* **2006**, *354*, 795–808. [CrossRef] [PubMed]

214. Wang, D.A.; Varghese, S.; Sharma, B.; Strehin, I.; Fermanian, S.; Gorham, J.; Fairbrother, D.H.; Cascio, B.; Elisseeff, J.H. Multifunctional chondroitin sulphate for cartilage tissue-biomaterial integration. *Nat. Mater.* **2007**, *6*, 385–392. [CrossRef] [PubMed]

215. Santo, V.E.; Gomes, M.E.; Mano, J.F.; Reis, R.L. Chitosan-chondroitin sulphate nanoparticles for controlled delivery of platelet lysates in bone regenerative medicine. *J. Tissue Eng. Regener. Med.* **2012**, *6*, S47–S59. [CrossRef] [PubMed]

216. Zhao, L.; Liu, M.; Wang, J.; Zhai, G. Chondroitin sulfate-based nanocarriers for drug/gene delivery. *Carbohydr. Polym.* **2015**, *133*, 391–399. [CrossRef] [PubMed]

217. Strehin, I.; Nahas, Z.; Arora, K.; Nguyen, T.; Elisseeff, J. A versatile pH sensitive chondroitin sulfate-PEG tissue adhesive and hydrogel. *Biomaterials* **2010**, *31*, 2788–2797. [CrossRef] [PubMed]

218. Guo, Y.M.; Shi, X.M.; Fang, Q.L.; Zhang, J.; Fang, H.; Jia, W.L.; Yang, G.; Yang, L. Facile preparation of hydroxyapatite-chondroitin sulfate hybrid mesoporous microrods for controlled and sustained release of antitumor drugs. *Mater. Lett.* **2014**, *125*, 111–115. [CrossRef]

219. Vitale, C.; Berutti, S.; Bagnis, C.; Soragna, G.; Gabella, P.; Fruttero, C.; Marangella, M. Dermatan sulfate: An alternative to unfractionated heparin for anticoagulation in hemodialysis patients. *J. Nephrol.* **2013**, *26*, 158–163. [CrossRef] [PubMed]

220. Mourao, P.A.; Pereira, M.S. Searching for alternatives to heparin: Sulfated fucans from marine invertebrates. *Trends Cardiovasc. Med.* **1999**, *9*, 225–232. [CrossRef]

221. Davenport, A. Alternatives to standard unfractionated heparin for pediatric hemodialysis treatments. *Pediatr. Nephrol.* **2012**, *27*, 1869–1879. [CrossRef] [PubMed]

222. Trowbridge, J.M.; Gallo, R.L. Dermatan sulfate: New functions from an old glycosaminoglycan. *Glycobiology* **2002**, *12*, 117R–125R. [CrossRef] [PubMed]

223. Kreuger, J.; Spillmann, D.; Li, J.P.; Lindahl, U. Interactions between heparan sulfate and proteins: The concept of specificity. *J. Cell. Biol.* **2006**, *174*, 323–327. [CrossRef] [PubMed]

224. Kovalszky, I.; Dudás, J.; Oláh-Nagy, J.; Pogány, G.; Továry, J.; Timár, J.; Kopper, L.; Jeney, A.; Iozzo, R.V. Inhibition of DNA topoisomerase I activity by heparin sulfate and modulation by basic fibroblast growth factor. *Mol. Cell. Biochem.* **1998**, *183*, 11–23. [CrossRef] [PubMed]

225. Sasisekharan, R.; Shriver, Z.; Venkataraman, G.; Narayanasami, U. Roles of heparan-sulphate glycosaminoglycans in cancer. *Nat. Rev. Cancer* **2002**, *2*, 521–528. [CrossRef] [PubMed]

226. Stewart, M.D.; Sanderson, R.D. Heparan sulfate in the nucleus and its control of cellular functions. *Matrix Biol.* **2014**, *35*, 56–59. [CrossRef] [PubMed]

227. Vlodavsky, I.; Ilan, N.; Naggi, A.; Casu, B. Heparanase: Structure, biological functions, and inhibition by heparin-derived mimetics of heparan sulfate. *Curr. Pharm. Des.* **2007**, *13*, 2057–2073. [CrossRef] [PubMed]

228. Lindahl, U.; Kjellen, L. Pathophysiology of heparan sulphate: Many diseases, few drugs. *J. Intern. Med.* **2013**, *273*, 555–571. [CrossRef] [PubMed]
229. Knelson, E.H.; Nee, J.C.; Blobe, G.C. Heparan sulfate signaling in cancer. *Trends Biochem. Sci.* **2014**, *39*, 277–288. [CrossRef] [PubMed]
230. Uchimura, K. Keratan sulfate: Biosynthesis, structures, and biological functions. In *Glycosaminoglycans*; Kuberan, B., Hiroshi, N., Desai, U.R., Eds.; Springer: Berlin/Heidelberg, Germany, 2015; pp. 389–400.
231. Funderburgh, J.L. Keratan sulfate biosynthesis. *IUBMB Life* **2002**, *54*, 187–194. [CrossRef] [PubMed]
232. Geisert, E.E., Jr.; Bidanset, D.J.; del Mar, N.; Robson, J.A. Up-regulation of a keratan sulfate proteoglycan following cortical injury in neonatal rats. *Int. J. Dev. Neurosci.* **1996**, *14*, 257–267. [CrossRef]
233. Ueno, R.; Miyamoto, K.; Tanaka, N.; Moriguchi, K.; Kadomatsu, K.; Kusunoki, S. Keratan sulfate exacerbates experimental autoimmune encephalomyelitis. *J. Neurosci. Res.* **2015**, *93*, 1874–1880. [CrossRef] [PubMed]
234. Usov, A.I. Structural analysis of red seaweed galactans of agar and carrageenan groups. *Food Hydrocoll.* **1998**, *12*, 301–308. [CrossRef]
235. Hoare, T.R.; Kohane, D.S. Hydrogels in drug delivery: Progress and challenges. *Polymer* **2008**, *49*, 1993–2007. [CrossRef]
236. Rossi, F.; Santoro, M.; Casalini, T.; Veglianese, P.; Masi, M.; Perale, G. Characterization and degradation behavior of agar-carbomer based hydrogels for drug delivery applications: Solute effect. *Int. J. Mol. Sci.* **2011**, *12*, 3394–3408. [CrossRef] [PubMed]

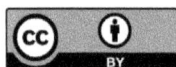

marine drugs

MDPI

Review

Fucoidans in Nanomedicine

Lucas Chollet [1,2,3,†], Pierre Saboural [1,2,†], Cédric Chauvierre [1,2], Jean-Noël Villemin [3], Didier Letourneur [1,2] and Frédéric Chaubet [1,2,*]

[1] Inserm, U1148, LVTS, University Paris Diderot, X Bichat Hospital, F-75877 Paris, France; lucas.chollet@algues-et-mer.com (L.C.); pierre.saboural@univ-paris13.fr (P.S.); cedric.chauvierre@inserm.fr (C.C.); didier.letourneur@inserm.fr (D.L.)
[2] Galilée Institute, University Paris 13, Sorbonne Paris Cité, F-93430 Villetaneuse, France
[3] Algues & Mer, Kernigou, F-29242 Ouessant, France; jn.villemin@algues-et-mer.com
* Correspondence: frederic.chaubet@univ-paris13.fr; Tel.: +33-1-4940-4090; Fax: +33-1-4940-3008
† These authors contributed equally to this work.

Academic Editor: Paola Laurienzo
Received: 17 June 2016; Accepted: 21 July 2016; Published: 29 July 2016

Abstract: Fucoidans are widespread cost-effective sulfated marine polysaccharides which have raised interest in the scientific community over last decades for their wide spectrum of bioactivities. Unsurprisingly, nanomedicine has grasped these compounds to develop innovative therapeutic and diagnostic nanosystems. The applications of fucoidans in nanomedicine as imaging agents, drug carriers or for their intrinsic properties are reviewed here after a short presentation of the main structural data and biological properties of fucoidans. The origin and the physicochemical specifications of fucoidans are summarized in order to discuss the strategy of fucoidan-containing nanosystems in Human health. Currently, there is a need for reproducible, well characterized fucoidan fractions to ensure significant progress.

Keywords: fucoidans; nanomedicine; sulfated polysaccharides; nanosystems; drug delivery; imaging agent; tissue regeneration

1. Introduction

Fucoidans are abundant cost-effective marine polysaccharides which exhibit a wide spectrum of biological activities with potential clinical applications. For more than half a century, extensive works have been published about the activities of these molecules; some of the most recent reviews are listed in Table 1. Recently, nanomedicine began to incorporate the use of fucoidans especially in the domains of cancer, regenerative medicine, and cardiovascular diseases, fields in which nanotechnologies are making progress every day. Since 2005, reports on fucoidans in nanomedicine have increased to represent about 7% of the overall works in 2014 related to both topics (Figure 1).

This review focuses on the progress at the interface of fucoidans and nanomedicine in the perspective of development of new diagnostic and therapeutic tools for human use. In the first part, fucoidans and their biological properties are briefly presented and in the second part the main studies of fucoidans with regard to developments in nanomedicine are given. In the last part, we discuss the relevance of these studies in light of the structural data of fucoidans and we question an appropriate strategy for the development of fucoidans for human applications.

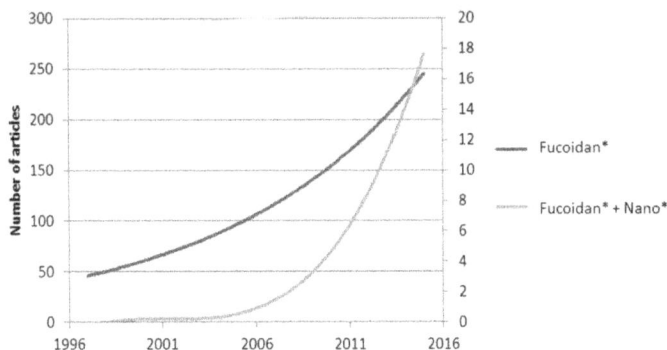

Figure 1. Evolution of published articles reporting fucoidans (from Web of Science). Left axis: number of articles for "Fucoidan*", right axis: number of articles for "Fucoidan* + Nano*".

2. What Are Fucoidans?

Fucoidans belong to a large family of marine sulfated polysaccharides named fucans mainly constituted of sulfated L-fucose, which include also ascophyllans (xylofucoglycuronan and xylofucomanuronan) and sargassans (glycuronofucogalactan) [1,2]. Fucoidans were first discovered in 1913 by Kylin in brown algae: *Ascophyllum nodosum, Fucus vesiculosus, Laminaria digitata* and *Laminaria saccharina* [3]. Since then, fucoidans have been identified in 70 more species of brown algae (*Phaeophyceae*) [4–12], in the body wall of some marine invertebrates such as sea cucumber (*Holothuroidae*), and in the egg jelly coat of sea urchins (*Echinoidea*) [4,13,14].

Fucoidans are contained in the extracellular matrix (ECM) of brown algae's cell walls [1]. Considering the eco-physiological influences (alga species, location and season of harvesting, the position on the intertidal zone, etc.) on the composition of fucoidans, they are implicated in the ionic and osmotic regulation and in the mechanical support of the cell wall [2,15]. Thus, the algae which have been most exposed to drying seem to contain the highest fucoidan content. In sea urchin, fucoidans play a role in the fertilization process since they are found in the surrounding coating of the female gamete (zona pellucida) and participate in the species-specific acrosome reaction [16,17]. In sea cucumber, fucoidans could be involved in the structural support of the body wall in the saline environment, as for algae [18].

The chemical composition of fucoidans is extremely variable depending on eco-physiological parameters. The first structure was elucidated in 1950 by Conchie and Percival from a fucoidan extracted from *Fucus vesiculosus* [19]. Kloareg et al. determined that fucoidans were composed of 50%–90% of L-fucose, 35%–45% of sulfate and less than 8% of uronic acid with a linear backbone based on an $\alpha(1{\rightarrow}2)$-glycosidic linkage of O-4 sulfated L-fucose and some oses like galactose, mannose, xylose, and glucose [1,2]. In 1993, Patankar et al. published a revised structure of a commercial fucoidan from *F. vesiculosus*: mainly an $\alpha(1{\rightarrow}3)$-L-fucose linear backbone with sulfate substitution at O-4 and some α-L-fucose branched at O-4 or O-2 [20]. Thereafter, studies on fucoidans' structure evidenced different repeating units for highly purified fucoidan fractions from different species [21–28]. Structures are based on an $\alpha(1{\rightarrow}3)$-L-fucose backbone with some alternating $\alpha(1{\rightarrow}4)$ linkages. The sulfation patterns are variable but sulfate groups are mainly found at O-2 and O-4 [29,30]. Fucoidans extracted from marine animals have a more regular chemical structure (Figure 2).

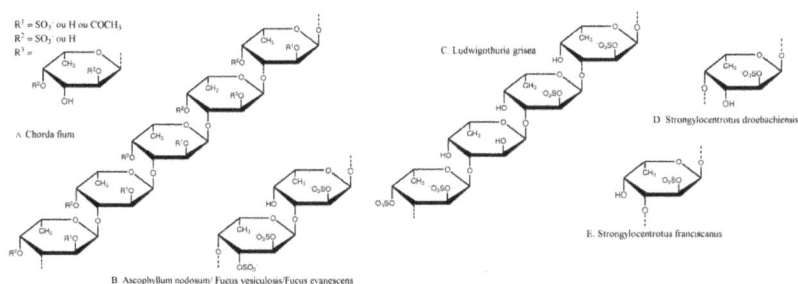

Figure 2. Repeating chemical structures of some fucoidans from brown algae (**A**) *Chorda filum* [28]; (**B**) *Ascophyllum* nodosum, *Fucus vesiculosus*, and *Fucus evanescens* [22,23,31] and from marine invertebrates: sea cucumber (*Holothuriodea*) (**C**) *Ludwigothuria grisea* [29]; (**D**) *Strongylocentrotus droebachiensis* [17], and (**E**) *Strongylocentrotus franciscanus* [30].

There are almost as many methods of extraction of fucoidans from brown algae as there are studies dealing with these polysaccharides. However a general pattern can be proposed: a first extraction with organic solvents (e.g., acetone, toluene, etc.) from the fresh materials provides dried extracts which can be treated with methanol, ethanol or formaldehyde to remove hydrophobic compounds like dyes and lipids. The remaining alginates are precipitated with calcium, followed by acidic and sometimes alkaline hydrolyses at temperatures ranging from ambient up to 100 °C, enabling both to discard non-fucoidan polysaccharides (in particular laminarin) and decrease the molecular weight of the fractions. More recently, microwave assisted extractions have been developed [32]. The extraction conditions influence the final chemical composition of the fucoidan fractions [9,12] which remain complex mixtures of macromolecular species with large molecular weight distributions (100–1000 kDa). Although it is now widely admitted that the term "fucoidan" refers to a sulfated-L-fucose based polymer, it is still not possible to speak of a single compound; "fucoidans" should always be used as a generic term as was first proposed by Larsen in 1966 [33] and a fraction specifically prepared should be referred to as "a fucoidan fraction"(FF). Both terms will be used in this review.

The bioactivities of low molecular weight FF were found to mimic those of heparin, a glycosaminoglycan of animal origin with a molecular weight of about 15 kDa. As a consequence, depolymerization methods of raw fucoidans were developed: by acid hydrolysis [9], by radical cleavage [34], by enzymatic degradation (fucoidanases) from bacteria as well as digestive secretion of mollusk [35–39], and by gamma irradiation [40–42]. These methods could often cause structural alteration (like debranching and desulfation) likely affecting the biological activities. An alternative approach to extraction methods is the synthesis of FF, either with enzymes or through a full chemical process. Fucoidanases, enzymes extracted from marine invertebrates, marine fungi or bacteria, are able to selectively degrade the fucose-based backbone of fucoidans offering structurally well-defined and biologically active fragments. Silchenko et al. isolated several fucoidanases [37,43] and developed a method for the screening and the detection of these enzymes in bacterial colonies [39]. Nifantiev et al. achieved the chemical synthesis of oligofucosides up to hexadecafucosides [44,45] with controlled sulfation patterns, allowing different types of FF to be obtained: some fractions were built up of (1→3)-linked α-L-fucose residues similar to the one found in *Laminaria saccharina* [24,27] or *Chorda filum* [28] and others were built up of alternating (1→3)- and (1→4)-linked α-L-fucose residues as found in *Ascophyllum nodosum* or *Fucus evanescens* as examples. These bottom-up approaches could be used to synthesize a wide range of FF with well-defined structures, improving the knowledge in the structure-biological activity relationships for these molecules. Although, tremendous progress in glycobiology and glycomedicine has driven the development in oligosaccharide synthesis [46], either with the aid of enzymes or by full synthesis, industrial preparation of tailor-made FF remains still hard to achieve due to low overall yields and the time needed to complete the process. Interestingly, there is currently no standard method to obtain reproducible bioactive well defined FF either from top-down or bottom-up strategies.

3. Biological Properties of Fucoidans

The interest of the scientific community in fucoidans and their low molecular weight fractions (i.e., below 30 kDa) is mainly driven by the wide spectrum of biological activities evidenced from their discovery up to now. Table 1 gathers the main biological effects reported and the identified targets. Over the last decades, new functions of polysaccharides and more specifically low molecular weight (LMW) fractions have attracted the interest of scientists for their ability to act in a wide variety of biological processes [47]. Structural variations such as degrees of substitution with chemical groups (in particular carboxylates, acetates or sulfates) are implicated in biological responses [48,49] and their activities are often attributed to their negative charges and sulfation degrees rather than to any specific carbohydrate structure as described for heparin [50]. Low molecular weight fractions from mammalian, glycosaminoglycans (GAGs) and more particularly low molecular weight-GAGs from heparin, heparan sulfate, hyaluronate, and chondroitin sulfate are implicated in a wide variety of biological processes as cofactors for growth factor, cytokines and chemokines production, tumorigenesis, signaling molecules in response to infection or other cellular damage, regulator of blood coagulation, and assisting viral and bacterial infections [51–53], the most active compounds being neutral or anionic structures partially acetylated or sulfated.

So far, multiple targets have been identified in blood and tissues to explain the biological activities of fucoidans. The anticoagulant activity, one of the most studied with reference to heparin, can be explained by the interactions of fucoidans towards natural thrombin inhibitors, serpins antithrombin, and heparin cofactor II, enhancing their activity [11]. P- and L-selectins, membrane proteins which play a role in the leukocyte rolling and extravasation process in vascular inflammatory response, have been reported and studied as the main targets in the anti-inflammatory activity of fucoidans [54,55]. Likewise, the inhibition of complement activation through classical and alternative pathways, also responsible for fucoidans anti-inflammatory activity, occurs by inhibiting formation or function of several complement's enzymes such as C4, C4b,2a, C3, and C3b,Bb [56].

Table 1. Biological properties of fucoidans and identified targets.

Biological Properties	Identified Targets	References
Anticoagulant/anti-thrombotic	Antithrombin, heparin cofactor II	[11,34,57–59]
Anti-complement	C4, C4b,2a, C3, and C3b,Bb	[56,59,60]
Anti-viral	CD4	[61–68]
Anti-inflammatory	P-selectin and L-selectin	[54,55,59,69–76]
Angiogenic effect	VEGFs, bFGF, FGF-2//α6, β1, and PECAM-1 integrin subunits	[10,11,54,59,77–87]
Anti-cancer	Capsases-3, -8 and -9, MAPK and their inhibitors, HIF-1	[29,88–110]
Anti-diabetic	α-glucosidase, α-amylase	[111–118]
Immune potentiating	NK cells, T-cells, dendritic cells	[119–123]
Antioxidant	-	[124–141]

Antiviral activity is ensured by the binding of fucoidans to the CD4 glycoprotein on T lymphocytes, an essential immunoglobulin in the infection process of host cells by the viruses [67]. Fucoidans, especially fucoidans with high sulfation content, inhibit α-glucosidase and α-amylase, two digestive enzymes, increasing or interrupting the absorption delay of glucose. The most sulfated fractions have an inhibitory effect more pronounced than the less sulfated ones and electrostatic interactions are likely involved [112,113]. In tissues, fucoidans have an effect on several enzymes responsible for mitosis or cellular apoptosis such as caspases-3, -8 and -9 or mitogen-activated protein kinase (MAPK) and their inhibitors [91,92,102], enhancing or silencing these factors in opposite ways in cancer cells or healthy cells (protective effect). Furthermore, LMW fucoidan fractions inhibit the accumulation of hypoxia-inducible factors-1 (HIF-1) which promote tumor angiogenesis in cancer cells [99].

The biological activities of fucoidans seem mainly modulated by their molecular weight and their sulfate content, which, as previously stated depend on the starting material and the method of preparation. One of the most striking examples is the anti/pro-angiogenic activity. Pomin et al. evidenced that fucoidans of various origins exhibit an anti-angiogenic activity due to their ability to interfere with vascular endothelial growth factors (VEGFs) and basic fibroblast growth factor (FGF-2) [11]. However, Matou et al. showed the pro-angiogenic effect of fucoidans, also extracted from *Ascophyllum nodosum*, by enhancing the expression of α6, β1, and PECAM-1 integrin subunits on the surface of endothelial cells, resulting in an increase of FGF-2-induced angiogenesis [85]. Nifantiev et al. reviewed numerous studies on the angiogenic activities of fucoidans from different brown algae to highlight structure-activity relationships. They could only conclude that FF from *Ascophyllum nodosum* with MW over 30 kDa exhibited anti-angiogenic activity whereas FF with MW lower than 30 kDa exhibited pro-angiogenic activity [10].

Fucoidans exhibit several bioactivities against a wide spectrum of pathological situations with a remarkable absence of adverse effects. On one hand, it is now widely accepted that levels of L-fucose and sulfate as well as the molecular weight are major structural parameters whose variation affect the biological properties. On the other hand, each algae species produces its own type of fucoidan whose composition also depends on the conditions of obtaining. Pharmaceutical grade fucoidans with well-defined molecular weight distributions and thoroughly defined chemical compositions are now needed. It is necessary to obtain proper structure-activity relationships in order to select the most relevant FF for human clinical trials.

4. Fucoidans in Nanomedicine

Nanomedecine, also defined as nanotechnology in the biomedical field, has gained considerably in interest in the last decade. Nanosystems, such as, in a non-exhaustive way, nanoparticles, polymeric carriers, nanotubes, micelles, and liposomes have size-dependent properties and nanometer-scale dimensions which play important roles in biological systems. For half a century, they have been developed for therapeutic and diagnostic purposes and more recently have found tremendous applications in regenerative medicine with the development of nanostructured biocompatible scaffolds for cell organization and proliferation [142]. Moreover, nanotheranostics or theranostic nanomedicines have also been developed combining diagnosis and therapy to monitor both the release and the bioavailability of the drug at the proper pathological site [143]. The major interest of nanomedicine remains for drug delivery and personalized medicine defined as "the right drug to the right patient at the right moment" [144,145]. Most of these new biomedical tools are currently employed for treatments via oral or parenteral administration to fight cancer, iron deficiency or multiple sclerosis as examples [142]. Lovrić et al. reviewed the marketed products and those with the greatest potential [142].

Sulfated polysaccharides, especially fucoidans have been included in nanosystems for diagnostic, drug delivery, and tissue engineering [146,147]. Fucoidans have also been used as stabilizers of nanoparticles (NPs) [148–152] or to study the behavior of the aqueous suspension of chitosan/fucoidan-based NPs [153–155]. These works will not be detailed here since this review is dedicated to FF-containing nanosystems with direct applications to diagnosis and therapy. Table 2 assembles such applications, mainly with fucoidan-containing nanoparticles (FNPs), and the most relevant are explained in the following text. Table 3 indicates the origin and physicochemical data of FF used in these 31 reported studies.

Table 2. Applications of fucoidan-containing nanosystems in nanomedicine.

Application	References
Imaging agent	[156–162]
Protein delivery	[163–167]
Small drug delivery	[168–176]
Anti-coagulant	[177,178]
Gene delivery	[179,180]
Regenerative medicine	[181–186]

Table 3. Features of the fucoidan fractions used in nanomedicine related studies.

Study	Objective	Origin of Fucoidans	Molecular Weight	Sulfate Content *	Other Data	Remarks
Bonnard et al. [157,159]	P-selectin targeting FMPs for SPECT imaging	*F. vesiculosus*	57 kDa/23 kDa	-	-	Commercial fucoidans from Sigma Aldrich Company
Changotade et al. [185]	Pretreatment of bone tissue substitute	-	-	-	-	-
Da Silva et al. [178]	FNPs preparation for therapeutic purposes	*F. vesiculosus*	-	-	-	Commercial fucoidans from Sigma Aldrich Company
Huang et al. [169]	Gentamicin controlled release	*F. vesiculosus*	-	-	-	Commercial fucoidans from Sigma Aldrich Company
Huang et al. [174]	Curcumin controlled release	*F. vesiculosus*	-	-	-	Commercial fucoidans from Sigma Aldrich Company
Huang et al. [165]	FGF-2 controlled release with FNPs	*F. vesiculosus*	80 kDa	-	-	Commercial fucoidans from Sigma Aldrich Company
Huang et al. [166]	SDF-1 controlled release with FNPs	*F. vesiculosus*	80 kDa	-	-	Commercial fucoidans from Sigma Aldrich Company
Jeong et al. [182]	Design of a scaffold for bone tissue regeneration		-	-	-	-
Jin et al. [186]	Design of a scaffold for bone tissue regeneration	*U. pinnatifida*	-	-	-	Commercial fucoidans from Haewon Biotech Company
Kimura et al. [172]	Evaluation of cytotoxic effects of FNPs	*C. okamuranus*	2–10 kDa	-	-	Fucoidans extracted and purified by the authors
Kurosaki et al. [180]	DNA delivery with FMPs	-	-	-	-	Commercial fucoidans from Sigma Aldrich Company
Lee et al. [171]	DOX controlled release with FNPs	*F. vesiculosus*	-	-	-	Commercial fucoidans from Sigma Aldrich Company
Lee et al. [187]	Electrospun mats for Tissue engineering	*U. pinnatifida*	-	34.2%	62.12% total polysaccharide	Commercial fucoidans from Haewon Biotech Company
Li et al. [162]	P-selectin targeting FMPs for PET imaging	-	-	-	-	Commercial fucoidans from Sigma Aldrich Company
Lira et al. [188]	Preparation and evaluation of FNPs	*S. cymosum*	53 kDa	-	-	Fucoidans extracted and purified by the authors

Table 3. *Cont.*

Study	Objective	Origin of Fucoidans	Molecular Weight	Sulfate Content *	Other Data	Remarks
Lowe et al. [183]	Design of a scaffold for bone tissue regeneration	*F. vesiculosus*	-	-	-	Commercial fucoidans from Sigma Aldrich Company
Nakamura et al. [164]	FGF-2 controlled release	*K. crassifolia*	-	-	-	Fucoidans extracted and purified by the authors
Park et al. [167]	ALA controlled release with FMNs	-	-	-	-	Commercial fucoidans from Haewon Biotech Company
Pinheiro et al. [176]	PLL controlled release	*F. vesiculosus*	57.26 kDa	-	40.2% Fuc, 2.98% Xyl, 0.55% Man, 3.6% Gal, 9.17% Ur.Ac, 0.11% Rha, 0.21% Glu	Commercial fucoidans from Sigma Aldrich Company
Puvaneswary et al. [184]	Design of a scaffold for bone tissue regeneration	*F. vesiculosus*	-	-	-	Commercial fucoidans from Sigma Aldrich Company
Sezer et al. [179]	DNA delivery with FMPs	*F. vesiculosus*	80 kDa	-	-	Commercial fucoidans from Sigma Aldrich Company
Sezer et al. [189,190]	FNPs for dermal burns treatment	*F. vesiculosus*	80 kDa	-	-	Commercial fucoidans from Sigma Aldrich Company
Suzuki et al. [191]	P-selectin targeting FNPs for MRI imaging	*A. nodosum*	8 kDa	27%	45% L-fucose, 25% D-glucuronic acid	Commercial fucoidans from Algues et Mer Company
Venkatesan et al. [181]	Design of a scaffold for bone tissue regeneration	-	-	-	-	-
Wu et al. [175]	Berberine controlled release	-	80 kDa	-	-	Commercial fucoidans from NOVA Pharma & Liposome Biotech Company
Yu et al. [168]	Berberine controlled release	*L. japonica*	-	24.3%	3.5% carboxyl groups	Commercial fucoidans from NOVA Pharma & Liposome Biotech Company
Yu et al. [96]	Oversulfated FF release via oral route	*F. vesiculosus*	80 kDa	41.7%	-	Commercial fucoidans from NOVA Pharma & Liposome Biotech Company

* g/100 g.

4.1. Fucoidans in Therapeutic Nanosystems

In 2006, Sezer and Akbuga were the first to design FNPs named "fucospheres" from mixtures of fucoidan and chitosan for drug delivery purposes [163]. Two years later, they demonstrated the efficacy of fucospheres from the same origin over chitosan-based NPs in the treatment of dermal burns in rabbits [189,190]. The fucospheres size ranged from 300 nm to 1000 nm with surface charges from +6 to +26 mV and were tested in vitro on freshly excised chicken back skin. Then, in vivo tests were conducted on rabbits with the most efficient FNPs and the authors observed the highest level of wound healing after 21 days in groups treated with fucospheres as compared to those treated with chitosan microspheres or FF solution. FF has been found to accelerate the healing effects on dermal burns when coupled with chitosan which is able to re-epithelize and encourage fibroblast migration to the burn sites.

At the same time, Nakamura et al. designed FF/chitosan microparticles loaded with fibroblast growth factor 2 (FGF-2) [164]. FF was purified from the starting material with calcium chloride. FGF-2-loaded microparticles were then subcutaneously injected and neovascularization was observed in ischemic tissue in a mice model.

In 2013, another group synthesized FGF-2-loaded spherical nanoparticles, by dripping a mixture of FF and FGF-2 into a solution of chitosan under stirring [165]. This study evaluated the release of the growth factor in vitro and its effect on the differentiation of PC12 neural progenitor cells evidencing a synergistic activity on nerve cell growth as compared to FGF-2 in solution alone.

Chitosan/FF/tripolyphosphate NPs were synthesized and loaded with stromal cell-derived factor-1 (SDF-1) as a therapeutic agent for tissue regeneration by Huang et al. [166]. FNPs were efficient in protecting SDF-1 from inactivation by proteolysis, heat, and pH and the released SDF-1 was able to improve the proliferation and the migration of rat mesenchymal stem cells for up to seven days.

In 2009, Sezer et al. also used fucospheres to encapsulate and to deliver plasmid DNA encoding GM-GSF [179]. The diameter ranged from 150 to 400 nm with a zeta potential from 8.3 mV to 17.1 mV depending on the chitosan molecular weight. The encapsulation capacity was evaluated between 84% and 95% depending on the chitosan molecular weight and the amount of plasmid added to the loading solution. Once encapsulated in fucospheres, the plasmid was released in vitro and its integrity was validated. No tests on cells or in vivo experiments have been published yet.

The same year, Kurosaki et al. developed a ternary complex FF/pDNA/Polyethylenimine [180]. The complexes had 72 nm mean diameter and -27 mV zeta potential. FNPs were tested on B16-F10 mouse melanoma cells to assess the uptake and the transfection efficiency in vitro. They showed no cytotoxicity as compared to the pDNA/PEI NPs after 2 h of incubation and a concentration of 10 mg/mL of pDNA. However, when added to the B16-F10 cells, FNPs showed significantly lower uptakes and gene expression as compared to fucoidan-free NPs.

Pinheiro et al. synthesized chitosan/fucoidan multilayer nanocapsules (FNCs) as a vector for the controlled release of poly-L-lysine (PLL), a polypeptide exhibiting strong antimicrobial activity, as a drug model [176]. Ten chitosan/fucoidan layers were formed over a polystyrene core removed after synthesis by repeated dipping in THF. The encapsulation of PLL was better when performed during the formation of the NCs. The encapsulation efficiency and the loading capacity of FNCs strongly depended on the initial PLL concentration used, with the highest values obtained at a PLL concentration of 1 mg·mL^{-1}. PLL release from the FNCs was found to be pH-dependent with a maximum at pH 2 due to a weakening of the nanocapsules interpolyelectrolyte structure and suggested a peculiar release behavior. Due to the bioactivities and non-cytotoxicity of FF and chitosan, FNCs were envisaged by the authors as nanocarriers to protect and release bioactive compounds for food and pharmaceutical applications.

Yu et al. prepared chitosan-based beads embedded with FNPs for oral delivery of berberine, an antimicrobial agent used to inhibit the growth of bacteria in the digestive system [168]. The NPs/beads complexes inhibited the growth of *Staphylococcus aureus* and *Escherichia coli* in simulated gastric or intestinal fluids. Complexes also demonstrated a delayed drug release over

24 h in simulated gastric fluid, which could be suitable for later drug delivery to the small intestine. Another group developed chitosan/fucoidan-taurine conjugate NPs to deliver berberine via the oral route to treat defective intestinal epithelial tight junction barrier [175]. The release of berberine was found to be pH-dependent with higher release at intestinal pH (7.4) than gastric pH (2.0). In vitro, the authors demonstrated the protective effect of the FNPs on Caco-2 cell monolayer, as a model of the epithelial barrier, co-cultured with LPS-treated RAW 264.7 cells. The results suggested the utility of such FNPs in allowing local delivery of berberine on bacterial-derived lipopolysaccharides intestinal epithelia tight junction disruption, to restore barrier function in inflammatory and injured intestinal epithelium.

Huang et al. developed antioxidant FNPs for antibiotic delivery to the lungs [169]. The use of FF was explained by their antioxidant and anti-inflammatory properties in order to treat pulmonary allergic inflammations. FNPs size ranged from 230 nm to 250 nm and their compactness and stability were maintained for 25 days. They exhibited highly potent antioxidant effects by scavenging 1,1-diphenyl-2-picrylhydrazyl (DPPH), and reducing the concentration of intracellular reactive oxygen species (ROS) as well as superoxide anion in stimulated macrophages. As an antibiotic model drug, Gentamicin (GM) was used for controlled release assays in vitro. The FNPs released 99% of GM over 72 h after an initial 10 h burst release. They were considered as potential carriers for antibiotics delivery to the lungs in the case of pulmonary infections and to be useful to treat airway inflammatory diseases.

In order to deliver drugs with low solubility and high pH sensitivity, Huang et al. developed O-carboxymethyl chitosan/fucoidan NPs to increase cellular curcumin uptake (Cur), a polyphenolic compound exhibiting several biological activities such as antitumor, antioxidant, inhibiting cardiovascular diseases, and inducing apoptosis [174]. Cur-loaded FNPs (Cur-FNPs) had an average diameter of 270 nm and encapsulated 92.8% of the drug. Cur-FNPs considerably decreased the cytotoxicity of Cur to mouse fibroblasts cells (L929), were stable in the gastric environment (pH 2.5), and allowed the release of Cur in the simulated intestinal environment (pH 7.4). The cellular uptake of Cur-FNPs was evaluated using Caco-2 cells. An internalization of Cur-FNPs by the cells through energy-dependent endocytic pathways was observed making O-carboxymethyl chitosan/fucoidan NPs potential carriers in oral delivery systems.

Park et al. prepared core/shell microparticles by co-axial electro-spray drying [167]. FF was mixed with the antioxidant α-lipoic acid (ALA). The size of the microparticles ranged from 5.4 to 8.4 μm. FF and ALA were detected within the core, and the chitosan within the shell of the microparticles. These composite microparticles were able to gel by water uptake and then swelled, contrary to the physical mixture of FF and chitosan; the swelling was found to depend on pH with a decrease for pH values higher than 7. In the same way, decreasing the chitosan/FF ratio lowered the swelling of the hydrogel. Finally, the release behavior of ALA from the gel was validated in vitro in different pH media by applying different electric potentials, inducing the drug release. The cumulative amounts of released ALA were quantified over 48 h to conclude that not only a declining concentration gradient occurred but also that the physical gelation between FF and chitosan over time reduced the diffusion of ALA, resulting in a unique release behavior with possible applications in drug delivery systems, wound healing dressings or scaffolds.

Lee et al. combined the immunotherapeutic activity of an acetylated FF with self-organized nanospheres loaded with doxorubicin (DOX) [171]. FNPs reached a 71% loading efficiency and the release followed a first order kinetic. FNPs were incubated for 24 h with RAW-264.7 macrophages, then tumor necrosis factor α (TNF-α) and granulocyte-macrophage colony-stimulating factor (GM-CSF) expression levels were measured. TNF-α expression was improved by a factor of 1.13 and GM-CSF by a factor of 1.86 as compared to unloaded FNPs and free DOX in a multidrug resistant cell model. Finally, these FNPs were considered as good candidates for combined immunotherapy and chemotherapy.

In the development of an oral drug delivery system, chitosan was found to modulate the opening of the tight junctions of epithelial cells [177]. Da Silva et al. prepared fucospheres with anti-coagulant properties for oral delivery by a nanocoacervation [178]. The size of FNPs ranged from 198 to 352 nm mean diameter and their zeta potential was measured between 35 and 53 mV. The anticoagulant activity of aqueous suspensions of these fucospheres was not found significantly different from that of FF, and FNPs did not show cytotoxicity for Caco-2 cells up to 1 mg/mL after 3 h of incubation.

At the same time, Yu et al. designed fucospheres to release an over sulfated FF via the oral route [96]. FNPs were able to go through a Caco-2 cell monolayer by opening the tight junctions. Eventually, it was found that released over sulfated FF had a higher anti-angiogenic activity than native FF.

By mixing FF and soybean lecithin in a homogenizer, Kimura et al. prepared unilamellar liposomes mixed with FF (FFL) of 100 nm and compared their cytotoxic effects with the native FF on osteosarcoma in vitro and in vivo [172]. FFL were found to reduce the viability of human osteosarcoma cell line 143B in vitro with a maximum inhibition for 2 mg/mL of liposome and 72 h of incubation. In addition, FFL were more potent than FF to induce apoptosis in cells. Mice were inoculated with murine osteosarcoma LM8 tumor cells and treated with FFL or native FF. FFL induced a reduction of the volume and the weight of the tumor compared to FF-treated mice.

Lira et al. compared in 2011 the cytotoxicity on macrophages and fibroblast murine cell lines of FNPs obtained by coating poly(isobutylcyanoacrylate) (PIBCA) with a blend of dextran and FF with two methods, a redox radical emulsion polymerization (RREP) and an anionic emulsion polymerization (AEP) [188]. FNPs prepared by the former were four times less toxic than those prepared by the latter. The authors also observed that FNPs obtained by RREP were not stable with a ratio FF/dextran of over 25, while FNPs obtained by AEP were stable in suspension with 100% FF as coating material.

4.2. Fucoidans in Diagnostic Nanosystems

Nanosystems for diagnosis must be blood compatible and non-toxic at concentrations sufficient for recording relevant images of the region of interest. To a large extent, sulfated polysaccharides could meet these criteria as vectors of imaging markers. Among these, fucoidans have been evidenced as good candidates to image atherothrombosis in vivo [156,191], and still awaited are studies evidencing their usefulness for cancer imaging.

In 2011, Rouzet et al. showed the direct complexation of ^{99m}Tc by a commercial FF allowing SPECT imaging of thrombosis and heart ischemia thanks to the interaction of FF with P-selectin overexpressed by activated platelet and activated endothelium [158]. Biodistribution studies of ^{99m}Tc-labelled FF in rat by SPECT imaging evidenced a urinary elimination and a moderate liver and spleen uptake which decreased with a fraction obtained from treatment with calcium ions of FF [160].

With the same FF, Suzuki et al. evidenced the capacity of superparamagnetic FNPs to detect in vivo the intraluminal thrombus of abdominal aortic aneurysm in a rat model with a 4.7 T MR Imager [191]. FNPs were obtained by linking FF to the carboxymethyldextran shell of Ultrasmall Superparamagnetic Iron oxide (USPIO). FNPs had a size of 50 nm and a zeta-potential of −14.3 mV. Surface Plasmon Resonance experiments evidenced an affinity of the FNPs for P-selectin in 1–10 nM range compared to NPs coated only with carboxymethyldextran, in accordance with previous work of Bachelet et al. [55]. Other in vitro studies showed the capacity of these FNPs to bind to activated human platelets [156].

Bonnard et al. developed polysaccharide-based NPs from dextran and pullulan cross-linked with sodium trimetaphosphate (STMP) in a water-in-oil emulsion [157,161]. FF was added to the emulsion to provide NPs functionalized with fucoidans (FNPs) with an average hydrodynamic diameter of 358 nm and a zeta-potential of −16 mV. MPFs contained about 1.6% (*w/w*) of FF and energy dispersive X-ray (EDX) spectrum showed the presence of FF at the surface of the particles. The interaction of MPFs with activated human platelets was validated in vitro. MPFs were radiolabeled with ^{99m}Tc [158] and used to image an aneurysmal thrombus in a rat model. Iron oxide embedded MPFs showed a high affinity for activated Human platelets in vitro and MR images of aneurysmal thrombus and activated endothelium were also obtained in murine models [159]. In another study, the authors developed MPFs containing

USPIO for magnetic resonance imaging [159]. On animal models a significant contrast enhancement of thrombus was obtained from 30 min to 2 h after the injection of MPFs.

In 2014, Li et al. developed a contrast agent for PET imaging [162]. FF was labelled with gallium 68 to image vulnerable active atherosclerosis plaques expressing P-selectin. After the validation with in vitro and ex vivo studies, they localized atherosclerotic plaques on an apolipoprotein E–deficient mice model using PET imaging. Anatomic structures of plaque were confirmed by 17.6 T MRI to correlate their results. The P-selectin affinity PET tracer was found to discriminate active and inactive atherosclerotic plaques.

4.3. Fucoidans in Regenerative Medicine

Marine polysaccharides have been used for years to design scaffolds for tissue engineering due to their interesting bioactivities and their biocompatibility. Senni et al. reviewed the studies in this field [192]. Particularly, fucoidans have raised interest in the design of biocomposites, especially for bone tissue engineering. So it is not surprising to find now the most advanced developments in this domain although there are still comparatively very few studies.

In 2008, Changotade et al. treated a commercial bone substitute (Lubboc®) with a low molecular weight FF (LMWF) to improve bone regeneration [185]. The authors found out that the pretreatment of the bone substitute with LMWF promotes human osteoblast proliferation, collagen type I expression and favors alkaline phosphatase activity enhancing the mineralization of the bone tissue. Regarding the origin and structure of LMWF used, the authors refer to older works without specifying any product parameter used in their study.

Three years later, Jin et al. developed polycaprolactone (PCL)/fucoidan composite scaffolds for bone tissue regeneration [186]. PCL/FF scaffolds with a 300 μm pore size dramatically increased the hydrophilic properties (with ⩾5 wt % of fucoidans). In addition mechanical properties were improved even with a low fucoidan/PCL ratio (as an example: a 22% increase of Young's modulus at 10 wt % of fucoidans). The biocompatibility of the scaffolds was assessed on osteoblast's-like-cells (MG63) evidencing a better cell adhesion to the surface of the FF-containing scaffolds with three times more mineralization compared to the pure PCL scaffold after 14 days of cell culture. At the same time, Lee et al. prepared a biocomposite of polycaprolactone (PCL) and FF [187]. The biocomposite showed a better distribution of osteoblast-like cells (MG63) compared to pure PCL mats. Furthermore, total protein content, alkaline phosphatase activity, and calcium mineralization were better and were higher with PCL/FF micro/nanofibrous mats suggesting that FF-complemented biocomposites would make good candidates for tissue engineering applications.

Since 2013, S. K. Kim's group has been developing scaffolds from hydroxyapatite/polysaccharide-based nanocrystals for bone tissue regeneration [181–183]. Chitosan/alginate scaffold (CAS) and chitosan/alginate/fucoidan scaffold (CAFFS) were first prepared. CAFFS with a pore size of 56–437 nm improved cytocompatibility, proliferation, and alkaline phosphatase secretion of MG63 osteosarcoma cells as compared to CAS. In addition, protein adsorption and mineralization were two times greater with CAFFS, which was attributed to the negative charges of FF sulfate groups. Then, they prepared scaffolds from hydroxyapatite (HapS) and hydroxyapatite mixed with FF (HapFFS) to induce FGF-2 activity and angiogenesis [182]. HapFFS showed a mineralization effect two times higher than HapS. Scaffolds obtained more recently by mixing HapFFS with chitosan evidenced a better mineralization as well as a good biocompatibility with mesenchymal stem cells (PMSCs) likely due to a suitable micro architecture for cell growth and nutrient supplementation [183]. Note that no data about the FF were provided for the two first studies.

In 2015, Puvaneswary et al. prepared tricalcium phosphate-chitosan-fucoidan biocomposite scaffold and demonstrated the benefic effect of FF [184]. They showed that the addition of FF in the scaffold increased the release of osteocalcin allowing the osteogenic differentiation of human mesenchymal stromal cells in vitro. Furthermore, FF was found to improve the compression strength and the biomineralization of the scaffolds.

5. Discussion

Fucoidan-containing nanosystems were first developed for the delivery of different therapeutic agents [147] followed by studies on regenerative medicine and more recently on diagnostics. Most of them focused on structures obtained from a mixture of FF and chitosan, a cationic polysaccharide with a random alternation of $\beta(1\rightarrow4)$-D-glucosamine, and N-acetyl-D-glucosamine. The formation of these nanosystems occurs from electrostatic interactions between sulfate and ammonium groups to generate multilayer architectures stable over a wide range of pH values and suitable for oral or parenteral administration. Different methods were used to obtain fucoidan-containing nanosystems such as emulsion, self-assembly, coacervation, polyelectrolyte complexing or ionic cross-linking, all without risks of modification of the polymer structure. Although, in some cases, fucoidans were used for their intrinsic biological properties, for most of these studies they appear to have been used more for an ability to form stable structures with chitosan, as well as for pre-supposed harmlessness. Interestingly, physicochemical data for chitosan are often more detailed than for FF for which they are in general limited and sometimes even absent. Indeed, as evidenced in Table 3, in most cases the origin of FF is the only information provided, and, as a consequence, it is difficult to compare the results. Only three studies provide sufficient characteristics to the readers, and additional works are needed for discussion [158,176,191]. On one hand, this lack of structural data does not allow drugs to be created based on these polysaccharides [193]. On the other hand, the developments for Human health improvements require well-defined reproducible fucoidan fractions. If not, the conclusions are unique for a particular fraction, and, as a consequence, the results cannot be reproduced.

Fucoidans are polysaccharides, one of the three families of natural macromolecules with proteins and nucleic acids. Scientists have been able to fully synthesize the latter two for several decades. However the complexity of fucoidan structures has significantly delayed this essential step in their development to Human health, and overall progress in this domain suffers from a lack of tools such as those that are readily available for studying nucleic acids and proteins. More generally, once a particular carbohydrate structure has been identified as being responsible for a biological effect, it often has to be synthesized in order to establish or confirm its structure assignment. Nevertheless, dedicated synthesis methods are time-consuming, limited to oligosaccharides, and practiced mostly by specialized laboratories using processes that may take months to years because of the structural complexity of these compounds. As a consequence, despite the prevalent role of polysaccharides and oligosaccharides in a wide range of biological processes, it is not surprising that there are so few carbohydrate based therapeutics and diagnostics on the market. In addition to monosaccharide-inspired drugs such as the influenza virus treatment Tamiflu (oseltamivir phosphate; Roche, Bâle, Switzerland), two drugs: acarbose (Precose, Glucobay; Bayer, Leverkusen, Germany) and heparin, stand out [194]. Note that both compounds were derived by isolation and reached the clinic before a detailed structure–activity relationship had been established. In particular, low molecular weight heparin (LMWH) (lovenox; Sanofi, Gentilly, France), mainly extracted from pig intestines and fractioned via chromatography, chemical cleavage or enzymatic hydrolysis, is still the only polysaccharide used in Human health since its first clinical trial reported in the early 80's [195–198]. FF production follows the same process but the raw material is from vegetal origin, thereby preventing all contaminations attributed to animal products. However Health agencies have hardened the legislation about new pharmaceuticals in the last decade due to health scandals (in particular implicating LMWH in 2008 [199]), making FF more difficult to reach the market or even impossible without a reliable source. Anyway, scientists and companies who want to develop fucoidan-containing nanosystems up to clinical use must provide robust data about their product.

Nanomedicine approaches have revolutionized the treatment of human pathologies, in particular cancer and cardiovascular diseases [200,201]. Drugs are entrapped within sterically stabilized, long-circulating vehicles (therapeutics). Imaging markers such as radiolabels, USPIO or quantum dots allow real-time visualization of pathological areas (diagnostics). The theranostic strategy associates both types in unique structures. These tailor-made nanosystems are built from polymers, carbon nanosheets, lipids, metal oxides etc., sometimes mixed to get hybrid structures, shaped as spheres, rods, capsules or more complicated geometry, and surface-modified to improve their efficacy and decrease side-toxicity. Ultimately they can be grafted with ligands to target cellular/molecular components of the diseases [200,201]. Bioactive carbohydrates, and in particular fucoidan fractions, are good candidates thanks to their overall biocompatibility, high versatility with regard to chemical modifications, and relatively low production costs. However the clinical development of fucoidan-based biospecific systems for nanomedicine remains a challenge because it requires not only a translational approach involving a partnership with pharmaceutical companies and respecting specifications approved by Health agencies [202] but also implementing a secure process to obtain reliable fractions.

In this context, we have considered a rational approach in order to develop a clinical contrast agent using FF (see [55,156,158,191]). From the pioneer works of Varki et al. [75], P-selectin was confirmed as a relevant molecular target of a commercial FF (Ascophyscient® from Algues & Mer, Ile d'Ouessant, France: a low molecular weight fucoidan fraction from *Ascophyllum nodosum*). In 2013, a joint laboratory was created with the Algues & Mer Company to secure the production of reproducible FF with well-defined composition and molecular weight. In 2015, these fucoidans were labeled by the French authorities as "raw materials for pharmaceutical uses". Today, they are part of the European project Nanoathero for the development of a SPECT marker for human atherothombosis [203] and clinical trials will start soon.

6. Conclusions

Fucoidans are abundant polysaccharides with remarkable biological properties. Their vegetal origins (considering that fucoidans extracted from marine animals are a tiny part of the total amount), the absence of adverse effects, and an affordable price due to easy-to-handle production processes make them promising for Human health. However these advantages are also the main bottlenecks for developments in nanomedicine due to the difficulty in obtaining reproducible chemical structures and molecular weights from one batch to another. Up to now, fucoidans in nanomedicine have been mainly used for protein or drug delivery with few studies about medical imaging; applications to regenerative medicine being still limited to bone tissue regeneration in animals. So far, isolation from natural sources is the only effective way to get fucoidans, but it is no longer possible to consider the molecular weight together with L-fucose and sulfate contents of a bioactive fraction as the only relevant parameters for further developments. The use of fucoidans in nanomedicine will be legitimated only by a translational strategy from a reproducible starting material with a defined and reproducible structure. This goal can be achieved only via two ways: (i) validation of an industrial production from natural extracts; or (ii) total synthesis with enzymes or chemical reactions. Currently, the first way is available; the second one is likely within the next decades [45]. The biomedical market represents an enormous opportunity for fucoidans, as their potential added value can, in principle, justify the inherent risk related with the development and approval of such products. Moreover, the possibility of developing a wide variety of chemically modified derivatives makes fucoidans versatile materials that could be applied in other fields of technological interest. This is a continuing challenge to polymer and biomaterial scientists, but it is already possible to anticipate that these strategic approaches will widen up perspectives and potential applications in the future.

Acknowledgments: This work was supported by Inserm and University Paris 13 and the competitiveness cluster Medicen Paris Region. P.S. is a recipient of the grant from University Paris 13 and IMOVA project founded by FUI/OSEO. L.C. is a recipient of a CIFRE grant from ANRT (ANR-13-RPIB-0006 "FucoThrombo"). The authors acknowledge the financial supports from FP7 NMP-LA-2012-309820 "NanoAthero", ANR-13-LAB1-0005-01 "FucoChem" and ANR-13-RPIB-0006 "FucoThrombo".

Conflicts of Interest: The founding sponsors had no role in the design of the study; in the collection, analyses, or interpretation of data; in the writing of the manuscript, and in the decision to publish the results.

References

1. Michel, G.; Tonon, T.; Scornet, D.; Cock, J.M.; Kloareg, B. The cell wall polysaccharide metabolism of the brown alga *Ectocarpus siliculosus*. Insights into the evolution of extracellular matrix polysaccharides in Eukaryotes. *New Phytol.* **2010**, *188*, 82–97. [CrossRef] [PubMed]
2. Kloareg, B.; Quatrano, R.S. Structure of the cell walls of marine algae and ecophysiological functions of the matrix polysaccharides. *Oceanogr. Mar. Biol.* **1988**, *26*, 259–315.
3. Kylin, H. Zur Biochemie der Meeresalgen. *Z. Physiol. Chem.* **1913**, *83*, 171–197. [CrossRef]
4. Berteau, O.; Mulloy, B. Sulfated fucans, fresh perspectives: Structures, functions, and biological properties of sulfated fucans and an overview of enzymes active toward this class of polysaccharide. *Glycobiology* **2003**, *13*, 29–40. [CrossRef] [PubMed]
5. Morya, V.K.; Kim, J.; Kim, E.K. Algal fucoidan: Structural and size-dependent bioactivities and their perspectives. *Appl. Microbiol. Biotechnol.* **2012**, *93*, 71–82. [CrossRef] [PubMed]
6. Li, B.; Lu, F.; Wei, X.; Zhao, R. Fucoidan: Structure and Bioactivity. *Molecules* **2008**, *13*, 1671–1695. [CrossRef] [PubMed]
7. Usov, A.I.; Bilan, M.I. Fucoidans—Sulfated polysaccharides of brown algae. *Russ. Chem. Rev.* **2009**, *78*, 785–799. [CrossRef]
8. Bilan, M.I.; Usov, A.I. Structural Analysis of Fucoidans. *Nat. Prod. Commun.* **2008**, *3*, 1639–1648.
9. Ale, M.T.; Meyer, A.S. Fucoidans from brown seaweeds: An update on structures, extraction techniques and use of enzymes as tools for structural elucidation. *RSC Adv.* **2013**, *3*, 8131–8141. [CrossRef]
10. Ustyuzhanina, N.E.; Bilan, M.I.; Ushakova, N.A.; Usov, A.I.; Kiselevskiy, M.V.; Nifantiev, N.E. Fucoidans: Pro- or antiangiogenic agents? *Glycobiology* **2014**, *24*, 1265–1274. [CrossRef] [PubMed]
11. Pomin, V.H. Fucanomics and galactanomics: Current status in drug discovery, mechanisms of action and role of the well-defined structures. *Biochem. Biophys. Acta* **2012**, *1820*, 1971–1979. [CrossRef] [PubMed]
12. Ale, M.T.; Mikkelsen, J.D.; Meyer, A.S. Important Determinants for Fucoidan Bioactivity: A Critical Review of Structure-Function Relations and Extraction Methods for Fucose-Containing Sulfated Polysaccharides from Brown Seaweeds. *Mar. Drugs* **2011**, *9*, 2106–2130. [CrossRef] [PubMed]
13. Vasseur, E.; Setälä, K.; Gjertsen, P. Chemical Studies on the Jelly Coat of the Sea-Urchin Egg. *Acta Chem. Scand.* **1948**, *2*, 900–913. [CrossRef]
14. Pomin, V.H. Fucanomics and Galactanomics: Marine Distribution, Medicinal Impact, Conceptions, and Challenges. *Mar. Drugs* **2012**, *10*, 793–811. [CrossRef] [PubMed]
15. Deniaud-Bouë, E.; Kervarec, N.; Michel, G.; Tonon, T.; Kloareg, B.; Hervé, C. Chemical and enzymatic fractionation of cell walls from Fucales: Insights into the structure of the extracellular matrix of brown algae. *Ann. Bot.* **2014**, *114*, 1203–1216. [CrossRef] [PubMed]
16. Alves, A.P.; Mulloy, B.; Diniz, J.A.; Mourao, P.A.S. Sulfated polysaccharides from the egg jelly layer are species-specific inducers of acrosomal reaction in sperms of sea urchins. *J. Biol. Chem.* **1997**, *272*, 6965–6971. [CrossRef] [PubMed]
17. Vilela-Silva, A.-C.E.S.; Castro, M.O.; Valente, A.-P.; Biermann, C.H.; Mourão, P.A.S. Sulfated fucans from the egg jellies of the closely related sea urchins *Strongylocentrotus droebachiensis* and *Strongylocentrotus pallidus* ensure species-specific fertilization. *J. Biol. Chem.* **2002**, *277*, 379–387. [CrossRef] [PubMed]
18. Mourão, P.A.; Bastos, I.G. Highly acidic glycans from sea cucumbers. Isolation and fractionation of fucose-rich sulfated polysaccharides from the body wall of *Ludwigothurea grisea*. *Eur. J. Biochem.* **1987**, *166*, 639–645. [CrossRef] [PubMed]
19. Conchie, J.; Percival, E.G.V. Fucoidin. Part II. The hydrolysis of a methylated fucoidin prepared from *Fucus vesiculosus*. *J. Chem. Soc.* **1950**, 827–832. [CrossRef]
20. Patankar, M.S.; Oehninger, S.; Barnett, T.; Williams, R.L.; Clark, G.F. A revised structure for fucoidan may explain some of its biological activities. *J. Biol. Chem.* **1993**, *268*, 21770–21776. [PubMed]
21. Nishino, T.; Nishioka, C.; Ura, H.; Nagumo, T. Isolation and partial characterization of a novel amino sugar-containing fucan sulfate from commercial *Fucus vesiculosus* fucoidan. *Carbohydr. Res.* **1994**, *255*, 213–224. [CrossRef]
22. Chevolot, L.; Mulloy, B.; Ratiskol, J.; Foucault, A.; Colliec-Jouault, S. A disaccharide repeat unit is the major structure in fucoidans from two species of brown algae. *Carbohydr. Res.* **2001**, *330*, 529–535. [CrossRef]

23. Bilan, M.I.; Grachev, A.A.; Ustuzhanina, N.E.; Shashkov, A.S.; Nifantiev, N.E.; Usov, A.I. Structure of a fucoidan from the brown seaweed *Fucus evanescens* C. Ag. *Carbohydr. Res.* **2002**, *337*, 719–730. [CrossRef]

24. Bilan, M.I.; Grachev, A.A.; Shashkov, A.S.; Kelly, M.; Sanderson, C.J.; Nifantiev, N.E.; Usov, A.I. Further studies on the composition and structure of a fucoidan preparation from the brown alga *Saccharina latissima*. *Carbohydr. Res.* **2010**, *345*, 2038–2047. [CrossRef] [PubMed]

25. Sinurat, E.; Peranginangin, R.; Saepudin, E. Purification and Characterization of Fucoidan from the Brown Seaweed *Sargassum binderi* Sonder. *Squalen Bull. Mar. Fish. Postharvest Biotechnol.* **2016**, *10*, 79–87. [CrossRef]

26. Luo, D.; Yuan, X.; Zeng, Y.; Nie, K.; Li, Z.; Wang, Z. Structure elucidation of a major fucopyranose-rich heteropolysaccharide (STP-II) from *Sargassum thunbergii*. *Carbohydr. Polym.* **2016**, *143*, 1–8. [CrossRef] [PubMed]

27. Usov, A.I.; Smirnova, G.P.; Bilan, M.I.; Shashkov, A.S. Polysaccharides of algae. 53. Brown alga *Laminaria saccharina* (L.) Lam. as a source of fucoidan. *Bioorg. Khim.* **1998**, *24*, 437–445.

28. Chizhov, A.O.; Dell, A.; Morris, H.R.; Haslam, S.M.; McDowell, R.A.; Shashkov, A.S.; Nifantiev, N.E.; Khatuntseva, E.A.; Usov, A.I. A study of fucoidan from the brown seaweed *Chorda filum*. *Carbohydr. Res.* **1999**, *320*, 108–119. [CrossRef]

29. Mulloy, B.; Ribeiro, A.C.; Alves, A.P.; Vieira, R.P.; Mourão, P.A. Sulfated fucans from echinoderms have a regular tetrasaccharide repeating unit defined by specific patterns of sulfation at the 0–2 and 0–4 positions. *J. Biol. Chem.* **1994**, *269*, 22113–22123. [PubMed]

30. Vilela-Silva, A.-C.E.S.; Alves, A.-P.; Valente, A.-P.; Vacquier, V.D.; Mourao, P.A.S. Structure of the sulfated alpha-L-fucan from the egg jelly coat of the sea urchin *Strongylocentrotus franciscanus*: Patterns of preferential 2-O- and 4-O-sulfation determine sperm cell recognition. *Glycobiology* **1999**, *9*, 927–933. [CrossRef] [PubMed]

31. Chevolot, L.; Foucault, A.; Chaubet, F.; Kervarec, N.; Sinquin, C.; Fisher, A.-M.; Boisson-Vidal, C. Further data on the structure of brown seaweed fucans: Relationships with anticoagulant activity. *Carbohydr. Res.* **1999**, *319*, 154–165. [CrossRef]

32. Yuan, Y.; Macquarrie, D.J. Microwave assisted step-by-step process for the production of fucoidan, alginate sodium, sugars and biochar from *Ascophyllum nodosum* through a biorefinery concept. *Bioresour. Technol.* **2015**, *198*, 819–827. [CrossRef] [PubMed]

33. Larsen, B.; Haug, A.; Painter, T.J. Sulphated Polysaccharides in Brown Algae. I. Isolation and Preliminary Characterisation of Three Sulphated Polysaccharides from *Ascophyllum nodosum*. *Acta Chem. Scand.* **1966**, *20*, 219–230. [CrossRef]

34. Nardella, A.; Chaubet, F.; Boisson-Vidal, C.; Blondin, C.; Durand, P.; Jozefonvicz, J. Anticoagulant low molecular weight fucans produced by radical process and ion exchange chromatography of high molecular weight fucans extracted from the brown seaweed *Ascophyllum nodosum*. *Carbohydr. Res.* **1996**, *289*, 201–208. [CrossRef]

35. Kusaykin, M.; Bakunina, I.; Sova, V.; Ermakova, S.; Kuznetsova, T.; Besednova, N.; Zaporozhets, T.; Zvyagintseva, T. Structure, biological activity, and enzymatic transformation of fucoidans from the brown seaweeds. *Biotechnol. J.* **2008**, *3*, 904–915. [CrossRef] [PubMed]

36. Kim, W.J.; Park, J.W.; Park, J.K.; Choi, D.J.; Park, Y.I. Purification and Characterization of a Fucoidanase (FNase S) from a Marine Bacterium *Sphingomonas paucimobilis* PF-1. *Mar. Drugs* **2015**, *13*, 4398–4417. [CrossRef] [PubMed]

37. Silchenko, A.S.; Kusaykin, M.I.; Kurilenko, V.V.; Zakharenko, A.M.; Isakov, V.V.; Zaporozhets, T.S.; Gazha, A.K.; Zvyagintseva, T.N. Hydrolysis of Fucoidan by Fucoidanase Isolated from the Marine Bacterium, *Formosa algae*. *Mar. Drugs* **2013**, *11*, 2413–2430. [CrossRef] [PubMed]

38. Martin, M.; Barbeyron, T.; Martin, R.; Portetelle, D.; Michel, G.; Vandenbol, M. The Cultivable Surface Microbiota of the Brown Alga *Ascophyllum nodosum* is Enriched in Macroalgal-Polysaccharide-Degrading Bacteria. *Front. Microbiol.* **2015**, *6*, 1487. [CrossRef] [PubMed]

39. Silchenko, A.S.; Khanh, H.H.N.; Hang, C.T.T.; Kurilenko, V.V.; Zakharenko, A.M.; Zueva, A.O.; Ly, B.M.; Kusaykin, M.I. A Simple Plate Method for the Screening and Detection of Fucoidanases. *Achiev. Life Sci.* **2015**, *9*, 104–106. [CrossRef]

40. Kim, H.-J.; Choi, J.-I.; Park, J.-G.; Song, B.-S.; Kim, J.-H.; Yoon, Y.; Kim, C.-J.; Shin, M.-H.; Byun, M.-W.; Lee, J.-W. Effects of Combined Treatment of Gamma Irradiation and Addition of Fucoidan/laminarin on Ready-to-eat Pork Patty. *Korean J. Food Sci. Anim. Resour.* **2009**, *29*, 34–39. [CrossRef]

41. Choi, J.; Kim, H.-J. Preparation of low molecular weight fucoidan by gamma-irradiation and its anticancer activity. *Carbohydr. Polym.* **2013**, *97*, 358–362. [CrossRef] [PubMed]

42. Choi, J.; Lee, S.G.; Han, S.J.; Cho, M.; Lee, P.C. Effect of gamma irradiation on the structure of fucoidan. *Radiat. Phys. Chem.* **2014**, *100*, 54–58. [CrossRef]

43. Silchenko, A.S.; Kusaykin, M.I.; Zakharenko, A.M.; Menshova, R.V.; Khanh, H.H.N.; Dmitrenok, P.S.; Isakov, V.V.; Zvyagintseva, T.N. Endo-1,4-fucoidanase from Vietnamese marine mollusk *Lambis* sp. which producing sulphated fucooligosaccharides. *J. Mol. Catal. B Enzym.* **2014**, *102*, 154–160. [CrossRef]

44. Gerbst, A.G.; Grachev, A.A.; Ustyuzhanina, N.E.; Khatuntseva, E.A.; Tsvetkov, D.E.; Usov, A.I.; Shashkov, A.S.; Preobrazhenskaya, M.E.; Ushakova, N.A.; Nifantiev, N.E. The Synthesis and NMR and Conformational Studies of Fucoidan Fragments: VI. Fragments with an α-(1→2)-Linked Fucobioside Unit. *Russ. J. Bioorg. Chem.* **2003**, *30*, 137–147. [CrossRef]

45. Krylov, V.B.; Kaskova, Z.M.; Vinnitskiy, D.Z.; Ustyuzhanina, N.E.; Grachev, A.A.; Chizhov, A.O.; Nifantiev, N.E. Acid-promoted synthesis of per-*O*-sulfated fucooligosaccharides related to fucoidan fragments. *Carbohydr. Res.* **2011**, *346*, 540–550. [CrossRef] [PubMed]

46. Hsu, C.H.; Hung, S.C.; Wu, C.Y.; Wong, C.H. Toward Automated Oligosaccharide Synthesis. *Angew. Chem. Int. Ed.* **2011**, *50*, 11872–11923. [CrossRef] [PubMed]

47. Delattre, C.; Michaud, P.; Courtois, B.; Courtois, J. Oligosaccharides engineering from plants and algae. Applications in biotechnology and therapeutic. *Minerva Biotechnol.* **2005**, *17*, 107–117.

48. Nugent, M.A. Heparin sequencing brings structure to the function of complex oligosaccharides. *Proc. Natl. Acad. Sci. USA* **2000**, *97*, 10301–10303. [CrossRef] [PubMed]

49. Lauder, R.M.; Huckerby, T.N.; Nieduszynski, I.A. A fingerprinting method for chondroitin/dermatan sulfate and hyaluronan oligosaccharides. *Glycobiology* **2000**, *10*, 393–401. [CrossRef] [PubMed]

50. Hricovini, M.; Guerrini, M.; Bisio, A. Structure of heparin-derived tetrasaccharide complexed to the plasma protein antithrombin derived from NOEs, *J*-couplings and chemical shifts. *Eur. J. Biochem.* **1999**, *261*, 789–801. [CrossRef] [PubMed]

51. Pineo, G.F.; Hull, R.D. Low-molecular-weight heparin: Prophylaxis and treatment of venous thromboembolism. *Annu. Rev. Med.* **1997**, *48*, 79–91. [CrossRef] [PubMed]

52. Liu, J.; Shriver, Z.; Pope, R.M.; Thorp, S.C.; Duncan, M.B.; Copeland, R.J.; Raska, C.S.; Yoshida, K.; Eisenberg, R.J.; Cohen, G.; et al. Characterization of a heparan sulfate octasaccharide that binds to herpes simplex virus type 1 glycoprotein D. *J. Biol. Chem.* **2002**, *277*, 33456–33467. [CrossRef] [PubMed]

53. Ghatak, S.; Misra, S.; Toole, B.P. Hyaluronan oligosaccharides inhibit anchorage-independent growth of tumor cells by suppressing the phosphoinositide 3-kinase/Akt cell survival pathway. *J. Biol. Chem.* **2002**, *277*, 38013–38020. [CrossRef] [PubMed]

54. Cumashi, A.; Ushakova, N.A.; Preobrazhenskaya, M.E.; D'Incecco, A.; Piccoli, A.; Totani, L.; Tinari, N.; Morozevich, G.E.; Berman, A.E.; Bilan, M.I.; et al. A comparative study of the anti-inflammatory, anticoagulant, antiangiogenic, and antiadhesive activities of nine different fucoidans from brown seaweeds. *Glycobiology* **2007**, *17*, 541–552. [CrossRef] [PubMed]

55. Bachelet, L.; Bertholon, I.; Lavigne, D.; Vassy, R.; Jandrot-Perrus, M.; Chaubet, F.; Letourneur, D. Affinity of low molecular weight fucoidan for P-selectin triggers its binding to activated human platelets. *Biochim. Biophys. Acta* **2009**, *1790*, 141–146. [CrossRef] [PubMed]

56. Blondin, C.; Fischer, E.; Boisson-Vidal, C.; Kazatchkine, M.D.; Jozefonvicz, J. Inhibition of complement activation by natural sulfated polysaccharides (fucans) from brown seaweed. *Mol. Immunol.* **1994**, *31*, 247–253. [CrossRef]

57. Springer, G.F.; Wurzel, H.A.; Mcneal, G.M.; Ansell, N.J.; Doughty, M.F. Isolation of anticoagulant fractions from crude fucoidin. *Proc. Soc. Exp. Biol. Med. Soc. Exp. Biol.* **1957**, *94*, 404–409. [CrossRef]

58. Zhao, X.; Guo, F.; Hu, J.; Zhang, L.; Xue, C.; Zhang, Z.; Li, B. Antithrombotic activity of oral administered low molecular weight fucoidan from *Laminaria Japonica*. *Thromb. Res.* **2016**, *144*, 46–52. [CrossRef] [PubMed]

59. Zaporozhets, T.; Besednova, N. Prospects for the therapeutic application of sulfated polysaccharides of brown algae in diseases of the cardiovascular system: Review. *Pharm. Biol.* **2016**, 1–10. [CrossRef] [PubMed]

60. Tissot, B.; Daniel, R. Biological properties of sulfated fucans: The potent inhibiting activity of algal fucoidan against the human complement system. *Glycobiology* **2003**, *13*, 29–30. [CrossRef] [PubMed]

61. Wang, W.; Wang, S.-X.; Guan, H.-S. The Antiviral Activities and Mechanisms of Marine Polysaccharides: An Overview. *Mar. Drugs* **2012**, *10*, 2795–2816. [CrossRef] [PubMed]

62. Schaeffer, D.J.; Krylov, V.S. Anti-HIV Activity of Extracts and Compounds from Algae and Cyanobacteria. *Ecotoxicol. Environ. Saf.* **2000**, *45*, 208–227. [CrossRef] [PubMed]
63. Vo, T.-S.; Kim, S.-K. Potential Anti-HIV Agents from Marine Resources: An Overview. *Mar. Drugs* **2010**, *8*, 2871–2892. [CrossRef] [PubMed]
64. Harrop, H.A.; Rider, C.C.; Coombe, D.R. Sulphated polysaccharides exert anti-HIV activity at differing sites. *Biochem. Soc. Trans.* **1992**, *20*, 163S. [CrossRef] [PubMed]
65. Dinesh, S.; Menon, T.; Hanna, L.E.; Suresh, V.; Sathuvan, M.; Manikannan, M. In vitro anti-HIV-1 activity of fucoidan from *Sargassum swartzii*. *Int. J. Biol. Macromol.* **2016**, *82*, 83–88. [CrossRef] [PubMed]
66. Baba, M.; Snoeck, R.; Pauwels, R.; De Clercq, E. Sulfated polysaccharides are potent and selective inhibitors of various enveloped viruses, including herpes simplex virus, cytomegalovirus, vesicular stomatitis virus, and human immunodeficiency virus. *Antimicrob. Agents Chemother.* **1988**, *32*, 1742–1745. [CrossRef] [PubMed]
67. McClure, M.O.; Moore, J.P.; Blanc, D.F.; Scotting, P.; Cook, G.M.W.; Keynes, R.J.; Weber, J.N.; Davies, D.; Weiss, R.A. Investigations into the mechanism by which sulfated polysaccharides inhibit HIV infection in vitro. *AIDS Res. Hum. Retrovir.* **1992**, *8*, 19–26. [CrossRef] [PubMed]
68. Ponce, N.M.A.; Pujol, C.A.; Damonte, E.B.; Flores, M.L.; Stortz, C.A. Fucoidans from the brown seaweed *Adenocystis utricularis*: Extraction methods, antiviral activity and structural studies. *Carbohydr. Res.* **2003**, *338*, 153–165. [CrossRef]
69. Kubes, P.; Jutila, M.; Payne, D. Therapeutic potential of inhibiting leukocyte rolling in ischemia/reperfusion. *J. Clin. Investig.* **1995**, *95*, 2510–2519. [CrossRef] [PubMed]
70. Omata, M.; Matsui, N.; Inomata, N.; Ohno, T. Protective effects of polysaccharide fucoidin on myocardial ischemia-reperfusion injury in rats. *J. Cardiovasc. Pharmacol.* **1997**, *30*, 717–724. [CrossRef] [PubMed]
71. Granert, C.; Raud, J.; Waage, A.; Lindquist, L. Effects of polysaccharide fucoidin on cerebrospinal fluid interleukin-1 and tumor necrosis factor alpha in pneumococcal meningitis in the rabbit. *Infect. Immun.* **1999**, *67*, 2071–2074. [PubMed]
72. Wu, G.J.; Shiu, S.M.; Hsieh, M.C.; Tsai, G.J. Anti-inflammatory activity of a sulfated polysaccharide from the brown alga *Sargassum cristaefolium*. *Food Hydrocoll.* **2016**, *53*, 16–23. [CrossRef]
73. Lasky, L.A. Selectin-carbohydrate interactions and the initiation of the inflammatory response. *Annu. Rev. Biochem.* **1995**, *64*, 113–139. [CrossRef] [PubMed]
74. Wen, Z.S.; Xiang, X.W.; Jin, H.X.; Guo, X.Y.; Liu, L.J.; Huang, Y.N.; OuYang, X.K.; Qu, Y.L. Composition and anti-inflammatory effect of polysaccharides from *Sargassum horneri* in RAW264.7 macrophages. *Int. J. Biol. Macromol.* **2016**, *88*, 403–416. [CrossRef] [PubMed]
75. Varki, A. Selectin ligands. *Proc. Nati. Acad. Sci. USA* **1994**, *91*, 7390–7397. [CrossRef]
76. Myers, S.P.; O'Connor, J.; Fitton, J.H.; Brooks, L.; Rolfe, M.; Connellan, P.; Wohlmuth, H.; Cheras, P.A.; Morris, C.A. A combined phase I and II open label study on the effects of a seaweed extract nutrient complex on osteoarthritis. *Biol. Targets Ther.* **2010**, *4*, 33–44. [CrossRef]
77. Liu, F.; Wang, J.; Chang, A.K.; Liu, B.; Yang, L.; Li, Q.; Wang, P.; Zou, X. Fucoidan extract derived from *Undaria pinnatifida* inhibits angiogenesis by human umbilical vein endothelial cells. *Phytomedicine* **2012**, *19*, 797–803. [CrossRef] [PubMed]
78. Koyanagi, S.; Tanigawa, N.; Nakagawa, H.; Soeda, S.; Shimeno, H. Oversulfation of fucoidan enhances its anti-angiogenic and antitumor activities. *Biochem. Pharmacol.* **2003**, *65*, 173–179. [CrossRef]
79. Soeda, S.; Kozako, T.; Iwata, K.; Shimeno, H. Oversulfated fucoidan inhibits the basic fibroblast growth factor-induced tube formation by human umbilical vein endothelial cells: Its possible mechanism of action. *Biochim. Biophys. Acta Mol. Cell Res.* **2000**, *1497*, 127–134. [CrossRef]
80. Luyt, C.-E.; Meddahi-Pellé, A.; Ho-Tin-Noe, B.; Colliec-Jouault, S.; Guezennec, J.; Louedec, L.; Prats, H.; Jacob, M.-P.; Osborne-Pellegrin, M.; Letourneur, D.; et al. Low-molecular-weight fucoidan promotes therapeutic revascularization in a rat model of critical hindlimb ischemia. *J. Pharmacol. Exp. Ther.* **2003**, *305*, 24–30. [CrossRef] [PubMed]
81. Purnama, A.; Aid-Launais, R.; Haddad, O.; Maire, M.; Mantovani, D.; Letourneur, D.; Hlawaty, H.; Le Visage, C. Fucoidan in a 3D scaffold interacts with vascular endothelial growth factor and promotes neovascularization in mice. *Drug Deliv. Transl. Res.* **2015**, *5*, 187–197. [CrossRef] [PubMed]

82. Bouvard, C.; Galy-Fauroux, I.; Grelac, F.; Carpentier, W.; Lokajczyk, A.; Gandrille, S.; Colliec-Jouault, S.; Fischer, A.M.; Helley, D. Low-Molecular-Weight Fucoidan Induces Endothelial Cell Migration via the PI3K/AKT Pathway and Modulates the Transcription of Genes Involved in Angiogenesis. *Mar. Drugs* **2015**, *13*, 7446–7462. [CrossRef] [PubMed]

83. Haddad, O.; Guyot, E.; Marinval, N.; Chevalier, F.; Maillard, L.; Gadi, L.; Laguillier-Morizot, C.; Oudar, O.; Sutton, A.; Charnaux, N.; et al. Heparanase and Syndecan-4 Are Involved in Low Molecular Weight Fucoidan-Induced Angiogenesis. *Mar. Drugs* **2015**, *13*, 6588–6608. [CrossRef] [PubMed]

84. Chabut, D.; Fischer, A.M.; Colliec-Jouault, S.; Laurendeau, I.; Matou, S.; Le Bonniec, B.; Helley, D. Low molecular weight fucoidan and heparin enhance the basic fibroblast growth factor-induced tube formation of endothelial cells through heparan sulfate-dependent alpha 6 overexpression. *Mol. Pharmacol.* **2003**, *64*, 696–702. [CrossRef] [PubMed]

85. Matou, S.; Helley, D.; Chabut, D.; Bros, A.; Fischer, A.M. Effect of fucoidan on fibroblast growth factor-2-induced angiogenesis in vitro. *Thromb. Res.* **2002**, *106*, 213–221. [CrossRef]

86. Giraux, J.-L.; Matou, S.; Bros, A.; Tapon-Bretaudiere, J.; Letourneur, D.; Fischer, A.-M. Modulation of human endothelial cell proliferation and migration by fucoidan and heparin. *Eur. J. Cell Biol.* **1998**, *77*, 352–359. [CrossRef]

87. Boisson-Vidal, C.; Zemani, F.; Caligiuri, G.; Galy-Fauroux, I.; Colliec-Jouault, S.; Helley, D.; Fischer, A.-M. Neoangiogenesis induced by progenitor endothelial cells: Effect of fucoidan from marine algae. *Cardiovasc. Hematol. Agents Med. Chem.* **2007**, *5*, 67–77. [CrossRef] [PubMed]

88. Kwak, J.-Y. Fucoidan as a marine anticancer agent in preclinical development. *Mar. Drugs* **2014**, *12*, 851–870. [CrossRef] [PubMed]

89. Han, Y.S.; Lee, J.H.; Lee, S.H. Antitumor Effects of Fucoidan on Human Colon Cancer Cells via Activation of Akt Signaling. *Biomol. Ther.* **2015**, *23*, 225–232. [CrossRef] [PubMed]

90. Atashrazm, F.; Lowenthal, R.M.; Woods, G.M.; Holloway, A.F.; Dickinson, J.L. Fucoidan and cancer: A multifunctional molecule with anti-tumor potential. *Mar. Drugs* **2015**, *13*, 2327–2346. [CrossRef] [PubMed]

91. Jin, J.-O.; Song, M.-G.; Kim, Y.-N.; Park, J.-I.; Kwak, J.-Y. The mechanism of fucoidan-induced apoptosis in leukemic cells: Involvement of ERK1/2, JNK, glutathione, and nitric oxide. *Mol. Carcinog.* **2010**, *49*, 771–782. [CrossRef] [PubMed]

92. Park, H.S.; Hwang, H.J.; Kim, G.-Y.; Cha, H.-J.; Kim, W.-J.; Kim, N.D.; Yoo, Y.H.; Choi, Y.H. Induction of apoptosis by fucoidan in human leukemia U937 cells through activation of p38 MAPK and modulation of Bcl-2 family. *Mar. Drugs* **2013**, *11*, 2347–2364. [CrossRef] [PubMed]

93. Zhang, Z.; Teruya, K.; Yoshida, T.; Eto, H.; Shirahata, S. Fucoidan Extract Enhances the Anti-Cancer Activity of Chemotherapeutic Agents in MDA-MB-231 and MCF-7 Breast Cancer Cells. *Mar. Drugs* **2013**, *11*, 81–98. [CrossRef] [PubMed]

94. Park, H.S.; Kim, G.-Y.; Nam, T.-J.; Kim, N.D.; Choi, Y.H. Antiproliferative activity of fucoidan was associated with the induction of apoptosis and autophagy in AGS human gastric cancer cells. *J. Food Sci.* **2011**, *76*, 77–83. [CrossRef] [PubMed]

95. Boo, H.-J.; Hyun, J.-H.; Kim, S.-C.; Kang, J.-I.; Kim, M.-K.; Kim, S.-Y.; Cho, H.; Yoo, E.-S.; Kang, H.-K. Fucoidan from *Undaria pinnatifida* induces apoptosis in A549 human lung carcinoma cells. *Phytother. Res.* **2011**, *25*, 1082–1086. [CrossRef] [PubMed]

96. Boo, H.-J.; Hong, J.-Y.; Kim, S.-C.; Kang, J.-I.; Kim, M.-K.; Kim, E.-J.; Hyun, J.-W.; Koh, Y.-S.; Yoo, E.-S.; Kwon, J.-M.; et al. The anticancer effect of fucoidan in PC-3 prostate cancer cells. *Mar. Drugs* **2013**, *11*, 2982–2999. [CrossRef] [PubMed]

97. Yang, L.; Wang, P.; Wang, H.; Li, Q.; Teng, H.; Liu, Z.; Yang, W.; Hou, L.; Zou, X. Fucoidan derived from *Undaria pinnatifida* induces apoptosis in human hepatocellular carcinoma SMMC-7721 cells via the ROS-mediated mitochondrial pathway. *Mar. Drugs* **2013**, *11*, 1961–1976. [CrossRef] [PubMed]

98. Shu, Z.; Shi, X.; Nie, D.; Guan, B. Low-Molecular-Weight Fucoidan Inhibits the Viability and Invasiveness and Triggers Apoptosis in IL-1beta-Treated Human Rheumatoid Arthritis Fibroblast Synoviocytes. *Inflammation* **2015**, *38*, 1777–1786. [CrossRef] [PubMed]

99. Chen, M.C.; Hsu, W.L.; Hwang, P.A.; Chou, T.C. Low Molecular Weight Fucoidan Inhibits Tumor Angiogenesis through Downregulation of HIF-1/VEGF Signaling under Hypoxia. *Mar. Drugs* **2015**, *13*, 4436–4451. [CrossRef] [PubMed]

100. Wei, C.; Xiao, Q.; Kuang, X.; Zhang, T.; Yang, Z.; Wang, L. Fucoidan inhibits proliferation of the SKM-1 acute myeloid leukaemia cell line via the activation of apoptotic pathways and production of reactive oxygen species. *Mol. Med. Rep.* **2015**, *12*, 6649–6655. [CrossRef] [PubMed]

101. Abu, R.; Jiang, Z.; Ueno, M.; Isaka, S.; Nakazono, S.; Okimura, T.; Cho, K.; Yamaguchi, K.; Kim, D.; Oda, T. Anti-metastatic effects of the sulfated polysaccharide ascophyllan isolated from *Ascophyllum nodosum* on B16 melanoma. *Biochem. Biophys. Res. Commun.* **2015**, *458*, 727–732. [CrossRef] [PubMed]

102. Cho, Y.; Yoon, J.H.; Yoo, J.J.; Lee, M.; Lee, D.H.; Cho, E.J.; Lee, J.H.; Yu, S.J.; Kim, Y.J.; Kim, C.Y. Fucoidan protects hepatocytes from apoptosis and inhibits invasion of hepatocellular carcinoma by up-regulating p42/44 MAPK-dependent NDRG-1/CAP43. *Acta Pharm. Sin. B* **2015**, *5*, 544–553. [CrossRef] [PubMed]

103. Li, J.; Chen, K.; Li, S.; Feng, J.; Liu, T.; Wang, F.; Zhang, R.; Xu, S.; Zhou, Y.; Zhou, S.; et al. Protective effect of fucoidan from *Fucus vesiculosus* on liver fibrosis via the TGF-beta1/Smad pathway-mediated inhibition of extracellular matrix and autophagy. *Drug Des. Dev. Ther.* **2016**, *10*, 619–630.

104. Ikeguchi, M.; Saito, H.; Miki, Y.; Kimura, T. Effect of Fucoidan Dietary Supplement on the Chemotherapy Treatment of Patients with Unresectable Advanced Gastric Cancer. *J. Cancer Ther.* **2015**, *6*, 1020–1026. [CrossRef]

105. Zhang, S.M.; Xie, Z.P.; Xu, M.L.; Shi, L.F. Cardioprotective effects of fucoidan against hypoxia-induced apoptosis in H9c2 cardiomyoblast cells. *Pharm. Biol.* **2015**, *53*, 1352–1357. [CrossRef] [PubMed]

106. Shimizu, J.; Wada-Funada, U.; Mano, H.; Matahira, Y.; Kawaguchi, M.; Wada, M. Proportion of murine cytotoxic T cells is increased by high molecular weight fucoidan extracted from *Okinawa mozuku* (*Cladosiphon okamuranus*). *J. Health Sci.* **2005**, *51*, 394–397. [CrossRef]

107. Yang, C.; Chung, D.; Shina, I.-S.; Lee, H.; Kim, J.; Lee, Y.; You, S. Effects of molecular weight and hydrolysis conditions on anticancer activity of fucoidans from sporophyll of *Undaria pinnatifida*. *Int. J. Biol. Macromol.* **2008**, *43*, 433–437. [CrossRef] [PubMed]

108. Azuma, K.; Ishihara, T.; Nakamoto, H.; Amaha, T.; Osaki, T.; Tsuka, T.; Imagawa, T.; Minami, S.; Takashima, O.; Ifuku, S.; et al. Effects of oral administration of fucoidan extracted from *Cladosiphon okamuranus* on tumor growth and survival time in a tumor-bearing mouse model. *Mar. Drugs* **2012**, *10*, 2337–2348. [CrossRef] [PubMed]

109. Cho, M.L.; Lee, B.Y.; You, S.G. Relationship between oversulfation and conformation of low and high molecular weight fucoidans and evaluation of their in vitro anticancer activity. *Molecules* **2010**, *16*, 291–297. [CrossRef] [PubMed]

110. Akihiro, K.; Shinsuke, A.; Nozomi, K.; Daisuke, T.; Kazunobu, T. Systematic synthesis of low-molecular weight fucoidan derivatives and their effect on cancer cells. *Org. Biomol. Chem.* **2015**, *13*, 10556–10568.

111. Liu, B.; Kongstad, K.T.; Wiese, S.; Jäger, A.K.; Staerk, D. Edible seaweed as future functional food: Identification of α-glucosidase inhibitors by combined use of high-resolution α-glucosidase inhibition profiling and HPLC–HRMS–SPE–NMR. *Food Chem.* **2016**, *203*, 16–22. [CrossRef] [PubMed]

112. Lakshmana, S.S.; Vinoth, K.T.; Geetharamani, D.; Suja, G.; Yesudas, R.; Chacko, A. Fucoidan—An alpha-amylase inhibitor from *Sargassum wightii* with relevance to NIDDM. *Int. J. Biol. Macromol.* **2015**, *81*, 644–647. [CrossRef] [PubMed]

113. Kim, K.T.; Rioux, L.E.; Turgeon, S.L. Molecular weight and sulfate content modulate the inhibition of α-amylase by fucoidan relevant for type 2 diabetes management. *PharmaNutrition* **2015**, *3*, 108–114. [CrossRef]

114. Chen, J.; Cui, W.; Zhang, Q.; Jia, Y.; Sun, Y.; Weng, L.; Luo, D.; Zhou, H.; Yang, L. Low molecular weight fucoidan ameliorates diabetic nephropathy via inhibiting epithelial-mesenchymal transition and fibrotic processes. *Am. J. Transl. Res.* **2015**, *7*, 1553–1563. [PubMed]

115. Heeba, G.H.; Morsy, M.A. Fucoidan ameliorates steatohepatitis and insulin resistance by suppressing oxidative stress and inflammatory cytokines in experimental non-alcoholic fatty liver disease. *Environ. Toxicol. Pharmacol.* **2015**, *40*, 907–914. [CrossRef] [PubMed]

116. Shan, X.; Liu, X.; Hao, J.; Cai, C.; Fan, F.; Dun, Y.; Zhao, X.; Li, C.; Yu, G. In vitro and in vivo hypoglycemic effects of brown algal fucoidans. *Int. J. Biol. Macromol.* **2015**. [CrossRef] [PubMed]

117. Wang, Y.; Wang, J.; Zhao, Y.; Hu, S.; Shi, D.; Xue, C. Fucoidan from sea cucumber *Cucumaria frondosa* exhibits anti-hyperglycemic effects in insulin resistant mice via activating the PI3K/PKB pathway and GLUT4. *J. Biosci. Bioeng.* **2016**, *121*, 36–42. [CrossRef] [PubMed]

118. Wang, J.; Hu, S.; Jiang, W.; Song, W.; Cai, L. Fucoidan from sea cucumber may improve hepatic inflammatory response and insulin resistance in mice. *Int. Immunopharm.* **2015**, *31*, 15–23. [CrossRef] [PubMed]

119. Thelen, T.; Hao, Y.; Medeiros, A.I.; Curtis, J.L.; Serezani, C.H.; Kobzik, L.; Harris, L.H.; Aronoff, D.M. The class A scavenger receptor, macrophage receptor with collagenous structure, is the major phagocytic receptor for *Clostridium sordellii* expressed by human decidual macrophages. *J. Immunol.* **2010**, *185*, 4328–4335. [CrossRef] [PubMed]

120. Hu, Y.; Cheng, S.C.-S.; Chan, K.-T.; Ke, Y.; Xue, B.; Sin, F.W.-Y.; Zeng, C.; Xie, Y. Fucoidin enhances dendritic cell-mediated T-cell cytotoxicity against NY-ESO-1 expressing human cancer cells. *Biochem. Biophys. Res. Commun.* **2010**, *392*, 329–334. [CrossRef] [PubMed]

121. Yang, M.; Ma, C.; Sun, J.; Shao, Q.; Gao, W.; Zhang, Y.; Li, Z.; Xie, Q.; Dong, Z.; Qu, X. Fucoidan stimulation induces a functional maturation of human monocyte-derived dendritic cells. *Int. Immunopharm.* **2008**, *8*, 1754–1760. [CrossRef] [PubMed]

122. Isnansetyo, A.; Fikriyah, A.; Kasanah, N. Non-specific immune potentiating activity of fucoidan from a tropical brown algae (Phaeophyceae), *Sargassum cristaefolium* in tilapia (*Oreochromis niloticus*). *Aquac. Int.* **2016**, *24*, 465–477. [CrossRef]

123. Myers, S.P.; O'Connor, J.; Fitton, J.H.; Brooks, L.; Rolfe, M.; Connellan, P.; Wohlmuth, H.; Cheras, P.A.; Morris, C. A combined Phase I and II open-label study on the immunomodulatory effects of seaweed extract nutrient complex. *Biol. Targets Ther.* **2011**, *5*, 45–60. [CrossRef] [PubMed]

124. Sharma, P. Cosmeceuticals: Regulatory scenario in US, Europe & India. *Int. J. Pharm. Technol.* **2012**, *3*, 1512–1535.

125. Rupérez, P.; Ahrazem, O.; Leal, J.A. Potential Antioxidant Capacity of Sulfated Polysaccharides from the Edible Marine Brown Seaweed *Fucus vesiculosus*. *J. Agric. Food Chem.* **2002**, *50*, 840–845. [CrossRef] [PubMed]

126. De Souza, M.C.R.; Marques, C.T.; Dore, C.M.G.; Da Silva, F.R.F.; Rocha, H.A.O.; Leite, E.L. Antioxidant activities of sulfated polysaccharides from brown and red seaweeds. *J. Appl. Phycol.* **2007**, *19*, 153–160. [CrossRef] [PubMed]

127. Costa, L.S.; Fidelis, G.P.; Telles, C.B.S.; Dantas-Santos, N.; Camara, R.B.G.; Cordeiro, S.L.; Costa, M.S.S.P.; Almeida-Lima, J.; Melo-Silveira, R.F.; Oliveira, R.M.; et al. Antioxidant and antiproliferative activities of heterofucans from the seaweed *Sargassum filipendula*. *Mar. Drugs* **2011**, *9*, 952–966. [CrossRef] [PubMed]

128. Wang, J.; Zhang, Q.; Zhang, Z.; Li, Z. Antioxidant activity of sulfated polysaccharide fractions extracted from *Laminaria japonica*. *Int. J. Biol. Macromol.* **2008**, *42*, 127–132. [CrossRef] [PubMed]

129. Li, B.; Liu, S.; Xing, R.; Li, K.; Li, R.; Qin, Y.; Wang, X.; Wei, Z.; Li, P. Degradation of sulfated polysaccharides from *Enteromorpha prolifera* and their antioxidant activities. *Carbohydr. Polym.* **2013**, *92*, 1991–1996. [CrossRef] [PubMed]

130. Hou, Y.; Wang, J.; Jin, W.; Zhang, H.; Zhang, Q. Degradation of *Laminaria japonica* fucoidan by hydrogen peroxide and antioxidant activities of the degradation products of different molecular weights. *Carbohydr. Polym.* **2012**, *87*, 153–159. [CrossRef]

131. Mak, W.; Hamid, N.; Liu, T.; Lu, J.; White, W.L. Fucoidan from New Zealand *Undaria pinnatifida*: Monthly variations and determination of antioxidant activities. *Carbohydr. Polym.* **2013**, *95*, 606–614. [CrossRef] [PubMed]

132. Hifney, A.F.; Fawzy, M.A.; Abdel-Gawad, K.M.; Gomaa, M. Industrial optimization of fucoidan extraction from *Sargassum* sp. and its potential antioxidant and emulsifying activities. *Food Hydrocoll.* **2016**, *54*, 77–88. [CrossRef]

133. Holdt, S.L.; Kraan, S. Bioactive compounds in seaweed: Functional food applications and legislation. *J. Appl. Phycol.* **2011**, *23*, 543–597. [CrossRef]

134. O'Doherty, J.V.; McDonnell, P.; Figat, S. The effect of dietary laminarin and fucoidan in the diet of the weanling piglet on performance and selected faecal microbial populations. *Livest. Sci.* **2010**, *134*, 208–210. [CrossRef]

135. Traifalgar, R.F.; Kira, H.; Tung, H.T.; Michael, F.R.; Laining, A.; Yokoyama, S.; Ishikawa, M.; Koshio, S.; Serrano, A.E.; Corre, V. Influence of Dietary Fucoidan Supplementation on Growth and Immunological Response of Juvenile *Marsupenaeus japonicus*. *J. World Aquac. Soc.* **2010**, *41*, 235–244. [CrossRef]

136. Lynch, M.B.; Sweeney, T.; Callan, J.J.; O'Sullivan, J.T.; O'Doherty, J.V. The effect of dietary Laminaria derived laminarin and fucoidan on intestinal microflora and volatile fatty acid concentration in pigs. *Livest. Sci.* **2010**, *133*, 157–160. [CrossRef]

137. Walsh, A.M.; Sweeney, T.; O'Shea, C.J.; Doyle, D.N.; O'Doherty, J.V. Effect of supplementing varying inclusion levels of laminarin and fucoidan on growth performance, digestibility of diet components, selected faecal microbial populations and volatile fatty acid concentrations in weaned pigs. *Anim. Feed Sci. Technol.* **2013**, *183*, 151–159. [CrossRef]

138. Zaporozhets, T.S.; Besednova, N.N.; Kuznetsova, T.A.; Zvyagintseva, T.N.; Makarenkova, I.D.; Kryzhanovsky, S.P.; Melnikov, V.G. The prebiotic potential of polysaccharides and extracts of seaweeds. *Russ. J. Mar. Biol.* **2014**, *40*, 1–9. [CrossRef]

139. Moroney, N.C.; O'Grady, M.N.; O'Doherty, J.V.; Kerry, J.P. Addition of seaweed (*Laminaria digitata*) extracts containing laminarin and fucoidan to porcine diets: Influence on the quality and shelf-life of fresh pork. *Meat Sci.* **2012**, *92*, 423–429. [CrossRef] [PubMed]

140. Moroney, N.C.; O'Grady, M.N.; Lordan, S.; Stanton, C.; Kerry, J.P. Seaweed polysaccharides (laminarin and fucoidan) as functional ingredients in pork meat: An evaluation of anti-oxidative potential, thermal stability and bioaccessibility. *Mar. Drugs* **2015**, *13*, 2447–2464. [CrossRef] [PubMed]

141. Fitton, H.; Irhimeh, M.; Falk, N. Macroalgal fucoidan extracts: A new oportunity for marine cometics. *Cosmet. Toil.* **2007**, *122*, 55–64.

142. Hafner, A.; Lovric, J.; Lakos, G.P.; Pepic, I. Nanotherapeutics in the EU: An overview on current state and future directions. *Int. J. Nanomed.* **2014**, *9*, 1005–1023.

143. Mura, S.; Couvreur, P. Nanotheranostics for personalized medicine. *Adv. Drug Deliv. Rev.* **2012**, *64*, 1394–1416. [CrossRef] [PubMed]

144. Bates, S. Progress towards personalized medicine. *Drug Discov. Today* **2010**, *15*, 115–120. [CrossRef] [PubMed]

145. Sadee, W.; Dai, Z. Pharmacogenetics/genomics and personalized medicine. *Hum. Mol. Gen.* **2005**, *2*, 207–214. [CrossRef] [PubMed]

146. Venkatesan, J.; Anil, S.; Kim, S.-K.; Shim, M. Seaweed Polysaccharide-Based Nanoparticles: Preparation and Applications for Drug Delivery. *Polymers* **2016**, *8*, 30. [CrossRef]

147. Cunha, L.; Grenha, A. Sulfated Seaweed Polysaccharides as Multifunctional Materials in Drug Delivery Applications. *Mar. Drugs* **2016**, *14*, 42. [CrossRef] [PubMed]

148. Silva, V.A.J.; Andrade, P.L.; Silva, M.P.C.; Bustamante, A.D.; De Los Santos Valladares, L.; Albino Aguiar, J. Synthesis and characterization of Fe3O4 nanoparticles coated with fucan polysaccharides. *J. Magn. Magn. Mater.* **2013**, *343*, 138–143. [CrossRef]

149. Andrade, P.L.; Silva, V.A.J.; Silva, M.P.C.; Albino Aguiar, J. Synthesis and Characterization of Fucan-Coated Cobalt Ferrite Nanoparticles. *J. Supercond. Novel Magn.* **2012**, *26*, 2511–2514. [CrossRef]

150. Leung, T.C.-Y.W. C.K.; Xie, Y. Green synthesis of silver nanoparticles using biopolymers, carboxymethylated-curdlan and fucoidan. *Mater. Chem. Phys.* **2010**, *121*, 402–405. [CrossRef]

151. Nagarajan, S.; Kuppusamy, K.A. Extracellular synthesis of zinc oxide nanoparticle using seaweeds of gulf of Mannar, India. *J. Nanobiotechnol.* **2013**, *11*, 39. [CrossRef] [PubMed]

152. Soisuwan, S.; Warisnoicharoen, W.; Lirdprapamongkol, K.; Svasti, J. Eco-friendly synthesis of fucoidan-stabilized gold nanoparticles. *Am. J. Appl. Sci.* **2010**, *7*, 1038–1042.

153. Lee, E.J.; Lim, K.H. Polyelectrolyte complexes of chitosan self-assembled with fucoidan: An optimum condition to prepare their nanoparticles and their characteristics. *Korean J. Chem. Eng.* **2014**, *31*, 664–675. [CrossRef]

154. Lee, E.J.; Lim, K.-H. Formation of chitosan-fucoidan nanoparticles and their electrostatic interactions: Quantitative analysis. *J. Biosci. Bioeng.* **2016**, *121*, 73–83. [CrossRef] [PubMed]

155. Ho, T.T. M.; Bremmell, K.E.; Krasowska, M.; Stringer, D.N.; Thierry, B.; Beattie, D.A. Tuning polyelectrolyte multilayer structure by exploiting natural variation in fucoidan chemistry. *Soft Matter* **2015**, *11*, 2110–2124. [CrossRef] [PubMed]

156. Bachelet-Violette, L.; Silva, A.K.A.; Maire, M.; Michel, A.; Brinza, O.; Ou, P.; Ollivier, V.; Nicoletti, A.; Wilhelm, C.; Letourneur, D.; et al. Strong and specific interaction of ultra small superparamagnetic iron oxide nanoparticles and human activated platelets mediated by fucoidan coating. *RSC Adv.* **2014**, *4*, 4864–4871. [CrossRef]

157. Bonnard, T.; Yang, G.; Petiet, A.; Ollivier, V.; Haddad, O.; Arnaud, D.; Louedec, L.; Bachelet-Violette, L.; Derkaoui, S.M.; Letourneur, D.; et al. Abdominal Aortic Aneurysms Targeted by Functionalized Polysaccharide Microparticles: A new Tool for SPECT Imaging. *Theranostics* **2014**, *4*, 592–603. [CrossRef] [PubMed]

158. Rouzet, F.; Bachelet-Violette, L.; Alsac, J.M.; Suzuki, M.; Meulemans, A.; Louedec, L.; Petiet, A.; Jandrot-Perrus, M.; Chaubet, F.; Michel, J.B.; et al. Radiolabeled fucoidan as a p-selectin targeting agent for in vivo imaging of platelet-rich thrombus and endothelial activation. *J. Nucl. Med.* **2011**, *52*, 1433–1440. [CrossRef] [PubMed]

159. Bonnard, T.; Serfaty, J.-M.; Journé, C.; Noe, B.H.T.; Arnaud, D.; Louedec, L.; Derkaoui, S.M.; Letourneur, D.; Chauvierre, C.; Le Visage, C. Leukocyte mimetic polysaccharide microparticles tracked in vivo on activated endothelium and in abdominal aortic aneurysm. *Acta Biomater.* **2014**, *10*, 3535–3545. [CrossRef] [PubMed]

160. Saboural, P.; Chaubet, F.; Rouzet, F.; Al-Shoukr, F.; Ben Azzouna, R.; Bouchemal, N.; Picton, L.; Louedec, L.; Maire, M.; Rolland, L.; et al. Purification of a Low Molecular Weight Fucoidan for SPECT Molecular Imaging of Myocardial Infarction. *Mar. Drugs* **2014**, *12*, 4851–4867. [CrossRef] [PubMed]

161. Desbree, A.; Bonnard, T.; Blanchardon, E.; Petiet, A.; Franck, D.; Chauvierre, C.; Le Visage, C. Evaluation of Functionalized Polysaccharide Microparticles Dosimetry for SPECT Imaging Based on Biodistribution Data of Rats. *Mol. Imaging Biol.* **2015**, *17*, 504–511. [CrossRef] [PubMed]

162. Li, X.; Bauer, W.; Israel, I.; Kreissl, M.C.; Weirather, J.; Richter, D.; Bauer, E.; Herold, V.; Jakob, P.; Buck, A.; et al. Targeting P-Selectin by Gallium-68-Labeled Fucoidan Positron Emission Tomography for Noninvasive Characterization of Vulnerable Plaques Correlation With In Vivo 17.6T MRI. *Arterioscler. Thromb. Vasc. Biol.* **2014**, *34*, 1661–1667. [CrossRef] [PubMed]

163. Sezer, A.D.; Akbuğa, J. Fucosphere—New microsphere carriers for peptide and protein delivery: Preparation and in vitro characterization. *J. Microencapsul.* **2006**, *23*, 513–522. [CrossRef] [PubMed]

164. Nakamura, S.; Nambu, M.; Ishizuka, T.; Hattori, H.; Kanatani, Y.; Takase, B.; Kishimoto, S.; Amano, Y.; Aoki, H.; Kiyosawa, T.; et al. Effect of controlled release of fibroblast growth factor-2 from chitosan/fucoidan micro complex-hydrogel on in vitro and in vivo vascularization. *J. Biomed. Mater. Res.* **2008**, *85*, 619–627. [CrossRef] [PubMed]

165. Huang, Y.-C.; Yang, Y.-T. Effect of basic fibroblast growth factor released from chitosan-fucoidan nanoparticles on neurite extension. *J. Tissue Eng. Regen. Med.* **2016**, *10*, 418–427. [CrossRef] [PubMed]

166. Huang, Y.-C.; Liu, T.-J. Mobilization of mesenchymal stem cells by stromal cell-derived factor-1 released from chitosan/tripolyphosphate/fucoidan nanoparticles. *Acta Biomater.* **2012**, *8*, 1048–1056. [CrossRef] [PubMed]

167. Park, S.; Hwang, S.; Lee, J. pH-responsive hydrogels from moldable composite microparticles prepared by coaxial electro-spray drying. *Chem. Eng. J.* **2011**, *169*, 348–357. [CrossRef]

168. Yu, S.H.; Wu, S.J.; Wu, J.Y.; Wen, D.Y.; Mi, F.L. Preparation of fucoidan-shelled and genipin-crosslinked chitosan beads for antibacterial application. *Carbohydr. Polym.* **2015**, *126*, 97–107. [CrossRef] [PubMed]

169. Huang, Y.C.; Li, R.Y. Preparation and Characterization of Antioxidant Nanoparticles Composed of Chitosan and Fucoidan for Antibiotics Delivery. *Mar. Drugs* **2014**, *12*, 4379–4398. [CrossRef] [PubMed]

170. Huang, Y.-C.; Lam, U.-I. Chitosan/fucoidan pH sensitive nanoparticles for oral delivery system. *J. Chin. Chem. Soc.* **2011**, *58*, 779–785. [CrossRef]

171. Lee, K.W.; Jeong, D.; Na, K. Doxorubicin loading fucoidan acetate nanoparticles for immune and chemotherapy in cancer treatment. *Carbohydr. Polym.* **2013**, *94*, 850–856. [CrossRef] [PubMed]

172. Kimura, R.; Rokkaku, T.; Takeda, S.; Senba, M.; Mori, N. Cytotoxic effects of fucoidan nanoparticles against osteosarcoma. *Mar. Drugs* **2013**, *11*, 4267–4278. [CrossRef] [PubMed]

173. Yu, S.H.; Tang, D.W.; Hsieh, H.Y.; Wu, W.S.; Lin, B.X.; Chuang, E.Y.; Sung, H.W.; Mi, F.L. Nanoparticle-induced tight-junction opening for the transport of an anti-angiogenic sulfated polysaccharide across Caco-2 cell monolayers. *Acta Biomater.* **2013**, *9*, 7449–7459. [CrossRef] [PubMed]

174. Huang, Y.C.; Kuo, T.H. O-carboxymethyl chitosan/fucoidan nanoparticles increase cellular curcumin uptake. *Food Hydrocoll.* **2016**, *53*, 261–269. [CrossRef]

175. Wu, S.J.; Don, T.M.; Lin, C.W.; Mi, F.L. Delivery of Berberine Using Chitosan/Fucoidan-Taurine Conjugate Nanoparticles for Treatment of Defective Intestinal Epithelial Tight Junction Barrier. *Mar. Drugs* **2014**, *12*, 5677–5697. [CrossRef] [PubMed]

176. Pinheiro, A.C.; Bourbon, A.I.; Cerqueira, M.A.; Maricato, E.; Nunes, C.; Coimbra, M.A.; Vicente, A.A. Chitosan/fucoidan multilayer nanocapsules as a vehicle for controlled release of bioactive compounds. *Carbohydr. Polym.* **2015**, *115*, 1–9. [CrossRef] [PubMed]

177. Yeh, T.-H.; Hsu, L.-W.; Tseng, M.T.; Lee, P.-L.; Sonjae, K.; Ho, Y.-C.; Sung, H.-W. Mechanism and consequence of chitosan-mediated reversible epithelial tight junction opening. *Biomaterials* **2011**, *32*, 6164–6173. [CrossRef] [PubMed]

178. Da Silva, L.C.G.T.; Mori, M.; Sandri, G.; Bonferoni, M.C.; Finotelli, P.V.; Cinelli, L.P.; Caramella, C.; Cabral, L.M. Preparation and characterization of polysaccharide-based nanoparticles with anticoagulant activity. *Int. J. Nanomed.* **2012**, *7*, 2975–2986. [CrossRef] [PubMed]

179. Sezer, A.D.; Akbuğa, J. Comparison on in vitro characterization of fucospheres and chitosan microspheres encapsulated plasmid DNA (pGM-CSF): Formulation design and release characteristics. *AAPS PharmSciTech* **2009**, *10*, 1193–1199. [CrossRef] [PubMed]

180. Kurosaki, T.; Kitahara, T.; Kawakami, S.; Nishida, K.; Nakamura, J.; Teshima, M.; Nakagawa, H.; Kodama, Y.; To, H.; Sasaki, H. The development of a gene vector electrostatically assembled with a polysaccharide capsule. *Biomaterials* **2009**, *30*, 4427–4434. [CrossRef] [PubMed]

181. Venkatesan, J.; Bhatnagar, I.; Kim, S.K. Chitosan-alginate biocomposite containing fucoidan for bone tissue engineering. *Mar. Drugs* **2014**, *12*, 300–316. [CrossRef] [PubMed]

182. Jeong, H.S.; Venkatesan, J.; Kim, S.K. Hydroxyapatite-fucoidan nanocomposites for bone tissue engineering. *Int. J. Biol. Macromol.* **2013**, *57*, 138–41. [CrossRef] [PubMed]

183. Lowe, B.; Venkatesan, J.; Anil, S.; Shim, M.S.; Kim, S.K. Preparation and characterization of chitosan-natural nano hydroxyapatite-fucoidan nanocomposites for bone tissue engineering. *Int. J. Biol. Macromol.* **2016**. [CrossRef] [PubMed]

184. Puvaneswary, S.; Talebian, S.; Raghavendran, H.B.; Murali, M.R.; Mehrali, M.; Afifi, A.M.; Kasim, N.H.; Kamarul, T. Fabrication and in vitro biological activity of betaTCP-Chitosan-Fucoidan composite for bone tissue engineering. *Carbohydr. Polym.* **2015**, *134*, 799–807. [CrossRef] [PubMed]

185. Changotade, S.I.; Korb, G.; Bassil, J.; Barroukh, B.; Willig, C.; Colliec-Jouault, S.; Durand, P.; Godeau, G.; Senni, K. Potential effects of a low-molecular-weight fucoidan extracted from brown algae on bone biomaterial osteoconductive properties. *J. Biomed. Mater. Res. A* **2008**, *87*, 666–675. [CrossRef] [PubMed]

186. Jin, G.; Kim, G.H. Rapid-prototyped PCL/fucoidan composite scaffolds for bone tissue regeneration: Design, fabrication, and physical/biological properties. *J. Mater. Chem.* **2011**, *21*, 17710–17718. [CrossRef]

187. Lee, J.S.; Jin, G.H.; Yeo, M.G.; Jang, C.H.; Lee, H.; Kim, G.H. Fabrication of electrospun biocomposites comprising polycaprolactone/fucoidan for tissue regeneration. *Carbohydr. Polym.* **2012**, *90*, 181–188. [CrossRef] [PubMed]

188. Lira, M.C.; Santos-Magalhaes, N.S.; Nicolas, V.; Marsaud, V.; Silva, M.P.; Ponchel, G.; Vauthier, C. Cytotoxicity and cellular uptake of newly synthesized fucoidan-coated nanoparticles. *Eur. J. Pharm. Biopharm.* **2011**, *79*, 162–70. [CrossRef] [PubMed]

189. Sezer, A.D.; Cevher, E.; Hatipoğlu, F.; Oğurtan, Z.; Baş, A.L.; Akbuğa, J. The use of fucosphere in the treatment of dermal burns in rabbits. *Eur. J. Pharm. Biopharm.* **2008**, *69*, 189–198. [CrossRef] [PubMed]

190. Sezer, A.D.; Cevher, E.; Hatipoglu, F.; Ogurtan, Z.; Bas, A.L.; Akbuga, J. Preparation of fucoidan-chitosan hydrogel and its application as burn healing accelerator on rabbits. *Biol. Pharm. Bull.* **2008**, *31*, 2326–2333. [CrossRef] [PubMed]

191. Suzuki, M.; Bachelet-Violette, L.; Rouzet, F.; Beilvert, A.; Autret, G.; Maire, M.; Menager, C.; Louedec, L.; Choqueux, C.; Saboural, P.; et al. Ultrasmall superparamagnetic iron oxide nanoparticles coated with fucoidan for molecular MRI of intraluminal thrombus. *Nanomedicine* **2015**, *10*, 73–87. [CrossRef] [PubMed]

192. Senni, K.; Pereira, J.; Gueniche, F.; Delbarre-Ladrat, C.; Sinquin, C.; Ratiskol, J.; Godeau, G.; Fischer, A.M.; Helley, D.; Colliec-Jouault, S. Marine polysaccharides: A source of bioactive molecules for cell therapy and tissue engineering. *Mar. Drugs* **2011**, *9*, 1664–1681. [CrossRef] [PubMed]

193. Ermakova, S.; Kusaykin, M.; Trincone, A.; Tatiana, Z. Ar multifunctional marine polysaccharides a myth or reality? *Front. Chem.* **2015**, *3*, 39. [CrossRef] [PubMed]

194. Seeberger, P.H.; Werz, D.B. Synthesis and medical applications of oligosaccharides. *Nature* **2007**, *446*, 1046–1051. [CrossRef] [PubMed]

195. Linhardt, R.J.; Gunay, N.S. Production and chemical processing of low molecular weight heparins. *Semin. Thromb. Hemost.* **1999**, *25*, 5–16. [PubMed]

196. Chavaroche, A.A.; van den Broek, L.A.; Eggink, G. Production methods for heparosan, a precursor of heparin and heparan sulfate. *Carbohydr. Polym.* **2013**, *93*, 38–47. [CrossRef] [PubMed]

197. Gray, E.; Mulloy, B.; Barrowcliffe, T.W. Heparin and low-molecular-weight heparin. *Thromb. Haemost.* **2008**, *99*, 807–818. [CrossRef] [PubMed]

198. Kakkar, V.V.; Djazaeri, B.; Fok, J.; Fletcher, M.; Scully, M.F.; Westwick, J. Low-molecular-weight heparin and prevention of postoperative deep vein thrombosis. *Br. Med. J.* **1982**, *284*, 375–379. [CrossRef]

199. Liu, H.; Zhang, Z.; Linhardt, R.J. Lessons learned from the contamination of heparin. *Nat. Prod. Rep.* **2009**, *26*, 313–321. [CrossRef] [PubMed]
200. Doshi, N.; Mitragotri, S. Designer Biomaterials for Nanomedicine. *Adv. Funct. Mater.* **2009**, *19*, 3843–3854. [CrossRef]
201. Gupta, A.S. Nanomedicine approaches in vascular disease: A review. *Nanomedicine* **2011**, *7*, 763–779. [CrossRef] [PubMed]
202. Sainz, V.; Conniot, J.; Matos, A.I.; Peres, C.; Zupancic, E.; Moura, L.; Silva, L.C.; Florindo, H.F.; Gaspar, R.S. Regulatory aspects on nanomedicines. *Biochem. Biophys. Res. Comm.* **2015**, *468*, 504–510. [CrossRef] [PubMed]
203. Chauvierre, C.; Letourneur, D. The European project NanoAthero to fight cardiovascular diseases using nanotechnologies. *Nanomedicine* **2015**, *10*, 3391–3400. [CrossRef] [PubMed]

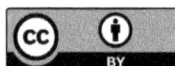

marine drugs

MDPI

Review

Therapies from Fucoidan; Multifunctional Marine Polymers

Janet Helen Fitton

Marinova Pty Ltd., 249 Kennedy Drive, Cambridge, Tasmania 7170, Australia; Helen.fitton@marinova.com.au;
Tel.: +61-3-62485800; Fax: +61-3-62484062

Received: 26 August 2011; in revised form: 22 September 2011; Accepted: 26 September 2011;
Published: 30 September 2011

Abstract: Published research on fucoidans increased three fold between 2000 and 2010. These algal derived marine carbohydrate polymers present numerous valuable bioactivities. This review discusses the role for fucoidan in the control of acute and chronic inflammation via selectin blockade, enzyme inhibition and inhibiting the complement cascade. The recent data on toxicology and uptake of fucoidan is detailed together with a discussion on the comparative activities of fractions of fucoidan from different sources. Recent *in vivo, in vitro* and clinical research related to diverse clinical needs is discussed. Targets include osteoarthritis, kidney and liver disease, neglected infectious diseases, hemopoietic stem cell modulation, protection from radiation damage and treatments for snake envenomation. In recent years, the production of well characterized reproducible fucoidan fractions on a commercial scale has become possible making therapies from fucoidan a realizable goal.

Keywords: fucoidan; inflammation; fibrosis; viral infection

1. Introduction

Fucoidans are a class of sulfated, fucose-rich polymers found in brown macroalgae [1,2]. They were identified in the first half of the last century by Kylin [3]. Subsequent research by researchers such as Bird [4] and Pervical [5] confirmed the basic identity of this class of compounds. Black reports the systematic isolation of fucoidan from a number of different British seaweeds [6]. Fucoidan was recognized as having a role in the biology of the seaweed, and examined over the next few decades for its activity in a number of biological systems. Current research interest in fucoidan is global. Research occurs in Australia, Japan, Korea, Russia and China in addition to Europe and the Americas. The intensity of biological activities of fucoidan varies with species, molecular weight, composition, structure and the route of administration.

Despite notable bioactivities and a lack of oral toxicity, fucoidans remain relatively unexploited as a source of therapeutics due to their plant source and heterogeneity. In recent decades pharmaceutical companies have preferred "druggable" well defined smaller molecules, leading to a neglect of the opportunities for larger and polydisperse entities. Older naturally occurring polymeric drugs such as heparin have held their place in the modern pharmacopeia despite recent concerns [7]. Carefully controlled sources of seaweed together with modern extraction and characterization methods to create reproducibly defined products together with new regulatory avenues mean that fucoidan fractions can be produced to standards suitable as ingredients in medical devices and even cross the threshold into drug development route [8]. There are also further potential applications for fucoidan products in complementary medicine and topical applications.

The reading of the literature can be confusing due to the diverse sources and fractions of fucoidan used. In general, fucoidans contain a high proportion of fucose in the sugar backbone of the polymer. They are sulfated, may be acetylated and may also contain uronic acids. The yield of a crude first fraction of fucoidan is generally 2–10% by weight, although *Cladosiphon* species may yield over 20% by dry weight. Fucoidans derived from seaweeds are all highly branched. A second source of linear rather than branched fucoidans is echinoderms, in particular sea cucumbers, which are largely outside of the scope of this review. Earlier reviews on the structure and significance of the fucoidans can be found in Fitton [9], Pomin [10] and Berteau [2] and also by Li [11].

The most common source of experimental fucoidan used in the literature is derived from *Fucus vesiculosis*, a common harvest crop of a northern hemisphere kelp. This fucoidan, like all primary fucoidan extracts, is heterodisperse and well characterized in an elegant paper by Nishino [12]. *Fucus vesiculosis* fucoidan is a high fucose sulfated fucoidan. Other common fucoidans are sourced from edible species such as *Cladosiphon okamuranus*, *Laminaria japonica* and *Undaria pinnatifida*. These seaweeds are harvested in significant quantities across Asia and have an excellent toxicity profile. The backbone sugars are different again. *Undaria pinnatifida* fucoidan contains a high proportion of galactose for example.

This review begins by identifying new research in uptake and toxicity of fucoidans. Secondly, this review limits the scope of potential therapeutic use of fucoidan in inflammation related areas; injury, infection, chronic inflammation and fibrosis, and lastly, protection of neuronal function. These areas represent areas of need for new approaches and perhaps greater potential for commercialization of new technology. It is not inferred that other areas of fucoidan bioactivity are not important, or indeed, any less likely to lead to real world therapeutic use. Research into the cancer inhibitory effects of fucoidan fractions is reviewed elsewhere [2,9] and not within the scope of this review.

2. Uptake and Fate of Fucoidan

The yet unanswered question is "Where does fucoidan go after oral, intraperitoneal or intravenous administration?" Although a number of research papers indicate biological effects after oral ingestion or systemic delivery, very little research has taken place on the uptake and fate of fucoidan. The expectation that large molecules are not orally absorbed causes difficulties in understanding how apparently systemic effects occur. Early work on digestion of fucoidan suggested that it was not changed by human bacterial flora and was wholly excreted [13,14]. Perhaps systemic observations are partly a result of prebiotic effects? Recent research indicates that there are favorable changes in intestinal flora after ingestion of fucoidan, including increased Lactobacilli [15,16].

There is however, a growing body of evidence for the absorption of larger polysaccharide molecules such as chondroitin sulfate [17] and polyethylene glycol [18], albeit in small quantities. The more recent research by Irhimeh [19], Tokita [20] and Nakazato [21] strengthens the case for small amounts of systemic uptake from oral dosing in which the fucoidan is unchanged in the serum.

Irhimeh used an antibody based method to detect small amounts of orally ingested Undaria derived fucoidan in serum in a human clinical study [19]. More recently, Tokita indicated that orally ingested *Cladosiphon* derived fucoidan can be detected in serum in a rat model [20] at levels two orders of magnitude lower than observed by Irhimeh. The differences in observations on the serum levels may be accounted for by differences in the source of fucoidan used, the time span over which the observations were taken (hours as opposed to days of ingestion) and the detection method (specific rather than cross reacting antibodies). Tokita also recorded molecular weight profiles of the fucoidan when absorbed, showing that fucoidan molecular weight was unchanged in serum or plasma. Lower molecular weight fucoidan was observed in the urine, which may indicate a hitherto unknown mammalian mechanism for the breakdown of fucoidan. The accumulation of sulfated polysaccharides in the kidney, and their urinary excretion was noted by Guimaraes in 1997 [22] although in this case, the fucoidan was delivered intravenously.

Nakazato [21] examined the fate of a crude (average 28 kDa) and a higher molecular weight subfraction (41.4 kDa) of *Cladosiphon okamuranus* derived fucoidan administered in the drinking water at 2% w/v in a rat model, determining the concentration of fucoidan in the liver. This study clearly demonstrated an inhibitory effect of orally delivered higher molecular weight fucoidan on induced fibrosis of the liver which was associated with decreased tissue expression of transforming growth factor beta (TGF beta) and stromal derived factor (SDF1 also known as CXCL12), the receptor for CXCR4. This research was important, not only because it illustrated the fibrosis inhibitory potential of fucoidan, but demonstrated systemic distribution of the molecule after oral ingestion in this animal model.

All of these studies have used antibody technology to either stain or quantify fucoidan. The increasing availability of antibodies will facilitate this type of research. Mizuno also prepared monoclonal antibodies that reacted with fucoidan isolated from *Laminaria japonica* and *Kjellmaniella gyrate*, but not with fucoidan from *Undaria pinnatifida* [23]. However, these were used only to stain for fucoidan in seaweed preparations. Earlier researchers also developed antibodies to *Fucus vesiculosis* fucoidan for botanical purposes [24]. The data are summarized in Table 1.

Table 1. Antibodies to fucoidan.

Specificity of antibody	Seaweed source	Trial	Route of administration	Use	Reference
Heparin and fucoidan	*Undaria pinnatifida*	Human	Oral	Estimation of serum uptake	Irhimeh 2005 [19]
Fucoidan	*Cladosiphon okamuranus*	Human	Oral	Estimation of serum, urine concentration	Tokita 2010 [20]
Fucoidan	*Cladosiphon okamuranus*	Rat	Oral	Staining in liver	Nakazato 2009 [21]
Fucoidan	*Laminaria japonica* and *Kjellmania gyrate*	Botanical stain	n/a	Staining	Mizuno 2009 [23]

3. Toxicology

Fucoidan derived from all species appears to lack toxicity *in vitro* and *in vivo*. In recent toxicology reports, fucoidan derived from *Undaria pinnatifida* and *Laminaria japonica* was found to be safe in animal models at very high levels of ingestion [25,26]. The oral safety of fucoidan is echoed in clinical studies. Human clinical studies using orally ingested fucoidan have shown no toxicity at a dose of 1 g per day up to three months [27], or 3 g per day for 12 days [19,28]. It is interesting- and important-to note that fucoidan has substantial coagulation modifying activity *in vitro*. This activity was echoed in Irhimeh 2009 [29] in which significant decreases in global clotting time were noted after ingestion of 3 g *Undaria pinnatifida* fucoidan although these stayed within the normal clinical range. Clotting times were increased at higher doses of 900 mg/kg body weight in a rat model with *Laminaria japonica* fucoidan [26], but intriguingly, no change in clotting time was noted in a rat model in which *Undaria pinnatifida* fucoidan at 1350 mg/kg body weight was ingested [30]. See Table 2 for details.

Table 2. Toxicology of fucoidan.

Fucoidan source	Characteristics	Studies	Dose	Species	Results	Ref.
Undaria pinnatifida	53% total sugar 7.4% sulfate 27% Uronic acid 54% fucose 35% galactose	Acute in vivo Ames test Bone marrow micronucleus	1000 mg/kg body weight per day for 28 days	Sprague Dawley rats	Not toxic to 1000 mg/kg bw; Increase in ALT at 200 mg/kg	Chung 2010 [25]
Laminaria japonica	Fucoidan Fraction MW average "10–300 kD"	Oral dosing in experimental model; Toxicity by clinical observation	Escalation doses up to 20 mg/kg	Dogs with hemophilia A; Rats	No clinical toxicity	Prasad 2008 [31]
Laminaria japonica	Fluorescent labeled fucoidan	Subcutaneous	5 mg/kg	Rat	Half life 83 min	Prasad 2008 [31]
Laminaria japonica	MW average 189 kDa Fucose 28% sulfate 29% total sugars 48%	Acute and sub-chronic toxicity	300, 900 and 2500 mg/kg bw to 6 months	Wistar Rats	Not toxic to 300 mg/kg bw Prolonged clotting at 900 and 1200 mg/kg bw	Li 2005 [26]
Undaria pinnatifida	64.4 ± 6.0% fucose, 31.9 ± 4.7% galactose, 3.6 ± 1.3% mannose, and 31.7 ± 2.2% sulfate	Genotoxicity Bacterial mutation Bone marrow Micronucleus formation	Up to 2000 mg/kg/bw orally	Sprague Dawley rats	Fucoidan presents no significant genotoxic concern.	Kim 2010 [32]
Undaria pinnatifida	64.4 ± 6.0% fucose, 31.9 ± 4.7% galactose, 3.6 ± 1.3% mannose, and 31.7 ± 2.2% sulfate	Toxicity measures—body weight, ophthalmoscopy urinalysis, hematology, and histopathology; Clotting parameters; Prothrombin time or activated partial thromboplastin time	1350 mg/kg bw/day for 4 weeks orally	Sprague Dawley rats	No changes to No change to prothrombin time or activated partial thromboplastin time	Kim 2009 [30]
Undaria pinnatifida	75% fucoidan	Full blood count, clinical biochemistry	3 g per day for 12 days	Human	No toxicity noted	Irhimeh 2005, 2007, 2009 [19,28,29]
Fucus vesiculosis Macrocystis pyrifera Laminaria japonica	75% total fucoidan	Full blood count, clinical biochemistry	0.1 and 1 g for 84 days	Human	No toxicity	Myers 2010 [27]
Fucus vesiculosis Macrocystis pyrifera Laminaria japonica	75% total fucoidan	Full blood count, clinical biochemistry	0.1 and 1 g for 28 days	Human	No toxicity	Myers 2011 [33]
Cladisiphon sp.	85% fucoidan	Patients with HTLV1 were treated clinically	6 g per day up to 13 months	Human	Four patients diarrhea; No other toxicity noted; Reduction in viral load	Araya 2011 [34]

4. Differences between Fucoidan Fractions

One difficulty in making comparisons within the literature lies in the many variations to molecular weight and composition of the fucoidan fractions used. Fractions vary widely in terms of purity, composition, weight and sulfation even from the same species of macroalga. As polyphenols and other components present in macroalgae also have bioactivity, less pure fractions can deliver confounding data [9,35].

A recent multi-author paper compared fucoidans from different sources in a suite of bioassays [36]. Cumashi and colleagues comprehensive study uses comparable preparation techniques to generate samples and concentrated on commercial (or potentially commercial) sustainable sources of seaweeds. Their data thoroughly illustrates the common bioactivities of fucoidans and yet their differences. All fucoidans tested inhibited *leukocyte* recruitment in an inflammation model in rats. The model used consisted of an induced acute peritonitis in female Wistar rats and the measurement of neutrophils into the peritoneal cavity. Test fucoidans were delivered intravenously. Fucoidans are well known as L-selectin blockage agents and were found to inhibit neutrophil extravasion into the peritoneal cavity. Clotting parameters were also assessed. The most active inhibitors were fucoidans from *Laminaria saccharina* and *Fucus evanescens*, which inhibited neutrophil extravasation by more than 90% whereas fucoidan from *Fucus distichus* and *Fucus spiralis* inhibited the neutrophil transmigration by only 60%. Other parameters investigated included P selectin inhibition in a platelet aggregation model, coagulation parameters and cancer cell adhesion to platelets *in vitro*. All fucoidans, except that from *Cladosiphon okamuranus*, exhibited anticoagulant activity *in vitro* and *in vivo*. Fucoidans from *Laminaria saccharina*, *Laminaria digitata*, *Fucus serratus*, *Fucus distichus*, and *Fucus vesiculosus* effectively inhibited breast carcinoma cell adhesion to platelets, an effect which may point to an inhibition of "platelet cloaking", a mechanism used by cancer cells to metastasise unchallenged throughout the body [37].

Others have investigated the relative effects of higher and lower molecular weight fractions of the same fucoidan source and found significant differences in their bioactivity. Firstly, Nakazato found that an orally delivered higher molecular weight fraction of fucoidan was more effective than an unfractionated crude fucoidan in inhibiting liver fibrosis [21]. Secondly, Maruyama confirmed that fucoidan is effective as an anti-tumor and immune modulating agent [38,39]. Shimizu then orally administered three different preparations of fucoidan from *Cladosiphon okamuranus* to mice [40]. The key findings were increases in CD8 expression in spleens of the highest molecular weight fucoidan fed mice. The CD4/CD8 ratio tended to decrease, and the number of cells expressing CD11b cells (NK, monocytes and macrophage cells) tended to increase as compared to the lower molecular weight fucoidan fed mice.

Thirdly, Park examined the differential effects of high and low molecular weight fractions of fucoidan in an arthritis model [41]. There was a marked contrast in the two preparations. The high molecular weight fraction activated the inflammatory process, whereas the low molecular weight fraction inhibited the disease.

Snake envenomation may be ameliorated by fucoidan (see Section 6.15. In a experiment to determine whether lower molecular weight would increase bioavailability of fucoidan and its effectiveness, Azofeifa found the reverse [42]. High molecular weight fucoidan was necessary to achieve the therapeutic effect against crude venom *in vivo*, whereas the lower molecular weight preparation was ineffective, despite being equally effective *in vitro*.

Lastly, the way in which fucoidan is administered may make a difference to activity. This is well illustrated in research presented by Yanase who describes the suppression of an IgE response to albumin by intraperitoneal fucoidan [43]. Elevated serum levels of IgE towards common environmental allergens are a feature of allergic diseases such as asthma and atopic dermatitis. Having found that fucoidan inhibited IgE production by B cells *in vitro*, they studied its effect in an allergic model in mice. In this study, the stimulated increase of plasma IgE was suppressed when fucoidan was delivered intraperitoneally at 100 mcg per mouse, but not when delivered orally at 10 mg per mouse. It is interesting to compare this to Hayashi's study in which orally delivered fucoidan was effective in reducing viral titres in mice after influenza infection [44].

These recent examples are illustrative of the variation in fucoidan and the care that needs to be taken when developing a fraction for a particular application. They also illustrate remarkable bioactivity by molecules with low toxicity profiles.

5. Inflammation and Fibrosis

Inflammation can be classified as either acute or chronic. Acute inflammation, which may occur as a result of infection or injury, is characterized by its rapid resolution, neutrophilic inflammation and edema. Chronic inflammation is a response that persists for several months and is characterized by simultaneous inflammation, tissue remodeling and repair processes without resolution. Whilst there are clinically distinct fibrotic disorders they commonly start off from a persistent aggravating inflammation that sustains the production of matrix degrading enzymes, growth factors and cytokines, which gradually obliterate normal tissue architecture and cause organ damage [45].

Acute inflammatory responses experienced after an ischemic event such as a heart attack, can be destructive to organs. Post ischemic organ damage results from inflammatory cascades pursuant to necrotic tissue. Diseases involving chronic inflammation are debilitating. Causes of inflammation are diverse, ranging from viral infection to systemic metabolic disorders. Chronic inflammation can enhance cancer metastasis and lead to increases in other disease processes. Non toxic, orally delivered therapeutics to address both short term and long term inflammation are highly desirable.

Fucoidan's potential lies in its pleiotropic anti-inflammatory effects. These include inhibition of selectins, inhibition of complement and enzyme inhibitory activity.

5.1. Inhibition of Selectins

Fucoidan is a well known research tool as a selectin blockade agent [36,46,54]. Selectins are cell surface receptors on white blood cells that perform a braking function for the cells, allowing them to roll on an organs endothelial surface and ultimately enter that tissue space. Fucoidan prevents P and L selectins and thus *leukocyte* adhesion and rolling thereby reducing inflammation in whole organs such as the heart, kidneys or liver. The relative selectin blocking effects of fucoidans from different sources was investigated by Cumashi and colleagues [36]. These are discussed earlier in this review. All fucoidans tested were effective at inhibiting neutrophil extravasion in a peritoneal inflammation model system.

The selectin blockade effect has been established *in vivo* as a potential therapy for the prevention of post ischemic reperfusion injury and autoimmune cardiac injury [51]. In Tanaka's surgical model, saline or fucoidan was delivered intraperitoneally to rats over 28 days with either a sham operation or with cardiac myosin injection to stimulate autoimmune myocarditis. The invasion of CD4-positive T cells into the myocardium is the initial pathology in this model. After 3 weeks, fucoidan treatment improved the function of the heart muscle and its weight when compared with the control. Fucoidan treatment decreased serum inflammatory markers, the myocarditis area and inhibited macrophage and CD4-positive T-cell infiltration into the myocardium.

In 2010, Thomes investigated the effects of *Cladosiphon okamuranus* fucoidan in a model of cardiac infarction (*i.e.*, a heart attack) induced by isoproterenol [52]. Oral dosing of *Cladosiphon* derived fucoidan at 150 mg/kg for 7 days had a marked protective effect on the sequelae of the infarction, including lowering cardiac enzymes and lipid profiles. Like many other researchers, Thomes debates whether the effects are via absorption or perhaps conferred via immune changes in the gut.

In well-designed research by Kubes and colleagues, the mechanism of post ischemic organ protection by *Fucus vesiculosis* fucoidan was shown not to be a simplistic one [47]. Kubes used intravital microscopy to look at reperfusion of the liver after an ischemic event or endotoxin exposure. Fucoidan effectively inhibited neutrophil entry after ischemia but not after endotoxin exposure. Kubes noted that liver ischemia also leads upstream to gut ischemia and hypothesized that the protection of the liver was actually a result of protection of the gut, preventing downstream inflammation of the liver. After rerouting the circulation and removing the intestines in the rat model, fucoidan did not protect against neutrophil adhesion in the liver to the same degree, confirming that the protective effect is partly due to inhibition of inflammation in the gut.

Most recently, experimental encephalomyelitis was reduced by administration of fucoidan [53]. Kim used 50 mg/kg, daily intraperitoneal administration of fucoidan into a rat to test whether it could either treat or prevent encephalomyelitis generated by immunization with guinea-pig myelin basic protein. Preventive dosing was carried out one day before immunization and the 6 days thereafter. Treatment dosing was carried out from the 8th to the 14th day of the disease. Surprisingly, prevention was not successful in contrast to treatment, which was highly effective. The lessening of clinical effects coincided with decreased infiltration of inflammatory cells in the affected spinal cord, probably partly by L selectin blockade and the suppression of specific CD4+ T cells.

P selectin is present on platelets and assists with aggregation. Xenografting (the transplant of an organ from one species to another) is often complicated by abnormal clotting responses. In an attempt to overcome this, Alwayn [54] investigated the effects of a number of agents on xenograft induced clotting in a baboon model. Fucoidan from *Fucus vesiculosis* was very successful in inhibiting the platelet aggregation although the perturbation of clotting was considered problematic. Alwayn did not consider the potential to inhibit complement activation, although this is known limiting factor in xenografts [55].

5.2. Inhibition of Complement

Complement is a cascade system of enzymatic proteins occurring in normal serum that help to regulate immunity and form part of the pathogen defense system [55]. It consists of "classical" and "alternative" pathways that are triggered by, and combine with antibody-antigen complexes, producing lysis in affected cells. Complement consists of approximately 30 proteins, known as C1 to C9, with subtypes for each protein. Components C3 and C5 are involved promotion of leukocyte chemotaxis whereas C1 and C4 are involved in the specific antibody response to viruses. The alternative complement pathway is sequence in which C3 and C5 to C9 are activated without participation by C1, C2 and C4 or the presence of an antibody-antigen complex. Fucoidan fractions are very effective inhibitors of this cascade [55,59] being at least 40 times more potent than heparin.

Fucoidan can block the formation of classical C3 convertase. This may prevent the production of the pro-inflammatory anaphylatoxins and further downstream in the cascade, the C3b fragment. Indeed, this is one of the possible mechanisms via which fucoidan exerts an anti-allergic effect, as observed in diverse experimental models.

Tissot demonstrated that fucoidan strongly binds to C1q and points out that inhibition of complement binding to C1q receptors present on endothelial cells could assist with xenograft (cross species transplants) rejection [56,57]. Indeed, fucoidan derived from *Ascophyllum nodosum* protected of porcine endothelial cells against the complement-mediated lysis that is responsible for rejection [56]. More recent research on xenograft protection found that *Fucus vesiculosis* fucoidan was useful inhibitor of platelet aggregation—as a result of selectin blockade, although concerns were raised over its temporary anticoagulant effect. Curiously, complement blockade was not considered in this research [54].

Fucoidans are known to be highly branched polysaccharides but the potential meaning of the branching structures in terms of bioactivity was not considered until Clement's research of 2010 [60]. In an elegant NMR study, Clement tackles the structural heterogeneity and the random sulfation of the polysaccharide chain with relation to how they affect complement binding and inhibition. The results suggest that branching of fucoidan oligosaccharides is a major factor in their anti-complementary activity at the conformational level. This work is significant as it demonstrates that not only molecular weight, sulfation and sugar composition affect bioactivity, but also three dimensional structure. When therapies from fucoidan are developed, a holistic approach to all of these parameters is essential.

5.3. Inhibition of Enzymes

Fucoidan also has significant enzyme inhibitory activity against a number of enzymes including matrix metalloproteases, hyaluronidases and elastases [61,62]. This inhibitory activity limits tissue breakdown in inflammatory settings caused by injury and disease and can even inhibit metastasis.

Ultraviolet radiation is a prominent cause of skin photoaging and even skin cancers. It causes marked increases in elastase activity, breaking down elastin fibers, which accelerates loss of skin condition [63]. Research reported in 2009 indicates that ultraviolet radiation injury to skin fibroblasts *in vitro*, which causes increase in matrix metalloproteases and reduces procollagen levels, is markedly reduced by the presence of *Fucus vesiculosis* fucoidan [64]. Senni reported a comprehensive study on the inhibitory effects of fucoidan. Using human skin in *ex vivo* experiments he showed that fucoidan was able to curtail human leukocyte elastase activity which protected the elastic fibers from degradation [62]. A clinical study also indicated good potential for amelioration of skin aging [65]. *Fucus vesiculosis* fucoidan was applied to skin at 1% w/v twice daily for five weeks. A significant decrease in skin thickness and improvement in elasticity was noted compared to controls.

According to new research by Hlawaty [66], matrix metalloprotease type 2 (MMP2) is responsible for intimal hyperplasia in a rat model. In this model, the aorta is damaged and the rats are treated via intramuscular injection with 5 mg/kg/day of a low molecular weight fucoidan derived from *Fucus vesiculosis* for two weeks. The proliferation of the smooth muscle walls which causes the narrowing of the lumen in the damaged vessel was measured and found to be considerably more open in the fucoidan treated rats. Previous research has shown that this fucoidan fraction can successfully inhibit smooth muscle proliferation [67]. This study then looked at the enzyme activity in the vessel, and found that fucoidan specifically inhibited MMP2, an enzyme which degrades type IV collagen, a major structural component of basement membranes.

6. Therapies from Fucoidan

Selected applications for fucoidan based therapies are discussed in this section. Clinical data together with promising *in vivo* and *in vitro* data is discussed with reference to a diverse set of therapeutic goals.

6.1. Osteoarthritis

Osteoarthritis is the most common and disabling form of arthritis experienced by an increasing number of people as the population ages. It is characterized by a slow and progressive degeneration of articular cartilage. Whilst it is often regarded as a disease of "wear and tear" through ageing, osteoarthritis has a strong genetic component and is also affected by injury and by diseases such as obesity. In addition to the cartilage itself, osteoarthritis also involves the surrounding tissues, including the synovium and the subchondral bone. Osteoarthritis has an inflammatory component, and undoubtedly, a powerful tissue breakdown component which result in pain and stiffness [68].

Several recent studies indicate a role of fucoidan in addressing the symptoms of osteoarthritis. Park *et al.* used an animal model of collagen induced arthritis, and showed that orally administered *Undaria pinnatifida* fucoidan successfully inhibited pain [41]. In a small human clinical study, osteoarthritis symptoms were significantly inhibited by oral administration of fucoidan rich seaweed extract. Over three months, symptoms were reduced by 52% [27]. This result is a marked improvement for osteoarthritis symptoms. There was no reduction in TNF alpha which was used as inflammation marker, but an accompanying study in healthy volunteers showed a decrease in Interleukin 6, a marker for chronic inflammation [33].

The mechanism for the clinically observed reduction in pain of osteoarthritis is unclear. Was pain decreased by the blockade of neutrophils? Cunha showed that fucoidan successfully blocked the accumulation of neutrophils and pain nociception in an animal model [69]. Cunha's study emphasized the importance of neutrophils as an originator of inflammatory hypernociception and confirmed that fucoidan blocks the accumulation of neutrophils by selectin blockade in their model. See Table 3.

Table 3. Arthritis and fucoidan.

Fucoidan	Model	Adminstration	Observation	Reference
Fucus vesiculosis *Macrocystis pyrifera* *Laminaria japonica*	Human clinical	Oral daily 100 mg or 1000 mg for three months	No toxicity Up to 52% reduction in symptoms	Myers 2010 [27]
Fucus fucoidan (Sigma)	Mouse with surgical destabilization of the medial meniscus	20 mg/kg intraperitoneal injection	Fucoidan suppressed cellular infiltration of joint and suppress post-operative (3 days), but not late (16 weeks) pain	Mcnamee 2010 [70]
Fucus fucoidan (Sigma)	Wistar rats with carrageenan induced local inflammation in the footpad	20 mg/kg intravenously	Fucoidan inhibits mechanical hypernociception and neutrophil migration	Cunha 2008 [69]
Undaria pinnatifida fucoidan	Collagen induced arthritis in mice	100 kDa, 3.5 kDa and 1 kDa fractions orally administered daily 300 mg/kg to 49 days	1 kDa fraction effectively inhibited whereas 100 kDa exacerbated disease	Park 2010 [41]

6.2. Surgical Adhesions

As identified earlier, fucoidan is a potent selectin blocker, and can therefore inhibit inflammatory damage, such as that caused by post-ischemic inflammation. A fibrotic reaction after the inflammation is responsible for a condition called "surgical adhesions". This condition is a disabling result of minor damage during abdominal surgery or sometimes after infections. Small injuries cause inflammatory responses on the external surfaces of the bowel which generate the fibrotic response, leading to areas in which the bowel becomes tied to the peritoneal wall or to other parts of the bowel. Products aimed at reducing post surgical adhesions have variable levels of success. Now techniques have been developed using fucoidan as an ingredient in a film format [71]. In Cashman's 2010 study, a *Fucus vesiculosis* fucoidan loaded film inhibited the number of adhesions in a rabbit model by up to 90%. The effective level of fucoidan loading in the film was in the range of 0.33% to 33% w/w and no toxicity was observed.

6.3. Liver Fibrosis

Liver fibrosis occurs after toxic or pathogen insult to the liver. The function of the liver is compromised as the fibrous tissue takes over from active liver cells and significant morbidity may ensue. Several recent publications indicate that fucoidan has protective effects against liver damage by inhibiting fibrosis and this can be achieved by oral dosing in the models tested.

In damaged or diseased livers, hepatic stellate cells proliferate into fibrous masses whereas functional hepatic cells expire. Hayashi's 2008 research into carbon tetrachloride induced liver injury showed that fucoidan was a highly effective inhibitor of this type of fibrosis [72]. Saito used an alternative liver damage model (Concanavalin A), but used the same type of *Fucus vesiculosis* fucoidan [73] intravenously to inhibit the damage.

Nakazato's research used a different model of liver damage, but illustrated a profound inhibition of damage by orally delivered high molecular weight fractions of *Cladosiphon okamuranus* fucoidan [21]. Both crude (28 kDa) and high molecular weight (41.4 kDa) fucoidan fractions were delivered at 2% w/v in drinking water over 12 weeks. The high molecular weight fraction was a powerful inhibitor of N-nitrosodiethylamine (DEN) induced liver fibrosis as measured by histology and staining. There was a strong down regulation of TGF beta and SDF1 expression in the liver as compared to the controls.

D-galactosamine-induced hepatopathy is used as a model for liver disease because it resembles acute viral hepatitis [74]. Kawano had previously identified therapeutic potential of edible whole seaweeds in the diet of experimental rats with this type of liver damage [75]. In his 2007 study he identified the components of the seaweeds that gave rise to the inhibition of liver disease. The elevated levels of aspartate and alanine aminotransferases were inhibited specifically by the fucoidan in the diet at levels equivalent to those in whole seaweed at 5% of the total diet [75,76]. Lastly, Hayakawa addressed the issue of hepatocarcinoma in *ex vivo* samples of chronic cirrhosis and hepatitis B and C from a clinical setting and found that *Fucus vesiculosis* fucoidan has a potentially therapeutic effect [77].

To conclude, fucoidan appears to have good potential as an orally delivered adjunct therapy for liver disease. See Table 4 for details.

Table 4. Liver disease and fucoidan.

Fucoidan	Model	Treatment	Result	Ref.
Fucus vesiculosis fucoidan (Sigma)	Concanavalin induced liver injury in mice	1–30 mg/kg intravenously 30 min before concanavalin A	Significantly inhibited raised levels of TNF-alpha and IFN-gamma. Increased endogenous IL-10 production	Saito 2006 [73]
Fucus vesiculosis fucoidan (Sigma)	CCl4 induced liver fibrosis in mice	fucoidan (50 mg/kg body weight) administered intraperitoneally for 8 weeks	Protection of normal hepatocytes. Inhibition of hepatic stellate cell proliferation	Hayashi 2008 [72]
Cladosiphon okamuranus fractions Crude (28 kDa) and HMW (41.4 kDa)	N-nitrosodiethylamine (DEN) induced liver fibrosis model in Sprague dawley rats	2% fucoidan in drinking water for 12 weeks	Protection from damage Increased metallothionein Down regulation of TGFbeta 1 and SDF1	Nakazato 2010 [21]
Fucus vesiculosis fucoidan (Sigma)	*Ex vivo* human hepatoma (hepatitis B and C) and Cirrhosis	Inhibition of biotidinase in tissue samples was assessed	Fucoidan decreased the disease elevated activity of biotinidase	Hayakawa 2009 [77]
Fucus vesiculosis fucoidan (Sigma)	Rats with D-galactosamine-induced hepatopathy	Dietary inclusion of ~1.2% fucoidan for 8 days	Fucoidan was protective against D-galactosamineinduced hepatopathy in rat	Kawano 2007 [75,76]

6.4. Radiation and Fucoidan

Radiation causes a number of potential harms. Firstly, uptake of radioactive substances into the body perpetuates radiation damage, especially in children. Secondly, radiation damage itself causes cell death. This is particularly dangerous in that immune cells can be completely eliminated. The hemopoeitic stem cells that repopulate the immune system arise in the bone marrow and are called bone marrow stem cells. The protection of this progenitor population is very important in both medical and emergency settings.

Whole seaweed and seaweed extracts, particularly alginate, have been ingested as moderators of radiation damage [78]. The decontaminating effects of alginate syrups and additions to breads and milks have been known about for many years [79]. Alginate is used as a syrup useful in both reducing uptake of radioactive elements and increasing their excretion or "decorporation" [80]. Whilst iodine is a naturally occurring component and regular ingestion would assist in maintaining thyroid saturation, well timed and high levels of iodine in the form of sodium iodide are required to prevent uptake of radioactive isotopes of iodine.

Fucoidan, although a chelating agent, has not been recognized as a decorporation agent for radionuclides. It has, however, been demonstrated to provide radiation protection in both *in vitro* and mouse models [81,82]. Fucoidan was known to stimulate the maturation of dendritic cells, which are potent antigen-presenting cells in the immune system [83]. Byon measured the expression levels of cell surface markers in bone marrow stem cells after radiation. In this study the fucoidan was delivered intraperitoneally prior to radiation. As bone marrow is the main cellular source for the hematopoietic and immune systems, it contains large numbers of lymphocytes, granulocytes, and stromal cells as precursors and mature cells. Their results suggested that a specific population of cells—granulocytes— may selectively survive in response to fucoidan treatment following irradiation [82].

In irradiated mice the optimal intraperitoneal pre-treatment dosage of fucoidan to maximise survival was determined to be 100 mg/kg delivered into the peritoneal cavity [81]. Rhee also demonstrated the potential for protection from gamma irradiation in mice and *in vitro* [83]. *Laminaria japonica* derived fucoidan delivered intraperitoneally at 100 mg/kg was found to protect against changes in the counts of blood cells. Several parameters indicated better recovery after irradiation. The erythrocyte count in the irradiated controls ranged from 64% to 67% but the fucoidan-treated group increased gradually, ranging from 75% to 80%. The mean number of survival days and the

50-day survival rate in this group was 29 days and 30% at the highest fucoidan dose of 100 mg/kg as compared to 9 days and 0% for the control group.

6.5. Stem Cells and Fucoidan

Fucoidan is a known stem cell mobilizer when delivered intravenously. It has also shown activity then delivered orally [28]. When delivered intravenously, *Fucus vesiculosis* fucoidan is highly effective in mobilizing stem cells into the peripheral circulation in baboons and mice. The mechanism of mobilization appears not to relate solely to the inhibition of selectin binding but also to fucoidan's ability to bind to SDF1 (CXCL12) [84,85]. Stem cell mobilization is used as a method of collecting sufficient immune repopulating cells from the peripheral circulation that are stored and re-engrafted after chemotherapy and radiotherapy in selected cancer patients.

SDF1 binds to the G protein coupled CXCR4 receptor, which has SDF1 as its unique ligand. CXCR4 is expressed by some hemopoietic stem cells, most leukocyte populations, endothelial cells, epithelial cells and some carcinoma cells. This SDF1/CXCR4 affiliation is thought to be involved not only in the regulation of stem cell release and homing, but also in some disease processes, including fibrogenesis [85].

The binding of fucoidan to SDF1 was found to block liver regeneration in an animal model [86]. This outcome contrasts with the marked radiation protection of hemopoietic stem cells by fucoidan described in Section 6.4 and the effective use of fucoidan in the inhibition of liver disease in a number of animal models as described in Section 6.3. In Mavier's example, *Fucus vesiculosis* fucoidan was delivered intraperitoneally to rats at 25 mg/kg body weight. The liver was entirely damaged, both chemically and physically, and regeneration was observed. Under less dramatic circumstances, the liver regenerates from mature differentiated cells but when injured or after partial hepatectomy combined with inhibition of mature hepatocyte proliferation, regeneration is achieved from liver stem cells, which are known as "oval cells". In the control damaged rats, oval cell accumulation could be seen, but in fucoidan treated rats, the oval cell numbers were severely depressed.

Oral delivery of *Undaria pinnatifida* fucoidan in a clinical observational study also resulted in an increase in the number of stem cells, of serum levels of SDF1 and the expression of CXCR4 on stem cells (CD34+) [28]. This observation correlates with the *in vitro* and animal studies showing that fucoidan mobilizes stem cells, although the degree of mobilization was not as large at the time point measured. The increase in CXCR4 expression could in some way reflect the binding of SDF1 by fucoidan.

Lastly, oral delivery of a seaweed extract in a clinical study consisting of a blend of *Fucus vesiculosis*, *Macrocystis pyrifera* and *Laminaria japonica* fucoidans increased phagocytosis by granulocytes and macrophages [33] in addition to NK and cytotoxic T cell numbers. Additionally the chronic inflammation marker interleukin 6 was lowered. This data has common features with an animal study carried out by Shimizu [38] and may point to the potential for radiation protection potential by orally delivered fucoidan.

6.6. Blood Homeostasis

It is beyond the scope of this review to consider the entire recent research on fucoidan fractions and blood homeostasis. In brief, fucoidan compounds have a retarding effect on coagulation in part due to interference with antithrombin III and heparin cofactor II [87]. The *in vivo* effects of intravenous delivery of most types of fucoidan are to extend global clotting time, an effect which is reversible [36]. Kwak recently investigated *Fucus vesiculosis* fucoidans inhibitory effect in a ferric chloride induced thrombosis model in mice [88]. Fucoidan showed a stronger antithrombotic effect than heparin. The anti-thrombin and anti-factor Xa activities of fucoidan *in vitro* were less than those of heparin, which implies that the antithrombotic activities are due to binding with heparin cofactor II rather than with antithrombin.

Pomin addresses the issues of strong anticoagulant activity of fucoidans by desulfation, producing fractions with desirable bioactivity unfettered by anticoagulant behaviors [89]. A linear sulfated fucoidan from sea urchin egg jelly required significantly longer chains than mammalian glycosaminoglycans to achieve the same anticoagulant activity. A slight decrease in the molecular size of the sulfated fucan dramatically reduced its effect on thrombin inactivation mediated by heparin cofactor II. A sulfated fucoidan with 45 tetrasaccharide repeating units was able to bind to heparin cofactor II but was unable to link efficiently the plasma inhibitor and thrombin, which required fucoidan with 100 or more tetrasaccharide repeating units.

A recent clinical study examined the effects of orally ingested fucoidan on clotting times. 3 g of *Undaria pinnatifida* fucoidan were ingested daily for 12 days by healthy subjects [29]. A significant prolongation of global clotting time was noted but this was within normal clinical parameters. Toxicological studies on *Undaria pinnatifida* fucoidan in rats showed no effect on clotting times, even at very high doses [25]. A toxicology study on *Laminaria japonica* fucoidan did show some pertubations in clotting at 900 mg/kg [26], far above the dose used in the clinical study.

More recent research into activity illustrates the somewhat counter-intuitive "procoagulant" effect of fucoidan in hemophilia model [31]. In hemophilia A dogs, orally delivered *Laminaria japonica* fucoidan fraction improved clotting times, perhaps by creating a bypass in the normally blocked clotting pathway.

6.7. Neuronal Protection

Increasing interest in reducing or reversing brain ageing and disease has seen many agents assessed for their effects on neurons and brain function. Alzheimer's is a brain disease that causes significant and highly distressing loss of function. It is characterized by the accumulation of beta amyloid plaques in the brain tissue. It has been hypothesized that Alzheimer's is associated with Herpes infections in the central nervous system [90]. The relatively large size of fucoidan precludes penetration of the blood brain barrier but as noted below, systemic administration was effective in maintaining neuronal function in a mouse model.

Fucoidan shows promise in protecting brain function in a number of ways. It has been comprehensively assessed by Jhamandas [91] for effects on current in whole rat brain neurons and also on the neurotoxic effects caused by beta amyloid in primary culture neuronal cells. *Fucus vesiculosis* fucoidan at one micromolar concentration could inhibit currents by 15%. It was also able to reverse the current blocking effects of beta amyloid. Fucoidan did not inhibit the aggregation of beta amyloid, but did protect primary cultures of rat basal forebrain cholinergic neurons, against amyloid induced cell death.

Cui's recent research centered on a lipopolysaccharide (LPS) activated microglial cells [92]. Microglia are usually resting cells in the brain, but if activated, for example by LPS, they change shape, become active and secrete inflammatory mediators and nitric oxide (NO). If too much activation takes place, surrounding neuronal cells die, instigating more inflammation and beginning a cycle of neurodegeneration. 62.5 mcg/mL fucoidan was able to prevent shape change in the LPS exposed microglial cultures, and 125 mcg/mL inhibited NO production. In 2004 Li demonstrated the characteristic fragmented DNA (fDNA) observed in neuronal nuclei in Alzheimer brain was taken up by adjacent activated microglia which then became activated [93]. Blocking the scavenger receptors on the microglial cells with *Fucus vesiculosis* fucoidan at 40 ng/mL suppressed this uptake.

Pei also demonstrated the scavenger receptors on microglial cells could be successfully blocked by fucoidan [94]. Huang [95] used time lapse recording to investigate how microglia are involved in the growth of amyloid plaques. *Fucus vesiculosis* fucoidan at 10 micromolar concentration was able to inhibit the amyloid induced microglical clustering effect that gave rise to plaques. Do presented a study on tumor necrosis factor alpha (TNF-alpha) and interferon gamma (IFN-gamma) induced NO production in glioma cells [96]. Fucoidan inhibited NO production in this model system via a number of signaling pathways.

Luo, from the same research team as Cui, investigated the effects of the same *Laminaria japonica* fucoidan fraction in a model of Parkinson's disease in mice [97]. Mice were given fucoidan at a dose rate of 12.5 mg/kg or 25 mg/kg, intraperitoneally daily for 18 days. The Parkinson's inducing agent was given on the 11th day an hour after injection of fucoidan. There was a clear dose dependent protection by fucoidan at 25 mg/kg body weight, including inhibition of lipid peroxidation, enzyme functions and glutathione levels. See Table 5.

Table 5. Brain cells and fucoidan.

Fucoidan type	Model	Effects	Reference
Fucus vesiculosis fuucoidan (Sigma)	Rat neuron *in vitro*	Inhibits neurotoxic effects of amyloid	Jhamandas 2005 [91]
Laminaria japonica fuucoidan average MW 7000	Lipopolysaccharide activated microglial cells *in vitro*	Inhibits NO production in LPS activated microglial cells	Cui 2010 [92]
Sea cucumber fucoidan	Neuronal stem cells *in vitro*	Protection from radiation	Zhang 2010 [98]
Laminaria japonica fuucoidan average MW 7000	MPTP-induced Parkinsonism in mice Fucoidan delivered IP	Protects against Parkinsons disease model of neuronal damage	Luo 2009 [97]
Fucus vesiculosis fucoidan (Sigma)	Microglial cells *in vitro*	Fucoidan completely blocks microglial uptake of fDNA at only 40 ng/mL	Li 2004 [93]
Fucus vesiculosis fucoidan (Sigma)	*In vitro* microglial clustering assay	Fucoidan inhibits beta amyloid induced microglial clustering at 10 μM	Huang 2009 [95]
Fucus vesiculosis fucoidan (Sigma)	Microglial cells *in vitro*	Inhibits LPS uptake into microglia by scavenger receptors	Pei 2007 [94]
Fucus vesiculosis fucoidan (Sigma)	Glioma cells *in vitro*	Fucoidan inhibits TNF-alpha- and IFN-gamma-stimulated NO production via p38 MAPK, AP-1, JAK/STAT and IRF-1	Do 2009 [96]
Fucus vesiculosis fucoidan (Sigma)	NO production in neuronal blastoma cells *in vitro*	Fucoidan has protective effect via inducible nitric oxide synthase (iNOS)	Lee 2007 [99]

6.8. Viruses: Influenza, Herpes and Dengue

Inhibitory effects of fucoidan on coated viruses are well known and were well reviewed a decade ago by Schaeffer [100]. Fucoidans have no direct pathogen killing activity but rather, they inhibit infection via receptor entry blocking and interference with replicative processes. Other sulfated polysaccharides in addition to fucoidans have been known to possess inhibitory activity against coated viruses such as Herpes and HIV [100,102]. In the case of viruses, receptor blocking activity prevents viral cell entry and there may also be inhibition of viral replication and syncytia (giant cell) formation. Drawbacks to using fucoidan as an orally delivered agent remain those of bioavailability. However, pathogens targetable from the lumen of the gut, such as viruses harbored in gut immune structures, may be particularly well targeted by oral fucoidan. As the following examples illustrate, oral dosing does have protective effects against viral infection.

Influenza epidemics have become topical in recent years with outbreaks of Influenza A causing significant global concern. Existing therapies can become useless as resistance develops. Several research groups have investigated inhibitory effect of fucoidan fractions on clinical strains of influenza [103] and para-influenza [104] *in vitro*. *Undaria pinnatifida* has a marked inhibitory effect on the recent H1N1 influenza A virus with half maximal effective inhibitory concentrations at less than 1 mcg/mL [44]. Notably, these effects can also be seen *in vivo* with orally delivered fucoidan. Hayashi reported mouse model data in which 5 mg per day orally delivered *Undaria pinnatifida* fucoidan strongly inhibited influenza A infection [44]. It had a marked synergistic effect with oseltamivir, a neuraminidase inhibitor effective in treating influenza. Even as a sole agent, fucoidan was able to significantly reduce viral titres in the lung of infected mice. At the time of writing, there are no clinical studies on Influenza using fucoidan reported in the available literature.

Herpes infections can be debilitating and recurrent. There is a need for a both treatment and prevention strategies for both Herpes 1 and 2. In a small clinical case study series, Herpes reactivation was inhibited by ingesting a fucoidan rich *Undaria pinnatifida* preparation [105]. *Undaria pinnatifida* fucoidan was shown to be a highly effective inhibitor of clinical strains of Herpes entry to cells in culture [102,106] at microgram concentrations. Interestingly, stains resistant to the common drug therapy, acyclovir, were equally well inhibited. Hayashi established that the inhibitory effect of fucoidan was carried over to *in vivo* setting in a mouse model [101]. In his research, orally delivered *Undaria pinnatifida* fucoidan exerted protective effects via direct inhibition of viral replication and stimulation of both innate and adaptive immune defense functions. Oral administration of the fucoidan at 5 mg/day every 8 h (three times per day) from 1 week before virus inoculation to 1 week post-inoculation (pretreatment), or for 1 week after virus inoculation protected mice from infection with HSV-1 and enhanced cytotoxic T cell activity. NK cell activity was improved in HSV-1-infected immunosuppressed mice. The production of neutralizing antibodies in the mice inoculated with HSV-1 was significantly promoted by the oral administration of the fucoidan for 3 weeks.

Dengue virus is a debilitating viral infection spread by mosquitoes. Sometimes known as 'bone crack fever' for its painful joint effects, it has four different subtypes. Infection by one does not confer protection from infection by another type. There are no treatments for dengue other than pain relief and good nursing. Fucoidan from *Cladosiphon* has been shown to inhibit type 2 dengue *in vitro* [107]. Given the effectiveness of oral fucoidan in inhibiting Herpes, there may be potential in further research into the inhibitory effects of fucoidan fractions on Dengue fever. At the time of writing, there are no clinical studies on dengue using fucoidan reported in the literature.

6.9. Viruses: HTLV1

In a clinical "first" this year, Araya presented data on orally delivered fucoidan to treat Japanese subjects infected with Human T lymphotropic virus type-1 (HTLV-1) [34]. This human retrovirus causes HTLV-1associated myelopathy/tropical spastic paraparesis (HAM/TSP) and is also responsible for adult T cell leukaemia in a small number of infected subjects. A higher viral load in individuals with HTLV-1 infection increases their risk of developing and the clinical progression of HAM/TSP and unpleasant and increasingly disabling condition. *In vitro* studies by Japanese and Brazilian researchers have indicated that fucoidan from *Cladosiphon okamuranus,* and fucoidan containing water extracts from *Sargassum vulgare* and *Laminaria abysslis* were effective at inhibiting HTLV-1 viral infection in cell culture [108,109]. Although the extracts were not selectively toxic to infected cells, syncytia formation and thus cell to cell transfer of the virus was inhibited. In Araya's 2011 study, the *in vitro* inhibitory effect of fucoidan on cell-to-cell HTLV-1 infection was confirmed by using luciferase reporter cell assays.

In Araya's open-label trial, 13 patients with HAM/TSP were treated with 6 g of a relatively pure (85%) *Cladosiphon okamuranus* derived fucoidan daily for 6–13 months. HTLV-1 proviral DNA load was measured and found to decrease by 42.4% on average over the trial period. Interestingly, there was variation in the trial subjects with some achieving much greater reductions. Araya also measured immune cell function, as fucoidans are known to modulate immune function in other animal [38,40,53] and clinical studies [33,53]. Frequencies of HTLV-1-specific CD8(+) T-cells, natural killer cells, invariant natural killer T-cells and dendritic cells in the peripheral blood were analyzed but did not show significant changes. This contrasts with research in which fucoidan intake did alter immune parameters [33,40]. In this clinical study, there were mild side effects. During the treatment four patients with HAM/TSP developed diarrhea, which improved immediately after stopping fucoidan administration.

6.10. Leishmaniasis

Leishmaniasis is a protozoan parasite spread by the bites of sandflies. As many as 12 million people are believed to be currently infected, with about 1–2 million estimated new cases occurring every year [110]. There are many different types of leishmaniasis, most being spread from animal to humans, but some species are also spread between humans. Leishmaniasis most commonly manifests as a skin disease causing ulcers but may also spread to organs, a condition known as "visceral leishmaniasis" and can be fatal. There are no vaccines for leishmaniasis, and one older treatment, sodium antimony gluconate, is no longer effective in India.

In 2011, Kar published research in which fucoidan was administered in a rat model to treat Leishmaniasis [111]. Whilst the authors are cautious about the extrapolation of their work to humans and to other types of leishmaniasis, the potential for an adjunct or even a sole therapy is strong. Their data showed inhibitory effects on amastigote (part of the life cycle of leishmaniasis) multiplication within macrophages. There was complete elimination of liver and spleen parasite burden at 200 mg/kg/day given orally, 3 times weekly, in a 6-week mouse model of both antimony-susceptible and -resistant strains. They noted switching of immune defense from a Th2 to Th1 mode and increased splenocyte superoxide and NO production. IL-10 and TGF beta, both Th1 suppressive cytokines, were found to be profoundly down-regulated in infected fucoidan-treated mice. TGF beta, was found to be significantly down-regulated in fucoidan-treated mice. Most importantly, fucoidan was thought to be curative when administered orally 15 days post-infection.

At the time of writing there are no published clinical studies involving fucoidan and leishmaniasis infections.

6.11. Malaria

According to the World Health Organization, in 2008, there were 247 million cases of malaria and nearly one million deaths. Malaria is caused by four different types of *Plasmodium* parasites. The parasites are spread to people through the bites of infected *Anopheles* mosquitoes, called "malaria vectors". If resistance to the currently effective artemisinin drugs develops and spreads to other large geographical areas, as has happened before with chloroquine and sulfacoxine-pyrimethamine the public health consequences could be grim, as no alternative antimalarial medicines will be available in the near future.

The malaria parasites (*Plasmodium* merozoites) enter the blood stream and must then penetrate a red blood cell (erythrocyte) in order to multiply. The cell bursts and the cycle begins again. Malaria leads to severe anemia and cycles of fever as the parasite takes hold. Fucoidan is one agent that shows some promise as an inhibitory agent for *Plasmodium* infection *in vitro* and in mouse models [112]. *Undaria pinnatifida* fucoidan significantly inhibited the invasion of erythrocytes by *Plasmodium falciparum* merozoites. Four-day suppressive testing in *Plasmodium berghei*-infected mice (a model system) with fucoidan resulted in a 37% suppressive effect *versus* the control group and a significant delay in the deaths from anemia.

At the time of writing, there are no clinical studies on malaria using fucoidan reported in the available literature.

6.12. Prions

Transmissible spongiform encephalopathies or "prion" diseases are a group of fatal neurodegenerative disorders. They include the human diseases "Kuru" and Creutzfeldt-Jakob disease (CJD), the sheep disease scrapie, and bovine spongiform encephalopathy which affects cattle. 'Kuru' occurs among people from New Guinea who practiced a form of cannibalism in which they ate the brains of dead people as part of a funeral ritual. This practice stopped in 1960, but cases of Kuru occurred for decades because of the long incubation period [113,114]. These diseases are characterized by accumulation of an abnormally folded prion protein in the central nervous system and the lympho-reticular system. Recently, variant CJD became a major health concern in Europe after infected meat entered the food chain.

Prions remain a therapeutic challenge with no approved preventative or curative drug therapy available. Doh-Ura and colleagues examined the effects of fucoidan ingestion on prion infection in a mouse model and illustrated that prior ingestion of fucoidan could inhibit the development of disease [115]. Fucoidan orally administered to the mice after the enteral inoculation delayed the disease onset for about half the time of the control incubation. However fucoidan administered before enteral inoculation did not affect the incubation time. As fucoidans are large molecules, the blood brain barrier is unlikely to allow passage into the central nervous system. It is perhaps more likely that fucoidan exerted effects via the gut immune system. To date there are no reported clinical studies with fucoidan to assess effects on prion infections.

6.13. Helicobacter and Stomach Ulcers

A recent encouraging clinical study was carried out in Indonesia to determine the effectiveness of fucoidan therapy for *Helicobacter pylori* affected patients [116]. This study was supported by considerable *in vitro* and *in vivo* evidence to suggest that fucoidan has inhibitory effects on *Helicobacter* infections, largely by inhibiting adhesion to mucosal surfaces [117]. Juffrie's study included patients with at least eight years of abdominal pain or dyspepsia. After endoscope confirmation of ulceration and *Helicobacter* infection, subjects took placebo or 100 mg *Cladosiphon okamuranus* fucoidan daily for three weeks before undergoing another endoscopy which included a biopsy. There was relief from symptoms such as pain and vomiting in the fucoidan treated patients from 5 days into the study. At biopsy, the majority of the patients with severe ulcers who received fucoidan at 100 mg per day for three weeks changed to the healing stage or scarring stage whereas only 37.5% patients who received placebo changed to the healing stage.

In animal models, aspirin induced ulceration (a model for gastric ulcers) could be inhibited by orally delivered *Fucus vesiculosis* fucoidan at dose rates of 20 mg/kg body weight/day for two weeks [118]. Aspirin treatment generated the expected rises aspartate and alanine transaminases (AST and ALT) and the serum cytokines IL6, IL10 and IFN gamma. Oral fucoidan showed considerable ($p < 0.05$) protection against ulceration by inhibiting the acute alterations of AST, ALT, cytokines and stomach glycogen. However, aggravated serum INF-gamma was observed in the fucoidan-pre-treated group [118].

6.14. Renal Disease and Hyperoxaluria

Fucoidan may act in several ways to protect against kidney damage. As for other organs in the post ischemic stage, reperfusion injury may be protected by *Fucus vesiculosis* fucoidan administration at 10 mg/kg intravenously on the basis of its ability to inhibit P selectin [119]. Zhang demonstrated the effects of up to 200 mg/kg body weight orally administered *Laminaria japonica* fucoidan in the prevention of chronic renal failure or Heymann nephritis (an autoimmune condition) in a rat model [120,121].

Elevated levels of oxalate in serum are commonly associated with the painful joint swellings known as gout. Elevated oxalate levels are also responsible for kidney stones. In 2007, Veena assessed *Fucus vesiculosis* fucoidan in Wistar rats in which hyperoxaluria and calcium oxalate deposition in the kidneys was induced by ethylene glycol [122]. Daily doses of 5mg/kg body weight were administered subcutaneously over 28 days, after which tissues were harvested for assessment. Fucoidan successfully normalized the disturbances associated with hyperoxaluria. Josephine, from the same research group, published additional research in which the effects of fucoidan on Cyclosporine A (CsA)-induced nephrotoxicity were assessed [123]. A dose of 5 mg/kg body weight fucoidan isolated from *Sargassum wightii* or *Fucus vesiculosis* was administered subcutaneously over 21 days. Both fucoidans protected mitochondrial function and other biological measures to the same degree. The reasoning behind the model was the therapeutic use of cyclosporine. Cyclosporine is a useful immunosuppressive during transplants yet its nephrotoxicity curtails the degree of its use.

6.15. Snake Envenomation

Snake bite is a seriously neglected issue affecting Central and South America, parts of Asia and Africa [124,126]. Existing therapy for snake bites consists of anti-venoms. These can be costly, have a limited shelf life and also require careful storage. They are not always available in areas of greatest need.

Snake venoms are a complex mixture that may cause swelling, bleeding, blistering, and ultimately skin and muscle necrosis. In bites from commonly occurring South American snakes these effects are caused by two major components of the venoms; zinc dependent metalloproteinases and myotoxic phospholipases (PLA2). The metalloproteases degrade extracellular matrix components, such as the collagens that make up microvessel structures. The myotoxic phospholipases break down the plasma membrane of skeletal muscle cells. A large inflammatory reaction ensues with infiltration of leukocytes. Swelling follows, which can cause restricted blood flow, ischemia and further tissue damage.

Fucoidan from *Ascophyllum nodosum* was been investigated by Costa Rican research teams and was found to be an effective inhibitor of PLA2 variants present in the venoms of crotalid snakes [124,127]. Crotalid snake venom damages the lymphatic system via the enzyme PLA2. Mora demonstrated that the potent PLA2 inhibitory effects of fucoidan could completely eliminate the myotoxic effects of the venom if preincubated with it prior to injection in a mouse model, but it did not change the hemorrhagic effects of the venom [125]. Angulo demonstrated that fucoidan forms complexes with the snake venom PLA2 and inactivates them [127].

In Rucavado's most recent study [124], the effect of fucoidan combined with batimastat (a peptidomimetic hydroxamate metalloproteinase inhibitor known to inhibit crotalid venom activity) was investigated in a mouse model. Fucoidan reduced the presence of intracellular proteins in exudates, whereas batimastat reduced the amount of relevant extracellular matrix proteins. The combination of these inhibitors resulted in the elimination of the most relevant pathological effects of this venom.

Curiously, lowering the molecular weight of the fucoidan to theoretically enhance bioavailability was not effective in inhibiting snake venom [42]. A study evaluated the ability of two fractions of *Ascophyllum nodosum* fucoidan to prevent muscle necrosis when rapidly administered after injection of a purified myotoxin or crude venom in a mouse model. The two preparations were standardized to the same neutralizing potency. Local administration into the muscle of either fraction after myotoxin injection prevented nearly 50% of muscle necrosis. However, when tested against crude venom (which contains several myotoxin isoforms), muscle injection of the higher molecular weight fraction inhibited myonecrosis by nearly 50% as compared to the untreated group. In contrast to expectations, the use of smaller fucoidan fragments reduced rather than increased the therapeutic response. This may relate to a particular structural feature in the high molecular weight fraction that is absent in the lower molecular weight fraction.

In 2003, Vasanthi described the successful inhibition of cobra snake venom in a mouse model by intraperitoneal administration of an extract from *Padina boergensii* [128]. However, the extract was prepared with methanol, and it is unclear whether fucoidan was a major component of the extract as fucoidan has limited solubility in alcohols.

The relative stability of fucoidan fractions compared to conventionally produced antivenoms means that no cold storage would be required and a long shelf life could be anticipated. The development of fucoidan for this application could potentially limit the complications and distress caused by snakebite in a cost effective and realistic manner.

7. Conclusions

This review covers some of the more recent research into the bioactivity and discusses potential therapies from fucoidan. The research field has increased in the last decade and has started to produce clinical studies. This review has spanned potential applications as diverse as prion infection and osteoarthritis. The development of fucoidan fractions requires attention to the source and the required characteristics of the fraction, in addition to consideration of the route of delivery. Oral delivery appears promising, with research indicating therapeutic potential in different areas. Increasing bioavailability is likely to be important for orally delivered fucoidan. Overall, the availability and safety of commercially available fucoidan preparations will lead to interesting adjunct and sole therapies for some neglected disease states in addition to providing new approaches to inflammation and fibrosis.

Acknowledgments: The author wishes to thank Vicki Gardiner for her valuable assistance with the manuscript. The author wishes to apologise to any authors whose valuable research was not mentioned in this review for space reasons.

References

1. Kiple, KF; Ornelas, KC. Important Vegetable Supplements. In *The Cambridge World History of Food*; Beck, SV, Ed.; Cambridge University Press: Cambridge, UK, 2000; Volume 1, pp. 231–249.
2. Berteau, O; Mulloy, B. Sulfated fucans, fresh perspectives: Structures, functions, and biological properties of sulfated fucans and an overview of enzymes active toward this class of polysaccharide. *Glycobiolog* **2003**, *13*, 29–40.
3. Kylin, H. Zur biochemie der meeresalgen. *Hoppe-Seyler's Z. Physiol. Chem* **1913**, *83*, 171–197.
4. Bird, GM; Haas, P. On the nature of the cell wall constituents of *Laminaria* spp. Mannuronic acid. *Biochem. J* **1931**, *25*, 403–411.
5. Percival, EGV; Ross, AG. Fucoidin. Part I. The isolation and purification of fucoidin from brown seaweeds. *J. Chem. Soc* **1950**, *145*, 717–720.
6. Black, WAP; Dewar, ET; Woodward, FN. Manufacture of algal chemicals. IV. Laboratory scale isolation of fucoidin from brown marine algae. *J. Sci. Food Agric* **1952**, *3*, 122–129.
7. Bairstow, S; McKee, J; Nordhaus, M; Johnson, R. Identification of a simple and sensitive microplate method for the detection of oversulfated chondroitin sulfate in heparin products. *Anal. Biochem* **2009**, *388*, 317–321.
8. US Department of Health and Human Services, FDA. *Center for Drug Evaluation and Research (CDER), Guidance for Industry Botanical Drug Products*. 2004. Available online: http://www.fda.gov/cder/guidance/index.htm accessed on 20 May 2011.
9. Fitton, JH; Irhimeh, MR; Teas, J. Marine Algae and Polysaccharides with Therapeutic Applications. In *Marine Nutraceuticals and Functional Foods*; Barrow, C, Shahidi, F, Eds.; CRC Press, Taylor & Francis Group: Boca Raton, FL, USA, 2008; pp. 345–366.
10. Pomin, VH; Mourao, PA. Structure, biology, evolution, and medical importance of sulfated fucans and galactans. *Glycobiology* **2008**, *18*, 1016–1027.
11. Li, B; Lu, F; Wei, X; Zhao, R. Fucoidan: Structure and bioactivity. *Molecules* **2008**, *13*, 1671–1695.
12. Nishino, T; Nishioka, C; Ura, H; Nagumo, T. Isolation and partial characterization of a novel amino sugar-containing fucan sulfate from commercial *Fucus vesiculosus* fucoidan. *Carbohydr. Res* **1994**, *255*, 213–224.
13. Michel, C; Lahaye, M; Bonnet, C; Mabeau, S; Barry, J-L. *In vitro* fermentation by human faecal bacteria of total and purified dietary fibres from brown seaweeds. *Br. J. Nutr* **1996**, *75*, 263–280.
14. Yamada, Y; Miyoshi, T; Tanada, S; Imaki, M. Digestibility and energy availability of Wakame (*Undaria pinnatifida*) seaweed in Japanese. *Nippon Eiseigaku Zasshi* **1991**, *46*, 788–794.
15. Lynch, MB; Sweeney, T; Callan, JJ; O'Sullivan, JT; O'Doherty, JV. The effect of dietary Laminaria-derived laminarin and fucoidan on nutrient digestibility, nitrogen utilisation, intestinal microflora and volatile fatty acid concentration in pigs. *J. Sci. Food Agric* **2010**, *90*, 430–437.
16. O'Sullivan, L; Murphy, B; McLoughlin, P; Duggan, P; Lawlor, PG; Hughes, H; Gardiner, GE. Prebiotics from marine macroalgae for human and animal health applications. *Mar. Drugs* **2010**, *8*, 2038–2064.
17. Barthe, L; Woodley, J; Lavit, M; Przybylski, C; Philibert, C; Houin, G. *In vitro* intestinal degradation and absorption of chondroitin sulfate, a glycosaminoglycan drug. *Arzneimittelforschung* **2004**, *54*, 286–292.
18. Elsenhans, B; Caspary, WF. Differential changes in the urinary excretion of two orally administered polyethylene glycol markers (PEG 900 and PEG 4000) in rats after feeding various carbohydrate gelling agents. *J. Nutr* **1989**, *119*, 380–387.
19. Irhimeh, MR; Fitton, JH; Lowenthal, RM; Kongtawelert, P. A quantitative method to detect fucoidan in human plasma using a novel antibody. *Methods Find Exp. Clin. Pharmacol* **2005**, *27*, 705–710.

20. Tokita, Y; Nakajima, K; Mochida, H; Iha, M; Nagamine, T. Development of a fucoidan-specific antibody and measurement of fucoidan in serum and urine by sandwich ELISA. *Biosci. Biotechnol. Biochem* **2010**, *74*, 350–357.

21. Nakazato, K; Takada, H; Iha, M; Nagamine, T. Attenuation of N-nitrosodiethylamine-induced liver fibrosis by high-molecular-weight fucoidan derived from *Cladosiphon okamuranus*. *J. Gastroenterol. Hepatol* **2010**, *25*, 1692–1701.

22. Guimaraes, MA; Mourao, PA. Urinary excretion of sulfated polysaccharides administered to Wistar rats suggests a renal permselectivity to these polymers based on molecular size. *Biochim. Biophys. Acta* **1997**, *1335*, 161–172.

23. Mizuno, M; Nishitani, Y; Tanoue, T; Matoba, Y; Ojima, T; Hashimoto, T; Kanazawa, K. Quantification and localization of fucoidan in Laminaria japonica using a novel antibody. *Biosci. Biotechnol. Biochem* **2009**, *73*, 335–338.

24. Eardley, DD; Sutton, C; Hempel, WM; Reed, DC; Ebeling, AW. Monoclonal antibodies specific for sulfated polysaccharides on the surface of *Macrocystis pyrifera*. *J. Phycol* **1990**, *26*, 54–62.

25. Chung, HJ; Jeun, J; Houng, SJ; Jun, HJ; Kweon, DK; Lee, SJ. Toxicological evaluation of fucoidan from *Undaria pinnatifida in vitro* and *in vivo*. *Phytother. Res* **2010**, *24*, 1078–1083.

26. Li, N; Zhang, Q; Song, J. Toxicological evaluation of fucoidan extracted from *Laminaria japonica* in wistar rats. *Food Chem. Toxicol* **2005**, *43*, 421–426.

27. Myers, SP; O'Connor, J; Fitton, JH; Brooks, L; Rolfe, M; Connellan, P; Wohlmuth, H; Cheras, PA; Morris, C. A combined phase I and II open label study on the effects of a seaweed extract nutrient complex on osteoarthritis. *Biologics* **2010**, *4*, 33–44.

28. Irhimeh, MR; Fitton, JH; Lowenthal, RM. Fucoidan ingestion increases the expression of CXCR4 on human CD34+ cells. *Exp. Hematol* **2007**, *35*, 989–994.

29. Irhimeh, MR; Fitton, JH; Lowenthal, RM. Pilot clinical study to evaluate the anticoagulant activity of fucoidan. *Blood Coagul. Fibrinolysis* **2009**, *20*, 607–610.

30. Kim, KJ; Lee, OH; Lee, HH; Lee, BY. A 4-week repeated oral dose toxicity study of fucoidan from the Sporophyll of *Undaria pinnatifida* in Sprague-Dawley rats. *Toxicology* **2009**, *267*, 154–158.

31. Prasad, S; Lillicrap, D; Labelle, A; Knappe, S; Keller, T; Burnett, E; Powell, S; Johnson, KW. Efficacy and safety of a new-class hemostatic drug candidate, AV513, in dogs with hemophilia A. *Blood* **2008**, *111*, 672–679.

32. Kim, KJ; Lee, OH; Lee, BY. Genotoxicity studies on fucoidan from Sporophyll of *Undaria pinnatifida*. *Food Chem. Toxicol* **2010**, *48*, 1101–1104.

33. Myers, SP; O'Connor, J; Fitton, JH; Brooks, L; Rolfe, M; Connellan, P; Wohlmuth, H; Cheras, PA; Morris, C. A combined Phase I and II open-label study on the immunomodulatory effects of seaweed extract nutrient complex. *Biologics* **2011**, *5*, 45–60.

34. Araya, N; Takahashi, K; Sato, T; Nakamura, T; Sawa, C; Hasegawa, D; Ando, H; Aratani, S; Yagishita, N; Fujii, R; *et al.* Fucoidan therapy decreases the proviral load in patients with human T-lymphotropic virus type-1-associated neurological disease. *Antivir. Ther* **2011**, *16*, 89–98.

35. Zhang, J; Tiller, C; Shen, J; Wang, C; Girouard, GS; Dennis, D; Barrow, CJ; Miao, M; Ewart, HS. Antidiabetic properties of polysaccharide- and polyphenolic-enriched fractions from the brown seaweed Ascophyllum nodosum. *Can. J. Physiol. Pharmacol* **2007**, *85*, 1116–1123.

36. Cumashi, A; Ushakova, NA; Preobrazhenskaya, ME; D'Incecco, A; Piccoli, A; Totani, L; Tinari, N; Morozevich, GE; Berman, AE; Bilan, MI; *et al.* A comparative study of the anti-inflammatory, anticoagulant, antiangiogenic, and antiadhesive activities of nine different fucoidans from brown seaweeds. *Glycobiology* **2007**, *17*, 541–552.

37. Laubli, H; Borsig, L. Selectins promote tumor metastasis. *Semin. Cancer Biol* **2010**, *20*, 169–177.

38. Maruyama, H; Tamauchi, H; Hashimoto, M; Nakano, T. Suppression of Th2 immune responses by Mekabu fucoidan from *Undaria pinnatifida* sporophylls. *Int. Arch. Allergy Immunol* **2005**, *137*, 289–294.

39. Maruyama, H; Tamauchi, H; Hashimoto, M; Nakano, T. Antitumor activity and immune response of Mekabu fucoidan extracted from sporophyll of *Undaria pinnatifida*. *In Vivo* **2003**, *17*, 245–249.

40. Shimizu, J; Wada-Funada, U; Mano, H; Matahira, Y; Kawaguchi, M; Wada, M. Proportion of murine cytotoxic T-cell is increased by high-molecular weight fucoidan extracted from Okinawa Mozuku (*Cladosiphon okamuranus*). *J. Health Sci* **2005**, *51*, 394–397.

41. Park, SB; Chun, KR; Kim, JK; Suk, K; Jung, YM; Lee, WH. The differential effect of high and low molecular weight fucoidans on the severity of collagen-induced arthritis in mice. *Phytother. Res* **2010**, *24*, 1384–1391.

42. Azofeifa, K; Angulo, Y; Lomonte, B. Ability of fucoidan to prevent muscle necrosis induced by snake venom myotoxins: Comparison of high- and low-molecular weight fractions. *Toxicon* **2008**, *51*, 373–380.

43. Yanase, Y; Hiragun, T; Uchida, K; Ishii, K; Oomizu, S; Suzuki, H; Mihara, S; Iwamoto, K; Matsuo, H; Onishi, N; Kameyoshi, Y; Hide, M. Peritoneal injection of fucoidan suppresses the increase of plasma IgE induced by OVA-sensitization. *Biochem. Biophys. Res. Commun* **2009**, *387*, 435–439.

44. Hayashi, T; Hayashi, K; Kanekiyo, K; Ohta, Y; Lee, J-B. Promising antiviral Glyco-molecules from an edible alga. In *Combating the Threat of Pandemic Influenza: Drug Discovery Approaches*; Torrence, PF, Ed.; John Wiley & Sons: Hoboken, NJ, USA, 2007; pp. 166–182.

45. Wynn, TA. Cellular and molecular mechanisms of fibrosis. *J. Pathol* **2008**, *214*, 199–210.

46. Preobrazhenskaya, ME; Berman, AE; Mikhailov, VI; Ushakova, NA; Mazurov, AV; Semenov, AV; Usov, AI; Nifant'ev, NE; Bovin, NV. Fucoidan inhibits leukocyte recruitment in a model peritoneal inflammation in rat and blocks interaction of P-selectin with its carbohydrate ligand. *Biochem. Mol. Biol. Int* **1997**, *43*, 443–451.

47. Kubes, P; Payne, D; Woodman, RC. Molecular mechanisms of leukocyte recruitment in postischemic liver microcirculation. *Am. J. Physiol. Gastrointest. Liver Physiol* **2002**, *283*, 139–147.

48. Gassmann, P; Kang, ML; Mees, ST; Haier, J. *In vivo* tumor cell adhesion in the pulmonary microvasculature is exclusively mediated by tumor cell-endothelial cell interaction. *BMC Cancer* **2010**, *10*, 177.

49. Frenette, PS; Weiss, L. Sulfated glycans induce rapid hematopoietic progenitor cell mobilization: Evidence for selectin-dependent and independent mechanisms. *Blood* **2000**, *96*, 2460–2468.

50. Mansson, P; Zhang, XW; Jeppsson, B; Johnell, O; Thorlacius, H. Critical role of P-selectin-dependent rolling in tumor necrosis factor-alpha-induced leukocyte adhesion and extravascular recruitment *in vivo*. *Naunyn Schmiedebergs Arch. Pharmacol* **2000**, *362*, 190–196.

51. Tanaka, K; Ito, M; Kodama, M; Tomita, M; Kimura, S; Hoyano, M; Mitsuma, W; Hirono, S; Hanawa, H; Aizawa, Y. Sulfated polysaccharide fucoidan ameliorates experimental autoimmune myocarditis in rats. *J. Cardiovasc. Pharmacol. Ther* **2011**, *16*, 79–86.

52. Thomes, P; Rajendran, M; Pasanban, B; Rengasamy, R. Cardioprotective activity of *Cladosiphon okamuranus* fucoidan against isoproterenol induced myocardial infarction in rats. *Phytomedicine* **2010**, *18*, 52–57.

53. Kim, H; Moon, C; Park, EJ; Jee, Y; Ahn, M; Wie, MB; Shin, T. Amelioration of experimental autoimmune encephalomyelitis in Lewis rats treated with fucoidan. *Phytother. Res* **2010**, *24*, 399–403.

54. Alwayn, IP; Appel, JZ; Goepfert, C; Buhler, L; Cooper, DK; Robson, SC. Inhibition of platelet aggregation in baboons: Therapeutic implications for xenotransplantation. *Xenotransplantation* **2000**, *7*, 247–257.

55. Tissot, B; Montdargent, B; Chevolot, L; Varenne, A; Descroix, S; Gareil, P; Daniel, R. Interaction of fucoidan with the proteins of the complement classical pathway. *Biochim. Biophys. Acta* **2003**, *1651*, 5–16.

56. Charreau, B; Blondin, C; Boisson-Vidal, C; Soulillou, JP; Anegon, I. Efficiency of fucans in protecting porcine endothelial cells against complement activation and lysis by human serum. *Transplant. Proc* **1997**, *29*, 889–890.

57. Tissot, B; Daniel, R. Biological properties of sulfated fucans: The potent inhibiting activity of algal fucoidan against the human compliment system. *Glycobiology* **2003**, *13*, 29G–30G.

58. Blondin, C; Chaubet, F; Nardella, A; Sinquin, C; Jozefonvicz, J. Relationships between chemical characteristics and anticomplementary activity of fucans. *Biomaterials* **1996**, *17*, 597–603.

59. Galebskaya, LV; Ryumina, EV; Bogomaz, TA; Preobrazhenskaya, ME. The mechanism of fucoidan action on human complement. *Biomeditsinskaya Khimiya* **2003**, *49*, 542–547.

60. Clement, MJ; Tissot, B; Chevolot, L; Adjadj, E; Du, Y; Curmi, PA; Daniel, R. NMR characterization and molecular modeling of fucoidan showing the importance of oligosaccharide branching in its anticomplementary activity. *Glycobiology* **2010**, *20*, 883–894.

61. Thring, TS; Hili, P; Naughton, DP. Anti-collagenase, anti-elastase and anti-oxidant activities of extracts from 21 plants. *BMC Complement. Altern. Med* **2009**, *9*, 27.

62. Senni, K; Gueniche, F; Foucault-Bertaud, A; Igondjo-Tchen, S; Fioretti, F; Colliec-Jouault, S; Durand, P; Guezennec, J; Godeau, G; Letourneur, D. Fucoidan a sulfated polysaccharide from brown algae is a potent modulator of connective tissue proteolysis. *Arch. Biochem. Biophys* **2006**, *445*, 56–64.

63. Tsuji, N; Moriwaki, S; Suzuki, Y; Takema, Y; Imokawa, G. The role of elastases secreted by fibroblasts in wrinkle formation: Implication through selective inhibition of elastase activity. *Photochem. Photobiol* **2001**, *74*, 283–290.

64. Moon, HJ; Lee, SH; Ku, MJ; Yu, BC; Jeon, MJ; Jeong, SH; Stonik, VA; Zvyagintseva, TN; Ermakova, SP; Lee, YH. Fucoidan inhibits UVB-induced MMP-1 promoter expression and down regulation of type I procollagen synthesis in human skin fibroblasts. *Eur. J. Dermatol* **2009**, *19*, 129–134.

65. Fujimura, T; Tsukahara, K; Moriwaki, S; Kitahara, T; Sano, T; Takema, Y. Treatment of human skin with an extract of *Fucus vesiculosus* changes its thickness and mechanical properties. *J. Cosmet. Sci* **2002**, *53*, 1–9.

66. Hlawaty, H; Suffee, N; Sutton, A; Oudar, O; Haddad, O; Ollivier, V; Laguillier-Morizot, C; Gattegno, L; Letourneur, D; Charnaux, N. Low molecular weight fucoidan prevents intimal hyperplasia in rat injured thoracic aorta through the modulation of matrix metalloproteinase-2 expression. *Biochem. Pharmacol* **2011**, *81*, 233–243.

67. Deux, J-F; Anne, M-P; Le Blanche, AF; Feldman, LJ; Colliec-Jouault, S; Bree, F; Boudghène, F; Michel, J-B; Letourneur, D. Low molecular weight fucoidan prevents neointimal hyperplasia in rabbits iliac artery in-stent restenosis model. *Arterioscler. Thromb. Vasc. Biol* **2002**, *22*, 1604–1609.

68. Goldring, MB; Goldring, SR. Articular cartilage and subchondral bone in the pathogenesis of osteoarthritis. *Ann. N. Y. Acad. Sci* **2010**, *1192*, 230–237.

69. Cunha, TM; Verri, WA, Jr; Schivo, IR; Napimoga, MH; Parada, CA; Poole, S; Teixeira, MM; Ferreira, SH; Cunha, FQ. Crucial role of neutrophils in the development of mechanical inflammatory hypernociception. *J. Leukoc. Biol* **2008**, *83*, 824–832.

70. McNamee, KE; Burleigh, A; Gompels, LL; Feldmann, M; Allen, SJ; Williams, RO; Dawbarn, D; Vincent, TL; Inglis, JJ. Treatment of murine osteoarthritis with TrkAd5 reveals a pivotal role for nerve growth factor in non-inflammatory joint pain. *Pain* **2010**, *149*, 386–392.

71. Cashman, JD; Kennah, E; Shuto, A; Winternitz, C; Springate, CM. Fucoidan film safely inhibits surgical adhesions in a rat model. *J Surg Res* **2010**. [CrossRef]

72. Hayashi, S; Itoh, A; Isoda, K; Kondoh, M; Kawase, M; Yagi, K. Fucoidan partly prevents CCl$_4$-induced liver fibrosis. *Eur. J. Pharmacol* **2008**, *580*, 380–384.

73. Saito, A; Yoneda, M; Yokohama, S; Okada, M; Haneda, M; Nakamura, K. Fucoidan prevents concanavalin A-induced liver injury through induction of endogenous IL-10 in mice. *Hepatol. Res* **2006**, *35*, 190–198.

74. Keppler, D; Lesch, R; Reutter, W; Decker, K. Experimental hepatitis induced by d-galactosamine. *Exp. Mol. Pathol* **1968**, *9*, 279–290.

75. Kawano, N; Egashira, Y; Sanada, H. Effects of various kinds of edible seaweeds in diets on the development of d-galactosamine-induced hepatopathy in rats. *J. Nutr. Sci. Vitaminol. (Tokyo)* **2007**, *53*, 315–323.

76. Kawano, N; Egashira, Y; Sanada, H. Effect of dietary fiber in edible seaweeds on the development of d-galactosamine-induced hepatopathy in rats. *J. Nutr. Sci. Vitaminol. (Tokyo)* **2007**, *53*, 446–450.

77. Hayakawa, K; Nagamine, T. Effect of fucoidan on the biotinidase kinetics in human hepatocellular carcinoma. *Anticancer Res* **2009**, *29*, 1211–1217.

78. Nesterenko, AV; Nesterenko, VB; Yablokov, AV. Chapter IV. Radiation protection after the Chernobyl catastrophe. *Ann. N. Y. Acad. Sci* **2009**, *1181*, 287–288.

79. Levitskaia, TG; Creim, JA; Curry, TL; Luders, T; Morris, JE; Peterson, JM; Thrall, KD. Biomaterials for the decorporation of (85)Sr in the rat. *Health Phys* **2010**, *99*, 394–400.

80. Hollriegl, V; Rohmuss, M; Oeh, U; Roth, P. Strontium biokinetics in humans: Influence of alginate on the uptake of ingested strontium. *Health Phys* **2004**, *86*, 193–196.

81. Lee, J; Kim, J; Moon, C; Kim, SH; Hyun, JW; Park, JW; Shin, T. Radioprotective effects of fucoidan in mice treated with total body irradiation. *Phytother. Res* **2008**, *22*, 1677–1681.

82. Byon, YY; Kim, MH; Yoo, ES; Hwang, KK; Jee, Y; Shin, T; Joo, HG. Radioprotective effects of fucoidan on bone marrow cells: Improvement of the cell survival and immunoreactivity. *J. Vet. Sci* **2008**, *9*, 359–365.

83. Rhee, KH; Lee, KH. Protective effects of fucoidan against gamma-radiation-induced damage of blood cells. *Arch. Pharm. Res* **2011**, *34*, 645–651.

84. Sweeney, EA; Priestley, GV; Nakamoto, B; Collins, RG; Beaudet, AL; Papayannopoulou, T. Mobilization of stem progenitor cells by sulfated polysaccharides does not require selectin presence. *Proc. Natl. Acad. Sci. USA* **2000**, *97*, 6544–6549.

85. Fermas, S; Gonnet, F; Sutton, A; Charnaux, N; Mulloy, B; Du, Y; Baleux, F; Daniel, R. Sulfated oligosaccharides (heparin and fucoidan) binding and dimerization of stromal cell-derived factor-1 (SDF-1/CXCL 12) are coupled as evidenced by affinity CE-MS analysis. *Glycobiology* **2008**, *18*, 1054–1064.

86.   Mavier, P; Martin, N; Couchie, D; Préaux, A-M; Laperche, Y; Serge Zafrani, E. Expression of stromal cell-derived Factor-1 and of its receptor CXCR4 in liver regeneration from oval cells in rat. *Am. J. Pathol* **2004**, *165*, 1969–1976.

87.   Fonseca, RJ; Santos, GR; Mourao, PA. Effects of polysaccharides enriched in 2,4-disulfated fucose units on coagulation, thrombosis and bleeding. Practical and conceptual implications. *Thromb. Haemost* **2009**, *102*, 829–836.

88.   Kwak, KW; Cho, KS; Hahn, OJ; Lee, KH; Lee, BY; Ko, JJ; Chung, KH. Biological effects of fucoidan isolated from *Fucus vesiculosus* on thrombosis and vascular cells. *Korean J. Hematol* **2010**, *45*, 51–57.

89.   Pomin, VH; Pereira, MS; Valente, A-P; Tollefsen, DM; Pavo, MSG; Mouro, PAS. Selective cleavage and anticoagulant activity of a sulfated fucan: Stereospecific removal of a 2-sulfate ester from the polysaccharide by mild acid hydrolysis, preparation of oligosaccharides and heparin cofactor II-dependent anticoagulant activity. *Glycobiology* **2005**, *15*, 369–381.

90.   Wozniak, MA; Itzhaki, RF. Antiviral agents in Alzheimer's disease: Hope for the future? *Ther. Adv. Neurol. Disord* **2010**, *3*, 141–152.

91.   Jhamandas, JH; wie, MB; Harris, K; Mactavish, D; Kar, S. Fucoidan inhibits cellular and neurotoxic effects of β-amyloid (Aβ) in rat cholinergic basal forebrain neurons. *Eur. J. Neurosci* **2005**, *21*, 2649–2659.

92.   Cui, YQ; Zhang, LJ; Zhang, T; Luo, DZ; Jia, YJ; Guo, ZX; Zhang, QB; Wang, X; Wang, XM. Inhibitory effect of fucoidan on nitric oxide production in lipopolysaccharide-activated primary microglia. *Clin. Exp. Pharmacol. Physiol* **2010**, *37*, 422–428.

93.   Li, Y; Liu, L; Liu, D; Woodward, S; Barger, SW; Mrak, RE; Griffin, WS. Microglial activation by uptake of fDNA via a scavenger receptor. *J. Neuroimmunol* **2004**, *147*, 50–55.

94.   Pei, Z; Pang, H; Qian, L; Yang, S; Wang, T; Zhang, W; Wu, X; Dallas, S; Wilson, B; Reece, JM; Miller, DS; Hong, JS; Block, ML. MAC1 mediates LPS-induced production of superoxide by microglia: The role of pattern recognition receptors in dopaminergic neurotoxicity. *Glia* **2007**, *55*, 1362–1373.

95.   Huang, WC; Yen, FC; Shiao, YJ; Shie, FS; Chan, JL; Yang, CN; Sung, YJ; Huang, FL; Tsay, HJ. Enlargement of Abeta aggregates through chemokine-dependent microglial clustering. *Neurosci. Res* **2009**, *63*, 280–287.

96.   Do, H; Pyo, S; Sohn, EH. Suppression of iNOS expression by fucoidan is mediated by regulation of p38 MAPK, JAK/STAT, AP-1 and IRF-1, and depends on up-regulation of scavenger receptor B1 expression in TNF-alpha- and IFN-gamma-stimulated C6 glioma cells. *J. Nutr. Biochem* **2009**, *21*, 671–679.

97.   Luo, D; Zhang, Q; Wang, H; Cui, Y; Sun, Z; Yang, J; Zheng, Y; Jia, J; Yu, F; Wang, X. Fucoidan protects against dopaminergic neuron death *in vivo* and *in vitro*. *Eur. J. Pharmacol* **2009**, *617*, 33–40.

98.   Zhang, Y; Song, S; Song, D; Liang, H; Wang, W; Ji, A. Proliferative effects on neural stem/progenitor cells of a sulfated polysaccharide purified from the sea cucumber *Stichopus japonicus*. *J. Biosci. Bioeng* **2010**, *109*, 67–72.

99.   Lee, H-R; Do, H; Lee, S-R; Sohn, E-S; Pyo, S; Son, E. Effects of fucoidan on neuronal cell proliferation: Association with NO production through the iNOS pathway. *J. Food Sci. Nutr* **2007**, *12*, 74–78.

100. Schaeffer, DJ; Krylov, VS. Anti HIV activity of extracts and compounds from algae and cyanobacteria. *Ecotoxicol. Environ. Saf* **2000**, *45*, 208–227.

101. Hayashi, K; Nakano, T; Hashimoto, M; Kanekiyo, K; Hayashi, T. Defensive effects of a fucoidan from brown alga *Undaria pinnatifida* against herpes simplex virus infection. *Int. Immunopharmacol* **2008**, *8*, 109–116.

102. Thompson, KD; Dragar, C. Antiviral activity of *Undaria pinnatifida* against herpes simplex virus. *Phytother. Res* **2004**, *18*, 551–555.

103. Makarenkova, ID; Deriabin, PG; L'Vov, DK; Zviagintseva, TN; Besednova, NN. Antiviral activity of sulfated polysaccharide from the brown algae *Laminaria japonica* against avian Influenza A (H5N1) virus infection in the cultured cells. *Vopr. Virusol* **2010**, *55*, 41–45.

104. Taoda, N; Shinji, E; Nishii, K; Nishioka, S; Yonezawa, Y; Uematsu, J; Hattori, E; Yamamoto, H; Kawano, M; Tsurudome, M; O'Brien, M; Yamashita, T; Komada, H. Fucoidan inhibits parainfluenza virus type 2 infection to LLCMK2 cells. *Biomed. Res* **2008**, *29*, 331–334.

105. Cooper, R; Dragar, C; Elliot, K; Fitton, JH; Godwin, J; Thompson, K. GFS, a preparation of Tasmanian *Undaria pinnatifida* is associated with healing and inhibition of reactivation of herpes. *BMC Complement. Altern. Med* **2002**, *2*, 11–17.

106. Hemmingson, J; Falshaw, R; Furneaux, R; Thompson, K. Structure and antiviral activity of the galactofucan sulfates extracted from *Undaria Pinnatifida* (Phaeophyta). *J. Appl. Phycol* **2006**, *18*, 185–193.

107. Hidari, KI; Takahashi, N; Arihara, M; Nagaoka, M; Morita, K; Suzuki, T. Structure and anti-dengue virus activity of sulfated polysaccharide from a marine alga. *Biochem. Biophys. Res. Commun* **2008**, *376*, 91–95.

108. Haneji, K; Matsuda, T; Tomita, M; Kawakami, H; Ohshiro, K; Uchihara, J-N; Masuda, M; Takasu, N; Tanaka, Y; Ohta, T; Mori, N. Fucoidan extracted from *Cladosiphon okamuranus* Tokida induces apoptosis of human T-cell leukemia virus type 1-infected T-cell lines and primary adult T-cell leukemia cells. *Nutr. Cancer* **2005**, *52*, 189–201.

109. Romanos, MTV; Andrada-Serpa, MJ; Matos dos Santos, MG; Ribeiro, ACF; Yoneshigue-Valentin, Y; Costa, SS; Wigg, MD. Inhibitory effect of extracts of Brazilian marine algae on human T-cell lymphotropic virus type 1 (HTLV-1)-induced syncytium formation *in vitro*. *Cancer Invest* **2002**, *20*, 46–54.

110. Organisation W.H. *Leishmaniasis*. 2011. Available online: http://www.who.int/leishmaniasis/en/ accessed on 20 May 2011.

111. Kar, S; Sharma, G; Das, PK. Fucoidan cures infection with both antimony-susceptible and -resistant strains of *Leishmania donovani* through Th1 response and macrophage-derived oxidants. *J. Antimicrob. Chemother* **2011**, *66*, 618–625.

112. Chen, JH; Lim, JD; Sohn, EH; Choi, YS; Han, ET. Growth-inhibitory effect of a fucoidan from brown seaweed *Undaria pinnatifida* on *Plasmodium* parasites. *Parasitol. Res* **2009**, *104*, 245–250.

113. Manuelidis, L; Chakrabarty, T; Miyazawa, K; Nduom, NA; Emmerling, K. The kuru infectious agent is a unique geographic isolate distinct from Creutzfeldt-Jakob disease and scrapie agents. *Proc. Natl. Acad. Sci. USA* **2009**, *106*, 13529–13534.

114. Liberski, PP; Brown, P. Kuru: Its ramifications after fifty years. *Exp. Gerontol* **2009**, *44*, 63–69.

115. Doh-Ura, K; Kuge, T; Uomoto, M; Nishizawa, K; Kawasaki, Y; Iha, M. Prophylactic effect of dietary seaweed Fucoidan against enteral prion infection. *Antimicrob. Agents Chemother* **2007**, *51*, 2274–2277.

116. Juffrie, M; Rosalina, I; Rosalina, A; Damayanti, W; Djumhana, A; Ahmad, H. The efficacy of fucoidan on gastric ulcer. *Indones. J. Biotechnol* **2006**, *11*, 908–913.

117. Lutay, N; Nilsson, I; Wadstrom, T; Ljungh, A. Effect of heparin, fucoidan and other polysaccharides on adhesion of enterohepatic *Helicobacter* species to murine macrophage. *Appl. Biochem. Biotechnol* **2010**, *164*, 1–9.

118. Choi, JI; Raghavendran, HR; Sung, NY; Kim, JH; Chun, BS; Ahn, DH; Choi, HS; Kang, KW; Lee, JW. Effect of fucoidan on aspirin-induced stomach ulceration in rats. *Chem. Biol. Interact* **2010**, *183*, 249–254.

119. Bojakowski, K; Abramczyk, P; Bojakowska, M; Zwolinska, A; Przybylski, J; Gaciong, Z. Fucoidan improves the renal blood flow in the early stage of renal ischemia/reperfusion injury in the rat. *J. Physiol. Pharmacol* **2001**, *52*, 137–143.

120. Zhang, Q; Li, N; Zhao, T; Qi, H; Xu, Z; Li, Z. Fucoidan inhibits the development of proteinuria in active Heymann nephritis. *Phytother. Res* **2005**, *19*, 50–53.

121. Zhang, Q; Li, Z; Xu, Z; Niu, X; Zhang, H. Effects of fucoidan on chronic renal failure in rats. *Planta Med* **2003**, *69*, 537–541.

122. Veena, CK; Josephine, A; Preetha, SP; Varalakshmi, P. Beneficial role of sulfated polysaccharides from edible seaweed *Fucus vesiculosus* in experimental hyperoxaluria. *Food Chem* **2007**, *100*, 1552–1559.

123. Josephine, A; Amudha, G; Veena, CK; Preetha, SP; Rajeswari, A; Varalakshmi, P. Beneficial effects of sulfated polysaccharides from *Sargassum wightii* against mitochondrial alterations induced by Cyclosporine A in rat kidney. *Mol. Nutr. Food Res* **2007**, *51*, 1413–1422.

124. Rucavado, A; Escalante, T; Shannon, J; Gutierrez, JM; Fox, JW. Proteomics of wound exudate in snake venom-induced pathology: Search for biomarkers to assess tissue damage and therapeutic success. *J. Proteome Res* **2011**, *10*, 1987–2005.

125. Mora, J; Mora, R; Lomonte, B; Gutierrez, JM. Effects of bothrops asper snake venom on lymphatic vessels: Insights into a hidden aspect of envenomation. *PLoS Negl. Trop. Dis* **2008**, *2*, e318.

126. Gutiérrez, JM; Theakston, RDG; Warrell, DA. Confronting the neglected problem of snake bite envenoming: The need for a global partnership. *PLoS Med* **2006**, *3*, e150.

127. Angulo, Y; Lomonte, B. Inhibitory effect of fucoidan on the activities of crotaline snake venom myotoxic phospholipases A(2). *Biochem. Pharmacol* **2003**, *66*, 1993–2000.
128. Vasanthi, HR; Jaswanth, A; Krishnaraj, V; Rajamanickam, GV; Saraswathy, A. *In vitro* snake venom detoxifying action of some marine algae of Gulf of Mannar, south-east coast of India. *Phytother. Res* **2003**, *17*, 1217–1219.

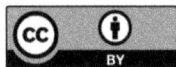

marine drugs

MDPI

Review

Chitosan: An Update on Potential Biomedical and Pharmaceutical Applications

Randy Chi Fai Cheung *, Tzi Bun Ng *, Jack Ho Wong and Wai Yee Chan

School of Biomedical Sciences, Faculty of Medicine, The Chinese University of Hong Kong, Hong Kong, China; jack1993@yahoo.com (J.H.W.); chanwy@cuhk.edu.hk (W.Y.C.)

* Authors to whom correspondence should be addressed; chifaicheung@cuhk.edu.hk (R.C.F.C.); b021770@mailserv.cuhk.edu.hk (T.B.N.); Tel.: +852-39438031 (R.C.F.C.); +852-39436872 (T.B.N.); Fax: +852-26035123 (R.C.F.C. & T.B.N.).

Academic Editor: Paola Laurienzo
Received: 1 June 2015; Accepted: 6 August 2015; Published: 14 August 2015

Abstract: Chitosan is a natural polycationic linear polysaccharide derived from chitin. The low solubility of chitosan in neutral and alkaline solution limits its application. Nevertheless, chemical modification into composites or hydrogels brings to it new functional properties for different applications. Chitosans are recognized as versatile biomaterials because of their non-toxicity, low allergenicity, biocompatibility and biodegradability. This review presents the recent research, trends and prospects in chitosan. Some special pharmaceutical and biomedical applications are also highlighted.

Keywords: chitosan; pharmaceutical applications; biomedical applications

1. Introduction

Chitosan, sometimes known as deacetylated chitin, is a natural polycationic linear polysaccharide derived from partial deacetylation of chitin [1]. Chitin is the structural element in the exoskeleton of insects, crustaceans (mainly shrimps and crabs) and cell walls of fungi, and the second most abundant natural polysaccharide after cellulose. The complexity of the chitin structure, difficulty in its extraction and insolubility in aqueous solution limited the research on this polymer until 1980s.

Chitosan is composed of β-(1-4)-linked D-glucosamine and N-acetyl-D-glucosamine randomly distributed within the polymer. The cationic nature of chitosan is rather special, as the majority of polysaccharides are usually either neutral or negatively charged in an acidic environment. This property allows it to form electrostatic complexes or multilayer structures with other negatively charged synthetic or natural polymers [2]. The interesting characteristics of chitosan such as biocompatibility, non-toxicity, low allergenicity and biodegradability allow it to be used in various applications [3]. Besides, chitosan is reported to have other biological properties, such as antitumor [4], antimicrobial [5], and antioxidant [6] activities. The degree of deacetylation, which is described by the molar fraction of deacetylated units or percentage of deacetylation, and the molecular weight of chitosan, were found to affect these properties [7]. Chitosan has been widely used for different biological and biomedical applications recently due to its unique properties. For instance, it can be used in water treatment [8], wound-healing materials [1], pharmaceutical excipient or drug carrier [9], obesity treatment [10] and as a scaffold for tissue engineering [11]. There is increased interest in pharmaceutical as well as biomedical applications of chitosan and its derivatives and significant development has been achieved. It can be reflected in the increasing number of related publications throughout the years. Figure 1 shows the number of Scopus indexed publications from 1985 to June 2015 related to chitosan and its derivatives.

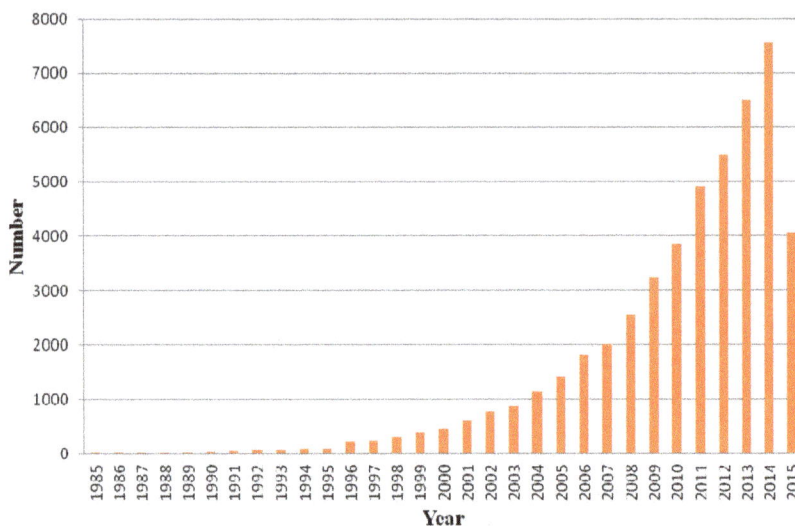

Figure 1. Scopus indexed publications related to chitosan and its derivatives.

2. Production and Characterization of Chitosan

The raw material for the production of chitosan is chitin. The main sources are the shells of crustaceans, mainly crabs and shrimps. The purification process is easier for shrimp shells which are thinner. Usually, shells of the same size and species are grouped, then cleaned, dried and ground into small shell pieces [12]. There is no standard purification method as different chitin sources require different treatments due to the diversity in their structures. Conventionally, the protocol is divided into demineralization, deproteinization and decolorization steps which can be carried out using chemical [13] or biological (enzymatic treatment or fermentation) [14] treatments. The end-products need to be highly purified if they are to be used for biomedical or pharmaceutical purposes, as residual proteins, minerals or pigments can cause serious side effects. Conversion of chitin to chitosan can be achieved by enzymatic [15] or chemical [16] deacetylation. Chemical deacetylation is more commonly used for commercial preparation because of economic issues and feasibility for mass production. No matter which method is used, depolymerization is inevitable [17]. The processes involved in chemical and biological preparation of chitosan from crustacean shells are illustrated in Figure 2.

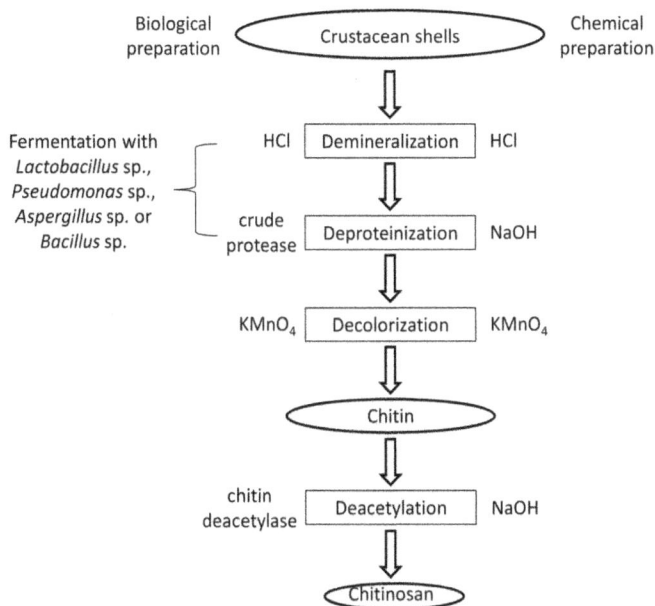

Figure 2. A schematic presentation of chitosan preparation from raw materials.

The quality of chitosan depends on the source of chitin and its method of isolation [18] and chitosan with different extents of deacetylation are commercially available today. The applications of the chitosan depend on the characteristics, such as appearance of polymer, turbidity of polymer solution, degree of deacetylation and molecular weight [19]. The degree of deacetylation can be determined by different techniques, such as infrared spectroscopy, potentiometric titration, and more advanced methods like ^{1}H liquid state and solid state ^{13}C-NMR. The average molecular weight of chitosan is usually obtained from steric exclusion chromatography equipped with a viscometer and light scattering detector or matrix-assisted laser desorption/ionization-mass spectrometer [12]. Different characterization techniques for determining molecular weight, degree of deacetylation and crystallinity are summarized in Table 1. Chitosan obtained from deacetylation of chitin becomes soluble in aqueous acidic solutions when the average degree of deacetylation is above 0.5, but not at an alkaline or physiological pH. The physical properties of chitosan in aqueous solution depend on the degree of deacetylation and the acetyl group distribution in the polymer chains. Uneven acetyl group distribution will lower its solubility and make them form aggregates easily [20]. The solubility problem hinders its applicability. Modification of chitosan at the molecular level increases its solubility and stability and thus makes it more versatile as a biopolymer. The presence of free amino groups on the chitosan chains allows modifications under mild conditions. Chitosan usually reacts with other small molecules or polymers and is transformed into derivatives or composites. Chitosan hydrogel is one of the various forms of its composites. It is composed of a cross-linked network of polymer chains with a high content of hydrophilic groups. Thus, it is a superabsorbent of water, but is water-insoluble because of the chemical or physical bonds formed between the polymer chains [21]. Typical examples are chitosan-poly (ethylene glycol) hydrogel [22], chitosan-hyaluronic hydrogel [23], chitosan-glycerophosphate hydrogel [24], chitosan-alginate composite [25], chitosan-collagen composite [26] chitosan-hydroxyapatite composite [27] and chitosan-tricalcium phosphate composite [28]. They can be molded into different shapes and forms (films, fibers, sponges, beads and solutions). These materials are mainly applied in bone tissue engineering scaffold [29], drug delivery system [30], wound healing materials [31] and metal and dye absorbent for polluted water [32].

Table 1. Physiochemical characteristics of chitosan and their methods of determination.

Physiochemical Characteristics	Method of Determination
molecular weight	viscometry; gel permeation chromatography; light scattering; high performance liquid chromatography; matrix-assisted laser desorption/ionization-mass spectrometer
degree of deacetylation	infrared spectroscopy; ultra violet spectrophotometry; nuclear magnetic resonance spectroscopy (^{1}H-NMR and ^{13}C-NMR); conductometric titration; potentiometric titration; differential scanning calorimetry
crystallinity	X-ray diffraction

3. Bioactivities of Chitosan

3.1. Antibacterial Activity

Many reports have shown that chitosan exhibited antimicrobial activity, but the actual mechanism has not yet been fully elucidated. Several hypotheses have been proposed based on its cationic nature. Low-molecular-weight chitosan can penetrate bacterial cell walls, bind with DNA and inhibit DNA transcription and mRNA synthesis [33], while high-molecular-weight chitosan can bind to the negatively charged components on the bacterial cell wall. It forms an impermeable layer around the cell, changes cell permeability and blocks transport into the cell [34]. This hypothesis was further supported by the studies from Muzzarelli *et al.* [35]. The hydrophilicity and negative charge on the cell surface were higher on gram-negative bacterial cell walls than those of gram-positive bacteria. Thus the gram-negative bacteria showed a stronger interaction with chitosan, which resulted in stronger antibacterial activity against them. It was also reported that the amount of chitosan binding to the bacterial cell wall was dependent on the environmental pH value, molecular weight and degree of acetylation of chitosan. Low environmental pH increases the positive charge in the chitosan polymer, which favors binding to the bacterial cell wall [36]. Younes *et al.* [37] reported that a lower degree of chitosan acetylation and a lower pH are favorable to the antibacterial activity of chitosan. A reduction in the molecular weight of chitosan increases the antibacterial activity of chitosan toward Gram-negative bacteria and reduces the activity on the Gram-positive bacteria. Chitosan has a wide spectrum of activity and high killing rate against Gram-positive and Gram-negative bacteria. The activity is the result of interactions between chitosan and its derivatives with bacterial cell wall molecules. The studies mentioned in this section demonstrated a close relationship between the antibacterial activity and the hydrophilicity of the cell wall, thus the action is specific and showed lower toxicity toward mammalian cells [38].

Eco-friendly, low-cost and biocompatible composites prepared by immobilizing ZnO nanoparticles on the chitosan matrix by an *in situ* sol-gel conversion of precursor molecules in a single step demonstrates more potent antimicrobial activity against the Gram positive bacterium *Staphylococcus aureus* and the Gram negative bacterium *Escherichia coli* than chitosan. [39]. Chitosan solution exhibited higher antibacterial potency than chitosan submicroparticles toward both planktonic and biofilm-related antibiotic-resistant *Pseudomonas aeruginosa* cells isolated from chronic diabetic foot infections [40]. Low-molecular-weight water-soluble β-chitosan (with molecular masses of 5 and 10 kDa, respectively) exhibited potent antibacterial activity, even at pH 7.4, targeting the bacterial membrane, bringing about calcein efflux in artificial mimetic bacterial membrane and morphological alterations on bacterial surfaces. Data from an *in vivo* experiment employing a mouse model of bacterial infection provided evidence that low-molecular-weight water-soluble β-chitosan may find anti-infective and wound healing applications [41]. Quaternary ammonium chitosan/polyvinyl alcohol/polyethylene oxide hydrogels prepared with the use of gamma radiation exhibited desirable swelling ability, water evaporation rate as well as mechanical characteristics and high antibacterial potency against *E. coli* and *S. aureus*. The hydrogels are promising for use as wound dressing [42]. Chitosan/lignosulfonates multilayers modified fibers with chitosan in the outermost layer exhibited higher antimicrobial activity against *E. coli* and higher antioxidant activity than that of original fibers under the same oxidation conditions [43]. A method for reductive aminating of chitosan biopolymers to produce *N,N*-dialkyl chitosan derivatives was developed by employing as a precursor 3, 6-O-di-tert-butyldimethylsilylchitosan. The corresponding mono *N*-alkyl derivatives were synthesized, and all alkyl compounds were then quaternized. These derivatives were studied for antibacterial activity against Gram positive *S. aureus* and *Enterococcus faecalis*, and Gram negative *E. coli* and *P. aeruginosa*, which could be correlated to the length of the alkyl chain, but the order was dependent on the bacterial strain. Toxicity against human red blood cells and human epithelial Caco-2 cells was proportional to the length of the alkyl chain. The most active chitosan derivatives were found to be more selective for killing bacteria than the quaternary ammonium disinfectants cetylpyridinium chloride and benzalkonium chloride, along with the antimicrobial peptides melittin and LL-37 [44]. Nontoxic honey-polyvinyl alcohol-chitosan nanofibers were constructed with high honey concentrations (up to 40%) in addition to high chitosan concentrations (up to 5.5% of the total fiber weight) employing biocompatible solvents (1% acetic acid), chemically cross-linked with the help of glutaraldehyde vapor, as well as physically cross-linked by heating and freezing/thawing. The nanofibers demonstrated potent antibacterial activity against *S. aureus* but meager antibacterial activity against *E. coli* [45].

3.2. Antifungal Activity

The effects of molecular weight and degree of acetylation of chitosan on its antifungal activity varies with the fungus [37]. Chitosan was also found to exhibit antifungal activity against several phytopathogenic fungi such as *Penicillium* sp. in citrus fruit [46], *Botrytis cinerea* in cucumber plants [47], *Phytophthora infestans* [48], *Alternaria solani* and *Fusarium oxysporum* [49] in tomatoes. The suggested mechanism involved a permeable chitosan film formed on the crop surface which interfered with the fungal growth and activated several defense processes like chitinase accumulation, proteinase inhibitor synthesis, callus synthesis and lignification [50].

Silver nanoparticles distributed superficially on and internally in chitosan spheres demonstrated a macroporous feature, and could find applications such as fungicidal agents [51].

Chitosan applied at a dosage of 100 μg/mL killed the bulk of fungal species pathogenic to human pathogens examined but did not express toxicity to HEK293 and COS7 mammalian cells. Survival of *Galleria mellonella* larvae after infection with *C. albicans* was elevated by chitosan [52].

Water-soluble chitosan was fungistatic to *Macrophomina phaseolina*. Fungal infection was suppressed and the activities of enzymes associated with defense including chitosanase and peroxidase in infected seedlings were upregulated following exposure to water-soluble chitosan [53].

The existence of cranberry and quince juice in the composition of chitosan and whey protein-chitosan films reinforced the elasticity and reduced the tensile strength of the films. Chitosan and whey proteins-chitosan films with quince and cranberry juice added are potentially useful for increasing the shelf life of apples [54].

The fungal inhibition indices of deacetylated chitosans generally increased with a rise in molecular weight. Nevertheless, high-molecular-weight chitosan derivatives with a low hydrophobicity and low-molecular-weight derivatives with a high hydrophobicity displayed the highest potency in suppressing growth in *Aspergillus flavus in vitro* [55].

Cu-chitosan nanoparticles impeded spore germination and mycelial proliferation in *Fusarium oxysporum* and *Alternaria solani in vitro* and controlled Fusarium wilt and early blight in pot experiments [49].

3.3. Anti-HIV-1 Activity and for Construction of Nanoparticles Loaded with Anti-HIV Drugs

QMW-chitosan oligomers and WMQ-chitosan oligomers (in which Q, M and W stand for glutamine, methionine and tryptophan, respectively) exerted a protective action on C8166 cells against cytolytic effects of HIV-1RF strain. The oligomers suppressed syncytium formation induced by HIV, and reduced the HIV load without any inhibitory effects on activities of HIV-1 reverse transcriptase and protease *in vitro*. Syncytium formation was suppressed when HIV-infected and uninfected C8166 cells were co-cultured. QMW-chitosan oligomers and WMQ-chitosan oligomers inhibit HIV-induced cytopathic effects by exerting their effects on HIV entry stage [56]. Chitooligosaccharides are nontoxic and water-soluble compounds derived from chitosans by enzymatic degradation. Sulfated chitooligosaccharide III with a molecular weight of 3–5 kDa potently suppressed HIV-1 replication, HIV-1-induced syncytium formation, lytic action, and p24 antigen production. Sulfated chitooligosaccharide III obstructed viral entry and virus-cell fusion probably by interfering with the binding of HIV-1 gp120 to CD4 cell surface receptor. Unsulfated chitooligosaccharides did not have similar actions [57].

Chitosan-thioglycolic acid-conjugated nanoparticles loaded with the anti-HIV drug tenofovir show better biophysical characteristics for mucoadhesion than native chitosan nanoparticles [58]. Lamivudine-PEGylated chitosan drug, with a low cytotoxicity and a high potency, suppresses replication of HIV more powerfully than lamivudine [59]. Stable intravaginal mucoadhesive microspheres of tenofovir disoproxil fumarate have been formulated using chitosan as the matrix-forming mucoadhesive polymer [60]. Chitosan nanoparticles loaded with the anti-HIV drug saquinavir had excellent drug loading potential with high cell targeting efficiency resulting in efficient control of HIV proliferation in target T-cells. The findings reveal the potential of chitosan nanocarriers as vehicles for anti-HIV-1 drugs [61]. Tenofovir, an acyclic nucleoside phosphonate analog employed for anti-HIV therapy embedded into a type of nanocarriers based on poly-(D,L-lactide-co-glycolide) and/or chitosan, is a good anti-HIV drug carrier for investigating cellular uptake and drug delivery in target cells like macrophages [62]. Chitosan based nanoparticles loaded with tenofovir did not exhibit cytotoxicity to vaginal epithelial cells and *Lactobacillus crispatus*. Mucoadhesion increased as the nanoparticle diameter was reduced. However, the combined action of drug encapsulation efficiency and percent mucoadhesion for larger size nanoparticles yielded the best results. Hence, large-sized chitosan nanoparticles loaded with an anti-HIV drug appeared to be promising for stopping HIV transmission [63]. Chitosan-*O*-isopropyl-5'-*O*-d4T monophosphate conjugate nano-prodrugs may be deployed as targeting and sustained polymeric prodrugs for improving anti-HIV treatment and curtailing side effects of the treatment [64]. Glutaraldehyde cross-linked chitosan microspheres have been utilized for controlled delivery of zidovudine [65].

Chitosan and its derivatives have been shown to have antimicrobial activities and the results are summarized in Table 2.

Table 2. The antimicrobial activities of chitosan and its derivatives

	Targets	Chitosan or Its Derivatives/MIC in μg/mL Reference
Gram-negative bacteria	*Escherichia coli*	chitosan 0.025% [38]; chitosan-Zn complex 0.00313% [38]; á-chitosan 9 μg/mL [41]; â-chitosan 9 μg/mL [41]; N,N-diethyl-N-methylchitosan 16 μg/mL [44]; N,N-dihexyl-N-methylchitosan 16 μg/mL [44]
	E. coli K88	chitosan 8 μg/mL [38]; chitosan nanoparticles 0.0625 μg/mL [38]; Cu loaded chitosan nanoparticles 0.0313 μg/mL [38]
	E. coli ATCC 25922	chitosan 8 μg/mL [38]; chitosan nanoparticles 0.0313 μg/mL [38]; Cu loaded chitosan nanoparticles 0.0313 μg/mL [38]
	E. coli O157	á-chitosan 9 μg/mL [41]; â-chitosan 9 μg/mL [41]
	Pseudomonas aeruginosa	chitosan 0.0125% [38]; chitosan-Zn complex 0.00625% [38]; á-chitosan 9 μg/mL [41]; â-chitosan 9 μg/mL [41]; N,N-diethyl-N-methylchitosan 32 μg/mL [44]
	Proteus mirabilis	chitosan 0.025% [38]; chitosan-Zn complex 0.00625% [38]
	Salmonella enteritidis	chitosan 0.05% [38]; chitosan-Zn complex 0.00625% [38]
	S. choleraesuis ATCC 50020	chitosan 16 μg/mL [38]; chitosan nanoparticles 0.0625 μg/mL [38]; Cu loaded chitosan nanoparticles 0.0313 μg/mL [38]
	S. typhimurium	á-chitosan 5 μg/mL [41]; â-chitosan 9 μg/mL [41]
	S. typhimurium ATCC 50013	chitosan 16 μg/mL [38]; chitosan nanoparticles 0.125 μg/mL [38]; Cu loaded chitosan nanoparticles 0.0625 μg/mL [38]
Gram-negative bacteria	*Enterobacter aerogenes*	chitosan 0.05% [38]; chitosan-Zn complex 0.00625% [38]
	Listeria monocytogenes	á-chitosan 9 μg/mL [41]; â-chitosan 9 μg/mL [41]
Gram-positive bacteria	*Staphylococcus aureus*	chitosan 0.05% [38]; chitosan-Zn complex 0.00625% [38]; á-chitosan 9 μg/mL [41]; â-chitosan 9 μg/mL [41]; N-ethyl-N,N-dimethylchitosan 4 μg/mL [44]
	S. aureus ATCC 25923	chitosan 8 μg/mL [38]; chitosan nanoparticles 0.125 μg/mL [38]; Cu loaded chitosan nanoparticles 0.0625 μg/mL [38]
	Corynebacterium	chitosan 0.025% [38]; chitosan-Zn complex 0.0313% [38]
	Staphylococcus epidermidis	chitosan 0.025% [38]; chitosan-Zn complex 0.0125% [38]; á-chitosan 5 μg/mL [41]; â-chitosan 5 μg/mL [41]
	Enterococcus faecalis	chitosan 0.05% [38]; chitosan-Zn complex 0.0125% [38]; N,N-diethyl-N-methylchitosan 16 μg/mL [44]
	Bacillus cereus	á-chitosan 9 μg/mL [41]; â-chitosan 9 μg/mL [41]
	Bacillus megaterium	á-chitosan 9 μg/mL [41]; â-chitosan 9 μg/mL [41]
Fungi	*Candida albicans*	chitosan 0.1% [38]; chitosan-Zn complex 0.1% [38]; chitosan 5 μg/mL [52]
	Candida parapsilosis	chitosan 0.1% [38]; chitosan-Zn complex 0.05% [38]; chitosan 40 μg/mL [52]
	Candida krusei	chitosan 5 μg/mL [52]
	Candida glabrata	chitosan 20 μg/mL [52]
	Penicillium digitatum	chitosan 65 μg/mL [46]
	Penicillium italicum	chitosan 57.5 μg/mL [46]
	Fusarium proliferatum	chitosan 2.5 μg/mL [52]
	Hamigera avellanea	chitosan 2.5 μg/mL [52]
	Aspergillus fumigatus	chitosan 1 μg/mL [52]
	Rhizopus stolonifer	chitosan 100 μg/mL [52]
	Cryptococcus neoformans	chitosan 5 μg/mL [52]
	Cryptococcus gatti	chitosan 2.5 μg/mL [52]
	Macrophomina phaseolina	chitosan 12.5 mg/mL [53]
Virus	IC_{50} of cytopathic effect by HIV-1_{RF}	QMW-chitosan oligomers 48.14 μg/mL [56]
	IC_{50} of cytopathic effect by HIV-1_{IIIB}	WMQ-chitosan oligomers 48.01 μg/mL [56]
	IC_{50} of p24 production by HIV-1_{IIIB}	QMW-chitosan oligomers 67.35 μg/mL [56]
	IC_{50} of p24 production by HIV-1_{Ba-L}	WMQ-chitosan oligomers 98.73 μg/mL [56]
	IC_{50} of p24 production by HIV-1_{RTMDR1}	QMW-chitosan oligomers 81.03 μg/mL [56]; WMQ-chitosan oligomers 144.02 μg/mL [56]
	IC_{50} of luciferase expression by HIV-1_{RF}	QMW-chitosan oligomers 68.13 μg/mL [56]; WMQ-chitosan oligomers 163.94 μg/mL [56]
	IC_{50} of interaction between gp41 and CD4 by HIV-1	QMW-chitosan oligomers 39.13 μg/mL [56]; WMQ-chitosan oligomers 51.48 μg/mL [56]
	IC_{50} of syncytia formation by HIV-1_{RF}	sulfated chitooligosaccharides 2.19 μg/mL [57]
	EC_{50} of protection of lytic effect by HIV-1	sulfated chitooligosaccharides 1.43 μg/mL [57]
	IC_{50} of p24 production by HIV-1_{RF}	sulfated chitooligosaccharides 4.33 μg/mL [57]
	IC_{50} of p24 production by HIV-1_{Ba-L}	sulfated chitooligosaccharides 7.76 μg/mL [57]

3.4. Antitumor Activity

Recent investigations revealed that chitosan and its derivatives exhibited antitumor activity in both *in vitro* and *in vivo* models. Tokoro *et al.* [66] observed that the antitumor effect of chitosan derivatives was due to the increase in secretion of interleukin-1 and 2 which caused maturation and infiltration of cytolytic T-lymphocytes. It was further supported by Dass and Choong [67] whose *in vivo* study demonstrated that chitosan elevated lymphokine production and proliferation of cytolytic T-lymphocytes. Other investigations showed that chitosan was involved in direct killing of tumor cells by inducing apoptosis. Chitosan was shown to inhibit adhesion of primary melanoma A375 cells and proliferation of primary melanoma SKMEL28 cells. It also exhibited strong pro-apoptotic effects against metastatic melanoma RPMI7951 cells through inhibition of specific caspases, up-regulation of Bax and down-regulation of Bcl-XL proteins. Besides, it induced CD95 receptor expression on RPMI7951 surface, making them more vulnerable to FasL-induced apoptosis [68]. He *et al.* [69] reported that carboxymethylated chitosan protected the peripheral nerves and inhibited the apoptosis of cultured Schwann cells. They used the hydrogen peroxide- induced apoptosis model. Decreases in caspase-3, -9 and Bax activities and increases in Bcl-2 activity were detected.

Carboxymethyl chitosan suppressed migration of human hepatoma cells BEL-7402 *in vitro* and murine hepatoma 22 cells *in vivo*. The expression of matrix metalloproteinase-9 (MMP-9) in BEL-7402 cells was downregulated and pulmonary metastases of hepatoma-22 in Kunming mice were curtailed. Reduction of the lung damage brought about by the metastasis of H22 cells was noted. The suppressive action of carboxymethyl chitosan could be ascribed partly to the attenuated vascular endothelial growth factor and E-selectin levels [70]. It has been reported how the degree of deacetylation and molecular mass of chitosan oligosaccharides, procured from enzymatic hydrolysis of high-molecular-weight chitosan, affected antitumor activity. Determination of the degree of deacetylation and molecular weights of chitosan oligosaccharides were conducted by means of matrix-assisted laser desorption/ionization-mass spectrometry. The chitosan oligosaccharides formed a mixture composed essentially of dimers (18.8%), trimers (24.8%), tetramers (24.9%), pentamers (17.7%), hexamers (7.1%), heptamers (3.3%), and octamers (3.4%). The chitosan oligosaccharides were resolved by gel filtration into two main fractions: (1) chitosan oligosaccharides, composed of glucosamine (n), $n = 3$–5 with 100% deacetylation; and (2) HOS, consisting of glucosamine (5) as the minimum residues and a varying number of N-acetylglucosamine (n), $n = 1$–2 with 87.5% deacetylation in random order. The concentrations required for chitosan oligosaccharides, chitooligosaccharides, and HOS to achieve 50% cell death in PC3 prostate cancer cells, A549 lung cancer cell, and HepG2 hepatoma cells, were 25 µg/mL, 25 µg/mL, and 50 µg/mL, respectively. The high- molecular-weight chitosan had about half the efficacy of chitosan oligosaccharides and chitooligosaccharides. These findings show that the molecular weight and degree of deacetylation of chitosanoligosaccharides are critical determinants for inhibiting growth of cancer cells [71]. Chitooligosaccharides, products of chitosan hydrolysis, manifest a diversity of biological functions. Proliferation of hepatocellular carcinoma HepG2 cells was attenuated, the percentage of cells in S-phase was diminished and the rate of DNA synthesis was reduced after treatment with chitooligosaccharides. Among the cycle-related genes, PCNA, cyclin A and CDK-2 were down-regulated whereas p21 was up-regulated. Chitooligosaccharides undermined the activity of metastatic related protein (MMP-9) in Lewis lung carcinoma cells. Chitooligosaccharides suppressed tumor growth of HepG2 xenografts in severe combined immune deficient mice. Chitooligosaccharides repressed tumor growth and reduced the number of lung metastasis colonies and prolonged the lifespan of Lewis lung carcinoma-bearing mice [72]. Table 3 summarizes the literature mentioned in this review.

Table 3. A summary of antitumor activities of chitosan and its derivatives.

Compound	Target Cell Lines or *in vivo* Model	Results	Ref.
chitosan	meth-A solid tumor transplanted into BALB/c mice	increased production of interleukins 1 and 2, sequentially, leading to the manifestation of antitumor effect through proliferation of cytolytic T-lymphocytes with the optimum inhibition ratio at the dose of 10 mg/kg	[66]
chitosan	aberrant crypt tumor lesions in the colon of mice	elevated lymphokine production and proliferation of cytolytic T-lymphocytes at the dose of 5 mg/kg	[67]
chitosan	A375, SKMEL28, and RPMI7951 cell lines	chitosan was coated in culture wells in which cultures with A375, SKMEL28, and RPMI7951 cells were carried out.	[68]
		decreased adhesion of A375 cells	
		decreased proliferation of SKMEL28 cells	
		inhibited specific caspases, upregulated Bax and downregulated Bcl-2 and Bcl-XL in RPMI7951 cells	
		induced CD95 receptor expression in RPMI7951 cell surface which renders them more susceptible to FasL-induced apoptosis	
carboxymethyl chitosan	hydrogen peroxide induced apoptosis models of Schwann cells	The cell viability was improved in a dose-dependent manner with maximum effect of 2.02 ± 0.16 fold at the dose of 200 µg/mL carboxymethyl chitosan	[69]
		decreased caspase-3, -9 and Bax activities and increased Bcl-2 activity	
carboxymethyl chitosan	BEL-7402 cell line	reduced the expression of MMP-9 in a dose-dependent manner	[70]
	hepatoma-22 cells in Kunming mice	inhibited the lung metastasis mouse model with the highest inhibition of 66.56% at the dose of 300 mg/kg	
chitosan	PC3 A549 and HepG2 cell line	suppressed cancer cell growth of PC3 A549 and HepG2 cells for 50% cell death at 25 µg/mL, 25 µg/mL and 50 µg/mL, respectively	[71]
chitosan	HepG2 and LCC cell line	inhibited MMP-9 expression, reduced cells in S-phase and decreased the rate of DNA synthesis, upregulated p21 and downregulated PCNA, cyclin A and CDK-2 with the highest inhibition at the dose of 1 mg/kg	[72]
chitosan	HepG2 and LCC xenografts in mouse model	inhibited tumor growth and decreased the number of metastatic colonies at the dose of 500 mg/kg	

3.5. Antioxidant Activity

Antioxidants are well-known for their beneficial effects on health. They protect the body against reactive oxygen species, which exert oxidative damage to membrane lipids, protein and DNA. Much effort has been invested to investigate the antioxidant activity of chitosan and its derivatives in recent years [6]. Park *et al.* [73] reported the *in vitro* oxygen radicals scavenging activity in chitosan and its derivatives. Low–molecular-weight chitosans are more active in scavenging free radicals, such as hydroxyl, superoxide, alkyl and 2,2-diphenyl-1-picrylhydrazyl radicals. It was proposed that the mechanism is due to the reaction of unstable free radicals with amino and hydroxyl groups on the pyranose ring, which form the stable radicals [12].

Nine kinds of hetero-chitooligosaccharides with relatively higher molecular weights, medium molecular weights, and lower molecular weights have been prepared from partially deacetylated hetero-chitosans (90%, 75% and 50% deacetylated chitosan), and their scavenging activities against 1,1-diphenyl-2-picrylhydrazyl, carbon-centered hydroxyl, superoxide and radicals were studied by employing electron spin resonance spin-trapping technique. Carbon-centered, hydroxyl, and superoxide radicals were generated from 2,2-azobis-(2-amidinopropane)-hydrochloride, hydrogen peroxide-ferrous sulfate (Fenton reaction), and hypoxanthine-xanthine oxidase reaction. The electron spin resonance data demonstrated that medium-molecular-weight hetero-chitooligosaccharides prepared from 90% deacetylated chitosan manifested the highest radical scavenging potency. The radical-scavenging activity of hetero-chitooligosaccharides was related to the degree of deacetylation values and the molecular weight [74]. Chitosan was prepared by alkaline *N*-deacetylation of â-chitin from squid pens, and *N*-carboxyethylated derivatives (*N*-CESC) with different degrees of carboxyethyl group substitution (*N*-CESC3 possessed the highest degree of substitution while *N*-CESC1 possessed the lowest degree of substitution) were synthesized. All three *N*-CESC samples displayed good water solubility at pH above 6.5. They manifested potent 2,2′-azinobis(3-ethylbenzothiazoline-6-sulfonic acid) (ABTS) radical scavenging activity, with EC_{50} values under 2 mg/mL. The ABTS radical scavenging activities of *N*-CECS with different degrees of substitution and concentrations are shown in Figure 3. It showed that the activity of *N*-CECS toward ABTS increased with concentration. Besides, the addition of carboxyethyl groups to chitosan enhanced its radical scavenging activity against ABTS. The scavenging ability of *N*-CESC against superoxide radicals showed a good correlation with the degree of substitution and concentration of *N*-CESC. The data suggested that *N*-CESC can be utilized to produce chitosan derivatives with good biochemical characteristics *in vitro* [75]. Graft chitosan derivatives with low grafting percentages, produced by graft copolymerization of methacrylic acid sodium and acrylic acid sodium onto the etherification product of chitosan-carboxymethyl chitosan, exhibit a relatively low 50% inhibition concentration (IC_{50}) for their radical scavenging activity, which could be attributed to their different contents of hydroxyl and amino groups in the polymer chains [76].

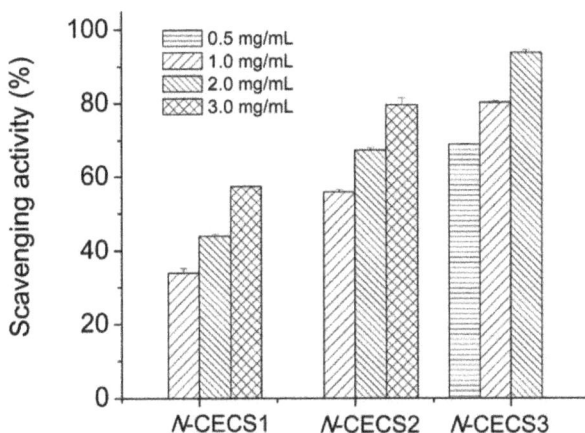

Figure 3. Scavenging effects of *N*-CECS with different degrees of substitution toward ABTS radicals. Reprinted with permission from [75] Copyright (2015) American Chemical Society.

4. Applications

Chitosan and its derivatives are recognized as versatile biomaterials because of their diverse bioactivities, non-toxicity, biocompatibility, biodegradability and low-allergenicity. They have superior physical properties such as high surface area, porosity, tensile strength and conductivity. In addition, they can be easily molded into different shapes and forms (films, fibers, sponges, beads, powder, gel and solutions) [77].

4.1. Tissue Engineering

Tissue engineering describes the use of a combination of cells, engineering materials, and suitable biochemical factors to improve or replace biological functions. It includes a wide range of applications such as repair or replacement of part of or whole tissues (for example, bone, cartilage, blood vessels, bladder, skin and muscle). Chitosan-based biomaterials have become a popular target in development for tissue engineering and significant progress has been made recently. It provides certain mechanical and structural properties for proper functioning for the repaired tissues [78].

N-methacryloyl chitosan, produced as a result of a single-step chemoselective *N*-acylation reaction, acquires the desirable features of hydrosolubility, UV crosslinkability and injectability. It facilitates quick and cost-effective construction of patterned cell-loaded polysaccharide microgels with distinctive amino groups as building materials for tissue engineering and quick transdermal curing hydrogel *in vivo* for localized and sustained protein delivery [79]. Chitosan-â-tricalcium phosphate composite exhibited histocompatibility with Beagle mesenchymal stem cells and was devoid of an effect on cellular growth and proliferation. It manifested efficacy in enhancing osteogenesis and vascularization and repair of bone defects in conjunction with mesenchymal stem cells [80]. Reinforcement of silk matrix with chitosan microparticles (silk:chitosan 1:1, 1:2 and 2:1) produced a visco-elastic matrix that promoted redifferentiation of caprine chondrocytes and retained more glycosaminoglycan which enhanced the aggregate modulus of the construct similar to native tissue. The data revealed one step forward in optimizing the construction of biomaterial scaffolds for cartilage tissue engineering [81]. Bone morphogenic protein 2/Chitosan microspheres were successively loaded onto a deproteinized bovine bone scaffold. BMP-2 underwent an initial burst release followed by a sustained release. The encapsulated bone morphogenetic protein 2 possessed biological activity. Biocompatibility was good. The microsphere scaffold system may find applications in tissue engineering [82]. A chitosan hollow tube employed for regeneration of the injured rodent transected sciatic nerve yielded results comparable to autologous nerve graft repair [83]. Implantation of chitosan nanofiber tube could partially restore the function of a damaged phrenic nerve in beagle dogs as seen in improvement of diaphragm movement, slow phrenic nerve conduction, connection of the damaged nerve by newly regenerating nerve fibers surrounded by granulation tissue within the chitosan nanofiber tube [84]. The loss of spinal cord tissue and cavity formation impedes the repair of damage to the spinal cord. The scaffold of chitosan+ECM+SB216763 enhanced neural stem cell differentiation into neurons, oligodendrocytes and astrocytes and hence is promising for repair of damaged spinal cords [85]. Chitosan/bioactive glass nanoparticles scaffolds possess the shape memory characteristics of chitosan and the biomineralization activity of bioactive glass nanoparticles for applications in bone regeneration [86].

4.2. Drug Delivery System

Chitosan has been widely used in pharmaceutical industry in drug delivery systems in different forms, like tablets, microspheres, micelles, vaccines, nucleic acids, hydrogels, nanoparticles and conjugates. Chitosan and its derivatives can be used in drug delivery systems in both implantable as well as injectable forms through oral, nasal and ocular routes. Besides, they facilitate transmucosal absorption which is important in nasal and oral delivery of some polar drugs like peptides along with protein vaccines for their administration [87]. It is commonly used as an excipient in tablet formulation for oral medication. High-molecular-weight chitosan is more viscous and delays the release of the active ingredient, prolongs the duration of drug activity, improves therapeutic efficiency as well as reducing the side effects of oral tablets [88]. Chitosan microspheres have been extensively investigated for controlled release of drugs and vaccines through oral and nasal delivery. They were prepared by complexation between the cationic chitosan in addition to the anionic compounds such as tripolyphosphate or alginates [89]. Different drugs or vaccines were loaded in the microspheres, they were protected, especially drugs which are protein in nature, in the digestive tract [90] and absorbed through the paracellular route on the epithelial layer [91]. The surface activity of chitosan is low as it does not possess any hydrophobic portions. It can be improved by chemical modifications at its glucosidic group with a hydrophobic substituent. The chitosan form micelles with an external hydrophilic shield and an internal hydrophobic center [92]. The hydrophobic drugs were protected in the center with improved solubility and bioavailability. The chitosan micelles were formed by the electrostatic repulsions between oppositely charged polymers [93]. The chitosan hydrogels are three-dimensionally structured hydrophilic polymers which can absorb and hold up to thousands of times more fluids than their dry weights and use in drug delivery. The drugs are loaded in the hydrogels by diffusion, entrapment, and tethering. Usually, the loaded hydrogel is injected into the body and the drug can diffuse into the neighboring tissues. The recent development of *in situ* forming depots using chitosan-based hydrogel has attracted much attention as a new method for controlled drug release [94]. The original thermosensitive chitosan-based polymer is in solution form at room temperature. When it is injected into the body, it forms semi-solid hydrogels at the physiological temperature. It showed protection for the drugs from physiological degradation, combined with prolonged and steady release of drugs [95]. Chitosan nanoparticles exhibit outstanding biodegradable and biocompatible properties which have been studied extensively as drug carriers. They can be administered through non-invasive means such as ocular, nasal, oral, and pulmonary routes. The drugs are protected from chemical and enzymatic degradation in the digestive system. Besides, they bind strongly to mucus which enhances the adsorption through intestinal epithelial cells [96]. They can be prepared by a number of methods such as ionotropic gelation, emulsion cross-linking, emulsion-solvent extraction, emulsification solvent diffusion, emulsion-droplet coalescence, complex coacervation, reverse microemulsion technique in addition to self-assembly [97]. The most common method is ionotropic gelation method in which the preparation conditions are mild and less time-consuming. It is based on spontaneous aggregation of positively-charged chitosan with a negatively-charged sodium polymer such as tripolyphosphate. The drugs are dissolved in either component. Then a nanoparticle suspension is formed upon addition of the other component under vigorous agitation [98]. The chitosan derivatives conjugate with antitumor agents to form a good partner for targeted drug delivery in cancer treatment. They manifest reduced side effects compared with the original drug because of a predominant distribution into the cancer cells and a progressive release of the free drug from the conjugates [99].

An intermolecular complex formed from a 1:1 ratio by weight of 30-kDa chitosan and sulfobutyl ether â-cyclodextrin was less soluble than either component. At pH 1.2, the drug famotidine was slowly released from the less-soluble chitosan/sulfobutyl ether â-cyclodextrin complex formed superficially on the tablet upon exposure to water, followed by dissolution of the interpolymer complex and, finally, breakdown of the tablet. At pH 6.8, gel formation by chitosan accounted for the gradual release. The slow release of the tablet was seen in the drug absorption *in vivo* following treatment of rats via the oral route [100]. Glycol chitosan nanogel uptake took place essentially by means of endocytosis mediated by flotillin-1 and Cdc42 and macropinocytosis with the participation of the actin cytoskeleton, and internalization mechanisms through the folate receptor. About half of the nanogel population was found in endolysosomal compartments, while the rest was located in undefined cytoplasmic compartments at the end of seven hours of incubation with HeLa cells. Glycol chitosan nanogels may be useful as drug delivery vectors for targeting different intracellular compartments [101]. Controlled-release, floating and mucoadhesive beads of glipizide were developed by polyionic complexation technique using chitosan as cationic and xanthan gum as anionic polymers. The beads displayed pH-dependent swelling kinetics, good bioadhesive strength and comparable floating capacity in the gastric fluids. Altering the chitosan to xanthan gum ratio did not affect the drug release [102]. Insulin was physically and chemically stable in a polyelectrolyte complex composed of insulin and 13-kDa low-molecular-weight chitosan in Tris-buffer (pH 6.5). Solubilization of the insulin-low-molecular-weight chitosan polyelectrolyte complex in a reverse micelle system, given to hyperglycemic rats, constituted an oral bioactive insulin delivery system [103]. The colon is a drug delivery target because of the long transit time and thus a prolonged drug absorption time. Progesterone has an abbreviated half-life, much first-pass metabolism, and low oral bioavailability. An oral Zn-pectinate/chitosan multiparticulate system prepared by ionotropic gelation, allowing increased oral bioavailability of progesterone as well as progesterone residence time in plasma for colonic-specific progesterone delivery, was developed. Negligible progesterone release in simulated gastric fluids was observed, but there was a burst release at pH 6.8 and sustained release at pH 7.4 [104]. Incorporation of glutaraldehyde augmented the drug entrapment efficacy of the Boswellia resin-chitosan polymer composites in phosphate buffer (pH 6.8). The drug release rate surged to 92% as the gum resin concentration in the composites was elevated to 80%. The composites released 60%–68% drug load in seven hours [105]. Water in oil nanosized systems containing low-molecular-weight chitosan-insulin polyelectrolyte complexes were constructed and their hypoglycemic activity was assayed in diabetic rats. The 1.3-kDa chitosan with 55% (among 55%, 80% and 100%) deacetylation possessed the most potent hypoglycemic activity among three molecular weights (namely, 1.3, 13 and 18 kDa) and different extents of deacetylation [106]. Higher retention of conjugate formed between chitosan and catechol derived from mussel adhesive proteins, in the gastrointestinal tract *versus* unmodified chitosan, owing to production of irreversible catechol mediated-crosslinking with mucin, may be advantageous for production of new mucoadhesive polymers to be employed for mucosal drug delivery [107]. Microcapsules loaded with fish oil were produced from oil-in-water emulsions by both membrane emulsification and ultrasonic emulsification employing *N*-stearoyl *O*-butylglyceryl chitosan as shell material. The microcapsules produced by membrane emulsification displayed a larger diameter and more desirable loading capacity and encapsulation efficiency. Microcapsules from both membrane emulsification and ultrasonic emulsification demonstrated sustained release of fish oil which had higher thermostability [108].

4.3. Wound Healing

Chitosan and its derivatives exhibit biodegradable, biocompatible, antimicrobial activity and low immunogenicity which are advantageous for development as biomaterials for wound healing [36]. They provide a three-dimensional tissue growth matrix, activate macrophage activity and stimulate cell proliferation [109]. Chitosan promotes activity of polymorphonuclear leukocytes, macrophages and fibroblasts that enhance granulation as well as the organization of the repaired tissues [110]. It will be slowly degraded into N-acetyl-β-D-glucosamine which stimulates fibroblast proliferation, aids regular collagen deposition in addition to stimulating hyaluronic acid synthesis at the wound site. It accelerates the healing progress along with preventing scar formation [111].

Nanofibrous and adhesive-based chitosan have been developed as wound dressing materials recently [112]. The electrospun chitosan nanofiber mats were found to be porous, have a high tensile strength, high surface area of the mats combined with ideal water vapor and oxygen transmission rate. It also showed compatibility with adipose derived stem cells, which is considered beneficial for wound healing [113]. The adhesive-based wound dressing was usually applied in surgery to enhance wound healing. The chitosan adhesive shows strong sealing strength as well as not requiring sutures or staples. It can effectively stop bleeding from blood vessels along with air leakage from the lung [114].

Several clinical studies have reported the favorable results of using chitosan for wound healing in patients undergoing plastic surgery [115], skin grafting [116,117] and endoscopic sinus surgery [118]. Currently, there are a number of chitosan-based wound dressings available in the market in the form of non-wovens, nanofibers, composites, films, and sponges. HemCon® hemostatic bandages which are chitosan-coated are the most famous. They were widely used in treating external hemorrhage in military operations as well as pre-hospital bleeding cases [119]. Similar products like GuardaCare®, ChitoFlex® and ChitoGauze® are temporary surgical dressings, stuffable dressings and gauze dressings, respectively, and are products from the same company. All of them offer an antibacterial barrier. Another chitosan-coated hemostatic gauze, Celox™ Gauze, has also been found to be effective in emergency bleeding control. They showed efficacious hemostasis in penetrating limb trauma when compared with the conventional pressure bandage in clinical trials [120]. Celox™ Granules, in the form of flakes, work in the same way as the gauze. When Celox™ gets into contact with blood, it swells and sticks together to form a gel-like clot. It works independently from the blood clotting mechanism and works well with hypothemic as well as heparinized blood. Celox™ and ChitoGauze® are approved for use by US military as hemostatic agents [119]. Chito-Seal™ and Clo-Sur^PLUS PAD are topical hemostasis chitosan-coated pads used for promoting vascular hemostasis following percutaneous catheters or tubes interventional. When put on the puncture site, the positively charged chitosan attracts the negatively charged red blood cells as well as platelets, thus shortening the clot formation in addition to hemostasis time [121]. Tegasorb™ and Tegaderm™ wound dressings are used for protective treatment of partial and full thickness dermal ulcers, leg ulcers, superficial wounds, abrasions, burns, as well as donor sites. The chitosan presented absorbs wound exudates, then swells up and produces a soft gel mass that enhances wound healing [122]. Other chitosan-containing wound-care products available on the market include ChiGel, Chitopack C® and TraumaStat™. Figure 4 shows a diagrammatic presentation of how the chitosan-based wound dressing works.

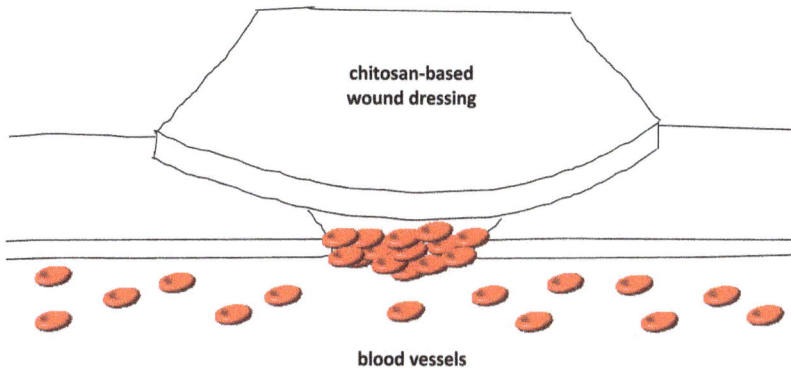

Figure 4. A diagrammatic presentation of how the chitosan-based wound dressing works.

Hydrogel films based on carboxyl-modified poly(vinyl alcohol) and chitosan were cross-linked through amide linkage formation. Their mechanical properties in dry and swollen state were greatly improved with high swelling ratio. They could maintain a moist environment over wound bed. Cross-linked hydrogel films loaded with gentamicin sulfate displayed sustained drug release, in addition to effectively suppressing bacterial proliferation along with protecting the wound from infection [123]. Curcumin-encapsulated bioglass-chitosan, which is promising for wound healing applications, displayed higher 1,1-diphenyl-2-picrylhydrazyl and superoxide free radical quenching activities compared with unmodified curcumin, antibacterial activity against *Staphylococcus aureus*, and reduction in tumor necrosis factor- â production [124].

4.4. Water Treatment

Chitosan is regarded as one of the most efficient materials for adsorption of pollutants in water treatment systems. The presence of amino and hydroxyl groups in chitosan allows its adsorption interactions with pollutants such as dyes [125], metals [126] and organic compounds [127], *etc.* Besides, these functional groups are subjected to modifications (cross-linking and grafting) which enhance the absorption efficiency and specificity [128]. For example, cross-linking the functional groups of chitosan improves the adsorption efficiency of chitosan at low pH. Grafting with sulphur or nitrogen improves specificity and capacity for some metal ions [129]. The dye adsorption performance by unmodified chitosan is good; however, its low stability has prompted many researchers to consider modifying them. Different modifications (grafted amino group, carboxyl group, sulfur group and alkyl group; cross-linked epichlorohydrin, ethylene glycol diglycidyl ether, glutaraldehyde and tripolyphosphate) were studied and employed to improve the adsorption efficiency as well as the mechanical and physical properties. The original properties of chitosan have been altered and are more suitable for the adsorption of different dyes [125]. Chitosan can act as a chelating polymer for binding toxic heavy metal ions. Metal cations can be chelated by the amine groups of chitosan in near-neutral conditions. For metal anions, the adsorption depends on electrostatic attraction on protonated amine groups in acidic conditions. Chitosan modified with different derivatives offers a wide range of properties for specific adsorption of metal ions [126]. Organic pollutants, including phenolic compounds, polycyclic aromatic hydrocarbons, organic pesticides and herbicides, cause health and environmental problems due to their toxic effects coupled with poor biodegradability. Chitosan adsorption for organic pollutants offer high adsorption capacities, insensitivity to toxic substances, good modifiability as well as recoverability. The mechanism depends on the characteristics along with the nature of the pollutants and is complicated. There is no simple theory or single mechanism to explain adsorption characteristics. Some interactions related to the adsorption mechanism include partition, diffusion, cation exchange, hydrogen bond, Van der Waals force, dipole–dipole interactions and electrostatic interaction [127].

Quaternary tetraalkylammonium chitosan derivatives can be utilized in the form of an inexpensive perchlorate-specific solid-phase extraction anion exchange cartridge in conjunction with colorimetric analysis for perchlorate removal or analysis [130]. Elevated initial fluoride concentrations, low dosages, combined with low ambient temperatures promoted, by ion exchange between chloride and fluoride, relatively selective fluoride adsorption from aqueous solutions on an Fe-impregnated chitosan granular adsorbent containing Fe-chelated to amino and hydroxyl groups on chitosan. At low fluoride concentrations, the adsorption characteristics followed the Langmuir model and at high initial fluoride concentrations, it followed the Freundlich model [131]. Magnetic hydroxypropyl chitosan/oxidized multiwalled carbon nanotubes composites were good for elimination of lead ions from aqueous solutions with pseudo-second-order kinetics. The optimal contact time and pH were 120 min and pH 5.0, respectively. Sips model is more appropriate than Langmuir, Freundlich and Dubinin-Radushkevich models for describing the adsorption process, which was endothermic and spontaneous [132]. Protonated polyamidoamine grafted chitosan beads loaded with Zr(IV) ions, produced by amination of chitosan beads by ethylenediamine through Michael addition and followed by protonation, eliminated fluoride ions from aqueous solutions with higher selectivity than other metal ions. The adsorption was spontaneous and endothermic [133]. Chitosan nanofibers formed by electrospinning with 5% chitosan in acetic acid as spinning solution were cross-linked with glutaraldehyde to eliminate chromium from water by adsorption with a pseudo-second order kinetic model, following a mixed isotherm of Freundlich and Langmuir. The maximum nanofiber adsorption capacity was more than double that of chitosan powders. Sodium, calcium magnesium, nitrate, and chloride, but not sulfate ions, had nil or negligible effect on adsorption which involved hydroxyl as well as amino groups of chitosan [134]. Chitosan along with polyphenol oxidase were used in conjunction for eliminaton of bisphenol derivatives from aqueous solutions based on adsorption of enzymatically generated quinine derivatives on chitosan beads or chitosan powders. The optimum temperature and pH conditions were 40 °C and pH 7 for bisphenols B, E, O, and Z; 30 °C and pH 7 for bisphenols C and F; and 40 °C and pH 8 for bisphenol T. The removal time could be reduced by using more chitosan beads or chitosan powders of a smaller size [135]. Sorption of Cd(II) ions onto cross-linked low-molecular-weight chitosan pyruvic acid derivative followed Langmuir isotherm model and displayed pseudo second-order kinetics. Two levels of Cd(II) concentration (1 or 3 mg/L, temperature (45 or 70 °C) and solution pH (6.0 or 10.0) were considered. The factors and their interaction effect on the efficacy of cadmium elimination followed the order: Cd(II) concentration > solution pH > interaction between solution pH and Cd(II) concentration > interaction between solution pH, temperature and Cd(II) concentration [136]. A procedure for concurrent elimination of cyanobacterial harmful algal blooms and microcystins, which may pose a public health threat, was devised by employing chitosan-modified local soil flocculation and microbe-modified soil capping. Breakdown of toxin was a consequence of the joint actions of flocculation and microcystin-degrading bacteria in the capping material, which inhibits dilution of bacterial biomass, enriches the algal cells, sequesters the liberated toxins, and promotes toxin biodegradation [137]. Chitosan nanorod with a minimum particle size smaller than 100 nm was produced by crosslinking chitosan of low molecular weight with polyanion sodium tripolyphosphate and was then physicochemically characterized (using AFM, DSC, FT-IR, SEM, TGA and XRD) for waste water treatment. Its sorption capacity and sorption isotherms for chromium were studied. How the initial concentration of chromium ions, sorbent amount, duration of shaking and solution pH affected sorption capacity were also examined. The findings disclosed that in the solid state nanochitosan was rod shaped and it effectively sorbed chromium (VI) to chromium (III) ions. The sorption capacity of chitosan nanoparticles is remarkably high; additionally the adsorbent favors multilayer adsorption based on the Langmuir, the Freundlich and the Temkin sorption isotherms. The adsorption follows pseudo-second-order kinetics, which infers transformation of chromium (VI) to chromium (III). Hence nanochitosan is a good biosorbent for chromium removal from water [138].

4.5. Obesity Treatment

Chitosan is marketed as a dietary supplement or nutraceutical for lowering serum cholesterol and controlling obesity. It is not specifically digested in our gastrointestinal tract. Chitosan swells up giving the feeling of satiety by physically filling the stomach [139]. By inhibiting pancreatic lipase activity, chitosan can reduce the absorption of dietary fat in intestines. Besides, it can bind and precipitate fat in the intestines so that it is not absorbed. The cationic chitosan binds with anionic carboxyl groups of fatty acids and bile acids, it also interferes with emulsification of neutral lipids like cholesterol and other sterols by binding them with hydrophobic interaction, thus fat and cholesterol absorption from gastrointestinal tract is reduced [140]. However, when it was evaluated in clinical trials, the results varied. There is some support that chitosan is more effective than placebo in the short-term treatment of obesity and hypercholesterolemia [141–144]. However, results obtained from larger and better-controlled trials showed that the effect of chitosan on body weight and serum cholesterol appeared to be ineffective, unconvincing and devoid of any clinical significance [145–147].

4.6. Other Applications

4.6.1. Cardiovascular Diseases Treatment

Administration of chitosan-oligosaccharides by gastric gavage to apolipoprotein E deficient mice (apoE-/-) fed a high fat diet for 12 weeks lowered triglyceride and cholesterol levels in non-high density lipoprotein fractions, undermined atherosclerosis, increased atherosclerotic plaque stability, upregulated hepatic expression of low density lipoprotein receptor, scavenger receptor BI and also the expression of macrophage scavenger receptor BI and ATP binding cassette transporter A1. There was no effect on the plasma lipid level in LDL-R mice with a deficiency of low density lipoprotein receptors and cholesterol absorption in wild-type mice [148].

4.6.2. Treatment of Age-Related Diseases

The potential utility of chitosan, chitooligosaccharides, their derivatives and chitosan-based functional food in forestalling and therapy of aging-associated diseases has been discussed and in this paper. The pathophysiological roles played by oxidative stress, oxidation of low density lipoprotein, increase of tissue stiffness, conformational changes of protein, aging-associated and chronic inflammation have been reviewed [149].

4.6.3. Mucosal Immunity Enhancer

Nasal administration of *Bacillus anthracis* protective antigen adsorbed on chitosan -C48/80 nanoparticles into mice produced elevated serum titers of antibodies against protective antigen and a more balanced Th1/Th2 pattern compared with C48/80 in solution or chitosan/alginate -C48/80 nanoparticles. The incorporation of C48/80 within chitosan nanoparticles promoted a stronger mucosal immunity than other adjuvanted groups examined. The findings indicate that chitosan nanoparticles could act in concert with a mast cell activator to effect nasal immunization [150].

4.6.4. Dry Mouth Syndrome Treatment

Chitosan-thioglycolic-mercaptonicotinamide conjugates, which were non-toxic against Caco-2 cells and synthesized by the oxidative S-S coupling of chitosan-thioglycolic acid with 6-mercaptonicotinamide, manifested improved swelling and cohesive characteristics compared with unmodified chitosan and were promising for therapy of dry mouth syndrome in which lubrication and mucoadhesiveness of the mucosa are wanting [151].

4.6.5. Food Industry

The use of electrospun chitosan fibers for wrapping during dry-aging of beef for up to three weeks yielded better results with regard to decrease of counts of microorganisms, molds and, yeasts, yield, lighter appearance, and less muscle denaturation in comparison with traditional dry-ageing. Regarding the wet-aging of beef, there were little weight and trimming losses but growth of lactic acid bacteria was detected [152].

4.6.6. Gene Silencing in Disease Vector Mosquito Larvae

Chitosan/interfering RNA nanoparticles mixed with food and consumed by larvae of *Aedes aegypti* (vector of the dengue and yellow fever) and *Anopheles gambiae* (vector of the primary African malaria vector) represented a methodology that can be applied to many insects and pests [153].

5. Conclusions

Chitosan is a biodegradable and inexpensive polymer which has numerous applications in biomedical as well as pharmaceutical industries. A large amount of research work has been done on chitosan and its derivatives for the purpose of tissue engineering, drug delivery, wound healing, water treatment, antitumor and antimicrobial effects.

Chitosan and its derivatives have been widely studied for potential tissue engineering biomaterials as they will be degraded at a reasonable rate without causing any inflammatory reaction or producing any toxic end-products when the new tissues are formed. They are porous in nature for diffusion of gases, nutrients, and metabolic wastes for the seeded cells along with increasing the surface area for cell attachment, migration and differentiation. They can be molded easily into anatomical shape and volume; are biocompatible with the surrounding biological fluids and tissues; as well as providing temporary mechanical support. All these properties fit the special properties use as tissue engineering scaffold.

Chitosan demonstrated antitumor activity in terms of as a therapeutic agent and as a drug carrier. As a therapeutic agent, it has been suggested that the antitumor activity related to their ability to induce cytokines production through increased T-cell proliferation. Other investigators reported that it involved MMP-9 inhibition and strong pro-apoptotic effects against tumor cells. The details of their actions are summarized in Table 3.

As a drug carrier, chitosan and its derivatives improve drug absorption, stabilize drug constituents for drug targeting in addition to drug release enhancement. Some studies showed that the antitumor agents/chitosan and its derivatives or conjugates exhibit better antitumor effects than the original form with a decrease in adverse effects. It is due to a predominant distribution in the cancer tissue and a gradual release of free drug from the conjugates.

Nowadays, the use of the wound-care products like hemostatic dressings is still uncommon due to the extra cost though they are more beneficial for fast recovery. However, using these products enables fewer changes of dressings and less attention to the patients, which can reduce the resources and workload required by the healthcare workers.

The recently developed nano-chitosan adsorbent gave new hope of commercializing chitosan into an alternative adsorbent. Chitosan, as an adsorbent, exhibited specific characteristics such as inexpensiveness, environmentally friendliness, versatility, biodegradability, high adsorption capability and selectivity. The nano-sized materials display the advantages of high specific surface area, low internal diffusion resistance, small size and quantum size effect that could enable them to exhibit higher capacities for pollutants. Up to now, adsorption of a number of dyes and heavy metal ions using nano-chitosan has been studied. In order to develop a multipurpose adsorbent for industrial

Mar. Drugs **2015**, *13*, 5156–5186

wastewater, organic pollutants and regeneration studies need to be done. These works can determine the reusability and versatility of nano-chitosan as an effective adsorbent.

For obesity treatment, chitosan appears to be safe for consumption and there is no known side-effect. However, its claim for obesity treatment seems to be lack of scientific support and more studies need to be done on testing the validity of such claim.

Quaternized chitosan, which introduces permanent positively charged quaternary groups to the hydroxyl group or amino group of the polymers, enhances antimicrobial activity over a wide pH range. In addition, the quaternized chitosan can also be used as an antimicrobial coating in orthopedic and dental implants and an antimicrobial wound dressing material for surgery.

Acknowledgments: We gratefully acknowledge the award of Health and Medical Research Fund, Hong Kong HMRF (grant number 12110672 and 12131221).

Author Contributions: Randy Chi Fai Cheung and Tzi Bun Ng were responsible for writing the review. Jack Ho Wong assisted in providing references, did the final editing and proofread the manuscript. Wai Yee Chan assisted in adding information to the first and second revision requested by the reviewers.

Conflicts of Interest: The authors declare no conflict of interest.

References

1. Chandy, T.; Sharma, C.P. Chitosan-as a biomaterial. *Biomater. Artif. Cells Artif. Organs* **1990**, *18*, 1–24. [CrossRef] [PubMed]
2. Venkatesan, J.; Kim, S.K. Chitosan composites for bone tissue engineering—An overview. *Mar. Drugs* **2010**, *8*, 2252–2266. [CrossRef] [PubMed]
3. Kumar, M.N.; Muzzarelli, R.A.; Muzzarelli, C.; Sashiwa, H.; Domb, A.J. Chitosan chemistry and pharmaceutical perspectives. *Chem. Rev.* **2004**, *104*, 6017–6084. [CrossRef] [PubMed]
4. Karagozlu, M.Z.; Kim, S.-K. Chapter Twelve—Anticancer effects of chitin and chitosan derivatives. In *Advances in Food and Nutrition Research*; Kim, S.K., Ed.; Academic Press: Waltham, MA, USA, 2014; Volume 72, pp. 215–225.
5. Martins, A.F.; Facchi, S.P.; Follmann, H.D.; Pereira, A.G.; Rubira, A.F.; Muniz, E.C. Antimicrobial activity of chitosan derivatives containing N-quaternized moieties in its backbone: a review. *Int. J. Mol. Sci.* **2014**, *15*, 20800–20832. [CrossRef] [PubMed]
6. Ngo, D.H.; Kim, S.K. Chapter Two—Antioxidant effects of chitin, chitosan, and their derivatives. In *Advances in Food and Nutrition Research*; Kim, S.K., Ed.; Academic Press: Waltham, MA, USA, 2014; Volume 73, pp. 15–31.
7. Aranaz, I.; Mengíbar, M.; Harris, R.; Paños, I.; Miralles, B.; Acosta, N.; Galed, G.; Heras, Á. Functional characterization of chitin and chitosan. *Curr. Chem. Biol.* **2009**, *3*, 203–230.
8. Onsosyen, E.; Skaugrud, O. Metal recovery using chitosan. *J. Chem. Technol. Biotechnol.* **1990**, *49*, 395–404. [CrossRef]
9. Felt, O.; Buri, P.; Gurny, R. Chitosan: A unique polysaccharide for drug delivery. *Drug Dev. Ind. Pharm.* **1998**, *24*, 979–993. [CrossRef] [PubMed]
10. Han, L.K.; Kimura, Y.; Okuda, H. Reduction in fat storage during chitin-chitosan treatment in mice fed a high-fat diet. *Int. J. Obes. Relat. Metab. Disord.* **1999**, *23*, 174–179. [CrossRef] [PubMed]
11. Zhang, Y.; Zhang, M. Three-dimensional macroporous calcium phosphate bioceramics with nested chitosan sponges for load-bearing bone implants. *J. Biomed. Mater. Res.* **2002**, *61*, 1–8. [CrossRef] [PubMed]
12. Younes, I.; Rinaudo, M. Chitin and chitosan preparation from marine sources. Structure, properties and applications. *Mar. Drugs* **2015**, *13*, 1133–1174. [CrossRef] [PubMed]
13. Percot, A.; Viton, C.; Domard, A. Optimization of chitin extraction from shrimp shells. *Biomacromolecules* **2003**, *4*, 12–18. [CrossRef] [PubMed]
14. Jung, W.J.; Jo, G.H.; Kuk, J.H.; Kim, K.Y.; Park, R.D. Extraction of chitin from red crab shell waste by cofermentation with *Lactobacillus paracasei* subsp. tolerans KCTC-3074 and *Serratia marcescens* FS-3. *Appl. Microbiol. Biotechnol.* **2006**, *71*, 234–237. [CrossRef] [PubMed]

15. Kafetzopoulos, D.; Martinou, A.; Bouriotis, V. Bioconversion of chitin to chitosan: Purification and characterization of chitin deacetylase from *Mucor rouxii*. *Proc. Natl. Acad. Sci. USA* **1993**, *90*, 2564–2568. [CrossRef] [PubMed]

16. No, H.K.; Meyers, S.P. Preparation and characterization of chitin and chitosan—A review. *J. Aquat. Food Prod. Technol.* **1995**, *4*, 27–52. [CrossRef]

17. Rege, P.R.; Block, L.H. Chitosan processing: Influence of process parameters during acidic and alkaline hydrolysis and effect of the processing sequence on the resultant chitosan's properties. *Carbohyd. Res.* **1999**, *321*, 235–245. [CrossRef]

18. Galed, G.; Miralles, B.; Inés Paños, I.; Santiago, A.; Heras, Á. N-Deacetylation and depolymerization reactions of chitin/chitosan: Influence of the source of chitin. *Carbohyd. Polym.* **2005**, *62*, 316–320. [CrossRef]

19. Nwe, N.; Furuike, T.; Tamura, H. Chapter One—Isolation and characterization of chitin and chitosan from marine origin. In *Advances in Food and Nutrition Research*; Se-Kwon, K., Ed.; Academic Press: Waltham, MA, USA, 2014; Volume 72, pp. 1–15.

20. Philippova, O.E.; Korchagina, E.V.; Volkov, E.V.; Smirnov, V.A.; Khokhlov, A.R.; Rinaudo, M. Aggregation of some water-soluble derivatives of chitin in aqueous solutions: Role of the degree of acetylation and effect of hydrogen bond breaker. *Carbohyd. Polym.* **2012**, *87*, 687–694. [CrossRef]

21. Bhattarai, N.; Gunn, J.; Zhang, M. Chitosan-based hydrogels for controlled, localized drug delivery. *Adv. Drug Deliv. Rev.* **2010**, *62*, 83–99. [CrossRef] [PubMed]

22. Tsao, C.T.; Leung, M.; Chang, J.Y.; Zhang, M. A simple material model to generate epidermal and dermal layers *in vitro* for skin regeneration. *J. Mater. Chem. B Mater. Biol. Med.* **2014**, *2*, 5256–5264. [CrossRef] [PubMed]

23. Lindborg, B.A.; Brekke, J.H.; Scott, C.M.; Chai, Y.W.; Ulrich, C.; Sandquist, L.; Kokkoli, E.; O'Brien, T.D. A chitosan-hyaluronan-based hydrogel-hydrocolloid supports *in vitro* culture and differentiation of human mesenchymal stem/stromal cells. *Tissue Eng. Part A* **2015**, *21*, 1952–1962. [CrossRef] [PubMed]

24. Salis, A.; Rassu, G.; Budai-Szucs, M.; Benzoni, I.; Csanyi, E.; Berko, S.; Maestri, M.; Dionigi, P.; Porcu, E.P.; Gavini, E.; et al. Development of thermosensitive chitosan/glicerophospate injectable *in situ* gelling solutions for potential application in intraoperative fluorescence imaging and local therapy of hepatocellular carcinoma: A preliminary study. *Expert Opin. Drug Deliv.* **2015**, *2*, 1–14. [CrossRef] [PubMed]

25. Rahaiee, S.; Shojaosadati, S.A.; Hashemi, M.; Moini, S.; Razavi, S.H. Improvement of crocin stability by biodegradeble nanoparticles of chitosan-alginate. *Int. J. Biol. Macromol.* **2015**, *79*, 423–432. [CrossRef] [PubMed]

26. Zeng, W.; Rong, M.; Hu, X.; Xiao, W.; Qi, F.; Huang, J.; Luo, Z. Incorporation of chitosan microspheres into collagen-chitosan scaffolds for the controlled release of nerve growth factor. *PLoS ONE* **2014**, *9*, e101300. [CrossRef] [PubMed]

27. Kiechel, M.A.; Beringer, L.T.; Donius, A.E.; Komiya, Y.; Habas, R.; Wegst, U.G.; Schauer, C.L. Osteoblast biocompatibility of premineralized, hexamethylene-1,6-diaminocarboxysulfonate cross-linked chitosan fibers. *J. Biomed. Mater. Res. A* **2015**. [CrossRef] [PubMed]

28. Kucharska, M.; Walenko, K.; Lewandowska-Szumiel, M.; Brynk, T.; Jaroszewicz, J.; Ciach, T. Chitosan and composite microsphere-based scaffold for bone tissue engineering: Evaluation of tricalcium phosphate content influence on physical and biological properties. *J. Mater. Sci. Mater. Med.* **2015**, *26*. [CrossRef] [PubMed]

29. Venkatesan, J.; Vinodhini, P.A.; Sudha, P.N.; Kim, S.K. Chitin and chitosan composites for bone tissue regeneration. *Adv. Food Nutr. Res.* **2014**, *73*, 59–81. [PubMed]

30. D'Ayala, G.G.; Malinconico, M.; Laurienzo, P. Marine derived polysaccharides for biomedical applications: Chemical modification approaches. *Molecules* **2008**, *13*, 2069–106. [CrossRef] [PubMed]

31. Tan, L.; Hu, J.; Huang, H.; Han, J.; Hu, H. Study of multi-functional electrospun composite nanofibrous mats for smart wound healing. *Int. J. Biol. Macromol.* **2015**, *79*, 469–476. [CrossRef] [PubMed]

32. Reddy, D.H.; Lee, S.M. Application of magnetic chitosan composites for the removal of toxic metal and dyes from aqueous solutions. *Adv. Colloid Interface Sci.* **2013**, *201–202*, 68–93. [CrossRef] [PubMed]

33. Sudarshan, N.R.; Hoover, D.G.; Knorr, D. Antibacterial action of chitosan. *Food Biotechnol.* **1992**, *6*, 257–272. [CrossRef]

34. Zheng, L.Y.; Zhu, J.F. Study on antimicrobial activity of chitosan with different molecular weights. *Carbohyd. Polym.* **2003**, *54*, 527–530. [CrossRef]

35. Muzzarelli, R.; Tarsi, R.; Filippini, O.; Giovanetti, E.; Biagini, G.; Varaldo, P.E. Antimicrobial properties of *N*-carboxybutyl chitosan. *Antimicrob. Agents Chemother.* **1990**, *34*, 2019–2023. [CrossRef] [PubMed]

36. Rhoades, J.; Roller, S. Antimicrobial actions of degraded and native chitosan against spoilage organisms in laboratory media and foods. *Appl. Environ. Microbiol.* **2000**, *66*, 80–86. [CrossRef] [PubMed]

37. Younes, I.; Sellimi, S.; Rinaudo, M.; Jellouli, K.; Nasri, M. Influence of acetylation degree and molecular weight of homogeneous chitosans on antibacterial and antifungal activities. *Int. J. Food Microbiol.* **2014**, *185*, 57–63. [CrossRef] [PubMed]

38. Kong, M.; Chen, X.G.; Xing, K.; Park, H.J. Antimicrobial properties of chitosan and mode of action: A state of the art review. *Int. J. Food Microbiol.* **2010**, *144*, 51–63. [CrossRef] [PubMed]

39. Mujeeb Rahman, P.; Muraleedaran, K.; Abdul Mujeeb, V.M. Applications of chitosan powder with *in situ* synthesized nano ZnO particles as an antimicrobial agent. *Int. J. Biol. Macromol.* **2015**, *77*, 266–272.

40. Machul, A.; Mikolajczyk, D.; Regiel-Futyra, A.; Heczko, P.B.; Strus, M.; Arruebo, M.; Stochel, G.; Kyziol, A. Study on inhibitory activity of chitosan-based materials against biofilm producing *Pseudomonas aeruginosa* strains. *J. Biomater. Appl.* **2015**. [CrossRef] [PubMed]

41. Park, S.C.; Nam, J.P.; Kim, J.H.; Kim, Y.M.; Nah, J.W.; Jang, M.K. Antimicrobial action of water-soluble beta-chitosan against clinical multi-drug resistant bacteria. *Int. J. Mol. Sci.* **2015**, *16*, 7995–8007. [CrossRef] [PubMed]

42. Fan, L.; Yang, J.; Wu, H.; Hu, Z.; Yi, J.; Tong, J.; Zhu, X. Preparation and characterization of quaternary ammonium chitosan hydrogels with significant antibacterial activity. *Int. J. Biol. Macromol.* **2015**, *79*, 830–836. [CrossRef] [PubMed]

43. Li, H.; Peng, L. Antimicrobial and antioxidant surface modification of cellulose fibers using layer-by-layer deposition of chitosan and lignosulfonates. *Carbohyd. Polym.* **2015**, *124*, 35–42. [CrossRef] [PubMed]

44. Sahariah, P.; Benediktssdottir, B.E.; Hjalmarsdottir, M.A.; Sigurjonsson, O.E.; Sorensen, K.K.; Thygesen, M.B.; Jensen, K.J.; Masson, M. Impact of chain length on antibacterial activity and hemocompatibility of quaternary *N*-alkyl and n,n-dialkyl chitosan derivatives. *Biomacromolecules* **2015**, *16*, 1449–1460. [CrossRef] [PubMed]

45. Sarhan, W.A.; Azzazy, H.M. High concentration honey chitosan electrospun nanofibers: Biocompatibility and antibacterial effects. *Carbohydr. Polym.* **2015**, *122*, 135–143. [CrossRef] [PubMed]

46. Tayel, A.A.; Moussa, S.H.; Salem, M.F.; Mazrou, K.E.; El-Tras, W.F. Control of citrus molds using bioactive coatings incorporated with fungal chitosan/plant extracts composite. *J. Sci. Food Agric.* **2015**. [CrossRef] [PubMed]

47. Ben-Shalom, N.; Ardi, R.; Pinto, R.; Aki, C.; Fallik, E. Controlling gray mould caused by *Botrytis cinerea* in cucumber plants by means of chitosan. *Crop. Prot.* **2003**, *22*, 285–290. [CrossRef]

48. Atia, M.M.M.; Buchenauer, H.; Aly, A.Z.; Abou-Zaid, M.I. Antifungal activity of chitosan against *Phytophthora infestans* and activation of defence mechanisms in tomato to late blight. *Biol. Agric. Hortic.* **2005**, *23*, 175–197. [CrossRef]

49. Saharan, V.; Sharma, G.; Yadav, M.; Choudhary, M.K.; Sharma, S.S.; Pal, A.; Raliya, R.; Biswas, P. Synthesis and *in vitro* antifungal efficacy of Cu-chitosan nanoparticles against pathogenic fungi of tomato. *Int. J. Biol. Macromol.* **2015**, *75*, 346–353. [CrossRef] [PubMed]

50. Bai, R.K.; Huang, M.Y.; Jiang, Y.Y. Selective permeabilities of chitosan-acetic acid complex membrane and chitosan-polymer complex membranes for oxygen and carbon dioxide. *Polym. Bull.* **1988**, *20*, 83–88. [CrossRef]

51. Wang, L.S.; Wang, C.Y.; Yang, C.H.; Hsieh, C.L.; Chen, S.Y.; Shen, C.Y.; Wang, J.J.; Huang, K.S. Synthesis and anti-fungal effect of silver nanoparticles-chitosan composite particles. *Int. J. Nanomedicine* **2015**, *10*, 2685–2696. [PubMed]

52. Lopez-Moya, F.; Colom-Valiente, M.F.; Martinez-Peinado, P.; Martinez-Lopez, J.E.; Puelles, E.; Sempere-Ortells, J.M.; Lopez-Llorca, L.V. Carbon and nitrogen limitation increase chitosan antifungal activity in *Neurospora crassa* and fungal human pathogens. *Fungal Biol.* **2015**, *119*, 154–169. [CrossRef] [PubMed]

53. Chatterjee, S.; Chatterjee, B.P.; Guha, A.K. A study on antifungal activity of water-soluble chitosan against *Macrophomina phaseolina*. *Int. J. Biol. Macromol.* **2014**, *67*, 452–457. [CrossRef] [PubMed]

54. Simonaitiene, D.; Brink, I.; Sipailiene, A.; Leskauskaite, D. The effect of chitosan and whey proteins-chitosan films on the growth of *Penicillium expansum* in apples. *J. Sci. Food Agric.* **2015**, *95*, 1475–1481. [CrossRef] [PubMed]

55. Gabriel Jdos, S.; Tiera, M.J.; Tiera, V.A. Synthesis, characterization, and antifungal activities of amphiphilic derivatives of diethylaminoethyl chitosan against *Aspergillus flavus*. *J. Agric. Food Chem.* **2015**, *63*, 5725–5731. [CrossRef] [PubMed]

56. Karagozlu, M.Z.; Karadeniz, F.; Kim, S.K. Anti-HIV activities of novel synthetic peptide conjugated chitosan oligomers. *Int. J. Biol. Macromol.* **2014**, *66*, 260–266. [CrossRef] [PubMed]

57. Artan, M.; Karadeniz, F.; Karagozlu, M.Z.; Kim, M.M.; Kim, S.K. *Anti*-HIV-1 activity of low molecular weight sulfated chitooligosaccharides. *Carbohydr. Res.* **2010**, *345*, 656–662. [CrossRef] [PubMed]

58. Meng, J.; Zhang, T.; Agrahari, V.; Ezoulin, M.J.; Youan, B.B. Comparative biophysical properties of tenofovir-loaded, thiolated and nonthiolated chitosan nanoparticles intended for HIV prevention. *Nanomedicine. (Lond.)* **2014**, *9*, 1595–1612. [CrossRef] [PubMed]

59. Aghasadeghi, M.R.; Heidari, H.; Sadat, S.M.; Irani, S.; Amini, S.; Siadat, S.D.; Fazlhashemy, M.E.; Zabihollahi, R.; Atyabi, S.M.; Momen, S.B.; *et al.* Lamivudine-PEGylated chitosan: A novel effective nanosized antiretroviral agent. *Curr. HIV Res.* **2013**, *11*, 309–320. [CrossRef] [PubMed]

60. Khan, A.B.; Thakur, R.S. Formulation and evaluation of mucoadhesive microspheres of tenofovir disoproxil fumarate for intravaginal use. *Curr. Drug Deliv.* **2014**, *11*, 112–122. [CrossRef] [PubMed]

61. Ramana, L.N.; Sharma, S.; Sethuraman, S.; Ranga, U.; Krishnan, U.M. Evaluation of chitosan nanoformulations as potent anti-HIV therapeutic systems. *Biochim. Biophys. Acta.* **2014**, *1840*, 476–484. [CrossRef] [PubMed]

62. Belletti, D.; Tosi, G.; Forni, F.; Gamberini, M.C.; Baraldi, C.; Vandelli, M.A.; Ruozi, B. Chemico-physical investigation of tenofovir loaded polymeric nanoparticles. *Int. J. Pharm.* **2012**, *436*, 753–763. [CrossRef] [PubMed]

63. Meng, J.; Sturgis, T.F.; Youan, B.B. Engineering tenofovir loaded chitosan nanoparticles to maximize microbicide mucoadhesion. *Eur. J. Pharm. Sci.* **2011**, *44*, 57–67. [CrossRef] [PubMed]

64. Yang, L.; Chen, L.; Zeng, R.; Li, C.; Qiao, R.; Hu, L.; Li, Z. Synthesis, nanosizing and *in vitro* drug release of a novel *anti*-HIV polymeric prodrug: Chitosan-*O*-isopropyl-5'-*O*-d4T monophosphate conjugate. *Bioorg. Med. Chem.* **2010**, *18*, 117–123. [CrossRef] [PubMed]

65. Nayak, U.Y.; Gopal, S.; Mutalik, S.; Ranjith, A.K.; Reddy, M.S.; Gupta, P.; Udupa, N. Glutaraldehyde cross-linked chitosan microspheres for controlled delivery of zidovudine. *J. Microencapsul.* **2009**, *26*, 214–222. [CrossRef] [PubMed]

66. Tokoro, A.; Tatewaki, N.; Suzuki, K.; Mikami, T.; Suzuki, S.; Suzuki, M. Growth-inhibitory effect of hexa-*N*-acetylchitohexaose and chitohexaose against Meth-A solid tumor. *Chem. Pharm. Bull. (Tokyo)* **1988**, *36*, 784–790. [CrossRef] [PubMed]

67. Lin, S.Y.; Chan, H.Y.; Shen, F.H.; Chen, M.H.; Wang, Y.J.; Yu, C.K. Chitosan prevents the development of AOM-induced aberrant crypt foci in mice and suppressed the proliferation of AGS cells by inhibiting DNA synthesis. *J. Cell Biochem.* **2007**, *100*, 1573–1580. [CrossRef] [PubMed]

68. Gibot, L.; Chabaud, S.; Bouhout, S.; Bolduc, S.; Auger, F.A.; Moulin, V.J. Anticancer properties of chitosan on human melanoma are cell line dependent. *Int. J. Biol. Macromol.* **2015**, *72*, 370–379. [CrossRef] [PubMed]

69. He, B.; Tao, H.Y.; Liu, S.Q. Neuroprotective effects of carboxymethylated chitosan on hydrogen peroxide induced apoptosis in Schwann cells. *Eur. J. Pharmacol.* **2014**, *740*, 127–134. [CrossRef] [PubMed]

70. Jiang, Z.; Han, B.; Li, H.; Li, X.; Yang, Y.; Liu, W. Preparation and anti-tumor metastasis of carboxymethyl chitosan. *Carbohydr. Polym.* **2015**, *125*, 53–60. [CrossRef] [PubMed]

71. Park, J.K.; Chung, M.J.; Choi, H.N.; Park, Y.I. Effects of the molecular weight and the degree of deacetylation of chitosan oligosaccharides on antitumor activity. *Int. J. Mol. Sci.* **2011**, *12*, 266–277. [CrossRef] [PubMed]

72. Shen, K.T.; Chen, M.H.; Chan, H.Y.; Jeng, J.H.; Wang, Y.J. Inhibitory effects of chitooligosaccharides on tumor growth and metastasis. *Food Chem. Toxicol.* **2009**, *47*, 1864–1871. [CrossRef] [PubMed]

73. Park, P.J.; Je, J.Y.; Kim, S.K. Free radical scavenging activity of chitooligosaccharides by electron spin resonance spectrometry. *J. Agric. Food Chem.* **2003**, *51*, 4624–4627. [CrossRef] [PubMed]

74. Je, J.Y.; Park, P.J.; Kim, S.K. Free radical scavenging properties of hetero-chitooligosaccharides using an ESR spectroscopy. *Food Chem. Toxicol.* **2004**, *42*, 381–387. [CrossRef] [PubMed]

75. Huang, J.; Xie, H.; Hu, S.; Xie, T.; Gong, J.; Jiang, C.; Ge, Q.; Wu, Y.; Liu, S.; Cui, Y.; *et al.* Preparation, characterization, and biochemical activities of *N*-(2-Carboxyethyl)chitosan from squid pens. *J. Agric. Food Chem.* **2015**, *63*, 2464–2471. [CrossRef] [PubMed]

76. Sun, T.; Xie, W.; Xu, P. Antioxidant activity of graft chitosan derivatives. *Macromol. Biosci.* **2003**, *3*, 320–323. [CrossRef]

77. Shukla, S.K.; Mishra, A.K.; Arotiba, O.A.; Mamba, B.B. Chitosan-based nanomaterials: A state-of-the-art review. *Int. J. Biol. Macromol.* **2013**, *59*, 46–58. [CrossRef] [PubMed]

78. Kim, I.Y.; Seo, S.J.; Moon, H.S.; Yoo, M.K.; Park, I.Y.; Kim, B.C.; Cho, C.S. Chitosan and its derivatives for tissue engineering applications. *Biotechnol. Adv.* **2008**, *26*, 1–21. [CrossRef] [PubMed]

79. Li, B.; Wang, L.; Xu, F.; Gang, X.; Demirci, U.; Wei, D.; Li, Y.; Feng, Y.; Jia, D.; Zhou, Y. Hydrosoluble, UV-crosslinkable and injectable chitosan for patterned cell-laden microgel and rapid transdermal curing hydrogel *in vivo*. *Acta. Biomater.* **2015**, *22*, 59–69. [CrossRef] [PubMed]

80. Yang, L.; Wang, Q.; Peng, L.; Yue, H.; Zhang, Z. Vascularization of repaired limb bone defects using chitosan-β-tricalcium phosphate composite as a tissue engineering bone scaffold. *Mol. Med. Rep.* **2015**, *12*, 2343–2347. [CrossRef] [PubMed]

81. Chameettachal, S.; Murab, S.; Vaid, R.; Midha, S.; Ghosh, S. Effect of visco-elastic silk-chitosan microcomposite scaffolds on matrix deposition and biomechanical functionality for cartilage tissue engineering. *J. Tissue Eng. Regen. Med.* **2015**. [CrossRef] [PubMed]

82. Li, Q.; Zhou, G.; Yu, X.; Wang, T.; Xi, Y.; Tang, Z. Porous deproteinized bovine bone scaffold with three-dimensional localized drug delivery system using chitosan microspheres. *Biomed. Eng. OnLine* **2015**, *14*. [CrossRef] [PubMed]

83. Shapira, Y.; Tolmasov, M.; Nissan, M.; Reider, E.; Koren, A.; Biron, T.; Bitan, Y.; Livnat, M.; Ronchi, G.; Geuna, S.; *et al.* Comparison of results between chitosan hollow tube and autologous nerve graft in reconstruction of peripheral nerve defect: An experimental study. *Microsurgery* **2015**. [CrossRef] [PubMed]

84. Tanaka, N.; Matsumoto, I.; Suzuki, M.; Kaneko, M.; Nitta, K.; Seguchi, R.; Ooi, A.; Takemura, H. Chitosan tubes can restore the function of resected phrenic nerves. *Interact. Cardiovasc. Thorac. Surg.* **2015**, *21*, 8–13. [CrossRef] [PubMed]

85. Jian, R.; Yixu, Y.; Sheyu, L.; Jianhong, S.; Yaohua, Y.; Xing, S.; Qingfeng, H.; Xiaojian, L.; Lei, Z.; Yan, Z.; *et al.* Repair of spinal cord injury by chitosan scaffold with glioma ECM and SB216763 implantation in adult rats. *J. Biomed. Mater. Res. A* **2015**. [CrossRef] [PubMed]

86. Correia, C.O.; Leite, A.J.; Mano, J.F. Chitosan/bioactive glass nanoparticles scaffolds with shape memory properties. *Carbohydr. Polym.* **2015**, *123*, 39–45. [CrossRef] [PubMed]

87. Jabbal-Gill, I.; Watts, P.; Smith, A. Chitosan-based delivery systems for mucosal vaccines. *Expert Opin. Drug Deliv.* **2012**, *9*, 1051–1067. [CrossRef] [PubMed]

88. Kofuji, K.; Qian, C.J.; Nishimura, M.; Sugiyama, I.; Murata, Y.; Kawashima, S. Relationship between physicochemical characteristics and functional properties of chitosan. *Eur. Polym. J.* **2005**, *41*, 2784–2791. [CrossRef]

89. Jiang, H.L.; Park, I.K.; Shin, N.R.; Kang, S.G.; Yoo, H.S.; Kim, S.I.; Suh, S.B.; Akaike, T.; Cho, C.S. *In vitro* study of the immune stimulating activity of an atrophic rhinitis vaccine associated to chitosan microspheres. *Eur. J. Pharm. Biopharm.* **2004**, *58*, 471–476. [CrossRef] [PubMed]

90. Borchard, G.; Lueβen, H.L.; de Boer, A.G.; Verhoef, J.C.; Lehr, C.M.; Junginger, H.E. The potential of mucoadhesive polymers in enhancing intestinal peptide drug absorption. III: Effects of chitosan-glutamate and carbomer on epithelial tight junctions *in vitro*. *J. Control. Release* **1996**, *39*, 131–138. [CrossRef]

91. Thanou, M.; Verhoef, J.C.; Junginger, H.E. Oral drug absorption enhancement by chitosan and its derivatives. *Adv. Drug Deliv. Rev.* **2001**, *52*, 117–126. [CrossRef]

92. Elsabee, M.Z.; Morsi, R.E.; Al-Sabagh, A.M. Surface active properties of chitosan and its derivatives. *Colloids Surf. B Biointerfaces* **2009**, *74*, 1–16. [CrossRef] [PubMed]

93. Harada, A.; Kataoka, K. Formation of polyion complex micelles in an aqueous milieu from a pair of oppositely-charged block copolymers with poly(ethylene glycol) segments. *Macromolecules* **1995**, *28*, 5294–5299. [CrossRef]

94. Supper, S.; Anton, N.; Boisclair, J.; Seidel, N.; Riemenschnitter, M.; Curdy, C.; Vandamme, T. Chitosan/glucose 1-phosphate as new stable *in situ* forming depot system for controlled drug delivery. *Eur. J. Pharm. Biopharm.* **2014**, *88*, 361–373. [CrossRef] [PubMed]

95. Supper, S.; Anton, N.; Seidel, N.; Riemenschnitter, M.; Curdy, C.; Vandamme, T. Thermosensitive chitosan/glycerophosphate-based hydrogel and its derivatives in pharmaceutical and biomedical applications. *Expert Opin. Drug Deliv.* **2014**, *11*, 249–267. [CrossRef] [PubMed]

96. Lai, P.; Daear, W.; Lobenberg, R.; Prenner, E.J. Overview of the preparation of organic polymeric nanoparticles for drug delivery based on gelatine, chitosan, poly(D,L-lactide-co-glycolic acid) and polyalkylcyanoacrylate. *Colloids Surf. B Biointerfaces* **2014**, *118*, 154–163. [CrossRef] [PubMed]

97. Hudson, D.; Margaritis, A. Biopolymer nanoparticle production for controlled release of biopharmaceuticals. *Crit. Rev. Biotechnol.* **2014**, *34*, 161–179. [CrossRef] [PubMed]

98. Calvo, P.; Remuñán-López, C.; Vila-Jato, J.L.; Alonso, M.J. Novel hydrophilic chitosan-polyethylene oxide nanoparticles as protein carriers. *J. Appl. Polym. Sci.* **1997**, *63*, 125–132. [CrossRef]

99. Kato, Y.; Onishi, H.; Machida, Y. Contribution of chitosan and its derivatives to cancer chemotherapy. *In Vivo* **2005**, *19*, 301–310. [PubMed]

100. Anraku, M.; Hiraga, A.; Iohara, D.; Pipkin, J.D.; Uekama, K.; Hirayama, F. Slow-release of famotidine from tablets consisting of chitosan/sulfobutyl ether beta-cyclodextrin composites. *Int. J. Pharm* **2015**, *487*, 142–147. [CrossRef] [PubMed]

101. Pereira, P.; Pedrosa, S.S.; Wymant, J.M.; Sayers, E.; Correia, A.; Vilanova, M.; Jones, A.T.; Gama, F.M. siRNA inhibition of endocytic pathways to characterize the cellular uptake mechanisms of folate-functionalized glycol chitosan nanogels. *Mol. Pharm.* **2015**, *12*, 1970–1979. [CrossRef] [PubMed]

102. Kulkarni, N.; Wakte, P.; Naik, J. Development of floating chitosan-xanthan beads for oral controlled release of glipizide. *Int. J. Pharm. Investig.* **2015**, *5*, 73–80. [CrossRef] [PubMed]

103. Al-Kurdi, Z.I.; Chowdhry, B.Z.; Leharne, S.A.; Al Omari, M.M.; Badwan, A.A. Low molecular weight chitosan-insulin polyelectrolyte complex: Characterization and stability studies. *Mar. Drugs* **2015**, *13*, 1765–1784. [CrossRef] [PubMed]

104. Gadalla, H.H.; Soliman, G.M.; Mohammed, F.A.; El-Sayed, A.M. Development and *in vitro/in vivo* evaluation of Zn-pectinate microparticles reinforced with chitosan for the colonic delivery of progesterone. *Drug Deliv.* **2015**, *8*, 1–14. [CrossRef] [PubMed]

105. Jana, S.; Laha, B.; Maiti, S. Boswellia gum resin/chitosan polymer composites: Controlled delivery vehicles for aceclofenac. *Int. J. Biol. Macromol.* **2015**, *77*, 303–306. [CrossRef] [PubMed]

106. Qinna, N.A.; Karwi, Q.G.; Al-Jbour, N.; Al-Remawi, M.A.; Alhussainy, T.M.; Al-So'ud, K.A.; Al Omari, M.M.; Badwan, A.A. Influence of molecular weight and degree of deacetylation of low molecular weight chitosan on the bioactivity of oral insulin preparations. *Mar. Drugs* **2015**, *13*, 1710–1725. [CrossRef] [PubMed]

107. Kim, K.; Ryu, J.H.; Lee, H. Chitosan-catechol: A polymer with long-lasting mucoadhesive properties. *Biomaterials* **2015**, *52*, 161–170. [CrossRef] [PubMed]

108. Chatterjee, S.; Judeh, Z.M. A. Encapsulation of fish oil with N-stearoyl O-butylglyceryl chitosan using membrane and ultrasonic emulsification processes. *Carbohyd. Polym.* **2015**, *123*, 432–442. [CrossRef] [PubMed]

109. Jayasree, R.S.; Rathinam, K.; Sharma, C.P. Development of artificial skin (Template) and influence of different types of sterilization procedures on wound healing pattern in rabbits and guinea pigs. *J. Biomater. Appl.* **1995**, *10*, 144–162. [PubMed]

110. Ueno, H.; Mori, T.; Fujinaga, T. Topical formulations and wound healing applications of chitosan. *Adv. Drug Deliv. Rev.* **2001**, *52*, 105–115. [CrossRef]

111. Muzzarelli, R.A.; Mattioli-Belmonte, M.; Pugnaloni, A.; Biagini, G. Biochemistry, histology and clinical uses of chitins and chitosans in wound healing. *EXS* **1999**, *87*, 251–264. [PubMed]

112. Azuma, K.; Izumi, R.; Osaki, T.; Ifuku, S.; Morimoto, M.; Saimoto, H.; Minami, S.; Okamoto, Y. Chitin, chitosan, and its derivatives for wound healing: Old and new materials. *J. Funct. Biomater.* **2015**, *6*, 104–142. [CrossRef] [PubMed]

113. Naseri, N.; Algan, C.; Jacobs, V.; John, M.; Oksman, K.; Mathew, A.P. Electrospun chitosan-based nanocomposite mats reinforced with chitin nanocrystals for wound dressing. *Carbohydr. Polym.* **2014**, *109*, 7–15. [CrossRef] [PubMed]

114. Ishihara, M.; Obara, K.; Nakamura, S.; Fujita, M.; Masuoka, K.; Kanatani, Y.; Takase, B.; Hattori, H.; Morimoto, Y.; Ishihara, M.; *et al.* Chitosan hydrogel as a drug delivery carrier to control angiogenesis. *J. Artif. Organs* **2006**, *9*, 8–16. [CrossRef] [PubMed]

115. Biagini, G.; Bertani, A.; Muzzarelli, R.; Damadei, A.; DiBenedetto, G.; Belligolli, A.; Riccotti, G.; Zucchini, C.; Rizzoli, C. Wound management with N-carboxybutyl chitosan. *Biomaterials* **1991**, *12*, 281–286. [CrossRef]

116. Stone, C.A.; Wright, H.; Devaraj, V.S.; Clarke, T.; Powell, R. Healing at skin graft donor sites dressed with chitosan. *Br. J. Plast. Surg.* **2000**, *53*, 601–606. [CrossRef] [PubMed]

117. Azad, A.K.; Sermsintham, N.; Chandrkrachang, S.; Stevens, W.F. Chitosan membrane as a wound-healing dressing: Characterization and clinical application. *J. Biomed. Mater. Res. B Appl. Biomater.* **2004**, *69*, 216–222. [CrossRef] [PubMed]

118. Valentine, R.; Athanasiadis, T.; Moratti, S.; Hanton, L.; Robinson, S.; Wormald, P.J. The efficacy of a novel chitosan gel on hemostasis and wound healing after endoscopic sinus surgery. *Am. J. Rhinol. Allergy* **2010**, *24*, 70–75. [CrossRef] [PubMed]

119. Bennett, B.L.; Littlejohn, L.F.; Kheirabadi, B.S.; Butler, F.K.; Kotwal, R.S.; Dubick, M.A.; Bailey, J.A. Management of external hemorrhage in tactical combat casualty care: Chitosan-based hemostatic gauze dressings—TCCC guidelines-change 13-05. *J. Spec. Oper. Med.* **2014**, *14*, 40–57. [PubMed]

120. Hatamabadi, H.R.; Asayesh Zarchi, F.; Kariman, H.; Arhami Dolatabadi, A.; Tabatabaey, A.; Amini, A. Celox-coated gauze for the treatment of civilian penetrating trauma: A randomized clinical trial. *Trauma Mon.* **2015**, *20*, e23862. [CrossRef] [PubMed]

121. Nguyen, N.; Hasan, S.; Caufield, L.; Ling, F.S.; Narins, C.R. Randomized controlled trial of topical hemostasis pad use for achieving vascular hemostasis following percutaneous coronary intervention. *Catheter. Cardiovasc. Interv.* **2007**, *69*, 801–807. [CrossRef] [PubMed]

122. Weng, M.H. The effect of protective treatment in reducing pressure ulcers for non-invasive ventilation patients. *Intensive Crit. Care Nurs.* **2008**, *24*, 295–259. [CrossRef] [PubMed]

123. Zhang, D.; Zhou, W.; Wei, B.; Wang, X.; Tang, R.; Nie, J.; Wang, J. Carboxyl-modified poly(vinyl alcohol)-cross-linked chitosan hydrogel films for potential wound dressing. *Carbohydr. Polym.* **2015**, *125*, 189–199. [CrossRef] [PubMed]

124. Jebahi, S.; Saoudi, M.; Farhat, L.; Oudadesse, H.; Rebai, T.; Kabir, A.; El Feki, A.; Keskes, H. Effect of novel curcumin-encapsulated chitosan-bioglass drug on bone and skin repair after gamma radiation: Experimental study on a Wistar rat model. *Cell Biochem. Funct.* **2015**, *33*, 150–159. [CrossRef] [PubMed]

125. Vakili, M.; Rafatullah, M.; Salamatinia, B.; Abdullah, A.Z.; Ibrahim, M.H.; Tan, K.B.; Gholami, Z.; Amouzgar, P. Application of chitosan and its derivatives as adsorbents for dye removal from water and wastewater: A review. *Carbohyd. Polym.* **2014**, *113*, 115–130. [CrossRef] [PubMed]

126. Boamah, P.O.; Huang, Y.; Hua, M.; Zhang, Q.; Wu, J.; Onumah, J.; Sam-Amoah, L.K. Sorption of heavy metal ions onto carboxylate chitosan derivatives-A mini-review. *Ecotoxicol. Environ. Saf.* **2015**, *116*, 113–120. [CrossRef] [PubMed]

127. Tran, V.S.; Ngo, H.H.; Guo, W.; Zhang, J.; Liang, S.; Ton-That, C.; Zhang, X. Typical low cost biosorbents for adsorptive removal of specific organic pollutants from water. *Bioresour. Technol.* **2015**, *182*, 353–363. [CrossRef] [PubMed]

128. Kyzas, G.Z.; Bikiaris, D.N. Recent modifications of chitosan for adsorption applications: A critical and systematic review. *Mar. Drugs* **2015**, *13*, 312–337. [CrossRef] [PubMed]

129. Yong, S.K.; Shrivastava, M.; Srivastava, P.; Kunhikrishnan, A.; Bolan, N. Environmental applications of chitosan and its derivatives. *Rev. Environ. Contam. Toxicol.* **2015**, *233*, 1–43. [PubMed]

130. Sayed, S.; Jardine, A. Chitosan derivatives as important biorefinery intermediates. Quaternary tetraalkylammonium chitosan derivatives utilized in anion exchange chromatography for perchlorate removal. *Int. J. Mol. Sci.* **2015**, *16*, 9064–9077. [CrossRef] [PubMed]

131. Zhang, J.; Chen, N.; Tang, Z.; Yu, Y.; Hu, Q.; Feng, C. A study of the mechanism of fluoride adsorption from aqueous solutions onto Fe-impregnated chitosan. *Phys. Chem. Chem. Phys.* **2015**, *17*, 12041–12050. [CrossRef] [PubMed]

132. Wang, Y.; Shi, L.; Gao, L.; Wei, Q.; Cui, L.; Hu, L.; Yan, L.; Du, B. The removal of lead ions from aqueous solution by using magnetic hydroxypropyl chitosan/oxidized multiwalled carbon nanotubes composites. *J. Colloid Interface Sci.* **2015**, *451*, 7–14. [CrossRef] [PubMed]

133. Prabhu, S.M.; Meenakshi, S. A dendrimer-like hyper branched chitosan beads toward fluoride adsorption from water. *Int. J. Biol. Macromol.* **2015**, *78*, 280–286. [CrossRef] [PubMed]

134. Li, L.; Li, Y.; Cao, L.; Yang, C. Enhanced chromium (VI) adsorption using nanosized chitosan fibers tailored by electrospinning. *Carbohyd. Polym.* **2015**, *125*, 206–213. [CrossRef] [PubMed]

135. Kimura, Y.; Takahashi, A.; Kashiwada, A.; Yamada, K. Removal of bisphenol derivatives through quinone oxidation by polyphenol oxidase and subsequent quinone adsorption on chitosan in the heterogeneous system. *Environ. Technol.* **2015**, 1–13. [CrossRef] [PubMed]

136. Boamah, P.O.; Huang, Y.; Hua, M.; Zhang, Q.; Liu, Y.; Onumah, J.; Wang, W.; Song, Y. Removal of cadmium from aqueous solution using low molecular weight chitosan derivative. *Carbohyd. Polym.* **2015**, *122*, 255–264. [CrossRef] [PubMed]

137. Li, H.; Pan, G. Simultaneous removal of harmful algal blooms and microcystins using microorganism- and chitosan-modified local Soil. *Environ. Sci. Technol.* **2015**, *49*, 6249–6256. [CrossRef] [PubMed]

138. Sivakami, M.S.; Gomathi, T.; Venkatesan, J.; Jeong, H.S.; Kim, S.K.; Sudha, P.N. Preparation and characterization of nano chitosan for treatment wastewaters. *Int. J. Biol. Macromol.* **2013**, *57*, 204–212. [CrossRef] [PubMed]

139. Heber, D. Herbal preparations for obesity: Are they useful? *Prim. Care* **2003**, *30*, 441–463. [CrossRef]

140. Ylitalo, R.; Lehtinen, S.; Wuolijoki, E.; Ylitalo, P.; Lehtimaki, T. Cholesterol-lowering properties and safety of chitosan. *Arzneimittelforschung* **2002**, *52*, 1–7. [CrossRef] [PubMed]

141. Gallaher, D.D.; Gallaher, C.M.; Mahrt, G.J.; Carr, T.P.; Hollingshead, C.H.; Hesslink, R., Jr.; Wise, J. A glucomannan and chitosan fiber supplement decreases plasma cholesterol and increases cholesterol excretion in overweight normocholesterolemic humans. *J. Am. Coll. Nutr.* **2002**, *21*, 428–433. [CrossRef] [PubMed]

142. Maezaki, Y.; Tsuji, K.; Nakagawa, Y.; Kawai, Y.; Akimoto, M.; Tsugita, T.; Takekawa, W.; Terada, A.; Hara, H.; Mitsuoka, T. Hypocholesterolemic effect of chitosan in adult males. *Biosci. Biotechnol. Biochem.* **1993**, *57*, 1439–1444. [CrossRef]

143. Wuolijoki, E.; Hirvela, T.; Ylitalo, P. Decrease in serum LDL cholesterol with microcrystalline chitosan. *Methods Find. Exp. Clin. Pharmacol.* **1999**, *21*, 357–361. [CrossRef] [PubMed]

144. Hernández-González, S.O.; Manuel González-Ortiz, M.; Martínez-Abundis, E.; Robles-Cervantes, J.A. Chitosan improves insulin sensitivity as determined by the euglycemic-hyperinsulinemic clamp technique in obese subjects. *Nutr. Res.* **2010**, *30*, 392–395. [CrossRef] [PubMed]

145. Pittler, M.H.; Abbot, N.C.; Harkness, E.F.; Ernst, E. Randomized, double-blind trial of chitosan for body weight reduction. *Eur. J. Clin. Nutr.* **1999**, *53*, 379–381. [CrossRef] [PubMed]

146. Mhurchu, C.N.; Poppitt, S.D.; McGill, A.T.; Leahy, F.E.; Bennett, D.A.; Lin, R.B.; Ormrod, D.; Ward, L.; Strik, C.; Rodgers, A. The effect of the dietary supplement, chitosan, on body weight: A randomised controlled trial in 250 overweight and obese adults. *Int. J. Obes. Relat. Metab. Disord.* **2004**, *28*, 1149–1156. [CrossRef] [PubMed]

147. Egras, A.M.; Hamilton, W.R.; Lenz, T.L.; Monaghan, M.S. An evidence-based review of fat modifying supplemental weight loss products. *J. Obes.* **2011**. [CrossRef] [PubMed]

148. Yu, Y.; Luo, T.; Liu, S.; Song, G.; Han, J.; Wang, Y.; Yao, S.; Feng, L.; Qin, S. Chitosan oligosaccharides attenuate atherosclerosis and decrease non-HDL in apoE-/- mice. *J. Atheroscler. Thromb.* **2015**. [CrossRef] [PubMed]

149. Kerch, G. The potential of chitosan and its derivatives in prevention and treatment of age-related diseases. *Mar. Drugs* **2015**, *13*, 2158–2182. [CrossRef] [PubMed]

150. Bento, D.; Staats, H.F.; Gonçalves, T.; Borges, O. Development of a novel adjuvanted nasal vaccine: C48/80 associated with chitosan nanoparticles as a path to enhance mucosal immunity. *Eur. J. Pharm. Biopharm.* **2015**, *93*, 149–164. [CrossRef] [PubMed]

151. Laffleur, F.; Fischer, A.; Schmutzler, M.; Hintzen, F.; Bernkop-Schnürch, A. Evaluation of functional characteristics of preactivated thiolated chitosan as potential therapeutic agent for dry mouth syndrome. *Acta Biomater.* **2015**, *21*, 123–131. [CrossRef] [PubMed]

152. Gudjónsdóttir, M.; Gacutan, M.D., Jr.; Mendes, A.C.; Chronakis, I.S.; Jespersen, L.; Karlsson, A.H. Effects of electrospun chitosan wrapping for dry-ageing of beef, as studied by microbiological, physicochemical and low-field nuclear magnetic resonance analysis. *Food Chem.* **2015**, *184*, 167–175. [CrossRef] [PubMed]

153. Zhang, X.; Mysore, K.; Flannery, E.; Michel, K.; Severson, D.W.; Zhu, K.Y.; Duman-Scheel, M. Chitosan/Interfering RNA nanoparticle mediated gene silencing in disease vector mosquito larvae. *J. Vis. Exp.* **2015**. [CrossRef] [PubMed]

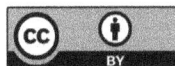

marine drugs

MDPI

Review

The Potential of Chitosan and Its Derivatives in Prevention and Treatment of Age-Related Diseases

Garry Kerch

Department of Materials Science and Applied Chemistry, Riga Technical University, Azenes 14/24, Riga, LV-1048, Latvia; garrykerch@inbox.lv; Tel.: +371-292-769-42

Academic Editor: Paola Laurienzo
Received: 19 February 2015; Accepted: 26 March 2015; Published: 13 April 2015

Abstract: Age-related, diet-related and protein conformational diseases, such as atherosclerosis, diabetes mellitus, cancer, hypercholesterolemia, cardiovascular and neurodegenerative diseases are common in the elderly population. The potential of chitosan, chitooligosaccharides and their derivatives in prevention and treatment of age-related dysfunctions is reviewed and discussed in this paper. The influence of oxidative stress, low density lipoprotein oxidation, increase of tissue stiffness, protein conformational changes, aging-associated chronic inflammation and their pathobiological significance have been considered. The chitosan-based functional food also has been reviewed.

Keywords: chitosan; chitooligosacharides; age-related diseases; protein conformations

1. Introduction

According to the recent report of The Department of Economic and Social Affairs of the United Nations Secretariat [1] globally, the number of elderly (aged 60 years or over) is expected to increase from 841 million people in 2013 to more than 2 billion in 2050. The global share of older persons increased from 9.2 per cent in 1990 to 11.7 per cent in 2013 and proportion of the world population will reach 21.1 per cent by 2050. The share of older people aged 80 years or over (the "oldest old") within the older population (aged 60 years or over) was 14 per cent in 2013 and is expected to reach 19 percent in 2050. There will be 392 million persons aged 80 years or over by 2050. Women live longer than men, so the older population will be mainly female.

The quality of life depends on the nutrition of the elderly population [2,3]. World Health Organization devoted special attention to nutrition for older people. Degenerative age-related diseases such as cardiovascular and cerebrovascular disease, diabetes, osteoporosis and cancer are the common diseases in older persons, and these diseases are also diet-affected [4]. Elevated serum cholesterol, a risk factor for cardiovascular diseases, is common in older people. It has been estimated that a 10% reduction in blood cholesterol concentration can reduce the risk of coronary heart disease by 30%. The decrease in salt and saturated fat intake can reduce blood pressure and blood cholesterol concentrations and can decrease the risk of cardiovascular disease. Increasing intake of fruit and vegetables by one to two servings daily could reduce cardiovascular risk by 30% [4].

Older people often suffer from impaired immunity [5–7]. Deficiency of trace elements zinc, iron, selenium, copper, Vitamins A, B, C, E have important impacts on immune responses. It has been reported [8] that chitooligosaccharide ascorbate is effective in compensation of deficiency in a number of minerals and vitamins. "The innate immune system is composed of a network of cells including neutrophils, NK and NKT cells, monocytes/macrophages, and dendritic cells that mediate the earliest interactions with pathogens. Age-associated defects are observed in the activation of all of these cell types, linked to compromised signal transduction pathways" [9]. Activation of intestinal T regulatory cells and homeostatic regulation of the gut microbiota may reduce low-grade inflammation in diet-related diseases [10] and, probably, also in age-related diseases.

Functional foods and nutraceuticals with antioxidant, anti-inflammatory, anti-diabetic and anticancer properties may prevent age-related and diet-related diseases. Decline in immune response with aging and the role of nutrition in enhancing immunity have been reviewed recently [11]. Dietary components have the potential to improve immunity in ageing. The molecular mechanism underlying effects of diet and functional food on immunity remain to be determined [12]. The herbal polysaccharides with antioxidant and anti-inflammatory properties that are able to inhibit protein aggregation and to prevent associated age-related diseases have been reviewed recently [13] as well as marine derived polysaccharides [14]. Chitosan is a linear natural nontoxic cationic polysaccharide that due to its biocompatibility, biodegradability and cationic nature has advantages in biomedical applications over other neutral or negatively charged polysaccharides. The properties and various applications of chitosan and its derivatives and composites have been described in a number of recent books [15–19]. The potential of chitosan and its derivatives to prevent age-related diseases is presented in Figure 1.

The structure, properties and applications of chitosan, chitooligosaccharides (COS) and their derivatives have been described in many review papers [20–30]. Chitosan is bioactive cationic polysaccharide with antibacterial, antifungal, antioxidant, antidiabetic, anti-inflammatory, anticancer, and hypocholesterolemic properties. Chitosan is used in biomedical and food applications. This review paper focuses on the ability of chitosan and COS to prevent age-related dysfunctions.

2. Oxidative Stress

Antioxidant effects of chitin, chitosan and their derivatives have been reviewed recently and it was concluded that their antioxidant properties play a vital role in human health and nutrition [31]. The studies on antioxidant properties that have not been included in this recent review are discussed here.

Increased risk of oxidative stress in elderly people has been reported [32]. Increased levels of reactive oxygen species (ROS) can cause oxidative modifications of lipids, proteins, and DNA. Oxidative stress and inflammation are involved in the pathology of age-related diseases such as cardiovascular diseases, cancer, neurodegenerative diseases, rheumatoid arthritis, and diabetes mellitus (Figure 1). It is important to protect the cells from oxidative damage by ROS [33–35].

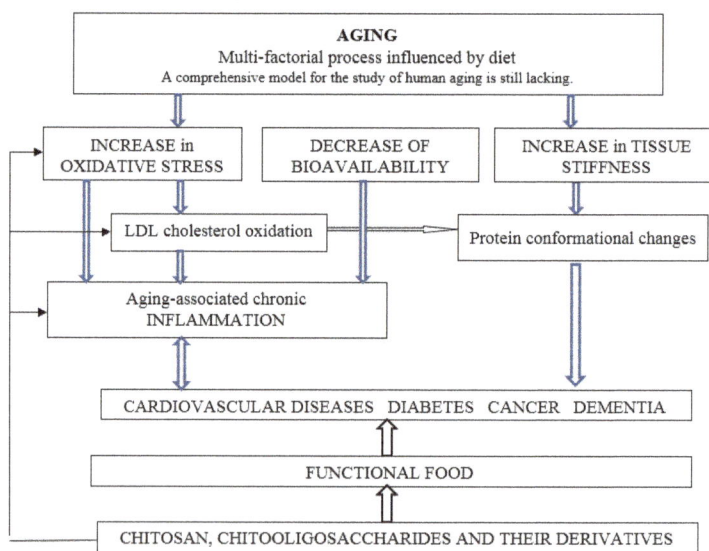

Figure 1. The potential effect of chitosan on age-related dysfunctions.

There is an urgent need to elucidate the role of oxidative stress in aging and to find promising perspectives on the efficacy of modulating agents for oxidative stress in treatment or prevention of age-related diseases. Perspectives on application of chitosan and its derivatives in the treatment of oxidative stress in age-related diseases have been considered in a number of research papers [31, 36–46]. Researchers from Fukuyama University, Japan [43] concluded that chitosan has a direct antioxidant activity in systemic circulation by lowering the indices of oxidative stress in both *in vitro* and *in vivo* studies.

Researchers from Hubei University of Medicine, China, reported that COS inhibit ethanol-induced lipid peroxidation and glutathione depletion via the transcriptional activation of nuclear factor erythroid-2-related factor-2 (Nrf2) and reduction of the ethanol-induced phosphorylation of p38 MAPK, JNK and ERK [47]. Dietary chitosan supplementation attenuates isoprenaline-induced oxidative stress in rat myocardium [48] and the antiaging effect of dietary chitosan supplementation on glutathione-dependent antioxidant system in young and aged rats has been reported [49]. COS protect mice from oxidative stress [50]. Sulfated COS decrease intracellular ROS production. The researchers from Xi'an Jiaotong University, China [51] have reported protective effects of sulfated COS against hydrogen peroxide-induced damage in pancreatic β-cells MIN6. Sulfated COS significantly suppress nitric oxide (NO) production [52], the activity and mRNA expression of inducible NO synthase (iNOS), and the protein level of nuclear factor NF-κB protein p65 [52], which were activated by hydrogen peroxide H_2O_2. These results indicated the good anti-oxidative capacity of sulfated COS and the possible mechanism via the blockade of the nuclear factor NF-κB signaling pathway. The protective effects of sulfated COS against oxidative injuries in MIN6 cells depend both on their degree of substitution and concentration. The antioxidant action of low molecular weight chitosan was more effective in preventing the formation of carbonyl groups in plasma protein than high molecular weight chitosan [53]. The antioxidant activity of chitosan was increased after media milling. Rats fed media-milled chitosan showed increased superoxide dismutase activity [54]. Antioxidant activities of novel chitosan-caffeic acid, chitosan-ferulic acid, and chitosan-sinapic acid conjugates with different grafting ratios were investigated. The antioxidant activities of the conjugates were increased compared to the unmodified chitosan [55]. Researchers of Korea University, Seoul [56] reported that antioxidant property of chitosan green tea polyphenols complex induces transglutaminase activation in wound healing. Caffeic and ferulic acids were grafted onto chitosan by a free radical mediated method [57]. The novel compounds had improved peroxidation inhibition effects and increased free radical scavenging. The antioxidant activity of the phenol acids grafted N,O-carboxymethyl chitosan increased in order of chitosan < N,O-carboxymethyl chitosan < ferulic acid—N,O-carboxymethyl chitosan < caffeic acid—N,O-carboxymethyl chitosan < gallic acid—N,O-carboxymethyl chitosan [58]. COS reduce oxidative damage of DNA by inhibiting hydrogen peroxide H_2O_2 and AAPH radicals [59–63] and block degradation of inhibitory kappa B alpha (IκB-α) protein and translocation of nuclear factor kappa B (NF-κB) [63]. NF-κB translocates to the nucleus from cytoplasm when activated by stress, bacteria, inflammatory stimuli, cytokines, free radicals, carcinogens, and other agents. NF-κB regulates the expression of enzymes (such as COX-2 and iNOS), cytokines (such as TNF, IL-1, IL-6, IL-8), adhesion molecules and has been linked with age-related diseases such as atherosclerosis, diabetes, osteoporosis, Alzheimer's disease, and cancer [64]. COS suppress NF-κB activation and so they are promising agents in prevention and treatment of age-related diseases.

The recent publications also show that grafting of natural antioxidant polyphenols on chitosan and COS derivatives, such as antioxidant sulfated COS [31], can result in the design of novel effective antioxidant nutraceuticals.

3. Inflammation

Oxidative stress and inflammation are involved in the pathology of age-related diseases such as cardiovascular diseases, cancer, neurodegenerative diseases, rheumatoid arthritis, and diabetes [33–35]. Chronic inflammation can be considered as a major risk factor for age-related diseases [65]. Oxidative stress results in upregulation of proinflammatory mediators (TNF-α, IL-1β, IL-6, COX-2, iNOS). Plasma TNF-α concentration is associated with aging and the risk of diabetes mellitus [66].

COS inhibit the expression of IL-6 in lipopolysaccharide (LPS)-induced human umbilical vein endothelial cells (HUVECs). The pre-treatment of HUVECs with COS inhibited the LPS-induced over-expression of phosphorylated p38 mitogen-activated protein kinase (MAPK), phosphorylated ERK1/2 and nuclear factor NF-κB. COS prevented degradation of inhibitory protein IκBα in nuclear factor NF-κB and translocation of NF-κB from cytoplasm to nucleus [67].

COS inhibit LPS-induced over-expression of inflammatory cytokines IL-6 and TNF-α also in RAW264.7 macrophage cells through blockade of MAPK and PI3K/Akt signaling pathways and suppress the activation of NF-κB and activator protein-1 (AP-1) [68]. The similar behavior has been reported for sulfated COS [52]. It has been suggested recently [69] that COS block LPS-induced *O*-GlcNAcylation (a dynamic modification of proteins by β-linked *N*-acetylglucosamine) of NF-κB and endothelial inflammatory response.

Adhesion molecules are involved in the adhesive interaction between endothelial cells and monocytes in inflammation. COS down regulate the expression of adhesion molecules E-selectin and ICAM-1 by inhibiting the phosphorylation of MAPKs and the activation of NF-κB in LPS-treated porcine iliac artery endothelial cells [70]. Sulfated chitosan inhibits P-selectin-mediated HL-60 leukocyte adhesion. Sulfochitosans exhibit inhibitory activity in the order: heparin > *N*-sulfated/6-*O*-sulfated chitosan $\geq$ 3-*O*,6-*O*-sulfated chitosan > 6-*O*-sulfated chitosan >> *N*-sulfated chitosan. So, it can be concluded that the sulfation of the double site in chitosan is essential for efficient inhibition of P-selectin-mediated HL-60 leukocyte adhesion [71].

The effects of chitosan and quaternized chitosan on production of IL-1β and TNF-α in LPS-stimulated human periodontal ligament cells has been studied [72]. Chitosan inhibited the production of IL-1β and TNF-α and quaternized chitosan increased IL-1β and TNF-α production.

COS attenuate ocular inflammation in rats with experimental autoimmune anterior uveitis [73] and prevented retinal ischemia and reperfusion injury via reduced oxidative stress and inflammation [74].

The elevated plasma glucose, TNF-α, and IL-6 in diabetic rats were decreased after 10 weeks of chitosan feeding [75]. Biomarkers provide insights into complex disease mechanisms and can help to develop novel nutraceuticals. Evidently, it does not mean that it is enough to decrease the content of inflammatory biomarkers to completely prevent and treat diabetes and other age-related diseases.

COS inhibited the release and expression levels of inflammatory cytokines TNF-α, IL-6 and IL-1β in LPS-stimulated BV2 microglia. COS also attenuated the production of NO and prostaglandin E2 (PGE2) by inhibiting iNOS and cyclooxygenase-2 (COX-2) expressions [76]. It has been confirmed recently that COS decrease the levels of NO, TNF-α and IL-1β, released from LPS-stimulated RAW264.7 cells by inhibiting the activation of the NF-κB pathway [77].

Chitosan decreased serum TNF-α and leptin levels in high fat fed rats [78]. NF-κB activation, and levels of TNF-α and IL-6 in colonic tissues, were suppressed in mice with inflammatory bowel disease receiving COS [79]. It has been reported that the oral intake of COS by elderly volunteers decreased inflammatory cytokines TNF-α and IL-1β levels [80]. COS added to diet have been reported as calcium fortifiers [81] in ovariectomised rats and this effect has been related to COS capacity to down-regulate mRNA and protein expression of COX-2, a key mediator linking inflammation and osteoporosis. It has been demonstrated *in vivo* that COS are able to induce an anti-inflammatory effect mediated by cyclooxygenase inhibition and reduction of prostaglandins [82].

The anti-inflammatory and anticancer properties of chitin oligosaccharide and chitosan oligosaccharide have been recently reviewed [83].

4. Diabetes Mellitus

Antidiabetic effects of chitin, chitosan and their derivatives have been reviewed recently [84]. It has been concluded that chitosan and its derivatives have the potential to be used in several antidiabetic therapeutic applications and future research should be directed to enhance the effectiveness of novel chitosan derivatives and chitosan-based compounds to be used as potent nutraceuticals for prevention of diabetes and diabetes-related complications. So, the studies on antidiabetic properties of chitosan, COS and their derivatives that have not been included in this recent review are discussed here with special attention given to application in age-related diabetes.

Protein-rich diet is recommended at present for the treatment of elderly malnutrition. However, it was demonstrated recently in a large population-based prospective study by scientists of Lund University [85] that high intakes of protein and processed meat are associated with increased incidence of type 2 diabetes. At the same time, the intake of fiber-rich bread and cereals was inversely associated with type 2 diabetes. Insulin independent diabetes mellitus, the type II diabetes, is a serious global problem getting worse every year. The team of researchers from University of Southern California led by Longo [86] also reported that high protein intake was associated with reduced cancer and overall mortality in respondents over 65, but a five-fold increase in diabetes mortality across all ages. It must be also taken into account that diabetes mellitus is a risk factor for incidence of age-related dementia, Alzheimer's disease, and cardiovascular diseases. So, a novel, complex balanced, more safe protein-rich diet and functional food to tackle malnutrition in elderly with lower risk of diabetes development must be designed.

The use of antioxidants reduces oxidative stress and alleviates diabetic complications [87]. Oxidative stress common for older people can lead to increased lipid peroxidation and development of diabetes mellitus [88,89]. TNF-α expression in the insulin resistant subjects and the diabetic patients was four-fold higher than in the insulin sensitive subjects [90]. Plasma TNF-α concentration is significantly associated with advancing age and it predicts the impairment in insulin action with advancing age [66]. Miura and coworkers [91] reported that chitosan had blood glucose-lowering and lipid-lowering effects in neonatal streptozotocin-induced diabetic mice. Hayashi and Ito [92] reported that low molecular-weight chitosan lactate had an antidiabetic effect also in obese diabetic KK-Ay mice. Chitosan may possess a potential for alleviating type-1 diabetic hyperglycemia through the decrease in liver gluconeogenesis and increase in skeletal muscle glucose uptake and use [93]. A randomized, double-blind, placebo-controlled clinical trial on 12 week supplementation of COS in subjects with prediabetes showed a significant decrease in the serum glucose level [94]. The effects of chitosan-oligosaccharide (GO2KA1) on postprandial blood glucose levels in adults with normal blood glucose levels have been recently reported [95,96]. GO2KA1 reduced postprandial blood glucose level due to the decrease of absorption of glucose in the small intestine as a result of carbohydrate hydrolyzing enzyme inhibition. Hsieh and coworkers [75] demonstrated that chitosan reduces plasma adipocytokines and lipid accumulation in liver and adipose tissues and ameliorates insulin resistance in diabetic rats. After 10 weeks of feeding, the elevated plasma glucose, TNF-α, and IL-6 and lower adiponectin levels caused by diabetes were effectively reversed by chitosan treatment. Chitosan feeding also reduced hepatic triglyceride and cholesterol contents. Hsieh and coworkers consider that long-term administration of chitosan may reduce insulin resistance through suppression of lipid accumulation in liver and adipose tissues and amelioration of chronic inflammation in diabetic rats.

5. Hypercholesterolemia

Low-density lipoprotein (LDL) oxidation is associated with coronary atherosclerosis. High levels of cholesterol oxidation products in oxidized LDL are toxic for endothelial cells [97,98]. Removal of oxidized LDL is an important part of the protective role of the macrophage in the inflammatory response [99]. Mediators of inflammation such as TNF-α, IL-1, and macrophage colony-stimulating factor increase binding of LDL to endothelium and smooth muscle. Antioxidants have an anti-inflammatory effect by preventing the up-regulation of adhesion molecules for monocytes. Antioxidants increase the resistance of human LDL to oxidation. High-density lipoproteins inhibit cytokine-induced expression of endothelial cell adhesion molecules [100].

Hypocholesterolemic effects of chitosan have been reported in many publications [101–111]. Recently, it has been demonstrated that the effect of media-milled chitosan on the decrease of serum triacylglycerol, total cholesterol and LDL cholesterol is higher compared to chitosan [54]. It has been also demonstrated recently that total cholesterol content in mice blood fed during 12 weeks with γ-irradiated chitosan (30–100 kGy) was significantly lower than that of the control [112]. The role of chitosan in lipid lowering treatment has been discussed recently by Patti and coworkers [113].

6. Cancer

In a recent review [31], it has been concluded that formation of cancer cells can be induced by free radicals. Hence, antioxidant properties of chitosan and its derivatives can be used to reduce the chance for the formation of cancer in the human body.

The anticancer properties of chitin and chitosan oligosaccharides have been recently reviewed [83]. Chitin and chitosan oligosaccharides have been evaluated as functional foods against cancer. The studies on anticancer properties that have not been included in this recent review are discussed here.

Polyphenols, such as curcumin or resveratrol, are effective natural antioxidants and their bioavailability can be essentially improved by encapsulation in chitosan-based nanoparticles [114] to be delivered to cancer cells. It has been also reported that novel cationic curcumin-chitosan poly (butyl cyanoacrylate) nanoparticles synthesized by emulsion polymerization, can improve the bioavailability of hydrophobic drug curcumin, suppress hepatocellular carcinoma growth and inhibit tumor angiogenesis efficiently *in vitro* and *in vivo* [115]. Rejinold and coworkers [116] fabricated curcumin with biodegradable thermoresponsive chitosan-g-poly (N-vinylcaprolactam) nanoparticles (TRC-NPs) for cancer drug delivery. Their results indicate that novel curcumin-loaded TRC-NPs could be a promising candidate for cancer drug delivery. The anticancer effect can be explained by activation of apoptosis signaling (curcumin inhibits Bcl2 and activates caspase 9 to induce apoptosis) and blockade of cell proliferation signaling pathways (such as MAP kinase pathway, AKT pathway and mTOR pathways) [117–121]. Researchers from Universidade Federal de Santa Catarina, Florianópolis, Brazil and Université Grenoble Alpes, Grenoble, France published a number of papers describing curcumin-loaded chitosan-coated nanoparticles. Curcumin-loaded chitosan-coated nanoparticles can be used for the local treatment of oral cavity cancer [122]. The mucoadhesive properties of chitosan due to its polycation nature have been used to prepare films containing chitosan-coated nanoparticles for buccal delivery of curcumin [123]. Xyloglucan-block-poly (ε-Caprolactone) copolymer nanoparticles coated with chitosan were developed as biocompatible mucoadhesive drug delivery system [124]. Chitosan interacts with mucin through electrostatic forces between protonated amino groups of chitosan and negatively charged groups of mucin [125].

It has been also reported that oral administration of chitosan based nanoformulated green tea polyphenol EGCG effectively inhibits prostate cancer cell growth [126]. EGCG has been encapsulated also into chitosan-coated nanoliposomes and anticancer effects are expected in the treatment of breast cancer [127].

The curcumin/5-fluorouracil loaded thiolated chitosan nanoparticles showed enhanced anticancer effects on colon cancer cells *in vitro* and improved the bioavailability of the drugs *in vivo* [128]. The 5-fluorouracil and curcumin released from the N,O-carboxymethyl chitosan nanoparticles also produced enhanced anticancer effects *in vitro* in colon cancer cells HT 29 and improved plasma concentrations under *in vivo* conditions in mouse model [129].

Chitosan-based nanoparticles for tumor-targeted drug delivery that display a range of useful properties such as biocompatibility, biodegradability, excellent cell membrane penetrability, high drug-carrying capacities, pH-dependent unloading and prolonged circulating time have been recently reviewed by Prabaharan [130]. The possible anticancer effect of chitosan and polyphenols encapsulated in chitosan nanoparticles is presented in Figure 2.

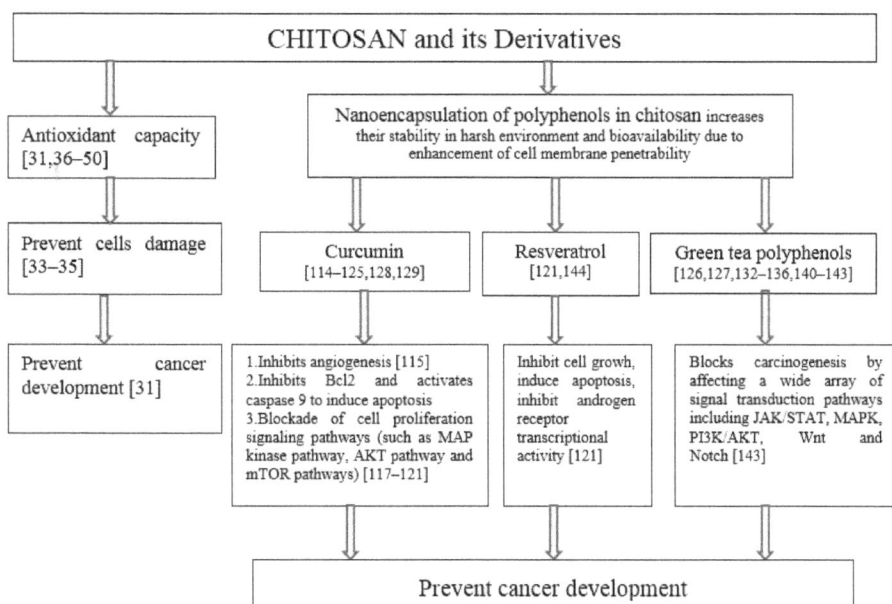

Figure 2. The possible anticancer effect of chitosan and polyphenols encapsulated in chitosan nanoparticles.

7. Nanomedicine

Application of chitosan as drug carriers has been reviewed [130,131]. Decrease of bioavailability of nutrients with aging is an important problem leading to age-related dysfunctions. So, it is a great challenge to use chitosan as carriers of nutraceuticals that are able to delay or prevent age-related dysfunctions.

Catechins found in green tea have demonstrated antioxidant, cardioprotective, neuroprotective and anticancer effects. However, the oral administration of these oxidation-sensitive compounds is limited by the harsh environment of the gastrointestinal tract, their poor stability and intestinal absorption. Encapsulation in chitosan nanoparticles enhance the intestinal absorption of the green tea catechins (+)-catechin and (−)-epigallocatechin gallate (EGCG) [132]. Researchers from Monash University, Australia, considered that the mechanism by which absorption was enhanced was not through an effect of chitosan nanoparticles on intestinal paracellular or passive transcellular transport or an effect on efflux proteins but was likely due to stabilization of catechins after encapsulation. Oral absorption of encapsulated EGCG has been evaluated in Swiss Outbred mice. Administration of the chitosan nanoparticles enhanced the plasma exposure of total EGCG by a factor of 1.5 relative to an EGCG solution [133]. Nanochemoprevention by encapsulation of (−)-epigallocatechin-3-gallate with bioactive peptides/chitosan nanoparticles for enhancement of its bioavailability also has been reported [134].

Tang and coworkers [135] consider that chitosan nanoparticles with a positive surface charge could transiently open the tight junctions between Caco-2 cells and thus increase the paracellular transport of tea catechins. They prepared nanoparticles composed of chitosan and an edible polypeptide, poly (γ-glutamic acid) (γ-PGA) for the delivery of tea catechins and demonstrated that chitosan/γ-PGA nanoparticles can be effective as a carrier for oral delivery of tea catechins with effective antioxidant activity.

It must be taken into account [136,137] that in comparison to the free-soluble polymers, the nanoparticles prepared by ionic gelation of the chitosan and its quaternized derivatives can have much lower effect on decreasing the transepithelial electrical resistance by opening of the tight junctions and on the permeability of cell layers in a Caco-2 cell system due to the reduced available amount of positive charge at the surface of the nanoparticles. However, no differences in cell permeability were detected between chitosan solution and chitosan nanoparticles on Calu-3 cells [138].

Chitosan coating prevents the aggregation of bovine serum albumin (BSA)—epigallocatechin gallate (EGCG) nanoparticles at pH 4.5–5.0 and may improve the absorption of EGCG [139]. Chitosan coating has been used also for (−)-epigallocatechin-3-gallate (EGCG) encapsulated nanostructured lipid carriers [140,141]. EGCG has been encapsulated into chitosan-coated nanoliposomes and a potential breakthrough in the prevention or even treatment of breast cancer has been expected [127]. Folate conjugated chitosan coated EGCG nanoparticles were prepared using the ionic gelation method with folic acid modified carboxymethyl chitosan and chitosan hydrochloride as carriers of catechin EGCG [142]. EGCG blocks carcinogenesis by affecting a wide array of signal transduction pathways including JAK/STAT, MAPK, PI3K/AKT, Wnt and Notch [143].

Chitosan/poly (D,L-lactic-co-glycolic acid) (PLGA) microcapsules were prepared by W/O/W double emulsion method and nutraceutical resveratrol was encapsulated into microcapsules [144].

8. Neurodegenerative Diseases

Cases of dementia and Alzheimer's are expected to almost double every 20 years to around 66 million in 2030 and over 115 million in 2050 [145].

A chronic inflammatory response associated with Aβ and IL-1β is responsible for the pathology of Alzheimer's disease. The polyphenol EGCG binds directly to a large number of proteins that are involved in protein misfolding diseases and inhibits their fibrillization [146]. Water-soluble chitosan inhibits the production of pro-inflammatory cytokine in human astrocytoma cells activated by Aβ and IL-1β and may reduce and delay the pathological events associated with Alzheimer's disease [147].

The effect of COS on NO production in LPS induced N9 microglial cells has been studied [148]. Pretreatment with COS could inhibit NO production by suppressing iNOS expression in activated microglial cells. COS inhibited LPS-induced phosphorylation of p38 MAPK and ERK1/2. COS pretreatment could also inhibit the activation of both NF-κB and activator protein-1 (AP-1). The possible effect of chitosan oligosaccharide on Alzheimer disease pathology is presented in Figure 3.

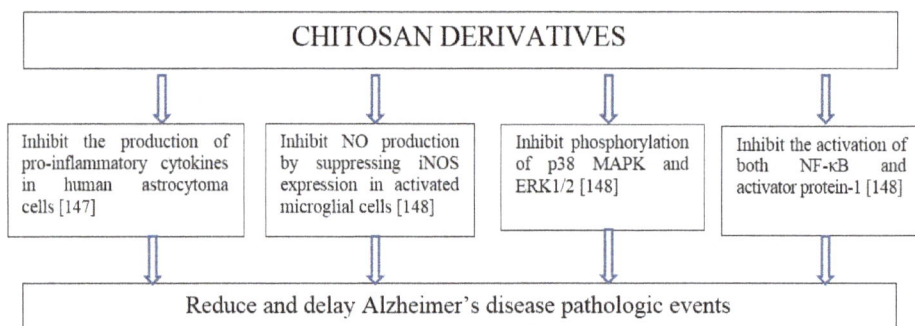

CHITOSAN DERIVATIVES			
Inhibit the production of pro-inflammatory cytokines in human astrocytoma cells [147]	Inhibit NO production by suppressing iNOS expression in activated microglial cells [148]	Inhibit phosphorylation of p38 MAPK and ERK1/2 [148]	Inhibit the activation of both NF-κB and activator protein-1 [148]
Reduce and delay Alzheimer's disease pathologic events			

Figure 3. The possible effect of chitosan oligosaccharide on Alzheimer disease pathology.

9. Protein Conformational Diseases

The changes in protein conformations lead to protein conformational diseases that are also age-related diseases—diabetes mellitus, cataract, Alzheimer's disease, dementia, and atherosclerosis. Protein oxidation or glycation induces protein unfolding, adhesion of unfolded proteins to the arterial wall with increased arterial stiffness and the initiation of vascular inflammation and atherosclerosis [149–154]. Atherosclerotic plaques contain oxidized LDL which has amyloid properties [155] and activates platelets [151]. Misfolded proteins support platelet activation and aggregation leading to protein conformational diseases [156,157].

The presence of water at the protein-lipid interface of membrane proteins can affect the changes in protein conformations. Cholesterol is known to reduce the water content of lipid bilayers. Changes in the degree of hydration can lead to changes in protein conformation [158]. Chitosan prevents formation of carbonyl and hydroperoxide groups in human serum albumin exposed to peroxyl radicals and inhibits conformational changes in the protein, assessed by absorption spectrum and intrinsic fluorescence [159].

Proteins can be denatured by various stresses. Various additives are known to minimize the damage and to enhance the stability of proteins [160]. So, the possible mechanism of beneficial effect of COS in protein conformational diseases can be also due to their ability to prevent conformational changes in proteins. Tissue dehydration with aging [161] can cause protein conformational changes. The possible effect of chitosan on protein conformational diseases is presented in Figure 4. The need for further research in this area is evident.

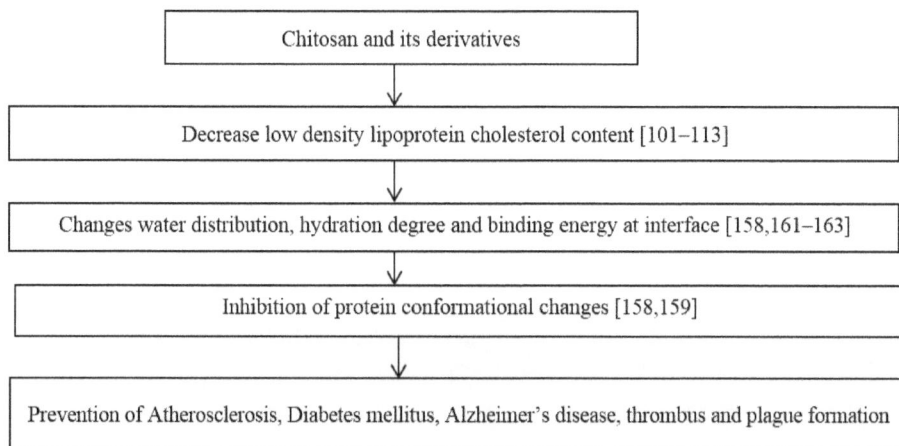

Figure 4. The possible influence of chitosan on low density lipoprotein cholesterol content, hydration, protein conformation, and protein conformational diseases.

It has been demonstrated that the presence of chitosan can change water migration and distribution in complex food systems such as bread [162] and can change interaction and water distribution between gluten and starch. Also, it has been shown that chitosan can prevent platelet adhesion to implants if water molecules are tightly bound to chitosan macromolecules and do not prevent platelet adhesion if water molecules at interface are free or loosely bound to the chitosan coated surface [163]. In both cases, interaction with protein depends on the water binding energy to chitosan macromolecules.

10. Chitosan Containing Food

It would be desirable if health promoting additives are used in everyday food and the elderly will not be forced to make drastic dietary changes. So, bread and dairy food containing chitosan and its derivatives could be the most appropriate functional food.

10.1. Bread Containing Chitosan and Its Derivatives

The papers published before 2007 have been reviewed by No *et al.* [164] and they reported that chitosan [165,166] and chitosan oligosaccharide [167] coatings extend shelf life of bread. The additives of chitosan [168] and carboxymethyl chitosan [169] also have been reported to extend shelf life of bread. The extension of bread shelf life has been explained by inhibiting microbial growth and by retarding starch retrogradation. Chitosans with higher molecular weight (30 and 120 kDa) have been reported to be more effective than chitosans with lower molecular weight (1 and 5 kDa) in extending the shelf life of bread.

The patients receiving chitosan-containing bread during 12 weeks decreased their mean levels of LDL-cholesterol and significantly increased their mean levels of HDL-cholesterol at the end of the study [101].

However, it has been also reported that chitosan increases the rate of bread staling [162]. Chitosan oligosaccharides and low molecular weight chitosan increase bread crumb staling rate to a much lesser extent than does middle molecular weight chitosan [170].

The addition of microcrystalline chitin increased specific loaf volume of white bread and protein fortified breads [171]. The properties of bread containing chitosan have been studied in a number of publications [172–177].

Chitosan has been approved as a food additive in Korea and Japan since 1995 and 1983, respectively. US FDA approved for chitosan GRAS status [154], so chitosan also can be used as a food additive.

10.2. Dairy Products Containing Chitosan and Its Derivatives

The use of chitosan in dairy products has been reported in a number of publications [164,178–190]. Microencapsulation with chitosan coating enhanced the survival of probiotic bacteria significantly in ice cream during storage compared to free cells [181]. Inhibitory effect of chitooligosaccharide on fermentation of sour cream [184] and inhibitory effect of chitosan on post-acidification of set yoghurt during cold storage [185] have been reported. Viscosity of sour cream increases with the increase of concentration of high molecular weight chitosan and anomalous viscosity decrease was observed with the increase in concentration of chitooligosaccharide [184].

11. Conclusions and Perspectives

Chitosan and COS due to their antioxidant, anti-inflammatory, antidiabetic, and anticancer properties show promising potential to be used in prevention, delay, mitigation and treatment of age-related dysfunctions and diseases. Hypocholesterolemic properties of chitosan decrease the risk of atherosclerosis and other cardiovascular dysfunctions common in elderly population. Chitosan ability to decrease serum total-cholesterol and LDL cholesterol levels, as well as to prevent their oxidation, changes water molecules distribution at biointerfaces and influences the conformation of proteins. So, chitosan has the potential to prevent protein conformational diseases that are also related with advanced aging. Mucoadhesive properties of chitosan can be applied in nanomedicine with potential to improve effectiveness of nutraceuticals and drug delivery systems. Combination of chitosan and COS with natural antioxidant polyphenols is promising. COS suppress nuclear factor NF-κB activation and translocation of NF-κB from cytoplasm to nucleus that has been linked with a number of age-related diseases.

Development of novel COS derivatives such as sulfated, carboxylated and phenolic acid conjugated COS and their application in novel nanoparticulated systems, functional foods, and nutraceuticals can essentially increase bioavailability and stability of bioactive components. Mucoadhesive films containing chitosan-coated nanoparticles can find novel applications in nanomedicine. Breakthrough results in delay and prevention of age-related dysfunctions can be expected in the future.

Acknowledgments: This work stemmed from an initiative of the author, and was not financially supported.

Conflicts of Interest: The author declares no conflict of interest.

References

1. United Nations, Department of Economic and Social Affairs, Population Division. *World Population Ageing 2013*; ST/ESA/SER.A/348; United Nations: New York, NY, USA, 2013.

2. Brownie, S. Why are elderly individuals at risk of nutritional deficiency? *Int. J. Nurs. Pract.* **2006**, *12*, 110–118. [CrossRef] [PubMed]

3. Wells, J.L.; Dumbrell, A.C. Nutrition and aging: assessment and treatment of compromised nutritional status in Frail elderly patients. *Clin. Interv. Aging* **2006**, *1*, 67–79. [CrossRef] [PubMed]

4. World Health Organization Media centre. Available online: http://www.who.int/mediacentre/factsheets/fs312/en/ (accessed on 16 November 2014).

5. Chandra, R.K. Nutrition and the immune system from birth to old age. *Eur. J. Clin. Nutr.* **2002**, *56*, 73–76. [CrossRef]

6. Chandra, R.K. Nutrition and the immune system: An introduction. *Am. J. Clin. Nutr.* **1997**, *66*, 460–463.

7. Chandra, R.K. Nutrition, immunity and infection: From basic knowledge of dietary manipulation of immune responses to practical application of ameliorating suffering and improving survival. *Proc. Natl. Acad. Sci. USA* **1996**, *93*, 14304–14307.

8. Kirilenko, Y.K.; Dushkova, Z.G.; Cherkasova, E.I.; Sigilietov, A.E. Chitosan oligomer and ascorbic acid salt in compensation of deficiency of some micronutrients. In *Advances in Chitin Science*; Senel, S., Varum, K.M., Sumnu, M.M., Hincal, A.A., Eds.; TUBITAK: Antalya, Turkey, 2007; Volume 10.

9. Shaw, A.C.; Joshi, S.; Greenwood, H.; Panda, A.; Lord, J.M. Aging of the innate immune system. *Curr. Opin. Immunol.* **2010**, *22*, 507–513. [CrossRef] [PubMed]

10. Magrone, T.; Perez de Heredia, F.; Jirillo, E.; Morabito, G.; Marcos, A.; Serafini, M. Functional foods and nutraceuticals as therapeutic tools for the treatment of diet-related diseases. *Can. J. Physiol. Pharm.* **2013**, *91*, 387–396. [CrossRef]

11. Pae, M.; Meydani, S.N.; Wu, D. The role of nutrition in enhancing immunity in aging. *Aging Dis.* **2012**, *3*, 91–129. [PubMed]

12. Maijó, M.; Clements, S.J.; Ivory, K.; Nicoletti, C.; Carding, S.R. Nutrition, diet and immunosenescence. *Mech. Ageing Dev.* **2014**, *136–137*, 116–128. [CrossRef] [PubMed]

13. Li, H.; Ma, F.; Hu, M.; Ma, C.W.; Xiao, L.; Zhang, J.; Xiang, Y.; Huang, Z. Polysaccharides from medicinal herbs as potential therapeutics for aging and age-related neurodegeneration. *Rejuvenation Res.* **2014**, *17*, 201–204. [CrossRef] [PubMed]

14. d'Ayala, G.G.; Malinconico, M.; Laurienzo, P. Marine derived polysaccharides for biomedical applications: Chemical modification approaches. *Molecules* **2008**, *13*, 2069–2106. [CrossRef] [PubMed]

15. *Chitin and Chitosan Derivatives: Advances in Drug Discovery and Developments*; Kim, S.K. (Ed.) CRC Press: Boca Raton, FL, USA, 2013; p. 527.

16. *Chitosan-Based Hydrogels: Functions and Applications*; Yao, K.; Li, J.; Yao, F.; Yin, Y. (Eds.) CRC Press: Boca Raton, FL, USA, 2011; p. 241.

17. *Chitosan for Biomaterials I*; Jayakumar, R.; Prabaharan, M.; Muzzarelli, R.A.A. (Eds.) Springer: Berlin Heidelberg, Germany, 2011; p. 243.

18. *Chitosan for Biomaterials II*; Jayakumar, R.; Prabaharan, M.; Muzzarelli, R.A.A. (Eds.) Springer: Berlin Heidelberg, Germany, 2011; p. 223.

19. *Green Biorenewable Biocomposites: From Knowledge to Industrial Applications*; Thakur, V.K.; Kessler, M.R. (Eds.) CRC Press: Boca Raton, USA, 2015; p. 568.

20. Xia, W.; Liu, P.; Zhang, J.; Chen, J. Biological activities of chitosan and chitooligosaccharides. *Food Hydrocolloids* **2011**, *25*, 170–179. [CrossRef]

21. Kumar, M.N.V.R. A review of chitin and chitosan applications. *React. Funct. Polym.* **2000**, *46*, 1–27. [CrossRef]

22. Rinaudo, M. Chitin and chitosan: Properties and applications. *Prog. Polym. Sci.* **2006**, *31*, 603–632. [CrossRef]

23. Kumar, M.N.V.R.; Muzzarelli, R.A.A.; Muzzarelli, C.; Sashiwa, H.; Domb, A.J. Chitosan chemistry and pharmaceutical perspectives. *Chem. Rev.* **2004**, *104*, 6017–6084. [CrossRef] [PubMed]

24. Dash, M.; Chiellini, F.; Ottenbrite, R.M.; Chiellini, E. Chitosan—A versatile semi-synthetic polymer in biomedical applications. *Prog. Polym. Sci.* **2011**, *36*, 981–1014. [CrossRef]

25. Anitha, A.; Sowmya, S.; Sudheesh Kumar, P.T.; Deepthi, S.; Chennazhi, K.P.; Ehrlich, H.; Tsurkan, M.; Jayakumar, R. Chitin and chitosan in selected biomedical applications. *Prog. Polym. Sci.* **2014**, *39*, 1644–1667. [CrossRef]

26. Zhang, J.; Xia, W.; Liu, P.; Cheng, Q.; Tahi, T.; Gu, W.; Li, B. Chitosan modification and pharmaceutical/biomedical applications. *Mar. Drugs* **2010**, *8*, 1962–1987. [CrossRef] [PubMed]

27. Jung, W.J.; Park, R.D. Bioproduction of chitooligosaccharides: Present and perspectives. *Mar. Drugs* **2014**, *12*, 5328–5356. [CrossRef] [PubMed]

28. Muzzarelli, R.A.A.; El Mehtedi, M.; Mattioli-Belmonte, M. Emerging biomedical applications of nano-chitins and nano-chitosans obtained via advanced eco-friendly technologies from marine resources. *Mar. Drugs* **2014**, *12*, 5468–5502. [CrossRef] [PubMed]

29. Laurienzo, P. Marine polysaccharides in pharmaceutical applications: An overview. *Mar. Drugs* **2010**, *8*, 2435–2465. [CrossRef] [PubMed]

30. Thakur, V.K.; Thakur, M.K. Recent advances in graft copolymerization and applications of chitosan: A review. *ACS Sustain. Chem. Eng.* **2014**, *2*, 2637–2652. [CrossRef]

31. Ngo, D.H.; Kim, S.K. Antioxidant effects of chitin, chitosan and their derivatives. In *Marine Carbohydrates: Fundamentals and Applications, Part B*; Kim, S.-K., Ed.; Elsevier Inc.: Oxford, UK, 2014; pp. 15–31.

32. Andriollo-Sanchez, M.; Hininger-Favier, I.; Meunier, N.; Venneria, E.; O'Connor, J.M.; Maiani, G.; Coudray, C.; Roussel, A.M. Age-related oxidative stress and antioxidant parameters in middle-aged and older European subjects: The ZENITH study. *Eur. J. Clin. Nutr.* **2005**, *59*, 58–62. [CrossRef]

33. Abdollahi, M.; Moridani, M.Y.; Aruoma, O.I.; Mostafalou, S. Oxidative stress in aging. *Oxidative Med. Cell. Longev.* **2014**, *2014*, 876834:1–876834:2. [CrossRef]

34. Aruoma, O.I. Free radicals, oxidative stress, and antioxidants in human health and disease. *J. Am. Oil Chem. Soc.* **1998**, *75*, 199–212. [CrossRef]

35. Saeidnia, S.; Abdollahi, M. Toxicological and pharmacological concerns on oxidative stress and related diseases. *Toxicol. Appl. Pharm.* **2013**, *273*, 442–455. [CrossRef]

36. Xie, W.; Xu, P.; Liu, Q. Antioxidant activity of water-soluble chitosan derivatives. *Bioorg. Med. Chem. Lett.* **2001**, *11*, 1699–1701. [CrossRef] [PubMed]

37. Jeon, T.I.; Hwang, S.G.; Park, N.G.; Jung, Y.R.; Shin, S.I.; Choi, S.D.; Park, D.K. Antioxidative effect of chitosan on chronic carbon tetrachloride induced hepatic injury in rats. *Toxicology* **2003**, *187*, 67–73. [CrossRef] [PubMed]

38. Chen, A.S.; Taguchi, T.; Sakai, K.; Kikuchi, K.; Wang, M.W.; Miwa, I. Antioxidant activities of chitobiose and chitotriose. *Biol. Pharm. Bull.* **2003**, *26*, 1326–1330. [CrossRef] [PubMed]

39. Sun, T.; Xie, W.; Xu, P. Superoxide anion scavenging activity of graft chitosan derivatives. *Carbohydr. Polym.* **2004**, *58*, 379–382. [CrossRef]

40. Huang, R.; Mendis, E.; Kim, S.K. Factors affecting the free radical scavenging behavior of chitosan sulfate. *Int. J. Biol. Macromol.* **2005**, *36*, 120–127. [CrossRef] [PubMed]

41. Feng, T.; Du, Y.; Li, J.; Wei, Y.; Yao, P. Antioxidant activity of half N-acetylated water-soluble chitosan *in vitro*. *Eur. Food Res. Technol.* **2007**, *225*, 133–138. [CrossRef]

42. Yen, M.T.; Tseng, Y.H.; Li, R.C.; Mau, J.L. Antioxidant properties of fungal chitosan from shiitake stipes. *LWT-Food Sci. Technol.* **2007**, *40*, 255–261. [CrossRef]

43. Anraku, M.; Fujii, T.; Furutani, N.; Kadowaki, D.; Maruyama, T.; Otagiri, M.; Gebicki, J.M.; Tomida, H. Antioxidant effects of a dietary supplement: Reduction of indices of oxidative stress in normal subjects by water-soluble chitosan. *Food Chem. Toxicol.* **2009**, *47*, 104–109. [CrossRef]

44. Anraku, M.; Michihara, A.; Yasufuku, T.; Akasaki, K.; Tsuchiya, D.; Nishio, H.; Maruyama, T.; Otagiri, M.; Maezaki, Y.; Kondo, Y.; *et al.* The antioxidative and antilipidemic effects of different molecular weight chitosans in metabolic syndrome model rats. *Biol. Pharm. Bull.* **2010**, *33*, 1994–1998. [CrossRef] [PubMed]

45. Friedman, M.; Juneja, V.K. Review of antimicrobial and antioxidative activities of chitosans in food. *J. Food Prot.* **2010**, *73*, 1737–1761. [PubMed]

46. Ngo, D.N. Chitin, Chitosan, and Their Derivatives against Oxidative Stress and Inflammation, and Some Applications. In *Seafood Processing By-Products*; Kim, S., Ed.; Springer: New York, NY, USA, 2014; pp. 389–405.

47. Luo, Z.; Dong, X.; Ke, Q.; Duan, Q.; Shen, L. Chitooligosaccharides inhibit ethanol-induced oxidative stress via activation of Nrf2 and reduction of MAPK phosphorylation. *Oncol. Rep.* **2014**, *32*, 2215–2222. [PubMed]

48. Anandan, R.; Ganesan, B.; Obulesu, T.; Mathew, S.; Kumar, R.S.; Lakshmanan, P.T.; Zynudheen, A.A. Dietary chitosan supplementation attenuates isoprenaline-induced oxidative stress in rat myocardium. *Int. J. Biol. Macromol.* **2012**, *51*, 783–787. [CrossRef] [PubMed]

49. Anandan, R.; Ganesan, B.; Obulesu, T.; Mathew, S.; Asha, K.K.; Lakshmanan, P.T.; Zynudheen, A.A. Antiaging effect of dietary chitosan supplementation on glutathione-dependent antioxidant system in young and aged rats. *Cell Stress Chaperon* **2013**, *18*, 121–125. [CrossRef]

50. Qiao, Y.; Bai, X.F.; Du, Y.G. Chitosan oligosaccharides protect mice from LPS challenge by attenuation of inflammation and oxidative stress. *Int. Immunopharmacol.* **2011**, *11*, 121–127. [CrossRef] [PubMed]

51. Lu, X.; Guo, H.; Sun, L.; Zhang, L.; Zhang, Y. Protective effects of sulfated chitooligosaccharides with different degrees of substitution in MIN6 cells. *Int. J. Biol. Macromol.* **2013**, *52*, 92–98. [CrossRef] [PubMed]

52. Kim, J.H.; Kim, Y.S.; Hwang, J.W.; Han, Y.K.; Lee, J.S.; Kim, S.K.; Jeon, Y.J.; Moon, S.H.; Jeon, B.T.; Bahk, Y.Y.; *et al.* Sulfated chitosan oligosaccharides suppress LPS-induced NO production via JNK and NF-κB inactivation. *Molecules* **2014**, *19*, 18232–18247. [CrossRef] [PubMed]

53. Tomida, H.; Fujii, T.; Furutani, N.; Michihara, A.; Yasufuku, T.; Akasaki, K.; Maruyama, T.; Otagiri, M.; Gebicki, J.M.; Anraku, M. Antioxidant properties of some different molecular weight chitosans. *Carbohydr. Res.* **2009**, *344*, 1690–1696. [CrossRef] [PubMed]

54. Zhang, W.; Xia, W. Effect of media milling on lipid-lowering and antioxidant activities of chitosan. *Int. J. Biol. Macromol.* **2015**, *72*, 1402–1405. [CrossRef]

55. Lee, D.S.; Woo, J.Y.; Ahn, C.B.; Je, J.Y. Chitosan–hydroxycinnamic acid conjugates: Preparation, antioxidant and antimicrobial activity. *Food Chem.* **2014**, *148*, 97–104. [CrossRef] [PubMed]

56. Qin, Y.; Guo, X.W.; Li, L.; Wang, H.W.; Kim, W. The antioxidant property of chitosan green tea polyphenols complex induces transglutaminase activation in wound healing. *J. Med. Food.* **2013**, *16*, 487–498. [CrossRef] [PubMed]

57. Liu, J.; Wen, X.; Lu, J.; Kan, J.; Jin, C. Free radical mediated grafting of chitosan with caffeic and ferulic acids: Structures and antioxidant activity. *Int. J. Biol. Macromol.* **2014**, *65*, 97–106. [CrossRef] [PubMed]

58. Liu, J.; Lu, J.; Kan, J.; Tang, Y.; Jin, C. Preparation, characterization and antioxidant activity of phenolic acids grafted carboxymethyl chitosan. *Int. J. Biol. Macromol.* **2013**, *62*, 85–93. [CrossRef] [PubMed]

59. Halder, S.K.; Jana, A.; Das, A.; Paul, T.; Mohapatra, P.K.D. Appraisal of antioxidant, anti-hemolytic and DNA shielding potentialities of chitosaccharides produced innovatively from shrimp shell by sequential treatment with immobilized enzymes. *Food Chem.* **2014**, *158*, 325–334. [CrossRef] [PubMed]

60. Fernandes, J.C.; Eaton, P.; Nascimento, H.; Gião, M.S.; Ramos, Ó.S.; Belo, L.; Santos-Silva, A.; Pintado, M.E.; Malcata, F.X. Antioxidant activity of chitooligosaccharides upon two biological systems: Erythrocytes and bacteriophages. *Carbohydr. Polym.* **2010**, *79*, 1101–1106. [CrossRef]

61. Ngo, D.N.; Kim, M.M.; Kim, S.K. Protective effects of aminoethyl-chitooligosaccharides against oxidative stress in mouse macrophage RAW 264.7 cells. *Int. J. Biol. Macromol.* **2012**, *50*, 624–631. [CrossRef] [PubMed]

62. Prashanth, K.V.H.; Dharmesh, S.; Rao, K.S.J.; Tharanathan, R.N. Free radical-induced chitosan depolymerized products protect calf thymus DNA from oxidative damage. *Carbohydr. Res.* **2007**, *342*, 190–195. [CrossRef] [PubMed]

63. Trinh, M.D.L.; Ngo, D.H.; Tran, D.K.; Tran, Q.T.; Vo, T.S.; Dinh, M.H.; Ngo, D.N. Prevention of H_2O_2-induced oxidative stress in Chang liver cells by 4-hydroxybenzyl-chitooligomers. *Carbohydr. Polym.* **2014**, *103*, 502–509. [CrossRef] [PubMed]

64. Ahn, K.S.; Aggarwal, B.B. Transcription factor NF-κB: A sensor for smoke and stress signals. *Ann. N. Y. Acad. Sci.* **2005**, *1056*, 218–233. [CrossRef] [PubMed]

65. Chung, H.Y.; Cesari, M.; Anton, S.; Marzetti, E.; Giovannini, S.; Seo, A.Y.; Carter, C.; Yu, B.P.; Leeuwenburgh, C. Molecular inflammation: Underpinnings of aging and age-related diseases. *Ageing Res. Rev.* **2009**, *8*, 18–30. [CrossRef] [PubMed]

66. Paolisso, G.; Rizzo, M.R.; Mazziotti, G.; Tagliamonte, M.R.; Gambardella, A.; Rotondi, M.; Carella, C.; Giugliano, D.; Varricchio, M.; D'Onofrio, F. Advancing age and insulin resistance: Role of plasma tumor necrosis factor-alpha. *Am. J. Physiol.* **1998**, *275*, E294–E299. [PubMed]

67. Liu, H.T.; Li, W.M.; Li, X.Y.; Xu, Q.S.; Liu, Q.S.; Bai, X.F.; Yu, C.; Du, Y.G. Chitosan oligosaccharides inhibit the expression of interleukin-6 in lipopolysaccharide-induced human umbilical vein endothelial cells through p38 and ERK1/2 protein kinases. *Basic Clin. Pharmacol. Toxicol.* **2010**, *106*, 362–371. [CrossRef] [PubMed]

68. Ma, P.; Liu, H.T.; Wei, P.; Xu, Q.S.; Bai, X.F.; Du, Y.G.; Yu, C. Chitosan oligosaccharides inhibit LPS-induced over-expression of IL-6 and TNF-α in RAW264.7 macrophage cells through blockade of mitogen-activated protein kinase (MAPK) and PI3K/Akt signaling pathways. *Carbohydr. Polym.* **2011**, *84*, 1391–1398. [CrossRef]

69. Li, Y.; Liu, H.; Xu, Q.S.; Du, Y.G.; Xu, J. Chitosan oligosaccharides block LPS-induced O-GlcNAcylation of NF-κB and endothelial inflammatory response. *Carbohydr. Polym.* **2014**, *99*, 568–578. [CrossRef] [PubMed]

70. Li, Y.; Xu, Q.; Wei, P.; Cheng, L.; Peng, Q.; Li, S.; Yin, H.; Du, Y. Chitosan oligosaccharides downregulate the expression of E-selectin and ICAM-1 induced by LPS in endothelial cells by inhibiting MAP kinase signaling. *Int. J. Mol. Med.* **2014**, *33*, 392–400. [PubMed]

71. Huang, J.; Wang, R.; Liu, X.; Zeng, X.; Wei, M. Sulfochitosan inhibits P-selectin-mediated HL-60 leukocyte adhesion under flow conditions. *Cell. Mol. Biol. Lett.* **2013**, *18*, 200–208. [CrossRef] [PubMed]

72. Ji, Q.; Deng, J.; Yu, X.; Xu, Q.; Wu, H.; Pan, J. Modulation of pro-inflammatory mediators in LPS-stimulated human periodontal ligament cells by chitosan and quaternized chitosan. *Carbohydr. Polym.* **2013**, *92*, 824–829. [CrossRef] [PubMed]

73. Fang, I.M.; Yang, C.H.; Yang, C.M. Chitosan oligosaccharides attenuate ocular inflammation in rats with experimental autoimmune anterior uveitis. *Mediat. Inflamm.* **2014**, *2014*, 827847.

74. Fang, I.M.; Yang, C.M.; Yang, C.H. Chitosan oligosaccharides prevented retinal ischemia and reperfusion injury via reduced oxidative stress and inflammation in rats. *Exp. Eye Res.* **2015**, *130*, 38–50. [CrossRef] [PubMed]

75. Hsieh, Y.L.; Yao, H.T.; Cheng, R.S.; Chiang, M.T. Chitosan reduces plasma adipocytokines and lipid accumulation in liver and adipose tissues and ameliorates insulin resistance in diabetic rats. *J. Med. Food* **2012**, *15*, 453–460. [CrossRef] [PubMed]

76. Pangestuti, R.; Bak, S.S.; Kim, S.K. Attenuation of pro-inflammatory mediators in LPS-stimulated BV2 microglia by chitooligosaccharides via the MAPK signaling pathway. *Int. J. Biol. Macromol.* **2011**, *49*, 599–606. [CrossRef] [PubMed]

77. Zhu, J.; Zhang, Y.; Wu, G.; Xiao, Z.; Zhou, H.; Yu, X. Inhibitory effects of oligochitosan on TNF-α, IL-1β and nitric oxide production in lipopolysaccharide-induced RAW264.7 cells. *Mol. Med. Rep.* **2015**, *11*, 729–733. [PubMed]

78. Mohamed, M.M. Effects of chitosan and wheat bran on serum leptin, TNF-α, lipid profile and oxidative status in animal model of non-alcoholic fatty liver. *Aust. J. Basic Appl. Sci.* **2011**, *5*, 1478–1488.

79. Yousef, M.; Pichyangkura, R.; Soodvilai, S.; Chatsudthipong, V.; Muanprasat, C. Chitosan oligosaccharide as potential therapy of inflammatory bowel disease: Therapeutic efficacy and possible mechanisms of action. *Pharmacol. Res.* **2012**, *66*, 66–79. [CrossRef] [PubMed]

80. Kim, H.M.; Hong, S.H.; Yoo, S.J.; Baek, K.S.; Jeon, Y.J.; Choung, S.Y. Differential effects of chitooligosaccharides on serum cytokine levels in aged subjects. *J. Med. Food* **2006**, *9*, 427–430. [CrossRef] [PubMed]

81. He, B.; Wang, J. Chitooligosaccharides prevent osteopenia by promoting bone formation and suppressing bone resorption in ovariectomised rats: Possible involvement of COX-2. *Nat. Prod. Res.* **2015**, *29*, 359–362. [CrossRef] [PubMed]

82. Fernandes, J.; Spindola, H.; de Sousa, V.; Alice Santos-Silva, A.; Pintado, M.E.; Malcata, F.X.; Carvalho, J.E. Anti-inflammatory activity of chitooligosaccharides *in Vivo*. *Mar. Drugs* **2010**, *8*, 1763–1768. [CrossRef] [PubMed]

83. Azuma, K.; Osaki, T.; Minami, S.; Okamoto, Y. Anticancer and anti-inflammatory properties of chitin and chitosan oligosaccharides. *J. Funct. Biomater.* **2015**, *6*, 33–49. [CrossRef] [PubMed]

84. Karadeniz, F.; Kim, S.K. Antidiabetic activities of chitosan and its derivatives: A mini review. In *Marine Carbohydrates: Fundamentals and Applications, Part B*; Kim, S., Ed.; Elsevier Inc.: Oxford, UK, 2014; pp. 15–31.

85. Ericson, U.; Sonestedt, E.; Gullberga, B.; Hellstrand, S.; Hindy, G.; Wirfält, E.; Orho-Melander, M. High intakes of protein and processed meat associate with increased incidence of type 2 diabetes. *Br. J. Nutr.* **2013**, *109*, 1143–1153. [CrossRef] [PubMed]

86. Levine, M.E.; Suarez, J.A.; Brandhorst, S.; Balasubramanian, P.; Cheng, C.W.; Madia, F.; Fontana, L.; Mirisola, M.G.; Guevara-Aguirre, J.; Wan, J.; *et al.* Low protein intake is associated with a major reduction in

IGF-1, cancer, and overall mortality in the 65 and younger but not older population. *Cell Metab.* **2014**, *19*, 407–417. [CrossRef] [PubMed]

87. Rahimi, R.; Nikfar, S.; Larijani, B.; Abdollahi, M. A review on the role of antioxidants in the management of diabetes and its complications. *Biomed. Pharmacother.* **2005**, *59*, 365–373. [CrossRef] [PubMed]

88. Maritim, A.C.; Sanders, R.A.; Watkins, J.B., III. Diabetes, oxidative stress, and antioxidants: A review. *J. Biochem. Mol. Toxicol.* **2003**, *17*, 24–38. [CrossRef] [PubMed]

89. Giacco, F.; Brownlee, M. Oxidative stress and diabetic complications. *Circ. Res.* **2010**, *107*, 1058–1070. [CrossRef] [PubMed]

90. Saghizadeh, M.; Ong, J.M.; Garvey, W.T.; Henry, R.R.; Kern, P.A. The expression of TNF alpha by human muscle. Relationship to insulin resistance. *J. Clin. Investig.* **1996**, *97*, 1111–1116. [CrossRef] [PubMed]

91. Miura, T.; Usami, M.; Tsuura, Y.; Ishida, H.; Seino, Y. Hypoglycemic and hypolipidemic effect of chitosan in normal and neonatal streptozotocin-induced diabetic mice. *Biol. Pharm. Bull.* **1995**, *18*, 1623–1625. [CrossRef] [PubMed]

92. Hayashi, K.; Ito, M. Antidiabetic action of low molecular weight chitosan in genetically obese diabetic KK-Ay mice. *Biol. Pharm. Bull.* **2002**, *25*, 188–192. [CrossRef] [PubMed]

93. Liu, S.H.; Chang, Y.H.; Chiang, M.T. Chitosan reduces gluconeogenesis and increases glucose uptake in skeletal muscle in streptozotocin-induced diabetic rats. *J. Agric. Food Chem.* **2010**, *58*, 5795–5800. [CrossRef] [PubMed]

94. Kim, H.J.; Ahn, H.Y.; Kwak, J.H.; Shin, D.Y.; Kwon, Y.I.; Oh, C.G.; Lee, J.H. The effects of chitosan oligosaccharide (GO2KA1) supplementation on glucose control in subjects with prediabetes. *Food Funct.* **2014**, *5*, 2662–2669. [CrossRef] [PubMed]

95. Jo, S.H.; Ha, K.S.; Lee, J.W.; Kim, Y.C.; Apostolidis, E.; Kwon, Y.I. The reduction effect of low molecular weight chitosan oligosaccharide (GO2KA1) on postprandial blood glucose levels in healthy individuals. *Food Sci. Biotechnol.* **2014**, *23*, 971–973. [CrossRef]

96. Kim, J.G.; Jo, S.H.; Ha, K.S.; Kim, S.C.; Kim, Y.C.; Apostolidis, E.; Kwon, Y.I. Effect of long-term supplementation of low molecular weight chitosan oligosaccharide (GO2KA1) on fasting blood glucose and HbA1c in db/db mice model and elucidation of mechanism of action. *BMC Complement. Altern. Med.* **2014**, *14*, 272. [CrossRef] [PubMed]

97. Rong, J.X.; Rangaswamy, S.; Shen, S.; Dave, R.; Chang, Y.H.; Peterson, H.; Hodis, H.N.; Chisolm, G.M.; Sevanian, A. Arterial injury by cholesterol oxidation products causes endothelial dysfunction and arterial wall cholesterol accumulation. *Arterioscl. Throm. Vas.* **1998**, *18*, 1885–1894. [CrossRef]

98. Sevanian, A.; Hodis, H.N.; Hwang, J.; McLeod, L.L.; Peterson, H. Characterization of endothelial cell injury by cholesterol oxidation products found in oxidized LDL. *J. Lipid Res.* **1995**, *36*, 1971–1986. [PubMed]

99. Ross, R. Atherosclerosis—An inflammatory disease. *N. Engl. J. Med.* **1999**, *340*, 115–149. [CrossRef] [PubMed]

100. Cockerill, G.W.; Rye, K.A.; Gamble, J.R.; Vadas, M.A.; Barter, P.J. High-density lipoproteins inhibit cytokine-induced expression of endothelial cell adhesion molecules. *Arterioscler. Thromb. Vasc. Biol.* **1995**, *15*, 1987–1994. [CrossRef] [PubMed]

101. Ausar, S.F.; Morcillo, M.; León, A.E.; Ribotta, P.D.; Masih, R.; Vilaro Mainero, M.; Amigone, J.L.; Rubin, G.; Lescano, C.; Castagna, L.F.; *et al.* Improvement of HDL- and LDL-cholesterol levels in diabetic subjects by feeding bread containing chitosan. *J. Med. Food* **2003**, *6*, 397–399. [CrossRef] [PubMed]

102. Wuolijoki, E.; Hirvela, T.; Ylitalo, P. Decrease in serum LDL cholesterol with microcrystalline chitosan. *Methods Find. Exp. Clin. Pharmacol.* **1999**, *21*, 357–361. [CrossRef] [PubMed]

103. Tai, T.S.; Sheu, W.H.H.; Lee, W.J.; Yao, H.T.; Chiang, M.T. Effect of chitosan on plasma lipoprotein concentrations in type 2 diabetic subjects with hypercholesterolemia. *Diabetes Care* **2000**, *23*, 1703–1704. [CrossRef] [PubMed]

104. Kanauchi, O.; Deuchi, K.; Imasato, Y.; Shizukuishi, M.; Kobayashi, E. Mechanism for the inhibition of fat digestion by chitosan and for the synergistic effect of ascorbate. *Biosci. Biotechnol. Biochem.* **1995**, *59*, 786–790. [CrossRef] [PubMed]

105. Rizzo, M.; Giglio, R.V.; Nikolic, D.; Patti, A.M.; Campanella, C.; Cocchi, M.; Katsiki, N.; Montalto, G. Effects of chitosan on plasma lipids and lipoproteins: A 4-month prospective pilot study. *Angiology* **2013**, *65*, 538–542. [CrossRef] [PubMed]

106. Liu, J.; Zhang, J.; Xia, W. Hypocholesterolaemic effects of different chitosan samples *in vitro* and *in vivo*. *Food Chem.* **2008**, *107*, 419–425. [CrossRef]

107. Choi, C.R.; Kim, E.K.; Kim, Y.S.; Je, J.Y.; An, S.H.; Lee, J.D.; Wang, J.H.; Ki, S.S.; Jeon, B.T.; Moon, S.H.; *et al.* Chitooligosaccharides decreases plasma lipid levels in healthy men. *Int. J. Food Sci. Nutr.* **2012**, *63*, 103–106. [CrossRef] [PubMed]

108. Park, J.H.; Hong, E.K.; Ahn, J.; Kwak, H.S. Properties of nanopowdered chitosan and its cholesterol lowering effect in rats. *Food Sci. Biotechnol.* **2010**, *19*, 1457–1462. [CrossRef]

109. Chiang, M.T.; Yao, H.T.; Chen, H.C. Effect of dietary chitosans with different viscosity on plasma lipids and lipid peroxidation in rats fed on a diet enriched with cholesterol. *Biosci. Biotechnol. Biochem.* **2000**, *64*, 965–971. [CrossRef] [PubMed]

110. Bokura, H.; Kobayashi, S. Chitosan decreases total cholesterol in women: A randomized, double-blind, placebo-controlled trial. *Eur. J. Clin. Nutr.* **2003**, *57*, 721–725. [CrossRef] [PubMed]

111. Zhang, J.; Zhang, W.; Mamadouba, B.; Xia, W. A comparative study on hypolipidemic activities of high and low molecular weight chitosan in rats. *Int. J. Biol. Macromol.* **2012**, *51*, 504–508. [CrossRef] [PubMed]

112. Rashid, T.U.; Shamsuddin, S.M.; Khan, M.A.; Rahman, M.M. Evaluation of Fat Binding Capacity of Gamma Irradiated Chitosan Extracted from Prawn Shell. *Soft Mater.* **2014**, *12*, 262–267. [CrossRef]

113. Patti, A.M.; Katsiki, N.; Nikolic, D.; Al-Rasadi, K.; Rizzo, M. Nutraceuticals in lipid-lowering treatment a narrative review on the role of chitosan. *Angiology* **2014**. [CrossRef]

114. Das, R.K.; Kasoju, N.; Bora, U. Encapsulation of curcumin in alginate-chitosan-pluronic composite nanoparticles for delivery to cancer cells. *Nanomedicine* **2010**, *6*, 153–160. [CrossRef] [PubMed]

115. Duan, J.; Zhang, Y.; Han, S.; Chen, Y.; Li, B.; Liao, M.; Chen, W.; Deng, X.; Zhao, J.; Huang, B. Synthesis and *in vitro/in vivo* anti-cancer evaluation of curcumin-loaded chitosan/poly(butyl cyanoacrylate) nanoparticles. *Int. J. Pharm.* **2010**, *400*, 211–220. [CrossRef] [PubMed]

116. Rejinold, N.S.; Muthunarayanan, M.; Divyarani, V.V.; Sreerekha, P.R.; Chennazhi, K.P.; Nair, S.V.; Tamura, H.; Jayakumar, R. Curcumin-loaded biocompatible thermoresponsive polymeric nanoparticles for cancer drug delivery. *J. Colloid Interface Sci.* **2011**, *360*, 39–51. [CrossRef] [PubMed]

117. Zaki, N. Progress and problems in nutraceuticals delivery. *J. Bioequivalence Bioavailab.* **2014**, *6*, 75–77. [CrossRef]

118. Tang, H.; Murphy, C.J.; Zhang, B.; Shen, Y.; van Kirk, E.A.; Murdoch, W.J.; Radosz, M. Curcumin polymers as anticancer conjugates. *Biomaterials* **2010**, *31*, 7139–7149. [CrossRef] [PubMed]

119. Shaikh, J.; Ankola, D.D.; Beniwal, V.; Singh, D.; Kumar, M.N. Nanoparticle encapsulation improves oral bioavailability of curcumin by at least 9-fold when compared to curcumin administered with piperine as absorption enhancer. *Eur. J. Pharm. Sci.* **2009**, *37*, 223–230. [CrossRef] [PubMed]

120. Prajakta, D.; Ratnesh, J.; Chandan, K.; Suresh, S.; Grace, S.; Meera, V.; Vandana, P. Curcumin loaded pH-sensitive nanoparticles for the treatment of colon cancer. *J. Biomed. Nanotechnol.* **2009**, *5*, 445–455. [CrossRef] [PubMed]

121. Narayanan, N.K.; Nargi, D.; Randolph, C.; Narayanan, B.A. Liposome encapsulation of curcumin and resveratrol in combination reduces prostate cancer incidence in PTEN knockout mice. *Int. J. Cancer* **2009**, *125*, 1–8. [CrossRef] [PubMed]

122. Mazzarino, L.; Loch-Neckel, G.; Bubniak, L.D.S.; Mazzucco, S.; Santos-Silva, M.C.; Borsali, R.; Lemos-Senna, E. Curcumin-loaded chitosan-coated nanoparticles as a new approach for the local treatment of oral cavity cancer. *J. Nanosci. Nanotechnol.* **2015**, *15*, 781–791. [CrossRef]

123. Mazzarino, L.; Borsali, R.; Lemos-Senna, E. Mucoadhesive films containing chitosan-coated nanoparticles: A new strategy for buccal curcumin release. *J. Pharm. Sci.* **2014**, *103*, 3764–3771. [CrossRef] [PubMed]

124. Mazzarino, L.; Otsuka, I.; Halila, S.; Bubniak Ldos, S.; Mazzucco, S.; Santos-Silva, M.C.; Lemos-Senna, E.; Borsali, R. Xyloglucan-block-Poly(ε-Caprolactone) Copolymer Nanoparticles Coated with Chitosan as Biocompatible Mucoadhesive Drug Delivery System. *Macromol. Biosci.* **2014**, *14*, 709–719. [CrossRef] [PubMed]

125. Mazzarino, L.; Coche-Guérente, L.; Lemos-Senna, E.; Borsali, R. On the mucoadhesive properties of chitosan-coated polycaprolactone nanoparticles loaded with curcumin using quartz crystal microbalance with dissipation monitoring. *J. Biomed. Nanotechnol.* **2014**, *10*, 787–794. [CrossRef] [PubMed]

126. Khan, N.; Adhami, V.M.; Siddiqui, I.A.; Bharali, D.J.; Mousa, S.A.; Mukhtar, H. Abstract 5438: Oral administration of naturally occurring chitosan based nanoformulated green tea polyphenol EGCG effectively inhibits prostate cancer cell growth in a xenograft model. In Proceedings of the 103rd Annual Meeting of the American Association for Cancer Research, Chicago, IL, USA, 31 March–4 April 2012; AACR: Philadelphia, PA, USA, 2012.

127. De Pace, R.C.; Liu, X.; Sun, M.; Nie, S.; Zhang, J.; Cai, Q.; Gao, W.; Pan, X.; Fan, Z.; Wang, S.; *et al.* Anticancer activities of (−)-epigallocatechin-3-gallate encapsulated nanoliposomes in MCF7 breast cancer cells. *J. Liposome Res.* **2013**, *23*, 187–196. [CrossRef] [PubMed]

128. Anitha, A.; Deepa, N.; Chennazhi, K.P.; Lakshmanan, V.K.; Jayakumar, R. Combinatorial anticancer effects of curcumin and 5-fluorouracil loaded thiolated chitosan nanoparticles towards colon cancer treatment. *Biochim. Biophys. Acta (BBA)—Gen. Subj.* **2014**, *1840*, 2730–2743. [CrossRef]

129. Anitha, A.; Sreeranganathan, M.; Chennazhi, K.P.; Lakshmanan, V.K.; Jayakumar, R. *In vitro* combinatorial anticancer effects of 5-fluorouracil and curcumin loaded N,O-carboxymethyl chitosan nanoparticles toward colon cancer and *in vivo* pharmacokinetic studies. *Eur. J. Pharm. Biopharm.* **2014**, *88*, 238–251. [CrossRef] [PubMed]

130. Prabaharan, M. Chitosan-based nanoparticles for tumor-targeted drug delivery. *Int. J. Biol. Macromol.* **2015**, *72*, 1313–1322. [CrossRef] [PubMed]

131. Wang, J.J.; Zeng, Z.W.; Xiao, R.Z.; T Xie, T.; Zhou, G.L.; Zhan, X.R.; Wang, S.L. Recent advances of chitosan nanoparticles as drug carriers. *Int. J. Nanomed.* **2011**, *6*, 765–774.

132. Dube, A.; Nicolazzo, J.A.; Larson, I. Chitosan nanoparticles enhance the intestinal absorption of the green tea catechins (+)-catechin and (−)-epigallocatechin gallate. *Eur. J. Pharm. Sci.* **2010**, *41*, 219–225. [CrossRef] [PubMed]

133. Dube, A.; Nicolazzo, J.A.; Larson, I. Chitosan nanoparticles enhance the plasma exposure of (−)-epigallocatechin gallate in mice through an enhancement in intestinal stability. *Eur. J. Pharm. Sci.* **2011**, *44*, 422–426. [CrossRef] [PubMed]

134. Hu, B.; Ting, Y.; Yang, X.; Tang, W.; Zeng, X.; Huang, Q. Nanochemoprevention by encapsulation of (−)-epigallocatechin-3-gallate with bioactive peptides/chitosan nanoparticles for enhancement of its bioavailability. *Chem. Commun.* **2012**, *48*, 2421–2423. [CrossRef]

135. Tang, D.W.; Yu, S.H.; Ho, Y.C.; Huang, B.Q.; Tsai, G.J.; Hsieh, H.Y.; Sung, H.W.; Mi, F.L. Characterization of tea catechins-loaded nanoparticles prepared from chitosan and an edible polypeptide. *Food Hydrocolloids* **2013**, *30*, 33–41. [CrossRef]

136. Oehlke, K.; Adamiuk, M.; Behsnilian, B.; Gräf, V.; Mayer-Miebach, E.; Walz, E.; Greine, R. Potential bioavailability enhancement of bioactive compounds using food-grade engineered nanomaterials: A review of the existing evidence. *Food Funct.* **2014**, *5*, 1341–1359. [CrossRef] [PubMed]

137. Sadeghi, A.M.; Dorkoosh, F.A.; Avadi, M.R.; Weinhold, M.; Bayat, A.; Delie, F.; Gurny, R.; Larijani, B.; Rafiee-Tehrani, M.; Junginger, H.E. Permeation enhancer effect of chitosan and chitosan derivatives: Comparison of formulations as soluble polymers and nanoparticulate systems on insulin absorption in Caco-2 cells. *Eur. J. Pharm. Biopharm.* **2008**, *70*, 270–278. [CrossRef] [PubMed]

138. Vllasaliu, D.; Exposito-Harris, R.; Heras, A.; Casettari, L.; Garnett, M.; Illum, L.; Stolnik, S. Tight junction modulation by chitosan nanoparticles: Comparison with chitosan solution. *Int. J. Pharm.* **2010**, *400*, 183–193. [CrossRef] [PubMed]

139. Li, Z.; Ha, J.; Zou, T.; Gu, L. Fabrication of coated bovine serum albumin (BSA)–epigallocatechin gallate (EGCG) nanoparticles and their transport across monolayers of human intestinal epithelial Caco-2 cells. *Food Funct.* **2014**, *5*, 1278–1285. [CrossRef] [PubMed]

140. Zhang, J.; Nie, S.; Wang, S. Nanoencapsulation Enhances Epigallocatechin-3-gallate Stability and Its Antiatherogenic Bioactivities in Macrophages. *J. Agric. Food Chem.* **2013**, *61*, 9200–9209. [CrossRef] [PubMed]

141. Hong, Z.; Xu, Y.Q.; Yin, J.F.; Jin, J.; Du, Q. Improving the Effectiveness of (−)-Epigallocatechin Gallate (EGCG) against Rabbit Atherosclerosis by EGCG-Loaded Nanoparticles Prepared from Chitosan and Polyaspartic Acid. *J. Agric. Food Chem.* **2014**, *62*, 12603–12609. [CrossRef] [PubMed]

142. Liang, J.; Cao, L.; Zhang, L.; Wan, X.C. Preparation, characterization, and *in vitro* antitumor activity of folate conjugated chitosan coated EGCG nanoparticles. *Food Sci. Biotechnol.* **2014**, *23*, 569–575. [CrossRef]

143. Singh, B.N.; Shankar, S.; Srivastava, R.K. Green tea catechin, epigallocatechin-3-gallate (EGCG): Mechanisms, perspectives and clinical applications. *Biochem. Pharmacol.* **2011**, *82*, 1807–1821. [CrossRef] [PubMed]

144. Sanna, V.; Roggio, A.M.; Pala, N.; Marceddu, S.; Lubinu, G.; Mariani, A.; Sechi, M. Effect of chitosan concentration on PLGA microcapsules for controlled release and stability of resveratrol. *Int. J. Biol. Macromol.* **2015**, *72*, 531–536. [CrossRef] [PubMed]

145. Alzheimer's Association. Alzheimer's disease facts and figures. *Alzheimers Dement.* **2012**, *8*, 131–168.

146. Bieschke, J. Natural compounds may open new routes to treatment of amyloid diseases. *Neurotherapeutics* **2013**, *10*, 429–439. [CrossRef] [PubMed]

147. Kim, M.S.; Sung, M.J.; Seo, S.B.; Yoo, S.J.; Lim, W.K.; Kim, H.M. Water-soluble chitosan inhibits the production of pro-inflammatory cytokine in human astrocytoma cells activated by amyloid beta peptide and interleukin-1beta. *Neurosci. Lett.* **2002**, *321*, 105–109. [CrossRef] [PubMed]

148. Wei, P.; Ma, P.; Xu, Q.S.; Bai, Q.H.; Gu, J.G.; Xi, H.; Du, Y.G.; Yu, C. Chitosan oligosaccharides suppress production of nitric oxide in lipopolysaccharide-induced N9 murine microglial cells *in vitro*. *Glycoconjugate J.* **2012**, *29*, 285–295. [CrossRef]

149. Howlett, G.J.; Moore, K.J. Untangling the role of amyloid in atherosclerosis. *Curr. Opin. Lipidol.* **2006**, *17*, 541–547. [CrossRef] [PubMed]

150. Herczenik, E.; Gebbink, M.F.B.G. Molecular and cellular aspects of protein misfolding and disease. *FASEB J.* **2008**, *22*, 2115–2133. [CrossRef] [PubMed]

151. Korporaal, S.J.; Gorter, G.; van Rijn, H.J.; Akkerman, J.W. Effect of oxidation on the platelet-activating properties of low-density lipoprotein. *Arterioscler. Thromb. Vasc. Biol.* **2005**, *25*, 867–872. [CrossRef] [PubMed]

152. Herczenik, E.; Bouma, B.; Korporaal, S.J.A.; Strangi, R.; Zeng, Q.; Gros, P.; van Eck, M.; van Berkel, T.J.C.; Gebbink, M.F.B.G.; Akkerman, J.W.N. Activation of Human Platelets by Misfolded Proteins. *Arterioscler. Thromb. Vasc. Biol.* **2007**, *27*, 1657–1665. [CrossRef] [PubMed]

153. Ursini, F.; Davies, K.J.; Maiorino, M.; Parasassi, T.; Sevanian, A. Atherosclerosis: Another protein misfolding disease? *Trends Mol. Med.* **2002**, *8*, 370–374. [CrossRef] [PubMed]

154. Hayden, M.R.; Tyagi, S.C.; Kerklo, M.M.; Nicolls, M.R. Type 2 diabetes mellitus as a conformational disease. *JOP* **2005**, *6*, 287–302. [PubMed]

155. Stewart, C.R.; Tseng, A.A.; Mok, Y.F.; Staples, M.K.; Schiesser, C.H.; Lawrence, L.J.; Varghese, J.N.; Moore, K.J.; Howlett, G.J. Oxidation of low-density lipoproteins induces amyloid-like structures that are recognized by macrophages. *Biochemistry* **2005**, *44*, 9108–9116. [CrossRef] [PubMed]

156. Kowalska, M.A.; Badellino, K. β-Amyloid protein induces platelet aggregation and supports platelet adhesion. *Biochem Biophys. Res. Commun.* **1994**, *205*, 1829–1835. [CrossRef] [PubMed]

157. Laske, C.; Sopova, K.; Stellos, K. Platelet activation in alzheimer's disease: From pathophysiology to clinical value. *Curr. Vasc. Pharmacol.* **2012**, *10*, 626–630. [CrossRef] [PubMed]

158. Ho, C.; Stubbs, C.D. Hydration at the membrane protein-lipid interface. *Biophys. J.* **1992**, *63*, 897–902. [CrossRef] [PubMed]

159. Anraku, M.; Kabashima, M.; Namura, H.; Maruyama, T.; Otagiri, M.; Gebicki, J.M.; Furutani, N.; Tomida, H. Antioxidant protection of human serum albumin by chitosan. *Int. J. Biol. Macromol.* **2008**, *43*, 159–164. [CrossRef] [PubMed]

160. Arakawa, T.; Prestrelski, S.J.; Kenney, W.C.; Carpenter, J.F. Factors affecting short-term and long-term stabilities of proteins. *Adv. Drug Deliv. Rev.* **1993**, *10*, 1–28. [CrossRef]

161. Lahm, D.; Lee, L.K.; Bettelheim, F.A. Age dependence of freezable and nonfreezable water content of normal human lenses. *Investig. Ophthalmol. Vis. Sci.* **1985**, *26*, 1162–1165.

162. Kerch, G.; Rustichelli, F.; Ausili, P.; Zicans, J.; Merijs Meri, R.; Glonin, A. Effect of chitosan on physical and chemical processes during bread baking and staling. *Eur. Food Res. Technol.* **2008**, *226*, 1459–1464. [CrossRef]

163. Kerch, G.; Zicans, J.; Merijs Meri, R.; Stunda-Ramava, A.; Jakobsons, E. The use of thermal analysis in assessing the effect of bound water content and substrate rigidity on prevention of platelet adhesion. *J. Therm. Anal. Calorim.* **2015**, *120*, 533–539. [CrossRef]

164. No, H.K.; Meyers, S.P.; Prinyawiwatkul, W.; Xu, Z. Applications of chitosan for improvement of quality and shelf life of foods: A review. *J. Food Sci.* **2007**, *72*, R87–R100. [CrossRef] [PubMed]

165. Park, I.K.; Lee, Y.K.; Kim, M.J.; Kim, S.D. Effect of surface treatment with chitosan on shelf-life of baguette. *J. Chitin Chitosan* **2002**, *7*, 208–213.

166. Ahn, D.H.; Choi, J.S.; Lee, H.Y.; Kim, J.Y.; Youn, S.K.; Park, S.M. Effects on preservation and quality of bread with coating high molecular weight chitosan. *Korean J. Food Nutr.* **2003**, *16*, 430–436.

167. Park, I.K.; Lee, Y.K.; Kim, M.J.; Kim, S.D. Effect of surface treatment with chito-oligosaccharide on shelf-life of baguette. *J. Chitin Chitosan* **2002**, *7*, 214–218.

168. Lee, H.Y.; Kim, S.M.; Kim, J.Y.; Youn, S.K.; Choi, J.S.; Park, S.M.; Ahn, D.H. Effect of addition of chitosan on improvement for shelf-life of bread. *J. Korean Soc. Food Sci. Nutr.* **2002**, *31*, 445–450. [CrossRef]

169. Lee, K.H.; Lee, Y.C. Effect of carboxymethyl chitosan on quality of fermented pan bread. *Korean J. Food Sci. Technol.* **1997**, *29*, 96–100.

170. Kerch, G.; Zicans, J.; Merijs Meri, R. The effect of chitosan oligosaccharides on bread staling. *J. Cereal Sci.* **2010**, *52*, 491–495. [CrossRef]

171. Knorr, D. Functional properties of chitin and chitosan. *J. Food Sci.* **1982**, *47*, 593–595. [CrossRef]

172. Lafarga, T.; Gallagher, E.; Walsh, D.; Valverde, J.; Hayes, M. Chitosan-containing bread made using marine shellfishery byproducts: Functional, bioactive, and quality assessment of the end product. *J. Agric. Food Chem.* **2013**, *61*, 8790–8796. [CrossRef] [PubMed]

173. Fadda, C.; Sanguinetti, A.M.; Del Caro, A.; Collar, C.; Piga, A. Bread staling: updating the view. *Compr. Rev. Food Sci. Food Saf.* **2014**, *13*, 473–492. [CrossRef]

174. Lafarga, T.; Hayes, M.; Valverde, J.; Walsh, D.; Gallagher, E. Prawn chitosan containing bread: assessment of functional, bioactive and sensory qualities. *J. Chitin Chitosan Sci.* **2013**, *1*, 150–156. [CrossRef]

175. Kerch, G.; Glonin, A.; Zicans, J.; Merijs Meri, R. A DSC study of the effect of ascorbic acid on bound water content and distribution in chitosan-enriched bread rolls during storage. *J. Therm. Anal. Calorim.* **2012**, *108*, 73–78. [CrossRef]

176. Rakcejeva, T.; Rusa, K.; Dukalska, L.; Kerch, G. Effect of chitosan and chitooligosaccharide lactate on free lipids and reducing sugars content and on wheat bread firming. *Eur. Food Res. Technol.* **2011**, *232*, 123–128. [CrossRef]

177. Kerch, G.; Glonin, A.; Zicans, J.; Merijs Meri, R. A DSC study of the effect of bread making methods on bound water content and redistribution in chitosan enriched bread. *J. Therm. Anal. Calorim.* **2012**, *108*, 185–189. [CrossRef]

178. Lee, J.W.; Lee, Y.C. The physico-chemical and sensory properties of milk with water soluble chitosan. *Korean J. Food Sci. Technol.* **2000**, *32*, 806–813.

179. El-Sisi, A.S. Impact of replacement of gelatin with chitosan on the physicochemical properties of ice-milk. *Int. J. Dairy Sci.* **2015**, *10*, 26–33.

180. Kwak, H.S.; Mijan, M.A.; Ganesan, P. *Application of Nanomaterials, Nano- and Microencapsulation to Milk and Dairy Products, in Nano- and Microencapsulation for Foods*; Kwak, H.-S., Ed.; John Wiley & Sons, Ltd: Chichester, UK, 2014. [CrossRef]

181. Zanjani, M.A.K.; Mohammadi, N.; Ahari, H.; Tarzi, B.G.; Bakhoda, H. Effect of microencapsulation with chitosan coating on survival of *Lactobacillus casei* and *Bifidobacterium bifidum* in ice cream. *Iran. J. Nutr. Sci. Food. Technol.* **2014**, *8*, 125–134.

182. Eduardo, M.F.; Correa De Mello, K.G.P.; Polakiewicz, B.; Da Silva Lannes, S.C. Evaluation of chocolate milk beverage formulated with modified chitosan. *J. Agric. Sci. Technol.* **2014**, *16*, 1301–1312.

183. Tasneem, M.; Siddique, F.; Ahmad, A.; Farooq, U. Stabilizers: Indispensable substances in dairy products of high rheology. *Crit. Rev. Food Sci. Nutr.* **2014**, *54*, 869–879. [CrossRef] [PubMed]

184. Zagorska, J.; Pelnik, A.; Kerch, G. Effect of the addition of chitosans with different molecular structure on fermentation process and viscosity changes during sour cream storage. *Biochem. Biophys. (BAB)* **2013**, *1*, 13–21.

185. Rajapaksha, D.S.W.; Kodithuwakku, K.A.H.T. Evaluation of chitosan for its inhibitory activity on post-acidification of set yoghurt under cold storage for 20 days. *J. Chitin Chitosan* **2014**, *2*, 16–20. [CrossRef]

186. Seo, M.H.; Chang, Y.H.; Lee, S.; Kwak, H.S. The physicochemical and sensory properties of milk supplemented with ascorbic acid-soluble nano-chitosan during storage. *Int. J. Dairy Technol.* **2011**, *64*, 57–63. [CrossRef]

187. Choi, H.J.; Ahn, J.; Kim, N.C.; Kwak, H.S. The Effects of Microencapsulated chitooligosaccharide on physical and sensory properties of the milk. *Asian Aust. J. Anim. Sci.* **2006**, *19*, 1347–1353. [CrossRef]

188. Krasaekoopt, W.; Bhandari, B.; Deeth, H.C. Survival of probiotics encapsulated in chitosan-coated alginate beads in yoghurt from UHT-and conventionally treated milk during storage. *LWT-Food Sci. Technol.* **2006**, *39*, 177–183. [CrossRef]

189. Seo, M.H.; Lee, S.Y.; Chang, Y.H.; Kwak, H.S. Physicochemical, microbial, and sensory properties of yogurt supplemented with nanopowdered chitosan during storage. *J. Dairy Sci.* **2009**, *92*, 5907–5916. [CrossRef] [PubMed]
190. Altieri, C.; Scrocco, C.; Sinigaglia, M.; del Nobile, M.A. Use of chitosan to prolong mozzarella cheese shelf life. *J. Dairy Sci.* **2005**, *88*, 2683–2688. [CrossRef] [PubMed]

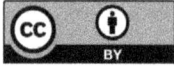

marine drugs

MDPI

Review

Stability of Chitosan—A Challenge for Pharmaceutical and Biomedical Applications

Emilia Szymańska * and Katarzyna Winnicka

Department of Pharmaceutical Technology, Faculty of Pharmacy, Medical University of Białystok,
Mickiewicza 2c, Białystok 15-222, Poland; kwin@umb.edu.pl
* Author to whom correspondence should be addressed; esz@umb.edu.pl;
  Tel.: +48-85-748-5893; Fax: +48-85-748-5616.

Academic Editor: Paola Laurienzo
Received: 25 February 2015; Accepted: 20 March 2015; Published: 1 April 2015

Abstract: Chitosan—one of the natural multifunctional polymers—due to its unique and versatile biological properties is regarded as a useful compound in medical and pharmaceutical technology. Recently, considerable research effort has been made in order to develop safe and efficient chitosan products. However, the problem of poor stability of chitosan-based systems restricts its practical applicability; thus, it has become a great challenge to establish sufficient shelf-life for chitosan formulations. Improved stability can be assessed by controlling the environmental factors, manipulating processing conditions (e.g., temperature), introducing a proper stabilizing compound, developing chitosan blends with another polymer, or modifying the chitosan structure using chemical or ionic agents. This review covers the influence of internal, environmental, and processing factors on the long-term stability of chitosan products. The aim of this paper is also to highlight the latest developments which enable the physicochemical properties of chitosan-based applications to be preserved upon storage.

Keywords: chitosan; drug delivery system; long-term stability; acidic hydrolysis; thermal degradation; storage conditions

1. Introduction

Nowadays, besides novel drug molecules discovery processes, the development of multifunctional drug delivery systems has become a current and attractive concept in pharmaceutical technology. Carbohydrate-based vehicles with a capability of reducing dosing frequency, improving drug pharmacological activity and delivering drugs at the specified site appear to be promising as pharmaceutical drug carriers [1–3]. Among various carbohydrate polymers, chitosan—a natural multifunctional polysaccharide—due to its biocompatibility, biodegradability, and mucoadhesiveness has been extensively studied for a number of biomedical and pharmaceutical applications, including prolonged or controlled release drug delivery systems [4], wound dressings [5], blood anticoagulants [6], cartilage and bone tissue engineering scaffolds [7,8], and space filling implants [9]. Chitosan is a polycationic copolymer, consisting of glucosamine and N-acetylglucosamine units, obtained by deacetylation of chitin derived from the exoskeleton of crustaceans, insects, or fungi [10,11]. It is available in a wide range of degrees of deacetylation and molecular weight, which are also the main factors influencing the nature and quality of the polymer. Chitosan—as an abundantly accessible and inexpensive biomaterial—can be easily formed into diverse semi-solid and solid structures under mild conditions. It is soluble only in diluted inorganic and organic acids with a pH lower than chitosan pK_a (about 6.3), forming a non-Newtonian, shear-thinning fluid [12]. At low pH, the free amino groups are protonated causing electrostatic repulsion between the polymer's chains and thus enabling polymer solvation. Chitosan possesses good mucoadhesive properties resulting from the cationic behavior and the presence of free hydroxyl and amino groups allowing the polymer to interact with mucin by hydrogen and electrostatic bonding. Hence, it is regarded as a suitable excipient to prepare buccal [13], nasal [14], ocular [15] and vaginal dosage forms [16]. In addition, chitosan is reported to show penetration enhancement properties by improving active agent transport through the epithelium layer containing tight junctions [17]. Due to its mucoadhesiveness and ability to cross epithelial barriers, chitosan has been widely studied as a vaccine adjuvant or co-adjuvant as it was shown to enhance bioavailability and immunogenicity of antigens after oral, nasal, or subcutaneous administration [18–20]. Superior hemostatic efficacy of chitosan through platelets activation and thrombin generation was also displayed [6] enabling its application in wound dressings [5]. The polymer is also considered as a promising candidate in obesity and hypercholesterolemia treatment as it is able to combine bile acids in the digestive tract and in consequence increase their excretion [21]. Numerous data have drawn attention to the use of chitosan as an antifungal and antibacterial agent [22–24]. Furthermore, chitosan has been recently employed as an adjunctive for an antimicrobial drug in order to increase its pharmacological activity [25,26]. Examples of chitosan-based delivery systems and biomedical devices are shown in Table 1.

Despite the fact that chitosan is a unique and versatile compound, widely used in the pharmaceutical and biomedical fields, there are hardly any available pharmaceutical products based on chitosan (only hemostatic dressings, preparations for wound-healing and nutraceutical products exist) (Table 2). This might be a result of the strong hygroscopic nature of chitosan and the fact that chitosan material extracted from various sources differs significantly in terms of its molecular weight and molecular weight distribution, degree of deacetylation, and purity level. Additionally, the high susceptibility of chitosan to environmental factors and processing conditions (such as heating or freezing) can impose stress on its structure and cause polymer degradation (Figure 1).

Table 1. Examples of chitosan (CS)-based drug delivery systems and biomedical devices.

Material	Active Substance	Dosage Form	Biomedical or Pharmaceutical Application	References
Composition of unmodified CS, ethyl cellulose and butylphthalate	Buspirone hydrochloride	Sustained release lyophilized sponges	Buccal treatment of anxiety	Kassem *et al.*, 2012 [13]
CS/xanthan polyelectrolyte complex	Promethazine hydrochloride	Mucoadhesive inserts	Nasal treatment of migraine	Dehghan *et al.*, 2014 [14]
Unmodified CS	Bimatoprost	Sustained release inserts	Ophthalmic treatment of glaucoma	Franca *et al.*, 2014 [15]
Unmodified CS and CS crosslinked with β-glycerophosphate	Clotrimazole	Prolonged release microgranules, tablets and hydrogel	Vaginal treatment of candidiasis	Szymańska *et al.*, 2012 [4] Szymańska *et al.*, 2014 [16,25]
Unmodified CS	Chloramphenicol	Sustained-release liposomal hydrogel	Topical, wound therapy	Hurler *et al.*, 2012 [5]
Unmodified CS	Metronidazole	Hydrogel	Periodontal therapy	Akncbay *et al.*, 2007 [22]
N-trimethyl CS	Ovalbumin	Nanoconjugates	Nasal and intradermal vaccination	Slütter *et al.*, 2010 [18]
N-trimethyl CS crosslinked with tripolyphosphate		Nanoparticles		Bal *et al.*, 2012 [19]
CS crosslikned with glucose-1-phosphate	Diclofenac potassium	*In situ* forming hydrogel	Injectable	Supper *et al.*, 2014 [27]
Composition of CS crosslinked with β-glycerophosphate and glucosamine	Articular chondrocytes	*In situ* forming hydrogel	Cartilage and bone tissue engineering	Hoemann *et al.*, 2005 [9]
CS crosslinked with citric acid	Cisplatin	Microspheres	Dry powder inhalation system for lung cancer	Singh *et al.*, 2012 [28]
Complexation of CS and dextran sulfate	Insulin	Nanoparticles	Oral delivery for insulin/diabetes therapy	Sarmento *et al.*, 2006 [29]
CS/alginate composite	Fucoidan	Freeze-dried scaffold	Bone tissue engineering	Venkatesan *et al.*, 2014 [8]

Table 2. Examples of commercial medical devices and oral nutraceuticals with chitosan (CS).

Product	Material	Usage/Application	Manufacturer
Wound-healing and hemostatic products			
Chitodine®	CS powder with adsorbed elementary iodine	Disinfection of wounded skin, surgical dressing	International Medical Services
ChitoPack C®	Cotton-like CS	Regeneration and reconstruction of body tissue, subcutaneous tissue and skin	Eisai Co.
Celox™	Gauze and granules with CS	Control of bleeding from non-cavitary grain wounds	MedTrade
ChitoFlex®	CS acetate sponge		HemCon Medical Technologies INC.
HemCon® Bandage Pro HemCon® Strip First Aid	Freeze-dried CS acetate salt		
PosiSep®	N,O-carboxymethyl CS sponge	Intranasal hemostatic splint for patients undergoing nasal/sinus surgery	Hemostatis LLC.
Syvek Excel™	Lyophilized three-dimensional CS fibers	Rapid control of bleeding for anticoagulated patients	Marine Polymer Technologies Inc.
Clo-Sur® PAD	Non-woven seal with a soluble CS	Control of moderate to severe bleeding	Scion Cardio-vascular
ChitoSeal®	Soluble chitosan salt		Abbott Vascular Devices
TraumaStat®	Porous polyethylene fibers filled with silica, coated with CS (ChitoClear®)		Ore-Medix
Tegasorb®	CS particles		Tesla-Pharma
Vulnosorb®	Composition of microcrystalline CS with fibrinogenic tissue glue		3M
Nutraceutical products			
Slim Med™	Non-animal CS	Prevention and treatment of overweight	KitoZyme S.A.
KiOcardio™	Non-animal CS	Maintenance of normal blood cholesterol level	KitoZyme S.A.
LipoSan Ultra®	Composition of CS (ChitoClear®) and succinic acid	Binding dietary fat and reducing its absorption in the intestine	Primex
Liposorb™	CS extracted from squid	Preventing irritable bowel syndrome; Binding dietary fat and reducing its absorption in the intestine	Good Health

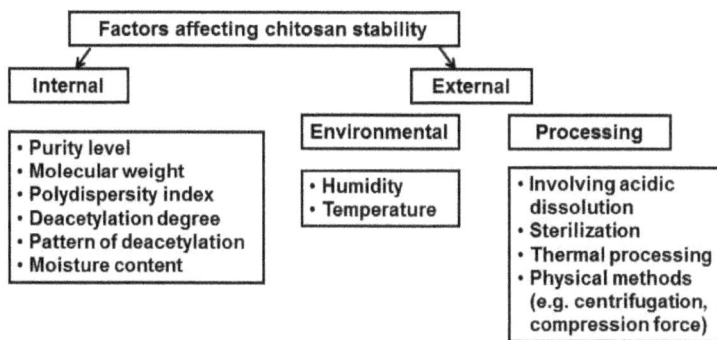

Figure 1. Factors affecting stability of chitosan-based products.

Chitosan as a natural biodegradable biopolymer undergoes enzymatic transformation to basic, non-toxic components. Chitosan is degraded *in vivo* by several enzymes, mainly by lysozyme—a non-specific protease present in all mammalian tissues—producing non-toxic oligosaccharides which can be then excreted or incorporated to glycosoaminoglycans and glycoproteins [30]. *In vitro* degradations of chitosan via oxidation, chemical, or enzymatic hydrolysis reactions are commonly used methods for the preparation of low molecular chitosan under controlled conditions [31]. The molecular weight, polydispersity, deacetylation degree, purity level and moisture content play a crucial role in determining the mechanism and the speed of polymer degradation. Regardless of the mode of degradation, the process usually begins with random splitting of β-1,4-glycosidic bonds (depolymerization) followed by N-acetyl linkage (deacetylation) (Figure 2). As a consequence, a decrease in average molecular weight and an increase in deacetylation degree are observed. Simultaneously with chitosan chain scission, cleavage and/or destruction of its functional groups (amino, carbonyl, amido, and hydroxyl) occur. In addition, chitosan depolymerization may lead to formation of free radicals which induce oxidation processes [32]. Strong intermolecular interactions between formed fragments of chitosan (interchain crosslinking) alter the polymer structure, thus leading to the irreversible loss of its physicochemical properties. Despite the fact, that numerous data have drawn attention to the chitosan-based applications in the pharmaceutical and biomedical field, only a limited number of studies and review articles have been devoted to long-term stability studies on chitosan-based assemblies [33–37].

This review considers the issue of chitosan's degradation mechanism and provides insight into internal, environmental and technological factors affecting the storage stability of chitosan-based systems. Furthermore, the focus of this paper is to describe different strategies and recent advancements implemented to preserve physicochemical properties of chitosan applications upon storage such as addition of stabilizer during the preparation process, formation of polymer blends, and use of ionic or chemical crosslinkers. Due to the wide range of this topic, improvement of the long-term stability of chitosan products by modification of chitosan's structure via grafting functional groups will be not considered in this review. As a high risk of uncontrolled chitosan decomposition arises from inappropriate storage conditions, the influence of temperature and humidity upon storage stability studies is also highlighted.

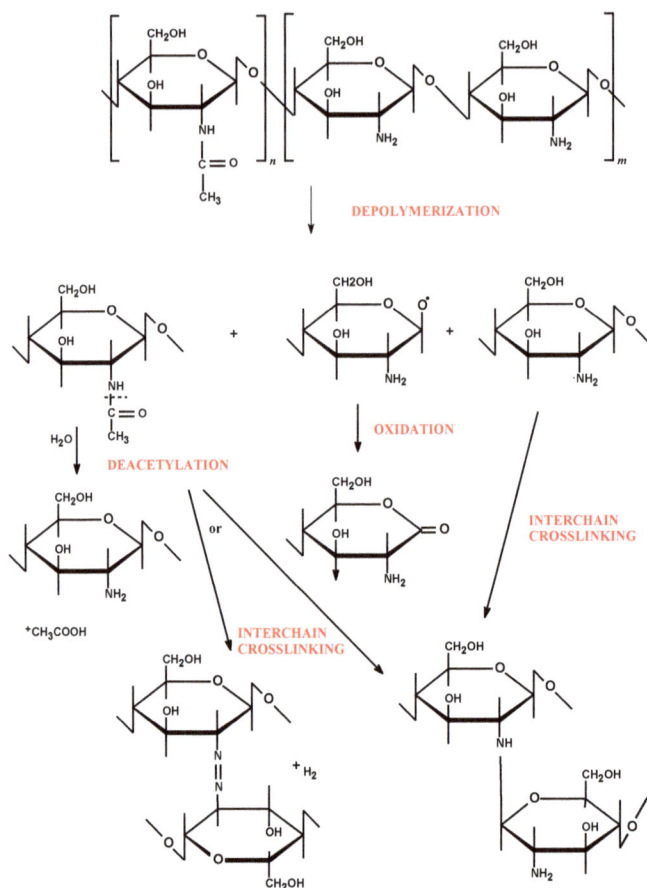

Figure 2. Possible degradation mechanisms of chitosan's structure (adapted from [32] with modifications).

2. Influence of Internal Factors on Chitosan's Stability

2.1. Purity Level

Although chitosan-based applications have been widely investigated in the biomedical field, there is still a lack of worldwide clear and definite requirements for chitosan as a pharmaceutical excipient. Monographs relating to chitosan and chitosan hydrochloride were first introduced into the European Pharmacopeia 6.0 and United States Pharmacopeia 34-NF 29th edition, respectively [38,39]. The chitosan pharmacopeial properties are summarized in Table 3. Chitosan is commercially available in various grades of purity, molecular weight, and degree of deacetylation. The wide range of chitosan sources and variety of its manufacturing processes lead to great differences in the quality and properties of chitosan products, which as a result might deviate from the pharmacopeial recommendations. Furthermore, the specification data provided by the chitosan suppliers are often incomplete, which may be misleading for pharmaceutical technologists. Although chitosan preparation involves basic purification methods like demineralization and deproteinization, chitosan material may contain some impurities, such as ash, heavy metals, or proteins. The purity level of chitosan is a factor which affects not only the biological properties like immunogenicity or biodegradability, but also has a profound effect on its solubility and stability. High ash and residual proteins content may cause difficulties in chitosan dissolution and impede preparation of chitosan-based drug delivery systems. On the other hand, microbiological contamination of the polymer may enhance chitosan degradation via enzymatic hydrolysis. Therefore, chitosan material should be of high purity and be free of contaminants (including the level of endotoxins where relevant).

Table 3. Chitosan and chitosan hydrochloride properties recommended by the European Pharmacopeia 6.0 and the United States Pharmacopeia 34-NF 29 [38,39].

Parameter	Acceptance Criteria	
	Eur. Ph. 6.0 *Chitosan hydrochloride*	**USP 34-NF 29** *Chitosan*
Appearance of solid product	White or almost white fine powder	n.d.
Degree of deacetylation	70.0%–95.0%	70.0%–95.0%
Distribution of molecular weight *	n.d.	0.85–1.15
pH of 1% (g/mL) solution	4.0–6.0	n.d.
Loss on drying *	n.d.	$\leq$5%
Insolubles/Impurities	$\leq$0.5%	$\leq$1.0%
Heavy metal	$\leq$40 ppm	$\leq$10 ppm
Iron	n.d.	$\leq$10 ppm
Sulphated ash *	$\leq$1%	n.d.
Protein	n.d.	$\leq$0.2%
Microbiological contamination	n.d.	Absence of *Pseudomonas aeruginosa* and *Staphylococcus aureus*
Aerobic microbials *	n.d.	10^3 cfu
Molds and yeasts *	n.d.	10^2 cfu

*: determined on 1.0 g sample; n.d.—not determined.

2.2. Molecular Weight and Molecular Weight Distribution (Polydispersity)

Chitosan is primarily characterized by its molecular weight, which is responsible for a number of its physicochemical and biological properties such as hydrophilicity, viscosity, water-uptake ability, biodegradability, and mucoadhesion [10,40]. The molecular weight (M_W) is expressed as an average of all the molecules present in the sample. With regard to the initial source material and the type of preparation method, the M_W of commercial chitosan varies between 10–100,000 kDa. The average molecular weight may be estimated by a number of techniques, such as osmometry, light scattering, NMR, viscometric assay of the polymer's intrinsic viscosity, or chromatographic techniques (size exclusion chromatography, gel permeation chromatography). All of these measurements display experimental difficulties and should be properly validated. Additionally, the M_W of chitosan samples may differ depending on the applied technique which can be misleading for technologists and complicate direct comparison between polymer materials obtained from different manufactures. The process of deacetylation may decrease the polymer M_W [41]. In order to ensure chitosan's uniformity and proper functionality in the final product, the molecular weight distribution (polydispersity index, PDI) should be determined [39,42]. PDI refers to the ratio of M_W to a number of average molecular weights (M_N) and a value between 0.85 and 1.15 is considered as having good polymer homogeneity [39]. Generally, high molecular weight chitosan is regarded as more stable. The M_W was found to affect the thermal stability of the polymer [32]. In addition, a number of factors, including strong acids, elevated temperature, mechanical shearing, or irradiation may influence the chitosan M_W. For instance, physical methods—high pressure homogenization, extensive shearing, or centrifugation—frequently used for preparation of biomedical chitosan devices, were noticed to decrease the polymer M_W and were responsible for the fluctuations of the PDI [43]. It should be also noted that the compression force during tablet preparation is responsible for heat generation and might influence the chitosan M_W distribution [44].

2.3. Degree of Deacetylation and the Pattern of Deacetylation

The degree of deacetylation (DD) is the ratio of glucosamine to *N*-acetylglucosamine units, while distribution of these groups along the polymer chain is described as the pattern of deacetylation (P_A). The degree of deacetylation of commercial chitosan is controlled by modifying the time and temperature of the de-*N*-acetylation process [41] and according to the pharmacopeial specifications, the parameter ranges from 70% to 95% [38,39]. Furthermore, with regard to deacetylation conditions, chitosan may show a characteristic P_A that varies from block to a random type [45]. It should be particularly important to accurately define the chitosan DD and P_A, as they are—similarly to M_W—crucial factors determining its physicochemical behavior and biological functionality. Recently, considerable research effort has been made to investigate the effect of DD on the potency and the rate of chitosan's degradation. Interestingly, polymer with low DD was found to induce an acute inflammatory response as a result of the fast rate of degradation, while chitosan with high DD caused minimal inflammation [30]. This is in agreement with observations made by Zhang *et al.*, who showed that chitosan with high DD possessed lower affinity to enzymes *in vitro* [46]. Moreover, the P_A was noticed to influence biodegradability, since homogenous distribution of acetylated groups (random type of P_A) resulted in a lower rate of enzymatic degradation [47]. The contamination level of chitosan material—which correlates with the DD—may also have an impact on the polymer immunogenic behavior. Yuan *et al.*, showed that the higher the DD, the higher the purity grade observed in the polymer sample [48]. Thus, careful selection of chitosan with proper DD should be of great interest, especially with regard to parenteral chitosan-based formulations.

Several studies revealed that chitosan DD affects both hydrolytic and thermal behavior of the polymer products [32,49–51]. It was found that the more extensive de-*N*-acetylated chitosan sample, the slower the rate of acidic hydrolysis observed during storage [49]. This phenomenon was explained by the fact that chitosan with higher DD has a less porous structure and lower water-uptake ability, which limits the rate of the degradation process in acidic environment. On the contrary, a slower rate of chitosan thermal depolymerization may be a result of interchain crosslinking between free amino groups, which exerts a stabilizing effect on the polymer's structure [32,50,51]. Nevertheless, chitosan with high DD was also shown to be more susceptible to photodegradation [52]. The P_A has a significant impact on the charge density, which in turn affects the solubility behavior of chitosan with the same M_W and DD [45]. For instance, chitosan with a block pattern of acetylated and deacetylated units was shown to aggregate in acidic environment impeding its dissolution process [53].

2.4. Moisture Content

Chitosan is hygroscopic in nature, having a greater capability to form hydrogen bonding (formed with both hydroxyl and amino groups) with water compared to chitin [54]. The amount of absorbed water depends on the initial moisture content as well as on the storage conditions, especially the environmental temperature and relative humidity. Rege *et al.*, found that the moisture level of chitosan powder ranged from 7% to 11% (w/w) and was independent of the polymer DD or M_W [55]. However, Mucha *et al.*, noticed that the water-uptake ability of chitosan films decreased on increasing their DD [56]. The presence of absorbed water plays a considerable role especially in solid chitosan-based formulations, affecting the flow properties and compressibility of the powders' or tablets' tensile strength. It was reported that moisture content up to 6% (w/w) may improve particle binding during compression as a result of formation of hydrogen bonds between the particles [57]. However, fluctuations in moisture levels of chitosan material upon storage may change the physicochemical and mechanical properties of chitosan-based systems. Studies conducted by No *et al.*, revealed that although the level of absorbed water in chitosan powder rose during storage, a decline in water binding capacity was observed [58]. Viljoen *et al.* showed that six-month storage of chitosan tablets caused a dehydration of the polymer, which resulted in a decrease in crushing strength followed by an increase in friability and disintegration time. In addition, the higher the water content in the chitosan structure, the faster and more pronounced was the damage of the polymer (via hydrolysis reactions) observed [59].

As initial moisture level and strong hygroscopic behavior may limit chitosan's applicability, the water content in chitosan material should be measured and optimized prior to preformulation studies and carefully controlled upon storage. Among various methods of moisture content determinations in solid forms, loss on drying technique is a simple and quick method, in which a material sample is weighed, heated in an oven, and reweighed after cooling [39]. The swelling index test is another commonly used method, which helps to investigate how the chitosan water-uptake ability changes upon long-term storage. The measurements, which can be applied for both semi-solid and solid formulations, consist in placing an accurately weighed sample in an acceptance medium (e.g., suitable body fluid simulant), usually at 37 °C. It is important to carefully select the type of the medium prior to the swelling studies, e.g., pure water usage should be excluded for experiments with unmodified chitosan-based formulations because of the impact of ionic strength on the chitosan's viscosity and swelling behavior and its poor solubility in water pH. At a predetermined time interval, the formulations are periodically weighed until a constant weight is obtained. The swelling ratio is then calculated using the following formula:

$$[SR] = \frac{W_S - W_O}{W_O} \tag{1}$$

where: SR—swelling ratio, W_O—initial weight of dosage form, W_S—weight of dosage form after swelling [60].

3. Influence of External Factors on Chitosan Stability

3.1. Environmental Factors

Chitosan is very sensitive to environmental conditions, hence it is recommended to store in closed containers at low temperatures (2–8 °C) [38]. In the preparation process of chitosan-based applications it is particularly important to establish the shelf-life of the product by conducting stability studies [27,59,61]. The purpose of the stability testing is to provide reliable evidence on how the quality of the chitosan product differs with time under the influence of environmental factors such as humidity and temperature. Type of stability studies (long-term, intermediate, or accelerated), storage conditions and frequency of testing should be selected with respect to the chitosan formulation properties [62]. The impact of the crucial environmental parameters—relative humidity and temperature—on the physicochemical properties of chitosan applications upon storage is presented below.

3.1.1. Humidity

The presence and distribution of moisture in the chitosan material strongly depends on the ambient relative humidity (RH). For relative low humidity (below 40%), water transport in chitosan material was shown to follow a Fickian process, whereas at higher values of humidity, an anomalous diffusion kinetic was observed [63]. The analysis of chitosan water sorption carried out under ambient conditions (25 °C, 60% RH) showed that chitosan absorbed 14%–16% (w/w) of water (within 100 min) and the process rate was dependent on the polymer DD [56]. In high humidity conditions (RH > 60%), water molecules were found to penetrate more intensively through chitosan chains, thus the chitosan moisture content increased significantly [58,63]. The environmental moisture content is responsible for a plasticizing or swelling effect of solid or semi-solid polymer assemblies, respectively. Long-term storage at high RH may not only accelerate the ratio of chitosan hydrolytic damage, but also alter the polymer's physicochemical and biological properties. Long-term stability studies revealed that chitosan tablets stored for six months at 70% RH possessed markedly lower mechanical properties compared to those kept at 60% RH [59]. Similar observations were made in the study on chitosan/amylose corn starch composite films which became mechanically weaker upon three-month storage at 40 °C/70% RH [64]. In the case of semi-solid chitosan applications, storing at high RH and changing its water-uptake ability alter the rate of drug release profile of the chitosan matrix. Kurek *et al.*, noticed that the increase of ambient humidity from 0% to 75% resulted in a greater swelling of chitosan films, which was responsible for a greater and faster release of active compound from the chitosan carrier [65]. In addition, excessive hydration at high relative humidity could weaken the mucoadhesive properties of chitosan carriers as a result of "dilution" of functional groups available for adhesive interactions with mucin [66].

3.1.2. Temperature

Apart from relative humidity, temperature is another variable which exerts an effect on the moisture content in chitosan-based systems. Exposure to elevated temperatures (40 °C) was found to cause a significant loss of moisture (dehydration of chitosan powder), which resulted in a decrease in hardness and mechanical tablet strength [59]. In addition, air temperature may affect the chitosan degradation ratio, especially in liquid and semi-solid products. Storage of chitosan solution, both at ambient and elevated temperatures, resulted in faster degradation of chitosan chains [49,67] and the rate of hydrolysis was found to follow first-order kinetics. Interestingly, no significant chain hydrolysis was noticed in the chitosan solution stored at 5 °C [67]. Furthermore, long-term stability studies established on chitosan/glucose 1-phosphate thermosensitive solution confirmed the necessity of their storage in a refrigerator (at 2–8 °C) [27].

3.2. Processing Factors

3.2.1. Processing Involving Acidic Dissolution

Chitosan degradation via hydrolysis is a particular problem in pharmaceutical technology because dissolution of chitosan in diluted acids is a routine stage in the pharmaceutical technology of chitosan-based formulations. During hydrolysis, acid acts as a catalyst which splits the polymer chains. As a result, a decrease in average M_W, viscosity, and weakness of mechanical properties is observed. It was reported that the rate of hydrolysis followed first-order kinetic and the main factors affecting this parameter were: DD, polymer concentration, type of acid and its concentration, treatment time, and temperature. There are several studies devoted to chitosan hydrolysis using several types of acids, namely acetic [34,67], formic [67], lactic [68], and hydrochloric [49]. Different acetic acid concentrations were found not to affect the degradation rate [67], whereas an accelerated rate of hydrolysis with increased concentration of hydrochloric acid was observed [49]. A faster rate of chain damage was noticed when chitosan with lower DD was used in the studies. This phenomenon can be explained by the fact that chitosan with low DD possesses a more porous structure and electrostatic repulsion between protonated amino groups is more pronounced thus promoting penetration of acid solution inside the polymer structure. Nevertheless, it should be pointed out that an increase in temperature (regardless of the type of acid used) is regarded as accelerating the degradation rate of the polymer [37]. Interestingly, studies accomplished by Nguyen *et al.*, revealed that the ratio of chitosan decomposition in acetic acid solutions could be slowed down by storage at 5 °C [67].

A simple and commonly used assay for stability testing of chitosan dispersions upon storage is a viscometric measurement of its intrinsic viscosity [η] using the Mark-Houwink equation:

$$[\eta] = k \times M_w^\alpha \tag{2}$$

where M_w—the viscosity-average molecular weight, η—the intrinsic viscosity, k and α (Mark-Houwink exponent) are empirical constants describing the polymer conformation [37].

The intrinsic viscosity of chitosan describes the ability to form viscous solution (under specific solvent and temperature conditions) and is directly proportional to the polymer average M_W. The Mark-Houwink exponent is suitable for indicating a specific chitosan conformation. When α = 0 the chitosan structure is referred to as a compact sphere, α = 0.5–0.8—random coil and α = 1.8—rigid coil. This exponent is useful when exploring alterations in polymer conformation with an increase in polymer chain length. The intrinsic viscosity is also a simple and quick method useful for determination of the average Mw of soluble macromolecules. This test requires calibration procedure development as the Mark-Houwink constants differ according to the type of solvent and temperature of measurement. Due to a lack of reference standards and validation data, this technique has not been incorporated into the pharmacopeias as an alternative method for the polymer average M_W measurements.

3.2.2. Sterilization

Chitosan-based drug delivery dosage forms intended for ocular or parenteral administration, and those which contact with wounds, require high microbiological purity and have to be sterilized. Commonly used sterilization methods of pharmaceutical products include filter sterilization, saturated steam sterilization, exposure to dry heat and ethylene oxide, or γ-radiation [38,39]. These methods act either physically or chemically and may lead to irreversible alteration in both chitosan structure and its function. The previous studies reported that sterilization of chitosan gels by saturated steam caused chain scission of the polymer which resulted in 20%–50% decrease in viscosity and almost 30% loss of M_W [69]. Similarly, Toffey et al., found that autoclaving was not suitable to sterilize chitosan films prepared in acetic acid, because harsh conditions which had been employed in the process reduced its tensile strength and diminished polymer solubility [70]. Moreover, Lim et al., noticed that chitosan heated at 160 °C for 2 h became insoluble in acidic solution, which may be related to interchain crosslinking involving the amino groups [71]. In addition, the experiments conducted by Lim et al., and Yang et al., showed that both dry heat (160 °C for 2 h) and autoclave sterilization (under the pressure 100 kPa, at 105–125 °C for 15–30 min) caused darkening of chitosan dried powder to a yellow color [71,72]. The authors suggested that the colored products which appeared as a probable consequence of the Maillard reaction between the amino and carbonyl groups, should be carefully examined in terms of their biocompatibility and cytotoxicity. On the contrary, some researchers did not notice significant changes in the chemical structure of chitosan suggesting autoclaving as a suitable sterilization method for solid chitosan devices [72]. San Juan *et al.*, found that the Mw of chitosan was unaltered after steam sterilization when the chitosan powder was dispersed in water prior to the autoclaving process [73].

Gamma irradiation—another potential sterilization technique—was found to cause significant main chain scissions of both powdered chitosan and its films, even when performed at −80 °C [72,74,75]. The studies also indicated a significant decrease in M_W followed with an increase in DD in a γ-radiation dose-dependent manner. In addition, chitosan films which had been exposed to irradiation, were shown to possess lower water sorption capacity [74] and higher value of tensile strength, probably due to polymer chain rearrangements [76]. Interestingly, several studies revealed that exposure to ethylene oxide (EO) caused relatively minor changes in the structure and physicochemical properties of chitosan dried powder or membranes, suggesting this method as the most appropriate for chitosan devices [72,76]. On the contrary, studies on the solid chitosan samples revealed that EO sterilization caused structural alterations in the polymer, irrespective of DD as a result of oxidation of its amine groups. Interestingly, observed chemical changes were restricted only to the polymer surface [77]. It should be also noted that chitosan products sterilized by ethylene oxide have to be quarantined prior to use in order to remove gas residues.

The influence of ultraviolet light (UV) radiation on chitosan films was also investigated [32,52]. Results of those studies displayed degradation of the polymer subjected to UV exposure mainly by formation of free radicals and destruction of polymer amino groups. The rate of degradation was more pronounced in the case of chitosan with higher DD [52].

To eliminate microbiological contamination and to guarantee a high purity level of heat-labile liquid chitosan formulations, filter sterilization could be applied. This quick and simple method appears not to influence the stability of chitosan-based products. However, filter sterilization has several obstacles resulting from the chitosan M_W and its concentration. For instance, highly viscous chitosan solutions are quite likely to clog the filter membrane and could not be sterilized by filtration. In addition, the type of the filter material should be carefully selected with regard to the solvent used for chitosan solution preparation (e.g., cellulose acetate or nylon membranes cannot be used for organic or/and acidic solutions).

Given these points, it is particularly important to investigate the effect of the sterilization process on the physicochemical properties and the end performance of chitosan material. Alternatively, preparation of chitosan-based formulations under aseptic conditions should be considered if the above mentioned sterilization methods failed. However, in such a situation application of ultrapure chitosan material is required.

3.2.3. Thermal Processing

Heating

Heat is often employed in preparation of chitosan-based formulations. Exposure to elevated temperatures might change a number of polymer properties, including aqueous solubility, viscosity, and appearance [37,71]. Chitosan decomposition during heating has been widely established and the rate and degree of the polymer damage was found to accelerate with rising temperature and duration of heating [70,71,78]. Thermal degradation of the chitosan structure, measured using the thermogravimetric method (TGA), is a complex reaction involving two or even three degradation stages [79–82]. The first stage occurs at temperature 30–110 °C and is assigned to the evaporation of the residual water present in the polymer sample. The second thermal event—attributed to the polymer decomposition—is observed over a wide temperature range, from 180 to 340 °C. The differences in glass transition temperatures were explained as a result of different M_W of the investigated chitosan [70] and the glass transition temperatures of chitosan samples were found to shift to a higher value with an increase in its M_W. Moreover, Diab *et al.*, presented the third stage observed at 470 °C with a subsequent weight loss of the chitosan sample [80]. On the basis of these results, it can be stated that chitosan may be heated up to temperatures below its glass transition temperature without affecting its physicochemical properties. Apart from the sterilization process (which was described in the previous section), preparation of pharmaceutical carriers or biomedical devices with chitosan usually does not involve heating above 100 °C. However, the time of gentle heating necessary to dissolve chitosan in acidic solution should be carefully controlled as overheating of a chitosan sample might not only cause polymer discoloration but also—as a result of the depolymerization process—change its rheological properties and/or, paradoxically, slow down its rate of dissolution [70]. In addition, the loss of water as a consequence of thermal treatment is regarded as being responsible for lowering the glass transition temperature, which makes the polymer more sensitive to temperature and subsequently reduces its stability during storage [83]. It should be noted, that the presence of a drug, plasticizer or other additives in chitosan-based systems tends to decrease the polymer glass transition temperature [60].

Currently, spray drying technique is an advanced thermal method of chitosan-based micro- and nanoparticles preparation widely used in the pharmaceutical technology [84,85]. The spray drying is an uncomplicated single phase process, in which dry particles are obtained from a fluid state by evaporating the solvent. In order to obtain chitosan micro- or nanoparticles with the desirable properties, understanding of the process and careful adjustment of the spray-drying conditions (e.g. the inlet temperature) are required [86]. With regard to active substance and excipients used in chitosan-based particles preparation, the inlet temperature can vary between 120 and 170 °C [84,85,87–89]. Although the fluid containing chitosan is exposed to high temperature for a very short period of time, the influence of this parameter on the end performance and the properties of chitosan product cannot be excluded. The large surface area of the chitosan micro- or nanoparticles is particularly exposed to a heat stream during spray-drying and thus it is most at risk of thermal decomposition and alteration of the polymer's physicochemical properties, especially its electrostatic charge. This might result in a higher content of hydrolysis products on the particles' surface and their accelerated aggregation [89].

Lyophilization

Lyophilization (freeze-drying) is a well-established drying method in which frozen material is dried by sublimation of ice. Lyophilization has many applications, especially for micro- and nanoparticles technology with the advantage of preventing not only particles aggregation but also the escape of encapsulated drug. Freeze-drying is also considered as a feasible strategy to improve the physicochemical stability of colloidal systems, including chitosan-based microparticulate delivery products over extended time periods [87,90]. Hafner *et al.*, established a freeze-drying process for melatonin-loaded lecithin/chitosan nanoparticles in order to improve their poor physicochemical stability in aqueous suspension [91]. After seven months storage, all lyophilisates remained in an amorphous state and the content of entrapped melatonin did not alter. Additionally, these nanoparticles were found to have re-dispersed easily with no particle aggregation after reconstitution. Nevertheless, lyophilization may impose stress on labile materials, such as unmodified chitosan and damage of the polymer can occur [92]. This is because chitosan undergoes strong inter- and intramolecular hydrogen bonding and hydrophobic interactions which might negatively affect physicochemical properties, such as viscosity, zeta potential, and water-uptake ability. In addition, too harsh removal of the residual water from chitosan material could result in destabilization of the polymer structure. Several reports consider the lyophilization process as an inappropriate drying method for chitosan-based formulations, even when modified chitosan was applied. The chitosan/polyol-phosphate thermogelling solutions after freeze-drying were found to be unable to maintain their viscoelastic properties [93]. In comparison to freshly prepared solutions, stored formulations were shown to possess higher viscosities, an increased gel strength, and shortened gelation time, which made them inconvenient as a ready-to-use product in pre-filled syringes [93]. In another study, Dehghan *et al.*, investigated the stability of lyophilized chitosan/xanthan polyelectrolyte complex for nasal delivery under accelerated conditions [14]. After three-month storage, the physical appearance of the nasal inserts did not alter and the drug content was within limits. However, a significant increase (26%) in weight as a result of moisture uptake was noticed, which was responsible for the acceleration of the drug release rate. The authors did not provide the stability data under either refrigerated or ambient conditions, which could have given a detailed insight into the stability of chitosan-based lyophilisates.

4. Strategies to Improve the Stability of Chitosan-Based Products

Over the last decades, chitosan has increasingly drawn attention as an attractive compound in the biomedical and pharmaceutical fields [4–8,47,69,87]. Despite the great potential of this polymer, its poor stability over time renders chitosan-based systems not applicable as final pharmaceutical products. Therefore, scientists have put an effort into improving the stability characteristics of chitosan products. Several strategies have been proposed to preserve the initial properties of chitosan by preventing polymer chain damage (Figure 3).

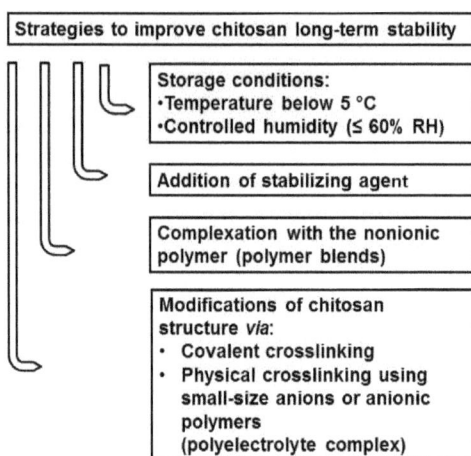

Figure 3. Strategies to improve the stability of chitosan-based products.

4.1. Stabilizing Agents

As pharmaceutical products with chitosan are highly susceptible to physicochemical degradation upon storage, one of the goals for technologists is to apply the proper excipients in order to improve the chitosan-based system's stability. It was previously explained that exposure to dry heat or steam sterilization has a marked effect on the properties and the end performance of the chitosan formulations [50,69–73]. Therefore, a number of stabilizing additives have been commonly tested in order to protect chitosan during thermal processing and/or sterilization treatment. Jarry *et al.*, showed that the addition of polyols (mannitol, sorbitol, glycerol) to chitosan and chitosan/β-glycerophosphate solutions prior to autoclaving markedly slowed down polymer degradation [75]. In addition, the incorporation of polyol additives to chitosan solutions was found to have a protective effect on M_W, viscosity, and thermogelling properties. This phenomenon could be attributed to creation of a protective hydration layer around the chitosan chains through interchain hydrogen bonds. Luangtana-Anan *et al.*, described the stability enhancement of chitosan microparticles prepared by ionotropic gelation and crosslinked with tripolyphosphate sodium in the presence of polyethylene glycol [94]. The addition of polyethylene glycol was shown to stabilize the zeta potential on the microparticles surface and prevent their aggregation over a period of one month. Conversely, the absence of the stabilizer resulted in a reduction in the particles' electrostatic charge and led to aggregation after one-week of storage.

A possible destabilizing influence of the freeze-drying process may be overcome by the addition of disaccharides (such as mannitol, sucrose, and trehalose), which protect chitosan material from freezing stress [91]. However, due to the risk of Maillard reaction and colored products formation, reducing sugars (e.g., lactose, maltose) should not be considered as bioprotectans. The stabilizing effect of the sugars is explained by the fact that disaccharides act as water replacement agents interacting by hydrogen bonding, similarly to the replaced water. In addition, they form highly viscous sugar glasses which hinder the labile materials from disruptive reactions occurring upon freezing. Chitosan-DNA nanoparticles conjugated with polyethylene glycol at the nanoparticles surface could be successively lyophilized in the presence of mannitol. The dried particles were found not to aggregate and to be easily re-suspended in both saline and PBS, upon one-month storage at either 4 °C or −20 °C [95]. In another study with chitosan nanoparticles cross-linked with tripolyphosphate, Rampino *et al.*, tested the influence of different bioprotectants—trehalose, mannitol and polyethylene glycol on the stability of the particles after drying by lyophilization or spray-drying technique [87]. The addition of trehalose to the suspension of nanoparticles significantly reduced particles aggregation enabling them to be re-dispersible after four-week storage and was the best protectant for both applied methods.

The addition of a plasticizer to chitosan films was found to influence the water-uptake and mechanical properties of chitosan formulations. Hermans *et al.*, revealed that glycerol decreased the swelling ratio of ophthalmic chitosan formulations with cyclosporine A, and as a consequence prolonged and more controlled drug release profile was achieved [96]. However, no stability tests were provided in the study, thus it is difficult to predict the long-term effect of glycerol on the behavior of chitosan films upon storage [96]. Cervera *et al.*, investigated the effect of different plasticizers—erythritol and glycerol—on the physical stability and sorption behavior of films prepared with chitosan and amylose corn starch blend [64]. The studies revealed the poor stability of films plasticized with erythritol as a result of liquefaction of the formulations in the presence of hygroscopic excipients—chitosan and erythritol. In contrast, composite films with glycerol were found to remain flexible and mechanically stable, although notable increase in water content upon three-month storage was observed.

Recently, metal ions have been used as agents which are able to increase the colloidal stability of chitosan polyelectrolyte complexes. Wu *et al.*, showed that the size and polydispersity index of chitosan/hyaluronate complex remained stable in PBS suspension at room conditions over 35 days in the presence of zinc ions [97]. The mode of the Zn (II) stabilization effect could be attributed to formation of co-ordinate bonds that tune the morphology of the hyaluronate/chitosan complex followed by alteration of their swelling properties [97].

4.2. Chitosan Blends

In recent years, chitosan blends with nonionic polymers have received much attention because they are characterized by improved physicochemical properties in comparison to the pure polymer. In order to enhance the material stability, numerous studies have been reported on the binary mixtures of chitosan with both natural (starch) or synthetic poly(vinyl alcohol), poly(ethylene oxide), and polyvinylopyrrolidone polymers [56,64,98]. The specific interactions in the chitosan blends may involve hydrogen, ionic bonds, or dipole interference and final properties strongly depend on the miscibility of the components [99]. The films composed of binary mixtures of chitosan and amylose-corn starch plasticized with glycerol were found to be flexible and remained amorphous during three-month storage at 25 °C/60% RH and 40 °C/75% RH [64]. Studies conducted on the miscible blends with poly(vinyl alcohol) displayed a significant decrease in moisture sensitivity of chitosan [56]. The modification of the polymer structure using poly(vinyl alcohol) was noticed to limit its water-uptake proportionally with the concentration of synthetic polymer as a result of the increase in structural packing of chitosan [56]. In another study, Khoo *et al.*, prepared homogenous chitosan/poly(ethylene oxide) and chitosan/polyvinylpyrrolidone films which were shown to possess higher initial temperature of thermal degradation compared to pure chitosan [98]. However, it should be noted that an improvement in thermal or hydrolytic stability might influence the biodegradability of chitosan blends which may become resistant to enzymatic degradation.

4.3. Chitosan Crosslinking

Chitosan modification through crosslinking is widely described in the literature and is a relatively easy method to prepare chitosan-based materials. On the basis of interaction between crosslinking agents and chitosan, chemical (covalent) and physical (ionic) crosslinking can be distinguished.

4.3.1. Chemical Crosslinking

Chemical (covalent) crosslinking can effectively guard the physicochemical stability of chitosan applications since the gelation is irreversible. The higher stability of such modified chitosan is based on the covalent bonds, but also other interactions—hydrogen or hydrophobic bonds—cannot be excluded. To date, the most common chemical crosslinkers of chitosan are dialdehydes (such as glutaraldehyde or glyoxal [100–102]) and genipin [103]. However, chemical crosslinking also changes biological properties of chitosan material which may limit its practical use in pharmaceutical applications. In addition, dialdehydes are considered to be toxic, thus it is particularly important to completely eliminate the unreacted crosslinkers during the preparation process. The influence of chitosan structure modification by covalent crosslinking has been widely investigated [104], but only limited data have focused on the impact of these modifications on chitosan long-term stability. Liu *et al.*, exhibited improved the physicochemical properties of chitosan/poly(acrylic acid) gel crosslinked with glutaraldehyde but the results were related only to freshly prepared formulations [105]. In another study, the stability of chitosan microspheres crosslinked with genipin in acidic conditions was investigated [103]. It was noted that the crosslinking level markedly influenced the swelling ability, mucoadhesiveness, and acidic stability of the prepared microparticles. However, besides improving the physicochemical properties, the crosslinking reaction between genipin and chitosan was found to be responsible for color alteration from transparent to blue [103,106]. Butler *et al.*, revealed that the formation of blue pigments was a result of genipin polymerization induced by oxygen radicals [107]. As the presence of free radicals may also affect the chitosan structure, the above observations might be indicative of the impaired stability of chitosan/genipin materials upon storage under environmental conditions.

4.3.2. Physical Crosslinking

In the ionic crosslinking process, a network of ionic bridges between negatively charged components and the positively charged chitosan chains is formed. Among ionic crosslinkers, small-size anions (as citrate, sulfate) or ionic molecules (e.g., phosphate-bearing groups) are commonly used. In addition, polyelectrolyte complexes (PEC) are included as a type of physical crosslinking, in which an additional natural or synthetic oppositely charged polymer is employed [108]. A list of the ionic crosslinkers commonly used for the modification of chitosan's structure is presented in Table 4.

Table 4. Examples of ionic crosslinkers used for chitosan-based drug delivery systems and biomedical devices.

Type of the Ionic Crosslinker		Examples of Agents	
metallic ions		Fe(III) Pt (II) Mo(VI)	
small-size anions or anionic molecules		citric acid succinic acid sulfate sodium	
	inorganic phosphate salts	tripolyphosphate pentasodium β-glycerophosphate disodium * glucose-1-phosphate disodium * glucose-6-phosphate disodium *	
anionic polymer	*natural*	carrageenan gelatin hyaluronic acid kondagogu gum pectin γ-poly(glutamic acid) sodium alginate sodium dextran sulfate xanthan gum	
	synthetic	poly(acrylic acid) poly(methacrylate) poly(N-isopropylacrylamide)	carbomer polycarbophil Eudragit poloxamer

*: the nature of interaction between polyol-phosphate agents and chitosan has not been clearly elucidated.

Physical modification of the chitosan structure, in contrast to chemical crosslinking, is a simple and mild process which requires neither the presence of catalysts nor the purification of the final product. The enhanced stability of the chitosan PEC can be attributed to the interaction between cationic chitosan and negatively charged complex polymer, which prevents the protonation of chitosan amino groups. In addition, the large anionic molecules are thought to buffer the solution and thus slow down the rate of chitosan hydrolysis.

However, chitosan crosslinked with small size ions is considered as unstable material over an extended time period because of the presence of the electrolytes and pH variations when stored in solution [109]. To our best knowledge, only a few attempts to improve long-term physicochemical stability of chitosan material by incorporation of the small-size ionic crosslinker have been reported. Chitosan co-crystals with acyclovir prepared by a solvent change method using sodium citrate as the salting out compound exhibited good physical stability with regard to the drug content and drug release profile upon three-month storage at 40 °C/75% RH [110]. Singh et al., studied the long-term stability of cisplatin-loaded chitosan glutamate microparticles, crosslinked with citric acid prepared by emulsification-ionotropic gelation [28]. No significant changes in physical appearance and drug content in all formulations stored in high-density polyethylene containers at 40 °C/75% RH and 25 °C/60% RH upon correspondingly 6- and 12-month periods were noticed. However, an approximately 17%–19% increase in moisture content and subsequent rise in the particle size during both long-term and accelerated stability studies were observed suggesting that chitosan microparticles might be still susceptible to physicochemical degradation over time [28].

Among a variety of chitosan applications, the stability of microparticulate-based delivery systems is extremely important as it strongly depends on the surface electrostatic charge, which alters upon storage. Several strategies have been proposed to prevent aggregation and changes in the zeta potential of chitosan micro- and nanoparticles. Insulin-loaded nanoparticles prepared by complexation of chitosan with dextran sulfate exhibited no significant differences in zeta potential and mean particle size up to 28 days at 4 °C [29]. Van der Lubben et al., demonstrated three-month physicochemical stability of chitosan microparticles crosslinked with sodium sulfate stored in PBS suspension under both refrigerated and ambient conditions [20]. No statistical differences in morphology and size of the particles, drug content and the drug release profile were displayed. Nevertheless, the improved stability of the microparticles could be attributed to the presence of the nonionic stabilizer—a polyoxyethylene sorbitan sodium monooleate (polysorbate)—used during preparation rather than the ionic crosslinking process. The potential stabilizing effect of freeze-drying step upon the microparticles elaboration process cannot be excluded as well. In another investigation, devoted to the polyelectrolyte complex nanoparticles composed of chitosan and hyaluronate, the authors noticed that prepared particles were stable in suspension up to four-week storage at room conditions. An increase in the amount of hyaluronate was found to be responsible for obtaining more stable formulations with minor fluctuations of zeta potential over storage period [111]. Mitra et al., revealed that introduction of succinic acid into chitosan/collagen PEC, notably improved the mechanical strength and thermal stability of the scaffold material [112].

A detailed stability analysis was also carried out on the chitosan/β-glycerophosphate (β-GP) *in situ* gels [113,114]. Those novel chitosan/polyol-phosphate compositions have gained great attention in the biomedical field due to the fact that modified chitosan becomes thermosensitive in diluted acids and can undergo gelation around body temperature [115]. These properties make chitosan/polyol-phosphate material a promising tool for a variety of applications, such as local drug delivery systems or injectable carriers for tissue-engineering. It should be noted that although the type of reaction between chitosan and polyol-phosphates is close to physical crosslinking, the nature of this interaction has not been clearly explained [27,116]. The fact that gelation appears even under refrigerated conditions is a substantial problem limiting thermoresponsive *in situ* chitosan/β-GP systems applications. Ruel-Gariepy *et al.*, investigated the viscosity changes of chitosan/β-GP solutions upon three-month storage [117]. The studies revealed that the solution/gel transition appeared under both refrigerated as well as under room conditions [117]. Similarly, Schuetz *et al.*, observed a gelation of the chitosan/β-GP within four-week storage at 4 °C confirming the instability of the systems under refrigerated conditions [93]. In contrast, the study on chitosan/β-GP gel formulation intended for periodontitis treatment—stored in closed containers at 30 °C/75% RH displayed no changes in color, consistency, pH, viscosity, and drug content over 90 days [113]. In order to overcome the poor stability of chitosan/β-GP thermogelling systems, Supper *et al.*, proposed application of glycerol-1-phosphate as an alternative gelling agent for chitosan. The chitosan/glycerol-1-phosphate solutions were found to maintain their thermogelling properties for two months under ambient conditions and over nine months in a refrigerator [27].

Regardless of the above mentioned methods, it is extremely important to set-up the most suitable storage conditions which ensure sufficient stability of chitosan products. Hafner *et al.*, in the long-term stability study of lyophilised lecithin/chitosan nanoparticles loaded with melatonin found that storage at 4 °C enabled their physicochemical properties to be retained without significant loss of encapsulated drug within a period of seven months [91]. The substantial changes in the rheological behavior of chitosan hydrogels with antifungal agent stored for a period of three months at 25 °C in comparison to hydrogels placed at 4 °C were reported [118]. A considerable (almost 50%) loss in viscosity values of the polymer-based formulation and a decrease in its pH at ambient temperature were found, whereas the physical stability of refrigerated formulations was shown not to statistically alter [118]. No *et al.*, noticed the differences in viscosity of chitosan solutions at 4 °C and 25 °C after 15-week storage [78]. Although a drop of viscosity was more pronounced in solutions stored at ambient temperature, all chitosan formulations were characterized by weaker antibacterial activity compared to the antibacterial effect of freshly prepared solutions. However, Supper *et al.*, indicated that the chitosan/β-GP thermogelling solutions intended for parenteral administration had poor physicochemical stability both under room and refrigerated conditions [114].

Selection of suitable humidity conditions is also important, especially for storage of solid chitosan-based products. Although no international requirements or standard references have been provided, several studies confirmed that the rate of hydration of chitosan products rose extensively at high RH [59,119]. Apart from selecting the most suitable storage conditions, proper air-tight containers, in order to protect hygroscopic chitosan products against environmental humidity should be also considered.

5. Conclusions

Despite the great potential of using chitosan in drug delivery or tissue engineering systems, its poor long-term stability is a substantial drawback in the scaling-up of chitosan pharmaceutical applications. Upon storage, chitosan undergoes gradual chain degradation followed by destruction of its functional groups which as a consequence leads to irreversible loss of its physicochemical properties. Both intrinsic (degree of deacetylation, molecular weight, purity, and moisture level) and extrinsic factors (environmental storage conditions, thermal processing, sterilization, and processing involving acidic dissolution) are acknowledged as crucial parameters affecting the stability of the chitosan-based formulations. To improve chitosan stability, several strategies (addition of the stabilizing agent during the preparation process, blending with hydrophilic polymer, and use of ionic or chemical crosslinkers) have also been reported. As there are no universal principles to preserve chitosan-based products upon storage, preformulation studies and selection of the most proper storage conditions are essential to provide their maximal stability.

Acknowledgments: This research was supported by Medical University of Białystok (grant 153-15553 F).

Author Contributions: The authors participated equally in the review concept. Emilia Szymańska collected the data and wrote the article whereas Katarzyna Winnicka revised the article.

Conflicts of Interest: The authors declare no conflict of interest.

References

1. D'Ayala, G.G.; Malinconico, M.; Laurienzo, P. Marine derived polysaccharides for biomedical applications: Chemical modification approaches. *Molecules* **2008**, *13*, 2069–2106. [CrossRef] [PubMed]

2. Laurienzo, P. Marine polysaccharides in pharmaceutical applications: An overview. *Mar. Drugs* **2010**, *8*, 2435–2465. [CrossRef] [PubMed]

3. Saravanakumar, G.; Jo, D.G.; Park, J.H. Polysaccharide-based nanoparticles: A versatile platform for drug delivery and biomedical imaging. *Curr. Med. Chem.* **2012**, *19*, 3212–3229. [CrossRef] [PubMed]

4. Szymańska, E.; Winnicka, K. Preparation and *in vitro* evaluation of chitosan microgranules with clotrimazole. *Acta Pol. Pharm. Drug Res.* **2012**, *69*, 509–513.

5. Hurler, J.; Škalko-Basnet, N. Potentials of chitosan-based delivery systems in wound therapy: Bioadhesion study. *J. Funct. Biomater.* **2012**, *3*, 37–48. [CrossRef] [PubMed]

6. Okamoto, Y.; Yano, R.; Miyatake, K.; Tomohiro, I.; Shigemasa, Y.; Minami, S. Effects of chitin and chitosan on blood coagulation. *Carbohydr. Polym.* **2003**, *53*, 337–342. [CrossRef]

7. Kim, I.Y.; Seo, S.J.; Moon, H.S.; Yoo, M.K.; Park, I.Y.; Kim, B.C.; Cho, C.S. Chitosan and its derivatives for tissue engineering applications. *Biotechnol. Adv.* **2008**, *26*, 1–21. [CrossRef] [PubMed]

8. Venkatesan, J.; Bhatnagar, I.; Kim, S.K. Chitosan-alginate biocomposite containing fucoidan for bone tissue engineering. *Mar. Drugs* **2014**, *12*, 300–316. [CrossRef] [PubMed]

9. Hoemann, C.D.; Sun, J.; Légaré, A.; McKee, M.D.; Buschmann, M.D. Tissue engineering of cartilage using an injectable and adhesive chitosan-based cell-delivery vehicle. *Osteoarthritis Cartilage* **2005**, *13*, 318–329. [CrossRef] [PubMed]

10. Dash, M.; Chiellini, F.; Ottenbrite, R.M.; Chiellini, E. Chitosan—A versatile semi-synthetic polymer in biomedical applications. *Prog. Polym. Sci.* **2011**, *36*, 981–1014. [CrossRef]

11. Ifuku, S. Chitin and chitosan nanofibers: Preparation and chemical modifications. *Molecules* **2014**, *19*, 18367–18380. [CrossRef] [PubMed]

12. Mucha, M. Rheological characteristics of semi-dilute chitosan solutions. *Macromol. Chem. Phys.* **1997**, *198*, 471–484. [CrossRef]

13. Kassem, M.A.; ElMeshad, A.N.; Fares, A.R. Lyophilized sustained release mucoadhesive chitosan sponges for buccal buspirone hydrochloride delivery: Formulation and *in vitro* evaluation. *AAPS Pharm. Sci. Tech.* **2014**, *6*, 1–11.

14. Dehghan, M.H.G.; Kazi, M. Lyophilized chitosan/xanthan polyelectrolyte complex based mucoadhesive inserts for nasal delivery of promethazine hydrochloride. *Iran. J. Pharm. Res.* **2014**, *13*, 769–784. [PubMed]

15. Franca, J.R.; Foureaux, G.; Fuscaldi, L.L.; Ribeiro, T.G.; Rodrigues, L.B.; Bravo, R.; Castilho, R.O.; Yoshida, M.I.; Cardoso, V.N.; Fernandes, S.O.; *et al.* Bimatoprost-loaded ocular inserts as sustained release drug delivery systems for glaucoma treatment: *in vitro* and *in vivo* evaluation. *PLoS ONE* **2014**, *9*, e95461–e95472. [CrossRef] [PubMed]

16. Szymańska, E.; Winnicka, K.; Amelian, A.; Cwalina, U. Vaginal chitosan tablets with clotrimazole-design and evaluation of mucoadhesive properties using porcine vaginal mucosa, mucin and gelatin. *Chem. Pharm. Bull.* **2014**, *62*, 160–167. [CrossRef] [PubMed]

17. Yeh, T.H.; Hsu, L.W.; Tseng, M.T.; Lee, P.L.; Sonjae, K.; Ho, Y.C.; Sung, H.W. Mechanism and consequence of chitosan-mediated reversible epithelial tight junction opening. *Biomaterials* **2011**, *32*, 6164–6173. [PubMed]

18. Slütter, B.; Bal, S.M.; Que, I.; Kaijzel, E.; Löwik, C.; Bouwstra, J.; Jiskoot, W. Antigen-adjuvant nanoconjugates for nasal vaccination: An improvement over the use of nanoparticles? *Mol. Pharm.* **2010**, *7*, 2207–2215. [CrossRef] [PubMed]

19. Bal, S.M.; Slütter, B.; Verheul, R.; Bouwstra, J.A.; Jiskoot, W. Adjuvanted, antigen loaded *N*-trimethyl chitosan nanoparticles for nasal and intradermal vaccination: Adjuvant- and site-dependent immunogenicity in mice. *Eur. J. Pharm. Sci.* **2012**, *45*, 475–481. [CrossRef] [PubMed]

20. Van der Lubben, I.M.; Kersten, G.; Fretz, M.M.; Beuvery, C.; Coos Verhoef, J.; Junginger, H.E. Chitosan microparticles for mucosal vaccination against diphtheria: Oral and nasal efficacy studies in mice. *Vaccine* **2003**, *21*, 1400–1408.

21. Baker, W.L.; Tercius, A.; Anglade, M.; White, C.M.; Coleman, C.I. A meta-analysis evaluating the impact of chitosan on serum lipids in hypercholesterolemic patients. *Ann. Nutr. Metabl.* **2009**, *55*, 368–374. [CrossRef]

22. Akncbay, H.; Senel, S.; Ay, Z.Y. Application of chitosan gel in the treatment of chronic periodontitis. *J. Biomed. Mater. Res. B Appl. Biomater.* **2007**, *80*, 290–296. [CrossRef] [PubMed]

23. Kong, M.; Chen, X.G.; Xing, K.; Park, H.J. Antimicrobial properties of chitosan and mode of action: A state of the art review. *Int. J. Food Microbiol.* **2010**, *144*, 51–63. [CrossRef] [PubMed]

24. Palmeira-de-Oliveira, A.; Ribeiro, M.P.; Palmeira-de-Oliveira, R.; Gaspar, C.; Costa-de-Oliveira, S.; Correia, I.J.; Pina, V.; Martinez-de-Oliveira, J.; Queiroz, J.A.; Rodrigues, A.G. Anti-Candida activity of a chitosan hydrogel: Mechanism of action and cytotoxicity profile. *Gynecol. Obstet. Invest.* **2010**, *70*, 322–327. [CrossRef] [PubMed]

25. Szymańska, E.; Winnicka, K.; Wieczorek, P.; Sacha, P.T.; Tryniszewska, E.A. Influence of unmodified and beta-glycerophosphate cross-linked chitosan on anti-Candida activity of clotrimazole in semi-solid delivery systems. *Int. J. Mol. Sci.* **2014**, *15*, 17765–17777. [CrossRef] [PubMed]

26. Perioli, L.; Ambrogi, V.; Pagano, C.; Scuota, S.; Rossi, C. FC90 chitosan as a new polimer for metronidazole mucoadhesive tablets for vaginal administration. *Int. J. Pharm.* **2009**, *377*, 120–127. [CrossRef] [PubMed]

27. Supper, S.; Anton, N.; Boisclair, J.; Seidel, N.; Riemenschnitter, M.; Curdy, C.; Vandamme, T. Chitosan/glucose 1-phosphate as new stable *in situ* forming depot system for controlled drug delivery. *Eur. J. Pharm. Biopharm.* **2014**, *88*, 361–373. [CrossRef] [PubMed]

28. Singh, D.J.; Lohade, A.A.; Parmar, J.J.; Hegde, D.D.; Soni, P.; Samad, A.; Menon, M.D. Development of chitosan-based dry powder inhalation system of cisplatin for lung cancer. *Indian J. Pharm. Sci.* **2012**, *74*, 521–526. [CrossRef] [PubMed]

29. Sarmento, B.; Ribeiro, A.; Veiga, F.; Ferreira, D. Development and characterization of new insulin containing polysaccharide nanoparticles. *Colloids Surf. B Biointerfaces* **2006**, *53*, 193–202. [CrossRef] [PubMed]

30. Kurita, K.; Kaji, Y.; Mori, T.; Nishiyama, Y. Enzymatic degradation of β-chitin: Susceptibility and the influence of deacetylation. *Carbohydr. Polym.* **2000**, *42*, 19–21. [CrossRef]

31. Ma, Z.; Wang, W.; Wu, Y.; He, Y.; Wu, T. Oxidative degradation of chitosan to the low molecular water-soluble chitosan over peroxotungstate as chemical scissors. *PLoS ONE* **2014**, *9*, e100743–e100750. [CrossRef] [PubMed]

32. Mucha, M.; Pawlak, A. Complex study on chitosan degradability. *Polymer* **2002**, *47*, 43–51.

33. Knapczyk, J. Antimycotic buccal and vaginal tablets with chitosan. *Int. J. Pharm.* **1992**, *88*, 9–14. [CrossRef]

34. Kam, H.M.; Khor, E.; Lim, L.Y. Storage of partially deacetylated chitosan films. *J. Biomed. Mater. Res.* **1999**, *48*, 881–888. [CrossRef] [PubMed]

35. Jones, C.; Crane, D.T.; Lemercinier, X.; Bolgiano, B.; Yost, S.E. Physicochemical studies of the structure and stability of polysaccharide-protein conjugate vaccines. *Dev. Biol. Stand.* **1996**, *87*, 143–151. [PubMed]

36. Soldi, V. Stability and degradation of polysaccharides. In *Polysaccharides: Structural Diversity and Functional Versatility*, 2nd ed.; Dumitriu, S., Ed.; CRC Press: London, UK, 2004; Chapter 14; pp. 395–409.

37. Howling, S.E. Some observations on the effect of bioprocessing on biopolymer stability. *J. Drug Target.* **2010**, *18*, 732–740. [CrossRef] [PubMed]

38. *The European Pharmacopeia*, 6th ed.; Council of Europe: Strasburg, France, 2007; Volume 2, pp. 1490–1491.

39. *The United States Pharmacopeia*; USP 34–NF 29; The United States Pharmacopeial Convention: Rockville, MD, USA, 2011; pp. 5361–5365. Second Supplement.

40. Aranaz, I.; Mengíbar, M.; Harris, R.; Paños, I.; Miralles, B.; Acosta, N.; Galed, G.; Heras, Á. Functional characterization of chitin and chitosan. *Curr. Chem. Biol.* **2009**, *3*, 203–230.

41. Tsaih, M.L.; Chen, R.H. The effect of reaction time and temperature during heterogenous alkali deacetylation on degree of deacetylation and molecular weight of resulting chitosan. *J. Appl. Polym. Sci.* **2003**, *88*, 2917–2923. [CrossRef]

42. Markland, P.; Yang, V.C. Biodegradable polymers as drug carriers. In *Encyclopedia of Pharmaeutical Technology*, 3rd ed.; Swarbrick, J., Ed.; Informa Healthcare: New York, NY, USA, 2007; Volume 1, pp. 176–193.

43. Dimonie, D.; Dima, S.O.; Petrache, M. Influence of centrifugation on the molecular parameters of chitosan solubilized in weakly acidic aqueous solutions. *Dig. J. Nanomater. Bios.* **2013**, *8*, 1799–1809.

44. Buys, G.M.; du Plessis, L.H.; Marais, A.F.; Kotze, A.F.; Hamman, J.H. Direct compression of chitosan: Process and formulation factors to improve powder flow and tablet performance. *Curr. Drug Deliv.* **2013**, *10*, 348–356. [CrossRef] [PubMed]

45. Weinhold, M.X.; Sauvageau, J.C.M.; Kumirska, J.; Thöming, J. Studies on acetylation patterns of different chitosan preparations. *Carbohydr. Polym.* **2009**, *78*, 678–684. [CrossRef]

46. Zhang, H.; Neau, S.H. *In vitro* degradation of chitosan by a commercial enzyme preparation: Effect of molecular weight and degree of deacetylation. *Biomaterials* **2001**, *22*, 1653–1658. [CrossRef] [PubMed]

47. Francis, S.; Matthew, J.K.; Howard, W.T. Application of chitosan-based polysaccharide biomaterials in cartilage tissue engineering: A review. *Biomaterials* **2000**, *21*, 2589–2598. [CrossRef] [PubMed]

48. Yuan, Y.; Chesnutt, B.M.; Haggard, W.O.; Bumgardner, J.D. Deacetylation of chitosan: Material characterization and *in vitro* evaluation via albumin adsorption and pre-osteoblastic cell cultures. *Materials* **2011**, *4*, 1399–1416. [CrossRef]

49. Vårum, K.M.; Ottøy, M.H.; Smisrød, O. Acid hydrolysis of chitosan. *Carbohydr. Polym.* **2001**, *46*, 89–98. [CrossRef]

50. Lopez, F.A.; Merce, A.L.R.; Alguacil, F.J.; Lopez-Delgado, A. A kinetic study on the thermal behaviour of chitosan. *J. Therm. Anal. Calorim.* **2008**, *91*, 633–639. [CrossRef]

51. Wanjun, T.; Cunxin, W.; Donghua, C. Kinetic studies on the pyrolysis of chitin and chitosan. *Polym. Degrad. Stab.* **2005**, *87*, 389–394.

52. Bajer, D.; Kaczmarek, H. Study of the influence on UV radiation on biodegradable blends based on chitosan and starch. *Progr. Chem. Appl. Chitin Deriv.* **2010**, *15*, 17–24.

53. Davydova, V.N.; Yermak, I.M.; Gorbach, V.I.; Krasikova, I.N.; Solov'eva, T.F. Interaction of bacterial endotoxins with chitosan. Effect of endotoxin structure, chitosan molecular mass, and ionic strength of the solution on the formation of the complex. *Biochemistry (Mosc.)* **2000**, *65*, 1082–1090.

54. Gocho, H.; Shimizu, H.; Tanioka, A.; Chou, T.J.; Nakajima, T. Effect of polymer chain end on sorption isotherm of water by chitosan. *Carbohydr. Polym.* **2000**, *41*, 87–90. [CrossRef]

55. Rege, P.R.; Shukla, D.J.; Block, L.H. Chitinosans as tableting excipients for modified release delivery systems. *Int. J. Pharm.* **1999**, *181*, 49–60. [CrossRef] [PubMed]

56. Mucha, M.; Ludwiczak, S.; Kawińska, M. Kinetics of water sorption by chitosan and its blends with poly(vinyl alcohol). *Carbohydr. Polym.* **2005**, *62*, 42–49. [CrossRef]

57. Garr, J.M.S.; Rubinstein, M.H. The influence of moisture content on the consolidation and compaction properties of paracetamol. *Int. J. Pharm.* **1992**, *81*, 187–192. [CrossRef]

58. No, H.K.; Prinyawiwatkul, W. Stability of chitosan powder during long-term storage at room temperature. *J. Agric. Food Chem.* **2009**, *57*, 8434–8438. [CrossRef] [PubMed]

59. Viljoen, J.M.; Steenekamp, J.H.; Marais, A.F.; Kotzé, A.F. Effect of moisture content, temperature and exposure time on the physical stability of chitosan powder and tablets. *Drug Dev. Ind. Pharm.* **2014**, *40*, 730–742. [CrossRef] [PubMed]

60. Hollenbeck, R.G. Moisture in pharmaceutical products. In *Encyclopedia of Pharmaceutical Technology*, 3rd ed.; Swarbrick, J., Ed.; Informa Healthcare: New York, NY, USA, 2007; Volume 4, pp. 2368–2383.

61. Chooi, K.W.; Simão Carlos, M.I.; Soundararajan, R.; Gaisford, S.; Arifin, N.; Schätzlein, A.G.; Uchegbu, I.F. Physical characterisation and long-term stability studies on quaternary ammonium palmitoyl glycol chitosan (GCPQ)-a new drug delivery polymer. *J. Pharm. Sci.* **2014**, *103*, 2296–2306. [CrossRef] [PubMed]

62. EMA: Stability testing of new drug substances and products. Available online: http://www.ema.europa. eu/docs/en_GB/document_library/Scientific_guideline/2013/01/WC500002651.pdf(ICHTopicQ1AR2) (accessed on 10 February 2015).

63. Despond, S.; Espuche, E.; Domard, A. Water sorption and permeation in chitosan films: Relation between gas permeability and relative humidity. *J. Polym. Sci. B Polym. Phys.* **2001**, *39*, 3114–3127. [CrossRef]

64. Cervera, M.F.; Karjalainen, M.; Airaksinen, S.; Rantanen, J.; Krogars, K.; Heinämäki, J.; Colarte, A.I.; Yliruusi, J. Physical stability and moisture sorption of aqueous chitosan-amylose starch films plasticized with polyols. *Eur. J. Pharm. Biopharm.* **2004**, *58*, 69–76. [CrossRef] [PubMed]

65. Kurek, M.; Guinault, A.; Voilley, A.; Galić, K.; Debeaufort, F. Effect of relative humidity on carvacrol release and permeation properties of chitosan based films and coatings. *Food Chem.* **2014**, *144*, 9–17. [CrossRef] [PubMed]

66. Smart, J.D. The basics and underlying mechanisms of mucoadhesion. *Adv. Drug Deliv. Rev.* **2005**, *57*, 1556–1568. [CrossRef] [PubMed]

67. Nguyen, T.T.B.; Hein, S.; Ng, C.H.; Stevens, W.F. Molecular stability of chitosan in acid solutions stored at various conditions. *J. Appl. Polym. Sci.* **2008**, *107*, 2588–2593. [CrossRef]

68. Il'ina, A.V.; Varlamov, V.P. Hydrolysis of chitosan in lactic acid. *Appl. Biochem. Microbiol.* **2004**, *40*, 300–303. [CrossRef]

69. Jarry, C.; Chaput, C.; Chenite, A.; Renaud, M.A.; Buschmann, M.; Leroux, J.C. Effects of steam sterilization on thermogelling chitosan-based gels. *J. Biomed. Mater. Res.* **2001**, *58*, 127–135. [CrossRef] [PubMed]

70. Toffey, A.; Samaranayake, G.; Frazier, C.E.; Glasser, W.G. Chitin derivatives. I. Kinetics of the heat-induced conversion of chitosan to chitin. *J. Appl. Polym. Sci.* **1996**, *60*, 75–85. [CrossRef]

71. Lim, L.Y.; Khor, E.; Ling, C.E. Effects of dry heat and saturated steam on the physical properties of chitosan. *J. Biomed. Mater. Res.* **1999**, *48*, 111–116. [CrossRef] [PubMed]

72. Yang, Y.M.; Zhao, Y.H.; Liu, X.H.; Ding, F.; Gu, X.S. The effect of different sterilization procedures on chitosan dried powder. *J. Appl. Polym. Sci.* **2007**, *104*, 1968–1972. [CrossRef]

73. San Juan, A.; Montembault, A.; Gillet, D.; Say, J.P.; Rouif, S.; Bouet, T.; Royaud, I.; David, L. Degradation of chitosan-based materials after different sterilization treatments. *IOP Conf. Ser. Mater. Sci. Eng.* **2012**, *31*, 1–5.

74. Lim, L.Y.; Khor, E.; Koo, O. Gamma irradiation of chitosan. *J. Biomed. Mater. Res.* **1998**, *43*, 282–290. [CrossRef] [PubMed]

75. Jarry, C.; Leroux, J.C.; Haeck, J.; Chaput, C. Irradiating or autoclaving chitosan/polyol solutions: Effect on thermogelling chitosan-beta-glycerophosphate systems. *Chem. Pharm. Bull.* **2002**, *50*, 1335–1340.

76. Marreco, P.R.; da Luz Moreira, P.; Genari, S.C.; Moraes, A.M. Effects of different sterilization methods on the morphology, mechanical properties, and cytotoxicity of chitosan membranes used as wound dressings. *J. Biomed. Mater. Res. B Appl. Biomater.* **2004**, *71*, 268–277. [CrossRef] [PubMed]

77. França, R.; Mbeh, D.A.; Samani, T.D.; le Tien, C.; Mateescu, M.A.; Yahia, L.; Sacher, E. The effect of ethylene oxide sterilization on the surface chemistry and *in vitro* cytotoxicity of several kinds of chitosan. *J. Biomed. Mater. Res. B Appl. Biomater.* **2013**, *101*, 1444–1455. [CrossRef] [PubMed]

78. No, H.K.; Kim, S.H.; Lee, S.H.; Park, N.Y.; Prinyawiwatkul, W. Stability and antibacterial activity of chitosan solutions affected by storage temperature and time. *Carbohydr. Polym.* **2006**, *65*, 174–178. [CrossRef]

79. Corazzari, I.; Nisticò, R.; Turci, F.; Faga, M.G.; Franzoso, F.; Tabasso, S.; Magnacca, G. Advanced physico-chemical characterization of chitosan by means of TGA coupled on-line with FTIR and GCMS: Thermal degradation and water adsorption capacity. *Polym. Degrad. Stabil.* **2015**, *112*, 1–9. [CrossRef]

80. Diab, M.A.; El-Sonbati, A.Z.; Bader, D.M. Thermal stability and degradation of chitosan modified by benzophenone. *Spectrochim. Acta A. Mol. Biomol. Spectrosc.* **2011**, *79*, 1057–1062. [CrossRef] [PubMed]

81. Pieróg, M.; Ostrowska-Czubenko, J.; Gierszewska-Drużyńska, M. Thermal degradation of double crosslinked hydrogel chitosan mebranes. *Progr. Chem. Appl. Chitin Deriv.* **2012**, *17*, 67–74.

82. Zawadzki, J.; Kaczmarek, H. Thermal treatment of chitosan in various conditions. *Carbohydr. Polym.* **2010**, *80*, 394–400. [CrossRef]

83. Dhawade, P.P.; Jagtap, R.N. Characterization of the glass transition temperature of chitosan and its oligomers by temperature modulated differential scanning calorimetry. *Adv. Appl. Sci. Res.* **2012**, *3*, 1372–1382.

84. Prata, A.S.; Grosso, C.R. Production of microparticles with gelatin and chitosan. *Carbohydr. Polym.* **2015**, *116*, 292–299. [CrossRef] [PubMed]

85. Keegan, G.M.; Smart, J.D.; Ingram, M.J.; Barnes, L.M.; Burnett, G.R.; Rees, G.D. Chitosan microparticles for the controlled delivery of fluoride. *J. Dent.* **2012**, *40*, 229–240. [CrossRef] [PubMed]

86. Cal, K.; Sollohub, K. Spray drying technique. I: Hardware and process parameters. *J. Pharm. Sci.* **2010**, *99*, 575–586. [PubMed]

87. Rampino, A.; Borgogna, M.; Blasi, P.; Bellich, B.; Cesàro, A. Chitosan nanoparticles: Preparation, size evolution and stability. *Int. J. Pharm.* **2013**, *455*, 219–228. [CrossRef] [PubMed]

88. Yonekura, L.; Sun, H.; Soukoulis, C.; Fisk, I. Microencapsulation of Lactobacillus acidophilus NCIMB 701748 in matrices containing soluble fibre by spray drying: Technological characterization, storage stability and survival after *in vitro* digestion. *J. Funct. Foods* **2014**, *6*, 205–214. [CrossRef] [PubMed]

89. Huang, Y.; Yeh, M.; Chiang, C. Formulation factors in preparing BTM-chitosan microspheres by spray drying method. *Int. J. Pharm.* **2002**, *242*, 239–242. [CrossRef] [PubMed]

90. Aranaz, I.; Gutiérrez, M.C.; Ferrer, M.L.; del Monte, F. Preparation of chitosan nanocomposites with a macroporous structure by unidirectional freezing and subsequent freeze-drying. *Mar. Drugs* **2014**, *12*, 5619–5642. [CrossRef] [PubMed]

91. Hafner, A.; Dürrigl, M.; Pepić, I.; Filipović-Grčić, J. Short- and long-term stability of lyophilised melatonin-loaded lecithin/chitosan nanoparticles. *Chem. Pharm. Bull.* **2011**, *59*, 1117–1123. [CrossRef] [PubMed]

92. Abdelwahed, W.; Degobert, G.; Stainmess, S.; Fessi, H. Freeze-drying of nanoparticles Formulation, process and storage considerations. *Adv. Drug Deliv. Rev.* **2006**, *58*, 1688–1713. [CrossRef] [PubMed]

93. Schuetz, Y.B.; Gurny, R.; Jordan, O. A novel thermoresponsive hydrogel based on chitosan. *Eur. J. Pharm. Biopham.* **2008**, *68*, 19–25. [CrossRef]

94. Luangtana-Anan, M.; Limmatvapirat, S.; Nunthanid, J.; Chalongsuk, R.; Yamamoto, K. Polyethylene glycol on stability of chitosan microparticulate carrier for protein. *AAPS Pharm. Sci. Tech.* **2010**, *11*, 1376–1382. [CrossRef]

95. Mao, H.-Q.; Roy, K.; Troung-Le, V.L.; Janes, K.A.; Lin, K.Y.; Wang, Y.; August, J.T.; Leong, K.W. Chitosan-DNA nanoparticles as gene carriers: Synthesis, characterization and transfection efficiency. *J. Control. Release* **2001**, *70*, 399–421. [CrossRef] [PubMed]

96. Hermans, K.; van den Plas, D.; Kerimova, S.; Carleer, R.; Adriaensens, P.; Weyenberg, W.; Ludwig, A. Development and characterization of mucoadhesive chitosan films for ophthalmic delivery of cyclosporine A. *Int. J. Pharm.* **2014**, *472*, 10–19. [CrossRef] [PubMed]

97. Wu, D.; Delair, T. Stabilization of chitosan/hyaluronate colloidal polyelectrolyte complexes in physiological conditions. *Carbohydr. Polym.* **2015**, *119*, 149–158. [CrossRef] [PubMed]

98. Khoo, C.G.; Frantzich, S.; Rosinski, A.; Sjöström, M.; Hoogstraate, J. Oral gingival delivery systems from chitosan blends with hydrophilic polymers. *Eur. J. Pharm. Biopharm.* **2003**, *55*, 47–56. [CrossRef] [PubMed]

99. El-Hefian, E.A.; Nasef, M.M.; Yahaya, A.H. Chitosan-based polymer blends: Current status and applications. *J. Chem. Soc. Pak.* **2014**, *36*, 11–28.

100. Gupta, K.C.; Jabrail, F.H. Glutaraldehyde and glyoxal cross-linked chitosan microspheres for controlled delivery of centchroman. *Carbohydr. Res.* **2006**, *341*, 744–756. [CrossRef] [PubMed]

101. Li, B.; Shan, C.L.; Zhou, Q.; Fang, Y.; Wang, Y.L.; Xu, F.; Han, L.R.; Ibrahim, M.; Guo, L.B.; Xie, G.L.; *et al.* Synthesis, characterization, and antibacterial activity of cross-linked chitosan-glutaraldehyde. *Mar. Drugs* **2013**, *11*, 1534–1552. [CrossRef] [PubMed]

102. Minet, E.P.; O'Carroll, C.; Rooney, D.; Breslin, C.; McCarthy, C.P.; Gallagher, L.; Richards, K.G. Slow delivery of a nitrification inhibitor (dicyandiamide) to soil using a biodegradable hydrogel of chitosan. *Chemosphere* **2013**, *93*, 2854–2858. [CrossRef] [PubMed]

103. Fernandes, M.; Gonçalves, I.C.; Nardecchia, S.; Amaral, I.F.; Barbosa, M.A.; Martins, M.C. Modulation of stability and mucoadhesive properties of chitosan microspheres for therapeutic gastric application. *Int. J. Pharm.* **2013**, *454*, 116–124. [CrossRef] [PubMed]

104. Kyzas, G.Z.; Bikiaris, D.N. Recent modifications of chitosan for adsorption applications: A critical and systematic review. *Mar. Drugs* **2015**, *13*, 312–337. [CrossRef] [PubMed]

105. Liu, C.; Thormann, E.; Claesson, P.M.; Tyrode, E. Surface grafted chitosan gels. Part II. Gel formation and characterization. *Langmuir* **2014**, *30*, 8878–8888. [CrossRef] [PubMed]

106. Mekhail, M.; Jahan, K.; Tabrizian, M. Genipin-crosslinked chitosan/poly-L-lysine gels promote fibroblast adhesion and proliferation. *Carbohydr. Polym.* **2014**, *108*, 91–98. [CrossRef] [PubMed]

107. Butler, M.F.; Clark, A.H.; Adams, S. Swelling and mechanical properties of biopolymer hydrogels containing chitosan and bovine serum albumin. *Biomacromolecules* **2006**, *7*, 2961–2970. [CrossRef] [PubMed]

108. Hamman, J.H. Chitosan Based Polyelectrolyte Complexes as Potential Carrier Materials in Drug Delivery Systems. *Mar. Drugs* **2010**, *8*, 1305–1322. [CrossRef] [PubMed]

109. Dautzenberg, H.; Kriz, J. Response of polyelectrolyte complexes to subsequent addition of salts with different cations. *Langmuir* **2003**, *19*, 5204–5211. [CrossRef]

110. Allam, A.N.; Naggar, V.F.; El Gamal, S.S. Formulation and physicochemical characterization of chitosan/acyclovir co-crystals. *Pharm. Dev. Technol.* **2013**, *18*, 856–865. [CrossRef] [PubMed]

111. Umerska, A.; Paluch, K.J.; Inkielewicz-Stępniak, I.; Santos-Martinez, M.J.; Corrigan, O.I.; Medina, C.; Tajber, L. Exploring the assembly process and properties of novel crosslinker-free hyaluronate-based polyelectrolyte complex nanocarriers. *Int. J. Pharm.* **2012**, *436*, 75–87. [CrossRef] [PubMed]

112. Mitra, T.; Sailakshmi, G.; Gnanamani, A.; Mandal, A.B. Studies on cross-linking of succinic acid with chitosan/collagen. *Materials Res.* **2013**, *16*, 755–765. [CrossRef]

113. Ruan, H.; Yu, Y.; Liu, Y.; Ding, X.; Guo, X.; Jiang, Q. Preparation and characteristics of thermoresponsive gel of minocycline hydrochloride and evaluation of its effect on experimental periodontitis models. *Drug Deliv.* **2014**, *25*, 1–7. [CrossRef]

114. Supper, S.; Anton, N.; Seidel, N.; Riemenschnitter, M.; Schoch, C.; Vandamme, T. Rheological study of chitosan/polyol-phosphate systems: Influence of the polyol part on the thermo-induced gelation mechanism. *Langmuir* **2013**, *29*, 10229–10237. [CrossRef] [PubMed]

115. Supper, S.; Anton, N.; Seidel, N.; Riemenschnitter, M.; Curdy, C.; Vandamme, T. Thermosensitive chitosan/glycerophosphate-based hydrogel and its derivatives in pharmaceutical and biomedical applications. *Expert Opin. Drug Deliv.* **2014**, *11*, 249–267. [CrossRef] [PubMed]
116. Chenite, A.; Chaput, C.; Wang, D.; Combes, C.; Buschmann, M.D.; Hoemann, C.D.; Leroux, J.C.; Atkinson, B.L.; Binette, F.; Selmani, A. Novel injectable neutral solutions of chitosan form biodegradable gels *in situ. Biomaterials* **2000**, *21*, 2155–2161. [CrossRef] [PubMed]
117. Ruel-Gariépy, E.; Chenite, A.; Chaput, C.; Guirguis, S.; Leroux, J. Characterization of thermosensitive chitosan gels for the sustained delivery of drugs. *Int. J. Pharm.* **2000**, *203*, 89–98. [CrossRef] [PubMed]
118. Celebi, N.; Ermiş, S.; Ozkan, S. Development of topical hydrogels of terbinafine hydrochloride and evaluation of their antifungal activity. *Drug Dev. Ind. Pharm.* **2014**. [CrossRef]
119. Murray, C.A.; Dutcher, J.R. Effect of changes in relative humidity and temperature on ultrathin chitosan films. *Biomacromolecules* **2006**, *7*, 3460–3465. [CrossRef] [PubMed]

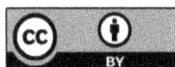

marine drugs

Review

Fucoidan as a Potential Therapeutic for Major Blinding Diseases—A Hypothesis

Alexa Klettner

Department of Ophthalmology, University Medical Center, University of Kiel, 24105 Kiel, Germany;
aklettner@auge.uni-kiel.de; Tel.: +0049-431-597-2401; Fax: +0049-431-597-3140

Academic Editor: Paola Laurienzo
Received: 30 November 2015; Accepted: 22 January 2016; Published: 3 February 2016

Abstract: Fucoidan is a heterogeneous group of sulfated polysaccharide with a high content of L-fucose, which can be extracted from brown algae and marine invertebrates. It has many beneficial biological activities that make fucoidan an interesting candidate for therapeutic application in a variety of diseases. Age-related macular degeneration and diabetic retinopathy are major causes for vision loss and blindness in the industrialized countries and increasingly in the developing world. Some of the characteristics found in certain fucoidans, such as its anti-oxidant activity, complement inhibition or interaction with the Vascular Endothelial Growth factor, which would be of high interest for a potential application of fucoidan in age-related macular degeneration or diabetic retinopathy. However, the possible usage of fucoidan in ophthalmological diseases has received little attention so far. In this review, biological activities of fucoidan that could be of interest regarding these diseases will be discussed.

Keywords: fucoidan; age-related macular degeneration; diabetic retinopathy; oxidative stress; VEGF; complement

1. Introduction

Fucoidans are sulfated polysaccharides found in the cell-wall matrix of phaeophyceae and in some marine invertebrates that contain high amounts of L-fucose [1]. The structure of fucoidans is highly complex and may differ substantially in composition and chemical structure between the species, depending also on regional and seasonal influences, and even on the method of extraction [1–3]. Because of a wide variety of beneficial biological activities, fucoidans have been considered as a potential treatment option for different diseases; however, so far no therapeutic application has been developed [3]. A field in which the therapeutic options of fucoidan have received little attention so far is ophthalmology. In this review, the activities of fucoidan will be discussed that might indicate a beneficial effect for two major blinding diseases in the industrialized countries, diabetic retinopathy (DR) and age-related macular degeneration (AMD).

1.1. Basic Structure of the Posterior Part of the Eye

In order to obtain visual input from the surroundings, the photoreceptors of the retina need to be stimulated by light. These photoreceptors are maintained by a single-layered epithelium located beneath them, the retinal pigment epithelium (RPE). These cells have many functions in order to maintain vision, as for example they comprise the outer blood-retinal barrier, transport nutrients and waste, recycle the visual pigment, and secrete growth factors [4]. The supply of nutrients and oxygen for photoreceptors is mainly provided by the choroid, a bed of vessels located beneath the retina [5]. The transduction of the signal is conducted by the neuroretinal layers downstream of the photoreceptors, culminating in the ganglion cells that transduce the information via the optic nerve to the brain. These retinal layers also contain vessels to supply them with oxygen and nutrients. In order to protect the retina from danger, specific cells of the monocytic lineage can be found in the retina, the so-called microglia, which convey innate immunity protection [6]. Interestingly, primates including humans, in contrast to other mammals, have a specific area in their retina, called the macula. This region is anatomically specified to facilitate high acuity vision [7].

1.2. Age-Related Macular Degeneration

Age-related macular degeneration is the major cause of blindness and severe visual impairment in the industrialized countries [8]. While the early forms of AMD are generally asymptomatic, the two late forms of AMD are associated with a devastating loss of vision. In the late "dry" form of the disease, geographic atrophy, extensive areas of the macula display a degeneration of the photoreceptors and the RPE. In the exudative "wet" form of AMD, vessels grow from the choroid beneath and into the retina. These vessels are immature and leaky, inducing tissue-destructive effects on photoreceptors and RPE. In addition, fluid accumulation under the macula occurs. The pathogenesis of AMD is so far not completely elucidated, but several factors have been implicated to contribute [9,10]. Environmental factors such as smoking and genetic susceptibilities have been shown to be significantly associated with the development of AMD. In addition, oxidative stress [11], as well as inflammatory factors, has been implicated [9]. Here, the complement system is of highest interest, as most genetic susceptibilities are connected to the complement system—mainly with the alternative pathway of the complement system [12,13].

In addition, activation of the resident microglia of the retina is currently discussed as a potential pathogenic factor in AMD, though its contribution is not clear [6]. Similarly, the migration of macrophage in the subretinal space is discussed as a possible pathogenic factor, as a healthy retina is devoid of macrophages [14].

For the development of exudative AMD, the Vascular Endothelial Growth Factor (VEGF) has been identified as the most important factor and considered to be prerequisite for the development of choroidal neovascularizations (CNV) (see below). Anti-VEGF therapies are the current gold standard for wet AMD treatment [8]. However, these treatments hold no cure for the disease, and the inhibitors, injected intravitreally, have to be given on a regular base. Visual decline is common even under therapy [15]. New treatment options are clearly warranted.

1.3. Diabetic Retinopathy

Diabetes is a chronic disease that is characterized by hyperglycemia, either resulting from a deficiency of insulin secretion, e.g., by autoimmunogenic destruction of the insulin producing pancreatic cells, or by an impaired insulin action. Diabetic retinopathy (DR) is the most frequent complication of diabetes, and one of the leading causes of visual impairment and blindness in the working population, both in the developed and the developing world [16].

Early signs of DR include microaneurysms, the loss of pericytes from retinal capillaries, and a breakdown of the blood-retinal-barrier, as well as retinal hemorrhages and exudates [17,18]. The most important factor in developing DR is the blood glucose level. In fact, early glycemic control may have lasting beneficial effects [19]. Hyperglycemia induces oxidative stress and low grade inflammation. [17]. Microangiopathy due to hyperglycemia leads to vascular leakage, causing edema. Another important risk factor for DR is hypertension [20]. In diabetic retinopathy, retinal pericytes and endothelial cells may die of apoptosis; here, reactive oxygen species concomitant with NFκB activation have been described to be of importance [16]. Leukostasis, in which immune cells become trapped in the retinal capillaries, induce a leukocyte-endothelial reaction. This may lead to an upregulation of pro-inflammatory cytokines and also to an occlusion of retinal capillaries [16]. Macrophages and neutrophils seem to be important for these processes [21,22]. The lack of perfusion induces ischemia, which, in turn, activates hypoxia-inducible factor (HIF)-1α and, consequently, VEGF. This can lead to the uncontrolled growth of new vessels, inducing proliferative diabetic retinopathy (PDR). In addition, the alteration of the retina in diabetes can disrupt the barrier function of the retinal endothelial cells and lead to fluid accumulation in the macular region (macular edema) [16]. A key element in the development both of PDR and macular edema is the growth factor VEGF.

1.4. Vascular Endothelial Growth Factor

VEGF (used synonymously for VEGF-A) is the most important angiogenic factor in development and disease [23,24]. The loss of one allele of its gene is embryonically lethal, and VEGF has been implicated in the development of cancer vascularization and of choroidal and retinal neovascularizations [25,26]. Of note, VEGF is also active in the healthy retina, where it exerts protective effects on neurons and the RPE, and where it maintains the endothelium of the choriocapillaris [27].

VEGF is expressed in different isoforms due to alternative splicing of the VEGF gene [28]. A wide variety of VEGF isoforms has been described; however, the most important are VEGF165 and VEGF121 [29,30]. The isoforms differ in their molecular weight and their ability to bind heparin-like molecules [31].

In order to regulate angiogenesis, different isoforms of VEGF can bind to its receptors, the tyrosine kinases VEGF-receptor (VEGFR-)1 and VEGFR-2, and, depending on the isoform, neuropilins (NRP1, NRP2) as co-receptors [32,33]. Several downstream pathways are involved in VEGF signaling, such as the mitogen activated protein kinase (MAPK) ERK1/2 in mitogenic signaling, phosphatidyl-inositol 3 kinase (PI3K) and Akt in survival signaling, and endothelial nitric oxide synthase (NOS) and p38 in permeability increase [34,35].

VEGF is regulated by a plethora of factors and inducible by many stimuli [32]. The major stimulus for VEGF upregulation is hypoxia, and the major transcription factor conveying this induction is HIF-1α [36]. Other transcription factors of importance for VEGF regulation include Sp1, Stat3 and NFκB [37,38]. Sp-1 and NFκB have been shown to be of particular importance in constitutive VEGF expression in the RPE [39,40]. A stimulus of high importance for VEGF expression, also considered a major factor in AMD and DR development [41,42], is oxidative stress. The retina is a location of high oxidative stress [11], and the oxidative burden accumulates over a lifetime. VEGF regulation of oxidative stress differs from constitutive VEGF expression. For oxidative stress, a role of the MAPK ERK1/2 has been described that was not found for constitutive VEGF expression [43].

2. Fucoidan

2.1. Fucoidan and VEGF

Fucoidan displayed several anti-VEGF functions in a variety of systems and seems to interfere with VEGF-induced signaling. Studies have shown that fucoidan can downregulate HIF-1α/VEGF signaling under hypoxia, as well as downregulate the phosphorylation of PI3K/Akt signaling [44–46]. Fucoidan has been shown to reduce the expression of the VEGF-receptors and even more of the VEGF co-receptors neuropilin [47]. In this setting, fucoidan inhibited the binding of VEGF to human umbilical vein endothelial cells (HUVEC) and inhibited HUVEC proliferation in response to VEGF [47]. This effect can be enhanced by oversulfation of fucoidan (*Fucus vesiculosus*) [48]. The authors show that both normal and oversulfated fucoidan with a molecular weight of 100–130 kDa prevent VEGF-induced phosphorylation of VEGFR-2, most likely by preventing binding of VEGF to its target [48]. Fucoidan from the same source (*Fucus vesiculosus*) reduced the expression of VEGF in tumor-bearing mice, concomitantly with a decrease in NFκB expression [49], a transcription factor shown to be important for VEGF expression [37,40]. Fucoidan from *Undaria pinnatifida* significantly reduced the expression of VEGF in HUVEC, suppressing its angiogenic activity [50]. Interestingly, while generally only an effect on VEGF165 is shown, as fucoidan does not bind to VEGF121, in this study, a reduction of expression is found also for VEGF121 [50]. Autoregulatory pathways involving VEGF binding to the VEGFR-2 have been described in VEGF regulation, with a positive feedback loop being induced by VEGF binding to its VEGFR-2 [39], which may offer an explanation as to how VEGF121 can be affected by an agent that does not bind to VEGF121. Cancer cells, such as HeLa, also show a reduced expression and secretion of VEGF under fucoidan treatment [51].

In a study of Chen *et al.*, low molecular weight (LMW) fucoidan reduced tube-like structure formation in HUVEC in hypoxic but not in normoxic conditions [44], which, considering the physiological role of VEGF in the retina, would be a big benefit compared to anti-VEGF molecules applied today, which do not discriminate between physiological and pathological VEGF.

It is important to note that the actions of fucoidan on VEGF are dependent on the molecular weight, the degree of sulfation, the source of the fucoidan and its concentration, and that pro-angiogenic activities of fucoidan have also been described [52]. For example, LMW fucoidan extracted from *Fucus vesiculosus* has been shown to induce endothelial cell migration by enhancing the binding of VEGF165 to its receptors VEGFR-2 and NRP1, which seemed to be a dose-dependent effect, as tube formation by HUVEC was increased at concentrations of 1 µg/mL and 10 µg/mL, while at 100 µg/mL the effect became inhibitory [53]. Indeed, fucoidan is used in scaffolds to load them with VEGF165 and to intensify the vascularization response [54].

It also must be noted that most of these studies were conducted in HUVEC cells or tumor-bearing mice. For the ophthalmological setting, neither of these models is appropriate to indicate beneficial effects. In the ophthalmological setting, VEGF expression and HIF-1α induction were reduced in retinas of diabetic mice treated with LMW fucoidan from *Laminaria japonica* [45]. VEGF is also reduced in a dose-dependent manner in brain microvascular endothelial cells treated with LMW fucoidan from *Laminaria japonica* [45]. Moreover, a study conducted with fucoidan from *Fucus vesiculosus* in different retinal pigment epithelium model systems clearly showed a reduction of VEGF secretion and expression over time [55]. Interestingly, a reduction of expression can be found even when coapplied with the anti-VEGF reagent bevacizumab. Moreover, the angiogenic potential induced by VEGF165 or RPE supernatant was reduced by fucoidan in this setting, clearly indicating a potential beneficial effect in choroidal neovascularizations [55].

These data implicate a possible potential effect of fucoidans in ophthalmology to treat VEGF induced pathologies; however, the bioactivity and concentration of the respective fucoidan used must be meticulously tested in order to eliminate potential unwanted adverse effects ameliorating VEGF-induced conditions.

2.2. Fucoidan and Oxidative Stress

An important feature of diabetic retinopathy and in age-related macular degeneration is the prevalence of oxidative stress [16,56]. Oxidative stress can be induced by the exposure to high energy wavelength of the visible light spectrum, especially combined with the high oxygen tension found in the retina [11]. In addition, hyperglycemia as encountered in diabetes can induce oxidative stress in the tissue, e.g., by upregulating the generation of superoxide radicals [57].

Fucoidan has been shown to have anti-oxidative properties [58], predominantly by scavenging superoxide radicals [59]. The antioxidative ability varies between fucoidans of different sources, with a positive correlation between sulfate content and radical scavenging ability [59–61]. The exact mechanisms of the scavenging abilities have not been elucidated so far, but have been suggested to be related to molecular weight (as small polysaccharides provide more reducing ends) and to uronic acid content [60]. In addition, fucoidan has also been shown to induce the expression of the transcription factor nuclear factor erythroid-2 related factor 2 (Nrf2) [61], an important transcription factor in anti-oxidant defense in the RPE [11], and its target gene superoxide dismutase [62]. Reduced Nrf2 activity may be involved in the development of AMD, as Nrf2 knock-out mice develop an AMD-like pathology [63], and the knock-out of Nrf2 renders RPE cells highly susceptible to oxidative stress-induced cell death [64].

Its anti-oxidant and protective effects have been shown in several biological systems. In tumor cells, fucoidan of *Cladosiphon* decreased both intracellular and released hydrogen peroxide (H_2O_2) levels [51]. Concomitantly, fucoidan suppressed the secretion of VEGF (see above). LMW fucoidan from *Undaria pinnatifida* suppressed oxidative stress in RAW264.7 cells, a macrophage cell line [65], and fucoidan from *Ecklonia cava* protected from oxidative stress in a zebrafish model [66] or, obtained from *Fucus vesiculosus*, from oxidative stress in liver fibroses [62]. In addition, fucoidan from *Cladosiphon okamuranus* prevented the disruption of the intestinal barrier function induced by H_2O_2 in Caco-2 cells [67]. This might be of special interest in diabetic retinopathy, where increased paracellular permeability of the retinal endothelial cells contributes strongly to the development of diabetic macular edema [68].

Little is known on the antioxidant properties of fucoidans in cells of the eye, but fucoidan was shown to protect ARPE19 cells, a human RPE cell line, from oxidative stress-induced by high glucose [69]. It protected the cells from cell death and normalized the generation of reactive oxygen species. In addition, it inhibited the activation of ERK1/2, a major factor in oxidative stress-induced VEGF upregulation [43,69]. These data indicate that the anti-oxidative properties of fucoidan may be beneficial in AMD or diabetic retinopathy.

2.3. Fucoidan and Complement

The complement system is an enzyme cascade of the innate immune system that protects the organism from harm by facilitating phagocytic uptake, activation of immune cells and lysis of harmful cells or microorganisms, and it links the innate immunity with adaptive defense. The complement system can be activated mainly via the classical pathway, induced by the binding of the factor C1q to microorganisms or antibody/antigen complexes, or the alternative pathway, induced mainly by a spontaneous activation of the factor C3 [13].

Fucoidan has been described to inhibit the activation of the classical, and, to a lesser extent, of the alternative pathway. Fucoidan has been shown to bind to C1q and C4, inhibiting the first steps of the classical pathway activation [70]. Additionally, a partial effect on the activation of C3 was observed, suppressing the C3 convertase [70,71]. Of note, the binding of CFB to C3b can be inhibited by fucoidan [70], which may be of particular interest since polymorphism of the CFB gene may contribute to a higher risk for AMD [72].

The action of fucoidan on the complement system is strongly dependent on its molecular composition. Sulfate groups have been described to be necessary but not sufficient for anti-complement activity, and the anti-complement activity to be dependent on the content of galactose and glucuronic acid, as shown for fucoidans of *Ascophyllum nodosum* [73]. In addition, molecular weight is an important factor, yet no simple correlation of weight and anti-complement activity can be postulated, with different molecular weight showing an optimum of inhibition concerning the classical and the alternative pathway [73]. The same authors show that the inhibitory effect on the formation of the C3 convertase cannot be shown for fucoidans with MW below 16,600 kDa [71].

These data indicate a potential beneficial effect of fucoidan on the pathogenesis of AMD. However, it must be noted that the effect of fucoidan is mainly on the pathway of classical activation, while it is the alternative pathway that is implicated for AMD pathogenesis. Moreover, the direct role of the complement system on the development of AMD has not been elucidated so far. In addition, as described above, the effect of fucoidan on the complement system is highly dependent on their chemical composition and needs to be elucidated thoroughly before preclinical or clinical testing can be considered.

2.4. Fucoidan and Monocyte-Likes Cells (Microglia, Macrophages)

Microglia activation in the retina has been discussed as a factor for the development of AMD [6]. The role of macrophages in the pathology of AMD is under debate and may depend on their polarization [14,74,75]. In DR, the involvement of microglia on the development of diabetic retinopathy is under debate [76], while macrophages are likely to be involved in its pathogenesis [21,22].

For activated microglia from the brain, it has been shown that fucoidan is able to reduce the activation following stimulation with lipopolysaccharide (LPS). In particular, fucoidan from *Fucus vesiculosus* reduced the activation of NFκB and the MAPK JNK, ERK1/2 and p38, as well as the expression of iNOS, Cox2 and the monocyte-chemoattractant factor MCP-1 [77]. Similarly, on macrophages activated with LPS, fucoidan from *Ecklonia cava* downregulated the expression of iNOS, Cox2, TNFα and IL-1β [78]. Conversely, however, fucoidans isolated from *Laminaria angustata* activated macrophages, inducing TNFα and IL-6 production [79]. Similar results were obtained with fucoidan isolated from *Agarum cribosum*, with activated macrophages expressing iNOS, Cox-2 and IL-10 [80]. This shows that the effect of fucoidans on monocyte-like cells is not uniform and depends on cell type and fucoidan origin. This needs to be considered regarding a possible use of fucoidan for AMD or diabetic retinopathy, as induction of pro-inflammatory macrophage activation is clearly not desirable in these diseases.

2.5. Fucoidan and Diabetic Retinopathy

Fucoidan from several different sources has been shown to reduce the blood-glucose levels in different models of diabetes. In insulin-resistant mice, fucoidan from *Cucumaria frondosa* increased the mRNA expression of the insulin receptor, as well as insulin receptor substrate 1, PI3K/Akt and Glut4, a glucose transporter protein [46]. Additionally, it reduced the weight of diabetic mice, reduced blood glucose and enhanced insulin sensitivity. In diabetic rats, in which diabetes was induced by alloxan, fucoidan from *Saccarina japonica* reduced blood glucose levels, which was accompanied by increased serum insulin levels and altered plasma lipid levels [81]. In another study, fucoidan from *Undaria pinnatifida* was used in three different fractions of different molecular weight. All three fractions suppressed blood glucose in db/db mice, a diabetic mouse model, and improved insulin sensitivity, depending on their sulfate content [82]. In addition, it has been shown that fucoidan from *Sargassum wightii* inhibited the enzyme alpha-D glucosidase, which is important for the provision of glucose into the blood stream [83]. However, this feature seems to be highly dependent on the source of fucoidan, since, e.g., fucoidans from *Fucus vesiculosus* were far less potent than fucoidans from *Ascophyllum nodosum* [84]. First line studies in obese but non-diabetic humans found that orally administered fucoidan elevated the insulin level in these patients; however, an increase in insulin resistance was noted [85]. Taken together, these results indicate that fucoidan could help regulating the blood glucose level in a non-toxic way and therefore help to prevent the onset of DR in diabetic patients.

Apart from its influence on blood glucose levels, fucoidan has been shown to attenuate diabetic retinopathy in the mouse model [45]. In this study, LMW fucoidan from *Laminaria japonica* reduces retinal damage and retinal neovascularization, most likely via inhibiting HIF-1α activation of VEGF (for more information on the influence of fucoidan on VEGF please see above). LMW fucoidan also inhibited the high-glucose induced proliferation of microvascular cells [45].

As described above, hypertension is a strong risk factor for developing and exacerbating diabetic retinopathy. In a model using Goto-Kakizaki rats, LMW fucoidan from *Laminaria japonica* could be found to ameliorate hypertension in these rats and protect the endothelium by inducing eNOS activity and NO production [86]. Indeed, a similar observation could be made in obese human patients, in which a daily oral supplementation of 500 mg/mL fucoidan reduced diastolic blood pressure [85].

Low grade inflammation has been implicated in the development of diabetic retinopathy [87], with inflammatory cytokines such as TNFα, IL-1β, or inflammatory mediators such as iNOS found in the aqueous humor or epiretinal membranes. In addition to the above-mentioned effects of fucoidan on microglia and macrophages, fucoidan has shown anti-inflammatory properties. In an ischemia-reperfusion model, fucoidan from *Laminaria japonica* reduced the levels of TNF-α [88], while, in C6 glioma cells treated with TNFα, fucoidan from *Fucus vesiculosus* has been shown to suppress the expression of iNOS [89]. However, similar to what has been described for macrophages, fucoidan from *Undaria pinnatifilda* activates neutrophils, leading to a pro-inflammatory TNF-α [90]. Again, the effect of fucoidan on inflammatory parameters is dependent on the source of fucoidan and the cell- and injury models used.

3. Future Directions

Taken together, these data give much indication for a potential beneficial effect of fucoidans on age-related macular degeneration and diabetic retinopathy. Yet it must be noted that the effects of fucoidan on the different features important for either AMD or DR are strongly dependent on molecular characteristics, extraction methods, and the source of the fucoidan. Furthermore, the use of unsuited fucoidans could have undesired, possibly even aggravating effects. Therefore, pre-clinical testing should be done to develop a database of different fucoidan fractions in order to identify those that combine various beneficial effects for the respective disease. In a second step, the most promising fucoidans should be tested in relevant *in vitro* systems, and, finally, these fucoidans should be tested in the appropriate animal models, such as streptozotocin-induced diabetes in mouse for diabetic retinopathy and Nrf2 knock-out mice in age-related macular degeneration. These data can then pave the way for clinical phase-one studies.

4. Conclusions

Fucoidans have many characteristics that render them interesting substances for the treatment of the major blinding diseases diabetic retinopathy and age-related macular degeneration. They can protect from oxidative stress, reduce VEGF activity, interfere with complement activation, have immune-modulating effects on microglia, reduce blood hyperglycemia, attenuate diabetic retinopathy in rodent models and ameliorate hypertension. A detailed list on the effects of fucoidan in the different experimental models can be found in Table 1 (*in vitro* models) and Table 2 (*in vivo* models). A schematic of the potential beneficial effects of fucoidan is depicted in Figure 1. However, most of the described features are highly dependent on the source, molecular weight, sulfation and even concentration. In order to investigate fucoidan further in this field, a thorough investigation of the bioactivity of the respective fucoidan fraction must be undertaken to identify the most promising candidate for preclinical and clinical testing and to avoid unwanted serious adverse events.

Table 1. Effect of different fucoidans in different cell culture models.

Cell Type	Disease Model	Concentration (µg)	Source	Effect	Ref.
HUVEC	Hypoxia	25–100/mL	*Sargassum hemiphyllum*	Reduced tube formation	[44]
HUVEC	VEGF165 application	8/mL 10/mL	*Fucus vesiculosus*	Blocks VEGF165 binding	[47] [48]
HUVEC	VEGF165 application	10/mL	*Fucus vesiculosus*	Reduces VEGFR-phosporylation	[48]
HUVEC	-	100, 200, 400/mL	*Undaria pinnatifida*	Reduces VEGF	[50]
T24 bladder cancer	Hypoxia	50, 100/mL	*Sargassum hemiphyllum*	Reduces VEGF	[44]
Microvascular endothelial cells	High glucose	12.5, 25, 50/mL	*Laminaria japonica*	Reduces VEGF	[45]
HeLa uterine carcinoma	-	10%, 20% extracts	*Cladosiphon novae-caledoniae kylin*	Reduces VEGF	[51]
Arpe19 RPE cell line	-	100/mL	*Fucus vesiculosus*	Reduces VEGF	[55]
Primary RPE cells	-	100/mL	*Fucus vesiculosus*	Reduces VEGF	[55]
Vero kidney fibroblasts	Oxidative stress	25–200/mL	*Ecklonia cava*	Scavenges ROS	[66]
Caco-2 intestinal epithelial	Oxidative stress	2.5/mL	*Cladosiphon okamuranus Tokida*	Protects barrier function	[67]
BV2 microglia	LPS stimulation	25–100/mL	*Fucus vesiculosus*	Reduces iNOS, Cox2, IL-1β, TNFα	[77]
C6 glioma cells	TNFα stimulation	50/mL	*Fucus vesiculosus*	Reduces iNOS	[89]
Neutrophils	-	10/mL	*Undaria pinnatifilda*	Induces TNFα	[90]
Raw 264.7 macrophages	LPS stimulation	12.5–100/mL	*Ecklonia cava*	Reduces iNOS, Cox-2, IL-1β, TNFα	[78]

Table 2. Effect of different fucoidans in different animal models.

Animal	Disease Model	Concentration (mg)	Source	Effect	Ref.
Nude mice (BALP/c)	Tumor growth	80, 160, 300/kg	*Sargassum hemiphyllum*	Reduces growth	[44]
C57BL/6 mice	Streptozotocin-induced diabetes	50, 100, 200/kg	*Laminaria japonica*	Reduces VEGF (retina)	[45]
C57BL/6J mice	Insulin resistance	80/kg	*Cucumaria frondosa*	Ameliorates insulin resistance	[46]
BALB/cAnNCr mice	Tumor angiogenesis assay	1/0.2 mL saline	*Fucus vesiculosus*	Reduces angiogenesis	[47]
C57BL/6J mice BALB/cAnNCr	VEGF Matrigel angiogenesis	1/0.2 mL saline	*Fucus vesiculosus*	Reduces angiogenesis	[47]
C57BL/6J mice	Lewis lung carcinoma cells inoculation	1, 3/mice	*Fucus vesiculosus*	Declines VEGF, MMP, NFκB	[49]
Zebrafish	Oxidative stress	100, 200 µg/mL	*Ecklonia cava*	Scavenges radicals	[66]
Sprague-Dawley rats	Liver fibrosis	100/kg	*Fucus vesiculosus*	Activates Nrf2	[62]
Sprague-Dawley rats	Ischemia-reperfusion injury	100, 200/kg	*Laminaria japonica*	Reduces TNFα, NFκB	[88]
Goto-Kakizaki rats	Diabetes	50, 100, 200/kg	*Laminaria japonica*	Reduces hypertension	[86]
Wistar rats	Alloxan-induced diabetes	50/kg	*Saccharina japonica*	Reduces blood glucose	[81]
C57BL/KSJ mice	Diabetes	200, 1200/kg	*Undaria pinnatifida*	Reduces blood glucose	[82]
Human	Obesity	500	*Laminaria japonica* and *Cystoseira canariensis*	Reduces hypertension	[85]

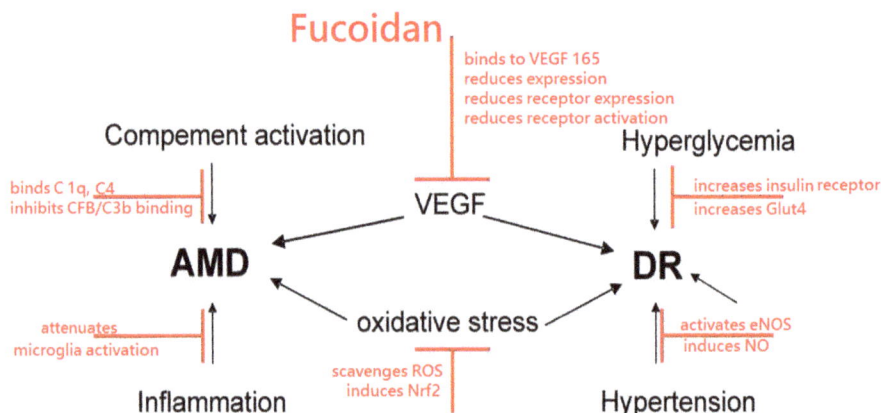

Figure 1. Schematic of potential beneficial effects of fucoidan, depicted in red, on age related macular degeneration (AMD) or diabetic retinopathy (DR). Additional abbreviations: complement component (C), complement factor B (CFB), endothelial nitric oxide synthase (eNOS), glucose transporter type 4 (Glut4), nitric oxide (NO), nuclear factor erythroid-2 related factor 2 (Nrf2), reactive oxygen species (ROS), Vascular Endothelial Growth Factor (VEGF).

Acknowledgments: The author is funded by the Hermann-Wacker foundation.

Conflicts of Interest: No conflicts of interest exist regarding this publication. Independently of this study, A.K. has been a consultant for, and received lecture fees and travel grants from, Novartis Pharma.

References

1. Li, B.; Lu, F.; Wei, X.; Zhao, R. Fucoidan: Structure and bioactivity. *Molecules* **2008**, *13*, 1671–1695. [PubMed]
2. Morya, V.K.; Kim, J.; Kim, E.K. Algal fucoidan: Structural and size-dependent bioactivities and their perspectives. *Appl. Microbiol. Biotechnol.* **2012**, *93*, 71–82. [CrossRef] [PubMed]
3. Fitton, J.H.; Stringer, D.N.; Karpiniec, S.S. Therapies from Fucoidan: An Update. *Mar. Drugs* **2015**, *13*, 5920–5946. [CrossRef] [PubMed]
4. Strauss, O. The retinal pigment epithelium in visual function. *Physiol. Rev.* **2005**, *85*, 845–881. [CrossRef] [PubMed]

5. Nickla, D.L.; Wallman, J. The multifunctional choroid. *Prog. Retin. Eye Res.* **2010**, *29*, 144–168. [CrossRef] [PubMed]
6. Karlstetter, M.; Scholz, R.; Rutar, M.; Wong, W.T.; Provis, J.M.; Langmann, T. Retinal microglia: Just bystander or target for therapy? *Prog. Retin. Eye Res.* **2015**, *45*, 30–57. [CrossRef] [PubMed]
7. Provis, J.M.; Penfold, P.L.; Cornish, E.E.; Sandercoe, T.M.; Madigan, M.C. Anatomy and development of the macula: Specialisation and the vulnerability to macular degeneration. *Clin. Exp. Optom.* **2005**, *88*, 269–281. [CrossRef] [PubMed]
8. Schmidt-Erfurth, U.; Chong, V.; Loewenstein, A.; Larsen, M.; Souied, E.; Schlingemann, R.; Eldem, B.; Monés, J.; Richard, G.; Bandello, F.; *et al.* Guidelines for the management of neovascular age-related macular degeneration by the European Society of Retina Specialists (EURETINA). *Br. J. Ophthalmol.* **2014**, *98*, 1144–1167. [CrossRef] [PubMed]
9. Miller, J.W. Age-related macular degeneration revisited—Piecing the puzzle: The LXIX Edward Jackson memorial lecture. *Am. J. Ophthalmol.* **2013**, *155*, 1–35. [CrossRef] [PubMed]
10. Klettner, A. Age-related macular degeneration—Biology and treatment. *Med. Monatsschr. Pharm.* **2015**, *38*, 258–264. [PubMed]
11. Klettner, A. Oxidative stress induced cellular signaling in RPE cells. *Front. Biosci. (Schol. Ed.)* **2012**, *4*, 392–411. [CrossRef] [PubMed]
12. Hageman, G.S.; Anderson, D.H.; Johnson, L.V.; Hancox, L.S.; Taiber, A.J.; Hardisty, L.I.; Hageman, J.L.; Stockman, H.A.; Borchardt, J.D.; Gehrs, K.M.; *et al.* A common haplotype in the complement regulatory gene factor H (HF1/CFH) predisposes individuals to age-related macular degeneration. *Proc. Natl Acad. Sci. USA* **2005**, *102*, 7227–7232. [CrossRef] [PubMed]
13. McHarg, S.; Clark, S.J.; Day, A.J.; Bishop, P.N. Age-related macular degeneration and the role of the complement system. *Mol. Immunol.* **2015**, *67*, 43–50. [CrossRef] [PubMed]
14. Cherepanoff, S.; McMenamin, P.; Gillies, M.C.; Kettle, E.; Sarks, S.H. Bruch's membrane and choroidal macrophages in early and advanced age-related macular degeneration. *Br. J. Ophthalmol.* **2010**, *94*, 918–925. [CrossRef] [PubMed]
15. Rofagha, S.; Bhisitkul, R.B.; Boyer, D.S.; Sadda, S.R.; Zhang, K.; SEVEN-UP Study Group. Seven-year outcomes in ranibizumab-treated patients in ANCHOR, MARINA, and HORIZON: A multicenter cohort study (SEVEN-UP). *Ophthalmology* **2013**, *120*, 2292–2299. [CrossRef] [PubMed]
16. Stitt, A.W.; Curtis, T.M.; Chen, M.; Medina, R.J.; McKay, G.J.; Jenkins, A.; Gardiner, T.A.; Lyons, T.J.; Hammes, H.P.; Simó, R.; *et al.* The progress in understanding and treatment of diabetic retinopathy. *Prog. Retin. Eye Res.* **2015**. [CrossRef] [PubMed]
17. Wan, T.T.; Li, X.F.; Sun, Y.M.; Li, Y.B.; Su, Y. Recent advances in understanding the biochemical and molecular mechanism of diabetic retinopathy. *Biomed. Pharmacother.* **2015**, *74*, 145–147. [CrossRef] [PubMed]
18. Nentwich, M.M.; Ulbig, M.W. Diabetic retinopathy—Ocular complications of diabetes mellitus. *World J. Diabetes* **2015**, *6*, 489–499. [CrossRef] [PubMed]
19. Friberg, T.R.; Rosenstock, J.; Sanborn, G.; Vaghefi, A.; Raskin, P. The effect of long-term near normal glycemic control on mild diabetic retinopathy. *Ophthalmology* **1985**, *92*, 1051–1058. [CrossRef]
20. Tuck, M.L. Diabetes and hypertension. *Postgrad. Med. J.* **1988**, *64* (Suppl. 3), 76–83 and 90–92. [CrossRef] [PubMed]
21. Schröder, S.; Palinski, W.; Schmid-Schönbein, G.W. Activated monocytes and granulocytes, capillary nonperfusion, and neovascularization in diabetic retinopathy. *Am. J. Pathol.* **1991**, *139*, 81–100. [PubMed]
22. Rangasamy, S.; McGuire, P.G.; Franco Nitta, C.; Monickaraj, F.; Oruganti, S.R.; Das, A. Chemokine mediated monocyte trafficking into the retina: Role of inflammation in alteration of the blood-retinal barrier in diabetic retinopathy. *PLoS ONE* **2014**, *9*, e108508. [CrossRef] [PubMed]
23. Carmeliet, P.; Ferreira, V.; Breier, G.; Pollefeyt, S.; Kieckens, L.; Gertsenstein, M.; Fahrig, M.; Vandenhoeck, A.; Harpal, K.; Eberhardt, C.; *et al.* Abnormal blood vessel development and lethality in embryos lacking a single VEGF allele. *Nature* **1996**, *4*, 435–439. [CrossRef] [PubMed]
24. Ferrara, N.; Davis-Smyth, T. The biology of vascular endothelial growth factor. *Endocr. Rev.* **1997**, *18*, 4–25. [CrossRef] [PubMed]
25. Marmé, D. Tumor angiogenesis: The pivotal role of vascular endothelial growth factor. *World J. Urol.* **1996**, *14*, 166–174. [CrossRef] [PubMed]

26. Witmer, A.N.; Vrensen, G.F.; Van Noorden, C.J.; Schlingemann, R.O. Vascular endothelial growth factors and angiogenesis in eye disease. *Prog. Retin. Eye Res.* **2003**, *22*, 1–29. [CrossRef]
27. Klettner, A. Physiological function of VEGF in the retina and its possible implications of prolonged anti-VEGF therapy. In *Vascular Endothelial Growth Factor—Biology, Regulation and Clinical Significance*; Parker, M.L., Ed.; Nova Biomedical: New York, NY, USA, 2013; pp. 117–136.
28. Tischer, E.; Mitchell, R.; Hartman, T.; Silva, M.; Gospodarowicz, D.; Fiddes, J.C.; Abraham, J.A. The human gene for vascular endothelial growth factor. Multiple protein forms are encoded through alternative exon splicing. *J. Biol. Chem.* **1991**, *266*, 11947–11954. [PubMed]
29. Kim, I.; Ryan, A.M.; Rohan, R.; Amano, S.; Agular, S.; Miller, J.W.; Adamis, A.P. Constitutive expression of VEGF, VEGFR-1, and VEGFR-2 in normal eyes. *Invest. Ophthalmol. Vis. Sci.* **1999**, *40*, 2115–2121. [PubMed]
30. Gerhardinger, C.; Brown, L.F.; Roy, S.; Mizutani, M.; Zucker, C.L.; Lorenzi, M. Expression of vascular endothelial growth factor in the human retina and in nonproliferative diabetic retinopathy. *Am. J. Pathol.* **1998**, *152*, 1453–1462. [PubMed]
31. Klettner, A.; Roider, J. Treating age-related macular degeneration—Interaction of VEGF-antagonists with their target. *Mini Rev. Med. Chem.* **2009**, *9*, 1127–1135. [CrossRef] [PubMed]
32. Klettner, A.; Roider, J. Mechanismen of pathological VEGF production in the retina and modifications with VEGF-antagonists. In *Studies on Retinal and Choriodal Disorders*; Stratton, R.D., Hauswirth, W.W., Gardner, T.W., Eds.; Humana Press: New York, NY, USA, 2012; pp. 277–306.
33. Guo, H.F.; Vander Kooi, C.W. Neuropilin function as an essential cell surface receptor. *J. Biol. Chem.* **2015**, *290*, 29120–29126. [CrossRef] [PubMed]
34. Gerber, H.P.; McMurtrey, A.; Kowalski, J.; Yan, M.; Keyt, B.A.; Dixit, V.; Ferrara, N. Vascular endothelial growth factor regulates endothelial cell survival through the phosphatidylinositol 3′-kinase/Akt signal transduction pathway. Requirement for Flk-1/KDR activation. *J. Biol. Chem.* **1998**, *273*, 30336–30343. [CrossRef] [PubMed]
35. Ehrlich, R.; Harris, A.; Ciulla, T.A.; Kheradiya, N.; Winston, D.M.; Wirostko, B. Diabetic macular oedema: Physical, physiological and molecular factors contribute to this pathological process. *Acta Ophthalmol.* **2010**, *88*, 279–291. [CrossRef] [PubMed]
36. Forsythe, J.A.; Jiang, B.H.; Iyer, N.V.; Agani, F.; Leung, S.W.; Koos, R.D.; Semenza, G.L. Activation of vascular endothelial growth factor gene transcription by hypoxia-inducible factor 1. *Mol. Cell. Biol.* **1996**, *16*, 4604–4613. [CrossRef] [PubMed]
37. Pagès, G.; Pouysségur, J. Transcriptional regulation of the Vascular Endothelial Growth Factor gene—A concert of activating factors. *Cardiovasc. Res.* **2005**, *65*, 564–573. [CrossRef] [PubMed]
38. Huang, S.; Robinson, J.B.; Deguzman, A.; Bucana, C.D.; Fidler, I.J. Blockade of nuclear factor-kappaB signaling inhibits angiogenesis and tumorigenicity of human ovarian cancer cells by suppressing expression of vascular endothelial growth factor and interleukin 8. *Cancer Res.* **2000**, *60*, 5334–5339. [PubMed]
39. Klettner, A.; Westhues, D.; Lassen, J.; Bartsch, S.; Roider, J. Regulation of constitutive vascular endothelial growth factor secretion in retinal pigment epithelium/choroid organ cultures: p38, nuclear factor κB, and the vascular endothelial growth factor receptor-2/phosphatidylinositol 3 kinase pathway. *Mol. Vis.* **2013**, *19*, 281–291. [PubMed]
40. Klettner, A.; Kaya, L.; Flach, J.; Lassen, J.; Treumer, F.; Roider, J. Basal and apical regulation of VEGF-A and placenta growth factor in the RPE/choroid and primary RPE. *Mol. Vis.* **2015**, *21*, 736–748. [PubMed]
41. Madsen-Bouterse, S.A.; Kowluru, R.A. Oxidative stress and diabetic retinopathy: Pathophysiological mechanisms and treatment perspectives. *Rev. Endocr. Metab. Disord.* **2008**, *9*, 315–327. [CrossRef] [PubMed]
42. Ding, X.; Patel, M.; Chan, C.C. Molecular pathology of age-related macular degeneration. *Prog. Retin. Eye Res.* **2009**, *28*, 1–18. [CrossRef] [PubMed]
43. Klettner, A.; Roider, J. Constitutive and oxidative-stress-induced expression of VEGF in the RPE are differently regulated by different Mitogen-activated protein kinases. *Graefes. Arch. Clin. Exp. Ophthalmol.* **2009**, *247*, 1487–1492. [CrossRef] [PubMed]
44. Chen, M.C.; Hsu, W.L.; Hwang, P.A.; Chou, T.C. Low molecular weight fucoidan inhibits tumor angiogenesis through downregulation of HIF-1/VEGF signaling under hypoxia. *Mar. Drugs* **2015**, *13*, 4436–4451. [CrossRef] [PubMed]

45. Yang, W.; Yu, X.; Zhang, Q.; Lu, Q.; Wang, J.; Cui, W.; Zheng, Y.; Wang, X.; Luo, D. Attenuation of streptozotocin-induced diabetic retinopathy with low molecular weight fucoidan via inhibition of vascular endothelial growth factor. *Exp. Eye Res.* **2013**, *115*, 96–105. [CrossRef] [PubMed]

46. Wang, Y.; Wang, J.; Zhao, Y.; Hu, S.; Shi, D.; Xue, C. Fucoidan from sea cucumber *Cucumaria frondosa* exhibits anti-hyperglycemic effects in insulin resistant mice via activating the PI3K/PKB pathway and GLUT4. *J. Biosci. Bioeng.* **2015**, *121*, 36–42. [CrossRef] [PubMed]

47. Narazaki, M.; Segarra, M.; Tosato, G. Sulfated polysaccharides identified as inducers of neuropilin-1 internalization and functional inhibition of VEGF165 and semaphorin3A. *Blood* **2008**, *111*, 4126–4136. [CrossRef] [PubMed]

48. Koyanagi, S.; Tanigawa, N.; Nakagawa, H.; Soeda, S.; Shimeno, H. Oversulfation of fucoidan enhances its anti-angiogenic and antitumor activities. *Biochem. Pharmacol.* **2003**, *65*, 173–179. [CrossRef]

49. Huang, T.H.; Chiu, Y.H.; Chan, Y.L.; Chiu, Y.H.; Wang, H.; Huang, K.C.; Li, T.L.; Hsu, K.H.; Wu, C.J. Prophylactic administration of fucoidan represses cancer metastasis by inhibiting vascular endothelial growth factor (VEGF) and matrix metalloproteinases (MMPs) in Lewis tumor-bearing mice. *Mar. Drugs* **2015**, *13*, 1882–1900. [CrossRef] [PubMed]

50. Liu, F.; Wang, J.; Chang, A.K.; Liu, B.; Yang, L.; Li, Q.; Wang, P.; Zou, X. Fucoidan extract derived from *Undaria pinnatifida* inhibits angiogenesis by human umbilical vein endothelial cells. *Phytomedicine* **2012**, *19*, 797–803. [CrossRef] [PubMed]

51. Ye, J.; Li, Y.; Teruya, K.; Katakura, Y.; Ichikawa, A.; Eto, H.; Hosoi, M.; Hosoi, M.; Nishimoto, S.; Shirahata, S. Enzyme-digested fucoidan extracts derived from seaweed *Mozuku* of *Cladosiphon novae-caledoniae kylin* inhibit invasion and angiogenesis of tumor cells. *Cytotechnology* **2005**, *47*, 117–126. [CrossRef] [PubMed]

52. Ustyuzhanina, N.E.; Bilan, M.I.; Ushakova, N.A.; Usov, A.I.; Kiselevskiy, M.V.; Nifantiev, N.E. Fucoidans: Pro- or antiangiogenic agents? *Glycobiology* **2014**, *24*, 1265–1274. [CrossRef] [PubMed]

53. Lake, A.C.; Vassy, R.; Di Benedetto, M.; Lavigne, D.; Le Visage, C.; Perret, G.Y.; Letourneur, D. Low molecular weight fucoidan increases VEGF165-induced endothelial cell migration by enhancing VEGF165 binding to VEGFR-2 and NRP1. *J. Biol. Chem.* **2006**, *281*, 37844–37852. [CrossRef] [PubMed]

54. Purnama, A.; Aid-Launais, R.; Haddad, O.; Maire, M.; Mantovani, D.; Letourneur, D.; Hlawaty, H.; Le Visage, C. Fucoidan in a 3D scaffold interacts with vascular endothelial growth factor and promote neovascularization in mice. *Drug Deliv. Transl. Res.* **2015**, *5*, 187–197. [CrossRef] [PubMed]

55. Dithmer, M.; Fuchs, S.; Shi, Y.; Schmidt, H.; Richert, E.; Roider, J.; Klettner, A. Fucoidan reduces secretion and expression of vascular endothelial growth factor in the retinal pigment epithelium and reduces angiogenesis *in vitro*. *PLoS ONE* **2014**, *9*, e89150. [CrossRef] [PubMed]

56. Zarbin, M.A. Current concepts in the pathogenesis of age-related macular degeneration. *Arch. Ophthalmol.* **2004**, *122*, 598–614. [CrossRef] [PubMed]

57. Behl, T.; Kotwani, A. Exploring the various aspects of the pathological role of vascular endothelial growth factor (VEGF) in diabetic retinopathy. *Pharmacol. Res.* **2015**, *99*, 137–148. [CrossRef] [PubMed]

58. Rupérez, P.; Ahrazem, O.; Leal, J.A. Potential antioxidant capacity of sulfated polysaccharides from the edible marine brown seaweed *Fucus vesiculosus*. *J. Agric. Food Chem.* **2002**, *50*, 840–845. [CrossRef] [PubMed]

59. Wang, J.; Zhang, Q.; Zhang, Z.; Li, Z. Antioxidant activity of sulfated polysaccharide fractions extracted from *Laminaria japonica*. *Int. J. Biol. Macromol.* **2008**, *42*, 127–132. [CrossRef] [PubMed]

60. Abu, R.; Jiang, Z.; Ueno, M.; Okimura, T.; Yamaguchi, K.; Oda, T. *In vitro* antioxidant activities of sulfated polysaccharide ascophyllan isolated from *Ascophyllum nodosum*. *Int. J. Biol. Macromol.* **2013**, *59*, 305–312. [CrossRef] [PubMed]

61. Marudhupandi, T.; Kumar, T.T.; Senthil, S.L.; Devi, K.N. *In vitro* antioxidant properties of fucoidan fractions from *Sargassum tenerrimum*. *Pak. J. Biol. Sci.* **2014**, *17*, 402–407. [CrossRef] [PubMed]

62. Hong, S.W.; Jung, K.H.; Lee, H.S.; Zheng, H.M.; Choi, M.J.; Lee, C.; Hong, S.S. Suppression by fucoidan of liver fibrogenesis via the TGF-β/Smad pathway in protecting against oxidative stress. *Biosci. Biotechnol. Biochem.* **2011**, *75*, 833–840. [CrossRef] [PubMed]

63. Zhao, Z.; Chen, Y.; Wang, J.; Sternberg, P.; Freeman, M.L.; Grossniklaus, H.E.; Cai, J. Age-related retinopathy in NRF2-deficient mice. *PLoS ONE* **2011**, *29*, e19456. [CrossRef] [PubMed]

64. Koinzer, S.; Reinecke, K.; Herdegen, T.; Roider, J.; Klettner, A. Oxidative stress induces biphasic ERK1/2 activation in the RPE with distinct effects on cell survival at early and late activation. *Curr. Eye Res.* **2015**, *40*, 853–857. [CrossRef] [PubMed]

65. Kim, K.J.; Yoon, K.Y.; Lee, B.Y. Low molecular weight fucoidan from the sporophyll of *Undaria pinnatifida* suppresses inflammation by promoting the inhibition of mitogen-activated protein kinases and oxidative stress in RAW264.7 cells. *Fitoterapia* **2012**, *83*, 1628–1635. [CrossRef] [PubMed]

66. Kim, E.A.; Lee, S.H.; Ko, C.I.; Cha, S.H.; Kang, M.C.; Kang, S.M.; Ko, S.C.; Lee, W.W.; Ko, J.Y.; Lee, J.H.; *et al.* Protective effect of fucoidan against AAPH-induced oxidative stress in zebrafish model. *Carbohydr. Polym.* **2014**, *102*, 185–191. [CrossRef] [PubMed]

67. Iraha, A.; Chinen, H.; Hokama, A.; Yonashiro, T.; Kinjo, T.; Kishimoto, K.; Nakamoto, M.; Hirata, T.; Kinjo, N.; Higa, F.; *et al.* Fucoidan enhances intestinal barrier function by upregulating the expression of claudin-1. *World J. Gastroenterol.* **2013**, *19*, 5500–5507. [CrossRef] [PubMed]

68. Felinski, E.A.; Antonetti, D.A. Glucocorticoid regulation of endothelial cell tight junction gene expression: Novel treatments for diabetic retinopathy. *Curr. Eye Res.* **2005**, *30*, 949–957. [CrossRef] [PubMed]

69. Li, X.; Zhao, H.; Wang, Q.; Liang, H.; Jiang, X. Fucoidan protects ARPE-19 cells from oxidative stress via normalization of reactive oxygen species generation through the Ca^{2+} -dependent ERK signaling pathway. *Mol. Med. Rep.* **2015**, *11*, 3746–3752. [PubMed]

70. Tissot, B.; Montdargent, B.; Chevolot, L.; Varenne, A.; Descroix, S.; Gareil, P.; Daniel, R. Interaction of fucoidan with the proteins of the complement classical pathway. *Biochim. Biophys. Acta* **2003**, *1651*, 5–16. [CrossRef]

71. Blondin, C.; Fischer, E.; Boisson-Vidal, C.; Kazatchkine, M.D.; Jozefonvicz, J. Inhibition of complement activation by natural sulfated polysaccharides (fucans) from brown seaweed. *Mol. Immunol.* **1994**, *31*, 247–253. [CrossRef]

72. Gold, B.; Merriam, J.E.; Zernant, J.; Hancox, L.S.; Taiber, A.J.; Gehrs, K.; Cramer, K.; Neel, J.; Bergeron, J.; Barile, G.R.; *et al.* Variation in factor B (BF) and complement component 2 (C2) genes is associated with age-related macular degeneration. *Nat. Genet.* **2006**, *38*, 458–462. [CrossRef] [PubMed]

73. Blondin, C.; Chaubet, F.; Nardella, A.; Sinquin, C.; Jozefonvicz, J. Relationships between chemical characteristics and anticomplementary activity of fucans. *Biomaterials* **1996**, *17*, 597–603. [CrossRef]

74. Cao, X.; Shen, D.; Patel, M.M.; Tuo, J.; Johnson, T.M.; Olsen, T.W.; Chan, C.C. Macrophage polarization in the maculae of age-related macular degeneration: A pilot study. *Pathol. Int.* **2011**, *61*, 528–535. [CrossRef] [PubMed]

75. Zandi, S.; Nakao, S.; Chun, K.H.; Fiorina, P.; Sun, D.; Arita, R.; Zhao, M.; Kim, E.; Schueller, O.; Campbell, S.; *et al.* ROCK-isoform-specific polarization of macrophages associated with age-related macular degeneration. *Cell. Rep.* **2015**, *10*, 1173–1186. [CrossRef] [PubMed]

76. Abcouwer, S.F. Neural inflammation and the microglial response in diabetic retinopathy. *J. Ocul. Biol. Dis. Inform.* **2012**, *4*, 25–33. [CrossRef] [PubMed]

77. Park, H.Y.; Han, M.H.; Park, C.; Jin, C.Y.; Kim, G.Y.; Choi, I.W.; Kim, N.D.; Nam, T.J.; Kwon, T.K.; Choi, Y.H. Anti-inflammatory effects of fucoidan through inhibition of NF-κB, MAPK and Akt activation in lipopolysaccharide-induced BV2 microglia cells. *Food Chem. Toxicol.* **2011**, *49*, 1745–1752. [CrossRef] [PubMed]

78. Lee, S.H.; Ko, C.; Ahn, G.; You, S.; Kim, J.S.; Heu, M.S.; Kim, J.; Jee, Y.; Jeon, Y.J. Molecular characteristics and anti-inflammatory activity of the fucoidan extracted from *Ecklonia cava*. *Carbohydr. Polym.* **2012**, *89*, 599–606. [CrossRef] [PubMed]

79. Teruya, T.; Takeda, S.; Tamaki, Y.; Tako, M. Fucoidan isolated from *Laminaria angustata* var. *longissima* induced macrophage activation. *Biosci. Biotechnol. Biochem.* **2010**, *74*, 1960–1962. [CrossRef] [PubMed]

80. Cho, M.; Lee, D.J.; Kim, J.K.; You, S. Molecular characterization and immunomodulatory activity of sulfated fucans from *Agarum cribrosum*. *Carbohydr. Polym.* **2014**, *113*, 507–514. [CrossRef] [PubMed]

81. Wang, J.; Jin, W.; Zhang, W.; Hou, Y.; Zhang, H.; Zhang, Q. Hypoglycemic property of acidic polysaccharide extracted from *Saccharina japonica* and its potential mechanism. *Carbohydr. Polym.* **2013**, *5*, 143–147. [CrossRef] [PubMed]

82. Kim, K.J.; Yoon, K.Y.; Lee, B.Y. Fucoidan regulate blood glucose homeostasis in C57BL/KSJ m+/+db and C57BL/KSJ db/db mice. *Fitoterapia* **2012**, *83*, 1105–1109. [CrossRef] [PubMed]

83. Vinoth Kumar, T.; Lakshmanasenthil, S.; Geetharamani, D.; Marudhupandi, T.; Suja, G.; Suganya, P. Fucoidan—A α-D-glucosidase inhibitor from *Sargassum wightii* with relevance to type 2 diabetes mellitus therapy. *Int. J. Biol. Macromol.* **2015**, *72*, 1044–1047. [CrossRef] [PubMed]

84. Kim, K.T.; Rioux, L.E.; Turgeon, S.L. Alpha-amylase and alpha-glucosidase inhibition is differentially modulated by fucoidan obtained from *Fucus vesiculosus* and *Ascophyllum nodosum*. *Phytochemistry* **2014**, *98*, 27–33. [CrossRef] [PubMed]

85. Hernández-Corona, D.M.; Martínez-Abundis, E.; González-Ortiz, M. Effect of fucoidan administration on insulin secretion and insulin resistance in overweight or obese adults. *J. Med. Food* **2014**, *17*, 830–832. [CrossRef] [PubMed]

86. Cui, W.; Zheng, Y.; Zhang, Q.; Wang, J.; Wang, L.; Yang, W.; Guo, C.; Gao, W.; Wang, X.; Luo, D. Low-molecular-weight fucoidan protects endothelial function and ameliorates basal hypertension in diabetic Goto-Kakizaki rats. *Lab. Investig.* **2014**, *94*, 382–393. [CrossRef] [PubMed]

87. Tang, J.; Kern, T.S. Inflammation in diabetic retinopathy. *Prog. Retin Eye Res.* **2011**, *30*, 343–358. [CrossRef] [PubMed]

88. Li, C.; Gao, Y.; Xing, Y.; Zhu, H.; Shen, J.; Tian, J. Fucoidan, a sulfated polysaccharide from brown algae, against myocardial ischemia-reperfusion injury in rats via regulating the inflammation response. *Food Chem. Toxicol.* **2011**, *49*, 2090–2095. [CrossRef] [PubMed]

89. Do, H.; Pyo, S.; Sohn, E.H. Suppression of iNOS expression by fucoidan is mediated by regulation of p38 MAPK, JAK/STAT, AP-1 and IRF-1, and depends on up-regulation of scavenger receptor B1 expression in TNF-alpha- and IFN-gamma-stimulated C6 glioma cells. *J. Nutr. Biochem.* **2010**, *21*, 671–679. [CrossRef] [PubMed]

90. Jin, J.O.; Yu, Q. Fucoidan delays apoptosis and induces pro-inflammatory cytokine production in human neutrophils. *Int. J. Biol. Macromol.* **2015**, *73*, 65–71. [CrossRef] [PubMed]

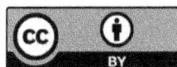

marine drugs

MDPI

Article

Production of Chondroitin Sulphate from Head, Skeleton and Fins of *Scyliorhinus canicula* By-Products by Combination of Enzymatic, Chemical Precipitation and Ultrafiltration Methodologies

María Blanco *, Javier Fraguas, Carmen G. Sotelo, Ricardo I. Pérez-Martín and José Antonio Vázquez

Marine Research Institute (IIM-CSIC), Eduardo Cabello, 6. Vigo, Galicia 36208, Spain; xavi@iim.csic.es (J.F.); carmen@iim.csic.es (C.G.S.); ricardo@iim.csic.es (R.I.P.-M.); jvazquez@iim.csic.es (J.A.V.)

* Author to whom correspondence should be addressed; mblanco@iim.csic.es;
 Tel.: +34-986-231-930; Fax: +34-986-292-762.

Academic Editor: Paola Laurienzo
Received: 20 February 2015; Accepted: 13 May 2015; Published: 27 May 2015

Abstract: This study illustrates the optimisation of the experimental conditions of three sequential steps for chondroitin sulphate (CS) recovery from three cartilaginous materials of *Scyliorhinus canicula* by-products. Optimum conditions of temperature and pH were first obtained for alcalase proteolysis of head cartilage (58 °C/pH 8.5/0.1% (v/w)/10 h of hydrolysis). Then, similar optimal conditions were observed for skeletons and fin materials. Enzymatic hydrolysates were subsequently treated with a combination of alkaline hydroalcoholic saline solutions in order to improve the protein hydrolysis and the selective precipitation of CS. Ranges of 0.53–0.64 M (NaOH) and 1.14–1.20 volumes (EtOH) were the levels for optimal chemical treatment depending on the cartilage origin. Finally, selective purification and concentration of CS and protein elimination of samples obtained from chemical treatment, was assessed by a combination of ultrafiltration and diafiltration (UF-DF) techniques at 30 kDa.

Keywords: chondroitin sulphate production; cartilage *S. canicula* wastes; by-products upgrade; process optimization; response surface methodology

---

1. Introduction

Seafood discards and by-products including whole dead individuals, skins, heads, viscera, bones, cartilage, *etc.* serve as a source for obtaining high value-added products with uses in biomedicine, nutraceutics, feed and cosmetics. In terms of availability of potential raw material for valorization purposes, *Scyliorhinus canicula* might be considered as an alternative source for obtaining valuable compounds. In this regard, *S. canicula* is one of the most discarded species in Northeast Atlantic fisheries. Previously reported data on this species, showed that the percentage of discards might reach 90%–100% in some fisheries [1,2]. In 2012 discards of the Bottom otter trawl (OTB) fleet, operating in the Bay of Biscay and Iberian Waters (ICES Division VIII) accounted for up to 900 t [3]. Besides the importance of *S. canicula* discards as a raw material for obtaining value-added compounds, there is also another fundamental factor contributing to the generation of large quantities of by-products: the onshore fish processing industry. As an example, sales of fresh *S. canicula* in one of the most important fishing ports of Europe, located in Vigo (North-West Spain), accounted for up to 60,700 in for 2013, with an average price of €1.2 per kg (data from http://www.pescadegalicia.com). From these, about 35%–75% of the total weight corresponds to by-products (heads, skin, cartilage, viscera, *etc.*) [4–6]. Although much of this waste is already being used, either for fish meal or oil production, it is considered that this kind of utilization produces very little added-value and that, with present technological development, a more valuable and profitable use is possible [7].

Cartilage for biomedical purposes was initially obtained from mammalian sources [8], however since the bovine spongiform encephalopathy outbreak, some concerns arose about the use of by-products from cattle, and more attention has been paid to the use of alternative sources, such as marine organisms for the production of added-value products. The preference for cartilage obtained from marine sources is also explained because previous studies found higher contents of cartilage in sharks in comparison to mammalian sources. Lee and Langer [9] have shown that cartilage in chondrichthyes represents 6%–8% of the total body weight, while mammalian cartilage represents scarcely 0.6%. Chondrichthyes such as *S. canicula* are characterised by a cartilage skeleton mainly composed of the polysaccharide chondroitin sulphate (CS). Chondroitin sulphate is a linear polysaccharide, characterized by a repeating disaccharide unit composed of glucuronic acid (GlcA) and *N*-acetylated galactosamine (GalNAc) sulphated in the carbon 4 (CS-A), 6 (CS-C), both 4 and 6 (CS-E) as well as positions 6 of GalNAc and 2 of GlcA (CS-D) [10]. The CS composition of *S. canicula* has been previously reported to be CS-A, CS-C, CS-D and CS unsulphated [11], whereas in other elasmobranchs such as skates, the composition of CS is different [12]. CS is covalently linked, together with other glycosaminoglycans (keratin sulphate: KS) to an axial protein creating the proteoglycan molecule. Proteoglycans are associated to a collagen matrix constituting the basis of the cartilage tissue. Chondroitin sulphate offers a wide range of applications in medicine such as antioxidant agent, ostheoarthritis treatments, connective tissue repair or anti-tumor drugs [9,13–15]. Recently, the combination of CS with other biopolymers such as collagen or hyaluronic acid has attracted much attention in the engineering of biological tissues [16–18].

One important aspect regarding the extraction of valuable compounds such as glycosaminoglycans from marine waste materials, is the selection of appropriate processes and the corresponding recovery conditions. Purification processes are commonly optimized using one-factor-at-a-time approaches. However, it is well-known that optimal conditions or interactions between variables cannot be predicted with this methodology. Both problems can be overcome by employing response surface methodology (RSM), a tool used by many researchers to maximize or minimize various independent variables and predict optimal experimental conditions [19,20].

The present work aims to optimize the extraction and purification of chondroitin sulphate from *S. canicula* cartilage wastes, using a set of environmental friendly processes. Firstly, the influence of pH and temperature (*T*) on cartilage hydrolysis with alcalase was studied, and optimized conditions were achieved. Secondly, the optimal concentration of NaOH and ethanol (EtOH) volume for alkaline proteolysis and selective precipitation of CS were obtained. Finally, ultrafiltration process and subsequent diafiltration were developed in order to achieve a high CS purity.

2. Results and Discussion

The average ($\pm$SD) chemical composition of cartilages from *S. canicula*, expressed as percentage of dry weight, was 52.47 ± 0.10, 55.17 ± 0.74, and 45.19 ± 0.14 of protein for heads, fins and skeletons respectively; 37.66 ± 1.19, 38.70 ± 0.62 and 51.28 ± 0.24 of ash for heads, fins and skeletons respectively; 1.50 ± 0.19, 0.45 ± 0.08 and 0.04 ± 0.01 of fat for heads, fins and skeletons respectively. By difference, the percentage of total carbohydrates was: 8.37 (heads), 5.68 (fins) and 3.45 (skeletons). The content of moisture (as percentage of total weight) was 78.09 ± 0.17, 76.06 ± 1.57 and 70.17 ± 0.25 for heads, fins and skeletons respectively. Similar moisture and fat content, and lower ash and protein content, has been previously described for fin shark cartilage [21].

2.1. Enzymatic Hydrolysis of Head Cartilages. Effect of pH and Temperature (T)

Alcalase hydrolysis of head cartilages from *S. canicula* using different conditions of pH and temperature (T) clearly showed non-linear patterns with various types of hyperbolic and sigmoid profiles (Figure 1). In this context, the Weibull Equation (4) is a well-known mathematical tool for simulating sigmoid and hyperbolic profiles as well as mixture of both curves [22]. It is also formulated with parameters of clear geometrical meaning and is routinely applied in the modelling of several systems and kinetics in toxicology, food technology and biotechnology [23].

The present experimental data were perfectly described, in all cases, by the equation proposed, obtaining determination coefficients of not less than 0.982. The values of the kinetic parameters and the statistical analysis performed on the numerical fittings are summarized in Table 1. All the parameters were statistically significant ($\alpha = 0.05$) and autocorrelation was not observed in the residuals distribution (data not shown). For the case (pH 6 and $T = 55$ °C), the values of parameters used as dependent variables (responses) in the subsequent surface response approach and calculation were established as zero.

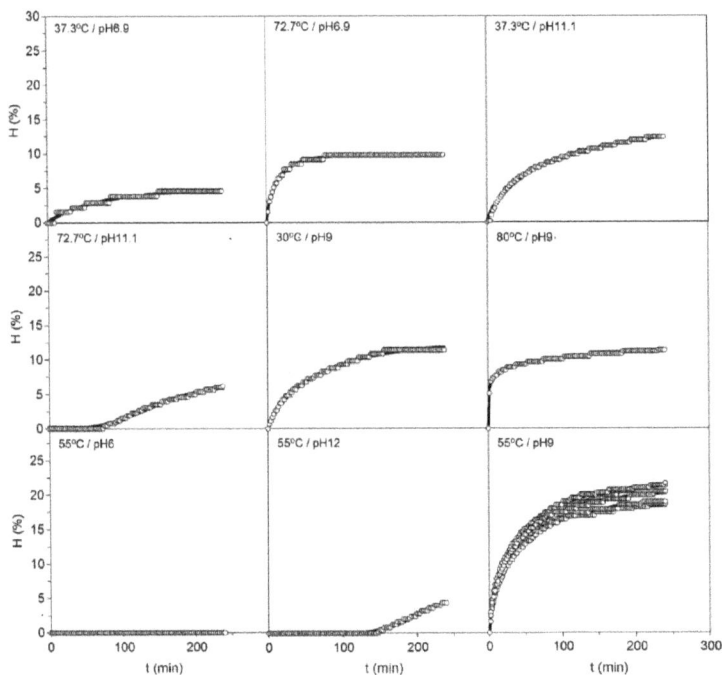

Figure 1. Kinetics of cartilage hydrolysis from *Scyliorhinus canicula* heads using alcalase in each one of the experimental conditions defined in Table 1. The experimental data (symbols) were fitted to the Weibull Equation (4) (continuous line).

Table 1. Parametric estimations corresponding to the Weibull Equation (4) applied to the enzymatic hydrolysis kinetics at the experimental conditions studied. Independent variables are expressed in natural values in brackets. Numerical values of the parameters are shown with their confidence intervals. Determination coefficients (R^2) and p-values from F-Fisher test are also summarized. H_m is the maximum degree of hydrolysis; β is a parameter related with the maximum slope of cartilage hydrolysis; τ is the time required to achieve the semi-maximum degree of hydrolysis and v_m is the maximum hydrolysis rate at the τ-time.

Experimental Conditions	H_m (%)	v_m (%·min^{-1})	τ (min)	β	R^2	p-value
T:−1 (37.3 °C)/pH:−1 (6.9)	5.05 ± 0.31	0.030 ± 0.004	51.51 ± 6.00	0.89 ± 0.10	0.982	<0.001
T:1 (72.7 °C)/pH:−1 (6.9)	9.85 ± 0.04	0.262 ± 0.007	9.82 ± 0.34	0.75 ± 0.03	0.993	<0.001
T:−1 (37.3 °C)/pH:1 (11.1)	14.04 ± 0.46	0.067 ± 0.005	54.65 ± 3.73	0.75 ± 0.03	0.996	<0.001
T:1 (72.7 °C)/pH:1 (11.1)	5.93 ± 0.21	0.045 ± 0.002	139.0 ± 3.17	3.03 ± 0.19	0.991	<0.001
T:−1.41 (30.0 °C)/pH:0 (9.0)	12.80 ± 0.33	0.079 ± 0.005	44.88 ± 2.32	0.80 ± 0.03	0.994	<0.001
T:1.41 (80.0 °C)/pH:0 (9.0)	15.81 ± 2.03	0.082 ± 0.071	14.11 ± 12.42	0.21 ± 0.02	0.992	<0.001
T:0 (55.0 °C)/pH:−1.41 (6.0)	-	-	-	-	-	-
T:0 (55.0 °C)/pH:1.41 (12.0)	4.34 ± 0.15	0.059 ± 0.003	190.23 ± 1.83	7.47 ± 0.44	0.993	<0.001
T:0 (55.0 °C)/pH:0 (9.0)	18.83 ± 0.14	0.225 ± 0.006	19.65 ± 0.45	0.68 ± 0.02	0.997	<0.001
T:0 (55.0 °C)/pH:0 (9.0)	23.44 ± 0.28	0.162 ± 0.006	30.10 ± 0.93	0.60 ± 0.01	0.999	<0.001
T:0 (55.0 °C)/pH:0 (9.0)	19.86 ± 0.16	0.179 ± 0.004	26.70 ± 0.52	0.69 ± 0.01	0.998	<0.001
T:0 (55.0 °C)/pH:0 (9.0)	22.67 ± 0.20	0.209 ± 0.006	23.80 ± 0.55	0.63 ± 0.01	0.998	<0.001
T:0 (55.0 °C)/pH:0 (9.0)	21.06 ± 0.18	0.206 ± 0.006	23.21 ± 0.53	0.66 ± 0.02	0.998	<0.001

The combined effect of pH and T on the kinetic parameters from Equation (4) was studied by means of surface response methodology (Figure 2). Two more dependent variables were also assessed: (1) the concentration of CS was obtained from each sample of hydrolysed cartilage and processed in suboptimal conditions of 0.2 M NaOH and 1 v/v EtOH, according to Murado *et al.* [12]; (2) the index of CS purity in relation to total proteins (I_p as %). The design and numerical responses of the 2-factor rotatable design are listed in Table 2. For these two responses, the average and corresponding errors (calculated as the intervals of confidence in the five replicated conditions) were: 9.01 ± 0.36 g/L of CS and 89.61% ± 0.53% for I_p.

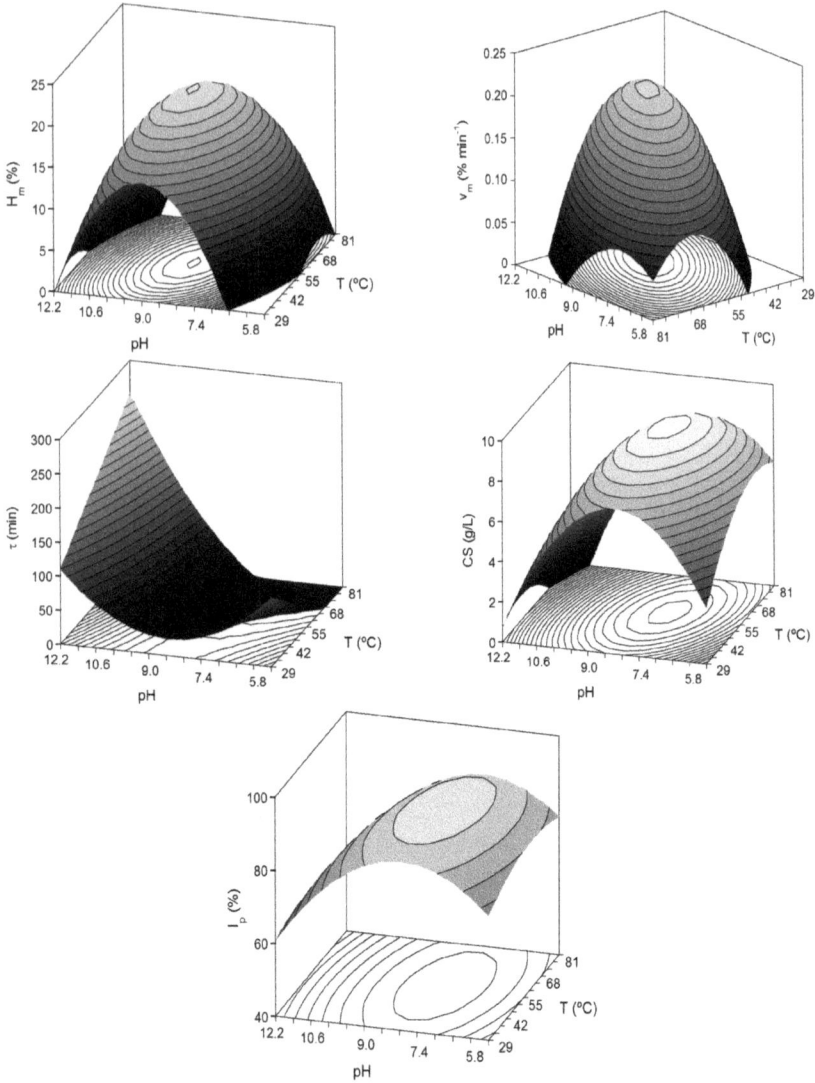

Figure 2. Predicted response surfaces by empirical equations summarized in Table 3 corresponding to the combined effect of pH and T on the different dependent variables evaluated for the study of head-cartilages proteolysis by alcalase.

Table 2. Summary of the independent variables (T, pH) in the response surface design with the corresponding experimental (Y_e) and predicted (Y_p) results of alcalase head-cartilage hydrolysis, CS production and CS purity regarding total protein (I_p). Natural values of experimental conditions are in brackets.* Determination of CS and I_p was only done at the end of the hydrolysis time (4 h).

Independent Variables		H_m (%)		v_m (% min^{-1})		τ (min)		CS (g/L) *		I_p (%) *	
X_1: T	X_2: pH	Y_e	Y_p	Y_e	Y_p	Y_e	Y_p	Y_e	Y_p	Y_e	Y_p
−1 (37.3)	−1 (6.9)	5.05	5.21	0.030	−0.018	51.5	41.7	7.09	6.86	85.12	84.64
1 (72.7)	−1 (6.9)	9.85	11.67	0.282	0.178	9.8	−21.3	9.21	8.35	89.43	86.33
−1 (37.3)	1 (11.1)	14.04	11.67	0.067	0.119	54.7	79.1	3.85	4.74	76.48	74.85
1 (72.7)	1 (11.1)	5.93	5.21	0.045	0.041	139.0	142.1	3.00	3.25	77.42	73.17
−1.41 (30)	0 (9.0)	12.80	14.58	0.079	0.065	44.9	24.7	7.45	7.40	85.25	86.01
1.41 (80)	0 (9.0)	15.81	14.58	0.082	0.148	14.1	24.7	7.38	7.40	82.02	86.01
0 (55)	−1.41 (6.0)	0.00	2.45	0.00	0.055	0.00	24.9	6.00	6.78	80.12	81.69
0 (55)	1.41 (12.0)	4.34	2.45	0.059	0.055	190.2	166.5	2.50	1.69	62.32	65.51
0 (55)	0 (9.0)	18.83	21.17	0.225	0.196	19.7	24.7	9.02	9.01	89.77	89.60
0 (55)	0 (9.0)	23.44	21.17	0.162	0.196	30.1	24.7	9.00	9.01	89.64	89.60
0 (55)	0 (9.0)	19.86	21.17	0.179	0.196	26.7	24.7	9.60	9.01	90.28	89.60
0 (55)	0 (9.0)	22.67	21.17	0.209	0.196	23.8	24.7	8.99	9.01	89.71	89.60
0 (55)	0 (9.0)	21.06	21.17	0.206	0.196	23.2	24.7	8.45	9.01	88.63	89.60

The polynomial models describing the correlation between the variables and response followed the general form defined by Equation (5) and is shown in Table 3.

Table 3. Second order equations describing the effect of T and pH on alcalase cartilage hydrolysis, CS production and I_p-index (coded values according to criteria defined in Table 1). The coefficient of adjusted determination (R_{adj}^2) and F-values (F_1, F_2, and F_3) is also shown. S: Significant; NS: Non-significant.

Parameters	H_m	v_m	τ	CS	I_p
b_0 (intercept)	21.17	0.196	24.69	9.01	89.60
b_1 (T)	-	0.029	-	-	-
b_2 (pH)	-	-	50.21	−1.80	−5.74
b_{12} (TxpH)	−3.23	−0.069	31.50	−0.74	−0.84
b_{11} (T^2)	−3.31	−0.045	-	−0.81	−1.80
b_{22} (pH^2)	−9.42	−0.071	35.73	−2.40	−8.05
R_{adj}^2	0.929	0.752	0.874	0.927	0.882
F_1	53.62 [$F_9^3 = 3.86$] ⇒ S	5.33 [$F_8^4 = 3.84$] ⇒ S	28.86 [$F_9^3 = 3.86$] ⇒ S	39.01 [$F_8^4 = 3.84$] ⇒ S	23.40 [$F_8^4 = 3.84$] ⇒ S
F_2	0.39 [$F_3^8 = 8.85$] ⇒ S	0.67 [$F_4^8 = 6.04$] ⇒ S	0.41 [$F_3^8 = 8.85$] ⇒ S	0.52 [$F_4^8 = 6.04$] ⇒ S	0.54 [$F_4^8 = 6.04$] ⇒ S
F_3	1.17 [$F_4^9 = 6.00$] ⇒ S	5.09 [$F_4^8 = 6.04$] ⇒ S	24.76 [$F_4^9 = 6.00$] ⇒ NS	2.71 [$F_4^9 = 6.04$] ⇒ NS	21.11 [$F_4^8 = 6.04$] ⇒ NS

A high proportion of variability (93% for H_m and CS) was successfully described by the second order equations. In any case, the agreement among experimental and predicted data was always greater than 75% and the robustness was good in all cases; it demonstrated the predictive capacity of the empirical equations in the range of T and pH here studied. The results of the multivariate analysis showed significant quadratic negative terms for pH and T ($p < 0.05$). This translates graphically in a dome (convex surface) with clear maximum points for the experimental domains of pH and T (Figure 2). The inverse response obtained for τ-parameter (concave surface) is in agreement with the fact that when the enzymatic hydrolysis is greater and faster (high H_m and v_m), the values of τ are shorter.

From the equations summarized in Table 3, the optima values of pH and T (pH$_{opt}$ and T_{opt}) that maximize the corresponding measured responses (Y_{max}) can be obtained by mathematical optimization using numerical or manual derivation [19] (Table 4). The optimal ranges depending on the variable of response were 55–62.6 °C and 8.14–9 for T and pH, respectively. Because all responses are equally important, it has been established the average of the values from Table 4 as the compromise option to select the best condition of pH_{opt} and T_{opt}. Thus, the values for the subsequent treatment in the alkaline hydroalcoholic solution were: pH = 8.5 and T = 58.1 °C.

Table 4. Optima values of the two independent variables (T_{opt} and pH_{opt}) to obtain the maximum responses from the equations defined in Table 3 and for the different dependent variables studied. [a] In this case, the optima values of T and pH are those that minimize the response of τ.

	H_m	v_m	τ	CS	I_p
T_{opt} (°C)	55.0	62.6	-	58.3	56.5
pH_{opt}	9.0	8.6	9.0 [a]	8.14	8.23
Y_{max}	21.17	0.204	-	9.38	90.6

In recent years, alcalase has shown excellent results in the hydrolysis of several fishing wastes, as for instance: Atlantic cod and cattle viscera [24,25], yellowfin tuna heads [26], salmon by-products [27] or cephalopods and shrimp wastewaters [28,29]. Kim *et al.* [30] performed a two-stage enzymatic hydrolysis for CS production from *Isurus oxyrinchus* using a combination of alcalase and flavourzyme. Other proteases have also been evaluated for cartilage hydrolysis in the purification of glycosaminoglycans. Lypaine was applied to the degradation of skate cartilage [31], papain was widely employed in the digestion of different tissues of several origins [11,21,32] and procolax obtained from ray pancreas and commercial papain were compared working on ray cartilage [12]. However, the high hydrolytic capacity, effectiveness on many different substrates and low cost, make alcalase a key enzyme for the recovery and pre-purification of CS from chondrichthyans discards and their by-products.

2.2. Enzymatic Hydrolysis of Skeletons and Fins Cartilages

In order to check whether the conditions described for heads were also suitable for the alcalase hydrolysis of other cartilages of *S. canicula* (skeletons and fins), two conditions of pH's (the initial obtained from the homogeneized cartilages and pH 8.5) at one temperature (58 °C) were assessed. Those modelled kinetics by Equation (4) are displayed in Figure 3 and estimations of the parameters are listed in Table 5.

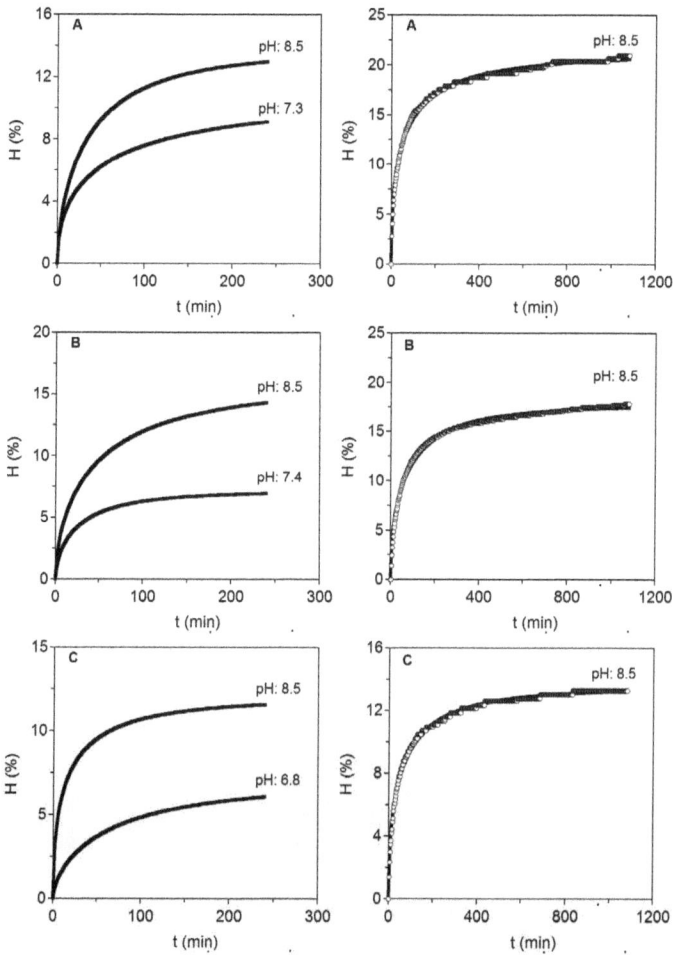

Figure 3. Enzymatic hydrolysis at two pH levels for different cartilages from *S. canicula* wastes (left). To the right, long hydrolysis at the best pH selected are additionally shown. Experimental data were fitted to the Weibull Equation (4). (**A**) Fins; (**B**) Heads and (**C**) Skeletons.

The results indicated that pH close to 8.5 was better than neutral pH for alcalase hydrolysis of cartilages. It suggests that the optimal conditions for heads can be also extrapolated to hydrolyse cartilages of skeleton and fins with similar positive results. In this context, higher maximum hydrolysis, maximum hydrolysis rate, CS production and CS purity index were significantly generated at alkaline pH. Moreover, the greatest hydrolysis (15.64%) and CS recovery (9.44 g/L) were produced in cartilaginous material from heads as substrate. Different extraction methods, including the use of high intense pulse fields (PEF), or a solvent-free mechanochemical extraction, have been tested for the production of CS from fish cartilage, reporting however, lower contents of CS, 6.92 g/L [33] and 9.33 g/L [34], than those obtained in this study for head shark cartilage. Longer kinetics of hydrolysis (18 h) at 58 °C and pH 8.5 were performed to establish more adequate time needed for enzyme catalysis. More than 8–10 h of proteolysis did not lead to significant increases in the degree of cartilages hydrolysis (less than 10% of variation).

Table 5. Parametric estimations corresponding to the Weibull Equation (4) applied to the enzymatic hydrolysis kinetics at the two pH indicated. Numerical values of the parameters are shown with their confidence intervals. In addition, CS concentrations and I_p-index obtained by selective precipitation under standard conditions are also summarized. [a] In this case, the kinetics were prolonged up to 18 h.

FINS	H_m (%)	v_m (%·min^{-1})	τ (min)	β	R^2	CS (g/L)	I_p (%)
pH: 7.3	10.73 ± 0.06	0.058 ± 0.001	31.82 ± 0.56	0.50 ± 0.00	0.991	5.65	77.5
pH: 8.5	13.59 ± 0.10	0.132 ± 0.003	22.84 ± 0.45	0.64 ± 0.01	0.999	6.50	83.7
[a] pH: 8.5	21.13 ± 0.10	0.110 ± 0.002	30.82 ± 0.65	0.46 ± 0.01	0.992	6.75	88.3
HEADS							
pH: 7.4	7.08 ± 0.01	0.094 ± 0.001	16.53 ± 0.09	0.64 ± 0.00	0.990	7.79	79.9
pH: 8.5	15.64 ± 0.02	0.111 ± 0.001	29.26 ± 0.10	0.60 ± 0.00	0.999	9.44	86.9
[a] pH: 8.5	17.72 ± 0.07	0.080 ± 0.001	42.60 ± 0.84	0.56 ± 0.01	0.992	9.68	89.6
SKELETONS							
pH: 6.8	6.85 ± 0.02	0.037 ± 0.001	42.54 ± 0.26	0.67 ± 0.00	0.997	4.79	76.7
pH: 8.5	11.93 ± 0.29	0.222 ± 0.021	9.25 ± 0.01	0.50 ± 0.04	0.969	6.07	80.4
[a] pH: 8.5	13.49 ± 0.04	0.074 ± 0.001	31.69 ± 0.84	0.50 ± 0.01	0.995	6.91	87.1

2.3. Optimisation of Alkaline Hydroalcoholic Treatment of Enzymatic Hydrolysates

Based on the optimised values described in the previous sections, the hydrolysates of cartilages from different origins (heads, skeletons and fins) were prepared under the following conditions: Hydrolysis time (10 h), $T = 58$ °C, pH = 8.5 (using Tris-HCl buffer 0.1 M), alcalase = 0.1% (v/w) (2.4 AU/kg), solid:liquid ratio (1:1), agitation = 200 rpm. The alcalase hydrolysates were centrifuged at 6000 rpm/20 min and the supernatants were employed in the subsequent treatment with alkaline hydroalcoholic solutions, as described here in the Experimental Section.

CS and I_p responses (experimental and predicted) from such treatments of *S. canicula* hydrolysates are summarized in Table 6.

Data from CS production and purities were converted into second-order polynomial equations as a function of two independent variables (E and N). The equations describing those effects and their statistical results are represented in Table 7.

The adjusted coefficients of determination were higher than 0.83 indicating a good correlation between experimental data and theoretical responses. In all cases, responses were significantly affected by positive E and N linear terms and negative quadratic coefficients of both variables ($p < 0.05$). The predicted response surfaces were very homogeneous displaying perfect domes (convex surfaces) in the experimental domain executed (Figure 4). Nevertheless, cases of over and under-estimation were observed (Table 6), which do not invalidate the results, and are due to not achieving coefficients of determination nearer to one (Table 7). As described previously, the present R^2_{adj} values revealed good but not perfect agreement among surfaces and experimental data; therefore little lack of fit is commonly obtained.

Table 6. Summary of the independent variables (NaOH: N, EtOH: E) in the response surface design with the corresponding experimental (Y_e) and predicted (Y_p) results of selective precipitation of CS from *S. canicula* wastes. Natural values of experimental conditions are in brackets.

		HEADS				FINS				SKELETONS			
		CS (g/L)		I_p (%)		CS (g/L)		I_p (%)		CS (g/L)		I_p (%)	
Independent Variables													
X_1: N	X_2: E	Y_e	Y_p	Y_e	Y_p	Y_e	Y_p	Y_e	Y_p	Y_e	Y_p	Y_e	Y_p
−1 (0.20)	−1 (0.46)	0.25	0.45	4.13	6.63	0.10	0.01	20.56	18.27	0.10	−0.45	22.20	15.48
1 (0.70)	−1 (0.46)	0.50	1.33	5.88	15.01	0.80	1.89	17.14	34.64	0.10	1.36	22.20	37.50
−1 (0.20)	1 (1.24)	0.70	1.75	8.24	19.74	5.74	4.75	86.05	72.17	5.26	4.00	83.63	68.67
1 (0.70)	1 (1.24)	7.32	9.00	87.04	105.17	5.72	5.90	86.34	92.25	5.39	5.81	85.13	90.69
−1.41 (0.10)	0 (0.85)	1.03	0.53	11.54	5.87	1.61	2.40	32.09	44.31	0.10	1.38	22.20	37.49
1.41 (0.80)	0 (0.85)	7.67	6.27	87.08	72.00	5.41	4.53	85.86	70.00	5.14	3.93	83.42	68.54
0 (0.45)	−1.41 (0.30)	0.10	−0.24	2.54	−1.46	0.44	−0.25	22.61	12.57	0.10	−0.40	22.20	16.02
0 (0.45)	1.41 (1.40)	7.62	6.08	88.09	71.34	5.32	5.92	84.78	91.18	5.30	5.88	84.43	91.02
0 (0.45)	0 (0.85)	7.68	7.71	87.44	86.77	5.76	5.67	85.71	85.33	5.26	5.47	84.00	84.19
0 (0.45)	0 (0.85)	7.54	7.71	86.79	86.77	5.46	5.67	85.22	85.33	5.70	5.47	84.71	84.19
0 (0.45)	0 (0.85)	7.70	7.71	86.43	86.77	5.74	5.67	85.91	85.33	5.45	5.47	83.59	84.19
0 (0.45)	0 (0.85)	7.72	7.71	86.19	86.77	5.72	5.67	85.19	85.33	5.47	5.47	84.73	84.19
0 (0.45)	0 (0.85)	7.89	7.71	86.77	86.77	5.66	5.67	84.57	85.33	5.49	5.47	83.93	84.19

Table 7. Second order equations describing the effect of N and E on selective precipitation of CS (coded values according to criteria defined in Table 6). The coefficient of adjusted determination (R^2_{adj}) and F-values (F_1 and F_2) is also shown. S: Significant.

	HEADS		FINS		SKELETONS	
Parameters	CS	I_p	CS	I_p	CS	I_p
b_0 (intercept)	7.71	86.77	5.67	85.33	5.47	84.19
b_1 (N)	2.04	23.45	0.76	9.11	0.91	11.01
b_2 (E)	2.24	25.81	2.19	27.88	2.23	26.59
b_{12} (N × E)	1.59	19.26	−0.18	0.93	NS	NS
b_{11} (N²)	−2.17	−24.06	−1.11	−14.17	−1.42	−15.68
b_{22} (E²)	−2.41	−26.07	−1.43	−16.83	−1.38	−15.43
R^2_{adj}	0.897	0.905	0.885	0.830	0.857	0.849
F_1	21.97 $[F^5_7 = 3.97]\,S$	23.88 $[F^5_7 = 3.97]\,S$	19.54 $[F^5_7 = 3.97]\,S$	12.71 $[F^5_7 = 3.97]\,S$	18.92 $[F^4_8 = 3.84]\,S$	17.85 $[F^4_8 = 3.84]\,S$
F_2	0.67 $[F^8_5 = 4.82]\,S$	0.66 $[F^8_5 = 4.82]\,S$	0.67 $[F^8_5 = 4.82]\,S$	0.69 $[F^8_5 = 4.82]\,S$	0.55 $[F^8_4 = 6.04]\,S$	0.56 $[F^8_4 = 6.04]\,S$

HEADS

FINS

SKELETONS

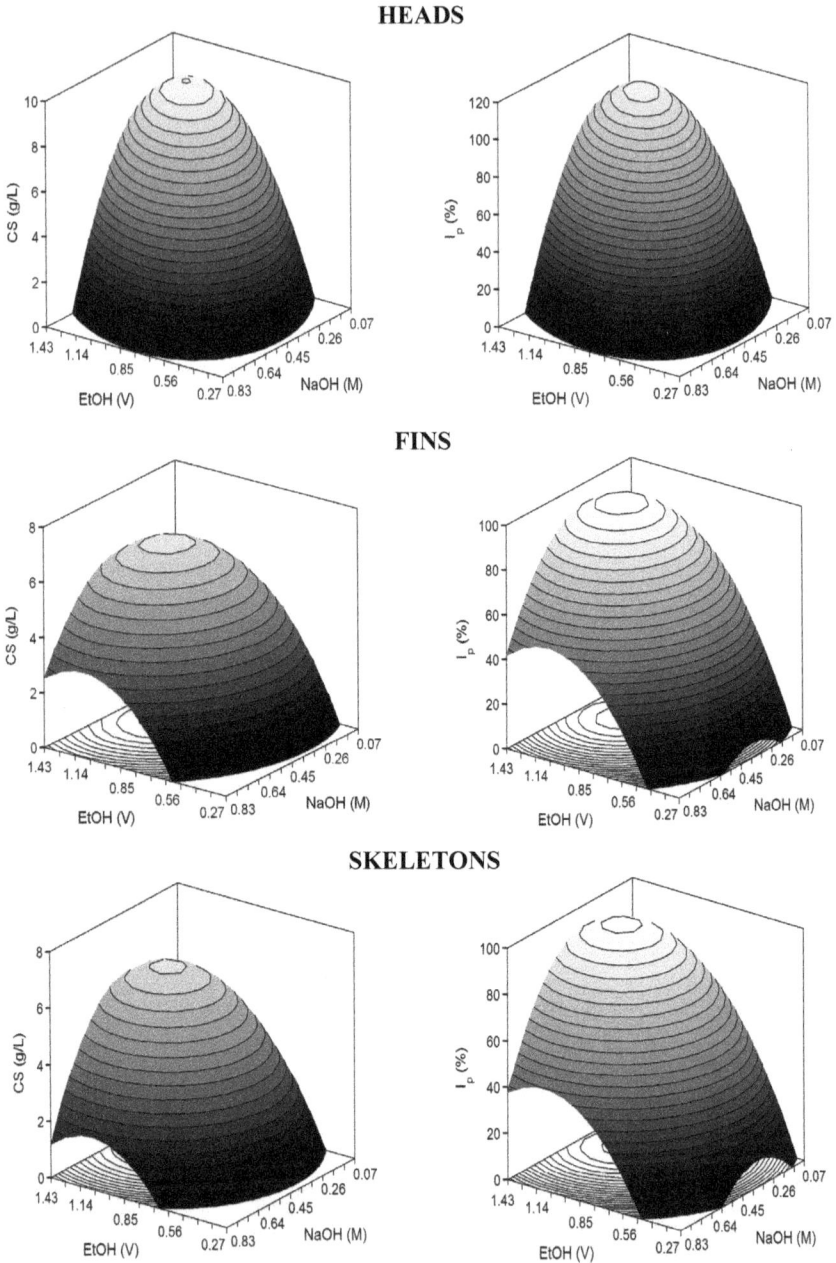

Figure 4. Predicted response surfaces by empirical equations summarized in Table 7 corresponding to the combined effect of NaOH and EtOH on the selective treatment of CS from hydrolysate cartilages of *S. canicula*.

The sequential combination of the two-stages for glycosaminoglycan recovery optimised until now led to almost 90% of CS purity against total protein. The best NaOH concentrations and volumes of ethanol for chemical treatment of hydrolysates were (averaging the two responses, CS concentration and purity): 0.64 M and 1.14 volumes for heads, 0.53 M and 1.16 volumes for fins and 0.54 M and 1.20 volumes for skeletons (Table 8). The aforementioned little lack of fit might be also the cause of the over-estimation of Y_{max} values showed in Table 8. The optima levels of alkali and alcohol were higher than those found for cartilages of *Raja clavata* [12]. Ethanol has been reported to be an excellent reagent for the selective precipitation of CS, removing the major protein presents in the extract [35]. However, increases in the quantity of ethanol used for the extraction of CS from shark cartilage, did not lead to increases in the yield of the CS obtained [34,36].

Table 8. Optima values of the two independent variables ($NaOH_{opt}$ and $EtOH_{opt}$) to obtain the best responses from the equations defined in Table 7 and for the two dependent variables studied (CS concentration and purity).

	HEADS		FINS		SKELETONS	
	CS	I_p	CS	I_p	CS	I_p
$NaOH_{opt}$ (M)	0.63	0.65	0.52	0.54	0.53	0.54
$EtOH_{opt}$ (V)	1.12	1.16	1.14	1.18	1.16	1.24
Y_{max}	9.24	106.4	6.59	98.6	6.52	97.6

2.4. Purification of CS by Ultrafiltration-Diafiltration Processes

The last stage of CS purification was carried out using membrane technologies at a 30 kDa cut-off. Four-liter batches of CS neutralized solutions obtained under the optimal experimental conditions described in previous sections, were purified by a sequence of UF and DF performances. The progress of CS and protein levels *versus* concentration factor by UF is displayed in Figure 5 (Top).

Perfect correlation agreement among theoretical and experimental concentration factor patterns (more than nine-fold in all cases) was reached after the initial 30 kDa UF where the CS concentration from skeletons and heads cartilages was concentrated up to 20–25 g/L. In contrast, the protein was mainly permeated (complete disagreement between predicted and real data) suggesting a lower molecular weight than 30 kDa of the peptidic fraction. The difference of CS recovery comparing origins of the cartilages was due to the lower initial CS content in the fins solutions prepared for UF-DF. The proportion in weight of such cartilage is much lower in comparison to the other fractions, therefore when 4 L of fin solution are obtained, in order to perform representative membrane experiments, the initial concentration of CS is indeed much lower. The filtrate flows during UF processes (concentration step) were maintained in average values of (mL/min): 755, 520 and 900 for fins, head and skeleton samples respectively. The flow falls were inferior to 15% of the average values.

Equation (6) accurately predicted the data of retention dynamics obtained by the DF process (Figure 5, bottom) with high statistical correlation ($R^2 > 0.988$) (Table 9). All the parameter determinations and the estimation of CS and protein rejection at three diavolumes (R_{3D}) are also defined in Table 9.

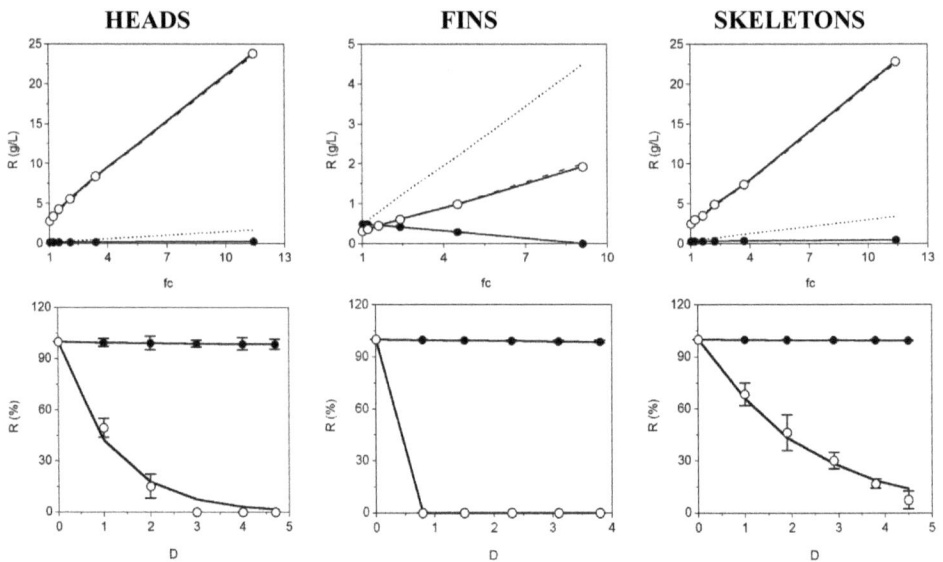

Figure 5. UF-DF process for CS purification from *S. canicula* cartilages of three origins at 30 kDa. Top: Concentration of retained protein (○) and CS (●) in linear relation with the factor of volumetric concentration (fc) showing experimental data (points) and theoretical profiles corresponding to a completely retained solute (discontinuous line). Bottom: Progress of protein (○) and CS (●) retention with the increase of diavolume from DF process (D). Equation (6) was used to fit the experimental data. Error bars are the confidence intervals ($\alpha = 0.05$; $n = 2$).

Table 9. Parametric estimates from DF purification data (with MWCO of 30 kDa) of CS and proteins fitted to the Equation (6). Determination coefficients (R^2) are also shown. NS: Non-significant.

		CS	Proteins
	R_0	2.52 ± 1.84	100.0 ± 22.6
	R_f	97.4 ± 1.91	0.0
HEADS	s	0.829 ± 0.189	0.134 (NS)
	R^2	0.996	0.988
	R_{3D}	1.01	92.6
	R_0	23.2 (NS)	-
	R_f	76.8 ± 41.8	-
FINS	s	0.985 ± 0.030	-
	R^2	0.999	-
	R_{3D}	1.02	-
	R_0	20 (NS)	100.0 ± 13.5
	R_f	80 (NS)	0.0
SKELETONS	s	0.994 ± 0.119	0.561 ± 0.115
	R^2	0.998	0.992
	R_{3D}	0.36	73.2

The values of the coefficients corresponding to CS, demonstrate that the retention was almost total ($s \sim 1$, $R_f > 76\%$ and $R_{3D} < 1.1\%$). In the case of proteins, the permeation of fin solutions was complete at the beginning of the DF and needed more than 3 or 4 relative diavolumes for the heads and skeletons samples, respectively. The complete desalination of retentates was also observed (data not shown). These results reveals the high efficiency of the 30 kDa UF-DF system as a final step to CS retention and recovery and protein discard from *S. canicula* wastes. The purity of CS retentates (in terms of I_p-values) after drying was: 98%, 97% and 96.2% for head, skeleton and fins. If an ulterior purification might be still required, dried samples could return to the alkaline-alcoholic treatment and UF-DF separation, in similar conditions to those described previously. The final yields of CS were (as % of wet weight cartilage): 4.8, 3.3 and 1.5 for heads, fins and skeleton materials, respectively. Membrane separation techniques have been used as the last step of purification of chondroitin sulphate from different cartilage sources, because of the high separation efficiency, different cut-off membranes, ease of scale-up and cost effectiveness [37]. Lignot *et al.* [31] using the UF technique showed lower concentration factors for CS in skate, than those found in this study (up to nine times).

Other methods for the separation/purification of CS are found in literature, including gel filtration [36] or ion-exchange chromatography [38], however the purity of the final CS did not showed any increase in comparison to our results. An initial analysis of chemical composition of sulphate groups indicated that all CS from different types of cartilage were similar with a proportion of sulphation in C6 (6S) and C4 (4S) of 40%–44% and 39%–43% respectively (unpublished data). It also confirmed the validity of the optimisation developed herein. Based on a similar proposal but obtaining different optimal conditions [12], the 6S proportion was 75% in ray cartilage (unpublished data).

3. Experimental Section

3.1. Cartilage Preparation and Compositional Analysis

Small-spotted catshark (*Scyliorhinus canicula*) individuals obtained approximately 12 h after capture from a local market in Vigo (North-West, Spain) were skinned, heads, skeletons and fins were separated from muscle and processed independently. These materials were heated in a water bath at 80 °C for 30 min to help the manual separation of muscular tissue from cartilage. The cartilages obtained were crushed and homogenized to a particle size of ~1 mm using a grinder and stored at −20 °C until use. The chemical composition of cartilaginous materials was evaluated in triplicate by analysing crude protein, ash, moisture and fat content. Total nitrogen content was determined according to the Kjeldahl method [38] in a DigiPREP HT digestor, DigiPREP 500 fully automatic steam distillation and a TitroLine easy titration unit, and crude protein content was calculated as total nitrogen multiplied by 6.25. Ash was obtained by calcination at 600 °C in a muffle furnace and moisture content determined after heating at 105 °C in an oven until constant weight. Lipid content was determined by the methodology of Bligh and Dyer [39]. Finally, the total carbohydrate content was estimated by the difference between total weight (subtracting protein, fat and ash) and moisture content.

3.2. Analytical Determinations

Total soluble proteins (Pr) of CS solutions were determined by the method of Lowry *et al.* [40]; CS, as glucuronic acid, was quantified by the method of Van den Hoogen *et al.* [41], according with the modifications of Murado *et al.* [42]. This modified method is mainly efficient and sensitive for glucuronic acid without sulphation. Thus, keratan sulphate (D-galactose + 6-sulphate-N-acetylglucosamine) is not detected and dermatan sulphate (also known as chondroitin sulphate B: Iduronic + 4-sulphate-N-acetylglucosamine) as well as heparan sulphate (2-sulphate-glucuronic or iduronic acid + 6-sulphate-N-sulphoglucosamine) proved to be less sensitive to that reaction (25% of the glucuronic acid sensitivity). Additionally, previous results [11,36] have indicated almost no presence of heparan sulphate in *S. canicula* and *Sphyrna Lewini* (another similar shark) and more than 80% of CS of the total glycosaminoglycans in the cartilage composition. The presence of hyaluronic acid (equally well determined by m-hydroxydifenyl reaction) in the proteoglycan matrix of fin cartilage from *S. Lewini* has not been demonstrated and its value is lower than 10% of total glycosaminglycans in *S. canicula* cartilage [11,36]. Therefore, quantification of CS as proposed is adequate and does not invalidate the results herein obtained. CS purity index (I_p), defined as I_p (%) = CS × 100/(CS + Pr), was also calculated in all purification stages.

3.3. Enzymatic Hydrolysis of Cartilages

Cartilages were hydrolysed using Alcalase 2.4 L from *Bacillus licheniformis* (Novozyme Nordisk, Bagsvaerd, Denmark). The enzyme/substrate ratio was 2.4 U/kg of fresh cartilage and the solid:liquid ratio was (1:1). Hydrolysis was prepared using a stirred (200 rpm) and thermostatted reactor (100 mL) connected to pH and temperature electrodes and coupled to an auto-titrator (Metrohm). T and pH conditions were established according to a full factorial design of second order, as it is described in the Experimental Section. pH levels of each point of the experimental design were adjusted by adding 0.2 M NaOH, and the pH was maintained constant during the hydrolysis reaction by automatic addition of 0.2 M NaOH. After 4 h of hydrolysis, samples were inactivated by boiling (10 min), cooled in an ice-water bath and centrifuged (6000× g, 20 min). Sediments were discarded and the supernatants stored at −20 °C until further analysis. The extent of enzymatic hydrolysis was determined by the pH-Stat method [43], which allows the estimation of degree of hydrolysis (H) based on amount of alkali needed to maintain the pH at the desired level. Thus, H (in %) could be obtained according to the following expression being the percent ratio between the total number of peptide bonds cleaved and the total number of peptide bonds in the original protein:

$$H = \frac{B\ N_b}{\alpha\ M_p\ h_{tot}} \tag{1}$$

where, B is the volume (mL) of 0.2 M NaOH consumed during hydrolysis; N_b is the normality of NaOH; M_p is the mass (g) of initial protein ($N \times 6.25$); h_{tot} is the total number of peptide bonds available for proteolytic hydrolysis (8.6 meq/g), and α is the average degree of dissociation of the amino groups in the protein substrate, and was calculated as follows:

$$\alpha = \frac{10^{pH-pK}}{1 + 10^{pH-pK}} \tag{2}$$

The pK value is dependent on the temperature of hydrolysis (in K degrees), therefore it can be also calculated according to the following expression:

$$pK = 2400\left(7.8 + \frac{298 - T}{298\ T}\right) \tag{3}$$

3.4. Mathematical Modelling of the Proteolysis Kinetics

The non-linear kinetics of *S. canicula* cartilage hydrolysis mediated by alcalase, under different pH and T conditions, were fitted to the Weibull equation [22,44]:

$$H = H_m\left\{1 - \exp\left[-\ln 2\left(\frac{t}{\tau}\right)^{\beta}\right]\right\} \text{ with } v_m = \frac{H_m\ \beta\ \ln 2}{2\ \tau} \tag{4}$$

where, H is the degree of hydrolysis (%); t is the time of hydrolysis (min); H_m is the maximum degree of hydrolysis (%); β is a parameter related with the maximum slope of cartilage hydrolysis (dimensionless); τ is the time required to achieve the semi-maximum degree of hydrolysis (min) and v_m is the maximum hydrolysis rate at the τ-time (% min^{-1}).

3.5. Experimental Designs and Statistical Analysis

Two different experimental designs were performed in the present work. First, the effect of temperature (T) and pH on the hydrolysis degree of head cartilages (according to kinetic parameters from Equation (4)) and catalyzed by alcalase, was studied. Then, the concentration of NaOH (N) and the volumes of ethanol (E) needed for the final alkaline proteolysis of proteoglycan and selective precipitation of CS against proteins, was optimized. In both cases, the factorial experiments were rotatable second order designs with five replicates in the centre of the experimental domains [45].

The conditions of the independent variables studied for the enzymatic hydrolysis of shark materials were: T in the range 30–80 °C and pH in the range 6–12. The rest of experimental conditions were kept constant (see enzymatic hydrolysis section). The experiments of CS recovery from the enzymatic hydrolysates obtained in the optimal conditions from previous design, were carried out by slow addition and with moderate agitation at room temperature, and hydroalcoholic solutions of NaOH in the required proportions to obtain reaction mixtures with the preestablished values of N and E in the following intervals: N (0.1–0.8 M) and E (0.3–1.4 v). In order to improve the subsequent CS recovery in water, 2.5% NaCl was added to all alkaline hydroalcoholic mixtures. After a period of 2 h in agitation, the suspensions were centrifuged ($6000 \times$ *g*; 20 min) and the sediments were redissolved with water and neutralized using 6 M HCl. The encoding procedure of the variables was performed by the following formulas:

Codification

$V_c = (V_n - V_0)/\Delta V_n$

V_n: Natural value of the variable to codify

V_0: Natural value in the centre of the domain

V_c: Codified value of the variable

ΔV_n: Increment of V_n per unit of V_c

Decodification

$V_n = V_0 + (\Delta V_n \times \Delta V_c)$

Both expressions of the independent variables, codified and natural values, in each experimental run are summarized in Tables 1, 2 and 6.

Orthogonal least-squares calculation on factorial design data, were used to obtain empirical equations describing the different dependent variables studied (Y), each one related to T and pH for enzymatic hydrolysis and N and E for CS production. The general form of the polynomial equations is:

$$Y = b_0 + \sum_{i=1}^{n} b_i X_i + \sum_{\substack{i=1 \\ j=2 \\ j>i}}^{n-1} \sum_{j=2}^{n} b_{ij} X_i X_j + \sum_{i=1}^{n} b_{ii} X_i^2 \tag{5}$$

where Y represents the response to be modelled; b_0 is a constant coefficient, b_i is the coefficient of linear effect, b_{ij} is the coefficient of interaction effect, b_{ii} the coefficients of squared effect, n is the number of variables and X_i and X_j define the independent variables. The statistical significance of the coefficients was verified by means of the Student t-test ($\alpha = 0.05$), goodness-of-fit was established as the adjusted determination coefficient (R_{adj}^2) and the model consistency by the Fisher F test ($\alpha = 0.05$) using the following mean squares ratios:

the model is acceptable when

F1 = Model/Total error $F1 \geq F_{den}^{num}$

F2 = (Model + Lack of fitting)/Model $F2 \leq F_{den}^{num}$

F3 = Total error/Experimental error $F3 \leq F_{den}^{num}$

F_{den}^{num} are the theoretical values to $\alpha = 0.05$ with the corresponding degrees of freedom for numerator (num) and denominator (den). All fitting procedures, coefficient estimates and statistical calculations were performed on a Microsoft Excel spreadsheet.

3.6. Ultrafiltration-Diafiltration Process

CS neutralized solutions were subjected to ultrafiltration-diafiltration (UF-DF) using a membrane (Prep/Scale-TFF: Spiral polyethersulfone membrane of 0.56 m^2, Millipore Corporation, Bedford, MA, USA) of 30 kDa molecular weight cut-off (MWCO). The operation mode was the following: An initial phase of ultrafiltration (UF) at 40 °C with total recirculation of retentate was performed, immediately followed by a diafiltration (DF) step. During UF, the inlet pressure remained constant (<1 bar) to determine the drops of flow rate due to the increased concentration of the retentate and to possible adhesions to the membrane. The final retentate (after DF) was lyophilized and stored at 4 °C for further analysis. Permeate of the UF step was analysed and finally discarded. For modelling the membrane process, we fixed a DF with constant volume (filtration flow = water intake flow), where the concentration of a permeable solute in the retentate was predicted by using the first-order equation [12]:

$$R = R_f + R_0 \exp[-(1-s)D] \tag{6}$$

where, R is the concentration of permeable protein or CS in the retentate (% from the level at initial DF), R_0 is the permeate concentration (%), R_f is the asymptotic and retentate concentration (%), D is the relative diavolume (volume of added water/constant retentate volume) and s is the specific retention of protein or CS with variation between 0 (the solute is filtered as the solvent) and 1 (the solute is totally retained). Thus, using normalized values (%): $R_0 + R_f = 100$, with $R_0 = 0$ if all protein or CS are permeable. In addition, the percentage of protein or CS eliminated by three diavolumes (R_{3D}) was calculated by substituting in Equation (6) the value of parameter D by 3.

3.7. Numerical Methods for Non-Linear Curves Modelling

Cartilage hydrolysis and UF-DF data were modelled by minimisation of the sum of quadratic differences between observed and predicted values, using the non-linear least-squares (quasi-Newton) method provided by the macro "Solver" of the Microsoft Excel spreadsheet. Confidence intervals from the parametric estimates (Student's *t* test) and consistence of mathematical models (Fisher's *F* test) and residual analysis (Durbin-Watson test) were evaluated by "SolverAid" macro [46].

4. Conclusions

A complete optimization of the different processes involved in the CS recovery and purification from cartilage wastes of *S. canicula* have been developed. Two experimental designs, incorporating kinetic approaches, were carried out to define the effect of pH and temperature on alcalase activity and the joint capacity of NaOH and EtOH on CS selective precipitation. Both proposals were successfully solved obtaining optimal conditions as follows: pH = 8.5 and T = 58 °C for enzymatic hydrolysis, and 0.53–0.64 M of NaOH and 1.14–1.20 volumes of EtOH for chemical treatment. In addition, we can indicate that the head wastes are the best source of CS production from *S. canicula*. Finally, the extracts from alkaline hydroalcoholic treatment were processed by UF-DF protocols at 30 kDa of MWCO for the differential retention of CS and concomitant rejection of protein material. Both objectives were successfully reached with total concentration and recoverability of CS as well as protein elimination using no more than 3–5 diavolumes in the DF step.

Our results showed that *S. canicula* is a good source of CS and such bioproduction is an excellent alternative for the valorization of discards and its by-products. However, further physicochemical studies are required to characterize completely the type of CS involved and the sulphation pattern presents in the glycosaminoglycan purified. These experiments exceed the objectives reported in the present work.

Acknowledgments: We are grateful to Ramón Novoa-Carballal (3B's Research Group, University of Minho, Portugal) for the determination of 6S sulphation pattern (data still unpublished). We also thank Ramiro Martínez (Novozymes A/S, Spain) for supplying us with Alcalase. Financial support from projects MARMED 2011-1/164 (Atlantic Area Programme, EU), 0687_NOVOMAR_1_P (POCTEP Programme, EU) and iSEAS LIFE13 ENV/ES/000131 (LIFE+ Programme, EU) is acknowledged.

Author Contributions: J.A.V. and M.B. conceived and designed the experiments; M.B. and J.F. performed the experiments; J.A.V. and M.B. analyzed the data; J.A.V. and M.B. wrote the paper, R.I.P.M. and C.G.S. participated regarding the interpretation of data and also critically revised the manuscript.

Conflicts of Interest: The authors declare no conflict of interest.

References

1. Olaso, I.; Velasco, F.; Pérez, N. Importance of discarded blue whiting (*Micromesistius poutassou*) in the diet of the lesser spotted dogfish (*Scyliorhinus canicula*) in the Cantabrian Sea. *ICES J. Mar. Sci.* **1998**, *55*, 331–341. [CrossRef]

2. Rodríguez-Cabello, C.; Fernández, A.; Olaso, I.; Sánchez, F.; Gancedo, R.; Punzón, A.; Cendrero, O. Overview of continental shelf elasmobranch fisheries in the Cantabrian Sea. *J. N. W. Atl. Fish. Sci* **2005**, *35*, 375–385. [CrossRef]

3. ICES. *Report of the Working Group on Elasmobranch Fishes (WGEF), 17–21 June 2013, Lisbon, Portugal*; International Council for the Exploration of the Sea: Copenhagen, Denmark, 2013; p. 680.

4. Chalamaiah, M.; Dinesh, K.; Hemalatha, R.; Jyothirmayi, T. Fish protein hydrolysates: Proximate composition, amino acid composition, antioxidant activities and applications: A review. *Food Chem.* **2012**, *135*, 3020–3038. [CrossRef] [PubMed]

5. Woo, J.; Yu, S.; Cho, S.; Lee, Y.; Kim, S. Extraction optimization and propertoes of collagen from yellowfin tuna (*Thunnus albacares*) dorsal skin. *Food Hydrocolloids* **2008**, *22*, 879–887. [CrossRef]

6. Bougatef, A.; Nedjar-Arroume, N.; Manni, L.; Ravallec, R.; Barkia, A.; Guillochon, D.; Nasri, M. Purification and identification of novel antioxidant peptides from enzymatic hydrolysates of sardinelle (*Sardinella aurita*) by-products proteins. *Food Chem.* **2010**, *118*, 559–565. [CrossRef]

7. Blanco, M.; Sotelo, C.G.; Chapela, M.J.; Perez-Martin, R.I. Towards sustainable and efficient use of fishery resources: Present and future trends. *Trends Food Sci. Technol.* **2007**, *18*, 29–36. [CrossRef]

8. Axelsson, I.; Heinegard, D. Characterization of chondroitin sulfate-rich proteoglycans from bovine corneal stroma. *Exp. Eye Res.* **1980**, *31*, 57–66. [CrossRef] [PubMed]

9. Lee, A.; Langer, R. Shark cartilage contains inhibitors of tumor aniogenesis. *Science* **1983**, *16*, 1185–1187. [CrossRef]

10. Malavaki, C.J.; Asimakopoulou, A.P.; Lamari, F.N.; Theocharis, A.D.; Tzanakakis, G.N.; Karamanos, N.K. Capillary electrophoresis for the quality control of chondroitin sulfates in raw materials and formulations. *Anal. Biochem.* **2008**, *374*, 213–220. [CrossRef] [PubMed]

11. Gargiulo, V.; Lanzetta, R.; Parrilli, M.; de Castro, C. Structural analysis of chondroitin sulfate from *Scyliorhinus canicula*: A useful source of this polysaccharide. *Glycobiology* **2009**, *19*, 1485–1491. [CrossRef] [PubMed]

12. Murado, M.A.; Fraguas, J.; Montemayor, M.I.; Vázquez, J.A.; González, P. Preparation of highly purified chondroitin sulphate from skate (*Raja clavata*) cartilage by-products. Process optimization including a new procedure of alkaline hydroalcoholic hydrolysis. *Biochem. Eng. J.* **2010**, *49*, 126–132. [CrossRef]

13. Pipitone, V.R. Chondroprotection with chondroitin sulphate. *Drugs Exp. Clin. Res.* **1991**, *17*, 3–7. [PubMed]

14. Vázquez, J.A.; Rodríguez-Amado, I.; Montemayor, M.I.; Fraguas, J.; González, M.P.; Murado, M.A. Chondroitin sulphate, hyaluronic acid and chitin/chitosan production using marine waste sources: Characteristics, applications and eco-friendly processes: A review. *Mar. Drugs* **2013**, *11*, 747–774. [CrossRef] [PubMed]

15. Yamada, S.; Sugahara, K. Potential therapeutic application of chondroitin sulfate/dermatan sulfate. *Curr. Drug Discov. Technol.* **2008**, *5*, 289–301. [CrossRef] [PubMed]

16. Kavya, K.C.; Dixit, R.; Jayakumar, R.; Nair, S.V.; Chennazhi, K.P. Synthesis and characterization of chitosan/chondroitin sulfate/nano-SiO_2 composite scaffold for bone tissue engineering. *J. Biomed. Nanotechnol.* **2012**, *8*, 149–160. [CrossRef] [PubMed]

17. Chang, C.H.; Liu, H.C.; Lin, C.C.; Chou, C.H.; Lin, F.H. Gelatin-chondroitin-hyaluronan tri-copolymer scaffold for cartilage tissue engineering. *Biomaterials* **2003**, *24*, 4853–4858. [CrossRef] [PubMed]

18. Leite, A.J.; Sher, P.; Mano, J.F. Chitosan/chondroitin sulfate multilayers as supports for calcium phosphate biomineralization. *Mater. Lett.* **2014**, *121*, 62–65.

19. Wardhani, D.H.; Vázquez, J.A.; Pandiella, S.S. Optimisation of antioxidants extraction from soybeans fermented by *Aspergillus oryzae*. *Food Chem.* **2010**, *118*, 731–739. [CrossRef]

20. Murado, M.A.; Montemayor, M.I.; Cabo, M.L.; Vázquez, J.A.; González, M.P. Optimization of extraction and purification process of hyaluronic acid from fish eyeball. *Food Bioprod. Process.* **2012**, *90*, 491–498. [CrossRef]

21. Garnjanagoonchorn, W.; Wongekalak, L.; Engkagul, A. Determination of chondroitin sulfate from different sources of cartilage. *Chem. Eng. Process.* **2007**, *46*, 465–471. [CrossRef]

22. Vázquez, J.A.; Lorenzo, J.M.; Fuciños, P.; Franco, D. Evaluation of non-linear equations to model different animal growths with mono and bisigmoid profiles. *J. Theor. Biol.* **2012**, *134*, 95–105. [CrossRef]

23. Prieto, M.A.; Vázquez, J.A.; Murado, M.A. A new mathematical model to quantify and characterize the response to pro- and anti-oxidants of the copper-induced oxidation of LDL assay. A tool for examination of potential preventive compounds and clinical risk prediction. *Food Res. Int.* **2014**, *66*, 501–513. [CrossRef]

24. Aspmo, S.I.; Horn, S.J.; Eijsink, V.G.H. Enzymatic hydrolysis of Atlantic cod (*Gadus morhua* L.) viscera. *Process Biochem.* **2005**, *40*, 1957–1966. [CrossRef]

25. Bhaskar, N.; Benila, T.; Radha, C.; Lalitha, R.G. Optimization of enzymatic hydrolysis of visceral waste proteins of Catla (*Catla catla*) for preparing protein hydrolysate using a commercial protease. *Bioresour. Technol.* **2008**, *99*, 335–343. [CrossRef] [PubMed]

26. Safari, R.; Motamedzadegan, A.; Ovissipour, M.; Regenstein, J.M.; Gildberg, A.; Rasco, B. Hydrolysates from yellowfin tuna (*Thunnus albacares*) heads as a complex nitrogen source for lactic acid bacteria. *Food Bioprocess Technol.* **2012**, *5*, 73–79. [CrossRef]

27. Ahn, C.B.; Kim, J.G.; Je, J.Y. Purification and antioxidant properties of octapeptide from salmon byproduct protein hydrolysate by gastrointestinal digestion. *Food Chem.* **2014**, *147*, 78–83. [CrossRef] [PubMed]

28. Amado, I.R.; Vázquez, J.A.; González, M.P.; Murado, M.A. Production of antihypertensive and antioxidant activities by enzymatic hydrolysis of protein concentrates recovered by ultrafiltration from cuttlefish processing wastewaters. *Biochem. Eng. J.* **2013**, *76*, 43–54. [CrossRef]

29. Amado, I.R.; Vázquez, J.A.; Murado, M.A.; González, M.P. Recovery of astaxanthin from shrimp cooking wastewater: Optimization of astaxanthin extraction by response surface methodology and kinetic studies. *Food Bioprocess Technol.* **2014**, *8*, 371–381. [CrossRef]

30. Kim, S.B.; Ji, C.I.; Woo, J.W.; Do, J.R.; Cho, S.M.; Lee, Y.B.; Nam, S. Simplified purification of chondroitin sulphate from scapular cartilage of shortfin mako shark (*Isurus oxyrinchus*). *Int. J. Food Sci. Technol.* **2012**, *47*, 91–99. [CrossRef]

31. Lignot, B.; Lahogue, V.; Bourseau, P. Enzymatic extraction of chondroitin sulfate from skate cartilage and concentration-desalting by ultrafiltration. *J. Biotechnol.* **2003**, *103*, 281–284. [CrossRef] [PubMed]

32. Muccia, A.; Schenettia, L.; Volpi, N. 1H and 13C nuclear magnetic resonance identification and characterization of components of chondroitin sulfates of various origin. *Carbohydr. Polym.* **2000**, *41*, 37–45. [CrossRef]

33. He, G.; Yin, Y.; Yan, X.; Yu, Q. Optimisation extraction of chondroitin sulfate from bone by high intensity pulsed electric fields. *Food Chem.* **2014**, *164*, 205–210. [CrossRef] [PubMed]

34. Wang, P.; Tang, J. Solvent-free mechanochemical extraction of chondroitin sulfate from shark cartilage. *Chem. Eng. Processs.* **2009**, *48*, 1187–1191. [CrossRef]

35. Shi, Y.; Meng, Y.; Li, J.; Chen, J.; Liu, Y.; Bai, X. Chondroitin sulfate: Extraction, purification, microbial and chemical synthesis. *J. Chem. Technol. Biotechnol.* **2014**, *89*, 1445–1465. [CrossRef]

36. Michelacci, Y.M.; Horton, D.S.P.Q. Proteoglycans from the cartilage of young hammerhead shark *Spyrna lewini*. *Compar. Biochem. Physiol.* **1989**, *92*, 651–658.

37. Liebezeit, G. Aquaculture of "non-feed organisms" for natural substance production. *Biochem. Eng. Biotechnol.* **2005**, *97*, 1–28.

38. *Methods of Analysis*, 15th ed.; Association of Official Analytical Chemistry: Washington, DC, USA, 1997.

39. Bligh, E.G.; Dyer, W.J. A rapid method of total lipid extraction and purification. *Can. J. Biochem. Physiol.* **1959**, *37*, 911–917. [CrossRef] [PubMed]

40. Lowry, O.H.; Rosebrough, N.J.; Farr, A.L.; Randall, R.J. Protein measurement with the folin phenol reagent. *J. Biol. Chem.* **1951**, *193*, 265–275. [PubMed]

41. Van den Hoogen, B.M.; van Weeren, R.; Lopes-Cardozo, M.; van Golpe, L.M.G.; Barneveld, A.; van de Lest, C.H.A. A microtiter plate assay for the determination of uronic acids. *Anal. Biochem.* **1998**, *257*, 107–111. [CrossRef] [PubMed]

42. Murado, M.A.; Vázquez, J.A.; Montemayor, M.I.; Cabo, M.L.; González, M.P. Two mathematical models for the correction of carbohydrate and protein interference in the determination of uronic acids by the m-hydroxydiphenyl method. *Biotechnol. Appl. Biochem.* **2005**, *41*, 209–216. [CrossRef] [PubMed]

43. Adler-Nissen, J. Enzymatic hydrolysis of food proteins. *Process Biochem.* **1977**, *12*, 18.

44. Murado, M.A.; Vázquez, J.A. Mathematical model for the characterization and objective comparison of antioxidant activities. *J. Agric. Food Chem.* **2010**, *58*, 1622–1629. [CrossRef] [PubMed]

45. Box, G.E.P.; Hunter, W.G.; Hunter, J.S. *Statistics for Experimenters: Design, Innovation, and Discovery*; John Wiley & Sons: Hoboken, NJ, USA, 2005.
46. Prikler, S. Robert de Levie: Advanced excel for scientific data analysis, 2nd ed. *Anal. Bioanal. Chem.* **2009**, *395*, 1945. [CrossRef]

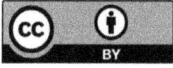

marine drugs

MDPI

Review

Chondroitin Sulfate, Hyaluronic Acid and Chitin/Chitosan Production Using Marine Waste Sources: Characteristics, Applications and Eco-Friendly Processes: A Review

José Antonio Vázquez [1,*], Isabel Rodríguez-Amado [1], María Ignacia Montemayor [2], Javier Fraguas [1], María del Pilar González [1] and Miguel Anxo Murado [1]

[1] Group of Recycling and Valorisation of Waste Materials (REVAL), Marine Research Institute (IIM-CSIC), r/Eduardo Cabello, 6. Vigo, Galicia 36208, Spain; sabelara@iim.csic.es (I.R.-A.); rvrlab@iim.csic.es (J.F.); pgonzalez@iim.csic.es (M.P.G.); reciclaa@iim.csic.es (M.A.M.)

[2] Research Centre of Vine and Wine Related Science (ICVV-CSIC), Scientific and Technical Complex of the University of La Rioja, Logroño 26006, Spain; nachi@iim.csic.es

* Author to whom correspondence should be addressed; jvazquez@iim.csic.es; Tel.: +34-986-214-468 or +34-986-231-930; Fax: +34-986-292-762.

Received: 17 December 2012; in revised form: 28 January 2013; Accepted: 6 February 2013; Published: 11 March 2013

Abstract: In the last decade, an increasing number of glycosaminoglycans (GAGs), chitin and chitosan applications have been reported. Their commercial demands have been extended to different markets, such as cosmetics, medicine, biotechnology, food and textiles. Marine wastes from fisheries and aquaculture are susceptible sources for polymers but optimized processes for their recovery and production must be developed to satisfy such necessities. In the present work, we have reviewed different alternatives reported in the literature to produce and purify chondroitin sulfate (CS), hyaluronic acid (HA) and chitin/chitosan (CH/CHs) with the aim of proposing environmentally friendly processes by combination of various microbial, chemical, enzymatic and membranes strategies and technologies.

Keywords: glycosaminoglycans; by-products upgrading; chondroitin sulphate; hyaluronic acid; chitin and chitosan; eco-friendly processes; clean production

---

1. Introduction

The world capture of marine organisms including aquaculture (mainly fish, mollusks and crustaceans) amounts to 132 million tons [1]. Among them, more than 35% of the total weight is handled as by-product and waste that include animal fractions (skeletons, heads, viscera) generated in seafood production or species, sizes or qualities without commercial value (discards and by-catch). Commonly, the production of such wastes is located in coastline areas with the corresponding problem associated with environmental pollution generated by an inefficient residue management [2,3]. In addition, the overexploitation of several species (e.g., sharks) has led to ecological risks derived from the reduction of biological resources [4]. To establish a more efficient control of fisheries, to increase the profitability of seafood operations and to satisfy environmental regulations, low cost and environmentally friendly technologies are being evolved by the necessity of recovering all the materials (polysaccharides, proteins, oils, minerals) [3,5–7]. Recently, alternative methods have been developed to obtain different products and molecules: enzymes, glycosaminoglycans, chitin, gelatin, biosilage, marine peptones, *etc.*, from skeletons, skins, viscera, heads, *etc.* [8–22]. Bearing in mind the number of applications and the economical value of final products, glycosaminoglycans and chitin are two of the most important and relevant compounds to upgrade from marine wastes [23].

Glycosaminoglycans (GAGs) are heteropolysaccharides defined by a repeating disaccharide unit without branched chains in which one of the two monosaccharides is always an amino sugar (*N*-acetylgalactosamine or *N*-acetylglucosamine) and the other one is a uronic acid. They are present on all animal cell surfaces and in the extracellular matrix where are known to bind and regulate different proteins (e.g., growth factors, enzymes, cytokines). After purification, they are used in numerous contexts from food, cosmetic and clinical areas [24–26].

Chemical structure of chitin is also a long linear chain formed by successive units of an amino monosaccharide (*N*-acetylglucosamine); however, it is not commonly classified as GAGs. It is the second most extended polysaccharide in nature after cellulose, forming part of microorganism cell walls, exoskeleton of insects and shells of crustaceans. Both chitin and its partially deacetylated form chitosan have been intensely studied in recent years with a promising potential for applications in pharmacy, alimentary and biomedicine devices [27–29].

Several methodologies have been developed to produce the mentioned biopolymers prepared with steps of hydrolysis and purification that are usually expensive and/or environmentally not friendly, for instance, to manage large volumes of alkalis and strong acids needed in hydrolysis and to use specific chromatographic techniques hardly scale-up in purification. The present review addresses an overview of different sustainable and clean processes to recover chondroitin sulfate (CS), hyaluronic acid (HA) and chitin/chitosan (CH/CHs) from marine waste materials.

2. Glycosaminoglycans

Traditionally, the production of GAGs is obtained from mammalian tissues mainly generated in slaughterhouse: Rooster combs, cartilage (tracheas and nasal from bovine and swine) and umbilical cords. However, as a consequence of the concern due to the bovine spongiform encephalopathy (BSE) and other food chain crisis, the exploration of microorganism and marine organisms as source of those glycoconjugates has received increasing attention. Marine organisms like sponges, sea cucumbers, squids, mollusks, invertebrates and mainly cartilaginous material from fishes (shark, salmon, ray, *etc.*) are well-documented as potential producers of them [30–32].

Cartilage is a tissue formed by a matrix of collagen associated with proteoglycans, macromolecules with a core protein to which the GAGs chondroitin sulfate, keratan sulfate, dermatan sulfate and heparan sulfate are covalently attached by means of a trisaccharide linked to a serine residue. HA is the only non-sulfated GAGs and is not covalently bound to the protein in any tissue, although specific HA-protein interaction is shown [33]. CS and HA are the most valued GAGs in market because of its abundance in mammalian tissues, physiological functions and high activity.

2.1. Characteristics and Applications of CS

CS is formed by only one type of repeating disaccharide units of glucuronic acid (GlcA) and *N*-acetylgalactosamine (GalNAc) linked by β-$(1\rightarrow3)$ glycosidic bonds and sulfated in different carbon positions (CS no-sulfated is CS-O). The classification and type of CS is dependent on sulfate group placing: carbon 4 (CS-A), 6 (CS-C, more common), both 4 and 6 (CS-E), positions 6 of GalNAc and 2 of GlcA (CS-D) and 4 of GalNAc/2 of GlcA (CS-B) [34]. Moreover, the composition and concentration of CS depends on the function of the organism and tissue, thus, CS from terrestrial and marine sources contains diverse chain lengths and oversulfated disaccharides (shark, CS-D; dogfish, CS-A and CS-D; squid and salmon, CS-E; crocodile, CS-E; chicken CS-A and CS-E; ray, CS-A and CS-C) [35,36] at different relative concentrations (e.g., 9% in shark fin and 14% in chicken keel).

In all cases, CS is an essential component of extracellular matrix of connective tissues in which plays a central role in various biological processes, such as the function and elasticity of the articular cartilage, hemostasis and inflammation, regulation of cell development, cell adhesion, proliferation and differentiation [37]. The number of commercial applications has been continuously increased, due to its high biocompatibility, mainly in the engineering of biological tissues associated with the processes of bone repair, cartilage and cutaneous wound. Moreover, its combination with other biopolymers (such as collagen, proteoglycans and HA) to formulate scaffolds with slow and controlled biodegradability that promote and accelerate the regeneration of damaged structures has been studied [38,39]. In these injuries, CS is involved in reepithelialization, in the stimulation of neovascularization and supplying growth factors and cytokines when it is included in hydrogels [40,41].

Recent studies have demonstrated that CS-E is a potent antiviral [42] whereas CS-proteoglycan is a potential target for the development of vaccines against malaria [43]. New findings about the sulfation pattern of CS related with cancer cell mechanisms have been also reported [44]. This feature revealed its ability and potential role as biomarker to early detection of diverse types of cancer [45]. Furthermore, fucosylated CS (CS-F) was obtained from sea cucumber has led to excellent results to inhibit adenocarcinoma growth in lungs using mouse model [46]. On the other hand, partially purified CS is also used as food preservative with emulsifying properties [47]. Nevertheless, the most successful commercial products of CS, by market volume and benefits, are those associated with cartilage regeneration, anti-inflammatory activity and osteoarthritis [48,49]. In this way, low/medium-molecular weight CS (inferior to 20 kDa) is orally administered in nutraceutical formulations to treat and prevent the osteoarthritis due to its inhibitory capacity of cartilage degradative enzymes [50].

From a marine perspective, shark fins have been the most commonly used source of CS but the increasing price of this substrate together with the irrational and non-controlled exploitation of shark stocks, as well other ecological aspects has led to the shark fishery on the brick of extinction [4,51]. The skeleton of ray is another attractive source of CS but similar bad habits on the stocks regulation have been also reported [51,52].

2.2. Characteristics and Applications of HA

HA is a linear, high molecular weight unbranched and non-sulfated GAG made by alternating disaccharide units of N-acetyl-D-glucosamine and D-glucuronic linked by β-(1→3) and β-(1→4) glycosidic bonds. It is ubiquitously distributed in connective tissues where is a major structural component of intercellular matrix. It has a fundamental role in controlling tissue permeation and hydration, macromolecular transport between cells and bacterial invasiveness [33]. The presence of HA is especially important in the umbilical cord, rooster comb, synovial fluid, vitreous humor (VH) and cell wall of *Streptococci* bacteria [53]. It holds a large number of water molecules in its molecular domain and occupies enormous hydrodynamic space in solution [54]. This characteristic ("swelling property") together with its chemical structure gives it a wide-ranging of physicochemical and biological properties and functions such as lubricity, viscoelasticity, biocompatibility, angiogenic and immunostimulatory. This polymer has great economical value with numerous applications in biotechnology, regenerative medicine and cosmetic fields such as plastic surgery, anti-aging cosmetics, arthritis treatment, joint injections, major burns and intra-ocular surgery [25,55]. The activity of HA is dependent on its size, hence all ranges of molecular weights are handled in specific usage area.

Originally, it has been obtained and commercialized from diverse mammalian substrates as rooster combs, synovial fluid, VH and umbilical cords [53]. Marine wastes have been also explored in the search of new sources of HA, being only found in VH of various fish species and in cartilage of chondrichthyes [56]. However, the most important alternative in recent years has been the development of microbial HA production by *Streptococcus* bacteria. This fermentation generates the best yields with higher concentrations of HA (>3 g/L) at lower costs and with more efficient downstream processes [57,58].

3. CS Production Processes

The types of applications for the formulations of CS or CS-derived, and therefore their market price, are dependent on the concentration and purity of this GAG in the commercial products. Different compounds including chemical solvents and detergents from isolation step and peptides, proteins, nucleic acids or organic compounds from tissues are commonly contaminating the samples; hence, they are reducing its commercial value and limiting its usage areas [49]. Clinical applications demand highly concentrated and pure CS in comparison with cosmetic, dietary supplements or food ingredients. Moreover, CS derived from fish (ray and shark) is referred as a better source than mammalian because of its sulfation pattern and safety. Therefore, it is especially important the development of highly yielded and low-cost extraction processes, maintaining the quality and great purity of CS in order to execute an optimum exploitation of marine sources.

In general, the methods of CS isolation from cartilage (the most interesting substrate from an industrial viewpoint) are defined for several years [59–61] and include various steps based on: (1) chemical hydrolysis of cartilage; (2) breakdown of proteoglycan core; (3) elimination of proteins and CS recovery; (4) purification of CS. The two first stages are mostly conducted by means of alkaline hydrolysis at high concentrations of NaOH, urea or guanidine HCl, subsequently combined with selective precipitation of GAG using cationic quaternary ammonium chemicals (as cetylpyridinium chloride), potassium thiocyanate, non-ionic detergents or alcoholic solutions [59,60], deproteinization by trichloroacetic acid and finally purification with gel filtration and/or ion-exchange and size-exclusion chromatography [62]. Unfortunately, those economically viable stages lead to unsatisfactory purity for clinical uses of CS. The techniques that improve final product quality need larger amounts of reagents and are time-consuming. In addition, costumers and manufactures try to develop more environmentally friendly and economical processes to obtain CS based on non contaminant solvent strategies.

Various alternative isolation methods have been recently developed to replace the classical methods for pursuing sustainability [63–66]. Those processes can be summarized as follows: digestion of cartilage and proteins mediated by enzymes, selective precipitations with alcoholic solutions, resuspension and neutralization with salt solutions and separation by molecular-weight using ultrafiltration-diafiltration technologies (UF-DF). Figure 1 shows a flow chart representing all the potential steps described for the downstream purification of marine CS. Firstly, the fishing by-products (e.g., ray skeletons or shark heads) are warmed separating the rests of flesh, excellent material for fish meal, and cartilage for CS production. Subsequently, dried and milled cartilage is hydrolyzed by proteases under controlled experimental conditions. Multiple enzymes have been studied, generally with successful results, with the objective of cartilage degradation, protein fraction breakdown and to obtain undamaged CS molecules. The proteolysis of proteoglycans from hammerhead shark fin cartilage was partially degraded by commercial papain but trypsin or superase were not effective [67]. Similar activity of papain digestion was also observed in adult zebrafish [68], ray [35] and dogfish tissues [69]. In all cases, the time of hydrolysis was superior to 18 h under optimal conditions of temperature (50–65 °C) and pH 7. Recently, a two-step enzymatic processing with alcalase and flavourzyme showed better yields of degradation with a significant reduction of time-processing [21]. Proteolytic and collagenolytic activities isolated from skate pancreas led to percentage of skate cartilage hydrolysis higher than 50% in 6 h [66]. The separation of hydrolysates is generally carried out by simple decantation or centrifugation removing the supernatant rich in CS and the rests of cartilage precipitated (useful as substrate for fish meal production). Tadashi [65] suggested a previous elimination stage of cartilage wastes based on the addition of activated charcoal at 55 °C.

The subsequent phase of alcoholic treatment is usually indicated by several authors as crucial for the selective precipitation of CS from the major protein presents in the hydrolysate [61,65,66,70]. The effectiveness of that process is dependent on the type and alcohol concentration and, in some cases, the influence of processing-temperature is also important [65]. Ethanol is the most commonly selected reagent for such precipitation, at concentrations of 40%–60%, due to its widespread use as a solvent of substances intended for human contact or consumption [65,66,70]. A recent report also proposed isopropanol at 40% for the purification of CS from scapular cartilage of shortfin mako shark [21]. In our lab, we have optimized the combination of alkaline proteolysis and selective precipitation of CS from ray cartilage by using alkaline hydroalcoholic solutions [66]. Under optimal conditions of NaOH 0.2 M and one volume of ethanol per volume of hydrolysate at room temperature with soft agitation for 1 h, more than 96% of CS recovery and CS purity were obtained. The repetition of this procedure, under the same experimental conditions, increased the CS purity up to 99%. The resuspension of CS sediment and pH neutralization is efficiently obtained by means of saline solutions as NaCl or sodium acetate, the salt excess can be subsequently removed by membrane dialysis method.

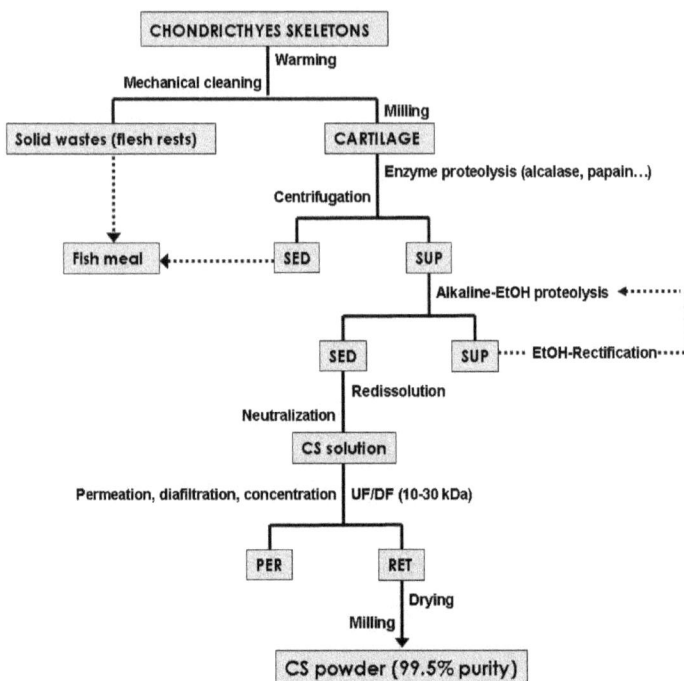

Figure 1. Overview of chondroitin sulfate (CS) recovery and purification processes from marine cartilage by-products. SED: sediment, SUP: supernatant, PER: permeate and RET: retentate.

The last step of purification by membrane technologies is widely performed in the majority of the biomacromolecules downstream processing (with higher sizes of 1 kDa) because of its separation effectiveness, easy scale-up, cost effective device, numerous types and cut-off membranes and simple operatory and control. However, the use of described methodology, to remove low-molecular-weight materials and salts from neutralized or resupended CS solution, has been poorly studied. Large quantities of CS from salmon tissues were extracted by alkali treatment and subsequent purified by repeating UF procedure, demonstrating superior efficient than using ion exchange resin [71]. A two-step process based on enzyme extraction of CS and concentration-desalting by UF-DF was studied using skate cartilage as substrate and ceramic membranes [63]. The authors advised that the desalting step by DF should be improved with a higher filtering area due to the 40% remaining of salts in the final solution of CS. This inconvenience was improved via polyethersulfone membranes with molecular-weight cut-off at 10 kDa and 6 diavolume [66]. The UF-DF system was assembled with total recirculation to obtain CS of 99.6% purity at final concentration of 35–45 g/L. Higher CS concentrated liquid generated excessive viscosities that reduced the filtrate flow and filled the membranes.

Finally, the powder of CS can be obtained by drying the concentrated solutions without adding chemical solvents using spray dryer equipment or evaporation in an oven, depositing CS in thin layers on trays followed by milling performance.

Microbial Production of CS

In order to avoid the health and ecological problems derived from the uses of mammalian and fishery wastes as substrate, different approximations to microbial production of CS-like polymers have been reported in recent years [37,72,73]. Initially, *Pasteurella multocida* was one of the bacteria selected as CS producer, but its well-known cholera pathogenicity has hindered and reduced its interest [74,75]. Excellent results were obtained in the production of capsular polysaccharide CS precursor (CSC) by *Escherichia coli* O5:K4:H4 under diverse experimental conditions and fermentation devices [37,73]. These authors have improved the CSC concentration of 0.2 g/L obtained in batch cultures [76] to 1.4 g/L with fed-batch operation [77] and more than 3 g/L using a membrane bioreactor [78]. Downstream processing finally yielded about 80% chondroitin with 90% purity [79]. Nevertheless, *E. coli* is a low virulent pathogen limiting its large scale production and CSC is an unsulphated structure of chondroitin (CS-O), with a furanose residue of fructose, which needs a subsequent step of chemical sulfation and hydrolysis of fructose monomer [80]. The production of CS by combined fermentation and chemical developments is a complementary alternative to achieve a global and sustainable control of chondrichthyes stocks.

4. HA Production Processes

The most conventional materials employed for HA extraction are selected for its feasibility and concentration, thus, umbilical cord presents an average level of 4 g/L, synovial fluid from pig (3 g/L) or bovine (18 g/L) and rooster combs (25 g/L) [56,81–83]. Nevertheless, the risk of animal-derived pathogens, inter-species viral or prionic contaminations (e.g., BSE, epizootic aphtha) has obligated to explore and optimize other alternatives of production.

In marine organisms, the only clear source of HA is the VH present in the eyeball of fish species. VH volume and HA concentration is different depending on the selected fish, for instance, HA is obtained from eyeballs of shark and swordfish at 0.3 g/L from 18 mL of VH and 0.055 g/L from 70 mL, respectively [56]. HA is also present in the cartilage matrix in which is very important as structural element of the aggrecan in cartilaginous fishes; however, its relatively low content makes it economically unavailable for any industrial extraction process [84].

The traditional protocols for extraction of HA from animal substrates (e.g., rooster comb) are developed according to the works reported by Swann [85] and Balazs [86] that include the preparation of the material, washing with water or alcohol, aqueous or organic solvent (mainly chloroform) extraction, precipitation by cetylpiridinium chloride, filtering and successive extractions with chloroform, centrifugation and occasional chromatographic purification. Other authors indicated that both procedures are costly, laborious, time-consuming and lead to contaminated HA solutions that limit their applications in biopharma formulations [87].

Different strategies have been proposed for the extraction of HA from mammalian VH including deproteinization of bovine substrate with xylenesulphonate-Na [88], extraction with water, precipitation with ethanol and purification by DEAE-cellulose [89] and fractional precipitation using ethanol combined with enzymatic protein hydrolysis [59]. The most exhaustive method was applied to tuna eyeball substrate [90], performing precipitation with overcooled acetone, actinase digestion, thermal coagulation, dialization by membrane and cetylpyridinium chloride precipitation. Similarly, we have addressed a method to recover and purify HA of VH from various fish eyeballs (tuna, shark, and swordfish) using easier, faster and cheaper stages [56]: (1) initial clarification of VH extracted from frozen eyeball (using centrifugation or glass wool filtration); (2) enzyme proteolysis; (3) concentration by UF; (4) precipitation and alkaline proteolysis in hydroalcoholic medium at low temperature; (5) selective redissolution and neutralization; (6) separation, purification and concentration by UF-DF; (7) removing of nucleic acids using absorption with hydroxyapatite obtained from fish bone. Medical-grade purity of 99.9% (molecular weight 2000 kDa) was thus reached (Figure 2). The lyophilization of final solutions is an excellent lab resource to avoid physical degradation and size reduction but they are too expensive for industrial scale.

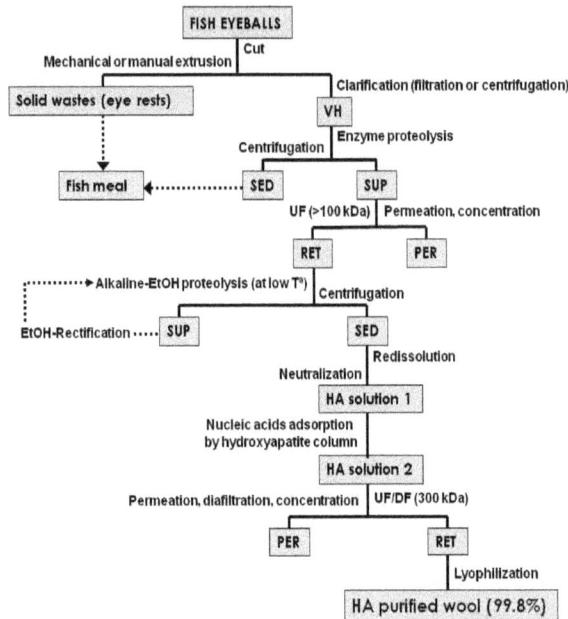

Figure 2. Flowchart of purification methods to extract hyaluronic acid (HA) from vitreous humor (VH) of fish eyeball. SED: sediment, SUP: supernatant, PER: permeate and RET: retentate.

Although prices of vitreous HA are commercially high, economic viability is unclear given the cost of vitreous humor (VH) removal (expensive labor) and the overdependence on raw materials (opportunistic prices of fish eyes) that usually tends to the overexploitation of this marine resource. Microbial production easily contains the concentration equivalent (3 g/L) to 660 eyes of shark or 900 of swordfish. Additionally, the presence of blood in the eyes supply should be avoided as much as possible because the iron from haemoglobin degrades HA molecule.

Microbial Production of HA on Marine Food Wastes

Bacterial production of HA using Lancerfield group A and C streptococci has been industrially developed to replace gradually the HA obtained from animal origin. Several culture variables have been studied and optimized such as lysozyme or hyaluronidase addition [91,92], agitation and aeration conditions [93–95], the type of bioreactor [96], effect of pH-gradient stress [97], continuous culture [98], medium optimization [99] and fed-batch operation [100]. Since no marine microorganisms have been discovered for HA production, the only marine approach for this bioproduction is derived from the substitution of commercial broths by alternative nutrients generated in the marine foodstuff manufacturing. Recently, the formulation of cultivation medium with mussel processing wastewaters (MPW), rich in glycogen as glucose substitutive, and peptones obtained from fish viscera by-products generated acceptable HA productions that were improved under fed-batch conditions [101,102]. Generally, HA downstream processes from post-incubated medium are easier than those reported for animal sources, especially if consumption of culture medium ingredients is complete at the end of fermentation. Cellular biomass precipitation (by means of detergent adding and centrifugation), deproteinization using proteases or specific adsorption to resin and membranes purification are the most conventional procedures. Other proposal includes silica gel filtration combined with active carbon treatment followed by diafiltration [58]. In Table 1, different alternatives and process conditions for CS and HA production from marine sources and some microbial cultivations are summarized.

Table 1. Summary of GAGs productionfrom marine sources (CS and HA), using marine culture broths for fermentation (HA) or by microbial fermentation (CS).

GAG	Type	Source	Process conditions	Yield (*Y*)/Production (*P*) Purity (*Pu*)	Ref.
CS	CS-C	shark cartilage	proteolysis, alcoholic precipitation, membrane purification	*Y* = 57% (w/v)	[21]
CS	CS-A, CS-C	ray and shark cartilage	proteolysis, cetylpyridinium HCl and NaCl precipitations, filtration and dialization	*Y* = 10%–11% (w/v)	[35]
CS	CS-A, CS-C	skate fin	proteolysis, cetylpyridinium HCl precipitation, electrophoresis and cromatographic purification	-	[62]
CS	CS-A, CS-C	skate cartilage	proteolysis, purification (UF-DF)	-	[63]
CS	CS-A, CS-C	ray cartilage	proteolysis, alkaline-hydroalcoholic precipitation, purification (UF-DF)	*Y* = 15% (w/w)/*Pu* > 99%	[66]
CS	CS-A, CS-C	shark fin	proteolysis, guanidine HCl extraction, electrophoresis and cromatographic purification	*Y* = 84%	[67]
CS	CS-A, CS-C, CS-O	zebrafish cartilage	proteolysis, electrophoresis and cromatographic purification	-	[68]
CS	CS-A, CS-C, CS-D, CS-O	dogfish cartilage	proteolysis, alcoholic precipitation, cromatographic purification	*Y* = 5% (w/w)	[69]
CS	CS-A, CS-C, CS-O, CS-E	salmon nasal cartilage	proteolysis, alkaline hydrolysis, alcoholic precipitation, cation exchange separation	*Y* = 24% (w/w)/*Pu* = 99%	[70]
CS	CS-A, CS-C, CS-O, CS-E	salmon nasal cartilage	proteolysis, alkaline hydrolysis, alcoholic precipitation, purification (UF)	-	[71]
CS	CS-O	*E. coli* O5:K4:H4	batch operation	*P* = 0.2 g/L	[76]
CS	CS-O	*E. coli* O5:K4:H4	fed-batch operation	*P* = 1.4 g/L	[77]
CS	CS-O	*E. coli* O5:K4:H4	membrane bioreactor, fed-batch, purification (UF-DF)	*Y* = 80%/*P* = 3 g/L *Pu* = 90%	[78]
HA	-	shark HV	proteolysis, concentration (UF), selective precipitation, purification (UF-DF)	*P* = 0.3 g/L/*Pu* > 99.5%	[56]
HA	-	swordfish HV	proteolysis, concentration (UF), selective precipitation, purification (UF-DF)	*P* = 0.06 g/L/*Pu* > 99.5%	[56]
HA	-	*S. zooepidemicus*	medium: shark or ray peptones, fed-batch	*P* = 2.5 g/L	[101]
HA	-	*S. zooepidemicus*	medium: tuna peptones and MPW, batch	*P* = 2.5 g/L	[102]

5. Chitin and Chitosan

During recent years, CH and CHs have attracted a great interest due to their distinctive biological and physicochemical properties [28], which make them interesting polymers, among others, for biotechnology, medicine, cosmetics, food technology and textile applications.

Marine organisms are principal source of CH since it is a constituent of the organic matrix of the exoskeletons of arthropods such as crustaceans (crabs, lobsters and shrimps) and of the endoskeleton of mollusks [103]. Although CH can also be found in many other organisms including fungi [104], yeasts [105], algae and squid pen [106], the shell of marine crustaceans is the preferred source of CH due to their high availability as waste from the seafood processing industry [28].

However, traditional methods involved in the recovery of CH from shellfish are extremely hazardous, energy consuming and environmentally polluting, due to the need of using high amounts of mineral acid and alkali [107]. In addition, the deacetylation of CH to produce CHs requires the use of very intense alkaline treatments. Hence, alternative environmentally friendly processes are being assessed including the use of proteases or proteolytic bacteria for deproteinization and demineralization of crustacean shells [108,109]. Alternatively, fermentation using lactic acid bacteria (LAB) has been widely applied for the extraction of CH from crab [110,111] and shrimp [112,113] biowastes. In case of CHs production, fungus *Mucor rouxii* has been widely studied as an alternative source of chitosan.

Characteristics and Applications of CH and CHs

CH is the most abundant biopolymer in nature after cellulose [27,28]. It is a linear polysaccharide composed of β-(1→4)-linked *N*-acetyl-D-glucosamine monomers. Its abundance in the environment is due to its role as major component in the supporting tissues of organisms such as crustacean, fungi and insects [114].

Depending on its source, CH can occur as either α, β or γ forms [115]. The α form has antiparallel microfibril orientation with strong intra and intermolecular hydrogen bonds and is the most abundant chitin in nature and the preferred form for industrial applications. The β-chitin form has parallel chains held by weak intra chain hydrogen bonds and occurs in squid pens [116]. A third and less characterized form, γ-chitin, has been described as a mixture of antiparallel and parallel chains, although there is controversy about the existence of this conformation [117,118].

Owing to the extensive hydrogen bonding in the solid state of α-chitin, it is insoluble in water, most organic acids and diluted acid and alkaline solutions [117]. However, it can be dissolved in concentrated hydrocloric, sulfuric and phosphoric acids as well as in dichloroacetic, trichloroacetic and formic acids [119]. In addition, special solvents such as hexafluoroacetone and *N,N*-dimethylacetamide containing 5%–8% lithium chloride have proved suitable for solubilizing CH [120]. Unlike α-chitin, β-chitin generally shows better solubility in most acids and swells in water considerably [28]. On the other hand, CHs is insoluble in either organic solvents or water [28], but it is soluble in diluted acid solutions below pH 6.0, due to the presence of free amino groups with a pKa value of 6.3 [121].

The lack of solubility of CH makes it necessary to modify the molecule for most of its applications. Among various reactions that can disrupt intra- and inter-molecular hydrogen bonds without cleaving glucosidic linkages, *N*-deacetylation is the simplest modification, which transforms CH to CHs [117]. The degree of *N*-acetylation (DA), *i.e.*, the ratio of 2-acetamido-2-deoxy-D-glucopyranose to 2-amino-2-deoxy-D-glucopyranose structural units has a remarkable effect on CH solubility and solution properties [115]. Chitosan is the *N*-deacetylated derivative of chitin with a typical DA of less than 0.35, therefore being a copolymer composed of glucosamine and *N*-acetylglucosamine [121].

CH, CHs and its derivatives are widely applied in different economical sectors, such as agriculture [122], water treatment [123], food and cosmetic industry [124], pharmaceutical and medicine [125]. Properties that make natural CH and CHs attractive polymers for various applications, mainly in pharmaceutics and medicine, are their antimicrobial activity, film-forming ability, high adsorption, biodegrability, biocompatibility and non-toxicity [126]. Among biomedical applications reported for CH and CHs are tissue engineering, wound healing, drug delivery and cancer diagnosis [127].

The use of CHs in the food industry is related to its functional properties, principally water- and fat-binding capacity [126] as well as emulsifying properties [128]. Also the antimicrobial activity of CHs has been exploited for the preparation of films as a packaging material for a preservation of a variety of foods [129]. Besides, CHs microparticles are being evaluated as carriers for essential oils in cosmetic formulations [130].

6. Traditional CH and CHs Production Processes

The most common sources of CH are crab and shrimp shell wastes. In the skeletal tissue of these species, CH is bound to proteins forming a chitin-protein matrix associated to mineral salts [11], principally calcium carbonate. In this regard, the main components of crustacean shells are on a dry weight basis and depending on the species and season, 30%–40% protein, 30%–50% mineral salts and 13%–42% CH [28]. Furthermore, small amounts of lipids from muscle or viscera residues [117] and carotenoids, mainly astaxanthin and is esters [131], associated with proteins of the exoskeleton can be found in crustacean shell waste.

The traditional method for the industrial recovery of CH from different crustacean shells consists of two steps (Figure 3), including a deproteinization with alkali treatment at high temperatures and a demineralization using diluted hydrochloric acid as the preferred reagent. Although it is considered that the order of these two phases is interchangeable depending on the source and proposed use of chitin [117], other authors suggest that demineralization should be performed first in order to decrease the residual mineral content [132].

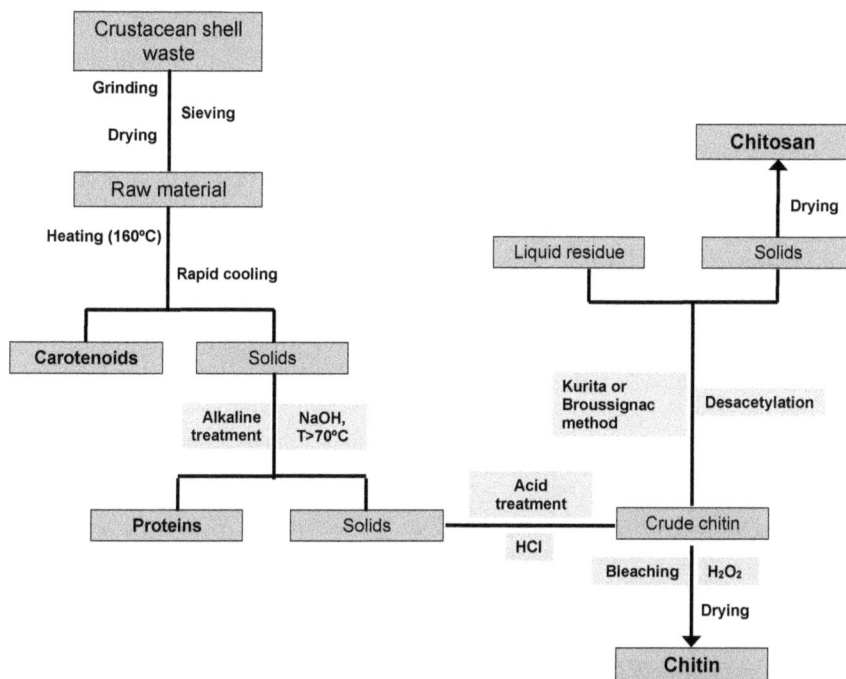

Figure 3. Scheme of CH and CHs preparation from crustacean shell waste using chemical methods.

After demineralization and deproteinization, CH isolated from crustacean sources has a lightly pink color and so a bleaching process using potassium permanganate, oxalic acid [133] or hydrogen peroxide [132] is usually carried out to yield a colorless product. On the contrary, CH isolated from squid pens is completely white and therefore, this final stage is unnecessary.

It is generally accepted that the processing conditions significantly affect the molecular weight and acetylation degree of CH. In this sense, the stronger the acidic conditions utilized for demineralization (pH, time and temperature), the lower molecular weight products are obtained [11]. Percot *et al.* studied the kinetics of demineralization of shrimp shells by following the pH variations in the reaction medium [11]. According to their results, they were able to define the optimal conditions necessary to perform a complete reaction, minimizing the hydrolysis of the glycosidic bonds. For this purpose, an excess of 0.25 M HCl, a solid-to-liquid ratio above 10 mL/g and 15 min of reaction at ambient temperature provided a final product with a DA above 95%.

In contrast, deproteinization by alkaline treatment has shown to be less damaging to the chitin structure compared to the acidic treatment involved in the demineralization [119]. In fact, Percot *et al.* reported that deproteinization using 1 M NaOH with a temperature and a reaction time below 70 °C and 24 h had no influence on both the molecular weight and DA, respectively [11]. Nevertheless, a large variation exists for the reported conditions of deproteinization for CH preparation. Chang and Tsai [134] analyzed protein removal from shrimp shell waste using NaOH by response surface methodology, reporting optimal conditions with 2.5 N NaOH, 75 °C and a minimal solution to solid ratio of 5 mL/g. According to their results, these authors also reported that kinetics of demineralization and deproteinization were pseudo-first order and two-stage first-order reactions, respectively. Tolaimate *et al.*, using a tailored isolation process according to the source of CH (shrimp, crab, lobster or squid), were able to obtain highly acetylated products (near 100%) preserving the crystalline structure of both α and β chitin [132]. These authors using low concentrated acid (0.55 M HCl) and base (0.3 M NaOH) solutions in a multi-stage process, highlighted the need to adapt the process conditions to the origin and specific characteristics of the CH source utilized.

On the other hand, the most commonly used methods for CHs production are the Broussignac [135] and Kurita [106] processes. The first procedure consists of a deacetylation of chitin in a nearly anhydrous reaction medium using a mixture of potassium hydroxide, ethanol and monoethylene glycol. On the other hand, the Kurita method proceeds in a stirred aqueous solution of sodium hydroxide, under a nitrogen stream at high temperatures (>80 °C).

Tolaimate *et al.* extensively compared both deacetylation methods and these studies indicated that the adjustment of different parameters related to the deacetylation process, the nature of the source, physical structure of the original CH and its isolation process allow to prepare CHs with controlled physico-chemical (molecular weight and DA) characteristics either from α or β-chitins [132,136]. Comparing the two processes for the production of CHs from a completely *N*-acetylated β-chitin prepared from squid pen (*Loligo vulgaris*), these authors concluded that the Kurita process enabled to obtain CHs with high molecular weights and a wide range of deacetylation degrees [136]. On the contrary, the Broussignac process could be carried out to obtain CHs with low degrees of acetylation and molecular weights, but in a faster way. Nevertheless, due to the high amounts of alkali and acid wastewaters generated in these production processes, there is a need to find alternatives to overcome the problem of wastewater neutralization. A possible way that has not been sufficiently explored to date is the reutilization of these effluents in the alkaline proteolysis step of CS isolation from cartilage (Figure 1). This strategy would allow the recycling of highly polluting wastewaters and goes towards the overall utilization of marine by-products.

7. Alternative CH and CHs Production Processes

Chemical CH purification is an energy consuming process and results in environmental problems with high waste processing costs, due to the need of neutralization of processing wastewaters [111]. Besides and as stated above, prolonged alkaline and acid treatments cause depolymerization and deacetylation of the polysaccharide. Furthermore, the low biological value of alkali-recovered proteins may limit its application in the animal feed industry, thus affecting the production costs of CH and CHs from crustacean by-products [117]. In recent years, several methods have been reported in the literature to solve chemical extraction problems (Figure 4). One of the biological alternatives proposed is the use of proteases for deproteinization of crustacean shells, avoiding alkaline treatments. Various commercial proteases have been assayed for protein removal from crustacean shells [137], being alcalase the most employed and effective enzyme [137–139]. In addition, the utilization of crude proteolytic extracts obtained from different microorganisms [140,141] or even from fish viscera [142] have been studied, leading to varying deproteinization yields depending on the conditions assayed. Although deproteinization levels achieved in such cases are generally lower than those obtained using alkaline treatments, this alternative has the advantage to produce nutritionally valuable protein hydrolysates in addition to chitin [138].

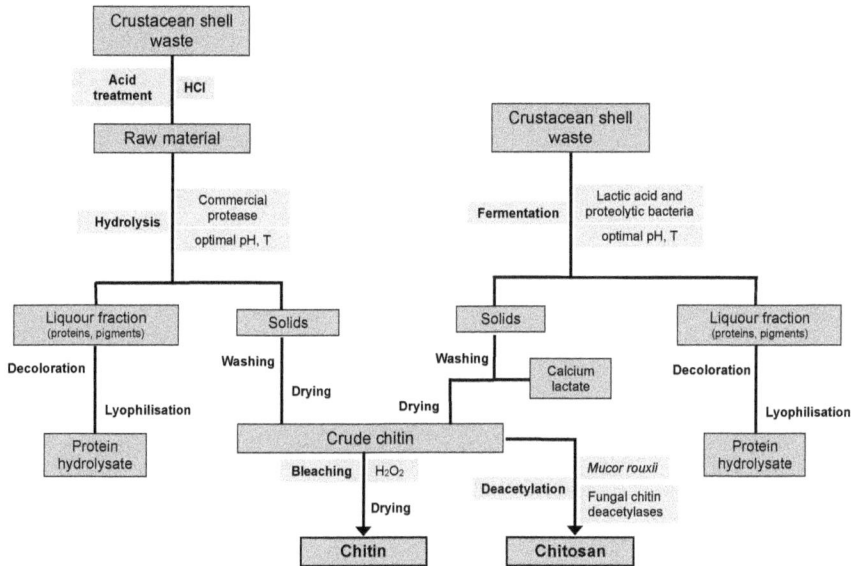

Figure 4. Scheme of chitin and chitosan preparation from crustacean shell waste using eco-friendly methods.

When using enzymatic deproteinization, previous demineralization is more convenient since it increases the permeability of the tissues and reduces the presence of potential enzyme inhibitors, favoring the subsequent action of the enzyme [138].

Another biotechnological approach for the production of CH from seafood wastes consists on their fermentation using lactic acid bacteria (LAB). The production of bio-silages from fish by-products consists on the ability of LAB strains to ferment the waste materials and to produce *in situ* organic acids, mainly lactic and acetic acids, in order to preserve and produce ingredients for animal feed production [18,102]. This methodology has also been applied for the recovery of other value-added by-products from ensilaged shrimp waste, such as carotenoids [143].

In the fermentation of crustacean by-products, two fractions are obtained: a solid phase containing crude chitin and a liquor fraction rich in proteins, minerals and pigments. This occurs because lactic acid produced during fermentation operates at two levels. On the one hand, it reacts with the calcium carbonate to produce calcium lactate, which precipitates and can be easily removed by washing [144]. In addition, lactic acid decreases pH values, leading to the activation of proteases. Deproteinization of the biowaste and simultaneous liquefaction of the proteins occurs mainly by proteolytic enzymes produced by the added LAB, by gut bacteria of the intestinal system of crustaceans, or by proteases present in the source byproduct [145].

Several LAB have been assayed in a wide range of raw materials of marine origin. Shrimp waste has been mainly fermented using *Lactobacillus plantarum* [113,146], but also with other lactic acid bacteria such as *Lactobacillus paracasei* [147], *Pediococcus acidolactici* [148] and *Lactobacillus helveticus* [149]. Non-LAB, including *Pseudomonas aeruginosa* K-187 [150] and *Bacillus subtilis* [151] have been assayed as inoculum source for the recovery of CH. Commercial bacterial inoculums containing a mixture of LAB have been utilized for the production of CH from waste shell of prawn (*Nephrops norvegicus*). Stabisil containing *Streptococcus faecium* M74, *L. plantarum*, and *P. acidilactici* [152] and a powdered grass silage inoculant consisting of a mixture of selected proteolytic enzyme producing bacteria [107] proved to be effective alternatives for the demineralization and deproteinization of prawn biowastes.

Duan *et al.* reported the production of CH from shrimp waste by fermentation with the epiphytic strain *Lactobacillus acidophilus* SW01 isolated from shrimp by-products [133]. Due to its high protease activity, the solid residue from fermented shrimp waste contained less than 1% minerals and proteins. Therefore, after 168 h of cultivation at 37 °C, pure CH could be easily recovered only following a bleaching treatment.

Co-fermentation using a LAB and a bacterium with proteolytic activity has also been investigated as an alternative for CH purification from marine by-products. The LAB *Lactococcus lactis* and *Teredinobacter turnirae*, a protease producer marine bacterium, were jointly utilized for the for biological CH extraction from prawn waste [153]. Both bacteria were cultivated individually and co-fermented in a culture medium prepared with 10% (w/v) shell solids in the presence of increasing concentrations of glucose (0%–15% w/v). Although the extraction of CH following this procedure was incomplete compared to the chemical method, the highest process yield (95.5%) was obtained when *T. turnirae* was first inoculated in co-fermentation. Similar results were obtained by Jung *et al.*, who co-cultivated the lactic acid bacterium *L. paracasei* subsp. tolerans KCTC-3074 and the protease producing bacterium *Serratia marcescens* FS-3 in crab shells [154]. These authors founded that the co-fermentation process was efficient, although highlighted the need to improve deproteinization.

In a later paper, Jung *et al.* reported for the first time successive two-step fermentation from red crab shell wastes using the same species than in the previous work [111,154]. This research concluded that the sequential order of inoculation is an important issue, since the best results in co-removal of CaCO$_3$ and proteins, 94.3% and 68.9%, respectively, from crab shells were obtained when successive fermentation was carried out in a first step with *S. marcescens* followed by a second cultivation with *L. paracasei*, and not *vice versa*.

Several process variables have been reported to influence the fermentation of marine wastes and therefore the efficiency of CH recovery from these sources, such as inoculum ratio [147], temperature [155] and initial pH [146]. Also carbon source and level, and the carbon on nitrogen ratio [147,156] were found to be important parameters for CH recovery from crustacean shells. Although the majority of the reports use the one-factor-at-a-time approach to study the effect of these variables on fermentation performances, other studies have attempted to optimize fermentation conditions for chitin recovery using response surface methodology [148,149,155].

Nevertheless, from the stated above it follows that demineralization and deproteinization occur simultaneously but incompletely in these biological processes [111]. This lower performance of LAB fermentation in deproteinization and demineralization of shell waste has been attributed to the compact structure of the shells [113]. For this reason, the fermentation of crustacean shells has been reported as a complementary strategy to chemical treatments, leading to a decrease in the amount of corrosive chemicals in the CH extraction process [112]. In addition to the reduction in the use of reagents, a major advantage of the fermentation process is obtaining a high-value by-product in the form of liquor rich in protein, minerals and asthaxanthin [113].

The same manner as chemical CH purification, the production of CHs by deacetylation of crustacean chitin with strong alkali appears to have limited potential for industrial acceptance, because of the large amounts of concentrated alkaline solution waste causing environmental pollution. Moreover, the conversion of CH to CHs, using a strong base solution at high temperature, causes variability of the product properties, decreases the CHs quality and increases the processing costs [157]. An alternative source of CHs is the cell wall of fungi, mainly zygomycetes. Among them, the fungus *M. rouxii* has been reported to contain significant amounts of CHs, CH and acidic polysaccharides as cell wall components [158]. For this reason, bioproduction of CHs from *M. rouxii* has been widely studied during recent years [117,159–162]. According to Chatterjee *et al.* culture media and fermentation conditions can be varied to provide CHs of more consistent physico-chemical properties compared to that obtained by chemical modification of chitin [159]. Among three fungal culture media, molasses salt medium (MSM), potato dextrose broth (PDB) and yeast extract peptone glucose (YPG), chitosan from MSM was less polydispersed and more crystalline compared to those from YPG and PDB, thus indicating a higher quality of the polymer.

Since CHs is a constituent of *M. rouxii* cell walls, its production is coupled to fungal growth, and therefore maximal productions are obtained when mycelial growth is maximal. CHs molecular weight was found to be dependent on the growth phase of *M. rouxii*, showing an increase of molecular weight with time of culture [160]. These authors also found a great influence of the pH on fungal growth and therefore on CHs production. Trutnau *et al.* found a higher CHs content with increasing time of cultivation in semi-continuous cultures, suggesting an adaption of the fungi to shear stress [162]. According to these authors, their results and model predictions of hyphal growth, suggest that repeated batch cultures might be optimal for CHs production.

Naturally occurring CHs is produced *in situ* by enzymatic deacetylation of chitin [163]. CH deacetylases were characterized in various fungi, such as *M. rouxii* [164], *Rhizopus nigricans* [165] and *Aspergillus nidulans* [166]. These enzymes have been also explored as an alternative to alkali treatment on chitin production from crustacean shells. Nevertheless, fungal CH deacetylases studied so far are only able to perform enzymatic deacetylation on their solid substrate to a 5%–10% of the total *N*-acetylglucosamine residues [167], preferring *N*-acetylglucosamine homopolymers as substrates [164]. Therefore pretreatment of crystalline CH would be necessary prior to enzyme hydrolysis, in order to improve the accessibility of acetyl groups to the enzyme. Several physical and chemical methods such as heating, sonicating, grinding, derivatization and interaction with saccharides have been assayed in order to improve the accessibility to the acetyl groups for the deacetylation [168]. Win and Stevens were successful at deacetylating CH to CHs (10% DA), using a chitin deacetylase from the fungus *Absidia coerulea* [167]. In this work a pretreatment of superfine CH, a decrystallized form with a very small particle size, with 18% formic acid resulted in the nearly complete enzymatic deacetylation.

Finally it is important to note that besides allowing the reduction in the use of chemicals, fungal CHs possesses two advantages that are interesting for medical applications: a lower molecular weight and lower contents of heavy metals [162]. In Table 2, different microbial processes studied for CH and CHs from marine sources are reported.

Table 2. Summary of procedures and conditions for CH and CHs productionfrom marine sources.

Final Product	Source	Procedure	Process conditions	Yield (Y)/Efficiency (DM, DP, DD)	Ref.
CH	prawn shell	anaerobic fermentation	Sil-Al 4 × 4 TM inoculant, glucose, 30 °C, 7 days	DP = 91%/Y = 20%	[107]
CH	red crab shell	successive two-step fermentation	*S. marcescens, L. paracasei,* glucose, 30 °C, 7 days	DM = 94.3%/DP = 68.9%/Y = 38.7%	[111]
CH	shrimp waste	anaerobic fermentation	*L. acidophilus* SW01, glucose, 37 °C, 168 h	DM = 99.3%/DP = 96.5%	[133]
CH	demineralised prawn shell	solid-state fermentation	Stabisil inoculant, lactose, 25 °C	DP = 40%	[152]
CH	prawn shell	co-fermentation	*L. lactis, T. turnirae,* glucose, 7 days	DM = 70%/DP = 70%/Y = 95.5%	[153]
CH	red crab shell	co-fermentation	*L. paracasei, S. marcescens,* glucose, 30 °C, 7 days	DM = 97.2%/DP = 52.6%	[154]
CHs	*M. rouxii*	semi-continuous fermentation	nutrient broth, 28 °C, 24 h	DD = 86%–88%/Y = 4.4%	[69]
CHs	*M. rouxii*	fermentation	MSM, PDB, YPG	DD(MSM) = 87.2%/DD(PDB) = 89.8%/DD(YPG) = 82.8%/Y(MSM) = 7.7%/Y(PDB) = 6%/Y(YPG) = 6.3%	[159]

DM, demineralization; *DP*, deproteinization; *DD*, deacetylation degree; *MSM*, molasses salt medium; *PDB*, potato dextrose broth; *YPG*, yeast extract peptone glucose.

8. Conclusions

CS, HA and CH/CHs have attracted increasing attention because of their beneficial effects on several ambits of the human health, in the formulation of cosmeceuticals and anti-aging products, nutraceuticals and food ingredients as well as their application in bio and nanotechnological processes.

From long time ago, extensive studies have been conducted on the clarification of the general aspects of the chemical structures, features, novel applications and more sustainable processes for their production. In this review, we have discussed a set of recent progresses in the definition of eco-friendly processes to extract and purify those biomacromolecules from marine by-products.

References

1. Food and Agriculture Organization, *Estadísticas de Pesca: Captura y Desembarques*; FAO: Roma, Italy, 2004.
2. Gildberg, A. Recovery of proteinases and protein hydrolysates from fish viscera. *Bioresour. Technol.* **1992**, *39*, 271–276. [CrossRef]
3. Blanco, M.; Sotelo, C.G.; Chapela, M.J.; Pérez-Martín, R.I. Towards sustainable and efficient use of fishery resources: Present and future trends. *Trends Food Sci. Technol.* **2007**, *18*, 29–36. [CrossRef]
4. European Community. On a European Community plan of action for the conservation and management of sharks. Available online: http://ec.europa.eu/fisheries/marine_species/wild_species/sharks/index_en.htm (accessed on 10 November 2012).
5. Arvanitoyannis, I.S.; Kassaveti, A. Fish industry waste: Treatments, environmental impacts, current and potential uses. *Int. J. Food Sci. Technol.* **2008**, *43*, 726–745. [CrossRef]
6. Senevirathne, M.; Kim, S.-K. Utilization of seafood processing by-products. Medicinal applications. *Adv. Food Nutr. Res.* **2012**, *65*, 495–512. [CrossRef]
7. Jayathilakan, K.; Sultana, K.; Radhakrishna, K.; Bawa, A.S. Utilization of byproducts and waste materials from meat, poultry and fish processing industries: A review. *J. Food Sci. Technol.* **2012**, *49*, 278–293. [CrossRef]
8. Kristinsson, H.G.; Rasco, B. Fish protein hydrolysates: Production, biochemical and functional properties. *Crit. Rev. Food Sci. Nutr.* **2000**, *40*, 43–81. [CrossRef]
9. Gómez-Guillén, M.C.; Turnay, J.; Fernández-Díaz, M.D.; Ulmo, N.; Lizarbe, M.A.; Montero, P. Structural and physical properties of gelatine extracted from different marine species: A comparative study. *Food Hydrocoll.* **2002**, *16*, 25–34. [CrossRef]
10. Gildberg, A. Enzymes and bioactive peptides from fish waste related to fish silage, fish feed and fish sauce preparation. *J. Aquat. Food Prod. Technol.* **2004**, *13*, 3–11. [CrossRef]
11. Percot, A.; Viton, C.; Domard, A. Optimization of chitin extraction from shrimp shells. *Biomacromolecules* **2003**, *4*, 12–18. [CrossRef]
12. Vázquez, J.A.; González, M.P.; Murado, M.A. A new marine medium. Use of different fish peatones and comparative study of selected species of marine bacteria. *Enzym. Microb. Technol.* **2004**, *35*, 385–392.
13. Aspmo, S.I.; Horn, S.J.; Eijsink, V.G.H. Hydrolysates from Atlantic cod (*Gadus morhua* L.) viscera as components of microbial growth media. *Process Biochem.* **2005**, *40*, 3714–3722. [CrossRef]
14. Vázquez, J.A.; Docasal, S.F.; Mirón, J.; González, M.P.; Murado, M.A. Proteases production by two *Vibrio* species on residuals marine media. *J. Ind. Microbiol. Biotechnol.* **2006**, *33*, 661–668. [CrossRef]
15. Vázquez, J.A.; Docasal, S.F.; Prieto, M.A.; González, M.P.; Murado, M.A. Growth and metabolic features of lactic acid bacteria in media with hydrolysed fish viscera. An approach to bio-silage of fishing by-products. *Bioresour. Technol.* **2008**, *99*, 6246–6257.
16. Murado, M.A.; González, M.P.; Vázquez, J.A. Recovery of proteolytic and collagenolytic activities from viscera by-products of rayfish (*Raja clavata*). *Mar. Drugs* **2009**, *7*, 803–815. [CrossRef]
17. Giménez, B.; Alemám, A.; Montero, P.; Gómez-Guillén, M.C. Antioxidant and functional properties of gelatine hydrolysates obtained from skin of sole and squid. *Food Chem.* **2009**, *114*, 976–983. [CrossRef]
18. Vázquez, J.A.; Nogueira, M.; Durán, A.; Prieto, M.A.; Rodríguez-Amado, I.; Rial, D.; González, M.P.; Murado, M.A. Preparation of marine silage of swordfish, ray and shark visceral waste by lactic acid bacteria. *J. Food Eng.* **2011**, *103*, 442–448. [CrossRef]
19. Herpandi, N.H.; Adzitey, F. Fish bone and scale as a potential source of halal gelatine. *J. Fish. Aquat. Sci.* **2011**, *6*, 379–389. [CrossRef]
20. Khaled, H.B.; Bougatef, A.; Balti, R.; Triki-Ellouz, Y.; Souissi, N.; Nasri, M. Isolation and characterisation of trypsin from sardinelle (*Sardinella aurita*) viscera. *J. Sci. Food Agric.* **2008**, *88*, 2654–2662. [CrossRef]

21. Kim, S.-B.; Ji, C.-I.; Woo, J.-W.; Do, J.-R.; Cho, S.-M.; Lee, Y.-B.; Kang, S.-N.; Park, J.-H. Simplified purification of chondroitin sulphate from scapular cartilage of shortfin mako shark (*Isurus oxyrinchus*). *Int. J. Food Sci. Technol.* **2012**, *47*, 91–99. [CrossRef]

22. Jayasinghe, P.; Hawboldt, K. A review of bio-oils from waste biomass: Focus on fish processing waste. *Renew. Sustain. Ener. Rev.* **2012**, *16*, 798–821.

23. Silva, T.H.; Alves, A.; Ferreira, B.M.; Oliveira, J.M.; Reys, L.L.; Ferreira, R.J.F.; Sousa, R.A.; Silva, S.S.; Mano, J.F.; Reis, R.L. Materials of marine origin: A review on polymers and ceramics of biomedical interest. *Int. Mat. Rev.* **2012**, *57*, 276–307. [CrossRef]

24. Ronca, F.; Palmieri, L.; Panicucci, P.; Ronca, G. Anti-inflammatory activity of chondroitin sulfate. *Osteoarthr. Cartil.* **1998**, *6* (Suppl. A), 14–21. [CrossRef]

25. Kogan, G.; Soltés, L.; Stern, R.; Gemeiner, P. Hyaluronic acid: A natural biopolymer with a broad range of biomedical and industrial applications. *Biotechnol. Lett.* **2007**, *29*, 17–25.

26. Zou, X.H.; Jiang, Y.Z.; Zhang, G.R.; Jin, H.M.; Nguyen, T.M.; Ouyang, H.W. Specific interactions between human fibroblasts and particular chondroitin sulphate molecules for wound healing. *Acta Biomater.* **2009**, *5*, 1588–1595. [CrossRef]

27. Kumar, M.N.V.R. A review of chitin and chitosan applications. *React. Funct. Polym.* **2000**, *46*, 1–27. [CrossRef]

28. Kurita, K. Chitin and chitosan: Functional biopolymers from marine crustaceans. *Mar. Biotechnol.* **2006**, *8*, 203–226. [CrossRef]

29. Mourya, V.K.; Inamdar, N.N. Chitosan-modifications and applications: Opportunities galore. *React. Funct. Polym.* **2008**, *68*, 1013–1051. [CrossRef]

30. Seno, N.; Meyer, K. Comparative biochemistry of skin the mucopolysaccharides of shark skin. *Biochim. Biophys. Acta* **1963**, *78*, 258–264. [CrossRef]

31. Vieira, R.P.; Mourao, P.A. Occurrence of a unique fucosebranched chondroitin sulfate in the body wall of a sea cucumber. *J. Biol. Chem.* **1988**, *263*, 18176–18183.

32. Kinoshita-Toyoda, A.; Yamada, S.; Haslam, S.M.; Khoo, K.-H.; Sugiura, M.; Morris, H.R.; Dell, A.; Sugahara, K. Structural determination of five novel tetrasaccharides containing 3-*O*-sulfated D-glucuronic acid and two rare oligosaccharides containing a β-D-glucose branch isolated from squid cartilage chondroitin sulfate E. *Biochemistry* **2004**, *43*, 11063–11074. [CrossRef]

33. Hardingham, T. Solution Properties of Hyaluronan. In *Chemistry and Biology of Hyaluronan*; Garg, H.G., Hales, C.A., Eds.; Elsevier Ltd.: Oxford, UK, 2004; pp. 1–16.

34. Malavaki, C.; Mizumoto, S.; Karamanos, N.; Sugahara, K. Recent advance in the structural study of functional chondroitin sulfate and dermatan sulphate in health and disease. *Connect. Tissue Res.* **2008**, *49*, 133–139. [CrossRef]

35. Garnjanagoonchorn, W.; Wongekalak, L.; Engkagul, A. Determination of chondroitin sulfate from different sources of cartilage. *Chem. Eng. Proc.* **2007**, *46*, 465–471. [CrossRef]

36. Lauder, R.M. Chondroitin sulphate: A complex molecule with potential impacts on a wide range of biological systems. *Complement. Ther. Med.* **2009**, *17*, 56–62. [CrossRef]

37. Schiraldi, C.; Cimini, D.; de Rosa, M. Production of chondroitin sulphate and chondroitin. *Appl. Microbiol. Biotechnol.* **2010**, *87*, 1209–1220. [CrossRef]

38. Pipitone, V.R. Chondroprotection with chondroitin sulphate. *Drugs Exp. Clin. Res.* **1991**, *17*, 3–7.

39. Chang, C.H.; Liu, H.C.; Lin, C.C.; Chou, C.H.; Lin, F.H. Gelatin–chondroitin–hyaluronan tri-copolymer scaffold for cartilage tissue engineering. *Biomaterials* **2003**, *24*, 4853–4858. [CrossRef]

40. Cai, S.; Liu, Y.; Shu, X.Z.; Prestwich, G.D. Injectable glycosaminoglycan hydrogels for controlled release of human basic fibroblast growth factor. *Biomaterials* **2005**, *26*, 6054–6067. [CrossRef]

41. Keskin, D.S.; Tezcaner, A.; Korkusuz, P.; Korkusuz, F.; Hasirei, V. Collagen-chondroitin sulfate-based PLLA-SAIB-coated rhBMP-2 delivery system for bone repair. *Biomaterials* **2005**, *6*, 4023–4034.

42. Yamada, S.; Sugahara, K. Potential therapeutic application of chondroitin sulfate/dermatan sulphate. *Curr. Drug Discov. Technol.* **2008**, *5*, 289–301. [CrossRef]

43. Alkhalil, A.; Achur, R.N.; Valiyaveettil, M.; Ockenhouse, C.F.; Gowda, D.C. Structural requirements for the adherence of *Plasmodium falciparum*-infected erythrocytes to chondroitin sulphate proteoglycans of human placenta. *J. Biol. Chem.* **2000**, *277*, 8882–8889.

44. Smetsers, T.F.; van de Westerlo, E.M.; ten Dam, G.B.; Overes, I.M.; Schalkwijik, J.; van Muijen, G.N.; van Kuppvelt, T.H. Human single-chain antibodies reactive with native chondroitin sulphate detect chondroitin sulphate alterations in melanoma and psoriasis. *J. Invest. Dermatol.* **2004**, *122*, 701–716.

45. Pothacharoen, P.; Siriaunkgul, S.; Ong-Chai, S.; Supabandhu, J.; Kumja, P.; Wanaphirak, C.; Sugahara, K.; Hardingham, T.; Kongtawelert, P. Raised serum chondroitin sulphate epitope level in ovarian epithelial cancer. *J. Biochem.* **2006**, *140*, 517–524. [CrossRef]

46. Borsig, L.; Wang, L.; Cavalcante, M.C.; Cardilo-Reis, L.; Ferreira, P.L.; Mourao, P.A.; Esko, J.D.; Pvao, M.S. Selectin blocking activity of a fucosylated chondroitin sulphate glycosaminoglycan from sea cucumber. Effect on tumor metastasis and neutrophil recruitment. *J. Biol. Chem.* **2007**, *282*, 14984–14991. [CrossRef]

47. Hamano, T.; Mitsuhashi, Y.; Acki, N.; Yamamoto, S.; Tsuji, S.; Ito, Y.; Oji, Y. High-performance liquid chromatography assay of chondroitin sulfate in food products. *Analyst* **1989**, *114*, 891–893. [CrossRef]

48. Conte, A.; Volpi, N.; Palmieri, L.; Bahous, I.; Ronca, G. Biochemical and pharmacokinetic aspects of oral treatment with chondroitin sulphate. *Arzneim. Forsch.* **1995**, *45*, 918–925.

49. Volpi, N. Quality of different chondroitin sulphate preparations in relation to their therapeutic activity. *J. Pharm. Pharmacol.* **2009**, *61*, 1271–1277. [CrossRef]

50. Michel, B.A.; Stucki, G.; Frey, D.; de Vathaire, F.; Vignon, E.; Bruehlmann, P.; Uebelhart, D. Chondroitins 4 and 6 sulfate in osteoarthritis of the knee: A randomized, controlled trial. *Arthritis Rheum.* **2005**, *52*, 779–786. [CrossRef]

51. Field, I.C.; Meekan, M.G.; Buckworth, R.C.; Bradshaw, C.J.A. Susceptibility of sharks, rays and chimaeras to global extinction. *Adv. Mar. Biol.* **2010**, *56*, 275–363.

52. García, V.B.; Lucifora, L.O.; Myers, R.A. The importance of habitat and life history to extinction risk in sharks, skates, rays and chimaeras. *Proc. R. Soc. B* **2008**, *275*, 83–89. [CrossRef]

53. Shiedlin, A.; Bigelow, R.; Christopher, W.; Arbabi, S.; Yang, L.; Maier, R.V.; Wainwright, N.; Childs, A.; Miller, R.J. Evaluation of hyaluronan from different sources *Streptococcus zooepidemicus*, rooster comb, bovine vitreous, and human umbilical cord. *Biomacromolecules* **2004**, *5*, 2122–2127. [CrossRef]

54. Beasley, K.L.; Weiss, M.A.; Weiss, M.D. Hyaluronic acid fillers: A comprehensive review. *Facial Plast. Surg.* **2009**, *25*, 86–94. [CrossRef]

55. Chong, B.F.; Blank, L.M.; Mclaughlin, R.; Nielsen, L.K. Microbial hyaluronic acid production. *Appl. Microbiol. Biotechnol.* **2005**, *66*, 341–351. [CrossRef]

56. Murado, M.A.; Montemayor, M.I.; Cabo, M.L.; Vázquez, J.A.; González, M.P. Optimization of extraction and purification process of hyaluronic acid from fish eyeball. *Food Bioprod. Proc.* **2012**, *90*, 491–498. [CrossRef]

57. Kim, S.J.; Park, S.Y.; Kin, C.W. A novel approach to the production of hyaluronic acid by *Streptococcus zooepidemicus*. *J. Microbiol. Biotechnol.* **2006**, *16*, 1849–1855.

58. Rangaswamy, V.; Jain, D. An efficient process for production and purification of hyaluronic acid from *Streptococcus equi* subsp. *zooepidemicus*. *Biotechnol. Lett.* **2008**, *30*, 493–496. [CrossRef]

59. Rodén, L.; Baker, J.R.; Cifonelli, J.A.; Mathews, M.B. Isolation and characterization of connective tissue polysaccharides. *Methods Enzymol.* **1972**, *28*, 73–140.

60. Chascall, V.; Calabro, A.; Midura, R.J.; Yanagishita, M. Isolation and Characterization of Proteoglycans. In *Methods in Enzymology*; Lennarz, W.J., Hart, G.W., Eds.; Academic Press: San Diego, CA, USA, 1994; Volume 230, pp. 390–417.

61. Sumi, T.; Ohba, H.; Ikegami, T.; Shibata, M.; Sakaki, T.; Salay, I.; Park, S.S. Method for the Preparation of Chondroitin Sulfate Compounds. U.S. Patent 6,342,367, 29 January 2002.

62. Patel, B.; Ehrlich, J.; Stivala, S.S.; Singh, N.K. Comparative studies of mucopolysaccharides from marine animals. I. *Raja eglanteria* Bosc. *J. Exp. Mar. Biol. Ecol.* **1980**, *46*, 127–135. [CrossRef]

63. Lignot, B.; Lahogue, V.; Bourseau, P. Enzymatic extraction of chondroitin sulfate from skate cartilage and concentration-desalting by ultrafiltration. *J. Biotechnol.* **2003**, *103*, 281–284. [CrossRef]

64. Mollard, L.; Montillet, A.; Horriere, C.; Legrand, J.; Nguyen, T.H. Method for Obtaining Avian Biological Products. U.S. Patent 6,844,424, 18 January 2005.

65. Tadashi, E. Sodium Chondroitin Sulfate,Chondroitin-Sulfate-Containing Material and Processes for Producing the Same. U.S. Patent Appl. 20,060,014,256, 19 January 2006.

66. Murado, M.A.; Fraguas, J.; Montemayor, M.I.; Vázquez, J.A.; González, M.P. Preparation of highly purified chondroitin sulphate from skate (*Raja clavata*) cartilage by-products. Process optimization including a new procedure of alkaline hydroalcoholic hydrolysis. *Biochem. Eng. J.* **2010**, *49*, 126–132.

67. Michelacci, Y.M.; Horton, D.S.P.Q. Proteoglycans from the cartilage of young hammerhead shark *Sphyrna lewini. Comp. Biochem. Physiol.* **1989**, *92B*, 651–658.

68. Souza, A.R.C.; Kozlowski, E.O.; Cerqueira, V.R.; Castelo-Branco, M.T.L.; Costa, M.L.; Pavão, M.S.G. Chondroitin sulfate and keratan sulfate are the major glycosaminoglycans present in the adult zebrafish *Danio rerio* (Chordata-Cyprinidae). *Glycoconj. J.* **2007**, *24*, 521–530. [CrossRef]

69. Gargiulo, V.; Lanzetta, R.; Parrilli, M.; de Castro, C. Structural analysis of chondroitin sulfate from *Scyliorhinus canicula*: A useful source of this polysaccharide. *Glycobiology* **2009**, *19*, 1485–1491. [CrossRef]

70. Takai, M.; Kono, H. Salmon-Origin Chondroitin Sulphate. U.S. Patent Appl. 20,030,162,744, 28 August 2003.

71. Nishigori, T.; Takeda, T.; Ohori, T. Method for Isolation and Purification of Chondroitin Sulfate. Jpn Patent 2000273102-A, 10 October 2000.

72. Jang, H.; Yoon, Y.K.; Kim, J.A.; Kim, H.S.; An, S.J.; Seo, J.H.; Cui, C.; Carbis, R. Optimization of Vi capsular polysaccharide production during growth of *Salmonella enterica* serotype Typhi Ty2 in a bioreactor. *J. Biotechnol.* **2008**, *135*, 71–77. [CrossRef]

73. Cimini, D.; de Rosa, M.; Schiraldi, C. Production of glucuronic acid-based polysaccharides by microbial fermentation for biomedical applications. *Biotechnol. J.* **2012**, *7*, 237–250. [CrossRef]

74. Rimler, R.B. Presumptive identification of *Pasteurella multocida* serogroups A, D and F by capsule depolymerisation with mucopolysaccharides. *Vet. Rec.* **1994**, *134*, 191–192.

75. Rimler, R.B.; Register, K.B.; Magyar, T.; Ackermann, M.R. Influence of chondroitinase on indirect hemagglutination titers and phagocytosis of *Pasteurella multocida* serogroups A, D and F. *Vet. Microbiol.* **1995**, *47*, 287–294. [CrossRef]

76. Cimini, D.; Restaino, O.F.; Catapano, A.; de Rosa, M.; Schiraldi, C. Production of capsular polysaccharide from *Escherichia coli* K4 for biotechnological applications. *Appl. Microbiol. Biotechnol.* **2010**, *85*, 1779–1787. [CrossRef]

77. Restaino, O.F.; Cimini, D.; de Rosa, M.; Catapano, A.; de Rosa, M.; Schiraldi, C. High cell density cultivation of *Escherichia coli* K4 in a microfiltration bioreactor: A step towards improvement of chondroitin precursor production. *Microb. Cell Fact.* **2011**, *10*, 1–10. [CrossRef]

78. Schiraldi, C.; Alfano, A.; Cimini, D.; de Rosa, M.; Panariello, A.; Restaino, O.F.; de Rosa, M. Application of a 22L scale membrane bioreactor and cross-flow ultrafiltration to obtain purified chondroitin. *Biotechnol. Prog.* **2012**, *28*, 1012–1018. [CrossRef]

79. Schiraldi, C.; Carcarino, L.I.; Alfano, A.; Restaino, O.F.; Panariello, A.; de Rosa, M. Purification of chondroitin precursor from *Escherichia coli* K4 fermentation broth using membrane processing. *Biotechnol. J.* **2011**, *6*, 410–419. [CrossRef]

80. Bedini, E.; de Castro, C.; de Rosa, M.; di Nola, A.; Iadonisi, A.; Restaino, O.F.; Schiraldi, C.; Parrilli, M. A microbiological-chemical strategy to produce chondroitin sulphate A,C. *Angew. Chem. Int. Ed.* **2011**, *50*, 6160–6163. [CrossRef]

81. Nakano, T.; Nakano, K.; Sim, J.S. A simple rapid method to estimate hyaluronic acid concentrations in rooster comb and wattle using cellulose acetate electrophoresis. *J. Agric. Food Chem.* **1994**, *42*, 2766–2768. [CrossRef]

82. Cullis-Hill, D. Preparation of Hyaluronic Acid from Synovial Fluid. U.S. Patent 4,879,375, 7 November 1989.

83. Marcellin, E.; Chen, W.; Nielsen, L.K. Microbial Hyaluronic Acid Biosynthesis. In *Microbial Production of Biopolymers and Polymer Precursors: Applications and Perspectives*; Rehm, B.H.A., Ed.; Caister Academic Press: Norwich, UK, 2009; pp. 163–180.

84. Imberty, A.; Lortat-Jacobb, H.; Pérez, S. Structural view of glycosaminoglycan–protein interactions. *Carbohydr. Res.* **2007**, *342*, 430–439. [CrossRef]

85. Swann, D.A. Studies on hyaluronic acid: I. The preparation and properties of rooster comb hyaluronic acid. *Biochim. Biophys. Acta* **1968**, *156*, 17–30. [CrossRef]

86. Balazs, E.A. Ultrapure Hyaluronic Acid and the Use Thereof. U.S. Patent 4,141,973, 27 February 1979.

87. O'Regan, M.; Martini, I.; Crescenzi, F.; de Luca, C.; Lansing, M. Molecular mechanisms and genetics of hyaluronan biosynthesis. *Int. J. Biol. Macromol.* **1994**, *16*, 283–286. [CrossRef]

88. Radulescu, G.; Lupescu, I.; Petrea, D.-M.; Scurei, H. Hyaluronic acid extraction from vitreous fluid. *Biotechnol. Lett.* **1997**, *2*, 147–152.

89. Gao, Y.-Q.; Liu, J.-H.; Huo, X.; Shan, Y.-L.; Xu, Z.-X. The purification and identification of hyaluronic acid isolated from various tissues. *Chin. Boichem. J.* **1996**, *12*, 215–218.

90. Mizuno, H.; Iso, N.; Saito, T.; Ogawa, H.; Sawairi, H.; Saito, M. Characterization of hyaluronic acid of yellowfin tuna eyeball. *Nippon Suisan Gakkaishi* **1991**, *57*, 517–519. [CrossRef]

91. Ogrodowski, C.S.; Hokka, C.O.; Santana, M.H.A. Production of hyaluronic acid by *Streptococcus*: The effects of the addition of lysozyme and aeration on the formation and the rheological properties of the product. *Appl. Biochem. Biotechnol.* **2005**, *5*, 121–124.

92. Liu, L.; Du, G.; Chen, J.; Wang, M.; Sun, J. Influence of hyaluronidase addition on the production of hyaluronic acid by batch culture of *Streptococcus zooepidemicus*. *Food Chem.* **2008**, *110*, 923–926. [CrossRef]

93. Johns, M.R.; Goh, L.T.; Oeggerli, A. Effect of pH, agitation and aeration on hyaluronic acid production by *Streptococcus zooepidemicus*. *Biotechnol. Lett.* **1994**, *16*, 507–512. [CrossRef]

94. Huang, W.C.; Chen, S.J.; Chen, T.L. The role of dissolved oxygen and function of agitation in hyaluronic acid fermentation. *Biochem. Eng. J.* **2006**, *32*, 239–243. [CrossRef]

95. Liu, L.; Du, G.; Chen, J.; Wang, M.; Sun, J. Comparative study on the influence of dissolved oxygen control approaches on the microbial hyaluronic acid production of *Streptococcus zooepidemicus*. *Bioprocess Biosyst. Eng.* **2009**, *32*, 755–763. [CrossRef]

96. Hiruta, O.; Yamamura, K.; Takebe, H.; Futamura, T.; Ilnuma, K.; Tanaka, H. Application of maxblend fermentor for microbial processes. *J. Ferm. Bioeng.* **1997**, *83*, 79–86. [CrossRef]

97. Liu, L.; Wang, M.; Du, G.; Chen, J. Enhanced hyaluronic acid production of *Streptococcus zooepidemicus* by an intermittent alkaline-stress strategy. *Lett. Appl. Microbiol.* **2008**, *46*, 383–388. [CrossRef]

98. Blank, L.M.; McLaughlin, R.L.; Nielsen, L.K. Stable production of hyaluronic acid in *Streptococcus zooepidemicus* chemostats operated at high dilution rate. *Biotechnol. Bioeng.* **2005**, *90*, 685–693. [CrossRef]

99. Zhang, J.; Ding, X.; Yang, L.; Kong, Z. A serum-free medium for colony growth and hyaluronic acid production by *Streptococcus zooepidemicus* NJUST01. *Appl. Microbiol. Biotechnol.* **2006**, *72*, 168–172. [CrossRef]

100. Liu, L.; Du, G.; Chen, J.; Wang, M.; Sun, J. Enhanced hyaluronic acid production by a two-stage culture strategy based on the modeling of batch and fed-batch cultivation of *Streptococcus zooepidemicus*. *Bioresour. Technol.* **2008**, *99*, 8532–8536. [CrossRef]

101. Vázquez, J.A.; Montemayor, M.I.; Fraguas, J.; Murado, M.A. High production of hyaluronic and lactic acids by *Streptococcus zooepidemicus* in fed-batch culture using commercial and marine peptones from fishing by-products. *Biochem. Eng. J.* **2009**, *44*, 125–130. [CrossRef]

102. Vázquez, J.A.; Montemayor, M.I.; Fraguas, J.; Murado, M.A. Hyaluronic acid production by *Streptococcus zooepidemicus* in marine by-products media from mussel processing wastewaters and tuna peptone viscera. *Microb. Cell Fact.* **2010**, *9*, 46. [CrossRef]

103. Yamada, T.; Kawasaki, T. Microbial synthesis of hyaluronan and chitin: New approaches. *J. Biosci. Bioeng.* **2005**, *99*, 521–528. [CrossRef]

104. Teng, W.L.; Khor, E.; Tan, T.K.; Lim, L.Y.; Tan, S.C. Concurrent production of chitin from shrimp shells and fungi. *Carbohydr. Res.* **2001**, *332*, 305–316. [CrossRef]

105. Roca, C.; Chagas, B.; Farinha, I.; Freitas, F.; Mafra, L.; Aguiar, F.; Oliveira, R.; Reis, M.A.M. Production of yeast chitin-glucan complex from biodiesel industry byproduct. *Process Biochem.* **2012**, *47*, 1670–1675. [CrossRef]

106. Kurita, K.; Tomita, K.; Tada, T.; Ishii, S.; Nishimura, S.-I.; Shimoda, K. Squid chitin as a potential alternative chitin source: Deacetylation behavior and characteristic properties. *J. Polym. Sci. A* **1993**, *31*, 485–491. [CrossRef]

107. Healy, M.; Green, A.; Healy, A. Bioprocessing of marine crustacean shell waste. *Acta Biotechnol.* **2003**, *23*, 151–160. [CrossRef]

108. Jo, G.H.; Jung, W.J.; Kuk, J.H.; Oh, K.T.; Kim, Y.J.; Park, R.D. Screening of protease-producing *Serratia marcescens* FS-3 and its application to deproteinization of crab shell waste for chitin extraction. *Carbohydr. Polym.* **2008**, *74*, 504–508. [CrossRef]

109. Manni, L.; Ghorbel-Bellaaj, O.; Jellouli, K.; Younes, I.; Nasri, M. Extraction and characterization of chitin, chitosan, and protein hydrolysates prepared from shrimp waste by treatment with crude protease from *Bacillus cereus* SV1. *Appl. Biochem. Biotechnol.* **2010**, *162*, 345–357. [CrossRef]

110. Bautista, J.; Jover, M.; Gutiérrez, J.F.; Corpas, R.; Cremades, O.; Fontiveros, E.; Iglesias, F.; Vega, J. Preparation of crayfish chitin by *in situ* lactic acid production. *Process Biochem.* **2001**, *37*, 229–234. [CrossRef]

111. Jung, W.J.; Jo, G.H.; Kuk, J.H.; Kim, Y.J.; Oh, K.T.; Park, R.D. Production of chitin from red crab shell waste by successive fermentation with *Lactobacillus paracasei* KCTC-3074 and *Serratia marcescens* FS-3. *Carbohydr. Polym.* **2007**, *68*, 746–750. [CrossRef]

112. Cira, L.A.; Huerta, S.; Hall, G.M.; Shirai, K. Pilot scale lactic acid fermentation of shrimp wastes for chitin recovery. *Process Biochem.* **2002**, *37*, 1359–1366. [CrossRef]

113. Rao, M.S.; Stevens, W.F. Chitin production by *Lactobacillus* fermentation of shrimp biowaste in a drum reactor and its chemical conversion to chitosan. *J. Chem. Technol. Biotechnol.* **2005**, *80*, 1080–1087. [CrossRef]

114. Muzzarelli, R.A.A. *Chitin*; Pergamon Press: Oxford, UK, 1977.

115. Rinaudo, M. Chitin and chitosan: Properties and applications. *Prog. Polym. Sci.* **2006**, *31*, 603–632. [CrossRef]

116. Minke, R.; Blackwell, J. The structure of β-chitin. *J. Mol. Biol.* **1978**, *120*, 167–181. [CrossRef]

117. Synowiecki, J.; Al-Khateeb, N.A. Production, properties, and some new applications of chitin and its derivatives. *Crit. Rev. Food Sci. Nutr.* **2003**, *43*, 145–171. [CrossRef]

118. Tharanathan, R.N.; Kittur, F.S. Chitin—The undisputed biomolecule of great potential. *Crit. Rev. Food Sci. Nutr.* **2003**, *43*, 61–87. [CrossRef]

119. Roberts, G.A.F. *Chitin Chemistry*; Macmillan Press Ltd.: London, UK, 1992; pp. 85–91.

120. Rutherford, F.A.; Austin, P.R. Marine Chitin Properties and Solvents. In Proceedings of the First International Conference on Chitin/Chitosan; Muzzarelli, R.A.A., Pariser, E.R., Eds.; MIT Sea Grant Program: Cambridge, MA, USA, 1978; pp. 182–191.

121. Pillai, C.K.S.; Paul, W.; Sharma, C.P. Chitin and chitosan polymers: Chemistry, solubility and fiber formation. *Prog. Polym. Sci.* **2009**, *34*, 641–678. [CrossRef]

122. Campaniello, D.; Bevilacqua, A.; Sinigaglia, M.; Corbo, M.R. Chitosan: Antimicrobial activity and potential applications for preserving minimally processed strawberries. *Food Microbiol.* **2008**, *25*, 992–1000. [CrossRef]

123. Huang, D.; Wang, W.; Kang, Y.; Wang, A. Chitin and chitosan as multipurpose natural polymers for groundwater arsenic removal and As_2O_3 delivery in tumor therapy. *J. Macromol. Sci. Pure Appl. Chem.* **2012**, *49*, 971–979.

124. Sánchez, R.; Stringari, G.B.; Franco, J.M.; Valencia, C.; Gallegos, C. Use of chitin, chitosan and acylated derivatives as thickener agents of vegetable oils for bio-lubricant applications. *Carbohydr. Polym.* **2011**, *85*, 705–714. [CrossRef]

125. Aam, B.B.; Heggset, E.B.; Norberg, A.L.; Sørlie, M.; Vårum, K.M.; Eijsink, V.G.H. Production of chitooligosaccharides and their potential applications in medicine. *Mar. Drugs* **2010**, *8*, 1482–1517. [CrossRef]

126. Zhang, J.; Xia, W.; Liu, P.; Cheng, Q.; Tahirou, T.; Gu, W.; Li, B. Chitosan modification and pharmaceutical/biomedical applications. *Mar. Drugs* **2010**, *8*, 1962–1987. [CrossRef]

127. Jayakumar, R.; Menon, D.; Manzoor, K.; Nair, S.V.; Tamura, H. Biomedical applications of chitin and chitosan based nanomaterials—A short review. *Carbohydr. Polym.* **2010**, *82*, 227–232. [CrossRef]

128. Rodríguez, M.S.; Albertengo, L.A.; Agulló, E. Emulsification capacity of chitosan. *Carbohydr. Polym.* **2002**, *48*, 271–276.

129. Fajardo, P.; Martins, J.T.; Fuciños, C.; Pastrana, L.; Teixeira, J.A.; Vicente, A.A. Evaluation of a chitosan-based edible film as carrier of natamycin to improve the storability of Saloio cheese. *J. Food Eng.* **2010**, *101*, 349–356. [CrossRef]

130. Anchisi, C.; Meloni, M.C.; Maccioni, A.M. Chitosan beads loaded with essential oils in cosmetic formulations. *J. Cosmet. Sci.* **2006**, *57*, 205–214.

131. Shahidi, F.; Synowiecki, J. Isolation and characterization of nutrients and value-added products from snow crab (*Chionoecetes opilio*) and shrimp (*Pandalus borealis*) processing discards. *J. Agric. Food Chem.* **1991**, *39*, 1527–1532. [CrossRef]

132. Tolaimate, A.; Desbrières, J.; Rhazi, M.; Alagui, A. Contribution to the preparation of chitins and chitosans with controlled physico-chemical properties. *Polymers* **2003**, *44*, 7939–7952. [CrossRef]

133. Duan, S.; Li, L.; Zhuang, Z.; Wu, W.; Hong, S.; Zhou, J. Improved production of chitin from shrimp waste by fermentation with epiphytic lactic acid bacteria. *Carbohydr. Polym.* **2012**, *89*, 1283–1288. [CrossRef]

134. Chang, K.L.B.; Tsai, G. Response surface optimization and kinetics of isolating chitin from pink shrimp (*Solenocera melantho*) shell waste. *J. Agric. Food Chem.* **1997**, *45*, 1900–1904. [CrossRef]

135. Broussignac, P. Unhaut polymere naturel peu connu dans l'industrie, Le chitosane. *Chim. Ind. Genie Chim.* **1968**, *99*, 1241–1247.

136. Tolaimate, A.; Desbrières, J.; Rhazi, M.; Alagui, A.; Vincendon, M.; Vottero, P. On the influence of deacetylation process on the physicochemical characteristics of chitosan from squid chitin. *Polymer* **2000**, *41*, 2463–2469. [CrossRef]

137. Valdez-Peña, A.U.; Espinoza-Pérez, J.D.; Sandoval-Fabian, G.C.; Balagurusamy, N.; Hernández-Rivera, A.; De-la-Garza-Rodríguez, I.M.; Contreras-Esquivel, J.C. Screening of industrial enzymes for deproteinization of shrimp head for chitin recovery. *Food Sci. Biotechnol.* **2010**, *19*, 553–557. [CrossRef]

138. Synowiecki, J.; Al-Khateeb, N.A.A.Q. The recovery of protein hydrolysate during enzymatic isolation of chitin from shrimp *Crangon crangon* processing discards. *Food Chem.* **2000**, *68*, 147–152. [CrossRef]

139. De Holanda, H.D.; Netto, F.M. Recovery of components from shrimp (*Xiphopenaeus kroyeri*) processing waste by enzymatic hydrolysis. *J. Food Sci.* **2006**, *71*, C298–C303. [CrossRef]

140. Giyose, N.Y.; Mazomba, N.T.; Mabinya, L.V. Evaluation of proteases produced by *Erwinia chrysanthemi* for the deproteinization of crustacean waste in a chitin production process. *Afr. J. Biotechnol.* **2010**, *9*, 707–711.

141. Haddar, A.; Hmidet, N.; Ghorbel-Bellaaj, O.; Fakhfakh-Zouari, N.; Sellami-Kamoun, A.; Nasri, M. Alkaline proteases produced by *Bacillus licheniformis* RP1 grown on shrimp wastes: Application in chitin extraction, chicken feather-degradation and as a dehairing agent. *Biotechnol. Bioprocess Eng.* **2011**, *16*, 669–678. [CrossRef]

142. Sila, A.; Nasri, R.; Bougatef, A.; Nasri, M. Digestive alkaline proteases from the goby (*Zosterisessor ophiocephalus*): Characterization and potential application as detergent additive and in the deproteinization of shrimp wastes. *J. Aquat. Food Prod. Technol.* **2012**, *21*, 118–133. [CrossRef]

143. Sachindra, N.M.; Bhaskar, N.; Siddegowda, G.S.; Sathisha, A.D.; Suresh, P.V. Recovery of carotenoids from ensilaged shrimp waste. *Bioresour. Technol.* **2007**, *98*, 1642–1646.

144. Hoffmann, K.; Daum, G.; Köster, M.; Kulicke, W.-M.; Meyer-Rammes, H.; Bisping, B.; Meinhardt, F. Genetic improvement of *Bacillus licheniformis* strains for efficient deproteinization of shrimp shells and production of high-molecular-mass chitin and chitosan. *Appl. Environ. Microbiol.* **2010**, *76*, 8211–8221. [CrossRef]

145. Woods, B. *Microbiology of Fermented Foods*, 2nd ed; Springer: New York, NY, USA, 1998.

146. Rao, M.S.; Muñoz, J.; Stevens, W.F. Critical factors in chitin production by fermentation of shrimp biowaste. *Appl. Microbiol. Biotechnol.* **2000**, *54*, 808–813. [CrossRef]

147. Shirai, K.; Guerrero, I.; Huerta, S.; Saucedo, G.; Castillo, A.; Gonzalez, R.O.; Hall, G.M. Effect of initial glucose concentration and inoculation level of lactic acid bacteria in shrimp waste ensilation. *Enzym. Microb. Technol.* **2001**, *28*, 446–452. [CrossRef]

148. Bhaskar, N.; Suresh, P.V.; Sakhare, P.Z.; Sachindra, N.M. Shrimp biowaste fermentation with *Pediococcus acidolactici* CFR2182: Optimization of fermentation conditions by response surface methodology and effect of optimized conditions on deproteination/demineralization and carotenoid recovery. *Enzym. Microb. Technol.* **2007**, *40*, 1427–1434. [CrossRef]

149. Arbia, W.; Adour, L.; Amrane, A.; Lounici, H. Optimization of medium composition for enhanced chitin extraction from *Parapenaeus longirostris* by *Lactobacillus helveticus* using response surface methodology. *Food Hydrocoll.* **2013**, *31*, 392–403. [CrossRef]

150. Ghorbel-Bellaaj, O.; Jellouli, K.; Younes, I.; Manni, L.; Ouled, S.M.; Nasri, M. A solvent-stable metalloprotease produced by *Pseudomonas aeruginosa* A2 grown on shrimp shell waste and its application in chitin extraction. *Appl. Biochem. Biotechnol.* **2011**, *164*, 410–425. [CrossRef]

151. Sini, T.K.; Santhosh, S.; Mathew, P.T. Study on the production of chitin and chitosan from shrimp shell by using *Bacillus subtilis* fermentation. *Carbohydr. Res.* **2007**, *342*, 2423–2429. [CrossRef]

152. Healy, M.G.; Romo, C.R.; Bustos, R. Bioconversion of marine crustacean shell waste. *Resour. Conserv. Recycl.* **1994**, *11*, 139–147. [CrossRef]

153. Aytekin, O.; Elibol, M. Cocultivation of *Lactococcus lactis* and *Teredinobacter turnirae* for biological chitin extraction from prawn waste. *Bioprocess Biosyst. Eng.* **2010**, *33*, 393–399. [CrossRef]

154. Jung, W.J.; Jo, G.H.; Kuk, J.H.; Kim, K.Y.; Park, R.D. Extraction of chitin from red crab shell waste by cofermentation with *Lactobacillus paracasei* subsp. tolerans KCTC-3074 and *Serratia marcescens* FS-3. *Appl. Microbiol. Biotechnol.* **2006**, *71*, 234–237. [CrossRef]

155. Pacheco, N.; Garnica-González, M.; Ramírez-Hernández, J.Y.; Flores-Albino, B.; Gimeno, M.; Bárzana, E.; Shirai, K. Effect of temperature on chitin and astaxanthin recoveries from shrimp waste using lactic acid bacteria. *Bioresour. Technol.* **2009**, *100*, 2849–2854. [CrossRef]

156. Choorit, W.; Patthanamanee, W.; Manurakchinakorn, S. Use of response surface method for the determination of demineralization efficiency in fermented shrimp shells. *Bioresour. Technol.* **2008**, *99*, 6168–6173. [CrossRef]

157. Synowiecki, J.; Al-Khateeb, N.A.A.Q. Mycelia of *Mucor rouxii* as a source of chitin and chitosan. *Food Chem.* **1997**, *60*, 605–610. [CrossRef]

158. Arcidiacono, S.; Kaplan, D.L. Molecular weight distribution of chitosan isolated from *Mucor rouxii* under different culture and processing conditions. *Biotechnol. Bioeng.* **1992**, *39*, 281–286. [CrossRef]

159. Chatterjee, S.; Adhya, M.; Guha, A.K.; Chatterjee, B.P. Chitosan from *Mucor rouxii*: Production and physico-chemical characterization. *Process Biochem.* **2005**, *40*, 395–400. [CrossRef]

160. Chatterjee, S.; Chatterjee, B.P.; Guha, A.K. Kinetics of *Mucor rouxii* fermentation in relation to chitosan production. *Res. J. Microbiol.* **2010**, *5*, 361–365.

161. Martinou, A.; Bouriotis, V.; Stokke, B.T.; Vårum, K.M. Mode of action of chitin deacetylase from *Mucor rouxii* on partially N-acetylated chitosans. *Carbohydr. Res.* **1998**, *311*, 71–78. [CrossRef]

162. Trutnau, M.; Suckale, N.; Groeger, G.; Bley, T.; Ondruschka, J. Enhanced chitosan production and modeling hyphal growth of *Mucor rouxii* interpreting the dependence of chitosan yields on processing and cultivation time. *Eng. Life Sci.* **2009**, *9*, 437–443. [CrossRef]

163. Kolodziejska, I.; Malesa-Ciecwierz, M.; Lerska, A.; Sikorski, Z. Properties of chitin deacetylase from crude extracts of *Mucor rouxii* mycelium. *J. Food Biochem.* **1999**, *23*, 45–57.

164. Araki, Y.; Ito, E. A pathway of chitosan formation in *Mucor rouxii*: Enzymatic deacetylation of chitin. *Biochem. Biophys. Res. Commun.* **1974**, *56*, 669–675. [CrossRef]

165. Jeraj, N.; Kunic, B.; Lenasi, H.; Breskvar, K. Purification and molecular characterization of chitin deacetylase from *Rhizopus nigricans*. *Enzyme Microb. Technol.* **2006**, *39*, 1294–1299. [CrossRef]

166. Alfonso, C.; Nuero, O.M.; Santamaria, F.; Reyes, F. Purification of a heat-stable chitin deacetylase from *Aspergillus nidulans* and its role in cell wall degradation. *Curr. Microbiol.* **1995**, *30*, 49–54.

167. Win, N.N.; Stevens, W.F. Shrimp chitin as substrate for fungal chitin deacetylase. *Appl. Microbiol. Biotechnol.* **2001**, *57*, 334–341. [CrossRef]

168. Zhao, Y.; Park, R.-D.; Muzzarelli, R.A.A. Chitin deacetylases: Properties and applications. *Mar. Drugs* **2010**, *8*, 24–46. [CrossRef]

Samples Availability: Available from the authors.

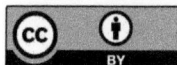

marine drugs

MDPI

Review

Biomedical Exploitation of Chitin and Chitosan via Mechano-Chemical Disassembly, Electrospinning, Dissolution in Imidazolium Ionic Liquids, and Supercritical Drying

Riccardo A. A. Muzzarelli

University of Ancona, IT-60100 Ancona, Italy; Muzzarelli.raa@gmail.it; Tel./Fax: +39-071-36206

Received: 26 July 2011; in revised form: 28 August 2011; Accepted: 31 August 2011; Published: 9 September 2011

Abstract: Recently developed technology permits to optimize simultaneously surface area, porosity, density, rigidity and surface morphology of chitin-derived materials of biomedical interest. Safe and ecofriendly disassembly of chitin has superseded the dangerous acid hydrolysis and provides higher yields and scaling-up possibilities: the chitosan nanofibrils are finding applications in reinforced bone scaffolds and composite dressings for dermal wounds. Electrospun chitosan nanofibers, in the form of biocompatible thin mats and non-wovens, are being actively studied: composites of gelatin + chitosan + polyurethane have been proposed for cardiac valves and for nerve conduits; fibers are also manufactured from electrospun particles that self-assemble during subsequent freeze-drying. Ionic liquids (salts of alkylated imidazolium) are suitable as non-aqueous solvents that permit desirable reactions to occur for drug delivery purposes. Gel drying with supercritical CO_2 leads to structures most similar to the extracellular matrix, even when the chitosan is crosslinked, or in combination with metal oxides of interest in orthopedics.

Keywords: chitin; chitosan; electrospinning; ionic liquids; nanofibrils; supercritical carbon dioxide

1. Introduction

A large body of knowledge exists today on the use of chitosans as safe biomaterials for a variety of applications: there are recent review articles in biomedical sciences [1,6] and in pharmaceutical sciences [7,15]. Besides the review articles most directly dealing with chemical approaches [16,21], some are focused on the preparation and applications of carboxymethyl and succinyl derivatives of chitin and chitosan with particular attention to their biomedical applications [22]; on the hydrophobic modifications of chitosans mainly for gene delivery in comparison with polyethyleneimine and polylysine [23], while more general treatments are also available [24,26]. Reviews on the safety of chitin have been published recently [27,28].

Chitins and chitosans and their beneficial characteristic properties could certainly be even further improved by more elaborate refinements of the technological approaches to enable further exploitation of the amply available chitin resources. The scope of the present review article is to provide technical details and evaluations of results, suitable for the appreciation of the immediate potential developments of the title technologies.

2. Chitin and Chitosan Nanofibrils

In the area of the isolation and characterization of nanofibrils (otherwise called chitin nanocrystals, or whiskers), significant scientific and technological advances have recently been made. In particular, articles were published dealing with: (i) disassembly of chitin for the isolation of nanochitin by

Mar. Drugs **2011**, *9*, 1510–1533

mechanical means in the presence of minor amounts of acetic acid; (ii) disassembly of chitosan; (iii) preparation of nanochitosan from partially deacetylated chitin.

2.1. Mechanical Disassembly of Chitin Nanofibrils

Chitin nanofibers were prepared by Kose and Kondo [29] by using the aqueous counter collision method that provided homogeneous aqueous dispersion of chitin nanofibers having a width of 10–20 nm. The mechanical disassembly of chitin has suddenly attracted much attention: in fact, suspensions of crude α-chitin were treated first with a blender, and then the slurry of 1% purified chitin was passed through a grinder at 1500 rpm, with a clearance gauge of 0.15 mm shift as demonstrated by Ifuku *et al.* [30].

The same team developed the concept that it would be advantageous to enhance the cationic repulsion existing between chitin fibers with the aid of partial protonation in order to disassemble the chitin: a protonation degree as small as 4% or less is sufficient to weaken the hydrogen bonds that protect the tight chitin structure [31]. Various industrial chitins, including the α-polymorphs, by this route yield nanofibrils having a high degree of crystallinity and 10–20 nm cross-section.

According to Shams *et al.* [32] several drops of acetic acid were added to the 1% slurry of purified wet chitin to adjust the pH value at 3–4 and to facilitate the fibrillation: the suspension was then blended for 10 min at a speed of 37,000 rpm, and kept in a never-dried condition. The neutralized disassembled nanofibrils were dispersed in water (0.1%) and a colloidal structure was obtained, indicating that the chitin fibrils were homogeneously dispersed: it was vacuum-filtered on a polytetrafluoroethylene membrane (0.1 μm porosity) to produce a dry sheet having diameter 9 cm, thickness 55 μm, and density 1.0 g/cm^3. The dried sheets were impregnated with neat acrylic resin (refractive index 1.536) in such a way as to obtain transparent nanocomposites, with 40% chitin content. The width distribution evaluated directly from the SEM images demonstrated that almost 70% of the nanofibril width was in the range 20–30 nm. The degree of *N*-acetylation 0.93 of the nanofibers was obtained by elemental analysis and indicated that no deacetylation occurred in the course of the treatment. Furthermore, the polysaccharide did not lose its transparency because fibers or particles which have such a small diameter do not produce light scattering; as a consequence it was claimed useful for optical devices. As an extension of that work, optically transparent chitin nanofibril composites were fabricated with 11 different types of (meth)acrylic resins. Chitin nanofibers significantly increased the Young's modulus and the tensile strength, and decreased the thermal expansion of all (meth)acrylic resins due to the reinforcement effect of chitin nanofibers endowed with extended crystal structure [33,34].

Incidentally, under the same conditions, ultrasonication was applied to the chitin slurries for 2 min using an ultrasonic homogenizer at 19.5 kHz and the 300 W output power (probe tip diameter 7 mm); the temperature increase was <5 °C during the ultrasonication [35].

The disadvantages of the earlier preparation methods were numerous and included low yield, dangerous handling of boiling HCl, disposal of the colored HCl solution, recovery of enormous quantities of slightly acidic water, difficult adjustment of the pH value because of the strength of HCl, scaling-up troubles and excessive costs. The new technology that permits today the treatment of industrial chitin dry powders instead of "never dried" chitins removes the most important limitation of the large-scale production of nanochitin. This technology provides a significant advantage towards chitin exploitation, in terms of transportation costs, stable supply, shelf life and storage space, since chitin nanofibers can be prepared from light, low volume, and non-perishable dry chitin.

2.2. Mechanical Disassembly of Chitosan Nanofibrils

High-pressure homogenization was combined with wet-grinding to disassemble suspended chitosan particles into nano-chitosan [36]. The chitosan slurry was forced to pass through the wet-grinding machine at the flow rate of 10 L/h and then it was poured into the stainless-steel tank of a Microfluidizer (M-100P, Microfluidics Corp. MA, USA) equipped with a pair of ceramic (200 μm) and diamond (87 μm) interaction chambers; it was cooled and then released back to the tank for the next cycle. Under the pressure of 207 MPa, the ground slurry passed 10 times through the interaction chambers at the flow rate of 8 L/h; then, the homogenized chitosan slurry was centrifuged at 1000 rpm for 5 min to remove the sediment and to yield a homogeneous chitosan suspension that was used to prepare a high strength liquid crystal thin film at relatively low temperature. There was no pattern or fingerprint found in the control cast films, meaning that chitosan nanofibrils self-assembled with cholesteric structure. Whilst the chitosan cast film possessed high tensile strength (about 35.8 ± 7.6 MPa) and Young's modulus (about 580.0 ± 21.8 MPa), the chitosan liquid crystal film had higher values up to 100.5 ± 4.0 MPa, and 2.2 ± 0.2 GPa, respectively, that are typical for liquid crystalline polymers [37].

2.3. Nanochitosan Obtained from Partially Deacetylated Chitin, or from Deacetylated Nanochitin

For this preparation, the deacetylation of chitin nanofibrils was made with 50% NaOH in the presence of borohydride; the molecular weight dropped to 59 kDa, much lower than the one of chitosan from chitin powder under the same conditions (422 kDa) [38]. The degree of deacetylation was 0.50 and the suspensions were colloidal at 1–13%. The new methods however opened new routes directly to nanofibrillar chitosan, which is more versatile than chitin. The fine chitin powder was also deacetylated in a relatively mild way, thus producing nano-chitosan that underwent homogeneous dispersion at pH 3–4 [39].

2.4. Applications

From the cell walls of five different types of mushrooms, chitin nanofibrils were isolated by removing glucans, minerals, and proteins, and subsequent grinding treatment under acidic conditions as described above. The chitin nanofibrils thus obtained by Ifuku *et al.* [40] were characterized by elemental analysis, FTIR spectrometry, and X-ray diffraction; they had uniform structure and were unusually long. The width of the nanofibers was in the range 20–28 nm and depended on the type of mushroom. The results showed that the α-chitin structure was maintained and glucans remained on the nanofiber surface. It was deemed that the said nanofibrils of fungal origin might have anti-tumor applications and immune-modulating activity.

Exhaustive studies were made by Muzzarelli *et al.* [41] who incorporated crustacean chitin nanofibrils into wound dressings made of chitosan glycolate and dibutyryl chitin that were applied in a variety of traumatic wounds with limited number of changes and excellent final healing; the nanofibrils were characterized with advanced instrumental analytical techniques (Figure 1).

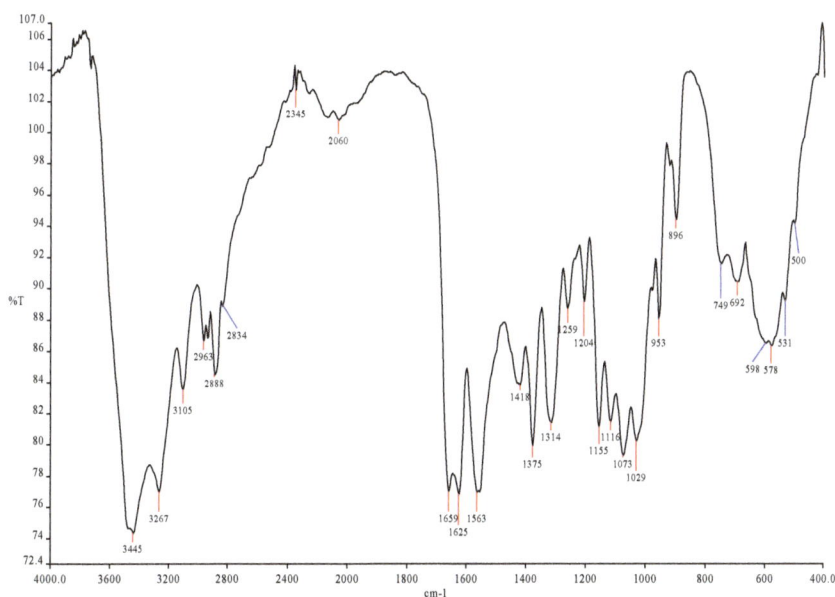

Figure 1. FTIR spectrum of spray-dried α-chitin nanofibrils ready for incorporation in a chitin + chitosan composite used for wound dressing. This spectrum showed for the first time unmatched resolution of all typical chitin bands. Reprinted from [41]. Copyright (2007) with permission from Elsevier.

Han *et al.* [42] investigated the influence of chitosan nanofiber scaffold on the production and infectivity of porcine endogenous retrovirus expressed by porcine hepatocytes. Freshly isolated porcine hepatocytes were cultured with a chitosan nanofiber scaffold, that prolonged the porcine endogenous retrovirus secreting time in pig hepatocytes, but did not appreciably influence its productive amount and infectivity, so it could be applied in the bioartificial liver without risk of virus transmission.

Chitin nanofibrils 5–10 nm diameter were employed by Ma *et al.* [43] as barrier layers in a new class of thin-film nanofibrous composite membranes for water purification. The very high surface-to-volume ratio leads to high virus adsorption capacity as verified by MS2 bacteriophage testing, and offers further opportunities in drinking water applications. The low cost of raw chitin, the environmentally friendly fabrication process, and the impressive high flux indicate that such ultrafine nanofibril-based membranes can surpass conventional-membranes in many water applications.

The chitin nanofibrils were effective in stabilizing oil-in-water emulsions against coalescence, presumably because of the adsorption of the nanofibrils at the oil–water interface. The rheological data provided evidence for network formation in the emulsions with increasing chitin nanocrystal concentration. Such a gel-like behavior was attributed to the formation of a chitin nanocrystal network in the continuous phase. The stability of the emulsions to creaming increased linearly with nanofibril concentration [44].

Several more applications of chitin nanofibrils have already been developed, for example, waterborne polyurethane-based nanocomposites were prepared by Huang *et al.* [45] by incorporating small quantities of chitin nanofibrils as the nanophase: the nanofibrils loading of 3% showed the maximum tensile strength (28.8 MPa) and enhanced the Young's modulus (6.5 MPa), ~1.8- and 2.2-fold over those of neat polyurethane. The active surface and rigidity of nanofibrils facilitated formation of the interface for stress transferring and provided endurance to stress. The incorporation of chitosan nanofibrils in alginate fibers was achieved by mixing homogenized chitosan nanofibrils colloidal suspension with 6% w/v sodium alginate aqueous solution, followed by wet spinning [38].

Porous bone scaffolds with enhanced physical, mechanical and biological performances were prepared with hyaluronan and gelatin (1:1 w/w blend), and the reinforcing filler was α-nanochitin; 1-ethyl-3-(3-dimethylaminopropyl) carbodiimide was used as a crosslinker [46]. The weight ratios of the nanochitin to the blend were up to 30%, the average pore size of the scaffolds ranged between 139 and 166 μm, regardless of the nanochitin content, but the incorporation of 2% nanochitin in the scaffolds doubled their tensile strength. The as-prepared nanochitin was in the form of slender rods with sharp ends (255 ± 56 × 31 ± 6 nm, with L/d aspect ratio ~8). Although the addition of 20–30% nanochitin improved thermal stability and resistance to biodegradation, the scaffolds with 10% were the best for supporting the proliferation of cultured human osteosarcoma cells.

Melatonin was adsorbed on the nanofibrils [47,48]; lipoic acid was likewise treated [49]. Glycerol plasticized-potato starch was mixed with chitin nanofibrils to prepare fully natural nano-composites by casting and evaporation: this led to improvements in tensile strength, storage modulus, glass transition temperature, and water vapor barrier properties of the composite. However, at >5% loading, aggregation of the nanofibrils took place with negative effects [50]. On the other hand, the effect of different concentrations of cellulose nanofibers, and plasticizer (glycerol) on tensile properties, water vapor permeability, and glass transition temperature of chitosan edible films were evaluated to work out a formulation that optimized their properties: the nanocomposite film with 15% cellulose nanofibers and 18% glycerol, comparable to some synthetic polymers in terms of strength and stiffness [51].

Chitin nanofibrils were acetylated to modify the fiber surface: the acetylation degree could be controlled from 0.99 to 2.96 by changing the reaction time. After a short acetylation (1 min), the moisture content of the nanocomposite decreased from 4.0 to 2.2%. The nanofibril shape was maintained and the thickness of the nanofibrils increased linearly with the acetylation degree. Composites containing the acetylated chitin nanofibrils (25%) in acrylic resin were fabricated [34]. Nanofibers based on poly(vinyl alcohol) as the matrix, and α-chitin nanofibrils (~31 nm × ~549 nm) were prepared [52]. Chitin nanofibrils were blended with polylactide to form organic composites, and with apatite or rectorite to form inorganic composites suitable for food-packaging applications [53,55].

3. Electrospun Nanofibers

Electrospun natural biopolymers are of great interest in the field of regenerative medicine due to their unique structure, biocompatibility, and potential to support controlled release of bioactive agents and/or the growth of cells near a site of interest. However, the scaling-up of chitosan nanofiber fabrication by electrospinning is problematic and challenging. First of all, solutions with a high concentration of chitosan are not injectable, while those with a very low concentration result in a low output rate. On the other hand, the large quantity of organic solvents used during the electrospinning process alters/denatures the structure and properties of the natural chitosan. Furthermore, due to its polyelectrolyte nature, chitosan cannot be continuously spun as droplets persistently form. It is well known that pore size and structure of a scaffold play a vital role in cell cultures because they are responsible not only for the adhesion, migration, and distribution of cells, but also for the exchange of nutrients and metabolic waste. Despite numerous efforts, issues relating to mechanical strength, uniformity, interconnections and porosity of nanofiber mats have not yet been solved.

3.1. Chitosan + Nylon Electrospun Nanofibers

The electrospun chitosan has been characterized by Nirmala *et al.* [56] with the aid of the most advanced analytical instrumentation: they found that the chitosan nanofibers had diameters ranging from 10 to 1200 nm, and anisotropic nature. Their stability was studied by Cooper *et al.* [57], while Jacobs *et al.* [58] optimized the electrospinning parameters for chitosan nanofibers.

Electrospinning offers unique possibilities when a single compound dissolves both chitosan and an artificial polymer, this being the case for chitosan and nylon, so that the biochemical properties of chitosan can be associated to the mechanical properties of nylon: outstanding performances can be expected from such a composite, as mentioned by Muzzarelli [59] for the recovery of metals from sea-water. A work by Nirmala *et al.* [60] focused on the preparation of chitosan blended polyamide-6 nanofibers by a single solvent via electrospinning, to be used for cultures of human osteoblasts. The nanofibers were well oriented and had good incorporation of chitosan. Infrared spectrometry indicated that the amino groups of chitosan still existed in the blended nanofibers. The morphological features of the cells attached to nanofibers were observed by SEM. The adhesion, viability and proliferation properties of osteoblast cells on the polyamide-6 + chitosan blended nanofibers were analyzed by *in vitro* cell compatibility test. In a further work, Nirmala *et al.* [61] reported that current-voltage measurements revealed interesting linear relation, including enhanced conductivity with respect to chitosan content. The electrical conductivity of the polyamide-6 + chitosan composite nanofibers increased with increasing content of chitosan due to the formation of ultrafine nanofibers. In addition, the sheet resistance of composite nanofibers decreased with increasing chitosan concentration.

A totally different approach was followed by Zhang *et al.* [62]: electrospun nylon-6 nanofibrous membrane with fiber diameters in the range of 50–200 nm were prepared and employed as affinity material for papain adsorption due to their excellent chemical and thermal resistance as well as high wettability. Covalent coupling of chitosan to activated nylon membrane was performed after the reaction of the nanofibrous nylon membrane with formaldehyde. The dye Cibacron Blue F3GA as a ligand was then covalently immobilized on the chitosan-coated membranes, to be used for papain collection, with adsorption capacity up to 133.2 mg/g.

3.2. Applications in Cardiology

Hussain *et al.* [63] explored electrospun chitosan-based nanofiber scaffolds for cardiac tissue engineering. In the 2D and 3D scaffolds, only the cardiomyocyte-fibroblasts co-cultures resulted in polarized cardiomyocyte morphology, and the expression of sarcomeric actin and connexin-43 was higher than under other culture conditions. Said fibroblasts co-cultures demonstrated synchronized contractions involving large tissue-like cellular networks. This was the first attempt to utilize 3D chitosan nanofibers as cardiomyocyte scaffolds with the result that cardiomyocyte retained their morphology and function. Other applications in cardiology were proposed by Cynthia *et al.* [64] who tested mechanical properties, biocompatibility and cell retention ability of gelatin-chitosan polyurethane. In fact, for a proper function of the cardiac valve the materials selected for the leaflets need to be biocompatible, robust, flexible, and have comparable mechanical properties to the natural ones. Native heart valve leaflets are subjected to continuous pulsatile and homodynamic forces and can be as thin as 300 μm. Endothelial cells, isolated from ovine carotid arteries were seeded onto these materials and exposed to a range of shear-stresses for a period of 1–3 h. Throughout the exposure time and the shear stress values tested, a mean cell retention of 80% was obtained in the gelatin-chitosan polyurethane group. Noticeably for the full range of physiological flow conditions tested, the electrospun gelatin-chitosan polyurethane demonstrated good biocompatibility and cell retention properties.

Likewise, scaffolds for blood vessel and nerve conduits, were designed on the basis of collagen-chitosan-thermoplastic polyurethane electrospun to mimic the components and the structural aspects of the native extracellular matrix. The scaffolds were crosslinked with glutaraldehyde vapor to prevent them from being dissolved in the culture medium. Cell viability studies with endothelial cells and Schwann cells demonstrated that the electrospun composite nanofibrous scaffolds had good biocompatibility, and that the aligned fibers could regulate cell morphology by inducing cell orientation. Vascular grafts and nerve conduits were electrospun or sutured based on the nanofibrous scaffolds: the results indicated that collagen-chitosan-polyurethane blended nanofibrous scaffolds might be suitable for vascular repair and nerve regeneration [45].

3.3. Other Preparations of Biomedical Interest

An alternative to the experiments described above is the esterification of chitosan with the use of lactide or polylactide: both chitosan and polylactide/polyglycolide have good biocompatibility and can be used to produce scaffolds for cultured cells. However the synthetic scaffolds lack groups that would facilitate their modification, whereas chitosan has extensive active amine and hydroxyl groups which would allow subsequent modification intended for the attachment of peptides, proteins and drugs. Moreover chitosan is very hydrophilic, whereas poly(D,L-lactide-co-glycolide) (PLGA) is relatively hydrophobic. Accordingly there are many situations where it would be ideal to have a copolymer of both, especially one that could be electrospun to provide a versatile range of scaffolds for tissue engineering. In a study by Xie *et al.* [65], chitosan was first modified with trimethylsilyl chloride, in the presence of dimethylamino pyridine. PLGA-grafted chitosan copolymers were prepared by reaction with end-carboxyl PLGA (PLGA-COOH). Elemental analysis showed segments with an average of 18-pyranose units when PLGA-COOH was grafted into the chitosan chain. Contact angle measurements demonstrated that copolymers became more hydrophilic than PLGA. The chitosan-g-PLGA copolymers were electrospun to produce either nano- or microfibers as desired. A 3D fibrous scaffold of the copolymers gave good fibroblast adhesion and proliferation which did not differ significantly from the performance of the cells on the chitosan or PLGA electrospun scaffolds.

Chitosan derivatives were prepared by Skotak *et al.* [66] following a "one pot" approach by grafting L-lactide oligomers. Chitosan was dissolved in methanesulfonic acid, followed by the addition of the L-lactide monomer. This reaction mixture was stirred for 4 h at 40 °C under an argon atmosphere. The side chain had values between 4.6 and 14 units. On average, there were two side chains of oligo-L-lactide per glucosamine ring, and their length depended on the initial reagents ratio. L-Lactide grafted chitosan samples display cytotoxicity over a range of substitution degree values, as demonstrated with fibroblast cultures. This synthetic route renders the esterified chitosans soluble in a broad range of organic solvents, facilitating formation of ultrafine fibers via electrospinning.

Likewise, from blended solutions of chitosan and poly(ethylene oxide) (PEO), chitosan-based defect-free nanofibers with average diameters from 62 ± 9 nm to 129 ± 16 nm were fabricated [67]. The use of polysorbate surfactant Tween 20 to improve the functionality of the nanofibers was studied by Ziani *et al.* [68] with two highly deacetylated chitosans (MW 148 and 68 kDa) dissolved with acetic acid and then mixed with PEO. Because pure chitosan dissolved in different acid concentrations did not form fibers but beads, addition of PEO was necessary to electrospin the chitosan solutions. Average fiber diameters and size distribution depended on acidity and molecular weight. Solutions of chitosan + PEO + surfactant were effectively electrospun. The presence of surfactant resulted in decrease of surface tension and in the formation of smooth fibers.

Cationic nanofibrous mats are expected to show improved cellular adhesion and stability. Caprolactone oligomers were grafted onto the hydroxyl groups of chitosan via ring-opening polymerization by using methanesulfonic acid as solvent and catalyst: then, nanofibrous mats were obtained by electrospinning. The content of amino groups on the nanofiber surface increased linearly with the quantity of grafted chitosan, as revealed by the increased zeta-potential of nanofibers. Chitosan-g-oligo(caprolactone) in poly(caprolactone) (2/8) mats with moderate surface zeta-potential (3 mV) were the best in promoting mouse fibroblast attachment and proliferation. Toluidine blue staining confirmed that said cells grew well and exhibited a normal morphology [69]. Chitosan/poly(caprolactone) nanofibrous scaffold was prepared in a single step by Shalumon *et al.* [70]. The presence of chitosan in the scaffold imparted improved hydrophilicity to the scaffold, as confirmed by decreased contact angle, which thereby enhanced bioactivity and protein adsorption on the scaffold, which was found to be cyto-compatible.

Feng *et al.* [71] developed a method to obtain high surface area nanofiber meshes composed of chitosan of various molecular weights. These chitosan nanofiber meshes were developed as a culture substrate for hepatocytes: they exhibited a uniform diameter distribution (average 112 nm) and stability. The chitosan nanofibers were biocompatible with hepatocytes and were expected to be useful for artificial liver and for liver regeneration.

Aligned and randomly oriented poly(D, L-lactide-co-glycolide) + chitosan nanofibrous scaffolds have been prepared by electrospinning [72]. The release of the drug fenbufen from the fenbufen-loaded aligned and randomly oriented PLGA and PLGA/chitosan nanofibrous scaffolds increased with the increase of chitosan content. Moreover, the nanofiber arrangement influenced the release behavior. Crosslinking in glutaraldehyde vapor contributed to decrease the burst release of the drug from the loaded PLGA/chitosan nanofibrous scaffold.

Gelatin and chitosan nanofibers were electrospun and then cross-linked by glutaraldehyde vapor at room temperature. The cross-linked mats kept their nanofibrous structure after being soaked in deionized water at 37 °C. The two main chemical reactions of cross-linking for chitosan and gelatin-chitosan complex are Schiff base reaction and acetalization. The mechanical properties of nanofibrous mats were improved after cross-linking. The biocompatibility of electrospun nanofibrous mats after cross-linking was investigated by the viability of porcine iliac endothelial cells [73].

Silk fibroin + hydroxybutyl chitosan nanofibrous scaffolds were fabricated by electrospinning by using hexafluoro-2-propanol and trifluoroacetic acid as solvents to mimic the extra-cellular matrix. Both tensile strength and elongation at break were remarkably improved when the weight ratio of fibroin to hydroxybutyl chitosan was 20:80. The use of genipin vapor not only induced conformation of fibroin to convert from random coil to beta-sheet structure but also acted as a cross-linking agent for fibroin + hydroxybutyl chitosan [74].

As an example of versatility of the chitosan derivatives, a new method was presented by Almodovar and Kipper [75] for functionalizing electrospun nanofibers with GAGs and growth factors by polyelectrolyte multilayers deposition. Chitosan nanofibers, electrospun from trifluoroacetic acid and dichloromethane, were coated with heparin and N,N,N-trimethyl chitosan. FGF-2 was adsorbed on the PEM-coated nanofibers.

Electrospun nanofibers can be mineralized. The chitosan/poly(vinyl alcohol) nanofibers produced thin $CaCO_3$ crystals that interlaced with the chitosan fiber not only on the surface of the membrane but also within it. The crystals developed into a continuous $CaCO_3$ membrane on the fibers at a late stage of mineralization: the crystals were mainly calcite with a small quantity of vaterite. The attachment and growth of mouse fibroblast occurred evenly on the surface of the mineralized composite membrane [76].

Espindola-Gonzalez *et al.* [77] studied structural and thermal properties of chitosan + starch + poly(ethylene terephthalate) (PET) fibers manufactured via electrospinning. Addition of PET to chitosan + starch systems resulted in improved thermal stability at elevated temperatures.

Kim and Lee [78] reported that the combination of electrospraying and subsequent freeze-drying can produce chitosan fibrous 3D network structures from low concentration chitosan solutions, well below fiber forming concentrations. Nanoparticle suspensions of chitosan were first fabricated by a controlled electrospraying process, and then the freeze-drying process promoted the assembly of the nanoparticles into fibrous networks. Figure 2 shows the typical fibrous structures obtained by electrospraying and subsequent freeze drying: the average diameter of a strand was 0.5–3 µm and the surface area of the fibers was 17.8 ± 0.39 m^2/g. The nanofibrils, showing interconnections with each other were exempt from the bead-string motifs often found in electrospun fibers. The surface of these nanofibrils is different from those of conventional fibers insofar as it has no significant textures resulting from stretching processes, as a point of difference from the surface of most chitosan fibers.

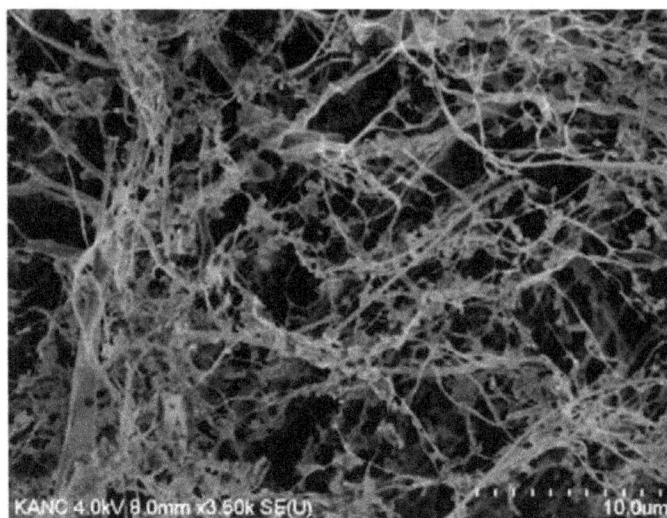

Figure 2. SEM micrograph of chitosan nonwoven fabrics obtained by electrospraying and subsequent freeze drying. Reprinted from [78]. Copyright (2011) with permission from Elsevier.

Chitosan, sodium chondroitin sulfate, and pectin-nanofibrous mats were prepared from the respective polysaccharide/poly(ethylene oxide) blend solutions by electrospray. Unblended polysaccharide solutions showed low processability; viz., the solutions could not be electrosprayed. The addition of 500 kDa poly(ethylene oxide) to chitosan solutions enhanced the formation of a fibrous structure. Sodium chondroitin sulfate/poly(ethylene oxide) and pectin/poly(ethylene oxide) blend solutions were generally too viscous to be sprayed at 25 °C, but at 70 °C the fibrous structure was formed [79].

Chitosan fibers showing narrow diameter distribution with a mean of 42 nm were produced by electrospinning and utilized for the sorption of Fe(III), Cu(II), Ag(I), and Cd(II) ions from aqueous solutions. By virtue of its mechanical integrity, the applicability of the chitosan mat in solid phase extraction under continuous flow looks interesting: the surface area calculated from the isotherms to be about $0.92 \text{ m}^2/\text{g}$ for the powder and $22.4 \text{ m}^2/\text{g}$ for the electrospun fibers, indicates that electrospinning introduced a 20-fold increase of the surface area of chitosan [80]. Of course this kind of data on the chelating capacity of nanofibrous mats endowed with large surface area can be extended to the enhancement of the antibacterial activity of silver chelates of this kind. In fact, electrospun chitosan + poly(vinyl alcohol) nanofibers functionalized with silver nanoparticles had 220–650 nm diameter, and the silver nanoparticles embedded into the fibers exerted high antibacterial activity against *E. coli* [81]. Data assessing the doping effects of monovalent, bivalent and trivalent metal ions on the morphological appearance of the electrospun chitosan + poly(ethylene oxide) blend nanofibers were made available by Su *et al.* [82].

Chitosan nano-powders were modified using hydrazine plasma produced at low pressure (26.66 Pa) with 13.56 MHz frequency at 100 W for 30 min. Chitosan and plasma-modified chitosan in poly(vinyl alcohol) (PVA) solutions were used to produce nanofibers by electrospinning, with average fiber diameters 480 and 280 nm, respectively. The antibacterial effect of the treated chitosan was enhanced [83]. The spinnability of chitosan with PVA was optimized by Huang *et al.* [84].

4. Ionic Liquids: New Reaction Media

The ionic liquids have emerged as a class of organic salts that can be used as components of polymeric matrices, templates for porous polymers and solvents for a wide variety of organic and inorganic compounds. They are liquids at room temperature and exhibit unique physico-chemical properties, namely no vapor pressure, excellent chemical and thermal stability, high ionic conductivity and easy recyclability. Their use as solvents or non-volatile reaction media instead of conventional organic solvents can minimize a number of environmental and safety problems. They have provided a new processing platform for the dissolution of cellulose, chitin, starch and lignin: the macromolecules can be dissolved, regenerated and functionalized, thus increasing their chances of exploitation.

Not so much information on the dissolution of chitin in ionic liquids is present in the literature yet, because attention was immediately captured by cellulose that is dissolved likewise: typical ionic liquids in this context are 1-allyl-3-methylimidazolium chloride (AmiCl); 1-butyl-3-methylimidazolium chloride (BmiCl), and 1-butyl-3-methylimidazolium acetate (BmiAc) [85].

Xie *et al.* [86] used BmiCl and declared that up to 10% of chitin could be dissolved within 5 h at 110 °C; however, this finding was questioned because results were not reciprocally comparable, presumably due to the diversity of chitin in terms of polymorphic form, different origin, molecular weight and degree of acetylation.

An acidic cellulose + chitin gel electrolyte made of cellulose, chitin, 1-butyl-3-methylimidazolium, 1-allyl-3-methylimidazolium bromide, and an aqueous H_2SO_4 solution was investigated for electric double layer capacitors with activated carbon fiber cloth electrodes. The acidic cellulose + chitin hybrid gel electrolyte has practical applicability to an advanced electric double-layer capacitor with excellent stability and working performance [87]. Rheological evaluations on the clear solution of 5% chitin in 1-allyl-3-methylimidazolium bromide (obtained at 100 °C for 48 h) showed that it behaved like weak gels [88]. Chitosan + cellulose composite fibers from an ionic liquid medium were obtained by electrospinning [89].

Another example was provided by Takegawa *et al.* [90] who prepared chitin + cellulose composite gels and films using the two ionic liquids, 1-allyl-3-methylimidazolium bromide and 1-butyl-3-methylimidazolium chloride. Both polysaccharides were dissolved separately and then the two liquids were mixed in various ratios at 100 °C to give homogeneous mixtures: gels were obtained after 4 days. Moreover, films made of chitin + cellulose were obtained by casting the mixtures on glass plates, followed by soaking in water and drying: the obtained gels and films were characterized by X-ray diffraction spectrometry and thermo-gravimetric analysis. The mechanical properties of the gels and films were evaluated under compressive and tensile modes, respectively [90]. More data by Wu *et al.* [91] and by Kadokawa *et al.* [92] relevant to the solubility of chitins and chitosans in said ionic liquids are collected in Table 1.

Table 1. Solubility of isolated chitins and chitosan in 4 ionic liquids. Based on data in [91,92].

Polymer	Origin and viscosity	Solubility (w/w%) at 110 °C			
		AmiCl	AmiBr	BmiAc	BmiCl
α-Chitin	Crab	n.a.	Soluble, 9.1	n.a	n.a.
α-Chitin	Crab, η 35 cp	Insoluble	n.a.	Soluble, 6	Partly soluble
β-Chitin	Squid pen, η 15 cp	Insoluble	n.a.	Soluble, 7	Partly soluble
β-Chitin	Squid pen, η 278 cp	Insoluble	n.a.	Soluble, 3	Insoluble
Chitosan	Crab, Mv 97 kDa	Soluble, 8	n.a.	Soluble, 12	Soluble, 10

AmiCl is 1-allyl-3-methylimidazolium chloride; BmiCl is 1-butyl-3-methylimidazolium chloride, BmiAc is 1-butyl-3-methylimidazolium acetate, and AmiBr is 1-allyl-3-methylimidazolium bromide. n.a. = not available.

The dissolution behavior of chitin in a series of ionic liquids containing alkylimidazolium chloride, alkylimidazolium dimethyl phosphate, and 1-allyl-3-methyl-imidazolium acetate has been studied by Wang *et al.* [93]. The dissolution behavior of chitin in ionic liquids was affected by the degree of acetylation, the degree of crystallinity, and the molecular weight of chitin, as well as by the nature of the anion of the ionic liquid. Moreover, 1-ethyl-3-methyl-imidazolium acetate dissolves raw crustacean shells completely, leading to the recovery of highly pure chitin of high molecular weight, in the form of powder, films and fibers directly spinnable from the extract solution [94].

Polyacrylamide was used by Zhou and Wu [95] as a matrix material for fabricating novel nanocomposite hydrogels reinforced with natural chitosan nanofibers via *in situ* free-radical polymerization. The chitosan nanofibers established hydrogen and covalent bonds with polyacrylamide, and acted as a multifunctional cross-linker and a reinforcing agent in the hydrogel system. The compression strength and storage modulus of the nanocomposite hydrogels were significantly higher than those of the pure polyacrylamide hydrogels. The 1.5% chitosan nanofibers loading showed the best combined swelling and mechanical properties of the hydrogels.

Chitin nanofibrils were easily formed by the gelation of commercial chitin powders with 1-allyl-3-methylimidazolium bromide followed by the regeneration with methanol, according to Kadokawa *et al.* [92]. By using poly(vinyl alcohol) prior to methanol, nanofibrils ~20–60 nm in width and several hundred nanometers in length were obtained. The key point of this facile preparation is that chitin was swollen with said ionic liquid at room temperature, followed by heating at 100 °C (Table 1). Then, a solution of PVA (1.25 mmol, 0.0750 g) in hot water (3.0 mL) was mixed to the gel at 80 °C with stirring; methanol (40 mL) was slowly added to the resulting mixture, and the system was left standing at room temperature for 24 h, followed by sonication to give a dispersion of chitin nanofibrils. Filtration of the dispersion was carried out to give a chitin film.

Hua D.B. *et al.* [96] reported the conjugation of hydrophobic drugs with chitosan, via Schiff reaction in an ionic liquid, which renders chitosan soluble in common organic solvents and amenable to further functional modifications. For example, thermo-responsive poly(*N*-isopropylacrylamide) was grafted to the chitosan-drug conjugate. The graft copolymer self-assembled in water at neutral pH into core-shell nanocarriers with size distribution ~142 ± 60 nm, favorable for intravenous administration. At 37 °C and pH 4.5 (conditions mimicking endosomal or lysosomal uptake) the nanocarriers formed reversed micelles (~8 ± 3 nm) favoring clearance by renal filtration, and 70% of the drug was liberated within 30 h through hydrolytic cleavage of the Schiff base conjugation. Based on the smart drug release profile said approach was deemed viable for the intravenous administration of hydrophobic drugs carried by chitosan-based vehicles.

1-Butyl-3-methyl-imidazolium chloride was used for auto-templating assembly of $CaCO_3$ and chitosan to produce well-defined hollow inorganic-organic nanoboxes and nanoframes. By varying the experimental conditions, size and shell-thickness of hollow nanostructures were adjusted in the ranges 200–400 nm and 15–75 nm, respectively [97].

The hybrid film of gold nanoparticles + ionic liquid + chitosan was used as an efficient immobilization matrix to fabricate an immunosensor. The film produced a well-defined voltammetric signal due to the synergistic effects of the ionic liquid and gold nanoparticles. By immobilizing an alkaline phosphatase-labeled antibody in said film, a sensitive amperometric immunosensor was developed for the prostate specific antigen (PSA). Under the optimized conditions, the immunosensor exhibited a linear range from 1.0 to 80 ng/mL of PSA [98]. In a similar fashion, Safavi *et al.* [99] prepared biosensors based on the electrocatalysed reduction or hydrogen peroxide at the electrode coated with cholesterol oxidase. The biosensor exhibited two wide linear ranges of response to cholesterol for concentrations of 0.05–6.2 and 6.2–11.2 mM. The sensitivity was 90.7 $\mu A \cdot mM^{-1} \cdot cm^{-2}$, the limit of detection was 101 μM of cholesterol, and the response time was <7 s.

Porous chitin-based materials were developed by Silva *et al.* [100] who combined the processing of chitin using ionic liquids together with the use of supercritical fluid technique, to provide a clean technology. Chitin was dissolved in 1-butyl-3-imidazolium acetate, followed by regeneration of the polymer in ethanol in specific moulds. The ionic liquid was removed using Soxhlet extraction and successive steps of extraction with supercritical fluid process using carbon dioxide/ethanol ratios of 50/50 and 70/30. Ultralight porous chitin structures were produced while the efficiency of the ionic liquid removal was measured by conductivity. The developed chitin matrices showed interesting features, such as: (i) low crystallinity resulting from loose hydrogen bonds in the chitin structure; (ii) wide mesoporous distribution; (iii) very low density (0.039–0.063 g/L); (iv) porosity between 84 and 90%, and (v) extremely low cytotoxicity for L929 fibroblasts.

5. Supercritical Drying

The popularity of supercritical carbon dioxide(sc-CO_2) stems from the fact that it is nontoxic, nonflammable, promptly available in large amounts, and that it is the second least expensive solvent after water. A special issue devoted to sc-CO_2 has been published in 2011 by the Journal of Supercritical Fluids. An interesting property associated with the critical state is that the density of the liquid and of the vapor becomes identical, and for this reason the interface between them disappears. Supercritical carbon dioxide is most widely used thanks to its easily accessible critical temperature and pressure (31.2 °C; 7.4 MPa). Supercritical fluid technology is a relatively new technique to obtain micro- and nano-particles: many drugs can be dissolved or liquefied in sc-CO_2 before being sprayed through a nozzle upon depressurization to produce fine drug particles. It is possible to take advantage from high supersaturation of drugs in sc-CO_2, which contributes to the particle size reduction; as an alternative, sc-CO_2 can be used as an antisolvent for the precipitation of drugs from organic solutions [101]. For polar and high MW polymers, the sc-CO_2 solvent power is unfortunately low, and the use of amphiphiles might be necessary: surfactants, ligands and phase transfer agents should be soluble in sc-CO_2 to assist in the dissolution process of polymers. Fluorinated polyacrylates, polyethers, and siloxane-based polymers are considered to be sc-CO_2-philic. The sc-fluid drying processes for preparing protein or polysaccharide-containing powders based on these concepts are described in detail by Jovanovic *et al.* [102]. Diez-Municio *et al.* [103] have investigated the impregnation of chitosan with lactulose using supercritical fluids under various operating conditions, in order to improve the solubility of this natural polymer at neutral or basic pH. The highest impregnation yield (8.6%) was obtained for chitosan scaffolds using the following parameters: continuous process, 60 min contact, 14% (v/v) of co-solvent ethanol:water (95:5), depressurization rate 3.3 bar/min, pressure 100 bar, and 100 °C. Under these conditions, the Maillard reaction took place as well. Biodegradable and mucoadhesive PLGA/chitosan microparticles were manufactured by Casettari *et al.* [104] by using scCO$_2$ with the addition of mPEG and chitosan in the absence of organic solvents, surfactants and crosslinkers. Analytical surface techniques, along with the interaction with mucin, demonstrated the presence of the chitosan (<100 µm) on the surface of the particles.

Chitosan solutions were prepared with acetic acid solution, poured in steel containers and frozen at −20 °C to obtain a hydrogel that was treated in different manners: (1) it was dried with air at 40 °C for 10 h; (2) it was put in a bath of acetone at ambient temperature for 24 h to allow the substitution of water with acetone and was dried with air at 40 °C for 8 h; (3) it was put in a bath of acetone at ambient temperature for 24 h and was dried by sc-CO_2; (4) it was put in a bath of acetone at −20 °C for 24 h and was dried by sc-CO_2 in the high-pressure vessel filled from the bottom with sc-CO_2. When the required pressure and temperature were obtained (200 bar and 35 °C), drying was performed for 4 h with the sc-CO_2 flow rate of about 1 kg/h, that corresponds to a residence time inside the vessel of about 4 min. The depressurization time of 20 min was allocated to bring back the system at atmospheric pressure [105].

When the preference was given to low temperature water substitution followed by supercritical gel drying to prevent the collapse of the chitosan gel, water substitution with acetone was performed at the same temperature of the gel formation (−20 °C for 24 h). Subsequently, sc-CO_2 gel drying was performed at the same processing conditions. In this case, the 3-D shape and the size of samples were preserved, as shown in Figure 3.

The obtained structures present a morphology very similar to the extracellular matrix, *i.e.*, a finely interconnected nano sub-structure, and therefore they can be suitable scaffolds. In fact, this kind of nanometric fibrous network is the ideal environment for cell adhesion and growth for the regeneration of cartilages, skin and bone [105]. The surface properties of biological materials are at the basis of phenomena like cell adhesion, formation of bacterial films, and recognition between biological units.

Surface polarity is a major parameter in controlling the adhesion of cells and bacteria, a relevant phenomenon in fields as different as safety of surgical devices, colonization of biomaterials, and sensitivity of biological sensors.

Based on these considerations, supercritically dried aerogels of several polysaccharides have been characterized by Robitzer *et al.* [106]. The nature of the functional groups of the polysaccharide significantly influences the adsorption of N_2 on the surface of the aerogel. Surface area values as high as 570 m^2g^{-1} have been measured. The net enthalpy of adsorption increases with the polarity of the chemical groups of the polymer, in the order: chitin < agar ≤ chitosan < carrageenan < alginic acid/alginate. The surface area and the mesopore distribution of the aerogels depend on the dispersion of the parent hydrogel and on the behavior of each polymer during the drying treatment. Aerogels retaining the dispersion of the parent hydrogel are mainly macroporous (pores larger than 50 nm) while materials liable to shrink upon solvent exchange form mesoporous structures.

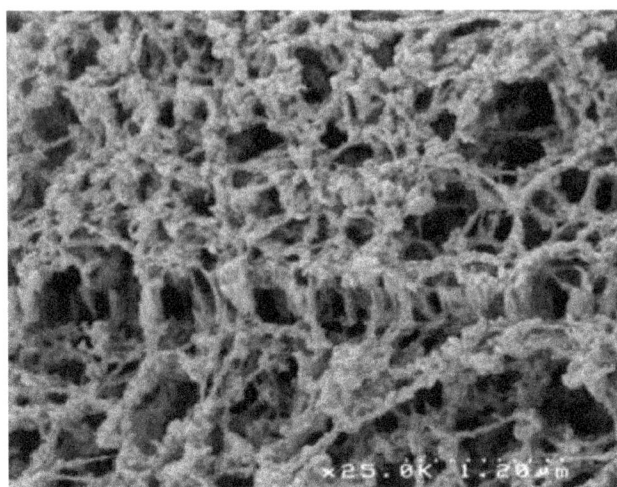

Figure 3. The chitosan fibers are replicated by titanium oxide: the SEM image shows the combined chitosan + titania fibers. Reprinted from [107]. Copyright (2011) with permission from Elsevier.

El Kadib *et al.* [107] described a versatile strategy for fabricating highly porous and nanofibrous titania, zirconia, alumina and tin oxide. By taking advantage from the favorable effect of scCO$_2$ drying to avoid the collapse of the transient hybrid material network, all targeted metal oxides were produced, after calcination, as fibrous filaments featuring dual meso- and macro-porous network with surface area ranging from 110 to 310 m^2g^{-1}, as shown in Figure 3 and .

Mar. Drugs **2011**, 9, 1510–1533

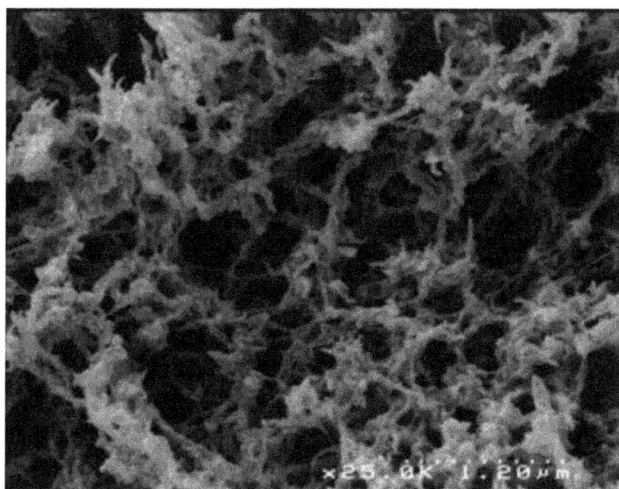

Figure 4. Removal of chitosan leads to pure titanium oxide with filamentous structure. Reprinted from [107]. Copyright (2011) with permission from Elsevier.

As far as silica is concerned, hydrophobic chitosan+silica hydrogels were prepared by Ayers *et al.* [108]: dried aerogels were exposed to hexamethyldisilazane vapors at 60 °C. After supercritical drying, uncracked monoliths with very little shrinkage were obtained. When exposed to water, said aerogels adsorbed a small amount of liquid at their outer surface, while maintaining their shape. The Brunauer–Emmett–Teller (BET) surface area of said aerogels was very large, 472–750 m^2/g, depending on the ratio chitosan/silica.

In a more elaborated preparation, a solution of chitosan (1%) was mixed with the crosslinker genipin solution (4%) [17]: stirring was continued until the solution turned into a viscous gel. Then the hydrogel was subjected to solvent exchange into acetone thrice to remove water from the structure. After solvent exchange, the chitosan–genipin derivative was placed inside a sealed chamber of the sc-CO$_2$ extractor at 40 °C and 200 bar. The reaction was left for 2 h and a flow of CO$_2$ was then applied through the sample in order to replace all the organic solvent with CO$_2$. The pressure was then released slowly to the atmosphere and the temperature was reduced to 20 °C. The chitosan derivative had BET surface area of 49 m^2/g, with a monolayer volume of 11 cm^3/g. The porosimetry result showed that genipin-crosslinked chitosan scaffold had adequate surface area to provide cell adhesion and proliferation. In fact the osteoblast proliferation on chitosan–genipin scaffolds was assessed using Almar Blue assay and found to be satisfactory considering that the number of cells attached to the genipin-crosslinked chitosan scaffolds after 1, 3, and 7 days of cell culture increased with time thus indicating the suitability of the material for tissue engineering applications [109,110].

The surface of chitin too can be expanded to large values: rapid expansion techniques with sc-CO$_2$ were used by Salinas-Hernandez *et al.* [111] to form chitin microstructures. Depending on the experimental conditions, they obtained either spherical microparticles with diameters 1.7–5.3 μm with the rapid expansion of sc-solution technique, or continuous microfibers with diameters 11.5–19.3 μm with the rapid expansion into water technique, possibly influenced, in the latter case, by the high forces in the hydrogen bond network of the molecular structure of chitin. It is important to mention that the present method makes it possible to produce much more uniform and thinner nanofibers on a larger scale than the electrospinning process, without using any hazardous chemicals.

6. Conclusion

This bibliographic survey shows the high viability of basic chemical and physical sciences that are promoting the applicability of chitin and chitosan in a number of demanding areas. Just in the most recent years a real interface of existing technologies and chitin science has taken place, and moreover new technologies are emerging in a few scattered articles (hot melt blending, processing, extrusion and stretching [112,115]; foaming [116]; electrofiltration [117]; decrystallization [118]; sonolysis, microfluidization and shearing [119]) that will certainly contribute to the exploitation of renewable chitin-bearing resources.

Acknowledgments: The author is grateful to Marilena Falcone, Central Library, Polytechnic University, Ancona, Italy, for assistance in handling the bibliographic information, and to Maria Weckx for the preparation of the manuscript. This work was not financially supported nor sponsored.

References

1. Muzzarelli, RAA. Chitosan composites with inorganics, morphogenetic proteins and stem cells, for bone regeneration. *Carbohydr. Polym* **2011**, *83*, 1433–1445.
2. Muzzarelli, RAA. Chitins and chitosans for the repair of wounded skin, nerve, cartilage and bone. *Carbohydr. Polym* **2009**, *76*, 167–182.
3. Jayakumar, R; Chennazhi, KP; Srinivasan, S; Nair, SV; Furuike, T; Tamura, H. Chitin scaffolds in tissue engineering. *Int. J. Mol. Sci* **2011**, *12*, 1876–1887.
4. Deng, C; Li, FF; Griffith, M; Ruel, M; Suuronen, EJ. Application of chitosan-based biomaterials for blood vessel regeneration. *Polym. Org. Chem* **2010**, *297*, 138–146.
5. Park, BK; Kim, MM. Applications of chitin and its derivatives in biological medicine. *Int. J. Mol. Sci* **2010**, *11*, 5153–5165.
6. Yang, TL. Chitin-based materials in tissue engineering: Applications in soft tissue and epithelial organ. *Int. J. Mol. Sci* **2011**, *12*, 1936–1963.
7. Muzzarelli, RAA; Boudrant, J; Meyer, D; Manno, N; DeMarchis, M; Paoletti, MG. Current views on fungal chitin/chitosan, human chitinases, food preservation, glucans, pectins and inulin: A tribute to Henri Braconnot, precursor of the carbohydrate polymers science, on the chitin bicentennial. *Carbohydr Polym* **2011**, in press.
8. Morris, GA; Kok, MS; Harding, SE; Adams, GG. Polysaccharide drug delivery systems based on pectin and chitosan. *Biotechnol. Genet. Eng. Rev* **2010**, *27*, 257–283.
9. Muzzarelli, RAA. Chitosans: New Vectors for Gene Therapy. In *Handbook of Carbohydrate Polymers: Development, Properties and Applications*; Ito, R, Matsuo, Y, Eds.; NOVA Publishers: Hauppauge, NY, USA, 2010; pp. 583–604.
10. Chaudhury, A; Das, S. Recent advancement of chitosan-based nanoparticles for oral controlled delivery of insulin and other therapeutic agents. *AAPS PharmSciTech* **2011**, *12*, 10–20.
11. Petkar, KC; Chavhan, SS; Agatonovik-Kustrin, S; Sawant, KK. Nanostructured materials in drug and gene delivery: A review of the state of the art. *Crit. Rev. Ther. Drug Carrier Syst* **2011**, *28*, 101–164.
12. Patel, MP; Patel, RR; Patel, JK. Chitosan mediated targeted drug delivery system: A review. *J. Pharm. Pharm. Sci* **2010**, *13*, 536–557.
13. Gupta, B; Agarwal, R; Alam, MS. Textile-based smart wound dressings. *Indian J. Fibre Textile Res* **2010**, *35*, 174–187.
14. Laurienzo, P. Marine polysaccharides in pharmaceutical applications: An overview. *Mar. Drugs* **2010**, *8*, 2435–2465.
15. Kean, T; Thanou, M. Biodegradation, biodistribution and safety of chitosan. *Adv. Drug Deliv. Rev* **2010**, *62*, 3–11.
16. Muzzarelli, RAA. Chitin Nanostructures in Living Organisms. In *Chitin Formation and Diagenesis*; Gupta, SN, Ed.; Springer: New York, NY, USA, 2011.
17. Muzzarelli, RAA. Genipin-chitosan hydrogels as biomedical and pharmaceutical aids. *Carbohydr. Polym* **2009**, *77*, 1–9.

18. Liu, Y; Shi, XW; Kim, E; Robinson, LM; Nye, CK; Ghodssi, R; Rubloff, GW; Bentley, WE; Payne, GF. Chitosan to electroaddress biological components in lab-on-a-chip devices. *Carbohydr. Polym* **2011**, *84*, 704–708.

19. Ngah, WSW; Teong, LC; Hanafiah, MAKM. Adsorption of dyes and heavy metal ions by chitosan composites: A review. *Carbohydr. Polym* **2011**, *83*, 1446–1456.

20. Quignard, F; Di Renzo, F; Guibal, E. From natural polysaccharides to materials for catalysis, adsorption, and remediation. *Top. Curr. Chem* **2010**, *294*, 165–197.

21. Sanchez, C; Belleville, P; Popall, M; Nicole, L. Applications of advanced hybrid organic-inorganic nanomaterials: from laboratory to market. *Chem. Soc. Rev* **2011**, *40*, 696–753.

22. Jayakumar, R; Prabaharan, M; Nair, SV; Tamura, H. Novel chitin and chitosan nanofibers in biomedical applications. *Biotechnol. Adv* **2010**, *28*, 142–150.

23. Liu, ZH; Zhang, ZY; Zhou, CR; Jiao, YP. Hydrophobic modifications of cationic polymers for gene delivery. *Prog. Polym. Sci* **2010**, *35*, 1144–1162.

24. Muzzarelli, RAA. Nanochitins and Nanochitosans, Paving the Way to Eco-Friendly and Energy-Saving Exploitation of Marine Resources. In *Comprehensive Polymer Science*, 2nd ed; Hoefer, R, Ed.; Elsevier: Amsterdam, the Netherlands, 2011; Volume 10.

25. Zhang, JL; Xia, WS; Liu, P; Cheng, QY; Tahirou, T; Gu, WX; Li, B. Chitosan modification and pharmaceutical/biomedical applications. *Mar. Drugs* **2010**, *8*, 1962–1987.

26. Kumari, A; Yadav, SK; Yadav, SC. Biodegradable polymeric nanoparticles based drug delivery systems. *Colloids Surf. B* **2010**, *75*, 1–18.

27. Muzzarelli, RAA. Chitins and chitosans as immunoadjuvants and non-allergenic drug carriers. *Mar. Drugs* **2010**, *8*, 292–312.

28. Baldrick, P. The safety of chitosan as a pharmaceutical excipient. *Regul. Toxicol. Pharmacol* **2010**, *56*, 290–299.

29. Kose, R; Kondo, T. Favorable 3D-network formation of chitin nanofibers dispersed in water prepared using aqueous counter collision. *Fiber* **2011**, *67*, 91–95.

30. Ifuku, S; Nogi, M; Abe, K; Yoshioka, M; Morimoto, M; Saimoto, H; Yano, H. Preparation of chitin nanofibers with a uniform width as alpha-chitin from crab shells. *Biomacromolecules* **2009**, *10*, 1584–1588.

31. Ifuku, S; Nogi, M; Yoshioka, M; Morimoto, M; Yano, H; Saimoto, H. Fibrillation of dried chitin into 10–20 nm nanofibers by a simple grinding method under acidic conditions. *Carbohydr. Polym* **2010**, *81*, 134–139.

32. Shams, MI; Ifuku, S; Nogi, M; Oku, T; Yano, H. Fabrication of optically transparent chitin nanocomposites. *Appl. Phys. A* **2011**, *102*, 325–331.

33. Ifuku, S; Morooka, S; Nakagaito, AN; Morimoto, M; Saimoto, H. Preparation and characterization of optically transparent chitin nanofiber/(meth)acrylic resin composites. *Green Chem* **2011**, *13*, 1708–1711.

34. Ifuku, S; Morooka, S; Morimoto, M; Saimoto, H. Acetylation of chitin nanofibers and their transparent nanocomposite films. *Biomacromolecules* **2010**, *11*, 1326–1330.

35. Fan, YM; Saito, T; Isogai, A. Preparation of chitin nanofibers from squid pen beta-chitin by simple mechanical treatment under acid conditions. *Biomacromolecules* **2008**, *9*, 1919–1923.

36. Liu, DG; Wu, QL; Chang, PR; Gao, GZ. Self-assembled liquid crystal film from mechanically defibrillated chitosan nanofibers. *Carbohydr. Polym* **2011**, *84*, 686–689.

37. Liu, DG; Chang, PR; Chen, MD; Wu, QL. Chitosan colloidal suspension composed of mechanically disassembled nanofibers. *J. Colloid Interface Sci* **2010**, *354*, 637–643.

38. Watthanaphanit, A; Supaphol, P; Tamura, H; Tokura, S; Rujiravanit, R. Wet-spun alginate/chitosan whiskers nanocomposite fibers: Preparation, characterization and release characteristic of the whiskers. *Carbohydr. Polym* **2010**, *79*, 738–746.

39. Fan, YM; Saito, T; Isogai, A. Individual chitin nano-whiskers prepared from partially deacetylated alpha-chitin by fibril surface cationization. *Carbohydr. Polym* **2010**, *79*, 1046–1051.

40. Ifuku, S; Nomura, R; Morimoto, M; Saimoto, H. Preparation of chitin nanofibers from mushrooms. *Materials* **2011**, *4*, 1417–1425.

41. Muzzarelli, RAA; Morganti, P; Morganti, G; Palombo, P; Palombo, M; Biagini, G; Mattioli-Belmonte, M; Giantomassi, F; Orlandi, F; Muzzarelli, C. Chitin nanofibrils with chitosan glycolate composites as wound medicaments. *Carbohydr. Polym* **2007**, *70*, 274–284.

42. Han, B; Shi, XL; Xiao, JQ; Zhang, Y; Chu, XH; Gu, JY; Tan, JJ; Gu, ZZ; Ding, YT. Influence of chitosan nanofiber scaffold on porcine endogenous retroviral expression and infectivity in pig hepatocytes. *World J. Gastroenterol* **2011**, *17*, 2774–2780.

43. Ma, HY; Burger, C; Hsiao, BS; Chu, B. Ultrafine polysaccharide nanofibrous membranes for water purification. *Biomacromolecules* **2011**, *12*, 970–976.
44. Tzoumaki, MV; Moschakis, T; Kiosseoglou, V; Biliaderis, CG. Oil-in-water emulsions stabilized by chitin nanocrystal particles. *Food Hydrocoll* **2011**, *25*, 1521–1529.
45. Huang, C; Chen, R; Ke, QF; Morsi, Y; Zhang, KH; Mo, XM. Electrospun collagen-chitosan-polyurethane nanofibrous scaffolds for tissue engineered tubular grafts. *Colloids Surf. B* **2011**, *82*, 307–315.
46. Hariraksapitak, P; Supaphol, P. Preparation and properties of alpha-chitin-whisker-reinforced hyaluronan-gelatin nanocomposite scaffolds. *J. Appl. Polym. Sci* **2010**, *117*, 3406–3418.
47. Yerlikaya, F; Aktas, Y; Capan, Y. LC-UV determination of melatonin from chitosan nanoparticles. *Chromatographia* **2010**, *71*, 967–970.
48. Hafner, A; Lovric, J; Voinovich, D; Filipovic-Grcic, J. Melatonin-loaded lecithin/chitosan nanoparticles: Physicochemical characterisation and permeability through Caco-2 cell monolayers. *Int. J. Pharm* **2009**, *381*, 205–213.
49. Kofuji, K; Nakamura, M; Isobe, T; Murata, Y; Kawashima, S. Stabilization of alpha-lipoic acid by complex formation with chitosan. *Food Chem* **2008**, *109*, 167–171.
50. Chang, PR; Jian, RJ; Yu, JG; Ma, XF. Starch-based composites reinforced with novel chitin nanoparticles. *Carbohydr. Polym* **2010**, *80*, 420–425.
51. Azeredo, HMC; Mattoso, LHC; Avena-Bustillos, RJ; Ceotto, G; Munford, ML; Wood, D; McHugh, TH. Nanocellulose reinforced chitosan composite films as affected by nanofiller loading and plasticizer content. *J. Food Sci* **2010**, *75*, N1–N7.
52. Junkasem, J; Rujiravanit, R; Supaphol, P. Fabrication of alpha-chitin whisker-reinforced poly(vinyl alcohol) nanocomposite nanofibres by electrospinning. *Nanotechnology* **2006**, *17*, 4519–4528.
53. Li, XX; Li, XY; Ke, BL; Shi, XW; Du, YM. Cooperative performance of chitin whisker and rectorite fillers on chitosan films. *Carbohydr. Polym* **2011**, *85*, 747–752.
54. Ezhova, ZA; Koval, EM; Zakharov, NA; Kalinnikov, VT. Synthesis and physicochemical characterization of nanocrystalline chitosan-containing calcium carbonate apatites. *Russ. J. Inorg. Chem* **2011**, *56*, 841–846.
55. Rizvi, R; Cochrane, B; Naguib, H; Lee, PC. Fabrication and characterization of melt-blended polylactide-chitin composites and their foams. *J. Cell. Plast* **2011**, *47*, 282–299.
56. Nirmala, R; Il, BW; Navamathavan, R; El-Newehy, MH; Kim, HY. Preparation and characterizations of anisotropic chitosan nanofibers via electrospinning. *Macromol. Res* **2011**, *19*, 345–350.
57. Cooper, A; Bhattarai, N; Kievit, FM; Rossol, M; Zhang, MQ. Electrospinning of chitosan derivative nanofibers with structural stability in an aqueous environment. *Phys. Chem. Chem. Phys* **2011**, *13*, 9969–9972.
58. Jacobs, V; Patanaik, A; Anandjiwala, RD; Maaza, M. Optimization of Electrospinning Parameters for Chitosan Nanofibres. *Curr. Nanosci* **2011**, *7*, 396–401.
59. Muzzarelli, RAA. Potential of chitin/chitosan-bearing materials for uranium recovery: An interdisciplinary review. *Carbohydr. Polym* **2011**, *84*, 54–63.
60. Nirmala, R; Navamathavan, R; Kang, HS; El-Newehy, MH; Kim, HY. Preparation of polyamide-6/chitosan composite nanofibers by a single solvent system via electrospinning for biomedical applications. *Colloids Surf. B* **2011**, *83*, 173–178.
61. Nirmala, R; Navamathavan, R; El-Newehy, MH; Kim, HY. Preparation and electrical characterization of polyamide-6/chitosan composite nanofibers via electrospinning. *Mater. Lett* **2011**, *65*, 493–496.
62. Zhang, HT; Han, J; Xue, Y; Nie, HL; Zhu, LM; Branford-White, CJ. Surface Modification of Electrospun Nylon Nanofiber Based Dye Affinity Membrane and Its Application to Papain Adsorption. Proceedings of 3rd International Conference on Bioinformatics and Biomedical Engineering, Beijing, China, 11–13 June 2009; 1, pp. 955–958.
63. Hussain, A; Collins, G; Cho, CH. Electrospun Chitosan-Based Nanofiber Scaffolds for Cardiac Tissue Engineering Applications. Proceedings of 2010 IEEE 36th Annual Northeast Bioengineering Conference, New York, NY, USA, 26–28 March 2010; pp. 62–63.
64. Cynthia, W; Shital, P; Rui, C; Owida, A; Morsi, Y. Biomimetic electrospun gelatin-chitosan polyurethane for heart valve leaflets. *J. Mech. Med. Biol* **2010**, *10*, 563–576.
65. Xie, DM; Huang, HM; Blackwood, K; MacNeil, S. A novel route for the production of chitosan/polylactide-co-glycolide) graft copolymers for electrospinning. *Biomed. Mater* **2011**, *5*, 159–167.

66. Skotak, M; Leonov, AP; Larsen, G; Noriega, S; Subramanian, A. Biocompatible and biodegradable ultrafine fibrillar scaffold materials for tissue engineering by facile grafting of l-lactide onto chitosan. *Biomacromolecules* **2008**, *9*, 1902–1908.

67. Klossner, RR; Queen, HA; Coughlin, AJ; Krause, WE. Correlation of chitosan's rheological properties and its ability to electrospin. *Biomacromolecules* **2008**, *9*, 2947–2953.

68. Ziani, K; Henrist, C; Jerome, C; Aqil, A; Mate, JI; Cloots, R. Effect of nonionic surfactant and acidity on chitosan nanofibers with different molecular weights. *Carbohydr. Polym* **2011**, *83*, 470–476.

69. Chen, HL; Huang, J; Yu, JH; Liu, SY; Gu, P. Electrospun chitosan-*graft*-poly (epsilon-caprolactone)/poly(epsilon-caprolactone) cationic nanofibrous mats as potential scaffolds for skin tissue engineering. *Int. J. Biol. Macromol* **2011**, *48*, 13–19.

70. Shalumon, KT; Anulekha, KH; Chennazhi, KP; Tamura, H; Nair, SV; Jayakumar, R. Fabrication of chitosan/poly(caprolactone) nanofibrous scaffold for bone and skin tissue engineering. *Int. J. Biol. Macromol* **2011**, *48*, 571–576.

71. Feng, ZQ; Leach, MK; Chu, XH; Wang, YC; Tian, TA; Shi, XL; Ding, YT; Gu, ZZ. Electrospun chitosan nanofibers for hepatocyte culture. *J. Biomed. Nanotechnol* **2010**, *6*, 658–666.

72. Meng, ZX; Zheng, W; Li, L; Zheng, YF. Fabrication, characterization and *in vitro* drug release behavior of electrospun PLGA/chitosan nanofibrous scaffold. *Mater. Chem. Phys* **2011**, *125*, 606–611.

73. Qian, YF; Zhang, KH; Chen, F; Ke, QF; Mo, XM. Cross-linking of gelatin and chitosan complex nanofibers for tissue-engineering scaffolds. *J. Biomater. Sci. Polym. Ed* **2011**, *22*, 1099–1113.

74. Zhang, KH; Qian, YF; Wang, HS; Fan, LP; Huang, C; Mo, XM. Electrospun silk fibroin-hydroxybutyl chitosan nanofibrous scaffolds to biomimic extracellular matrix. *J. Biomater. Sci. Polym. Ed* **2011**, *22*, 1069–1082.

75. Almodovar, J; Kipper, MJ. Coating electrospun chitosan nanofibers with polyelectrolyte multilayers using the polysaccharides heparin and *N,N,N*-trimethyl chitosan. *Macromol. Biosci* **2010**, *11*, 72–76.

76. Yang, DZ; Yu, K; Ai, YF; Zhen, HP; Nie, J; Kennedy, JF. The mineralization of electrospun chitosan/poly(vinyl alcohol) nanofibrous membranes. *Carbohydr. Polym* **2010**, *84*, 990–996.

77. Espindola-Gonzalez, A; Martinez-Hernandez, AL; Fernandez-Escobar, F; Castano, VM; Brostow, W; Datashvili, T; Velasco-Santos, C. Natural-synthetic hybrid polymers developed via electrospinning: the effect of PET in chitosan/starch system. *Int. J. Mol. Sci* **2010**, *12*, 1908–1920.

78. Kim, MY; Lee, J. Chitosan fibrous 3D networks prepared by freeze drying. *Carbohydr. Polym* **2011**, *84*, 1329–1336.

79. Seo, H; Matsumoto, H; Hara, S; Minagawa, M; Tanioka, A; Yako, H; Yamagata, Y; Inoue, K. Preparation of polysaccharide nanofiber fabrics by electrospray deposition: Additive effects of polyethylene oxide. *Polym. J* **2005**, *37*, 391–398.

80. Horzum, N; Boyaci, E; Eroglu, AE; Shahwan, T; Demir, MM. Sorption efficiency of chitosan nanofibers toward metal ions at low concentrations. *Biomacromolecules* **2010**, *11*, 3301–3308.

81. Zhuang, XP; Li, Z; Kang, WM; Cheng, BW. Electrospun antibacterial chitosan/poly(vinyl alcohol) nanofibers containing silver nanoparticles. *New Mater Adv Mater* **2011**, *152–153*, 1333–1336.

82. Su, P; Wang, CJ; Yang, XY; Chen, XY; Gao, CY; Feng, XX; Chen, JY; Ye, JA; Gou, ZR. Electrospinning of chitosan nanofibers: The favorable effect of metal ions. *Carbohydr. Polym* **2011**, *84*, 239–246.

83. Uygun, A; Kiristi, M; Oksuz, L; Manolache, S; Ulusoy, S. Hydrazine plasma modification of chitosan for antibacterial activity and nanofiber applications. *Carbohydr. Res* **2011**, *346*, 259–265.

84. Huang, CC; Lou, CW; Lu, CT; Huang, SH; Chao, CY; Lin, JH. Evaluation of the Preparation and Biocompatibility of Poly(vinyl alcohol)(PVA)/chitosan Composite Electrospun Membranes. *Adv Mater Res* **2010**, *123–125*, 975–978.

85. Swatloski, RP; Spear, SK; Holbrey, JD; Rogers, RD. The dissolution of cellulose in ionic liquids. *J. Am. Chem. Soc* **2002**, *124*, 4974–4975.

86. Xie, HB; Zhang, SB; Li, SH. Chitin and chitosan dissolved in ionic liquids as reversible sorbents of CO_2. *Green Chem* **2006**, *8*, 630–633.

87. Yamazaki, S; Takegawa, A; Kaneko, Y; Kadokawa, J; Yamagata, M; Ishikawa, M. Performance of electric double-layer capacitor with acidic cellulose-chitin hybrid gel electrolyte. *J. Electrochem. Soc* **2010**, *157*, A203–A208.

88. Prasad, K; Murakami, M; Kaneko, Y; Takada, A; Nakamura, Y; Kadokawa, J. Weak gel of chitin with ionic liquid, 1-allyl-3-methylimidazolium bromide. *Int. J. Biol. Macromol* **2009**, *45*, 221–225.

89. Park, TJ; Jung, YJ; Choi, SW; Park, H; Kim, H; Kim, E; Lee, SH; Kim, JH. Native chitosan/cellulose composite fibers from an ionic liquid via electrospinning. *Macromol. Res* **2011**, *19*, 213–215.

90. Takegawa, A; Murakami, M; Kaneko, Y; Kadokawa, J. Preparation of chitin/cellulose composite gels and films with ionic liquids. *Carbohydr. Polym* **2010**, *79*, 85–90.

91. Wu, Y; Sasaki, T; Irie, S; Sakurai, K. A novel biomass-ionic liquid platform for the utilization of native chitin. *Polymer* **2008**, *49*, 2321–2327.

92. Kadokawa, J; Takegawa, A; Mine, S; Prasad, K. Preparation of chitin nanowhiskers using an ionic liquid and their composite materials with polyvinyl alcohol. *Carbohydr. Polym* **2011**, *84*, 1408–1412.

93. Wang, WT; Zhu, J; Wang, XL; Huang, Y; Wang, YZ. Dissolution behavior of chitin in ionic liquids. *J. Macromol. Sci. B* **2010**, *49*, 528–541.

94. Qin, Y; Lu, XM; Sun, N; Rogers, RD. Dissolution or extraction of crustacean shells using ionic liquids to obtain high molecular weight purified chitin and direct production of chitin films and fibers. *Green Chem* **2010**, *12*, 968–971.

95. Zhou, CJ; Wu, QL. A novel polyacrylamide nanocomposite hydrogel reinforced with natural chitosan nanofibers. *Colloids Surf. B* **2011**, *84*, 155–162.

96. Hua, DB; Jiang, JL; Kuang, LJ; Jiang, J; Zheng, W; Liang, HJ. Smart chitosan-based stimuli-responsive nanocarriers for the controlled delivery of hydrophobic pharmaceuticals. *Macromolecules* **2011**, *44*, 1298–1302.

97. Chen, AN; Luo, ZP; Akbulut, M. Ionic liquid mediated auto-templating assembly of $CaCO_3$-chitosan hybrid nanoboxes and nanoframes. *Chem. Commun* **2011**, *47*, 2312–2314.

98. Lin, JH; He, CY; Pang, XJ; Hu, KC. Amperometric immunosensor for prostate specific antigen based on gold nanoparticles/ionic liquid/chitosan hybrid film. *Anal. Lett* **2011**, *44*, 908–921.

99. Safavi, A; Farjami, F. Electrodeposition of gold-platinum alloy nanoparticles on ionic liquid-chitosan composite film and its application in fabricating an amperometric cholesterol biosensor. *Biosens. Bioelectron* **2011**, *26*, 2547–2552.

100. Silva, SS; Duarte, ARC; Carvalho, AP; Mano, JF; Reis, RL. Green processing of porous chitin structures for biomedical applications combining ionic liquids and supercritical fluid technology. *Acta Biomater* **2011**, *7*, 1166–1172.

101. Moribe, K; Tozuka, Y; Yamamoto, K. Supercritical carbon dioxide processing of active pharmaceutical ingredients for polymorphic control and for complex formation. *Adv. Drug Deliv. Rev* **2008**, *60*, 328–338.

102. Jovanovic, N; Bouchard, A; Hofland, GW; Witkamp, GJ; Crommelin, DJA; Jiskoot, W. Stabilization of proteins in dry powder formulations using supercritical fluid technology. *Pharm. Res* **2004**, *21*, 1955–1969.

103. Diez-Municio, M; Montilla, A; Herrero, M; Olano, A; Ibanez, E. Supercritical CO_2 impregnation of lactulose on chitosan: A comparison between scaffolds and microspheres form. *J. Supercrit. Fluids* **2011**, *57*, 73–79.

104. Casettari, L; Castagnino, E; Stolnik, S; Lewis, A; Howdle, SM; Illum, L. Surface Characterisation of Bioadhesive PLGA/Chitosan Microparticles Produced by Supercritical Fluid Technology. *Pharm. Res* **2011**, *28*, 1668–1682.

105. Cardea, S; Pisanti, P; Reverchon, E. Generation of chitosan nanoporous structures for tissue engineering applications using a supercritical fluid assisted process. *J. Supercrit. Fluids* **2010**, *54*, 290–295.

106. Robitzer, M; Tourrette, A; Horga, R; Valentin, R; Boissiere, M; Devoisselle, JM; Di Renzo, F; Quignard, F. Nitrogen sorption as a tool for the characterisation of polysaccharide aerogels. *Carbohydr. Polym* **2011**, *85*, 44–53.

107. El Kadib, A; Molvinger, K; Cacciaguerra, T; Bousmina, M; Brunel, D. Chitosan templated synthesis of porous metal oxide microspheres with filamentary nanostructures. *Microporous Mesoporous Mater* **2011**, *142*, 301–307.

108. Ayers, MR; Hunt, AJ. Synthesis and properties of chitosan-silica hybrid aerogels. *J. Non-Cryst Solids* **2001**, *285*, 123–127.

109. Rinki, K; Dutta, PK; Hunt, AJ; Clark, JH; Macquarrie, DJ. Preparation of chitosan based scaffolds using supercritical carbon dioxide. *Macromol. Symp* **2009**, *277*, 36–42.

110. Rinki, K; Dutta, PK. Physicochemical and biological activity study of genipin-crosslinked chitosan scaffolds prepared by using supercritical carbon dioxide for tissue engineering applications. *Int. J. Biol. Macromol* **2010**, *46*, 261–266.

111. Salinas-Hernandez, R; Ruiz-Trevino, FA; Ortiz-Estrada, CH; Luna-Barcenas, G; Prokhorov, Y; Alvarado, JFJ; Sanchez, IC. Chitin microstructure formation by rapid expansion techniques with supercritical carbon dioxide. *Ind. Eng. Chem. Res* **2009**, *48*, 769–778.

112. Rizvi, R; Cochrane, B; Naguib, H; Lee, PC. Fabrication and characterization of melt-blended polylactide-chitin composites and their foams. *J. Cell. Plast* **2011**, *47*, 282–299.

113. Correlo, VM; Costa-Pinto, AR; Sol, P; Covas, JA; Bhattacharya, M; Neves, NM; Reis, RL. Melt processing of chitosan-based fibers and fiber-mesh scaffolds for the engineering of connective tissues. *Macromol. Biosci* **2010**, *10*, 1495–1504.

114. Jeung, S; Mishra, MK. Hot melt reactive extrusion of chitosan and poly(acrylic acid). *Int. J. Polym. Mater* **2011**, *60*, 102–113.

115. Thuaksuban, N; Nuntanaranont, T; Pattanachot, W; Suttapreyasri, S; Cheung, LK. Biodegradable polycaprolactone-chitosan three-dimensional scaffolds fabricated by melt stretching and multilayer deposition for bone tissue engineering: Assessment of the physical properties and cellular response. *Biomed. Mater* **2011**, *6*, 100–116.

116. Ji, CD; Annabi, N; Khademhosseini, A; Dehghani, F. Fabrication of porous chitosan scaffolds for soft tissue engineering using dense gas CO_2. *Acta Biomater* **2011**, *7*, 1653–1664.

117. Gozke, G; Posten, C. Electrofiltration of biopolymers. *Food Eng. Rev* **2010**, *2*, 131–146.

118. Beckham, GT; Crowley, MF. Examination of the α-chitin structure and decrystallization thermodynamics at the nanoscale. *J. Phys. Chem. B* **2011**, *115*, 4516–4522.

119. Chen, RH; Huang, JR; Tsai, ML; Tseng, LZ; Hsu, CH. Differences in degradation kinetics for sonolysis, microfluidization and shearing treatments of chitosan. *Polym. Int* **2011**, *60*, 897–902.

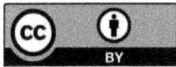

marine drugs

MDPI

Review

Seaweed Hydrocolloid Production: An Update on Enzyme Assisted Extraction and Modification Technologies

Nanna Rhein-Knudsen, Marcel Tutor Ale and Anne S. Meyer *

Center for Bioprocess Engineering, Department of Chemical and Biochemical Engineering, Technical University of Denmark (DTU), Søltofts Plads, Building 229, DK-2800 Lyngby, Denmark; nark@kt.dtu.dk (N.R.-K.); mta@kt.dtu.dk (M.T.A.)

* Author to whom correspondence should be addressed; am@kt.dtu.dk; Tel.: +45-4525-2800; Fax: +45-4593-2906.

Academic Editor: Paola Laurienzo

Received: 28 February 2015; Accepted: 13 May 2015; Published: 27 May 2015

Abstract: Agar, alginate, and carrageenans are high-value seaweed hydrocolloids, which are used as gelation and thickening agents in different food, pharmaceutical, and biotechnological applications. The annual global production of these hydrocolloids has recently reached 100,000 tons with a gross market value just above US$ 1.1 billion. The techno-functional properties of the seaweed polysaccharides depend strictly on their unique structural make-up, notably degree and position of sulfation and presence of anhydro-bridges. Classical extraction techniques include hot alkali treatments, but recent research has shown promising results with enzymes. Current methods mainly involve use of commercially available enzyme mixtures developed for terrestrial plant material processing. Application of seaweed polysaccharide targeted enzymes allows for selective extraction at mild conditions as well as tailor-made modifications of the hydrocolloids to obtain specific functionalities. This review provides an update of the detailed structural features of κ-, ι-, λ-carrageenans, agars, and alginate, and a thorough discussion of enzyme assisted extraction and processing techniques for these hydrocolloids.

Keywords: seaweed; carrageenan; alginate; agar; hydrocolloid; enzymatic extraction

1. Introduction

Hydrocolloids can be defined as substances that interact with water to form colloid systems either in the form of a gel or a sol system of solubilized particles. In practice, the viscosity of the system will generally increase as a result of the interaction between the hydrocolloid and water. Hydrocolloid polysaccharides have significant importance, both technologically and economically, since they are used in the food, pharmaceutical, medicinal, and biotechnological industries due to their distinct physico-chemical properties. The currently used hydrocolloid polysaccharides are derived from plant, microbial, and seaweed sources: pectin is, for example, extracted from apple pomace and citrus peel; xanthan gum is prepared by aerobic fermentation from *Xanthomonas campestris*, and agar, alginates, and carrageenans are obtained from brown and red seaweeds. Seaweed-derived hydrocolloids currently have a global value of approximately US$ 1.1 billion, which is prospected to increase [1]. Seaweeds, thus, constitute a unique source of high-value hydrocolloid polysaccharides: agars have the highest retail price per kg (18 US$/kg), whereas carrageenans currently have the highest commercial total production (60,000 ton/year) and contribute the highest total value of US$ 626 million per year, Table 1 [1].

Table 1. The market for seaweed-derived hydrocolloids, agars, alginates, and carrageenans [1].

Product	Global Production (ton/year)	Retail Price (US$/kg)	Approximate Gross Market Value (US$ million/year)
Agars	10,600	18	191
Alginates	30,000	12	339
Carrageenans	60,000	10.4	626

The Asia-Pacific region dominates seaweed cultivation production, followed by countries such as, Chile, Tanzania, and Madagascar [2]. In these countries, seaweed farming has had positive socio-economic benefits on the coastal communities by improving the economic and social livelihood for the people living in the coastal areas and has reduced overfishing [3].

This review describes the chemistry, properties, and applications of the three seaweed-derived hydrocolloids, carrageenans, agar, and alginate, with a focus on novel enzyme-assisted processing techniques. Enzyme technology is a tool for targeted extractions and modifications that has recently gained increased attention in relation to preserving specific structural traits and functional properties of the target products. The use of enzymes, moreover, allows for reduction of chemicals in seaweed hydrocolloid extraction and thus holds enormous potential for creation of sustainable processing of seaweed polysaccharides.

2. Carrageenans

2.1. Common Carageenan Sources

Commercial carrageenans are extracted from the carrageenophyte red seaweed genera *Kappaphycus*, *Gigartina*, *Eucheuma*, *Chondrus*, and *Hypnea*, in which the carrageenans comprise up to 50% of the dry weight [4]. κ-Carrageenan is mostly extracted from *Kappaphycus alvarezii*, known in the trade as *Eucheuma cottonii*, while ι-carrageeman is predominantly produced from *Eucheuma denticulatum*, also known as *Eucheuma spinosum*. λ-Carrageenan is obtained from seaweeds within the *Gigartina* and *Chondrus* genera, which as sporophytic plants produce λ-carrageenan while they make a κ/ι-hybrid as gametophytic plants [4,5]. Southeast Asia and Tanzania are the main producers of seaweed derived carrageenans from *Kappaphycus alvarezii* and *Eucheuma spinosum* [6].

Table 2. Summary of seaweed sources, hydrocolloid carbohydrate products, chemical structures (main structural units), and applications of the seaweed derived hydrocolloids carrageenans, agars, and alginates.

Seaweed Source	Products	Main Chemical Structures	Applications	Research Conducted
Kappaphycus alvarezii	κ-Carrageenan		Gelling agent (stiff and brittle gel)	[7]
Eucheuma spinosum	ι-Carrageenan		Gelling agent (flexible soft gel)	[7]
Gigartina spp. *Chondrus* spp.	λ-Carrageenan		Thickener	[7]
Kappaphycus alvarezii	μ-Carrageenan		κ-Carrageenan precursor	[8]
Eucheuma spinosum	ν-Carrageenan		ι-Carrageenan precursor	[8]
Gelidiella spp. *Gelidium* spp.	Agar/Agarose		Microbiology Gelling agent (strong and rigid)	[9]
Porphyra umbilicalis	Porphyran		Agar precursor	[8]
Laminaria spp. *Sargassum* spp.	Alginate		Gelling agent	[10,11]

2.2. Carrageenan Chemical Structure

Carrageenans are hydrophilic sulfated linear galactans that mainly consist of D-galactopyranose units bound together with alternating α-1,3 and β-1,4 linkages. This base structure is consistent in the three main commercially used carrageenans, κ-, ι-, and λ-carrageenan, Table 2. The presence of 4-linked 3,6-anhydro-α-D-galactopyranose varies among the different carrageenans, as do the substitutions with sulfates, which are ester-linked to C2, C4, or C6 of the galactopyranose units, depending on the specific carrageenan: κ-, ι-, or λ-carrageenan. κ-Carrageenan has one sulfate ester, while ι-and λ-carrageenan contain two and three sulfates per dimer, respectively, Table 2. In addition, the galactopyranose units may also be methylated or substituted with e.g., monosaccharide residues, such as D-xylose, 4-O-methyl-L-galactose, and D-glucuronic acid [12,13]. Acid hydrolysis, infrared spectroscopy, and NMR analyses of commercial carrageenan typically show sulfate content of 25%–30% for κ-carrageenan, 28%–30% for ι-carrageenan, and 32%–39% for λ-carrageenan, although large differences can occur [7,14,15]. The differences in sulfate levels are explained by the fact that carrageenans are very heterogeneous carbohydrates, with structural differences coexisting within the specific type of carrageenan depending on the algal source, life-stage, and extraction method [16]. In addition, naturally occurring carrageenans contain traces of their biosynthetic precursors, μ- and ν-carrageenan, adding further to the complexity of these polysaccharides, Figure 1 [7]. Likewise, hybrid carrageenans exist, representing a mixture of the different carrageenan repeating units [5].

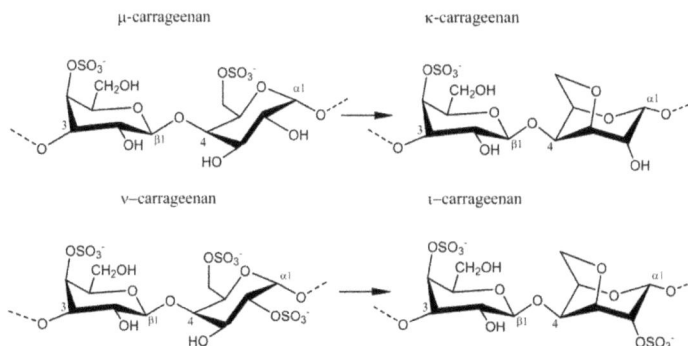

Figure 1. Conversion of the pre cursors µ- and ν-carrageenan into κ- and ι-carrageenan.

2.3. Physico-Chemical Properties of Carrageenans

Carrageenans are soluble in water, but the solubility depends on the content of hydrophilic sulfates, which lowers the solubility temperature, and the presence of potential associated cations, such as sodium, potassium, calcium, and magnesium, which promote cation-dependent aggregation between carrageenan helices [17]. Another factor affecting the physico-chemical properties in relation to viscosity and gelation is the presence of anhydro-bridges: κ- and ι-carrageenans have 3,6-anhydro-galactopyranose units, while λ-carrageenan is composed exclusively of α-1,3 galactopyranose and β-1,4 galactopyranose, Table 2.

The presence of anhydro-bridges in κ- and ι-carrageeenan is proposed to be a result of elimination of a sulfate ester present on their respective precursors, *i.e.*, in µ- and ν-carrageenan, and subsequent spontaneous anhydro-bridge formation in the desulfated monomer residue, Figure 1. The removal of the sulfate esters in µ- and ν-carrageenan reduces the hydrophilicity of the sugar residue and inverts the chair conformation from $^1C_4$ to $^4C_1$, Figure 1. The conformation change allows the polysaccharide to undergo conformational transitions which are conducive to the gelation properties of the anhydro-bridge containing carrageenans [8].

The thermo-reversible gel formation is proposed to occur in a two-step mechanism, dependent on temperature and gel-inducing agents. At high temperatures, *i.e.*, above 75–80 °C, the carrageenans exist as random coil structures as a result of electrostatic repulsions between adjacent polymer chains. Upon cooling, the polymeric chains change conformation to helix structure. Further cooling and presence of cations (K^+, Ca^{2+}, Na^{2+}) lead to aggregation of the helical dimers and formation of a stable three dimensional network, which forms through intermolecular interactions between the carrageenan chains [18,19]. The molecular details of carrageenan gelation are still uncertain. The formation of double helices prior to gelation is not fully proven, and, in principle, the formation of a duplex via chain-chain interactions may not necessarily be an unequivocal evidence for double helix formation. Nevertheless, based on the available literature data and theoretical explanations, we interpret that for the stiff κ-carrageenan gels to form, the cations, typically potassium for κ-carrageenan, function to stabilize the junction zones between the two helixes by binding to the negatively charged sulfate groups without hindering cross-linking of the two helices, Figure 2. According to this model, calcium, typically for ι-carrageenan, analogously function to cross-link the two helices through ionic salt bridges [20]. The charged sulfate esters on the other side of the monomer though, present on ι-carrageenan, encourage an extensive conformation via a repulsion effect of the negative SO_3^- groups and inhibit gelation while promoting viscosity in the solution [17]. The differences in sulfate position, their proportion, and the presence of anhydro-bridges, thus, give the carrageenans distinctive gel profiles: κ-carrageenan forming strong and rigid gels, ι-carrageenan forming soft gels, and λ-carrageenan that does not gel, but still provides elevated viscosity in solution, due to a structure that does not allow helix formation, Table 2. Is has to be emphasized that natural carrageenans are heterogenous, *i.e.*, have heteropolymeric structures. In practice, the rheological properties of carrageenans reflect that hybrid structures exist.

2.4. Enzyme Technology for Carrageenans Extraction

Carrageenans are produced as semi-refined or refined carrageenans. In the production of semi-refined carrageenans, the carrageenans are not extracted from the seaweed, but instead heated (to around 75 °C) with an alkaline solution of potassium hydroxide. The hydroxide reacts with the sulfate esters at the precursors μ- and ν-carrageenan to produce κ- and ι-carrageenan, which improves the gel strength of the product, while potassium binds to the carrageenans and promotes gel formation by preventing the hydrocolloid chains from dissolving. The seaweed containing the potassium bound carrageenan is washed, dried, and minced to powder [21]. When producing refined carrageenans, the process of semi-refined carrageenan extraction is continued further by heating (95–110 °C) the alkali treated seaweed in order to dissolve the gel matrix in the seaweed frond. The carrageenans are recovered by alcohol precipitation or gel pressing [4]. The preparation of semi-refined carrageenans is considerably cheaper than extraction of refined carrageenans, since costs associated with alcohol recovery and/or carrageenan recovery is avoided. In order to avoid the use of chemicals and the negative impacts they have on the environment, it could be of interest to process the seaweed by enzymes for the extraction of carrageenans. Apart from that, as shown for fucoidan, a non-hydrocolloid seaweed polysaccharide present in brown seaweed, the polysaccharides can also undergo degradation under severe conditions like pressure extraction, high temperatures, and high alkali concentrations [22,23].

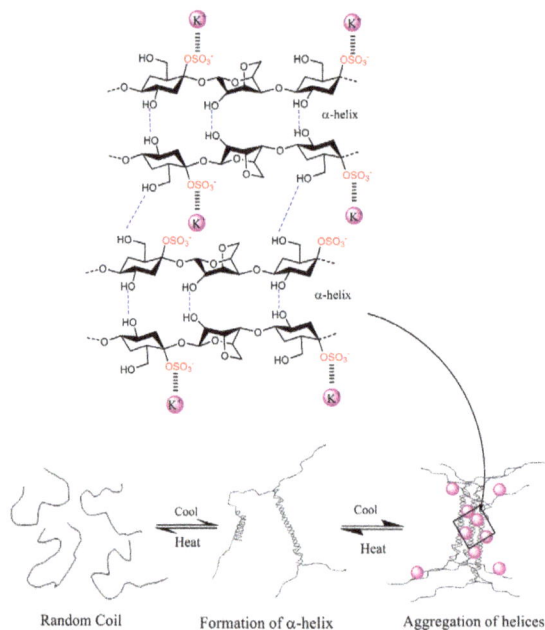

Figure 2. The gelation mechanism of κ-carrageenan in the presence of potassium ions.

Mar. Drugs **2015**, *13*, 3340–3359

The literature reports several examples of enzymatic extraction of carrageenans from red seaweed; Blanco-Pascual *et al.*, (2014) obtained a carrageenan yield of 28.65% by using an alcalase (a commercially available protease) for the extraction of a κ/ι-hybrid from *Mastocarpus stellatus*. Their product showed good gelling properties and in addition, they extracted other valuable components such as polyphenols, thereby adding value to the seaweed extraction [24]. This example emphasizes that hybrid carrageenans may be selectively extracted by use of enzymes, and that enzymes may allow for targeted production of specific gelation properties since hybrid carrageenans may exhibit unique, desirable physical properties. De Araújo *et al.*, (2012) have performed ι-carrageenan extraction experiments from *Soliera filiformis* by use of papain (a protease derived from papaya fruits). Their results showed lower yield when compared to extraction by hot water (approximately 19% compared to 33%), but by enzymatic extraction, they avoided the presence of contaminant proteins, which were present when extracting by the traditional method [25]. Varadarajan *et al.*, (2009) have compared the use of a cellulase, *Aspergillus niger*, and traditional boiling extraction of carrageenan from *Eucheuma cottonii*. They got the highest carrageenan yield when using the cellulase Novozyme NS50013: 45% by weight compared to 37% and 37.5%, respectively. The viscosity of the cellulase-extracted carrageenan was lower than the one extracted by the traditional method though. The decrease in viscosity could be explained by the presence of impurities bound to the carrageenans as the cellulase attacks the cell walls in the seaweed to release the carrageenans and thus does not degrade the carrageenan structure itself. Likewise, the fungal treatment of the seaweed with *A. niger* resulted in the extraction of low viscosity carrageenans, most likely because the organism may have used the carrageenans as carbon source [26].

It should be added that in addition to enzymatic polysaccharide extraction from seaweed, the literature also reports aims at improving protein and metabolites extraction by enzymatic degradation: These studies have targeted enzymatic degradation of the seaweed cell wall carbohydrates simultaneously with targeted enzyme-assisted degradation of seaweed hydrocolloids. Fleurence *et al.*, (1995) thus used used κ-carrageenase and agarase in combination with cellulase for the extraction of proteins from red seaweeds. In their experiment, they showed that the highest protein yield was achieved when combining cellulase with the seaweed specific enzymes: a 10-fold increase for protein extraction from *Chondrus crispus* and a 3-fold increase from *Gracilaria verrucosa* compared to the use of cellulase alone [27]. Kulshreshtha *et al.*, used commercial carbohydrases and proteases and reported a significant improvement in extraction efficiency of bioactive materials from *Chondrus crispus* compared to aqueous extraction [28]. As stated above, the current enzymatic carrageenan extraction methods have not aimed at modifying the target polysaccharides during the extraction. However, when extracting carrageenans by enzymatic reactions, the precursors µ- and ν-carrageenan have to be converted into κ- and ι-carrageenan for achievement of purer product and better gelling abilities. Genicot-Joncour *et al.*, (2009) [8] have identified and purified sulfurylases that are capable of converting ν-carrageenan into ι-carrageena, Figure 1 and Table 3. Likewise, sulfurylases responsible for catalyzing the sulfate removal causing the conversion of µ-carrageenan into κ-carrageenan, Figure 1 and Table 3, have been identified [8].

Intensive research has been conducted on the hydrolysis of carrageenans and by far the most studied microorganism in respect to this is the marine bacterium *Pseudoalteromonas carrageenovora*—and the enzymes produced by this organism. From this bacterium, Potin *et al.*, (1995) purified and analyzed a κ-carrageenase (EC 3.2.1.83) responsible for cleavage of the β-1,4 linkages, belonging to the glycoside hydrolase (GH) 16 family, along with several β-agarases responsible for the degradation of agarose, Table 3 [29]. In 2000, Barbeyron *et al.*, purified a ι-carrageenase (EC 3.2.1.157) from *Zolbellia galactanivorans*—the enzyme belongs to GH family 82 along with other reported ι-carrageenase, Table 3 [30]. In 2007, Guibet *et al.*, isolated yet another carrageenase from *P. carrageenovora*, but this enzyme acts only on λ-carrageenan, Table 3 (EC 3.2.1.162). Comparisons of sequences, catalytic sites, and mechanisms have revealed that this latter enzyme belongs to another family of glycoside hydrolases, a new family yet to be specified [31].

Digestion by carrageenases generates oligo-galactans of various sizes, most likely carbohydrates with a degree of polymerization (DP) of 2, 4, and 6. The reason for the production of different DPs is a result of the heterogenous carrageenan structure and the mechanisms that the enzymes follow. The alternating α-1,3 and β-1,4 linkages in the carrageenans results in successive β-1,4 linkages to be in opposite orientations and hence only every second disaccharide is in the right position for cleavage [30,32]. The three carrageenases all have an endo-lytic mode of action, in which they act on linkages in the middle of the chains, resulting in the formation of DP6s [31,33,34]. The main products from κ- and ι-carrageenase digestion are DP4s and DP2s, indicating a processive mechanism, in which the enzyme does not dissociate from the substrate and instead slides along the polysaccharide, cleaving all possible bonds. The tunnel-shaped active sites, found in both κ- and ι-carrageenases, further indicate a processive mechanism, where the substrate is enclosed in the active site of the enzyme. This processive behavior favors the formation of DP4s and DP2s [30,33,35]. λ-Carrageenase on the other hand, proceeds in a more random manner, resulting in higher amounts of DP6s (and possible other higher DPs as products) compared to the products from κ- and ι-carrageenase hydrolysis. Enzymes responsible for the conversion of smaller carrageenan oligosaccharides have, to our knowledge, only been reported for κ-carrageenan DP4, which is converted into κ-carrageenan DP2 by a carratetraose 4-*O* monosulfate β-hydrolase, Table 3 [36]. However, some studies indicate that the carrageenases can attack the last β-1,3 linkages for the formation of monosaccharides with prolonged incubation time [31,32,34]. Several carrageenases have been identified so far, which all degrade carrageenan substrates, but differ in their substrate specificity, mechanism, processivity, structure, sequence, and enzyme family. The molecular mechanism for hydrolysis of the β-1,3 bonds differs between the different carrageenases. Hence, κ-carrageenases retain the anomeric configuration, while ι- and λ-carrageenases invert the anomeric [29,34]. From the strict substrate specificity it seems that carrageenases recognize the sulfation pattern, which indicates that cleavage of the internal β-1,4 linkages is the first step in the degradation of carrageenans.

Desulfation of carrageenans causes them to lose their gelling properties and is thus a less studied area, when their main application is exactly due to these qualities. Nevertheless, McLean and Williamson (1979) have identified a sulfatase from *P. carrageenovora* capable of removing the sulfate group on κ-carrageenan oligosaccharides, Table 3 [37]. An ι-carrageenan sulfatase removing the sulfate ester at position 4 in ι-carrageenan has only been identified recently from a *Pseudomonas* sp. [38]. This enzyme does not act on the sulfate at position 4 in κ-carrageenan or the sulfate at position 2 in ι-carrageenan, indicating that it specifically recognizes the sulfate on 3,6-anhydro-D-galactopyranoses [38]. These results indicate that the sulfatases are highly specific, as is the case for the carrageenases, but with limited knowledge about the topic, a great deal of research is still required to fully understand and control enzyme catalyzed desulfation of carrageenans. Research on other polysaccharide-acting sulfatases supports the assumption on substrate specificity: As an example, the 2S-heparan sulfatase from *Flavobacterium heparinum* is inactive on 6S-heparan sulfates and reciprocally the 6S-heparan sulfatase does not recognize 2S-heparan sulfates [39].

2.5. Carrageenans Applications

Due to the physico-chemical properties of carrageenans, they are often used as stabilizers, gelling agents, emulsifiers, and thickeners in the food and baking industries (ice-cream, cheese, jam, bread dough). Other applications include their use as binders in toothpaste, thickeners and stabilizers in cosmetics, and as smoothers in pet food. The semi-refined carrageenan flour is colored, and may have a high bacterial count, and is thus not appropriate for human consumption but is used in canned pet food, where the canning process destroys any living organisms [40]. More recently, carrageenans have attracted attention in the pharmaceutical industry, since it has been shown, that carrageenan can inhibit attachment of viruses such as the human papillomavirus, dengue virus, and herpes virus. In addition, carrageenans are used in several drug delivery systems as matrixes to control drug release, microcapsules, and microspheres [41].

Table 3. Summary of enzymes reported in relation to modification of carrageenans, agar, and alginate.

Hydrocolloids	Enzymes	Organisms	Catalytic Reaction	Research Conducted
κ-Carrageenan	κ-Carrageenase EC 3.2.1.83 GH 16	*Pseudoalteromonas carrageenovora*	Endohydrolysis of (1,4)-β-D-linkages between D-galactose 4-sulfate and 3,6-anhydro-D-galactose	[29]
κ-Carrageenan	Sulfatase	*Pseudomonas carrageenovora*	Eliminates sulfate from D-galactose 4-sulfate, producing D-galactose	[37]
κ-Carrageenan	Carratetraose-4-O monosulfate-β-hydrolase	*Pseudomonas carrageenovora*	Hydrolysis of (1,4)-β-D-linkages between D-galactose 4-sulfate and 3,6-anhydro-D-galactose in κ-carrageenan DP4	[36]
κ-Carrageenan	Sulfurylase I and II	*Chondrus crispus*	Eliminates sulfate from D-galactose 6-sulfate of μ-carrageenan, producing 3,6 anhydro-D-galactose residues	[42]
ι-Carrageenan	ι-Carrageenase EC 3.2.1.157 GH 82	*Zolbellia galacta*	Endohydrolysis of (1,4)-β-D-linkages between D-galactose 4-sulfate and 3,6-anhydro-D-galactose-2-sulfate	[30]
ι-Carrageenan	Sulfatase	*Pseudoalteromonas atlantica*	Eliminates sulfate from D-galactose 4-sulfate, producing D-galactose	[38]
ι-Carrageenan	Sulfurylases I and II	*Chondrus crispus*	Eliminates sulfate from D-galactose 6-sulfate of ν-carrageenan, producing 3,6 anhydro-D-galactose residues	[8]
λ-Carrageenan	λ-Carrageenase EC 3.2.1.162	*Pseudoalteromonas carrageenovora*	Endohydrolysis of (1,4)-β-D-linkages between D-galactose 2-sulfate and D-galactose 2,6-sulfate	[31]
Agar	Gal-6-sulfurylase EC 2.5.1.5	*Porphyra umbilicalis*	Eliminates sulfate from L-galactose 6-sulfate of porphyran, producing 3,6-L-anhydrogalactose	[43]
Agar	α-Agarase EC 3.2.1.158	*Thalassomonas agarivorans* JAMP-A33	Endohydrolysis of (1,3)-α-L-linkages between D-galactose and 3,6-anhydro-L-galactose	[44]
Agar	β-Agarase EC 3.2.1.81	*Alteromonas* sp. SY37-12	Hydrolysis of (1,4)-β-D-linkages between 3,6-anhydro-L-galactose and D-galactose in agar	[45]
Alginate	Mannuronate lyase EC 4.2.2.3 PL5	*Azotobacter chroococcum*	Cleavage of polysaccharides with β-D-mannuronate	[46]
Alginate	Guluronate lyase EC 4.2.2.11 PL7	*Klebsiella aerogenes*	Cleavage of polysaccharides containing α-L-guluronate	[47]
Alginate	Mannuronan C5 epimerase	*Azotobacter vinelandii*	Epimerisation of β-D-mannuronic acid residues at C5	[48]

3. Agars

3.1. Common Red Seaweed Sources

Agars are industrially produced from the agarophytes red seaweed genera *Gelidium*, *Gracilaria*, and *Gelidiella* [2]. *Gelidium* seaweed is harvested in large quantities on the north coast of Spain, at the southern coast of Portugal, and at the west coast of Morocco. *Gracilaria* species are widely distributed in colder waters such as southern Chile and the Atlantic coast of Canada, with some species adapted to tropical waters, e.g., around Indonesia. Commercial cultivation of *Gracilaria* was established using *Gracilaria chilensis*, which is a native red seaweed species originating from the southern coast of Chile. Significant quantities of *Gracilaria* sp. is now cultivated in ponds and estuaries in Asia, notably in China, in the southern provinces of Guangxi and Hainan, and also in Indonesia, and Vietnam, whereas *Gelidiella acerosa* is the main source of agar in India [2] The global production of agar was approximately 10,600 ton/year, with an estimated worth of US$ ~191 million in 2014, Table 1.

3.2. Chemical Structure of Agar

Like carrageenans, agars are hydrophilic galactans consisting of galactopyranose units with alternating α-1,3 and β-1,4 linkages, but, whereas the α-linked galactopyranose is in the D-configuration in carrageenans, agar is made up of L-galactopyranose units. Some agars contain traces of its precursor porphyran: D-galactose and L-galactopyranose 6-sulfate [12]. The presence of 3,6-anhydro-L-galactopyranose was first proposed by Rees (1961) [49] via enzymatically synthesized 3,6-anhydro-L-galactopyranose with porphyran from L-galactose 6-sulfate units. Later on, various substitutions in which the most frequent are methylated galactose units such as 6-O-methyl-D-galactose and 4-*O*-methyl-L-galactose, L-galactose, methyl-pentose, and xylose were described for agar by Araki *et al.*, (1967) [50]. Agar extracted from the red seaweed *Laurencia pinnatifida* Lamour was identified to contain 2-*O*-methyl-3,6-anhydrogalactose, 2-*O*-methyl-L-galactose 6-sulfate, and D-galactose 2-sulfate [51]. The 2-*O*-methylated anhydro-sugar has now been confirmed to be the major sugar in agar from *Gracilaria eucheumoides* Harvey, where it coexists with 6-*O*-methyl-D-galactose and galactose 4-sulfate [14,52]. Craigie and Jurgens (1989) established that 4-*O*-methyl-L-galactose occurs as a branch on galactose in the polymer backbone. Methylated agar is found mostly on the commercial agarose which contain some 6-*O*- and/or 2-*O*-methylated repeating units [53].

Agarose refers to the neutral unmodified backbone of agar, of which around 20% of the dimers carry methyl or sulfate groups, while agaropectin is the modified part of agar [19]. The complexity of the agar structure is a challenge in relation to establishing a standard processing technology for agar. Nevertheless, most of the natural chemical modifications, except the biological precursor, do not affect the helical conformation of the agar polysaccharides, but they may have an effect on aggregation of helices and as a consequence affect the gelation properties [54].

3.3. Physico-Chemical Properties of Agar

The gelling and solubility properties of agar polysaccharides are outstanding among the hydrocolloid polysaccharides because of their relative hydrophobicity: The basic structure is made up of repeating units of alternating 1,3-linked β-D-galactopyranose and 1,4-linked 3,6-anhydro-α-L-galactopyranose that allows agar to form helical dimers according to a mechanism similar to that of the carrageenans described above (Section 2.3). When 3,6-anhydrogalactose is replaced by its biological precursors, L-galactose 6-sulfate or L-galactose, helix formation and gel formation is partially prevented because of "kinks", *i.e.*, the helix has breaking units that lack the 3,6-anhydride bridge [49].

A comparison of the physico-chemical properties of agar and carrageenan (presumably κ-carrageenan) shows that the gel strength of agar is 2–10 times higher than that of carrageenan, and that the melting point of agar is close to the boiling point of water, whereas the melting point of a carrageenan gel is 50–70 °C, Table 4. The increased gel strength and the higher melting point of agar gels are believed to be associated with the lower content of the anionic sulfates. However, the viscosity of agar in solution at 60 °C is lower than that of carrageenan, Table 4. The difference is due to the lower molar mass of the agar polysaccharides as compared to carrageenan, for commercial agar preparations, the average molecular weight typically ranges from 36 kDa to 144 kDa; in contrast, the solubility of agar depends on the ability of the solvent to disrupt and melt the ordered conformations, not the molecular weight [55].

In addition, high concentration of methoxyl and 3,6-anhydrogalactose in agar increases its hydrophobic properties, allowing agar solubility in hot solutions of 40%–80% aqueous ethanol [52]. The physico-chemical properties makes agar gels strong and rigid [56], but as for carrageenans, the natural products are hybrid heteropolymers and may harbor different heteropolymeric subunits.

Table 4. Physico-chemical properties for agar and carrageenans. The numbers are estimates. Viscosity values are given as (centipoise, cP) that is equivalent to $N \cdot s \cdot m^{-2}$ [56].

Properties	Agar	Carrageenan
Solubility	Boiling water	Boiling water
Gel Strength (1.5% at 20 °C)	700–1000 g/cm^3	100–350 g/cm^3
Viscosity (1.5% at 60 °C)	10–100 centipoise	30–300 centipoise
Melting point	85–95 °C	50–70 °C
Gelling point	32–45 °C	30–50 °C

3.4. Extraction and Processing of Agar

The extraction procedure for agar is dependent on the specific seaweed species, but generally consists of an alkali treatment followed by hot-water extraction. As described above for carrageenans, the alkali treatment causes a chemical change in agar (formation of the 3,6-anhydro-galactopyranose) resulting in increased gel strength. The hot-water extraction is done at temperatures around 100 °C for around 2–4 h, sometimes under pressure. The agar dissolves in the water, seaweed residuals are removed by filtration, and the agar is recovered by alcohol precipitation [41]. Agarose preparation is done by fractional precipitation methods with e.g. polyethylene glycol 6000 [42], adsorption methods with e.g., aluminum hydroxide [43], or chromatography methods such as ion-exchange chromatography [44].

For extraction of agar there is a need for mild extraction conditions that can promote solubility and gel strength and avoid harmful effects on the environment and destruction of the valuable carbohydrates. As is the case for carrageenans, the anhydrogalactose accounts for the gelling capacities of agar, thus the precursor porphyran having L-galactose 6-sulfate has to be converted into 3,6-anhydrogalactose. The synthesis of 3,6-anhydro-L-galactose has been carried out using a Gal-6-sulfurylase whose activities have been demonstrated by Rees (1961) [49]. When incubating the enzyme (0.2%) and substrate (porphyran, 1%, w/v; 10 mL.) at 35 °C, the reaction leading to the formation of 3,6-anhydrogalactose, by liberation of sulfate from the ester linkages of porphyran, occurs. The detailed mechanisms of this "double reaction" desulfation and 3,6-anhydrogalactose formation is not yet fully elucidated, since 3,6-anhydrogalactose is usually combined in polysaccharides through position 4 and in a linkage. It is likely that the L-galactose 6-sulfate precursor units are similarly linked. The de-esterification of the L-galactose 6-sulfate residues, which are known to be present in porphyran, could proceed simultaneously with 3,6-anhydro-L-galactose formation, since an analogous chemical reaction is known [57].

No attempts on enzymatic extraction of agar from red seaweed have been reported, but enzymatic hydrolysis of agars has been demonstrated several times. This hydrolysis requires agarases, which are classified according to their mode of action: β-agarases that catalyze hydrolysis of the β-1,4 linkages and α-agarases that catalyze hydrolysis of the α-1,3 linkages, Table 3 [30]. The enzyme α-agarase (EC 3.2.1.158) from *Thalassomonas* sp. can use agarose, agarohexaose and neo-agarohexaose as substrates. The products of agarohexaose hydrolysis are dimers and tetramers, with agarotetraose being the predominant product, whereas hydrolysis of neo-agarohexaose gives rise to two types of trimer. While this enzyme can also hydrolyse the highly sulfated agarose porphyran very efficiently, it cannot hydrolyse the related compounds κ-carrageenan (see EC 3.2.1.83) and ι-carrageenan (see EC 3.2.1.157) [30]. The agarose 4-glycanohydrolase (*i.e.*, β-agarase, EC 3.2.1.18) catalyzes the cleavage of the β-(1→4) linkages in agarose in a random manner with retention of the anomeric-bond configuration, producing β-anomers that progressively give rise to α-anomers when mutarotation takes place [6]. The end products of the hydrolysis are neo-agarotetraose and neo-agarohexaose in the case of AgaA (β-agarase genes A), from the marine bacterium *Zobellia galactanivorans*, and neo-agarotetraose and neo-agarobiose in the case of (AgaB β-agarase gene B) [58].

3.5. Commercial Applications of Agar

Due to its physiochemical properties, agar is used in the food industry as a gelling agent in, e.g., ice-cream and jam, in cosmetics as, e.g., a thickener in creams, and in pharmaceuticals as, e.g., an excipient in pills [56]. In addition, agar is widely used in growth media for culturing bacteria for scientific research. Agarose is also used in biotechnological applications, notably in gel electrophoresis and agarose-based chromatography. The reason for using agarose and not agar lies in the fact that agaropectin holds unsaturated chemical bonds in the sulfate and pyruvate substitutions that bestow high UV absorption in agarose gels and interfere with the detection of nucleic acids after electrophoresis [9].

4. Alginates

4.1. Common Brown Seaweed Sources of Alginate

Alginates or alginic acids are distinguished from the other seaweed hydrocolloids because they are extracted from brown seaweeds. In brown seaweeds, alginate constitutes a key component of the seaweed cell walls and also appears to be present in the intercellular space matrix. Alginate therefore appears to be present in most brown seaweed species, but the amounts vary. The main species used for commercial alginate extraction are *Laminaria* spp., *Macrocystis* spp., *Ascophyllum* spp., *Sargassum* spp., and *Fucales* spp.—in these species, alginate comprises up to 40% of the dry matter [2,4,59]. *Laminaria japonica* (a.k.a. *Saccharina japonica*) is abundant in China and can compete with the western alginate producers. However, the low guluronic to mannuronic acid ratio (M:G) of *L. japonica* from China yields weakly gelling alginates (see below). This issue prompts Chinese alginate producers to import *Lessonia nigrescens* from Chile and Peru [60]. It has been postulated that *Sargassum* spp. are only used when no other brown seaweed is available because its alginate is usually borderline quality and the yields are low [2]. Nonetheless, it was shown that different species of *Sargassum* and extraction technology employed provide very different yields and quality of alginates [61]. Alginates can also be isolated from bacteria such as *Azotobacteria* and *Pseudomonas* [62], but at present bacterial alginate production is not employed commercially.

Europe, USA and Japan were the main producers of alginates 30 years ago, but the emergence of Chinese alginate producers has changed the alginate industry in the last decades. The global market value for alginates is currently estimated to be US$ 339 million/year, Table 1. The alginates market share by application has increased by 20% for food/pharmaceutical segments. The world production capacity has expanded by 25%, mainly in China, during the last decade [60] (although reliable figures from China are difficult to obtain).

4.2. Chemical Structure and Physico-Chemical Properties of Alginate

Alginates are linear polymers build up by the two monomeric uronic acids, β-D-mannuronic acid (M) and α-L-guluronic acid (G). The two uronic acids are arranged in an irregular blockwise pattern of varying proportions of MM, MG, and GG blocks, depending on algal source, extraction technique, and harvest time. The mannuronic acids form β-1,4 linkages, which gives the MM-blocks a linear and flexible conformation, while guluronic acid gives rise to α-1,4 linkages, and introduces a steric hindrance around the carboxyl groups, thereby providing a folded and rigid structure that ensures the stiffness in the polymer chain [59].

Like the other seaweed-derived hydrocolloids described in this paper, alginate has gel-formation capacities as well. In the presence of divalent cations, mostly Ca^{2+}, the ions can bind to the carboxyl groups in alginate and act as cross-linkers that stabilize the alginate chains by formation of a gel-network. As shown by Grant *et al.* (1973), the gelation process predominantly involves cooperative binding of the divalent ions across the GG-blocks of aligned alginate chains, hence the M:G ratio has a major impact on the physico-chemical properties of alginate: Alginates with low M:G ratios (*i.e.*, having relatively high numbers of guluronic acid residues) generally form dense and brittle gels, whereas alginates with high M:G ratios (*i.e.*, with a relatively low number of guluronic acid residues) produce more elastic gels [10,11].

The M:G ratio varies amongst brown seaweed taxonomic ranks (*i.e.*, order); typically *Ascophyllum nodosum* (*Fucales*) have alginates with an M:G ratio of approximately 1.2; whereas *Laminaria japonica* (*Laminariales*) have higher M:G ratios of approximately 2.2, while many *Sargassum* (*Fucales*) alginates have M:G ratios ranging from 0.8 to 1.5 [61].

4.3. Alginates Extraction and Processing

Alginates are extracted in different ways depending on the application, but the most commonly used procedure is the one described by Calumpong *et al.* (1999), which relies on extracting the alginate as sodium alginate. The method is based on converting the insoluble calcium- and magnesium-alginates present within the brown seaweed cell walls to soluble sodium alginates that are subsequently recovered as alginic acid or calcium alginate. This conversion is done by sequential addition of acid, alcohol, and sodium carbonate [63]. The extraction techniques available for alginate extraction face some difficulties in, e.g., relation to separation of the seaweed residuals that do not dissolve. As the alginate dissolves as sodium alginate, the thickness of the solution hinders filtration and the solution has to be diluted with large quantities of water. As the seaweed residuals are very fine and can clog the filter, filter aids must be provided making the process expensive. In addition, the chemicals used for extraction are believed to influence the physico-chemical properties of alginates [64]. To avoid the difficulties encountered in the traditional extraction techniques and the destructive effects they have on the functional properties there is a need for alternative extraction and processing techniques.

Enzymatic hydrolysis of alginates has been intensively studied and both β-D-mannuronate and α-L-guluronate lyases that catalyze the degradation of alginate have been isolated from marine algae, marine mollusks, and a wide range of microorganisms, Table 3 [46,47].

The two alginate lyases catalyze the degradation of alginate by a β-elimination mechanism targeting the 1,4 glycosidic bond connecting the two uronic acid monomers. A double bond is formed between the carbon atoms at position 4 and 5 in the uronic acid ring, from which the 1,4 glycosidic bond is eliminated, resulting in the production of a 4-deoxy-L-erythro-hex-4-enopyranosyluronic acid. Although the enzymes are classified according to their specificity, they usually have moderate to low processivity for the other epimer [65]. As mentioned above, lab scale studies have demonstrated that alginate can be synthesized by bacteria belonging to the genera *Azotobacter* and *Pseudomonas* where alginates are synthesized as mannuronan, and varying amounts of the M residues in the polymer are then epimerized to G residues by mannuronan C-5-epimerases [66]. In an early study conducted by Haug and Larsen (1971), mannuronan C-5-epimerases isolated from liquid cultures of *Azotobacter vinelandii* were examined to epimerize D-mannuronic acid residues to L-guluronic acid residues of calcium alginate prepared from brown algae. The results showed that both homopolymeric blocks of L-guluronic acid and blocks having an alternating sequence of M- and G-residues are formed by this enzymatic epimerization reaction [48]. Since the gel-forming, water-binding, and immunogenic properties of the polymer are dependent on the relative amount and sequence distribution of M and G residues, the available studies indicate that certain enzymes can be used for production of alginates with specialized properties. However, to our knowledge, there are no reports available that examine the addition of epimerase during extraction and processing of alginates.

To our knowledge, no attempts on enzymatic extraction of alginate from brown seaweed have been reported, but as previously described for red seaweeds, proteins and bioactive components have been isolated from brown seaweed by enzyme-assisted extraction techniques as well. These experiments have aimed at degrading the cell walls in order to release the desirable compounds from the seaweed cells. Hardouin *et al.*, (2013) have used carbohydrases and proteases for the extraction of antiviral compounds from the brown seaweed *Sargassum muticum* and showed that the yield could be increased by the use of enzymes when compared to the traditional extraction [67]. Anticoagulant compounds have been extracted from seven brown seaweed sources using five carbohydrases by Athukorala *et al.*, (2006) [68] and Heo *et al.*, (2005) used five commercial carbohydrases and proteases for the extraction of antioxidants from brown seaweed [69].

4.4. Common Applications for Alginates

Alginates are used in the food industry as stabilizers and thickeners in e.g., jelly, drinks, and desserts. In addition, alginates are important in the healthcare and pharmaceutical industry where they are being used as wound dressings and as matrices to encapsulate and/or release cells and medicine [70–72].

Alginate has also been reported as a suitable substrate for heavy-metal adsorption and several studies reason that brown seaweed therefore could be used for absorption of heavy metal. This application could be considered implemented as a strategic removal of toxic substances from wastewaters when cultivating seaweed for alginate extraction [73].

5. Conclusions

Seaweed is a unique source of valuable hydrocolloids that due to their functional properties have significant importance in the food, medicinal, and biotechnological industries. The traditional extraction techniques rely on the use of chemicals under harsh conditions. In order to maintain the functional properties of the valuable hydrocolloid polysaccharides and to avoid the use of chemicals, there is a need for milder and more selective extractions techniques.

Current literature mainly focuses on hydrolysis of the hydrocolloids, and several seaweed specific enzymes have been identified which degrade the hydrocolloid polysaccharides and thereby change the solubility and gel strength. A few studies have covered the use of commercial, microbially-derived cellulases and proteases, as well as combinations of the two with seaweed specific enzymes, for seaweed hydrocolloid extraction. Such enzyme mixtures have also been used for extraction of protein and other components from selected seaweed species. However, the commercial enzyme mixtures employed have generally been developed for terrestrial plant biomass processing, and not for seaweed carbohydrates, and some enzyme treatments increased the carbohydrates yield while maintaining the gelling properties and others decreased the hydrocolloid yield and interfered with the gelling abilities of the hydrocolloids. There is a need for developing better enzymes designed for seaweed polysaccharides processing, since the use of enzymes allows for reduction of chemicals in seaweed hydrocolloid extraction while allowing for tailor-made functional properties and thus holds enormous potential for creation of sustainable processing of seaweed polysaccharides.

Acknowledgments: This review paper is part of the Seaweed Biorefinery Research Project in Ghana (SeaBioGha) supported by Denmark's development cooperation (Grant DANIDA-14-01DTU), The Ministry of Foreign Affairs of Denmark.

Author Contributions: N.R.K., M.T.A., A.M.: Presentation, interpretation and discussion of the data presented in the manuscript.

Conflicts of Interest: The authors declare no conflict of interest.

References

1. The Sea Weed Site: Information on Marine Algae. Available online: http://seaweed.ie/uses_general/industrialgums.php (accessed on 18 May 2015).
2. Mchugh, D.J. *A Guide to the Seaweed Industry*; FAO Fisheries Technical Paper 441; Food and Agriculture Organization of the United Nations: Rome, Italy, 2003.
3. Msuya, F. The impact of seaweed farming on the socioeconomic status of coastal communities in Zanzibar, Tanzania. *World Aquac.* **2011**, *42*, 45–48.
4. McHugh, D. *Production and Utilization of Products from Commercial Seaweeds*; FAO Fisheries Technical Paper 288; Food and Agriculture Organization of the United Nations: Rome, Italy, 1987.
5. Van De Velde, F.; Peppelman, H.A.; Rollema, H.S.; Hans, R. On the structure of κ/ι-hybrid carrageenans. *Carbohydr. Res.* **2001**, *331*, 271–283.
6. Valderrama, D.; Cai, J.; Hishamunda, N.; Ridler, N. *Social and Economic Dimensions of Carrageenan Seaweed Farming*; Fisheries and Aquaculture Technical Paper 580; Food and Agriculture Organization of the United Nations: Rome, Italy, 2013.
7. De Ruiter, G.A.; Rudolph, B. Carrageenan biotechnology. *Trends Food Sci. Technol.* **1997**, *8*, 389–395.
8. Genicot-Joncour, S.; Poinas, A.; Richard, O.; Potin, P.; Rudolph, B.; Kloareg, B.; Helbert, W. The cyclization of the 3,6-anhydro-galactose ring of iota-carrageenan is catalyzed by two D-galactose-2,6-sulfurylases in the red alga *Chondrus crispus*. *Plant Physiol.* **2009**, *151*, 1609–1616. [CrossRef] [PubMed]

9.   Wang, T.P.; Chang, L.L.; Chang, S.N.; Wang, E.C.; Hwang, L.C.; Chen, Y.H.; Wang, Y.M. Successful preparation and characterization of biotechnological grade agarose from indigenous *Gelidium amansii* of Taiwan. *Process. Biochem.* **2012**, *47*, 550–554. [CrossRef]

10. Grant, G.T.; Morris, E.R.; Rees, D.A.; Smith, P.J.C.; Thom, D. Biological interactions between polysaccharides and divalent cations: The egg-box model. *FEBS Lett.* **1973**, *32*, 195–198. [CrossRef]

11. Torres, M.R.; Sousa, A.P.A.; Silva Filho, E.A.T.; Melo, D.F.; Feitosa, J.P.A.; de Paula, R.C.M.; Lima, M.G.S. Extraction and physicochemical characterization of *Sargassum vulgare* alginate from Brazil. *Carbohydr. Res.* **2007**, *342*, 2067–2074. [CrossRef] [PubMed]

12. Usov, A.I. Polysaccharides of the red algae. *Adv. Carbohydr. Chem. Biochem.* **2011**, *65*, 115–217. [PubMed]

13. Knutsen, S.H.; Myslabodski, D.E.; Larsen, B.; Usov, A.I. A modified system of nomenclature for red algal galactans. *Bot. Mar.* **1994**, *37*, 163–169. [CrossRef]

14. Rochas, C.; Lahaye, M.; Yaphe, W. Sulfate content of carrageenan and agar determined by infrared spectroscopy. *Bot. Mar.* **1986**, *29*, 335–340. [CrossRef]

15. Van de Velde, F.; Knutsen, S.H.; Usov, A.I.; Rollema, H.S.; Cerezo, A.S. ^{1}H and ^{13}C high resolution NMR spectroscopy of carrageenans: Application in research and industry. *Trends Food Sci. Technol.* **2002**, *13*, 73–92. [CrossRef]

16. Craigie, J.S. Cell walls. In *Biology of the Red Algae*; Cole, K., Sheath, R., Eds.; Cambridge University Press: Cambridge, UK, 1990; pp. 221–257.

17. Montero, P.; Pe, M. Effects of Na$^+$, K$^+$ and Ca^{2+} on gels formed from fresh mince containing a carrageenan or alginate. *Food Hydrocoll.* **2002**, *16*, 375–385. [CrossRef]

18. Gulrez, S.K.H.; Al-Assaf, S.; Phillips, G.O. Hydrogels: Methods ofpPreparation, characterisation and application. In *Progress in Molecular and Environmental Bioengineering—From Analysis and Modeling to Technology Applications*; InTech: Rijeka, Croatia, 2011; Chapter 5.

19. Rees, D. Structure, conformation and mechanism in the formation of polysaccharide gels and networks. *Adv. Carbohydr. Chem. Biochem.* **1969**, *24*, 267–332. [PubMed]

20. Wu, P.; Imai, M. *Novel Biopolymer Composite Membrane Involved with Selective Mass Transfer and Excellent Water Permeability*; InTech: Rijeka, Croatia, 2012.

21. Bono, A.; Anisuzzaman, S.M.; Ding, O.W. Effect of process conditions on the gel viscosity and gel strength of semi-refined carrageenan (SRC) produced from seaweed (*Kappaphycus alvarezii*). *J. King Saud Univ. Eng. Sci.* **2012**, *26*, 3–9.

22. Ale, M.T.; Mikkelsen, J.D.; Meyer, A.S. Important determinants for fucoidan bioactivity: A critical review of structure-function relations and extraction methods for fucose-containing sulfated polysaccharides from brown seaweeds. *Mar. Drugs* **2011**, *9*, 2106–2130. [CrossRef] [PubMed]

23. Ale, M.T.; Meyer, A.S. Fucoidans from brown seaweeds: An update on structures, extraction techniques and use of enzymes as tools for structural elucidation. *RSC Adv.* **2013**, *3*, 8131–8141. [CrossRef]

24. Blanco-Pascual, N.; Alemán, A.; Gómez-Guillén, M.C.; Montero, M.P. Enzyme-assisted extraction of κ/ι-hybrid carrageenan from *Mastocarpus stellatus* for obtaining bioactive ingredients and their application for edible active film development. *Food Funct.* **2014**, *5*, 319. [CrossRef] [PubMed]

25. De Araújo, I.W.F.; Rodrigues, J.A.G.; Vanderlei, E.D.S.O.; de Paula, G.A.; Lima, T.D.B.; Benevides, N.M.B. Iota-carrageenans from *Solieria filiformis* (Rhodophyta) and their effects in the inflammation and coagulation. *Acta Sci. Technol.* **2012**, *34*, 127–135. [CrossRef]

26. Varadarajan, S.A.; Ramli, N.; Ariff, A.; Said, M.; Yasir, S.M. Development of high yielding carragenan extraction method from *Eucheuma Cotonii* using cellulase and *Aspergillus niger*. In Proceedings of Prosiding Seminar Kimia Bersama UKM-ITB VIII, Bangi, Malaysia, 9–11 Jan 2009; pp. 461–469.

27. Fleurence, J.; Massiani, L.; Guyader, O.; Mabeau, S. Use of enzymatic cell wall degradation for improvement of protein extraction from *Chondrus crispus, Gracilaria verrucosa* and *Palmaria palmata*. *J. Appl. Phycol.* **1995**, *7*, 393–397. [CrossRef]

28. Kulshreshtha, G.; Burlot, A.-S.; Marty, C.; Critchley, A.; Hafting, J.; Bedoux, G.; Bourgougnon, N.; Prithiviraj, B. Enzyme-assisted extraction of bioactive material from *Chondrus crispus* and *Codium fragile* and its effect on Herpes simplex virus (HSV-1). *Mar. Drugs* **2015**, *13*, 558–580. [CrossRef] [PubMed]

29. Potin, P.; Richard, C.; Barbeyron, T.; Henrissat, B.; Gey, C.; Petillot, Y.; Forest, E.; Dideberg, O.; Rochas, C.; Kloareg, B. Processing and hydrolytic mechanism of the cgkA-encoded κ-carrageenase of *Alteromonas carrageenovora*. *Eur. J. Biochem.* **1995**, *228*, 971–975. [CrossRef] [PubMed]

30. Barbeyron, T.; Michel, G.; Potin, P.; Henrissat, B.; Kloareg, B. Iota-carrageenases constitute a novel family of glycoside hydrolases, unrelated to that of kappa-carrageenases. *J. Biol. Chem.* **2000**, *275*, 35499–35505. [CrossRef] [PubMed]

31. Guibet, M.; Barbeyron, T.; Genicot, S.; Kloareg, B.; Michel, G. Degradation of λ-carrageenan by *Pseudoalteromonas carrageenovora* λ-carrageenase: A new family of glycoside hydrolases unrelated to κ- and ι-carrageenases. *Biochem. J.* **2007**, *114*, 105–114.

32. Lemoine, M.; Nyvall Collén, P.; Helbert, W. Physical state of kappa-carrageenan modulates the mode of action of kappa-carrageenase from *Pseudoalteromonas carrageenovora*. *Biochem. J.* **2009**, *419*, 545–553. [CrossRef] [PubMed]

33. Michel, G.; Chantalat, L.; Duee, E.; Barbeyron, T.; Henrissat, B.; Kloareg, B.; Dideberg, O. The kappa-carrageenase of *P. carrageenovora* features a tunnel-shaped active site: A novel insight in the evolution of Clan-B glycoside hydrolases. *Structure* **2001**, *9*, 513–25. [CrossRef] [PubMed]

34. Henares, B.M.; Enriquez, E.P.; Dayrit, F.M.; Rojas, N.R.L. Iota-carrageenan hydrolysis by *Pseudoalteromonas carrageenovora* IFO12985. *Philipp. J. Sci.* **2010**, *139*, 131–138.

35. Ma, S.; Duan, G.; Chai, W.; Geng, C.; Tan, Y.; Wang, L.; Le Sourd, F.; Michel, G.; Yu, W.; Han, F. Purification, cloning, characterization and essential amino acid residues analysis of a new ι-carrageenase from *Cellulophaga* sp. QY3. *PLoS ONE* **2013**, *8*, e64666. [CrossRef] [PubMed]

36. McLean, M.W.; Williamson, F.B. Neocarratetraose 4-*O*-monosulphate *P*-hydrolase from *Pseudomonas carrageenovora*. *Eur. J. Biochem.* **1981**, *456*, 447–456. [CrossRef]

37. McLean, M.W.; Williamson, F.B. Glycosulphatase from *Pseudomonas carrageenovora*. *Eur. J. Biochem.* **1979**, *101*, 497–505. [CrossRef] [PubMed]

38. Préchoux, A.; Genicot, S.; Rogniaux, H.; Helbert, W. Controlling carrageenan structure using a novel formylglycine-dependent sulfatase, an *endo*-4S-iota-carrageenan sulfatase. *Mar. Biotechnol.* **2013**, *15*, 265–274. [CrossRef] [PubMed]

39. Raman, R.; Myette, J.R.; Shriver, Z.; Pojasek, K.; Venkataraman, G.; Sasisekharan, R. The heparin/heparan sulfate 2-*O*-sulfatase from *Flavobacterium heparinum*: A structural and biochemical study of the enzyme active site and saccharide substrate specificity. *J. Biol. Chem.* **2003**, *278*, 12167–12174. [CrossRef] [PubMed]

40. Renn, D. Biotechnology and the red seaweed polysaccharide industry: Status, needs and prospects. *Trends Biotechnol.* **1997**, *15*, 9–14. [CrossRef]

41. Li, L.; Ni, R.; Shao, Y.; Mao, S. Carrageenan and its applications in drug delivery. *Carbohydr. Polym.* **2014**, *103*, 1–11. [CrossRef] [PubMed]

42. Wong, K.F.; Craigie, J.S. Sulfohydrolase activity and carrageenan biosynthesis in *Chondrus crispus* (*Rhodophyceae*). *Plant Physiol.* **1978**, *61*, 663–666. [CrossRef] [PubMed]

43. Rees, D.A. Enzymic desulphation of porphyran. *Biochem. J.* **1961**, *80*, 449–453. [PubMed]

44. Ohta, Y.; Hatada, Y.; Miyazaki, M.; Nogi, Y.; Ito, S.; Horikoshi, K. Purification and Characterization of a novel a-agarase from a *Thalassomonas* sp. *Curr. Microbiol.* **2005**, *50*, 212–216. [CrossRef] [PubMed]

45. Wang, J.; Mou, H.; Jiang, X.; Guan, H. Characterization of a novel β-agarase from marine *Alteromonas* sp. SY37-12 and its degrading products. *Appl. Microbiol. Biotechnol.* **2006**, *71*, 833–839. [CrossRef] [PubMed]

46. Haraguchi, K.; Kodama, T. Purification and propertes of poly(β-D-mannuronate) lyase from *Azotobacter chroococcum*. *Appl. Microbiol. Biotechnol.* **1996**, *44*, 576–581. [CrossRef]

47. Boyd, J.; Turvey, J.R. Isolation of poly-alpha-L-guluronate lyase from *Klebsiella aerogenes*. *Carbohydr. Res.* **1977**, *57*, 163–171. [CrossRef] [PubMed]

48. Haug, A.; Larsen, B. Biosynthesis of Alginate: Part II. Polymannuronic acid C-5-epimerase from *Azotobacter vinelandii*. *Carbohydr. Res.* **1971**, *17*, 297–308.

49. Rees, D.A. Enzymic synthesis of 3:6-anhydro-L-galactose within porphyran from L-galactose 6-sulphate units. *Biochem. J.* **1961**, *81*, 347–352. [PubMed]

50. Araki, C.; Arai, K.; Hirase, S. Studies on the chemical constitution of agar-agar. *Bull. Chem. Soc. Jpn.* **1967**, *40*, 1452–1456. [CrossRef] [PubMed]

51. Bowker, D.M.; Turkey, J.R. Water-soluble polysaccharides of the red alga *Laurencia pinnatifida* Part I. Constituents Units. *J. Chem. Soc.* **1968**, *1968*, 983–988.

52. Lahaye, M.; Yaphe, W.; Viet, M.T.P.; Rochas, C. ^{13}C-NMR spectroscopic investigation of methylated and charged agarose oligosaccharides and polysaccharides. *Carbohydr. Res.* **1989**, *190*, 249–265. [CrossRef]

53. Craigie, J.S.; Jurgens, A. Structure of agars from *Gracilaria tikvahiae rhodophyta*: Location of 4-*O*-methyl-L-galactose and sulphate. *Carbohydr. Polym.* **1989**, *11*, 265–278. [CrossRef]

54. Lahaye, M.; Rochas, C. Chemical structure and physico-chemical properties of agar. *Hydrobiologia* **1991**, *221*, 137–148. [CrossRef]

55. Rochas, C.; Lahaye, M. Average molecular weight and molecular weight distribution of agarose and agarose-type polysaccharides. *Carbohydr. Polym.* **1989**, *10*, 289–298. [CrossRef]

56. Agargel. Available online: http://www.agargel.com.br/index-en.html (accessed on 18 May 2015).

57. Duff, R.B.; Perciaval, E.G. Carbohydrate Sulphuric Ester. Part II. The isolation of 3:6-anhydromethylhexosides from methylhexopyranoside sulphatases. *J. Chem. Soc.* **1941**, *1941*, 830–833. [CrossRef]

58. Jam, M.; Flament, D.; Allouch, J.; Potin, P.; Thion, L.; Kloareg, B.; Czjzek, M.; Helbert, W.; Michel, G.; Barbeyron, T. The *endo*-beta-agarases AgaA and AgaB from the marine bacterium *Zobellia galactanivorans*: Two paralogue enzymes with different molecular organizations and catalytic behaviours. *Biochem. J.* **2005**, *385*, 703–713. [CrossRef] [PubMed]

59. Draget, K.I.; Moe, S.T.; Skjåk-Bræk, G.; Smidsrød, O. Alginates. In *Food Poolysaccharrides and Their Applications*; CRC Press, Taylor & Francis Group: Boca Raton, FL, USA, 2006.

60. Bixler, H.J.; Porse, H. A decade of change in the seaweed hydrocolloids industry. *J. Appl. Phycol.* **2011**, *23*, 321–335. [CrossRef]

61. Davis, T.A.; Ramirez, M.; Mucci, A.; Larsen, B. Extraction, isolation and cadmium binding of alginate from *Sargassum* spp. *J. Appl. Phycol.* **2004**, *16*, 275–284. [CrossRef]

62. Chèze-Lange, H.; Beunard, D.; Dhulster, P.; Guillochon, D.; Cazé, A.M.; Morcellet, M.; Saude, N.; Junter, G.A. Production of microbial alginate in a membrane bioreactor. *Enzyme Microb. Technol.* **2002**, *30*, 656–661. [CrossRef]

63. Calumpong, H.P.; Maypa, A.P.; Magbanua, M. Population and alginate yield and quality assessment of four *Sargassum* species in Negros Island, central Philippines. *Hydrobiologia* **1999**, *398–399*, 211–215. [CrossRef]

64. Vauchel, P.; Kaas, R.; Arhaliass, A.; Baron, R.; Legrand, J. A new process for the extraction of alginates from *Laminaria digitata*: Reactive extrusion. *Food Bioprocess Technol.* **2008**, *1*, 297–300. [CrossRef]

65. Haug, A.; Larsen, B.; Smidsrød, O.; Eriksson, G.; Blinc, R.; Paušak, S.; Ehrenberg, L.; Dumanović, J. Studies on the sequence of uronic acid residues in alginic acid. *Acta Chem. Scand.* **1967**, *21*, 691–704. [CrossRef]

66. Ertesvåg, H.; Høidal, H.K.; Schjerven, H.; Svanem, B.I.; Valla, S. Mannuronan C-5-epimerases and their application for *in vitro* and *in vivo* design of new alginates useful in biotechnology. *Metab. Eng.* **1999**, *1*, 262–269. [CrossRef] [PubMed]

67. Hardouin, K.; Burlot, A.S.; Umami, A.; Tanniou, A.; Stiger-Pouvreau, V.; Widowati, I.; Bedoux, G.; Bourgougnon, N. Biochemical and antiviral activities of enzymatic hydrolysates from different invasive French seaweeds. *J. Appl. Phycol.* **2014**, *26*, 1029–1042. [CrossRef]

68. Athukorala, Y.; Jung, W.K.; Vasanthan, T.; Jeon, Y.J. An anticoagulative polysaccharide from an enzymatic hydrolysate of *Ecklonia cava*. *Carbohydr. Polym.* **2006**, *66*, 184–191. [CrossRef]

69. Heo, S.J.; Park, E.J.; Lee, K.W.; Jeon, Y.J. Antioxidant activities of enzymatic extracts from brown seaweeds. *Bioresour. Technol.* **2005**, *96*, 1613–1623. [CrossRef] [PubMed]

70. Paul, W.; Sharma, C. Chitosan and alginate wound dressings: A short review. *Trends Biomater. Artif. Organs* **2004**, *18*, 18–23.

71. Finotelli, P.V.; da Silva, D.; Sola-Penna, M.; Rossi, A.M.; Farina, M.; Andrade, L.R.; Takeuchi, A.Y.; Rocha-Leão, M.H. Microcapsules of alginate/chitosan containing magnetic nanoparticles for controlled release of insulin. *Colloids Surf. B Biointerfaces* **2010**, *81*, 206–211. [CrossRef] [PubMed]

72. Leslie, S.K.; Cohen, D.J.; Sedlaczek, J.; Pinsker, E.J.; Boyan, B.D.; Schwartz, Z. Controlled release of rat adipose-derived stem cells from alginate microbeads. *Biomaterials* **2013**, *34*, 8172–8184. [CrossRef] [PubMed]

73. Davis, T.A.; Llanes, F.; Volesky, B.; Mucci, A. Metal selectivity of *Sargassum* spp. and their alginates in relation to their a-L-guluronic acid content and conformation. *Environ. Sci. Technol.* **2003**, *37*, 261–267. [CrossRef] [PubMed]

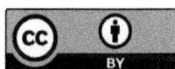

Article

Toxicological Evaluation of Low Molecular Weight Fucoidan in Vitro and in Vivo

Pai-An Hwang [1], Ming-De Yan [2], Hong-Ting Victor Lin [3], Kuan-Lun Li [4] and Yen-Chang Lin [4,*]

[1] Department of Bioscience and Biotechnology, National Taiwan Ocean University, Keelung 20246, Taiwan; amperehwang@gmail.com
[2] Cancer Center, Wan Fang Hospital, Taipei Medical University, Taipei 11696, Taiwan; yanmd717@gmail.com
[3] Department of Food Science, National Taiwan Ocean University, Keelung 20246, Taiwan; HL358@ntou.edu.tw
[4] Graduate Institute of Biotechnology, Chinese Culture University, Taipei 11114, Taiwan; noodleplusalan@gmail.com
* Correspondence: lyc10@ulive.pccu.edu.tw; Tel.: +886-2-2861-0511 (ext. 31832); Fax: +886-2-2861-8266

Academic Editor: Paola Laurienzo
Received: 25 April 2016; Accepted: 17 June 2016; Published: 24 June 2016

Abstract: For a long time, fucoidan has been well known for its pharmacological activities, and recently low molecular weight fucoidan (LMF) has been used in food supplements and pharmaceutical products. In the present study, LMF was extracted from *Laminaria japonica* by enzyme hydrolysis. The toxicity of LMF in mouse and rat models was determined by many methods, such as total arsenic content, bacterial reverse mutation assay, chromosome aberration assay, and in vivo micronucleus assay. The present findings showed that LMF at 5000 µg/mL exhibited no mutagenicity. It also produced no formatting disruption of red blood cells in vivo. At 2000 mg/kg BW/day there were no toxicological indications. LMF is expected to be used as a safe food supplement.

Keywords: low molecular weight fucoidan; toxicity; *Laminaria japonica*

---

1. Introduction

Prior to the 1950s, seaweeds were used as traditional and folk medicines [1]. Biologically active compounds from brown seaweed, however, were not discovered until the 1990s. Fucoidan is the general term for a class of sulfated and fucosylated polysaccharides found in brown seaweed; it was identified by Kylin [2]. The intensity of fucoidan's biological activities varies with species, molecular weight, composition, structure, and method of extraction [3], and its non-animal origin has been related to particular pharmacological activities [4]. Fucoidan has been well studied concerning its antitumor [5–7], antiviral [8], anti-inflammatory [9,10], anticoagulant [11], and osteogenic-enhancing differentiation activities [12]. Those activities, however, are closely related to molecular weight [13] and sulfate content [14]. Low molecular weight fucoidan (LMF) shows greater potency in its bioactivities than does high molecular weight fucoidan (HMF) [15]. Previous studies have demonstrated that LMF has high bioactivities in vitro and in vivo [5–7,12]. In this study, LMF has therefore been investigated for its toxicity at various concentrations.

Laminaria japonica is known as sea kelp and is one of the popular edible brown seaweeds in many countries. In recent years, *L. japonica* has been cultured extensively and different strains have been bred to improve its production for commercial use [16]. Fucoidan extracted from *L. japonica* has been studied extensively for its diverse biological activities [17]. Only Li et al., however, have reported on its acute and sub-chronic toxicity [18]. Furthermore, brown seaweed accumulates arsenic (As) during its growth and its total arsenic content is relatively higher than that of green or red seaweed [19]. The As compounds in brown seaweed include major organic forms, such as monomethylarsonic acid (MMA), dimethlarsinic acid (DMA), arsenobetaine (AsB), and arsenocholine (AsC). These are significantly less toxic than inorganic forms, such as arsenite (AsIII) and arsenate (AsV) [20,21]. Organic arsenic, however, can be a cancer promoter [22].

The demand for fucoidan has increased, driven by its use in food supplements, recent bioactive studies of LMF, and the pharmaceutical industry in general. Because of that increased demand, we tested the toxicity of LMF prepared from *L. japonica* by enzyme hydrolysis. The tests included bacterial reverse mutation assay, chromosome aberration assay, in vivo mouse micronucleus assay, and in vivo rat repeated dose 28-day oral toxicity assay.

2. Results and Discussion

2.1. Total Arsenic and Inorganic Arsenic Content of Laminaria japonica and LMF-LJ

Arsenic is one of the five identified industrial metals with strong neurotoxicity, the inorganic forms of AsIII and AsV are highly toxic, and the organic forms have varying degrees of toxicity [23]. Epidemiological studies have indicated that there are significant dose-response relationships between inorganic arsenic ingestion and cancer incidences [24,25]. In addition, organic arsenic has been revealed as a clastogenic agent in vitro [26] and a promoter of carcinogenesis in vivo [22]. We therefore carefully investigated the total arsenic content and arsenic species in raw *L. japonica* and LMF.

The total arsenic in the *L. japonica* of our study was 61.100 ± 3.110 mg/kg, a slightly higher value than the 30–54 mg/kg reported by [27]. It is believed that the seaweed accumulates arsenic from seawater and the arsenic concentration in the seaweed is related to the environmental conditions, growth, and metabolic rate [27]. According to the LC-ICP-MS results, the concentrations of the species of arsenic in *L. japonica* were as follows: AsB (34.31 ± 1.21 mg/kg) > MMA (9.27 ± 0.96 mg/kg) > DMA (9.23 ± 0.83 mg/kg) > AsC (59.00 ± 1.65 mg/kg). The species AsIII and AsV were not detected. The total arsenic in LMF-LJ was 6.200 ± 2.005 mg/kg, which showed a significant reduction in the concentration of organic arsenic (89.85%), and AsIII and AsV were not detected either (Table 1). Fortunately, no inorganic arsenic was detected in *L. japonica* and LMF-LJ. This is because the bioaccessibility of inorganic arsenic significantly increases after processing [19], which represents a toxicological risk of seaweed products. Reduction of organic arsenic is also an important issue for food safety, however, since significant liver tumor induction has been observed in rats that were treated with 200 ppm or more DMA [22].

Table 1. Total arsenic and inorganic arsenic content of *Laminaria japonica* and LMF-LJ.

Species	*Laminaria japonica* (mg/kg)	LMF-LJ (mg/kg)
AsIII	ND [a]	ND
AsV	ND	ND
MMA	9.27 ± 0.96	1.35 ± 0.63
DMA	9.23 ± 0.83	ND
AsB	34.31 ± 1.21	4.77 ± 0.88
AsC	6.19 ± 2.17	ND
Total arsenic (sum)	59.00 ± 1.65	6.12 ± 2.14
Total arsenic (direct)	61.100 ± 3.110	6.200 ± 2.005

[a] Detection limit was 0.02 ppm. LMF-LJ: low molecular weight fucoidan from *L. japonica*; ASIII: arsenite; ASV: arsenate; MMA: monomethylarsonic acid; DMA: dimethlarsinic acid; AsB: arsenobetaine; AsC: arsenocholine; ND: Not detected.

International limits on inorganic arsenic content have been adopted to protect people. The concentration of inorganic arsenic in LMF-LJ measured in this study (<0.02 mg/kg) was in line with Taiwan (<1 mg/kg) [28], China (<1.5 mg/kg) [29], Australia (<1 mg/kg) [30], New Zealand (<1 mg/kg) [30], and the USA (<3 mg/kg) [31]. It is therefore suggested that the total arsenic content of the experimental LMF-LJ carried no toxicological concern.

2.2. Bacterial Reverse Mutation Assay

The bacterial reverse mutation assay is a widely employed method that uses bacteria to test whether a given chemical can cause mutations in the DNA of the test organism. Li et al. have demonstrated the toxicity of fucoidan from *L. japonica* in vivo but none have tested its genotoxicity in vitro [18]. We therefore tested, for the first time, the genotoxicity of LMF-LJ. No dose-dependent effect in revertant colonies was observed at LMF-LJ levels up to 5000 μg/mL. LMF-LJ did not cause more than a twofold increase in revertants per plate with or without S9 compared to the negative control. The positive control for each strain resulted in the expected significant increase in the number of revertant colonies (Table 2). Our data indicated no evidence of mutagenic potential under the conditions used in this assay for LMF-LJ. It has been reported that fucoidan and LMF of *Undaria pinnatifida* showed no mutagenicity up to 5000 μg/mL in the Ames test [32,33], results similar to those in our study.

Table 2. Results of the definitive bacterial reverse mutation assay on LMF-LJ.

| LMF-LJ (μg/mL) | S9 | Average Number of Revertants (Number of Colonies/Plate) | | | | |
| | | Frameshift | | Base Pair Substitution | | Transition |
		TA97a	TA98	TA100	TA1535	TA102
Negative control	−	109.7 ± 7.2 [a]	17.3 ± 2.9	102.0 ± 9.5	11.7 ± 1.5	475.0 ± 27.7
312.5	−	111.0 ± 5.5	14.3 ± 0.6	101.7 ± 11.5	12.3 ± 0.5	536.0 ± 31.4
625	−	123.3 ± 13.5	16.3 ± 4.5	101.7 ± 8.3	13.0 ± 2.6	541.3 ± 38.4
1250	−	128.3 ± 11.6	15.3 ± 5.8	109.0 ± 6.9	12.0 ± 3.0	494.7 ± 37.4
2500	−	114.0 ± 13.0	9.7 ± 1.5	103.0 ± 11.5	11.0 ± 3.0	480.7 ± 56.1
5000	−	112.0 ± 7.0	14.3 ± 1.1	104.0 ± 2.6	14.0 ± 3.0	432.0 ± 31.4
Positive control						
NPD	−	524.7 ± 104.5 *	836.0 ± 72.6 *			
NaN$_3$	−			1209.7 ± 263.3 *	352.3 ± 45.6 *	
MMC	−					1970.7 ± 113.4 *
Negative control	+	138.3 ± 7.3	24.7 ± 1.5	122.0 ± 20.8	11.7 ± 1.5	503.0 ± 70.5
312.5	+	128.3 ± 16.0	27.0 ± 2.0	105.3 ± 8.1	12.0 ± 2.6	538.0 ± 14.0
625	+	136.0 ± 15.6	18.0 ± 4.3	123.0 ± 5.0	11.3 ± 4.6	516.7 ± 36.0
1250	+	152.3 ± 6.6	23.7 ± 1.5	121.7 ± 8.5	13.7 ± 0.5	510.7 ± 32.3
2500	+	123.3 ± 11.1	24.0 ± 3.4	108.0 ± 11.7	12.7 ± 3.2	485.3 ± 19.4
5000	+	128.0 ± 11.5	17.3 ± 4.9	111.3 ± 15.3	15.3 ± 2.5	452.0 ± 26.0
Positive control						
2-AF	+	367.3 ± 28.3 *		287.3 ± 22.6		
BP	+		59.7 ± 10.2 *			
2-AA	+				108.7 ± 15.5 *	1009.3 ± 56.05 *

[a] Values were expressed as mean ± SD, *n* = 3; * The number of revertant colonies was two-fold greater than the negative control. NPD: 4-nitro-o-phenylenediamine; MMC: mitomycin C; 2-AF: 2-aminofluorene; BP: benzo[α]pyrene; 2-AA: 2-aminoanthracene.

2.3. Chromosome Aberration Assay

LMF-LJ gene mutagenicity was determined with the chromosome aberration assay. The highest dose tested in the chromosome aberration assay was 5000 μg/mL. No increases in structural or numerical chromosomal aberrations were observed at any dose of LMF-LJ (312.5–5000 μg/mL) with or without S9 compared to the negative control. The positive control, MMC, with or without S9, increased the frequency of cells with >10% chromosome aberration (Table 3). LMF-LJ therefore does not induce chromosome aberrations according to our study, as with LMF of *U. pinnatifida* [33].

Table 3. Results of chromosomal aberrations in CHO-K1 cells after 3 h treated with LMF-LJ, absence and non-absence of S9.

LMF-LJ (µg/mL)	S9	Cell Viability (×10⁶ cells)	Number of Aberrations													Aberrant Cell (% ± SD) [a]
			SG	TG	SB	SD	TB	TD	TR	QR	R	CR	DC	PP	PC	
Negative control [b]	−	3.45 ± 0.02	0	0	0	0	0	0	0	0	0	0	0	0	0	0.0
Positive control [c]	−	2.78 ± 0.09	0	0	0	0	2	0	8	2	0	0	0	0	0	12.6 ± 1.1 *
312.5	−	3.58 ± 0.01	0	0	0	0	0	0	0	0	0	0	0	0	0	0.0
625	−	3.70 ± 0.01	0	0	0	0	0	0	0	0	0	0	0	0	0	0.0
1250	−	3.85 ± 0.03	0	0	0	0	0	0	0	0	0	0	0	0	0	0.0
2500	−	3.63 ± 0.02	0	0	1	0	0	0	0	0	0	0	0	0	0	1.4 ± 0.5
5000	−	3.53 ± 0.04	0	0	0	0	0	0	0	0	0	0	0	0	0	0.0
Negative control	+	3.68 ± 0.03	0	0	0	0	0	0	0	0	0	0	0	0	0	0.0
Positive control	+	2.60 ± 0.12	0	0	0	0	7	0	7	5	0	0	0	0	2	21.3 ± 1.4 *
312.5	+	3.90 ± 0.01	0	0	0	0	0	0	0	0	0	0	0	0	0	0.0
625	+	3.73 ± 0.04	0	0	0	0	0	0	0	0	0	0	0	0	0	0.0
1250	+	3.88 ± 0.02	0	0	0	0	0	0	0	0	0	0	0	0	0	0.0
2500	+	3.58 ± 0.02	0	0	0	0	0	0	0	1	0	0	0	0	0	1.2 ± 0.3
5000	+	3.80 ± 0.01	0	0	0	0	0	0	0	0	0	0	0	1	0	1.5 ± 1.0

[a] Frequency of aberrant cells in 100 mataphases scored; [b] Culture medium with FBS; [c] 2 µM MMC was used as a mutagen; * $p < 0.05$ as compared with negative control; SG: chromosome gap; TG: chromatid gap; SB: chromosome break; SD: chromosome deletion; TB: chromatid break; TD: chromatid deletion; TR: triradial; QR: quadriradial; R: ring; CR: complex rearrangement; DC: dicentric; PP: polyploidy; PC: pulverized cell.

3. Materials and Methods

3.1. Low Molecular Weight Fucoidan

The LMF from *L. japonica* (LMF-LJ) named Hi-Q Oligo-fucoidan®, was provided by Hi-Q Marine Biotech International Ltd. (New Taipei City, Taiwan). It was obtained by enzyme hydrolysis of the original fucoidan. The characteristics of LMF-LJ were as follows: average molecular weight of <667 Da with a 85.9% fucose content (127.2 ± 1.3 µmol/g), sulfate content 28.4% ± 2.1% (*w/w*), protein content 4.3% ± 0.3% (*w/w*), fat content 0.6% ± 0.1% (*w/w*), ash 4.1% ± 0.1% (*w/w*), and moisture content 3.9% ± 0.8% (*w/w*). The LMF-LJ was a light brownish-white powder and well soluble below the highest concentration.

3.2. Determination of Total Arsenic and Inorganic Arsenic Species

The methodology for the determination of total arsenic and inorganic arsenic species followed that of [21]. Briefly, milled samples of *L. japonica* and LMF-LJ were digested using an ETHOS 1 laboratory microwave system (Milestone, Leutkirch, Germany). Total arsenic determinations were carried out with an Agilent 7700e ICP-MS (Agilent Technologies, Santa Clara, CA, USA) with a microflow nebulizer; the detection limit was 0.010 mg/kg. LC-ICP-MS was used for the determination of arsenic species in sample extracts; the detection limit was 0.02 mg/kg. An Agilent 1260 Infinity Quaternary LC System (Agilent Technologies, Waldbronn, Germany) consisting of a solvent degassing unit, a binary pump, an autosampler, and a thermostatted column compartment was used. The 10 µ Hamilton PRP-X100 column (250 mm × 4.1 mm) was protected by a guard column filled with the same stationary phase. The outlet of the LC column was connected via PEEK capillary tubing (0.125 mm i.d.) to the nebulizer, which served as the arsenic-selective detector. The stock solutions of arsenic compounds were prepared from AsIII oxide (Sigma Aldrich, St. Louis, MO, USA) by dissolution in 0.2% NaOH and from AsV oxide hydrate (Sigma Aldrich, St. Louis, MO, USA). MMA, DMA, AsB, and AsC were purchased from Arcos-Organics (Fair Lawn, NJ, USA).

3.3. Bacterial Reverse Mutation Assay

The bacterial reverse mutation assay was conducted by the pre-incubation method in the presence and absence of S9 metabolic activation [34,35]. Tester strains included *Salmonella typhimurium* TA97a, TA98, TA100, TA102, and TA1535 with and without S9 and corresponding positive control agents such as 4-nitro-o-phenylenediamine (NPD), NaN_3, mitomycin C (MMC), 2-aminofluorene (2-AF), benzo[α]pyrene (BP), and 2-aminoanthracene (2-AA). LMF and positive controls were dissolved in DMSO as a vehicle. A preliminary range-finding study was conducted for all tester strains at LMF-LJ concentrations of 100, 500, 1000, and 5000 µg/plate. Results of that study indicated the definitive study concentrations of 312.5, 625, 1250, 2500, and 5000 µg LMF-LJ /plate. For each treatment, 0.1 mL of LMF-LJ or control preparation was introduced into a sterilized test tube, to which 0.1 mL of bacterial suspension was added. For preparations with S9, 0.5 mL of S9 mix was also added; for preparations without S9, 0.5 mL of 0.1 M sodium phosphate buffer solution was added. Mixtures were then incubated with gentle shaking for 20 min at 37 °C, 120 rpm. After incubation, 4 mL of top agar (45 °C) containing 0.5 mm histidine/biotin was added, and then all substances were spread evenly on minimal glucose agar plates. After the top agar solidified, the plates were inverted and incubated for 48 h at 37 °C. The numbers of revertant colonies were counted by either an automatic colony analyzer or manual counting. The test substance was judged positive for mutagenicity when (1) substances induced a dose-dependent increase in the number of revertant colonies to a level greater than twofold of the negative control value and (2) the dose-dependent increase was reproducible.

3.4. Chromosome Aberration Assay

The experiment was carried out in triplicate to determine the effects of LMF-LJ (at concentrations of 312.5, 625, 1250, 2500, and 5000 µg/mL) on the induction of chromosomal aberrations in Chinese hamster ovary cells (CHO-K1, CCRC 60006). Cells were cultured in reconstituted minimum essential medium supplemented with 2.2 g sodium bicarbonate, 292 mg L-glutamine, streptomycin sulfate (100 µg/mL), penicillin G-Na (105 units), and 10% (*v*/*v*) fetal bovine serum (FBS) per liter. The cells were grown as monolayers in culture flasks and incubated in a humidified atmosphere of 5% CO_2 in air at 37 °C [36].

The LMF-LJ was added after 1 h incubation in 4.0 mL of fresh culture medium with or without S9. The negative control was treated with FBS only; 2 µM mitomycin C was used as a positive control. After 22 h, 5 mg/mL colchicine was added for 2 h. Chromosomes were prepared according to standard procedures. Hypotonic treatment with 0.4% KCl (37 °C) was applied for 20 min. The cells were fixed with methanol and acetic acid (3:1) and the fixative was changed twice. Air-dried slides were stained with Giemsa (5%) and scored for chromosome aberrations according to [37]. The structural aberrations recorded were chromosome gap, chromatid gap, chromosome break, chromosome deletion, chromatid break, chromatid deletion, triradial, quadriradial, ring, complex rearrangement, dicentric, polyploidy, and pulverized cell. Each slide was scanned systematically and each set of metaphases was examined under 1000× magnification. After each type of aberration was recorded, the number of aberrant metaphases and total aberrations were calculated.

3.5. In Vivo Mouse Micronucleus Assay

Some 25 healthy male Imprinting Control Region (ICR) mice (six weeks of age) were used in this study; they were purchased from National Taiwan University College of Medicine Laboratory Animal Center (Taipei, Taiwan). All animals were seven weeks of age at the start of the experiment and were housed in a normal, environmentally controlled animal room with free access to pathogen-free feed and water *ad libitum*. Over three consecutive days, the mice were treated by gavage with 500, 1000, and 2000 mg/kg body weight (BW) LMF-LJ dissolved in saline. The negative control (0 mg/kg BW LMF-LJ) mice were treated identically with equal volumes of normal saline also via gavage throughout the study. MMC (2 mg/kg, i.p.) was administered as a positive control.

Whole blood smears were collected on the day following the last LMF-LJ administration or one day after MMC treatment. Whole blood smears were prepared on clean microscope slides, air dried, fixed in methanol, and stained with 1% brilliant cresyl blue (BCB) (Lot No. MKBH8545V, Sigma, St. Louis, MO, USA) for 10 min just before the evaluation with a fluorescence microscope (Nikon ECLIPSE E600, Tokyo, Japan). The frequency of reticulocytes (RETs) per total erythrocytes was determined using a sample size of 1000 erythrocytes per animal. The number of micronuclei (MNs) was determined using 2000 RET per animal. Briefly, immature erythrocytes (i.e., RETs) were identified by their orange-red color; MNs were identified by their yellow-green color (Kirkland, 1994).

All experimental procedures, including the use of experimental animals, were approved by Institutional Animal Care and Use Committee (IACUC), Chinese Culture University, Taiwan, Republic of China with permission number CCU-IACUC-104011 and CCU-IACUC-10509.

3.6. In Vivo Rat Repeated-Dose 28-Day Oral Toxicity Assay

40 male and 40 female Sprague-Dawley (SD) rats (four weeks of age) were used in this study; they were purchased from National Taiwan University College of Medicine Laboratory Animal Center (Taipei, Taiwan). All animals were six weeks of age at the start of the experiment and were housed in a normal, environmentally controlled animal room with free access to pathogen-free feed and water *ad libitum*. These 80 SD rats were randomly divided into a control and three dose levels (500, 1000, and 2000 mg/kg BW LMF-LJ) with 10 males and 10 females in each group. Concentrations of 500, 1000, and 2000 mg/kg BW LMF-LJ were dissolved in saline and then administered by oral gavage in 10 mL/kg of BW on a daily basis for 28 days. The control (0 mg/kg BW LMF-LJ) rats were treated identically with equal volumes of normal saline also via gavage throughout the study. Rats were anesthetized with diethyl ether followed by cervical decapitation. Blood samples were collected for evaluation of clinical hematology and biochemistry [38,39].

3.6.1. Body Weight, Food Intake, and Water Consumption

Body weights and food and water intake were measured at 0 days before treatment and at 7, 14, and 28 days after treatment. Food and water intake was measured in mg/kg BW/day; the amount of food and water was measured before supplying them to the cage and the remainder was measured the next day.

3.6.2. Observation of Clinical Signs

All abnormal clinical signs were noted and measured before and after dosing, at least twice a day based on the functional observational battery test.

3.6.3. Urinalysis

Before sacrifice, a 16-h (17:00 to next day 9:00) urine sample was collected and the urine parameters were determined by a Clinitek 500 urine chemistry analyzer (Bayer Health Care, Cambridge, MA, USA) and a Multistix 10SG reagent strip (Bayer, Elkhart, IN, USA).

3.6.4. Hematology

A hematological examination was conducted at the end of the study. Hematological parameters were determined by an automated hematology analyzer (XT-1800i, Sysmex Corporation, Kobe, Japan). Prothrombin time (PT) and activated partial thromboplastin time (APTT) were determined by an automated coagulation analyzer (CA-1500, Sysmex Corporation, Kanagawa, Japan).

3.6.5. Serum Biochemistry

The animals fasted for more than 8 h before being sacrificed. Blood was collected and centrifuged at $1500 \times g$ for 15 min to collect serum. Serum was then analyzed by an automated biochemistry analyzer (Vitros 5.1 FS, Johnson & Johnson, New Brunswick, NJ, USA) for serum biochemistry parameters such as alanine aminotransferase, aspartate aminotransferase, alkaline phosphatase, total bilirubin, total protein, albumin, globulin, blood urea, nitrogen, creatinine, total cholesterol, triglyceride, prothrombin time, and activated partial thromboplastin time.

3.6.6. Organ Weight

All organs were carefully examined macroscopically and the brain, heart, kidneys, liver, spleen, adrenals, testes (males), and ovaries (females) were weighed relative to total body weight.

3.6.7. Histopathology

All organs were fixed in 10% neutral buffered formalin solution for pathologic examination. The organs from the control and test groups were further processed, embedded in paraffin, sectioned at 2 μm by microtome (Finesse 325, Thermo Shandon Ltd., Cheshire, UK), stained with hematoxylin and eosin (H&E), and evaluated for histopathology under a microscope (BX-51, Olympus, Tokyo, Japan).

3.7. Statistical Analysis

Numerical data are presented as means ± standard deviation. The data was analyzed by a one-way analysis of variance (ANOVA), which was followed by the least significant difference test using SPSS (Chicago, IL, USA) version 10 software. A *p*-value of <0.05 was considered a significant difference.

4. In Vivo Mouse Micronucleus Assay

The micronucleus test is a mammalian in vivo test that detects damage of the chromosomes or mitotic apparatus by chemicals. It is based on an increase in the frequency of micronucleated polychromatic erythrocytes in the bone marrow of treated animals. No significant clinical symptoms were observed during the experiment, and no mouse died.

LMF-LJ administration at 500, 1000, and 2000 mg/kg BW caused no significant change in RETs/1000 erythrocytes% and MNs/2000 RETs%, while the positive control, MMC, significantly changed in RETs/1000 erythrocytes% and MNs/2000 RETs%, as expected (Table 4). None of the fucoidan or LMF levels changed significantly in the micronucleus assay [38–40]. These results suggested that the oral administration of LMF-LJ did not disrupt the normal formation of erythrocytes and that the intake of less than 2000 mg/kg BW was safe.

Table 4. Results of micronucleus assay in peripheral blood erythrocytes of mice treated with LMF-LJ.

Sample	Dose (mg/kg BW)	Body Weight (g)		RETs/1000 Erythrocytes (%)	MNs/2000 RET (%)	Clinical Signs	Mortalities (Dead/Total)
		First treatment	Sacrifice			ND	0/5
Negative control		31.44 ± 1.49 [a]	30.5 ± 1.9	30.5 ± 1.9	1.2 ± 0.8	ND	0/5
Positive control [b]	1	30.50 ± 1.76	10.9 ± 4.6 *	10.9 ± 4.6 *	29.3 ± 5.4 *	ND	0/5
LMF	500	31.70 ± 1.56	26.4 ± 3.2	26.4 ± 3.2	1.0 ± 0.7	ND	0/5
	1000	31.64 ± 1.80	24.8 ± 3.9	24.8 ± 3.9	1.8 ± 1.3	ND	0/5
	2000	32.12 ± 1.43	28.5 ± 3.6	28.5 ± 3.6	1.4 ± 1.5	ND	0/5

[a] Values were expressed as mean $\pm$ SD, $n = 5$; [b] MMC was used as a mutagen; * $p < 0.05$ as compared with negative control; RETs: reticulocytes, MNs: micronucleus.

5. In Vivo Rat Repeated Dose 28-Day Oral Toxicity Assay

5.1. Body Weights, Food Intake, Water Consumption, and Clinical Signs

The Organisation for Economic Co-operation Development (OECD) (2001)-recommended guideline for the highest dose of test material is 2000 mg/kg BW; the highest dose of LMF-LJ was therefore selected as 2000 mg/kg, which was repeated daily for the 28-day oral toxicity assay [41]. No significant changes in body weight, food intake, or water intake were detected in all groups (500, 1000, and 2000 mg/kg BW) tested compared to the normal saline control (Figure 1). No significant clinical symptoms were observed during the experiment, and no rat died.

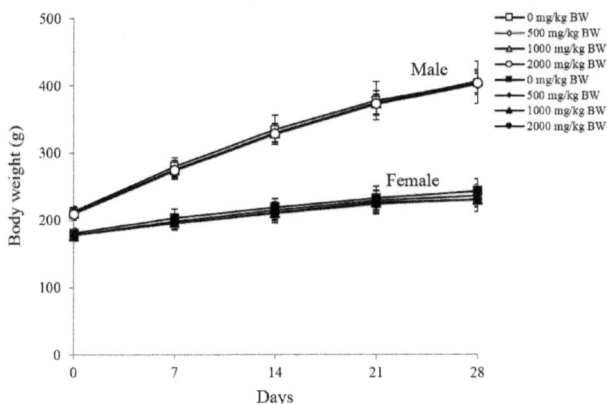

Figure 1. Growth curves for male (open symbols) and female (solid symbols) rats treated with LMF-LJ for 28 days. Values were expressed as mean $\pm$ SD, $n = 10$.

5.2. Urinalysis Results

The urinary volume of the control rats was 6.3 ± 0.3 mL/16 h in the male groups and 5.9 ± 0.8 mL/16 h in the female groups; there was no significant increase in urine production after treating with LMF-LJ. There was no significant difference between dosed groups and normal saline control in levels of urine SG, pH, protein, Uro, and ketone; Glu and Nit were absent in the urine of all groups. Although there were trace levels of Oc. blood in 2000 mg/kg BW of only one mouse in the male groups, there were no significant abnormalities to note (Table 5). Rats that received fucoidan of *U. pinnatifida* for 28 days also showed 80 Ery/μL in urine [27]. This variation was therefore considered within the normal physiological changes for rats and not a dose-related effect.

5.3. Hematological, Blood Clotting, and Serum Biochemistry Results

LMF-LJ did not increase the activity of serum toxicity marker enzymes (alanine aminotransferase (ALT), aspartate aminotransferase (AST)) up to 2000 mg/kg BW, indicating normal liver function. LMF-LJ administration also did not affect hematological parameters (red blood cell (RBC), white blood cell (WBC), platelet count (PLK), neutrophil (NEUT), lymphocyte (LYMPH)), blood clotting time (prothrombin time (PT), activated partial thromboplastin time (APTT)), and some serum biochemical parameters (alkaline phosphatase (ALP), total bilirubin (T-BIL), total protein (TP), albumin (ALB), globulin (GLO), blood urea nitrogen (BUN), total cholesterol (TC), Na, K, Ca, and P), but creatinine (CRE) and triglyceride (TG) showed significant decreases compared to the control (Table 6). Creatinine levels fluctuated after treatment with different concentrations of fucoidan from *Cladosiphon okamuranus* in Wistar rats [18,42]. In another study, creatinine levels were reduced in a male rat but increased in a female one when treated with fucoidan from *Undaria pinnatifida*. That may suggest that the fucoidan extract from different sources may have different effects on creatinine levels [27]. In agreement with those studies, the fucoidan extract from *Laminaria japonica* also correlated with decreased plasma creatinine levels in the Active Heymann Nephritis rat model [43]. From our findings, the fucoidan extract from *L. japonica* reduced creatinine levels in male and female rats. These results are consistent with previously reports [27].

Triglyceride level has been suggested as causal factor for cardiovascular disease and type 2 diabetes mellitus [44,45]. Fucoidan polysaccharide sulfuric acid ester extract from *Laminaria japonica* at concentrations ranging from 0.1 to 0.4 g/kg has been known to significantly reduce total serum triglycerides in hyperlipidemic rats [46]. Fucoidan extract from *Cladosiphon okamuranu* (150 mg/kg/day for seven days) can reduce the triglyceride level in myocardial infarction rats [47]. Fucoidan from *Undaria pinnatifida* (concentrations ranging from 150 to 1350 mg/kg) has been correlated with an increased level of triglycerides in male rats and a decreased level of triglycerides in female rats relative to controls. In our study, we found that fucoidan from *L. japonica* correlated with an increased level of triglycerides in male rats and a decreased level in female rats, which is consistent with the previous study [46].

Although there were significant changes in CRE, the values remained within the normal range (0.4–1.4 mg/dL) [48]. Similar effects were also observed by [27] and [49], namely that fucoidan can decrease CRE slightly in serum. LMF-LJ significantly reduced TG in serum; this might have been caused by an increase in levels of lipid metabolizing enzymes [46,50]. Li et al. studied fucoidan from *L. japonica* in Wistar rats for six months and reported no significant toxicological changes with 300 mg/kg BW/day, though prolonged clotting times were seen at doses of 900 and 2500 mg/kg BW/day [18]. Gideon and Rengasamy demonstrated similar results in prolonged clotting times when Wistar rats received 1500 mg/kg BW fucoidan from *Cladosiphon okamuranus* [42]. This phenomenon, however, was not observed in our study.

5.4. Organ Weight and Histopathological Results

Absolute and relative organ weights of male and female rats are summarized in Table 7. There were no meaningful changes in the gross findings of eight principal organs in all experimental groups. No histopathological results were observed in any of the LMF-LJ experimental groups (data not shown).

Table 5. Urinalysis results of male and female rats treated with LMF-LJ for 28 days.

Sex	Dose (mg/kg BW)	Volume (mL)	SG	pH	Protein (mg/dL)	Uro (EU/dL)	Glu N	Bilirubin N	Bilirubin ±	Ketone [a] +1	Ketone [a] +2	Nit N	Oc. Blood N	Oc. Blood ±
Male	0	6.7 ± 0.3 [b]	1.024 ± 0.001	7.1 ± 0.1	86.2 ± 8.3	0.32 ± 0.03	10 [c]	5	5	2	8	10	10	0
	500	6.7 ± 0.8	1.019 ± 0.004	7.2 ± 0.4	97.7 ± 10.2	0.28 ± 0.02	10	4	6	3	7	10	10	0
	1000	6.4 ± 0.6	1.025 ± 0.002	7.0 ± 0.2	92.4 ± 9.6	0.30 ± 0.03	10	5	5	2	8	10	10	0
	2000	6.8 ± 0.2	1.024 ± 0.006	6.9 ± 0.1	98.1 ± 11.4	0.30 ± 0.01	10	5	5	1	9	10	9	1
Female	0	5.9 ± 0.8	1.019 ± 0.005	7.2 ± 0.6	75.6 ± 6.5	0.26 ± 0.01	10	7	3	8	2	10	10	0
	500	6.5 ± 0.3	1.021 ± 0.003	7.1 ± 0.4	83.1 ± 8.9	0.31 ± 0.08	10	6	4	3	7	10	10	0
	1000	5.8 ± 0.7	1.022 ± 0.007	6.8 ± 0.3	79.5 ± 10.0	0.30 ± 0.01	10	9	1	7	3	10	10	0
	2000	6.2 ± 0.4	1.027 ± 0.006	6.9 ± 0.2	89.2 ± 7.8	0.29 ± 0.02	10	7	3	6	4	10	10	0

[a] +1: 5–15 mmol/l; +2: 15–30 mmol/l; [b] Values were expressed as mean ± SD, *n* = 10; [c] Number of rats with each result; SG: specific gravity; Uro: urobilinogen; Glu: glucose; Nit: nitrite; Oc. blood: occult blood; N: negative; ±: trace.

Table 6. Hematological, blood clotting and serum biochemical results of male and female rats treated with LMF-LJ for 28 days.

Sex	Male				Female			
Dose (mg/kg BW)	0	500	1000	2000	0	500	1000	2000
RBC (M/µL)	7.82 ± 0.19 [a]	7.59 ± 0.26	7.87 ± 0.35	7.70 ± 0.15	7.90 ± 0.31	8.08 ± 0.34	8.10 ± 0.56	8.16 ± 0.55
WBC (K/µL)	8.96 ± 1.51	9.61 ± 0.94	10.43 ± 1.99	9.51 ± 1.38	6.85 ± 0.99	6.44 ± 1.97	6.04 ± 2.57	6.49 ± 1.68
PLT (K/µL)	1050.2 ± 66.7	1043.0 ± 102.0	1030.9 ± 93.8	957.9 ± 61.2	1025.9 ± 87.0	976.0 ± 108.9	1039.5 ± 77.2	1050.1 ± 109.1
NEUT (%)	16.97 ± 2.44	15.97 ± 5.30	14.29 ± 5.00	17.89 ± 5.58	14.82 ± 3.75	11.70 ± 4.57	10.11 ± 3.73	15.80 ± 6.70
LYMPH (%)	77.85 ± 2.75	80.17 ± 5.59	81.55 ± 5.44	76.90 ± 5.88	79.83 ± 3.97	80.17 ± 4.77	81.91 ± 3.67	79.87 ± 8.18
PT (sec)	14.12 ± 1.84	12.77 ± 0.97	13.46 ± 1.42	12.94 ± 0.97	9.97 ± 0.27	9.91 ± 0.12	9.84 ± 0.38	9.85 ± 0.14
APTT (sec)	18.13 ± 1.39	16.91 ± 1.06	17.29 ± 1.22	17.48 ± 1.01	15.33 ± 0.66	15.56 ± 0.84	16.35 ± 2.25	15.54 ± 0.27
ALT (U/L)	31.0 ± 4.1	32.5 ± 5.3	35.2 ± 8.5	35.8 ± 8.1	26.1 ± 3.0	29.1 ± 8.2	27.1 ± 6.6	31.0 ± 5.7
AST (U/L)	102.9 ± 17.6	106.3 ± 9.3	104.0 ± 17.3	118.3 ± 12.8	148.9 ± 21.7	130.5 ± 21.9	138.5 ± 21.3	146.7 ± 19.6
ALP (U/L)	171.6 ± 34.8	177.1 ± 28.6	181.2 ± 32.9	184.5 ± 25.2	98.4 ± 20.8	102.4 ± 25.8	101.3 ± 19.7	109.6 ± 21.02
T-BIL (mg/dL)	0.055 ± 0.016	0.045 ± 0.016	0.05 ± 0.000	0.05 ± 0.000	0.05 ± 0.000	0.05 ± 0.000	0.055 ± 0.016	0.05 ± 0.000
TP (g/dL)	6.46 ± 0.34	6.24 ± 0.30	6.46 ± 0.28	6.30 ± 0.24	6.93 ± 0.38	7.12 ± 0.46	6.90 ± 0.39	6.89 ± 0.62
ALB (g/dL)	4.12 ± 0.20	3.97 ± 0.13	4.04 ± 0.15	3.98 ± 0.14	4.42 ± 0.24	4.56 ± 0.28	4.38 ± 0.29	4.38 ± 0.35
GLO (g/dL)	2.34 ± 0.22	2.27 ± 0.18	2.42 ± 0.16	2.32 ± 0.13	2.51 ± 0.17	2.56 ± 0.18	2.52 ± 0.21	2.51 ± 0.29

Table 6. Cont.

Sex	Male				Female			
	0	500	1000	2000	0	500	1000	2000
BUN (mg/dL)	15.26 ± 2.42	15.00 ± 1.86	15.05 ± 1.18	15.57 ± 1.58	17.43 ± 2.77	16.45 ± 2.25	17.36 ± 2.64	17.60 ± 3.31
CRE (mg/dL)	0.54 ± 0.09	0.47 ± 0.02 *	0.47 ± 0.05 *	0.50 ± 0.04	0.62 ± 0.06	0.53 ± 0.06 *	0.52 ± 0.04 *	0.55 ± 0.04 *
TC (mg/dL)	64.2 ± 13.9	66.3 ± 13.0	56.4 ± 7.4	61.5 ± 7.7	77.4 ± 15.6	74.7 ± 15.0	84.4 ± 19.5	67.8 ± 12.1
TG (mg/dL)	53.5 ± 10.4	37.9 ± 9.5 *	35.8 ± 6.9 *	41.4 ± 8.1 *	46.4 ± 8.1	37.7 ± 13.4 *	37.6 ± 10.8 *	31.3 ± 9.4 *
Na (mmol/L)	147.4 ± 1.0	146.2 ± 1.3	147.2 ± 1.5	147.2 ± 1.0	145.1 ± 1.4	145.7 ± 2.0	144.6 ± 2.1	146.1 ± 1.5
K (mmol/L)	7.21 ± 1.07	7.83 ± 0.71	7.71 ± 0.70	7.01 ± 1.06	7.38 ± 0.64	7.33 ± 0.51	7.23 ± 0.89	7.34 ± 1.36
Ca (mg/dL)	10.80 ± 0.36	11.08 ± 0.23	11.21 ± 0.50	11.15 ± 0.36	11.38 ± 0.39	11.67 ± 0.27	11.32 ± 0.43	11.51 ± 0.59
P (mg/dL)	13.32 ± 2.79	13.70 ± 0.90	14.03 ± 1.30	14.04 ± 1.00	13.09 ± 1.11	12.65 ± 1.04	12.00 ± 0.85	13.87 ± 1.28

[a] Values were expressed as mean ± SD, n = 10; * $p < 0.05$ as compared with negative control; RBC: red blood cell; WBC: white blood cell; PLT: platelet count; NEUT: neutrophil; LYMPH: lymphocyte; ALT: alanine aminotransferase; AST: aspartate aminotransferase; ALP: alkaline phosphatase; T-BIL: total bilirubin; TP: total protein; ALB: albumin; GLO: globulin; BUN: blood urea nitrogen; CRE: creatinine; TC: total cholesterol; TG: triglyceride; PT: prothrombin time; APTT: activated partial thromboplastin time.

Table 7. Absolute and relative organ weights of male and female rats treated with LMF-LJ for 28 days.

Sex	Male				Female			
Dose (mg/kg BW)	0	500	1000	2000	0	500	1000	2000
Brain Weight (g)	1.99 ± 0.09 [a]	1.95 ± 0.08	1.98 ± 0.07	1.95 ± 0.06	1.82 ± 0.07	1.75 ± 0.10	1.82 ± 0.05	1.81 ± 0.09
Heart Weight (g)	1.39 ± 0.11	1.34 ± 0.07	1.36 ± 0.07	1.36 ± 0.09	0.81 ± 0.07	0.83 ± 0.08	0.82 ± 0.08	0.80 ± 0.03
Ratio [b]	0.69 ± 0.07	0.69 ± 0.03	0.69 ± 0.04	0.70 ± 0.05	0.44 ± 0.04	0.47 ± 0.03	0.45 ± 0.04	0.44 ± 0.02
Kidneys Weight (g)	3.09 ± 0.23	2.99 ± 0.24	2.97 ± 0.25	3.06 ± 0.29	1.66 ± 0.06	1.66 ± 0.18	1.56 ± 0.14	1.66 ± 0.12
Ratio	1.55 ± 0.14	1.52 ± 0.08	1.50 ± 0.16	1.57 ± 0.14	0.91 ± 0.05	0.95 ± 0.08	0.85 ± 0.07	0.92 ± 0.07
Liver Weight (g)	13.24 ± 1.71	12.45 ± 1.19	12.82 ± 0.64	12.66 ± 0.64	6.97 ± 0.61	7.29 ± 0.76	7.23 ± 0.89	6.97 ± 0.55
Ratio	6.65 ± 0.97	6.38 ± 0.67	6.48 ± 0.44	6.50 ± 0.39	3.82 ± 0.38	4.17 ± 0.39	3.96 ± 0.45	3.86 ± 0.34
Spleen Weight (g)	0.72 ± 0.11	0.70 ± 0.08	0.71 ± 0.06	0.74 ± 0.11	0.43 ± 0.06	0.42 ± 0.06	0.49 ± 0.08	0.42 ± 0.05
Ratio	0.36 ± 0.06	0.36 ± 0.04	0.36 ± 0.03	0.38 ± 0.06	0.23 ± 0.03	0.23 ± 0.02	0.26 ± 0.04	0.23 ± 0.02
Adrenals Weight (g)	0.050 ± 0.006	0.053 ± 0.004	0.055 ± 0.005	0.050 ± 0.008	0.060 ± 0.006	0.059 ± 0.007	0.058 ± 0.008	0.059 ± 0.008
Ratio (%) [c]	2.514 ± 0.347	2.733 ± 0.225	2.785 ± 0.281	2.579 ± 0.410	3.320 ± 0.380	3.386 ± 0.385	3.223 ± 0.463	3.271 ± 0.511
Testes Weight (g)	2.98 ± 0.16	3.13 ± 0.28	3.03 ± 0.31	2.92 ± 0.21	-	-	-	-
Ratio	1.49 ± 0.09	1.60 ± 0.15	1.53 ± 0.19	1.50 ± 0.09	-	-	-	-
Ovaries Weight (g)	-	-	-	-	0.067 ± 0.010	0.076 ± 0.008	0.074 ± 0.016	0.072 ± 0.013
Ratio (%)	-	-	-	-	3.680 ± 0.471	4.397 ± 0.562	4.072 ± 0.886	4.031 ± 0.822

[a] Values were expressed as mean ± SD, n = 10; [b] Organ weight/brain weight; [c] Organ weight/brain weight × 100%.

6. Conclusions

In conclusion, LMF-LJ at 5000 μg/mL displayed no mutagenicity by either the bacterial reverse mutation or the chromosomal aberration assay in vitro. Moreover, LMF-LJ caused no formatting disruption of erythrocytes in vivo. Through 28 days of repeated oral administration to SD rats, it was found that up to 2000 mg/kg BW/day of LMF-LJ caused no toxicological indications. The use of LMF-LJ is presently expected to be safe and may prove to be a useful bioactive agent after further toxicity research.

Acknowledgments: We thank the National Science Council (NSC) of the Executive Yuan, Taiwan [NSC 104-2320-B-034-003 (to Yen-Chang Lin); NSC 105-2320-B-034-001 (to Yen-Chang Lin)] for their support and the grant funding.

Author Contributions: Conceived and designed the experiments: P.-A.H., M.-D.Y., H.-T.V.L.; Performed the experiments: K.-L.L., P.-A.H., M.-D.Y.; Analyzed the data: P.-A.H., M.-D.Y.; Contributed reagents/materials/analysis tools: Y.-C.L., K.-L.L.; wrote the manuscript: P.-A.H., M.-D.Y., H.-T.V.L., Y.-C.L.

Conflicts of Interest: The authors declare no conflict of interest.

References

1. Lincoln, R.A.; Strupinski, K.; Walker, J.M. Bioactive compounds from algae. *Life Chem. Rep.* **1991**, *8*, 97–183.
2. Kylin, H. Zur biochemie der meeresalgen. *HoppeSeylers Z. Physiol. Chem.* **1913**, *83*, 171–197. [CrossRef]
3. Fitton, J.H. Therapies from fucoidan; multifunctional marine polymers. *Mar. Drugs* **2011**, *9*, 1731–1760. [CrossRef] [PubMed]
4. Senni, K.; Gueniche, F.; Foucault-Bertaud, A.; Igondjo-Tchen, S.; Fioretti, F.; Colliec-Jouault, S.; Durand, P.; Guezennec, J.; Godeau, G.; Letourneur, D. Fucoidan a sulfated polysaccharide from brown algae is a potent modulator of connective tissue proteolysis. *Arch. Biochem. Biophys.* **2006**, *445*, 56–64. [CrossRef] [PubMed]
5. Hsu, H.-Y.; Lin, T.-Y.; Hwang, P.-A.; Tseng, L.-M.; Chen, R.-H.; Tsao, S.-M.; Hsu, J. Fucoidan induces changes in the epithelial to mesenchymal transition and decreases metastasis by enhancing ubiquitin-dependent TGFβ receptor degradation in breast cancer. *Carcinogenesis* **2013**, *34*, 874–884. [CrossRef] [PubMed]
6. Chen, M.-C.; Hsu, W.-L.; Hwang, P.-A.; Chou, T.-C. Low molecular weight fucoidan inhibits tumor angiogenesis through downregulation of HIF-1/VEGF signaling under hypoxia. *Mar. Drugs* **2015**, *13*, 4436–4451. [CrossRef] [PubMed]
7. Hsu, H.-Y.; Lin, T.-Y.; Wu, Y.-C.; Tsao, S.-M.; Hwang, P.-A.; Shih, Y.-W.; Hsu, J. Fucoidan inhibition of lung cancer in vivo and in vitro: Role of the Smurf2-dependent ubiquitin proteasome pathway in TGFβ receptor degradation. *Oncotarget* **2014**, *5*, 7870–7885. [CrossRef] [PubMed]
8. Tengdelius, M.; Lee, C.-J.; Grenegård, M.; Griffith, M.; Påhlsson, P.; Konradsson, P. Synthesis and biological evaluation of fucoidan-mimetic glycopolymers through cyanoxyl-mediated free-radical polymerization. *Biomacromolecules* **2014**, *15*, 2359–2368. [CrossRef] [PubMed]
9. Hwang, K.-A.; Yi, B.-R.; Choi, K.-C. Molecular mechanisms and in vivo mouse models of skin aging associated with dermal matrix alterations. *Lab. Anim. Res.* **2011**, *27*, 1–8. [CrossRef] [PubMed]
10. Hwang, P.-A.; Hung, Y.-L.; Chien, S.-Y. Inhibitory activity of sargassum hemiphyllum sulfated polysaccharide in arachidonic acid-induced animal models of inflammation. *J. Food Drug Anal.* **2015**, *23*, 49–56. [CrossRef]
11. Irhimeh, M.R.; Fitton, J.H.; Lowenthal, R.M. Pilot clinical study to evaluate the anticoagulant activity of fucoidan. *Blood Coagul. Fibrinolysis* **2009**, *20*, 607–610. [CrossRef] [PubMed]
12. Hwang, P.-A.; Hung, Y.-L.; Phan, N.N.; Hieu, B.-T.-N.; Chang, P.-M.; Li, K.-L.; Lin, Y.-C. The in vitro and in vivo effects of the low molecular weight fucoidan on the bone osteogenic differentiation properties. *Cytotechnology* **2015**. [CrossRef] [PubMed]
13. Yang, C.; Chung, D.; Shin, I.-S.; Lee, H.; Kim, J.; Lee, Y.; You, S. Effects of molecular weight and hydrolysis conditions on anticancer activity of fucoidans from sporophyll of *Undaria pinnatifida*. *Int. J. Biol. Macromol.* **2008**, *43*, 433–437. [CrossRef] [PubMed]
14. Soeda, S.; Sakaguchi, S.; Shimeno, H.; Nagamatsu, A. Fibrinolytic and anticoagulant activities of highly sulfated fucoidan. *Biochem. Pharmacol.* **1992**, *43*, 1853–1858. [CrossRef]

15. Park, S.-B.; Chun, K.-R.; Kim, J.-K.; Suk, K.; Jung, Y.-M.; Lee, W.-H. The differential effect of high and low molecular weight fucoidans on the severity of collagen-induced arthritis in mice. *Phytother. Res. PTR* **2010**, *24*, 1384–1391. [CrossRef] [PubMed]

16. Li, D.; Zhou, Z.-G.; Liu, H.; Wu, C. A new method of laminaria japonica strain selection and sporeling raising by the use of gametophyte clones. *Hydrobiologia* **1999**, *398*, 473–476. [CrossRef]

17. Wijesinghe, W.A.J.; Jeon, Y.J.P. Biological activities and potential industrial applications of fucose rich sulfated polysaccharides and fucoidans isolated from brown seaweeds: A review. *Carbohydr. Polym.* **2012**, *88*, 13–20. [CrossRef]

18. Li, N.; Zhang, Q.; Song, J. Toxicological evaluation of fucoidan extracted from *Laminaria japonica* in wistar rats. *Food Chem. Toxicol.* **2005**, *43*, 421–426. [CrossRef] [PubMed]

19. Laparra, J.M.; Velez, D.; Montoro, R.; Barbera, R.; Farré, R. Estimation of arsenic bioaccessibility in edible seaweed by an in vitro digestion method. *J. Agric. Food Chem.* **2003**, *51*, 6080–6085. [CrossRef] [PubMed]

20. Dopp, E.; Hartmann, L.; Florea, A.-M.; von Recklinghausen, U.; Pieper, R.; Shokouhi, B.; Rettenmeier, A.; Hirner, A.; Obe, G. Uptake of inorganic and organic derivatives of arsenic associated with induced cytotoxic and genotoxic effects in chinese hamster ovary (cho) cells. *Toxicol. Appl. Pharmacol.* **2004**, *201*, 156–165. [CrossRef] [PubMed]

21. Han, C.; Cao, X.; Yu, J.-J.; Wang, X.-R.; Shen, Y. Arsenic speciation in sargassum fusiforme by microwave-assisted extraction and LC-ICP-MS. *Chromatographia* **2009**, *69*, 587–591. [CrossRef]

22. Yamamoto, S.; Konishi, Y.; Matsuda, T.; Murai, T.; Shibata, M.-A.; Matsui-Yuasa, I.; Otani, S.; Kuroda, K.; Endo, G.; Fukushima, S. Cancer induction by an organic arsenic compound, dimethylarsinic acid (cacodylic acid), in F344/DuCrj rats after pretreatment with five carcinogens. *Cancer Res.* **1995**, *55*, 1271–1276. [PubMed]

23. Grandjean, P.; Landrigan, P.J. Neurobehavioural effects of developmental toxicity. *Lancet Neurol.* **2014**, *13*, 330–338. [CrossRef]

24. Chen, C.-J.; Wang, C.-J. Ecological correlation between arsenic level in well water and age-adjusted mortality from malignant neoplasms. *Cancer Res.* **1990**, *50*, 5470–5474. [PubMed]

25. Bates, M.N.; Smith, A.H.; Hopenhayn-Rich, C. Arsenic ingestion and internal cancers: A review. *Am. J. Epidemiol.* **1992**, *135*, 462–476. [PubMed]

26. Endo, G.; Kuroda, K.; Okamoto, A.; Horiguchi, S.I. Dimethylarsenic acid induces tetraploids in Chinese hamster cells. *Bull. Environ. Contam. Toxicol.* **1992**, *48*, 131–137. [CrossRef] [PubMed]

27. Zhao, Y.; Shang, D.; Ning, J.; Zhai, Y. Arsenic and cadmium in the marine macroalgae (porphyra yezoensis and *Laminaria japonica*)—Forms and concentrations. *Chem. Speciat. Bioavailab.* **2012**, *24*, 197–203. [CrossRef]

28. *Taiwan's "Act Governing Food Sanitation"*. Algae food hygiene standards issue, Taipei, Taiwan, 2013.

29. Sha, J.H.H.C.X.; Li, S.Q.; Ni, M.Z.; Deng, X.Y.; Cai, Y.P.; Yuan, B.J. *Hygienic Standard for Marine Algae and Algae Products*; Standardization Administration of China: Beijing, China, 2005.

30. Food Standards Australia New Zealand. *Food Standards Code*; Australian Government Publishing Service: Kingston, Australia, 1994.

31. Mabeau, S.; Fleurence, J. Seaweed in food products: Biochemical and nutritional aspects. *Trends Food Sci. Technol.* **1993**, *4*, 103–107. [CrossRef]

32. Kim, K.-J.; Lee, O.-H.; Lee, B.-Y. Genotoxicity studies on fucoidan from sporophyll of *Undaria pinnatifida*. *Food Chem. Toxicol.* **2010**, *48*, 1101–1104. [CrossRef] [PubMed]

33. Song, M.Y.; Ku, S.K.; Han, J.S. Genotoxicity testing of low molecular weight fucoidan from brown seaweeds. *Food Chem. Toxicol.* **2012**, *50*, 790–796. [CrossRef] [PubMed]

34. Claxton, L.D.; Allen, J.; Auletta, A.; Mortelmans, K.; Nestmann, E.; Zeiger, E. Guide for the *Salmonella typhimurium*/mammalian microsome tests for bacterial mutagenicity. *Mutat. Res./Genet. Toxicol.* **1987**, *189*, 83–91. [CrossRef]

35. Organisation for Economic Co-operation Development (OECD). *Test No. 471: Bacterial Reverse Mutation Test*; Organisation for Economic Co-operation Development Publishing: Paris, France, 1997.

36. Galloway, S.; Armstrong, M.; Reuben, C.; Colman, S.; Brown, B.; Cannon, C.; Bloom, A.; Nakamura, F.; Ahmed, M.; Duk, S. Chromosome aberrations and sister chromatid exchanges in chinese hamster ovary cells: Evaluations of 108 chemicals. *Environ. Mol. Mutagen.* **1987**, *10*, 1–35. [CrossRef] [PubMed]

37. Galloway, S. International workshop on standardisation of genotoxicity test procedures. Commentary. *Mutat. Res.* **1994**, *312*, 201. [CrossRef]

38. Kim, K.-J.; Lee, O.-H.; Lee, H.-H.; Lee, B.-Y. A 4-week repeated oral dose toxicity study of fucoidan from the sporophyll of *Undaria pinnatifida* in sprague-dawley rats. *Toxicology* **2010**, *267*, 154–158. [CrossRef] [PubMed]
39. Organisation for Economic Co-operation Development (OECD). *407: Repeated Dose 28-Day Oral Toxicity Study in Rodents*; Organisation for Economic Co-operation Development Guidelines For the Testing of Chemicals, Section 4; OECD Publishing: Paris, France, 2008.
40. Chung, H.J.; Jeun, J.; Houng, S.J.; Jun, H.J.; Kweon, D.K.; Lee, S.J. Toxicological evaluation of fucoidan from *Undaria pinnatifida*in vitro and in vivo. *Phytother. Res.* **2010**, *24*, 1078–1083. [PubMed]
41. Organisation for Economic Co-operation Development (OECD). *423: Acute Oral Toxicity-Acute Toxic Class Method*; Organisation for Economic Co-operation Development Guidelines for the Testing of Chemicals; OECD Publishing: Paris, France, 2001; pp. 1–14.
42. Gideon, T.P.; Rengasamy, R. Toxicological evaluation of fucoidan from *Cladosiphon okamuranus*. *J. Med. Food* **2008**, *11*, 638–642. [CrossRef] [PubMed]
43. Zhang, Q.; Li, N.; Zhao, T.; Qi, H.; Xu, Z.; Li, Z. Fucoidan inhibits the development of proteinuria in active heymann nephritis. *Phytother. Res.* **2005**, *19*, 50–53. [CrossRef] [PubMed]
44. Toth, P.P. Triglyceride-rich lipoproteins as a causal factor for cardiovascular disease. *Vasc. Health Risk Manag.* **2016**, *12*, 171. [CrossRef] [PubMed]
45. Wang, S.; Song, K.; Srivastava, R.; Fathzadeh, M.; Li, N.; Mani, A. The protective effect of transcription factor 7-like 2 risk allele rs7903146 against elevated fasting plasma triglyceride in type 2 diabetes: A meta-analysis. *J. Diabetes Res.* **2015**, *2015*. [CrossRef] [PubMed]
46. Huang, L.; Wen, K.; Gao, X.; Liu, Y. Hypolipidemic effect of fucoidan from *Laminaria japonica* in hyperlipidemic rats. *Pharm. Biol.* **2010**, *48*, 422–426. [CrossRef] [PubMed]
47. Thomes, P.; Rajendran, M.; Pasanban, B.; Rengasamy, R. Cardioprotective activity of *Cladosiphon okamuranus* fucoidan against isoproterenol induced myocardial infarction in rats. *Phytomedicine* **2010**, *18*, 52–57. [CrossRef] [PubMed]
48. Sharp, P.; Villano, J.S. *The Laboratory Rat*; CRC Press: Boca Raton, FL, USA, 2012.
49. Abe, S.; Hiramatsu, K.; Ichikawa, O.; Kawamoto, H.; Kasagi, T.; Miki, Y.; Kimura, T.; Ikeda, T. Safety evaluation of excessive ingestion of mozuku fucoidan in human. *J. Food Sci.* **2013**, *78*, T648–T651. [CrossRef] [PubMed]
50. Yokota, T.; Nagashima, M.; Ghazizadeh, M.; Kawanami, O. Increased effect of fucoidan on lipoprotein lipase secretion in adipocytes. *Life Sci.* **2009**, *84*, 523–529. [CrossRef] [PubMed]

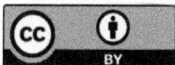

marine drugs

MDPI

Article

Purification and Characterization of a New Alginate Lyase from Marine Bacterium *Vibrio* sp. SY08

Shangyong Li [1,†], Linna Wang [1,†], Jianhua Hao [1,2,*], Mengxin Xing [1], Jingjing Sun [1] and Mi Sun [1,2,*]

[1] Key Laboratory of Sustainable Development of Marine Fisheries, Ministry of Agriculture, Yellow Sea Fisheries Research Institute, Chinese Academy of Fishery Sciences, 106 Nanjing Road, Qingdao 266071, China; lshywln@163.com (S.L.); wlnwfllsy@163.com (L.W.); 15865506157@126.com (M.X.); sunjj@ysfri.ac.cn (J.S.)

[2] Laboratory for Marine Drugs and Bioproducts, Qingdao National Laboratory for Marine Science and Technology, Qingdao 266237, China

* Correspondence: haojh@ysfri.ac.cn (J.H.); sunmi0532@yahoo.com (M.S.); Tel./Fax: +86-532-8581-9525 (J.H. & M.S)

† These authors contributed equally to this paper.

Academic Editor: Paola Laurienzo

Received: 24 November 2016; Accepted: 19 December 2016; Published: 23 December 2016

Abstract: Unsaturated alginate disaccharides (UADs), enzymatically derived from the degradation of alginate polymers, are considered powerful antioxidants. In this study, a new high UAD-producing alginate lyase, AlySY08, has been purified from the marine bacterium *Vibrio* sp. SY08. AlySY08, with a molecular weight of about 33 kDa and a specific activity of 1070.2 U/mg, showed the highest activity at 40 °C in phosphate buffer at pH 7.6. The enzyme was stable over a broad pH range (6.0–9.0) and retained about 75% activity after incubation at 40 °C for 2 h. Moreover, the enzyme was active in the absence of salt ions and its activity was enhanced by the addition of NaCl and KCl. AlySY08 resulted in an endo-type alginate lyase that degrades both polyM and polyG blocks, yielding UADs as the main product (81.4% of total products). All these features made AlySY08 a promising candidate for industrial applications in the production of antioxidants from alginate polysaccharides.

Keywords: alginate lyase; thermostability; unsaturated alginate disaccharides; *Vibrio* sp.

1. Introduction

Alginate is a linear hetero-polyuronic acid polymer, composed of β-D-mannuronate (M) and its C5 epimer α-L-guluronate (G), which can be arranged as polyM blocks, polyG blocks, and alternating or random polyMG blocks [1–3]. It is the most abundant carbohydrate in brown algae and approximately 30,000 tons of alginate are produced worldwide annually [3–5]. The alginate polymer is a commercially valuable polysaccharide widely used in the food and pharmaceutical industries mainly due to its high viscosity and gelling properties [1,3,6].

Alginate lyases catalyze the depolymerization of alginate through a β-elimination reaction between uronic acids in the linear polymer, thus producing unsaturated alginate oligosaccharides (UAOs) with double bonds between C4 and C5 at the non-reducing ends [7,8]. UAOs are endowed with an excellent antioxidant activity, superior to ascorbic acid in lipid oxidation treatment [9,10]. Their antioxidant activity is dependent on the conjugated alkene acid structure occurring in UAOs from the enzymatic depolymerization of alginate [9]. Neither acid hydrolysis of alginate nor alginate monosaccharides present conjugated alkene acid structures, thus exhibiting a lower antioxidant activity in comparison with UAOs [11–13]. Moreover, the antioxidant activity is inversely related to the molecular weight of UAOs: the smaller the size of the UAOs, the higher the antioxidant activity [14].

As the minimum unit endowed with the peculiar antioxidant structure, the unsaturated alginate disaccharides (UADs) are thought to be the best antioxidants [9].

Thus far, hundreds of alginate lyases have been isolated and characterized from marine microorganisms, brown seaweeds and mollusks [7,8]. According to their action mechanism, alginate lyases are generally classified into endo- or exo-lytic enzymes [15,16]. The product of exo-type alginate lyases consists of alginate monosaccharides, while the main product of endo-type alginate lyases is a mixture of unsaturated alginate disaccharides, trisaccharides and tetrasaccharides [16,17]. High levels of UADs in the product are beneficial for their antioxidant activity. However, UADs are generally present in low proportions (less than 50% of the total) in the products of most alginate lyases, except for AlyL2 from *Agarivorans* sp. L11 [18–27]. Although the full-length alginate lyase, AlyL2-FL, is able to produce a high ratio of UADs (64.6% of the total product), the activity strictly depends on the NaCl concentration [22]. The desalting of UAOs, especially for UADs, is very difficult and represents an important limitation on UAD production and application [28]. Therefore, the discovery of new alginate lyases yielding high levels of UADs is of the utmost importance.

Here, we report the isolation and characterization of a new endo-type alginate lyase, AlySY08, from the marine bacterium *Vibrio* sp. SY08. AlySY08 is an enzyme yielding UADs as the main product (81.4% of the total) and its activity is independent of NaCl.

2. Results and Discussion

2.1. Isolation and Identification of Strain SY08

Through screening the sole carbon source, we detected 29 strains with alginate lyase activities in their culture supernatants. Among these strains, SY08 showed the highest activity and was selected it for further research. A 1411 bp fragment of the 16S rDNA gene of the strain SY08 (Genbank accession number: KY214288) was cloned and sequenced. The alignment of 16S rDNA gene sequences revealed that strain SY08 was 99% identical to the *Vibrio* strain. According to the phylogenetic position of its 16S rDNA (Figure 1), SY08 was assigned to the genus *Vibrio* and named *Vibrio* sp. SY08.

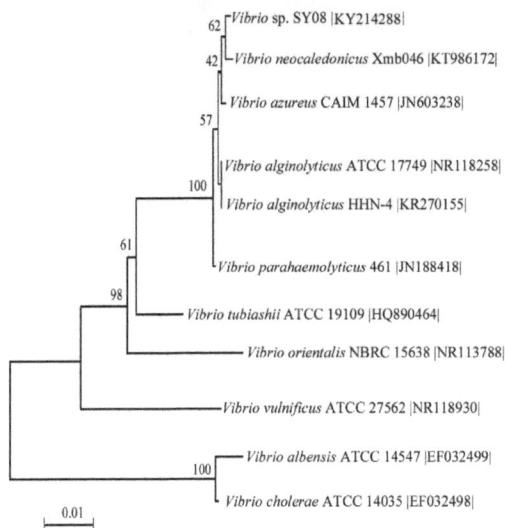

Figure 1. Phylogenetic tree of strain SY08 and related bacteria. The tree ID is based on a maximum parsimony analysis of the 16S rDNA sequences. The obtained 16S rDNA sequence was searched for and aligned by using the BLASTn and ClustalX programs, respectively. The phylogenetic tree was obtained by using MEGA 4.0 software.

2.2. Purification and Biochemical Characterization of AlySY08

The enzyme was purified to 13.1-fold homogeneity with a specific activity of 1070.2 U/mg. The purification was achieved through ammonia sulfate precipitation and only one hydrophobic interaction chromatography step (Table S1). The activity recovery of alginate lyase was 43.6%, and about 2.1 mg of purified AlySY08 could be obtained from 1 L of strain SY08 culture supernatant. The purity of AlySY08 was evaluated by SDS-PAGE, along with the molecular weight, estimated to be approximately 33 kDa (Figure 2).

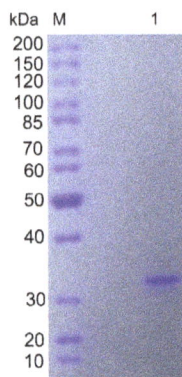

Figure 2. SDS-PAGE analysis of purified AlySY08. The purified AlySY08 was resolved by 10% acrylamide (*w/v*) SDS-PAGE followed by staining with Coomassie Blue G-250. Lane M, molecular weight markers; Lane 1, purified AlySY08.

AlySY08 showed the highest activity in phosphate buffer at pH 7.6 (Figure 3a), remaining stable in a range of pH 6.0–9.0 (Figure 3c). The optimal temperature of AlySY08 was 40 °C (Figure 3b). AlySY08 retained ~90% and ~75% of its activity after incubation at 30 °C and 40 °C for 120 min, respectively. It still retained ~40% of its activity after being incubated at 45 °C for 90 min or 50 °C for 40 min (Figure 3d). Because of the long half-life, high temperature stability and low production costs, thermostable enzymes are widely used in industrial applications. As previously reported, alginate lyases from the genera *Pseudoalteromonas*, *Agarivorans*, *Microbulbifer* and most of *Vibrio* are stable only at temperatures below 40 °C for less than 60 min [23,24,27,29,30]. Only few alginate lyases are thermostable, such as AlyV5 from *Vibrio* sp. QY105 which retains 40% of its activity after incubation at 60 °C for 60 min or 90 °C for 10 min [25]; the alginate lyase from *Isoptericola halotolerans* CGMCC 5336 which retains 60% of its activity after incubation at 40 °C for 180 min [18]; and AlyL2-FL from *Agarivorans* sp. L11 which retains 50% of its activity after incubation at 40 °C for 120 min or 50 °C for 70 min [22]. The main products of AlyV5 and the alginate lyase from *I. halotolerans* CGMCC 5336 consist of a mixture of hard-to-separate disaccharides, trisaccharides, tetrasaccharides and pentasaccharides [18,25,31]. In addition, both AlyV5 and AlyL2 are NaCl-dependent enzymes, since very low levels of enzymatic activities have been detected in the absence of NaCl [22,25].

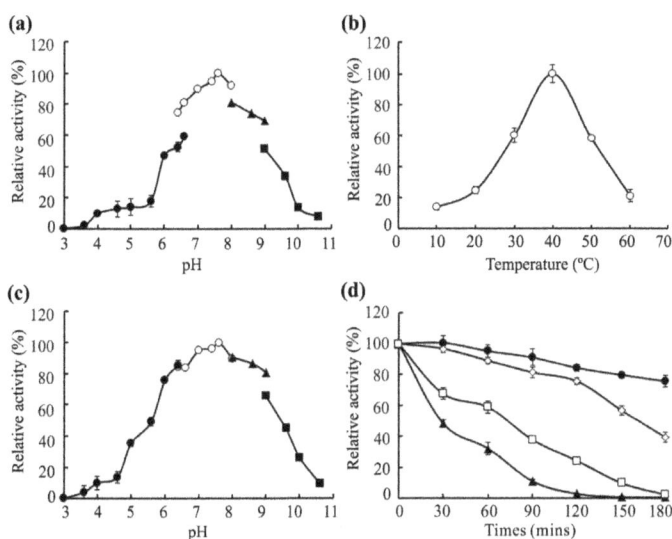

Figure 3. Effects of pH and temperature on the activity and stability of AlySY08. (**a**) The optimum pH for AlySY08 was determined by measuring its activity at 40 °C in 50 mM Na_2HPO_4-citric acid buffer (filled circle), 50 mM Na_2HPO_4-NaH_2PO_4 buffer (open circle), 50 mM Tris-HCl buffer (filled triangle) and 50 mM Gly-NaOH buffer (filled square); (**b**) The optimal temperature for AlySY08 was determined by measuring its activity at various temperatures (10–60 °C); (**c**) pH stability of AlySY08. The residual activity was measured at 40 °C in 50 mM phosphate buffer (pH 7.6) after incubation in the buffers reported above at 4 °C for 6 h; (**d**) Thermostability of AlySY08. The enzyme was incubated at 30 °C (filled circle), 40 °C (open rhombus), 45 °C (open square) and 50 °C (filled triangle) for various times. The residual activity was then determined at 40 °C. The activity of control (100% relative activity) is 12.6 U/mL.

Although the activity of AlySY08 could be enhanced by the addition of NaCl and KCl, the enzyme was still active in the absence of NaCl and KCl (Figure 4 and Table S2). In more detail, Cu^{2+}, Zn^{2+}, Mn^{2+}, Al^{3+} and Fe^{3+} inhibited the activity of AlySY08, while Mg^{2+} and Ca^{2+} enhanced its activity. Both of the chelating agents (EDTA and SDS) and the reducing agent (2-Mercaptoethanol) significantly inhibited the activity of AlySY08 (Table S2).

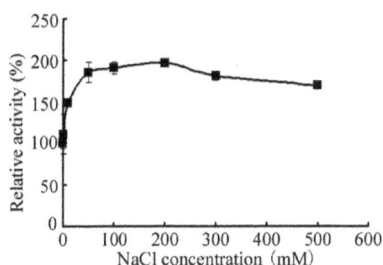

Figure 4. Effect of NaCl on enzymatic activity of AlySY08. The activity of AlySY08 in the absence of NaCl was retained at 100%. All the experiments were conducted in triplicate.

2.3. Substrate Specificity and Kinetic Parameters of AlySY08

The substrate specificity of AlySY08 was evaluated by using alginate, polyG blocks and polyM blocks as substrates. Among the assayed polymeric substrates, AlySY08 was revealed to be more active towards polyG blocks with respect to polyM blocks and alginate (Table 1).

Table 1. The substrate specificity and kinetic parameters of AlySY08.

Substrate	Relative Activity (%)	K_m (mg/mL)	V_{max} (U/mg)
Sodium alginate	100.0 ± 0.8	0.36 ± 0.04	1183.7 ± 21.5
PolyG blocks	123.8 ± 2.8	0.34 ± 0.02	1255.5 ± 14.7
PolyM blocks	28.2 ± 1.3	0.85 ± 0.16	512.9 ± 8.3

The activity towards sodium alginate was determined as the 100% relative activity. All the experiments were conducted in triplicate. The data are expressed as the mean $\pm$ SD.

The kinetic parameters of AlySY08 relative to the cleavage of various alginate polymers are also shown in Table 1. The apparent K_m of AlySY08 against sodium alginate, polyG blocks, and polyM blocks was 0.36, 0.34 and 0.85 mg/mL, respectively. The Vmax of AlySY08 against alginate, polyG blocks, and polyM blocks was 1183.7, 1255.5 and 512.9 U/mg, respectively. Both the specific activity and kinetic parameters indicated that AlySY08 is active towards both polyG and polyM blocks, but degrades the former more efficiently. As previously reported, most of the alginate lyases are polyM-preferred alginate lyases. Only few alginate lyases are polyG-preferred alginate lyases, including AlyV5 from *Vibrio* sp. QY105 [25], alginate lyase from *Vibrio* sp. 510-64 [28] and alginate lyase from *Streptomyces* sp. ALG-5 [30].

2.4. Mode of Enzyme Action and Reaction Products of AlySY08

The mode of the enzyme action was monitored by size-exclusion chromatography (Figure 5). The rapid degradation of the substrate, the increase in polydispersity and the production of intermediate oligosaccharides suggested that AlySY08 acts in an endo-lytic mode [23]. Moreover, as shown in the viscometric assay (Figure S1), after adding AlySY08, the viscosity of the alginate solution decreased rapidly in first 5 min, but changed little in the following 25 min. The amount of reducing sugar (A235) increased steadily during the whole observation period (Figure S1). All of these findings suggested that the enzyme is an endo-type enzyme.

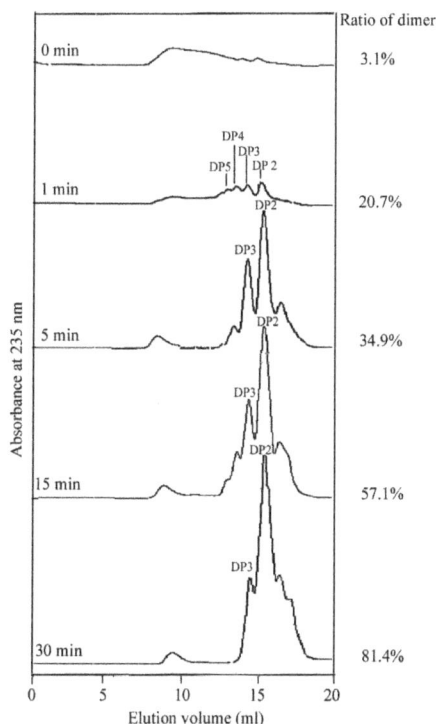

Figure 5. Size-exclusion chromatography of the alginate degradation products by AlySY08. The elution volumes of the dimer (DP2), trimer (DP3), tetramer (DP4), and pentamer (DP5) are 16.1 mL, 14.9 mL, 14.1 mL and 13.7 mL, respectively. The ratios of dimers present in the degradation products were analyzed by the peak integration function on the UNICORN 5.31 software (GE Healthcare, Madison, WI, USA).

Degradation products obtained from the most common endo-type alginate lyases are usually determined by TLC [7], clearly indicating that the main products are a mixture of alginate penta-, tetra-, tri- and di-saccharides [7,24–27,29]. However, when we analyzed the reaction products of AlySY08 by TLC, we observed only one spot on the TLC plate. The migration rate of this spot was in good agreement with the UAD marker (Figure 6a). When the reaction products of AlySY08 were analyzed by size-exclusion chromatography with a Superdex peptide 10/300 column, UADs were revealed as the main product (81.4% of the total product). The reaction products were further identified by negative ESI-MS. As reported in Figure 6b, the main peaks at 351.05 m/z [ΔDP2-H]$^{-}$ and 175.02 m/z [ΔDP2-2H]$^{2-}$ corresponded with the UAD [26]. All of these results indicated that the main product of AlySY08 consists of UADs.

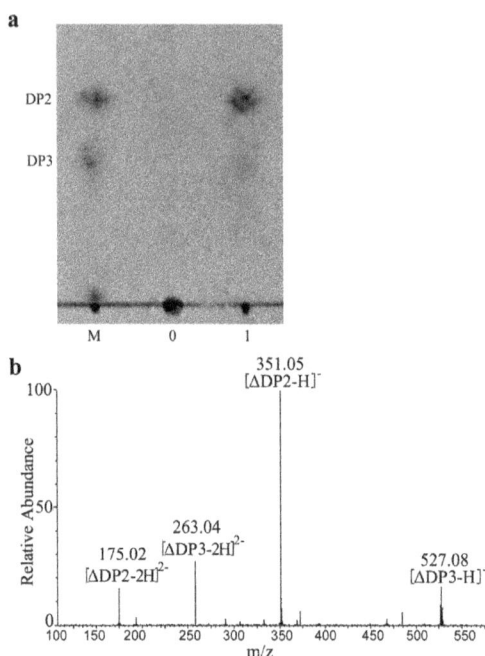

Figure 6. TLC and ESI-MS analysis of the main products of AlySY08. (**a**) TLC analysis. The reaction products were separated on a HPTLC plate with *n*-butanol/formic acid/water (2:1:1, by vol) and visualized with a diphenylamine/aniline/phosphate reagent. Lane M: standard UAOs mixture, disaccharide (DP2) and trisaccharide (DP3); Lane 0 sodium alginate; Lane 1 reaction products; (**b**) ESI-MS analysis of the main products by AlySY08.

If compared with other alginate lyases, AlySY08 shows the highest UAD-yielding levels (Table 2). A high ratio of UADs in the mixture of products is beneficial for antioxidant activity. Recently, depolymerization products of many other alginate lyases were also characterized by using size-exclusion chromatography (Table 2). Although the full-length alginate lyase AlyL2-FL produces a high ratio of UADs (64.6% of the total), its activity is strictly dependent on the NaCl concentration [22]. The concentration of UADs produced by the mutated alginate lyase MJ3-Arg236Ala, from *Sphingomonas* sp. MJ-3 is about 80.6% towards polyM blocks, about 47.1% towards polyMG blocks and only 37.5% towards alginate [17].

Table 2. Comparison of the main products of AlySY08 with other alginate lyases.

Enzyme	Source	Main Products (DP)	Ratio of Dimer (%) [a]	Reference
AlySY08	*Vibrio* sp. SY08	2	81.4	This study
AlyL2-FL	*Agarivorans* sp. L11	2–3	64.6	[22]
AlyL2-CM	*Agarivorans* sp. L11	2–3	52.6	[22]
AlyL1	*Agarivorans* sp. L11	2–3	47.3	[23]
MJ3-Arg236Ala	*Sphingomonas* sp. MJ-3	2–5	37.9	[17]
AlgMsp	*Microbulbifer* sp. 6532A	2–5	37.5	[26]
AlyA1	*Zobellia galactanivorans*	2–6	19.0	[24]
Aly5	*Flammeovirga* sp. MY04	2–7	15.7	[19]

[a] The ratio of dimers was determined by the peak integration function of the UNICORN 5.31 software.

3. Materials and Methods

3.1. Isolation and Identification of Strain SY08

Decayed brown seaweed samples were collected from the coastal zone of Jiaozhou Bay, Qingdao, China. They were immersed, diluted, and spread on the fermentation medium agar plate (5 g sodium alginate, 30 g NaCl, 0.01 g $MgSO_4$, 2 g $(NH_4)_2SO_4$, 0.02 g $FeSO_4$, 3 g K_2HPO_4, 7 g KH_2PO_4, 15 g agar in 1 L distilled water, pH 6.5). The plates were incubated at 25 °C for two days to form the detectable colonies. At least 300 strains were inoculated into selective medium without agar and assayed for alginate lyase activity in the culture supernatant. The 16S rDNA gene was amplified according to the method described by Wang et al. 2013 [25]. The obtained 16S rDNA gene sequence was searched and aligned with its closely related sequences retrieved from GenBank using the BLASTn (National Center of Biotechnology Information, Bethesda, MD, USA) and Clustal W programs (Conway Institute UCD Dublin, Dublin, Ireland). Multiple sequence alignments were obtained using ClustalX 1.83 (Conway Institute UCD Dublin, Dublin, Ireland), and the phylogenetic tree was constructed with the MEGA 4.0 software (Biodesign Institute, Arizona State University, Tempe, AZ, USA).

3.2. Purification of AlySY08

Strain SY08 was inoculated in 1 L selective medium and cultured at 25 °C for 48 h with shaking at 120 rpm. The culture supernatant of strain SY08 was obtained by centrifugation at 12,000× *g* for 10 min. Then, ammonium sulfate was added to a final saturation of 40% and incubated for 2 h. After centrifugation (12,000× *g*, 30 min), the supernatant was loaded onto a Phenyl-Sepharose column (1.6 cm × 20 cm) equilibrated with 50 mM phosphate buffer (pH 7.6), then eluted with a linear gradient of $(NH_4)_2SO_4$ (1.5–0 M, 100 mL) at a flow rate of 1 mL/min. All steps of enzyme purification were carried out at 4 °C. The active fractions were stored at −20 °C. The molecular weight of purified AlySY08 was determined by SDS-PAGE. The protein concentration was determined by the Bradford method with bovine serum albumin (BSA) as standard.

3.3. Alginate Lyase Activity Assay

Alginate lyase activity was measured as the increase in the absorbance at 235 nm. In brief, the enzymatic reaction was conducted with 100 µL of enzyme solution and 900 µL of substrate solution (0.3% (*w*/*v*) alginate, 50 mM phosphate buffer, pH 7.6) at 40 °C for 10 min. One unit (U) was defined as the amount of the enzyme required to increase by 0.1 the absorbance at 235 nm per minute. For the study of substrate specificities, polyM blocks and polyG blocks were used as substrates in the same conditions.

3.4. Effects of Temperature, pH, Metal Ions and Chelators

The optimum pH of the enzyme was determined by measuring its activity in different buffers at 40 °C for 10 min [23]. Its optimal temperature was determined by measuring its activity in a range of 10–60 °C in 50 mM phosphate buffer (pH 7.6). To determine pH stability of AlySY08, the residual activity was measured after enzyme was incubated in different buffers for 6 h at 4 °C. The thermostability of the enzyme was evaluated by measuring the residual activity after the enzyme in 50 mM phosphate buffer (pH 7.6) was incubated at 30 °C, 40 °C, 45 °C and 50 °C for different times (0, 30, 60, 90, 120, 150, 180 min). The effects of metal ions and chelators on AlySY08 activity were examined by monitoring the enzymatic activity in the presence of various cation ions or chelators.

3.5. Enzymatic Kinetic Parameters Assay

To measure the kinetic parameters of AlySY08, 10 different concentrations (ranging from 0.1 to 8 mg/mL) of alginate, polyM blocks and polyG blocks in 50 mM phosphate buffer (pH 7.6) were incubated at 40 °C for 10 min. AlySY08 was then added to a final concentration of 10 nM, and incubated at 40 °C for 3 min. The K_m and V_{max} values were calculated by double-reciprocal plots of Lineweaver and Burk [27].

3.6. Analysis of Reaction Mode and Products

The reaction mixture containing 0.5 mL (20 U) of purified AlySY08 and 2 mL of sodium alginate (1 mg/mL) in 50 mM phosphate buffer (pH 7.6) was incubated at 40 °C for 1, 5, 15 or 30 min. Reaction products were analyzed by the fast protein liquid chromatography (FPLC) with a Superdex peptide 10/300 gel filtration column (GE Healthcare, Madison, WI, USA) as previously described by Li et al. 2015 [22,23]. Then, products obtained from the enzymatic action (30 min) of AlySY08 on alginate were further characterized by using thin-layer chromatography (TLC) and negative-ion electrospray ionization mass spectrometry (ESI-MS), as previously reported [26,28]. To further determine its action mode, the viscometric assay was done using as Ostwald viscometer (No. 1; Shibata Scientific Technology LTD., Soka-City, Saitama, Japan) [32]. Briefly, mixtures of 5 mL AlySY08 (5 U/mL) and 50 mL sodium alginate (2 g/L in 20 mM phosphate buffer, pH 7.6) were incubated at 40 °C for up to 30 min. An aliquot of enzymatic product (0.5 mL) was taken out at different times (1, 5, 10, 15 and 30 min) in order to determine the viscosity and degradation products.

4. Conclusions

In this study, AlySY08, an alginate lyase from the marine bacterium *Vibrio* sp. SY08, was purified and characterized. AlySY08 showed the highest activity at 40 °C in phosphate buffer at pH 7.6. The enzyme was stable over a broad pH range (6.0–9.0) and active in the absence of salt ions. AlySY08 yielded UADs, a promising class of molecules with powerful antioxidant activity, as the main product (81.4% of the total product), thus representing an interesting candidate for industrial applications. Further works will be focused on gene cloning and elucidating the molecular mechanism of action of AlySY08, along with the determination of its three-dimensional structure.

Supplementary Materials: The following are available online at www.mdpi.com/1660-3397/15/1/1/s1, Table S1: Summary of AlySY08 purification, Table S2: Effect of metal ions, chelators and detergents on the activity of AlySY08, Figure S1: Viscosity reduction during enzymatic degradation of alginate. The initial viscosity of the reaction mixture without enzyme was taken as 100%. Open circles with solid line rate of viscosity reduction; filled circles with dotted line absorbance at 235 nm.

Acknowledgments: This project was funded by the National Science Foundation-Joint Fund (U1406402-5); the International Science and Technology Cooperation and Exchanges (2014DFG30890); The Scientific and Technological Innovation Project Financially Supported by the Qingdao National Laboratory for Marine Science and Technology (2015ASKJ02-06); the National High-tech R&D Program of China (2014AA093516); the National Natural Science Foundation of China (41506218 and 41376175); the Postdoctoral Science Foundation of China (2015M582170 and 2016M590673); the Postdoctoral Science Foundation of Shandong; the Postdoctoral Researcher Applied Research Project of Qingdao (Q51201613 and Q51201601).

Author Contributions: S.L., J.H. and M.S. conceived and designed the experiments. S.L., L.W., J.S. and M.X. performed the experiments. S.L., L.W. and J.H. analyzed the data. S.L., L.W. and M.S. wrote the main manuscript text. All authors reviewed the manuscript.

Conflicts of Interest: The authors declare no conflict of interest.

References

1. Lee, K.Y.; Mooney, D.J. Alginate: Properties and biomedical applications. *Prog. Polym. Sci.* **2012**, *37*, 106–126. [CrossRef] [PubMed]
2. Momoh, F.U.; Boateng, J.S.; Richardson, S.C.; Chowdhry, B.Z.; Mitchell, J.C. Development and functional characterization of alginate dressing as potential protein delivery system for wound healing. *Int. J. Biol. Macromol.* **2015**, *81*, 137–150. [CrossRef] [PubMed]
3. Pawar, S.N.; Edgar, K.J. Alginate derivatization: A review of chemistry, properties and application. *Biomaterials* **2012**, *33*, 3279–3305. [CrossRef] [PubMed]

4. Enquist-Newman, M.; Faust, A.M.; Bravo, D.D.; Santos, C.N.; Raisner, R.M.; Hanel, A.; Sarvabhowman, P.; Le, C.; Regitsky, D.D.; Cooper, S.R.; et al. Efficient ethanol production from brown macroalgae sugars by a synthetic yeast platform. *Nature* **2014**, *505*, 239–243. [CrossRef] [PubMed]

5. Wargacki, A.J.; Leonard, E.; Win, M.N.; Regitsky, D.D.; Santos, C.N.; Kim, P.B.; Cooper, S.R.; Raisner, R.M.; Herman, A.; Sivitz, A.B.; et al. An engineered microbial platform for direct biofuel production from brown macroalgae. *Science* **2012**, *335*, 308–313. [CrossRef] [PubMed]

6. Formo, K.; Aarstad, O.A.; Skjåk-Bræk, G.; Strand, B.L. Lyase-catalyzed degradation of alginate in the gelled state: Effect of gelling ions and lyase specificity. *Carbohydr. Polym.* **2014**, *110*, 100–106. [CrossRef] [PubMed]

7. Kim, H.S.; Chu, Y.J.; Park, C.H.; Lee, E.Y.; Kim, H.S. Site-directed mutagenesis-based functional analysis and characterization of endolytic lyase activity of N- and C-terminal domains of a novel oligoalginate lyase from *Sphingomonas* sp. MJ-3 possessing exolytic lyase activity in the intact enzyme. *Mar. Biotechnol.* **2015**, *17*, 782–792. [CrossRef] [PubMed]

8. Wong, T.; Preston, L.; Schiller, N. Alginate lyase: Review of major sources and enzyme characteristics, structure-function analysis, biological roles, and applications. *Annu. Rev. Microbiol.* **2000**, *54*, 289–340. [CrossRef] [PubMed]

9. Falkeborg, M.; Cheong, L.Z.; Gianfico, C.; Sztukiel, K.M.; Kristensen, K.; Glasius, M.; Xu, X.; Guo, Z. Alginate oligosaccharides: Enzymatic preparation and antioxidant property evaluation. *Food Chem.* **2014**, *164*, 185–194. [CrossRef] [PubMed]

10. Ueno, M.; Hiroki, T.; Takeshita, S.; Jiang, Z.D.; Kim, D.; Yamaguchi, K.; Oda, T. Comparative study on antioxidative and macrophage-stimulating activities of polyguluronic acid (PG) and polymannuronic acid (PM) prepared from alginate. *Carbohydr. Res.* **2012**, *352*, 88–93. [CrossRef] [PubMed]

11. Küpper, F.C.; Müller, D.G.; Peters, A.F.; Kloareg, B.; Potin, P. Oligoalginate recognition and oxidative burst play a key role in natural and induced resistance of sporophytes of laminariales. *J. Chem. Ecol.* **2002**, *28*, 2057–2081. [CrossRef] [PubMed]

12. Trommer, H.; Neubert, R.H. The examination of polysaccharides as potential antioxidative compounds for topical administration using a lipid model system. *Int. J. Pharm.* **2005**, *298*, 153–163. [CrossRef] [PubMed]

13. Wang, P.; Jiang, X.L.; Jiang, Y.H.; Hu, X.K.; Mou, H.J.; Li, M.; Guan, H. In vitro antioxidative activities of three marine oligosaccharides. *Nat. Prod. Res.* **2007**, *21*, 646–654. [CrossRef] [PubMed]

14. Zhou, X.X.; Xu, J.; Ding, Y.T. Alginate-derived oligosaccharides product by alginate lyase and detection of the antioxidant activity. *Food. Fement. Ind.* **2014**. [CrossRef]

15. Wang, L.N.; Li, S.Y.; Yu, W.G.; Gong, Q.H. Cloning, overexpression and characterization of a new oligoalginate lyase from a marine bacterium, *Shewanella* sp. *Biotechnol. Lett.* **2015**, *37*, 665–671. [CrossRef] [PubMed]

16. Li, S.Y.; Wang, L.N.; Han, F.; Gong, Q.H.; Yu, W.G. Cloning and characterization of the first polysaccharide lyase family 6 oligoalginate lyase from marine *Shewanella* sp. Kz7. *J. Biochem.* **2015**. [CrossRef]

17. Kim, H.S.; Lee, C.G.; Lee, E.Y. Alginate lyase: Structure, property, and application. *Biotechnol. Bioprocess Eng.* **2011**, *16*, 843–851. [CrossRef]

18. Dou, W.F.; Wei, D.; Li, H.; Rahman, M.M.; Shi, J.S.; Xu, Z.H.; Xu, Z.; Ma, Y. Purification and characterisation of a bifunctional alginate lyase from novel *Isoptericola halotolerans* CGMCC 5336. *Carbohydr. Polym.* **2013**, *98*, 1476–1482. [CrossRef] [PubMed]

19. Han, W.J.; Gu, J.Y.; Cheng, Y.Y.; Liu, H.H.; Li, Y.Z.; Li, F.C. A novel alginate lyase (Aly5) from a polysaccharide-degrading marine bacterium *Flammeovirga* sp. MY04: Effects of module truncation to the biochemical characteristics, alginate-degradation patterns, and oligosaccharide-yielding properties. *Appl. Environ. Microbiol.* **2015**, *82*, 364–374. [CrossRef] [PubMed]

20. Hu, X.K.; Jiang, X.L.; Hwang, H.M. Purification and characterization of an alginate lyase from marine bacterium *Vibrio* sp. mutant strain 510-64. *Curr. Microbiol.* **2006**, *53*, 135–140. [CrossRef] [PubMed]

21. Ertesvåg, H. Alginate-modifying enzymes: Biological roles and biotechnological uses. *Front. Microbiol.* **2015**. [CrossRef] [PubMed]

22. Li, S.Y.; Yang, X.M.; Bao, M.M.; Yu, W.G.; Han, F. Family 13 carbohydrate-binding module of alginate lyase from *Agarivorans* sp. L11 enhances its catalytic efficiency and thermostability, and alters its substrate preference and product distribution. *FEMS. Microb. Lett.* **2015**. [CrossRef] [PubMed]

23. Li, S.Y.; Yang, X.M.; Zhang, L.; Yu, W.G.; Han, F. Cloning, expression, and characterization of a cold-adapted and surfactant-stable alginate lyase from marine bacterium *Agarivorans* sp. L11. *J. Microbiol. Biotechnol.* **2015**, *25*, 681–686. [CrossRef] [PubMed]

24. Thomas, F.; Lundqvist, L.C.; Jam, M.; Jeudy, A.; Barbeyron, T.; Sandström, C.; Michel, G.; Czjzek, M. Comparative characterization of two marine alginate lyases from *Zobellia galactanivorans* reveals distinct modes of action and exquisite adaptation to their natural substrate. *J. Biol. Chem.* **2013**, *288*, 23021–23037. [CrossRef] [PubMed]

25. Wang, Y.; Guo, E.W.; Yu, W.G.; Han, F. Purification and characterization of a new alginate lyase from marine bacterium *Vibrio* sp. *Biotechnol. Lett.* **2013**, *35*, 703–708. [CrossRef] [PubMed]

26. Swift, S.M.; Hudgens, J.W.; Heselpoth, R.D.; Bales, P.M.; Nelson, D.C. Characterization of AlgMsp, an alginate lyase from *Microbulbifer* sp. 6532A. *PLoS ONE* **2014**, *9*, e112939. [CrossRef] [PubMed]

27. Zhu, B.W.; Tan, H.D.; Qin, Y.Q.; Xu, Q.S.; Du, Y.G.; Yin, H. Characterization of a new endo-type alginate lyase from *Vibrio* sp. W13. *Int. J. Biol. Macromol.* **2015**, *75*, 330–337. [CrossRef] [PubMed]

28. Hu, T.; Li, C.X.; Zhao, X.; Yu, G.L.; Guan, H.S. Preparation and characterization of guluronic acid oligosaccharides degraded by a rapid microwave irradiation method. *Carbohydr. Res.* **2013**, *373*, 53–58. [CrossRef] [PubMed]

29. Huang, L.S.X.; Zhou, J.G.; Li, X.; Peng, Q.; Lu, H.; Du, Y.G. Characterization of a new alginate lyase from newly isolated *Flavobacterium* sp. S20. *J. Ind. Microbiol. Biotechnol.* **2013**, *40*, 113–122. [CrossRef] [PubMed]

30. Kim, D.E.; Lee, E.Y.; Kim, H.S. Cloning and characterization of alginate lyase from a marine bacterium *Streptomyces* sp. ALG-5. *Mar. Biotechnol.* **2009**, *11*, 10–16. [CrossRef] [PubMed]

31. Li, J.W.; Dong, S.; Song, J.; Li, C.B.; Chen, X.L.; Xie, B.B.; Zhang, Y.-Z. Purification and characterization of a bifunctional alginate lyase from *Pseudoalteromonas* sp. SM0524. *Mar. Drugs* **2011**, *9*, 109–123. [CrossRef] [PubMed]

32. Kobayashi, T.; Uchimura, K.; Miyazaki, M.; Nogi, Y.; Hori-koshi, K. A new high-alkaline alginate lyase from a deep-sea bacterium *Agarivorans* sp. *Extremophiles* **2009**, *13*, 121–129. [CrossRef] [PubMed]

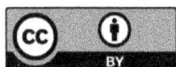

Article

Preparation, Characterization and Properties of Alginate/Poly(γ-glutamic acid) Composite Microparticles

Zongrui Tong [1], Yu Chen [1,*], Yang Liu [1], Li Tong [2,*], Jiamian Chu [3], Kecen Xiao [1], Zhiyu Zhou [1], Wenbo Dong [1] and Xingwu Chu [3]

[1] School of Material Science and Engineering, Beijing Institute of Technology, Beijing 100081, China; zrtong@163.com (Z.T.); lyang425@yeah.net (Y.L.); xiaokecen@163.com (K.X.); zhouzhiyuandy@163.com (Z.Z.); dwb194413@126.com (W.D.)
[2] Department of Biochemistry and Molecular Biology, Beijing Normal University, Beijing 100875, China
[3] Taizhou Roosin Medical Co., Ltd., Taizhou 225300, China; jameschu@roosin.com (J.C.); rongxingchu@roosin.net (X.C.)
*   Correspondence: cylsy@163.com (Y.C.); tongli29@bnu.edu.cn (L.T.); Tel.: +86-136-8318-3781 (Y.C.)

Academic Editors: Paola Laurienzo and Anake Kijjoa
Received: 27 November 2016; Accepted: 20 March 2017; Published: 11 April 2017

Abstract: Alginate (Alg) is a renewable polymer with excellent hemostatic properties and biocapability and is widely used for hemostatic wound dressing. However, the swelling properties of alginate-based wound dressings need to be promoted to meet the requirements of wider application. Poly(γ-glutamic acid) (PGA) is a natural polymer with high hydrophility. In the current study, novel Alg/PGA composite microparticles with double network structure were prepared by the emulsification/internal gelation method. It was found from the structure characterization that a double network structure was formed in the composite microparticles due to the ion chelation interaction between Ca^{2+} and the carboxylate groups of Alg and PGA and the electrostatic interaction between the secondary amine group of PGA and the carboxylate groups of Alg and PGA. The swelling behavior of the composite microparticles was significantly improved due to the high hydrophility of PGA. Influences of the preparing conditions on the swelling behavior of the composites were investigated. The porous microparticles could be formed while compositing of PGA. Thermal stability was studied by thermogravimetric analysis method. Moreover, in vitro cytocompatibility test of microparticles exhibited good biocompatibility with L929 cells. All results indicated that such Alg/PGA composite microparticles are a promising candidate in the field of wound dressing for hemostasis or rapid removal of exudates.

Keywords: alginate; poly(γ-glutamic acid); emulsification/internal gelation method; microparticle; swelling behavior

1. Introduction

Wound healing is a complex process with sequential phases and demands a proper environment. Because hydrogels keep the wound surface in a moist environment, they could promote healing, according to the early work by Winters [1]. Advanced dressings should possess ideal swelling behavior to absorb exudates quickly, keep proper moisture in the covering areas and be easily removed [2,3]. Numerous super-absorbent materials have been investigated and applied for wound healing [4–6]. Furthermore, natural polysaccharides were studied to produce super-absorbent composites as substitutes of non-biodegradable synthetic polymers [7,8]. Among them, alginate has been widely investigated for wound dressings [9,10].

Alginate is a renewable resource and widely derived from brown algae [10,11]. Due to its non-toxicity, biocompatibility and ability to promote cell proliferation [12–15], it is widely used in tissue engineering, drug delivery and wound dressing, etc. The alginate-based wound dressings could absorb water up to several times their own weight [16–18]. However, wound dressings with higher swelling behavior are required as reported in the literature to help hemostasis, autolytic debridement, increased collagenase production and the moisture content of necrotic wounds. For example, Burn shield hydrogel dressing (Levtrade International) is polyurethane foam that can absorb more than 30 times its own weight in water [19,20]. A hemostatic wound dressing for severe artery hemorrhage could absorb massive water [21].

In previous studies, a natural hydrophilic polymer like poly(γ-glutamic acid) (PGA) was chosen for a composite with alginate instead of synthetic super-absorbent polymers. Alg/PGA composite hydrogel was prepared with improved swelling property [22]. Layered hydrogel with poly(γ-glutamic acid), sodium alginate and chitosan was prepared and characterized [23]. Poly(γ-glutamic acid) is a unique natural anionic homo-polyamide which can be produced by the fermentations by common *Bacillus* microbes [24]. It has been widely used in food and cosmetics industries due to its biocompatiblity and biodegradability. In addition, its potential application as microcapsules for drug delivery has also attracted considerable interest in recent years [25,26]. PGA is highly hydrophilic and could promote the absorption behavior of composite biomaterials by mixing it with another matrix [27].

Recently, preparation of highly hydrophilic Alg/PGA microparticles has attracted considerable attention. Suzuki et al. prepared core-shell Alg/PGA microparticles by dropping alginate solution into $CaCl_2$ solution and coating the alginate microparticles with PGA [28]. Wang et al. dropped Alg/PGA mixture solution directly into $CaCl_2$ solution to prepare Alg/PGA microparticles [29]. All the above works used the coacervation method to prepare Alg/PGA microparticles. In a typical coacervation process, an alginate solution is dropped into a calcium chloride solution to form microparticles by a crosslinking reaction [30]. The reaction occurs rapidly and the structure of the microparticle product is uncontrollable. In contrast, the emulsification/internal gelation technique is an effective way to prepare the microparticles with the controllable structure with the aid of the moderate crosslinking reaction in the emulsion droplets [31–35]. However, this method was still not used in the preparation of the Alg/PGA composite microparticles.

In the present study, the Alg/PGA composite microparticles with controllable structure were prepared using the emulsification/internal gelation method, and then the conditions to control the structure and properties of the composite microparticles were studied and discussed. The emulsification/internal gelation method could promote the properties and widen the application of these microparticles.

2. Results and Discussion

2.1. Characterization of Alg/PGA Composite Microparticles

Figure 1 shows the FT-IR spectra of alginate, PGA and Alg/PGA microparticles prepared under different conditions. The stretching vibrations of the O–H in alginate and PGA led to broad absorption bands centered at 3446 cm^{-1} and 3444 cm^{-1} respectivley [36]. The corresponding absorption band of microparticles shifted to 3420 cm^{-1}, indicating the presence of hydrogen bonds between alginate and PGA.

The asymmetric stretching vibration peak of the C=O in the carboxylate (COO^-) was observed at 1631 cm^{-1} and belongs to PGA. The corresponding peak was blue-shifted in the spectrum of the composite microparticles due to the chelating action between the COO^- and Ca^{2+}. A maximum shift to 1614 cm^{-1} was observed in the spectra of the composite microparticles prepared with $m_{Alg}:m_{PGA}$ = 7:3 and 8:2, indicating that the strongest chelation interaction occurred in these composites. Alginate is a water-soluble anionic polysaccharide consisting of repeat units of mannuronic acid and glucuronic acid. The electrostatic interaction occurs between the carboxylate groups of alginate and high valent cations [35]. The chelating interaction between Ca^{2+} and carboxylate groups of glucuronic acid and PGA is also a possible interaction in the emulsification/internal gelation method.

The absorption peak at 1126 cm^{-1} in the spectrum of PGA was assigned to the C–N stretching vibration of the secondary amine. The corresponding peak of the composite microparticles was shifted dramatically to 1095 cm^{-1} due to a strong electrostatic interaction between the amide group of PGA and the carboxylate group of alginate. In full, a double network structure (Figure 1b) was formed in the Alg/PGA microparticles via two kinds of interaction: the ion chelation between Ca^{2+} and carboxylate groups of PGA and Alginate and the electrostatic interaction between the secondary amine group of PGA and carboxylate groups of alginate and PGA.

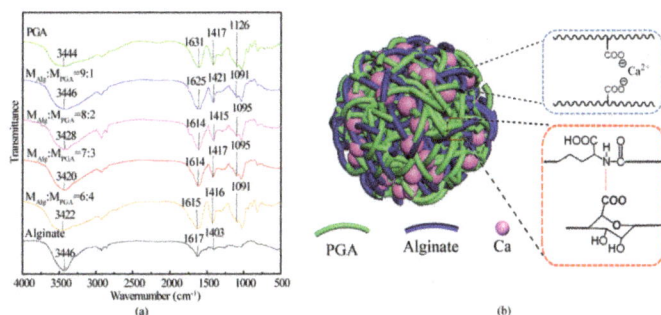

Figure 1. (a) FT-IR spectra of alginate, PGA and composite microparticles with various contents; (b) double-network structure scheme of the composite microparticle.

To further investigate the structure of the Alg/PGA microparticles, their surface chemical bonds were determined with the wide scan XPS. As shown in Figure 2, the binding energy (B.E.) peaks at 283.4, 284.9 and 286.7 eV can be assigned to C–C, C–O and C=O, respectively [37]. The relative content ratio of C to O (C/O) in the microparticles is higher than that in Alg and is increased with the increase of the PGA content in feeding materials (Table 1). In addition, the content of C=O group in the composite microparticles is significantly higher than that in alginate and is also increased with the increase of PGA content in the microparticles. These results indicate the presence of PGA and Alg in the composite microparticles.

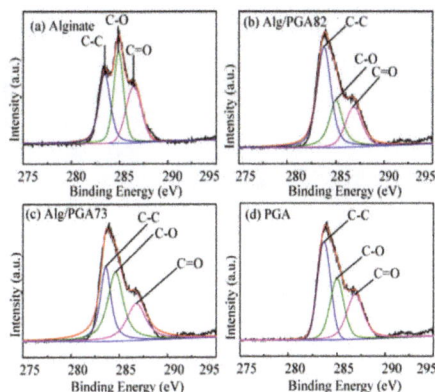

Figure 2. XPS C1s spectra of alginate (**a**), Alg/PGA82 (composite microparticles whose mass ratio is $m_{Alg}:m_{PGA}$ = 8:2) (**b**), Alg/PGA73 (composite microparticles whose mass ratio is $m_{Alg}:m_{PGA}$ = 7:3) (**c**) and PGA (**d**).

Table 1. Relative content of O and C in alginate, PGA and microparticles.

Samples	Relative Content Ratio of C/O	C–O		C=O	
		B.E. (eV)	Relative Content	B.E. (eV)	Relative Content
Alginate	1.6	531.37	81.1%	529.84	18.9%
Alg/PGA82 (m_{Alg}:m_{PGA} = 8:2)	1.9	531.40	69.7%	530.00	30.3%
Alg/PGA73 (m_{Alg}:m_{PGA} = 7:3)	2.1	531.45	51.4%	530.19	48.6%
PGA	2.2	531.50	45.1%	530.25	54.9%

Figure 3 shows the X-ray diffraction (XRD) patterns of Alg, PGA and Alg/PGA microparticles. Alg exhibited two typical crystalline diffraction peaks at 13.73° and 21.71°. One crystalline diffraction peak was found at 21.43° in the XRD spectrum of PGA [38,39]. The Alg/PGA composite microparticles exhibited two broad diffuse diffraction peaks centered at 14.10° and 26.61°, indicating its poor crystallinity after the gelation. This can be explained by the fact that the original polymer crystal structures of Alg and PGA were destructed during the formation of the full-interpenetrating composite polymer, resulting in decreased lattice density. Meanwhile, the aggregation degree of the microparticles was increased due to the chelation between the COO$^-$ and Ca^{2+} and electrostatic interaction between polyelectrolytes. Therefore, the crystalline diffraction peaks of the composite were diffused and a network structure was established in the composite microparticles.

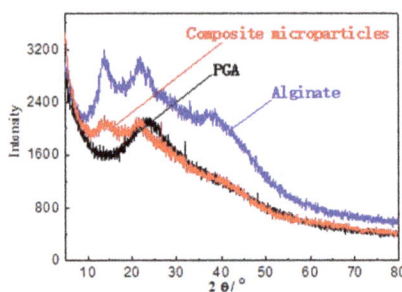

Figure 3. XRD patterns of Alginate, PGA and composite microparticles.

2.2. Morphology of the Alg/PGA Composite Microparticles

The surface morphology of the composite microparticles prepared with different mass ratios of Alg and PGA were observed by SEM (Figure 4) and particles size distributions were shown in Supplementary Figure S1 and Table S1. A fluctuating microparticle size (Mean size from 148.8 ± 13.0 to 9.4 ± 0.5 μm) can be observed in Figure 4a–e (×500) with an increase of PGA content. According to Supplementary Figure S1 and Table S1, the microparticle sizes decreased at first, increased later with increasing PGA content, and reach the turning point when m_{Alg}:m_{PGA} = 8:2 (9.4 ± 0.5 μm). The porous structure of composite microparticles is obvious in Figure 4 (×20,000) with the involvement of PGA compared with alginate microparticles. Relatively concentrated pores with nanoscale microparticles prepared with m_{Alg}:m_{PGA} = 8:2 could be found.

Higher feeding ratio of PGA leads to bigger composite microparticles and more irregular particle surface. Clusters on the surface of microparticles prepared with m_{Alg}:m_{PGA} = 6:4 were also detected. When compared with other types of microparticles, the PGA microparticles contain rare and larger pores.

In all, the fluctuating changes of microparticles with PGA content increase and different porous surfaces could be concluded via SEM images. The microparticles prepared with m_{Alg}:m_{PGA} = 8:2 are smallest, and the microparticles prepared with m_{Alg}:m_{PGA} = 8:2 and 7:3 own concentrated pores on their surfaces.

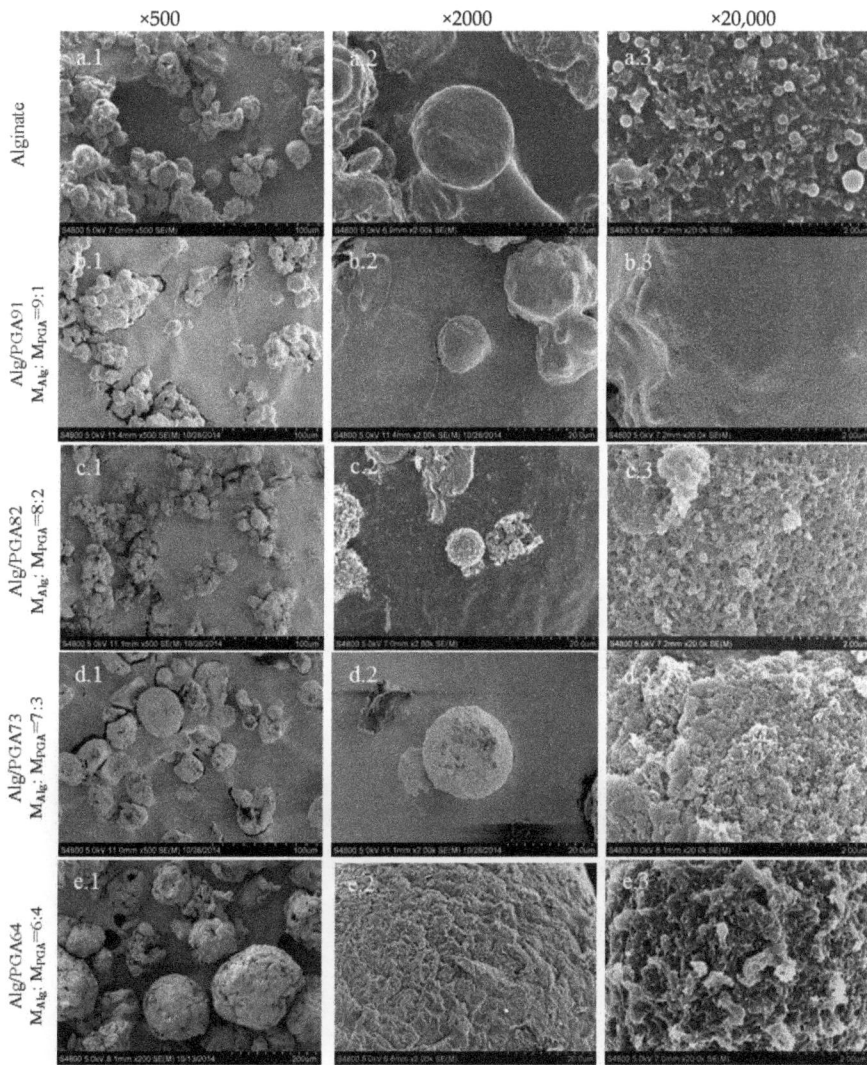

Figure 4. Morphology of the Alg/PGA Composite Microparticles. Note: SEM images of various microparticles at 500, 2000 and 20,000 magnification scales (**a–e** belongs to alginate microparticles and Alg/PGA composite microparticles with mass ratio is m_{Alg}:m_{PGA} = 9:1, 8:2, 7:3, 6:4 respectively).

2.3. Swelling Behavior of Alg/PGA Composite Microparticles

Figure 5 shows the swelling behavior of various composite microparticles prepared under different conditions. The swelling kinetics of microparticles was fitted by Voigt model and the kinetic parameters are listed in Table 2. It can be seen that both maximum water up-take ratio (σ_0/E) and swelling rate (k_i) were increased with the increase of the PGA amount in the composite and reached the maximum in the composite A2 prepared with m_{Alg}:m_{PGA} = 8:2. Further increasing PGA content leads to decreased σ_0/E and k_i. Relatively low τ_0, t_c of composite A2 could also represent the relatively fast swelling rate. However, the maximum water up-take ratio and swelling rate of sample A4 prepared with a m_{Alg}:m_{PGA} = 6:4 are still higher than those of pure alginate microparticles.

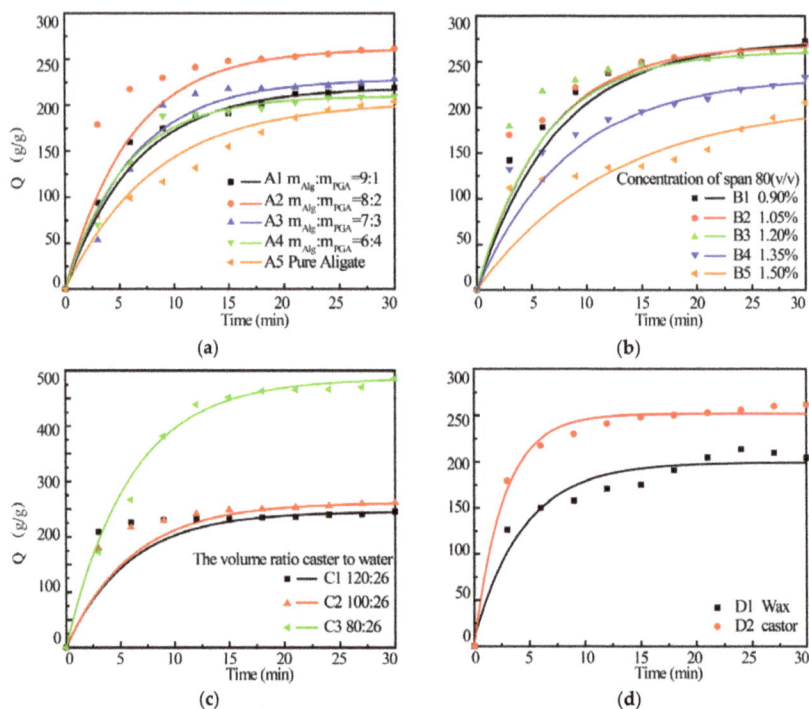

Figure 5. Effect of feeding ratio (**a**), concentration of span 80 (**b**), W/O ratio (**c**) and oil phase (**d**) on the swelling behavior of Alg/PGA composite microparticles.

Table 2. Swelling kinetic parameter of various microparticles.

Group	Sample	$(\sigma_0/E)/g\cdot g^{-1}$	τ_0/min	$k_i/g\cdot min^{-1}$	t_c/min
	A1	219.3	6.5	19.5	7.9
	A2	261.6	6.1	25.0	7.3
A	A3	228.6	6.3	22.8	7.0
	A4	210.0	5.5	21.6	6.8
	A5	204.1	8.3	14.2	10.0
	B1	272.6	7.3	21.9	8.7
	B2	268.3	6.3	24.8	7.6
B	B3	261.6	6.1	25.0	7.3
	B4	233.3	8.3	16.4	10.0
	B5	205.5	12.3	9.81	14.7
	C1	236.0	1.4	25.9	6.4
C	C2	261.6	6.1	25.0	7.3
	C3	482.7	6.0	47.8	7.1

As discussed above, PGA was incorporated into the composite microparticles and the interaction between PGA and alginate is very strong. The swelling capacity and rate of the composite were increased with the increasing of PGA content in the microparticles. Therefore, the better swelling behavior of the composite microparticles is largely attributed to a good hydrophility of PGA. In addition, the porous surface of the microparticles (Figure 4) can increase the contact area between the microparticles and water, which promotes the water absorption rate due to the capillary water absorption effect. However, the microparticles with extreme high PGA content become larger and thus the specific area of the microparticles decreased sharply, leading to low swelling capacity and rate. The maximum swelling capacity and rate were obtained in the Alg/PGA composite prepared with m_{Alg}:m_{PGA} = 8:2.

The emulsifier can influence the formation of the composite microparticles by reducing the surface tension of the system and promoting the stability of water/oil (W/O) emulsion [31]. As shown in Figure 5b, both water absorption ratio and swelling rate were slightly decreased as the concentration of non-ionic surfactant span 80 was increased to 1.2%. Theoretically, the size of composite microparticle is decreased with the increase of the emulsifier concentration due to the improved dispersion. However, the extremely high concentration of span 80 may cause decreased emulsions and increased composite drop size, leading to decreased swelling capacity and rate [32,40]. Therefore, concentration of span 80 was optimized as 1.2% (v/v) for the preparation of composite microparticles with stable structure and proper swelling behavior.

The effects of the oil to water ratio in the reaction medium on the swelling behavior were further studied. The results indicate sample C5 prepared in a medium with V_{castor}:V_{water} = 80:26 showed the fastest absorption rate and highest water absorption ratio at the same time (Figure 5c and Table 2). The oil content can also significantly affect the droplet size of the composite. Higher oil phase content leads to a reduction in specific surface area and an increased droplet size, resulting in undesired swelling behavior [41].

The swelling behaviors of the microparticles prepared with different dispersing phases were also investigated. The water absorption ratio and rate of the composite microparticles prepared in castor oil are higher than those of the microparticles prepared in wax. It has been reported that the emulsion size and composite particle size decreased with the increase of the reaction medium viscosity [42]. Therefore, the higher viscosity of castor oil leads to smaller emulsion, higher specific surface areas and better swelling behavior of the composite microparticles.

In all, the optimum conditions for preparation of Alg/PGA composite microparticles with excellent swelling behavior are a reaction medium with castor oil as oil phase and V_{castor}:V_{water} = 80:26, 1.2% (v/v) span 80 as emulsifier and the feeding ratio of m_{Alg}:m_{PGA} is 8:2.

2.4. Thermal Stability of Alg/PGA Composite Microparticles

The TGA and DTG curves of alginate, PGA and the composite microparticles, prepared under different conditions, are shown in Supplementary Figure S2. The thermal degradation process of alginate occures in three stages. At the first stage, the coordinated water in alginate was removed due to the dehydration and breaking of the glycosidic bonds at temperatures below 200 °C. During the second stage, in the temperature range of 200–280 °C, alginate skeleton was fractured. Further increasing the temperature causes the degradation of carboxylate group and the release of CO_2 [43,44]. The weight loss of PGA at temperatures lower than 250 °C may be attributed to the desorption of free water and surface hydroxyl groups. The weight loss at temperatures higher than 250 °C is caused by decomposition [45]. Similarly, the thermal degradation process of Alg/PGA composite microparticles occurs in three stages in the temperature ranges of 50–200 °C, 200–280 °C and 280–450 °C respectively. The parameters at each thermal degradation stage are listed in Table 3. The weight loss at the first stage is attributed to the water loss. The primary decomposition of alginate skeleton and degradation of PGA occurred during the second stage. The third degradation stage can be assigned to the secondary decomposition of alginate skeleton and degradation of PGA. The weight loss of the composite microparticles in the temperature range of 200–280 °C was lower than that of Alg at the corresponding temperature. The temperatures required for 5% and 50% weight loss in the composite microparticles are higher than those required for the corresponding weight loss in Alg and lower than those required for the corresponding weight loss in PGA. Among all the composites, the microparticles prepared with m_{Alg}:m_{PGA} = 8:2 required the highest temperatures for 5% and 50% weight loss.

Compared with alginate, the thermal stablity of composite microparticles was promoted by the ionic crosslinking, hydrogen bonding and the electrostatic binding between the polyelectrolytes.

It can be concluded that the introduction of PGA promotes the thermal stablity of the composite microparticles and the composite with strongest intermolecular interactions shows the highest thermal stablity.

Table 3. Thermogravimetric analysis of SA, PGA and various SA/PGA composite microparticles from TG-DTG analysis.

Sample	Stage	Temperature Range (°C)	T_{max} (°C)	Weight Loss (%)	Weight Loss 5% (°C)	Weight Loss 50% (°C)
PGA	1	50–250	55	11.84	155	Above 450
	2	250–450	345	35.74		
Alginate	1	50–200	184	12.03	77	287
	2	200–280	252	36.20		
	3	280–450	361	10.71		
m_{Alg}:m_{PGA} = 9:1	1	50–200	116	12.57	80	312
	2	200–280	263	31.32		
	3	280–450	405	15.22		
m_{Alg}:m_{PGA} = 8:2	1	50–200	79	9.04	104	341
	2	200–280	252	32.01		
	3	280–450	349	19.62		
m_{Alg}:m_{PGA} = 7:3	1	50–200	79	10.67	88	336
	2	200–280	250	32.06		
	3	280–450	354	17.20		
m_{Alg}:m_{PGA} = 6:4	1	50–200	122	11.56	75	338
	2	200–280	279	26.94		
	3	280–450	319	27.95		

2.5. In Vitro Cytotoxicity and Compatibility

Cytotoxicity is one of the most important methods for biological safety evaluation [45]. The cytotoxicity of Alg/PGA composite microparticles was evaluated with cellular morphology and relative cell viability (RCV). As shown in Figure 6, the cytotoxicity of the leach liquors of the composite microparticles are 0 grade or 1 grade according to the RCV after 24, 48 and 72 h cultures, which means that the cytotoxicity evaluation is valid. There was no significant difference between experimental groups and control group after 24 and 48 h cultures ($p > 0.05$). After the 72 h culture, obvious enhanced cell viability of all three experimental groups was observed compared with control group according to the CCK-8 assay. As shown in Figure 6b, no pronounced cell debris or changes in morphology, such as cell lysis, loss of spindle shape or detachment from the bottom, were observed in the samples. The above results confirm good cytocompatibility of the leach liquors of the composite microparticles.

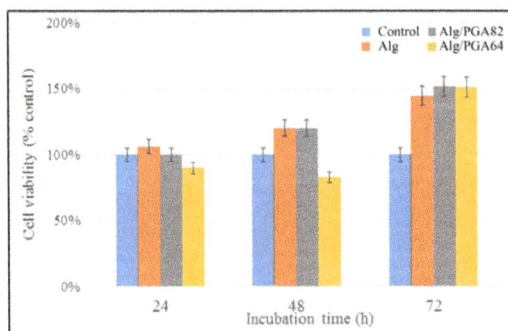

(a)

Figure 6. *Cont.*

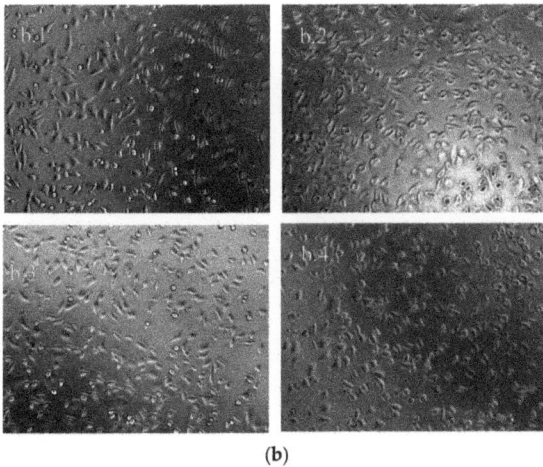

(b)

Figure 6. (a) Cytotoxicity assay of leach liquors. (b) Micrographs of cells cultured in leach liquors of samples Alg (**b.1**), Alg/PGA82 (**b.2**), Alg/PGA64 (**b.3**) and control group (**b.4**). Note: Samples Alg, Alg/PGA82 and Alg/PGA64 represent alginate microparticles, composite microparticles prepared with $m_{Alg}{:}m_{PGA} = 8{:}2$ and composite microparticles prepared with $m_{Alg}{:}m_{PGA} = 6{:}4$ respectively.

3. Materials and Methods

3.1. Materials

Sodium Alginate (NaAlg), with a viscosity of 200 ± 20 Mpa·S, was purchased from Aladdin Industrial Corporation (Los Angeles, CA, USA). Span 80 was provided by Tianjin Guangfu Fine Chemical Research Institute (Tianjin, China). Castor oil was purchased from Tianjin Chemical Reagent Factory (Tianjin, China). Liquid paraffin was acquired from Beijing Chemical Factory (Beijing, China). All of these materials were analytical grade. PGA (>92.0%) with a molecular weight of 1000 kDa was purchased from Nanjing Saitaisi Biotechnology Co., Ltd. (Nanjing, China), MEM-EBSS (Minimum Essential Medium; Sigma–Aldrich, St. Louis, MO, USA).

3.2. Preparation of Alg/PGA Composite Microparticles

A 6 mL suspension of 0.5% (w/v) $CaCO_3$ and 1.0% (w/v) polyvinylpyrrolidone (PVP) was dispersed uniformly into 20 mL 2% (w/v) Alg/PGA aqueous solution with specific weight ratio between Alg and PGA. The mixture was added into 50 mL castor oil containing 1.2% (v/v) Span 80 under stirring and was mechanically stirred for 15 min. Another 50 mL castor oil containing 2% (v/v) acetic acid was added slowly into the mixture prepared above. The reaction mixture was stirred at 40 °C for 1 h, kept stand for 24 h and vacuum filtered. The residue was washed with 200 mL ethanol at 60 °C for 2 h and dried at 60 °C for 24 h.

3.3. Characterization of Alg/PGA Composite Microparticles

FTIR spectra were obtained by a Thermo-Nicolet NEXUS 470 Spectroscopy (ThermoFish, Waltham, MA, USA) equipped with a KBr beam splitter. The test samples were prepared as KBr pellets.

X-ray Photoelectron Spectroscopy (XPS) spectra were obtained by a PHI QUANTERA-II instrument (Ulvac-PHI Inc. Chigasaki, Kanagawa, Japan) equipped with a monochromatized Al KRX-ray source operated at 25 W and 15 kV. For wide-scan spectra, an energy range of 0–1100 eV was used with pass energy of 280.00 eV and a step size of 1.00 eV. High-resolution spectra were collected at

26.00 eV pass energy using a step size of 0.025 eV. The XPS results were interpreted as binding energies that were further fitted in a nonlinear least squares curve fitting program (XPS-peak-41 software).

XRD diffractograms were recorded in the 2θ range of $5.0°$–$80.0°$ on a Rigaku D/Max-1200 instrument (Rigaku, Tokyo, Japan) equipped with Ni-filtered Cu Kα radiation (40 kV, 40 mA) to determine the crystallinity of Alg/PGA composite microparticles.

SEM was used to examine the structure and surface morphology of the produced microparticles. Microparticles were dusted onto a double-sided tape on an aluminum stub, coated with a gold layer using a gold sputter coater and imaged on an S-4800 SEM instrument (Hitachi, Tokyo, Japan) with a 5 kV electron beams.

3.4. Determination of the Swelling Behavior of Composite Microparticles

The swelling behavior of the composite microparticles was investigated by the filtering bag test method. A certain amount of sample was put in a nylon bag and immersed into the liquid to be absorbed at room temperature. The mass of the swollen sample was weighed every 3 min after the excess water removed. The water uptake ratio (Q) of the microparticle was calculated as the following:

$$Q = ((W_1 - W_0 - W_2)/W_0) \times 100\%$$

where, W_1 is the weight of the test sample and bag at a given swelling time, W_2 is the weight of nylon bag and W_0 is the initial weight of the sample.

The swelling process of the composite microparticles is similar to the creeping response of polymer. It is caused by the combination of hydrophilic interactions, the repulsion force between the anions and the osmotic pressures between inside and outside of the networks. Therefore, the swelling kinetic parameters of the composite microparticles can be fitted by the Voigt model [46]. Assuming that the force σ_0 is applied to the model at time t_0 and the corresponding response ε was produced at time t, the model can be expressed as the following:

$$\varepsilon(t) = \sigma_0/E\{1 - \exp[(t_0 - t)/\tau_0]\} = \varepsilon(\infty)\{1 - \exp[(t_0 - t)/\tau_0]\}$$

where, τ_0 is the relaxation time that is theoretically inversely proportional to the swelling ratio of the microparticles and E is Young's modulus that represents the resistance to deformation. σ_0/E equals to $\varepsilon_{(\infty)}$, representing the maximum swelling ratio. The slope of forward straight part of the curve (k_i) with $Q = 0.7\varepsilon_{(\infty)}$ and the time (t_c) when the swelling becomes slow can be calculated accordingly. The swelling rate is directly proportional to k_i and inversely proportional to t_c.

3.5. Thermal Stability Study of Composite Microparticles

Thermogravimetric analysis (TGA) was carried out on a DTG-60 Thermogravimetry Analyzer (SHIMADZU, Kyoto, Japan). Samples with weights of 3–5 mg were heated from 50 to 450 °C with heating rate of 10 °C /min in a nitrogen atmosphere with the flow rate of 50 mL/min.

3.6. In Vitro Cytotoxicity and Compatibility

The preliminary investigation of indirect in vitro cytotoxicity and cytocompatibility with L929 cells (provided by Cell Bank of Chinese Academy of Sciences, Beijing, China) was performed. The microparticles were sterilized by irradiation with ^{60}Co (at the room temperature, dose rate was 100 Gy/min and the irradiation dose was 15 kGy), and leached in MEM-EBSS for 24 to swell completely. The supernatant was leached at polymer concentration of 1/400 (g/mL) and collected after centrifuged at 3000 r/min for 5 min for further use. The leach liquor of the microparticles was diluted with the cell culture fluid to final concentration of 50% for CCK-8 assays.

The culture was maintained in the incubator (Zhongxing Co. Ltd., Beijing, China) at 37 °C under a wet atmosphere containing 5% CO_2. MEM-EBSS supplemented with 10% horse serum, together with non-essential amino acid was used as cell culture fluid. The cell suspension was injected into a 96-well culture plate with 6 wells for each group and 5×10^4 cells in each well and cultured in the incubator for 4 h. Then 100 μL of the leach liquors and diluted leach liquors with the concentration of 50% were respectively added into the wells of the experimental groups and 100 μL of the control solutions were respectively added to the control groups. The cells were then cultured in the incubator for 48 h. Micrographs of cell cultured in leach liquors were taken before the addition of CCK-8 with Axio Vert A1 light microscope. 20 μL CCK-8 soultion was injected into every well, then kept in incubator for 2 h. The absorbance of each well at 570 nm was determined with a POLARstar Omega analyzer. The relative cell viability (RCV) was calculated with the following Equation:

$$RCV = \frac{[Abs]_{Sample}}{[Abs]_{Control}} \times 100\%$$

And the average value was reported.

The cytotoxicity was evaluated according to the following standard [47]: the cytotoxicity is zero grade for RCV higher than 100%, 1st grade for RCV in the range of 75%–99%, 2nd grade for RCV in the range of 50%–74%, 3rd grade for RCV in the range of 25%–49%, 4th grade for RCV in the range of 1%–24%, and 5th grade for RCV = 0%. The 1st grade or less cytotoxicity is acceptable. If the cells showed 2nd grade response to the polymer, the cell morphology should be analyzed for comprehensive evaluation. The response level equal to or higher than 3rd grade indicates that the polymer is off specification for cytotoxicity evaluation.

3.7. Statistical Analysis

Statistical analysis was performed using SPSS version 20 (Statistical Package). Value of $p \leq 0.05$ was considered to be significant. All the values are expressed as means ± SD.

4. Conclusions

Alg/PGA composite microparticles with controllable structure were successfully prepared through the emulsification/internal gelation method and then characterized. Inside the microparticles, a double network structure was formed by ion-chelating interaction between carboxylate groups and Ca^{2+} and electrostatic interaction between carboxylate groups and secondary amine group. The swelling behavior of microparticles was promoted by the introduction of PGA. The conditions for the preparation of Alg/PGA microparticles with excellent swelling behavior were optimized. These Alg/PGA microparticles could absorb hundreds of times their weight in water. A porous surface could be observed on composite microparticles. The morphological structure could also influence the variation of swelling behavior. The composite microparticles also showed better thermal stability compared with alginate. Alg/PGA composite microparticles also possess good biocompatibility. Alg/PGA composite microparticles are promising candidates in the field of wound dressing for hemostasis as well as for rapidly removing exudates.

Supplementary Materials: The following are available online at www.mdpi.com/1660-3397/15/4/91/s1, Figure S1: Particles size distribution of alginate microparticles and various composite microparticles (Alg/PGA91, Alg/PGA82, Alg/PGA73, Alg/PGA64 represent composite microparticles whose mass ratio is m_{Alg}:m_{PGA} = 9:1, 8:2, 7:3, 6:4 respectively), Figure S2: TG (a) and DTG (b) curves of Alginate, PGA and Alg/PGA microparticles prepared at different weight ratio, Table S1: Size distribution statistic data of various microparticles.

Acknowledgments: The authors gratefully acknowledge the financial support of The National Undergraduate Innovative Experiment Program of China.

Author Contributions: Zongrui Tong and Yu Chen designed and performed the experiments and wrote the paper; Yang Liu, Kecen Xiao, Zhiyu Zhou and Wenbo Dong performed the preparation and data analysis; Li Tong contributed to the cell culture and biological evaluation; Jiamian Chu, Shengwu Chu contributed to the conception and design of the experiments. All authors reviewed the manuscript and approved the final version.

Conflicts of Interest: The authors declare no conflict of interest.

References

1. Winter, G.D. Formation of the scab and the rate of epithelization of superficial wounds in the skin of the young domestic pig. *J. Wound Care* **1995**, *4*, 368–371. [CrossRef]
2. Liakos, I.; Rizzello, L.; Bayer, I.S.; Pompa, P.P.; Cingolani, R.; Athanassiou, A. Controlled antiseptic release by alginate polymer films and beads. *Carbohydr. Polym.* **2013**, *92*, 176–183. [CrossRef] [PubMed]
3. Albertini, B.; Di, S.M.; Calonghi, N.; Rodriguez, L.; Passerini, N. Novel multifunctional platforms for potential treatment of cutaneous wounds: Development and in vitro characterization. *Int. J. Pharm.* **2013**, *440*, 238–249. [CrossRef] [PubMed]
4. Tadej, M. The use of flivasorb in highly exuding wounds. *B. J. Nurs.* **2009**, *18*, 38–42. [CrossRef] [PubMed]
5. Mignon, A.; Graulus, G.J.; Snoeck, D.; Martins, J.; Belie, N.D.; Dubruel, P.; Vlierberghe, S.V. Ph-sensitive superabsorbent polymers: A potential candidate material for self-healing concrete. *J. Mater. Sci.* **2015**, *50*, 970–979. [CrossRef]
6. Islam, M.S.; Rahaman, M.S.; Yeum, J.H. Electrospun novel super-absorbent based on polysaccharide–polyvinyl alcohol–montmorillonite clay nanocomposites. *Carbohydr. Polym.* **2015**, *115*, 69–77. [CrossRef] [PubMed]
7. Sharma, S.; Dua, A.; Malik, A. Polyaspartic acid based superabsorbent polymers. *Eur. Polym. J.* **2014**, *59*, 363–376. [CrossRef]
8. Rashidzadeh, A.; Olad, A. Slow-released NPK fertilizer encapsulated by NaAlg-g-poly(AA-co-AAm)/mmt superabsorbent nanocomposite. *Carbohydr. Polym.* **2014**, *114*, 269–278. [CrossRef] [PubMed]
9. Hrynyk, M.; Martins-Green, M.; Barron, A.E.; Neufeld, R.J. Alginate-peg sponge architecture and role in the design of insulin release dressings. *Biomacromolecules* **2012**, *13*, 1478–1485. [CrossRef] [PubMed]
10. Andersen, T.; Melvik, J.E.; Gåserød, O.; Alsberg, E.; Christensen, B.E. Correction to ionically gelled alginate foams: Physical properties controlled by operational and macromolecular parameters. *Biomacromolecules* **2012**, *13*, 3703–3710. [CrossRef] [PubMed]
11. Fischer, F.G.; Dorfel, H. Polyuronic acids in brown algae. *Hoppe-Seyler's Z. Physiol. Chem.* **1955**, *302*, 186–203. [CrossRef] [PubMed]
12. Haug, A.; Claeson, K.; Hansen, S.E.; Sömme, R.; Stenhagen, E.; Palmstierna, H. Fractionation of alginic acid. *Acta Chem. Scand.* **1959**, *13*, 601–603. [CrossRef]
13. Kost, J.; Langer, R. Responsive polymeric delivery systems. *Adv. Drug Deliv. Rev.* **2001**, *46*, 19–50. [CrossRef]
14. Urbanska, A.M.; Karagiannis, E.D.; Guajardo, G.; Langer, R.S.; Anderson, D.G. Therapeutic effect of orally administered microencapsulated oxaliplatin for colorectal cancer. *Biomaterials* **2012**, *33*, 4752–4761. [CrossRef] [PubMed]
15. Fang, A.; Cathala, B. Smart swelling biopolymer microparticles by a microfluidic approach: Synthesis, in situ encapsulation and controlled release. *Colloids Surf. B Biointerfaces* **2011**, *82*, 81–86. [CrossRef] [PubMed]
16. Jin, S.G.; Yousaf, A.M.; Kim, K.S.; Kim, D.W.; Kim, D.S.; Kim, J.K.; Yong, C.S.; Youn, Y.S.; Kim, J.O.; Choi, H.G. Influence of hydrophilic polymers on functional properties and wound healing efficacy of hydrocolloid based wound dressings. *Int. J. Pharm.* **2016**, *501*, 160–166. [CrossRef] [PubMed]
17. Cicco, F.D.; Russo, P.; Reverchon, E.; Garcíagonzález, C.A.; Aquino, R.P.; Gaudio, P.D. Prilling and supercritical drying: A successful duo to produce core-shell polysaccharide aerogel beads for wound healing. *Carbohydr. Polym.* **2016**, *147*, 482–489. [CrossRef] [PubMed]
18. Karri, V.V.S.R.; Kuppusamy, G.; Talluri, S.V.; Mannemala, S.S.; Kollipara, R.; Wadhwani, A.D. Curcumin loaded chitosan nanoparticles impregnated into collagen-alginate scaffolds for diabetic wound healing. *Int. J. Biol. Macromol.* **2016**, *93*, 1519–1529. [CrossRef] [PubMed]
19. Caló, E.; Khutoryanskiy, V.V. Biomedical applications of hydrogels: A review of patents and commercial products. *Eur. Polym. J.* **2015**, *65*, 252–267. [CrossRef]
20. Morgado, P.I.; Aguiar-Ricardo, A.; Correia, I.J. Asymmetric membranes as ideal wound dressings: An overview on production methods, structure, properties and performance relationship. *J. Membr. Sci.* **2015**, *490*, 139–151. [CrossRef]
21. Chen, Y.; Zhang, Y.; Wang, F.J.; Meng, W.W.; Yang, X.L.; Jiang, J.X.; Tan, H.M.; Zheng, Y.F. Preparation of the porous carboxymethyl chitosan grafted poly (acrylic acid) superabsorbent by solvent precipitation and its application as a hemostatic wound dressing. *Mater. Sci. Eng. C* **2016**, *63*, 18–29. [CrossRef] [PubMed]
22. Inbaraj, B.S.; Wang, J.S.; Lu, J.F.; Siao, F.Y.; Chen, B.H. Adsorption of toxic mercury(II) by an extracellular biopolymer poly(gamma-glutamic acid). *Bioresour. Technol.* **2009**, *100*, 200–207. [CrossRef] [PubMed]

23. Lee, Y.H.; Chang, J.J.; Lai, W.F.; Yang, M.C.; Chien, C.T. Layered hydrogel of poly(γ-glutamic acid), sodium alginate, and chitosan: Fluorescence observation of structure and cytocompatibility. *Colloids Surf. B Biointerfaces* **2011**, *86*, 409–413. [CrossRef] [PubMed]

24. Huang, M.H.; Yang, M.C. Swelling and biocompatibility of sodium alginate/poly (γ-glutamic acid) hydrogels. *Polym. Adv. Technol.* **2010**, *21*, 1099–1581. [CrossRef]

25. Stojkovska, J.; Kostić, D.; Jovanović, Ž.; Vukašinovićsekulić, M.; Mišković́stanković, V.; Obradović, B. A comprehensive approach to in vitro functional evaluation of ag/alginate nanocomposite hydrogels. *Carbohydr. Polym.* **2014**, *111*, 305–314. [CrossRef] [PubMed]

26. Yan, S.; Zhang, X.; Sun, Y.; Wang, T.; Chen, X.; Yin, J. In situ preparation of magnetic Fe_3O_4 nanoparticles inside nanoporous poly(l-glutamic acid)/chitosan microcapsules for drug delivery. *Colloids Surf. B Biointerfaces* **2014**, *113*, 302–311. [CrossRef] [PubMed]

27. Akagi, T.; Higashi, M.; Kaneko, T.; Kida, T.; Akashi, M. In vitro enzymatic degradation of nanoparticles prepared from hydrophobically-modified poly(gamma-glutamic acid). *Macromol. Biosci.* **2005**, *5*, 598–602. [CrossRef] [PubMed]

28. Shih, I.L.; Van, Y.T. The production of poly-(gamma-glutamic acid) from microorganisms and its various applications. *Bioresour. Technol.* **2001**, *79*, 207–225. [CrossRef]

29. Suzuki, S.; Asoh, T.A.; Kikuchi, A. Design of core–shell gel beads for time-programmed protein release. *J. Biomed. Mater. Res. A* **2013**, *101A*, 1345–1352. [CrossRef] [PubMed]

30. Wang, F.; Zhao, J.; Wei, X.; Huo, F.; Li, W.; Hu, Q.; Liu, H. Adsorption of rare earths (III) by calcium alginate–poly glutamic acid hybrid gels. *J. Chem. Technol. Biotechnol.* **2014**, *89*, 969–977. [CrossRef]

31. Guan, H.; Chi, D.; Yu, J.; Li, H. Encapsulated ecdysone by internal gelation of alginate microspheres for controlling its release and photostability. *Chem. Eng. J.* **2011**, *168*, 94–101. [CrossRef]

32. Paques, J.P.; Van, d.L.E.; van Rijn, C.J.; Sagis, L.M. Preparation methods of alginate nanoparticles. *Adv. Colloid Interface Sci.* **2014**, *209*, 163–171. [CrossRef] [PubMed]

33. Silva, C.M.; Ribeiro, A.J.; Figueiredo, I.V.; Gonçalves, A.R.; Veiga, F. Alginate microspheres prepared by internal gelation: Development and effect on insulin stability. *Int. J. Pharm.* **2006**, *311*, 1–10. [CrossRef] [PubMed]

34. Lupo, B.; Maestro, A.; Porras, M.; Gutiérrez, J.M.; González, C. Preparation of alginate microspheres by emulsification/internal gelation to encapsulate cocoa polyphenols. *Food Hydrocoll.* **2014**, *38*, 56–65. [CrossRef]

35. Lee, K.Y.; Mooney, D.J. Alginate: Properties and biomedical applications. *Prog. Polym. Sci.* **2012**, *37*, 106–126. [CrossRef] [PubMed]

36. Mundargi, R.C.; Shelke, N.B.; Babu, V.R.; Patel, P.; Rangaswamy, V.; Aminabhavi, T.M. Novel thermo-responsive semi-interpenetrating network microspheres of gellan gum-poly(n -isopropylacrylamide) for controlled release of atenolol. *J. Appl. Polym. Sci.* **2010**, *116*, 1832–1841. [CrossRef]

37. Beamson, G.; Briggs, D. *High Resolution XPS of Organic Polymers: The Scienta Esca300 Database*; Wiley: Hoboken, NJ, USA, 1992.

38. Paşcalău, V.; Popescu, V.; Popescu, G.L.; Dudescu, M.C.; Borodi, G.; Dinescu, A.; Perhaiţa, I.; Paul, M. The alginate/k-carrageenan ratio's influence on the properties of the cross-linked composite films. *J. Alloys Compd.* **2012**, *536*, 418–423. [CrossRef]

39. Lee, H.Y.; Jeong, Y.; Choi, K.C. Hair dye-incorporated poly-γ-glutamic acid/glycol chitosan nanoparticles based on ion-complex formation. *Int. J. Nanomed.* **2011**, *6*, 2879–2888.

40. Santini, E.; Liggieri, L.; Sacca, L.; Clausse, D.; Ravera, F. Interfacial rheology of span 80 adsorbed layers at paraffin oil–water interface and correlation with the corresponding emulsion properties. *Colloids Surf. A Physicochem. Eng. Asp.* **2007**, *309*, 270–279. [CrossRef]

41. Hadnađev, T.D.; Dokić, P.; Krstonošić, V.; Hadnađev, M. Influence of oil phase concentration on droplet size distribution and stability of oil-in-water emulsions. *Eur. J. Lipid Sci. Technol.* **2013**, *115*, 313–321. [CrossRef]

42. Bouchemal, K.; Briançon, S.; Perrier, E.; Fessi, H. Nano-emulsion formulation using spontaneous emulsification: Solvent, oil and surfactant optimisation. *Int. J. Pharm.* **2004**, *280*, 241–251. [CrossRef] [PubMed]

43. Dong, Y.; Dong, W.; Cao, Y.; Han, Z.; Ding, Z. Preparation and catalytic activity of fe alginate gel beads for oxidative degradation of azo dyes under visible light irradiation. *Catal. Today* **2011**, *175*, 346–355. [CrossRef]

44. Cao, H.; Gao, Y.J.; Ren, W.H.; Li, T.T.; Duan, K.Z.; Cui, Y.H.; Cao, X.H.; Zhao, Z.Q.; Ji, R.R.; Zhang, Y.Q. Influence of cation on the pyrolysis and oxidation of alginates. *J. Anal. Appl. Pyrolysis* **2011**, *91*, 344–351.

45.	Shan, Z.; Yang, W.-S.; Zhang, X.; Huang, Q.-M.; Ye, H. Preparation and characterization of carboxyl-group functionalized superparamagnetic nanoparticles and t he potential for bio-applications. *J. Braz. Chem. Soc.* **2007**, *18*, 1329–1335. [CrossRef]
46.	Chen, Y.; Liu, Y.; Tang, H.; Yan, R.; Tan, H. Preparation of cmcts-g-paa macroporous superabsorbent polymer by foaming method. *CIESC J.* **2008**, *59*, 785–789.
47.	Wilsnack, R.E. Quantitative cell culture biocompatibility testing of medical devices and correlation to animal tests. *Biomater. Med. Devices Artif. Organs* **1976**, *4*, 235–261. [CrossRef] [PubMed]

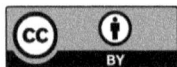

marine drugs

MDPI

Article

Electrospinning of Nanodiamond-Modified Polysaccharide Nanofibers with Physico-Mechanical Properties Close to Natural Skins

Mina Mahdavi [1], Nafiseh Mahmoudi [1], Farzad Rezaie Anaran [1] and Abdolreza Simchi [1,2,*]

[1] Department of Materials Science and Engineering, Sharif University of Technology, Azadi Avenue, 14588 Tehran, Iran; mina_m1372@yahoo.com (M.M.); Nafiseh_Mahmoudi@mehr.sharif.ir (N.M.); fd_rezaieanaran@dena.sharif.ir (F.R.A.)

[2] Institute for Nanoscience and Nanotechnology, Sharif University of Technology, P.O. Box 11365-9466, Azadi Avenue, 14588 Tehran, Iran

*   Correspondence: simchi@sharif.edu; Tel.: +98-21-6616-5226; Fax: +98-21-6600-5717

Academic Editor: Paola Laurienzo
Received: 30 May 2016; Accepted: 29 June 2016; Published: 7 July 2016

Abstract: Electrospinning of biopolymers has gained significant interest for the fabrication of fibrous mats for potential applications in tissue engineering, particularly for wound dressing and skin regeneration. In this study, for the first time, we report successful electrospinning of chitosan-based biopolymers containing bacterial cellulous (33 wt %) and medical grade nanodiamonds (MND) (3 nm; up to 3 wt %). Morphological studies by scanning electron microscopy showed that long and uniform fibers with controllable diameters from 80 to 170 nm were prepared. Introducing diamond nanoparticles facilitated the electrospinning process with a decrease in the size of fibers. Fourier transform infrared spectroscopy determined hydrogen bonding between the polymeric matrix and functional groups of MND. It was also found that beyond 1 wt % MND, percolation networks of nanoparticles were formed which affected the properties of the nanofibrous mats. Uniaxial tensile testing of the woven mats determined significant enhancement of the strength (from 13 MPa to 25 MP) by dispersion of 1 wt % MND. The hydrophilicity of the mats was also remarkably improved, which was favorable for cell attachment. The water vapor permeability was tailorable in the range of 342 to 423 $\mu g \cdot Pa^{-1} \cdot s^{-1} \cdot m^{-1}$. The nanodiamond-modified mats are potentially suitable for wound healing applications.

Keywords: nanodiamond; chitosan nanofiber; bacterial cellulose; electrospinning; wound dressing

1. Introduction

Structural disruption in basement membranes of skin due to different types of injuries have to be cared and repaired as the skin is the largest organ of the body with many vital functions [1]. Elastic, biocompatible, and non-allergenic wound dressing materials are commonly utilized with an aim to keep the injured environment moist while protecting it from new infections [2]. With the same morphology and structure as the natural extracellular matrix (ECM), polymeric fibers are the most suitable materials that can be utilized for skin regeneration [3]. The porosity, oxygen permeability, mechanical durability, and hydrophilicity of fibrous membranes can be adjusted to practical needs by chemical and structural modifications [4].

So far, chitosan (CS) and CS-based fibers have been the most studied natural polymeric materials for wound healing and skin tissue engineering applications [5]. Not surprisingly, this natural polysaccharide offers a number of advantages over other natural and synthetic polymers. As a derivate of chitin [6], CS has proved to be biocompatible with non-allergenic activity and bactericidal capacity [7–9]. Perhaps the main drawback of CS is in regard to its relatively low mechanical durability, low structural stability in a physiological environment, and its degradation products [10]. From a processing point of view, high viscosity of CS solution may insert some restrictions on the fabrication of long and uniform fibers with controllable sizes [11]. Although electrospinning is one of the most versatile techniques to fabricate fibrous mats of various biopolymers in a cost-effective way [12], viscous CS solution is hard to be electrospun without utilizing co-surfactants and organic solvents (which may not be biocompatible) [13]. Recent studies have shown that CS fibers can be electrospun through blending with synthetic polymers; examples include PVA, PEO, PCL, and PVP [14,15]. The synthetic polymers reduce the viscosity of CS solution making it spinnable while improving the mechanical durability of fibrous mats. Recent advances are focused on utilizing natural polymers in order to tailor the properties of CS fibers. Bacterial cellulose (BC), which is produced by the bacterium *Acetobacter xylinum*, is a good candidate. This is because the ultrafine network of uniaxial cellulose nanofibers (3–8 nm) [16] terminates as a large surface area that can hold a large amount of water (up to 200 times of its dry mass) while providing a great elasticity, wet mechanical durability, and conformability [17]. The hydrophilicity [18], biocompatibility [19], and non-toxicity [20] of BC have also made this natural polymer a promising candidate for many biomedical applications [21,22]. Transparency and flexibility of CS/BC films prepared by solvent casting methods were studied by Fernandes et al. [23]. Phisalaphong et al. [24] added CS to the culture medium of BC during biosynthesis to attain CS/BC blends. Enhanced mechanical properties and water absorption capacity of the composite blend was shown. Additionally, the blends did not exhibit an adverse effect on in vitro cell viability [25]. The fabrication of CS/BC nanofibers has recently been attempted [26]. Very recently, Azarnia et al. [27] utilized the surface methodology approach to determine a set of optimum parameters to attain long, uniform, and fine CS/BC fibers. They showed how electrospinning parameters affected the morphology and size of the fibers and examined the physico-mechanical properties of the woven mats.

Although CS-based fibrous mats are promising candidates for wound dressing, the mechanical properties of the membranes do not meet the requirements of natural skin. In order to improve the mechanical durability and to tailor physical properties (permeability and hydrophilicity) of the electrospun membranes, the addition of secondary (reinforcing) particles to the polymer network has been studied [28,29]. Particular attention has been paid to carbon nanostructures [27,30,31]. Graphene-modified nanofibers have gained much interest in recent years [32]. It has been shown that graphene oxide and reduced graphene oxide nanosheets can be embedded in or folded around the polymer fibers to boost the mechanical strength of biopolymers, while providing bactericidal capacity along with enhanced cell attachment [27,33]. In the present work, biomedical grade nanodiamonds (MND) were utilized for the modification of CS/BC fibers. To the best knowledge of the authors, MND has not been utilized in wound dressing applications so far, despite the high potential of the material for biomedical applications. Nanodiamonds have been shown to be biocompatible in various cell lines and some animal models with minimal or no cytotoxicity [34,35]. The particular feature of MND that distinguishes them from other carbon nanostructures is related to their ultrafine sizes with many surface functional groups that have made them excellent carriers for drug delivery [36]. The functional groups provide stable colloids in aqueous solutions with an ability to conjugate to various drugs and growth factors. Therefore, the main objective of this work is to introduce MND to biopolymers in order to: (a) ease electrospinning of concentrated CS solutions; (b) decrease fiber diameters to nano-scale range; (c) enhance the mechanical durability of the membranes to be closer to that of the natural skin in the back area; and (d) provide a platform to conjugate drugs and growth factors to the nanoparticles for controlled release. In this first stage, and within this paper, we present experimental results on the electrospinning of MND-modified CS/BC nanofibers. The effects of MND on the spinnability, mechanical properties, hydrophilicity, water vapor permeability, and cytocompatibility are also shown. It is worthwhile to mention that this work is particularly focused on materials processing and characterizations, but further studies are underway to investigate the drug-loading ability of the MND-modified nanofibers structure.

2. Results and Discussion

2.1. Size and Morphology of Electrospun Fibers

Figure 1 shows representative SEM micrographs of electrospun fibers containing different amounts of MND. The size distribution of the fibers was determined by image analysis and is shown in Figure 1 and Table 1. Randomly oriented fibers with diameters ranging from 80 to 300 nm were obtained by electrospinning the polysaccharide suspension (Figure 1a,b). Some mini-jets were also visible, which could be due to the high viscosity of the suspension, i.e., the electrical field could not overcome surface tension forces [37]. Introduction of diamond nanoparticles reduced the fiber diameters and yielded more uniform fibers with narrower size distribution (Table 1). It is possible that the effect of MND on the fiber diameters is related to the enhanced viscosity and conductivity of the suspension from which the fibers are drawn. At a given electric field strength, the higher liquid viscosity typically results in a weaker stretching of liquid jet while higher conductivity changes the shape of meniscus [38]. The balance between the effect of nanoparticles on the viscosity and conductivity determines the size of the fibers that leads to the formation of coarser fibers [39]. As it will be shown in the next section, no strong chemical interactions between MND and polymer occurs, but agglomeration of the nanoparticles are favorable, particularly at high concentrations. For instance, Figure 2 shows the formation of MND clusters in electrospun fibers. Rakha et al. [40] related particles' agglomeration to their surface functional groups. As the effective size of ultrafine MND increased, their effect on the viscosity decreased, so that finer fibers were attained [41].

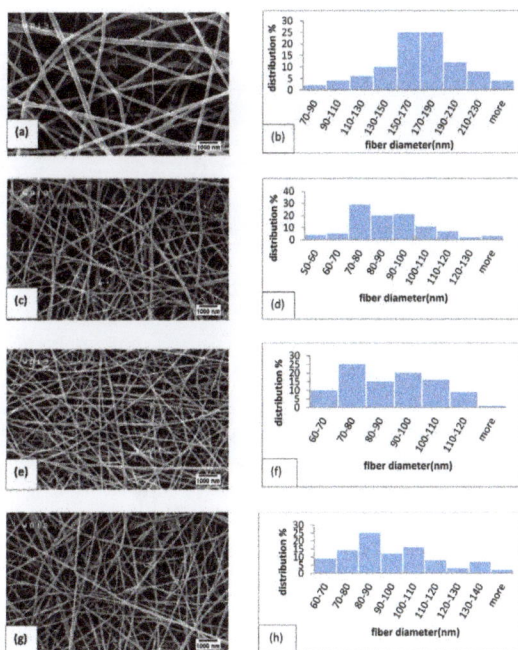

Figure 1. Effect of medical grade nanodiamonds (MND) on the morphology and size distribution of electrospun fibers: (**a**) chitosan/bacterial cellulose (CS/BC) without MND; (**c**) contain 1%; (**e**) 2% and (**g**) 3% MND particles, respectively. (**b**), (**d**), (**f**) and (**h**) show the fiber diameter distribution diagrams of each specimen.

(a)

(b)

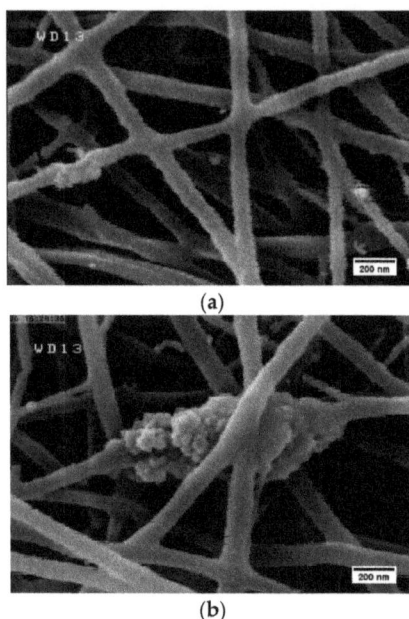

Figure 2. Formation of large nanoparticle clusters upon electrospinning. The concentration of MND (%) is (**a**) 2 and (**b**) 3.

Table 1. Effect of medical grade nanodiamonds (MND) particles on size and size distribution of fibers.

Concentration	Average Fiber Diameter (nm)	Size Range (nm)
0	173 ± 44	73–308
1	88 ± 18	57–160
2	89 ± 14	61–128
3	95 ± 22	60–157

2.2. Interactions between Nanoparticles and Polymer

In order to figure out the possible interactions between CS, BC, and MND particles, FT-IR spectroscopy was employed. Figure 3 shows FT-IR spectrum of the polymer blend, pristine MND particles, and electrospun fibers containing 3 wt % MND. The –OH stretching vibration of CS occurs at 3000–3500 cm^{-1} [25,42]. The peak around 2965 cm^{-1} is assigned to aliphatic C–H stretching vibration [31]. The N–H peak is for CS which overlaps the wide absorption peak of –OH group in range of 3000–3500 cm^{-1}. The peaks at 1343 cm^{-1} and 1467 cm^{-1} are attributed to symmetric and bending vibration of C-H group, respectively. Another peak at 1050 cm^{-1} is due to the stretching vibration of C–O–C group. As to the PEO, triplet peaks of the C–O–C stretching vibrations appear at 1148, 1101, and 1062 cm^{-1}. An absorption band at 2885 cm^{-1} is attributed to CH_2 stretching vibration in PEO [43,44]. The peak of the glucose carbonyl of cellulose is detected at 1643 cm^{-1}. The peak at around 1045 cm^{-1} shows the C–O–C stretching vibration. Overall, the results are in a good agreement with previous studies on CS and BC composite films and firmly verify the presence of many intermolecular hydrogen and ionic bonds, as well as a few covalent bonds [24,25,42]. The absorption peaks of MND are seen at 3426 cm^{-1}, 1626 cm^{-1}, and 1107 cm^{-1} which are attributed to stretching vibration of –OH, –C=O, and the overlap of C–O groups with nitrogen groups, respectively. The peak at 1735 cm^{-1} indicates stretching vibration of functional groups of C=O and –COOH and the peak at 2341 cm^{-1} is related to the absorption of CO_2 [45–47]. The FT-IR results determined there was no formation of new peaks as a result of blending the polymers with MND; only a slight red shift in characteristics peaks were observed that could be due to hydrogen bonding [48].

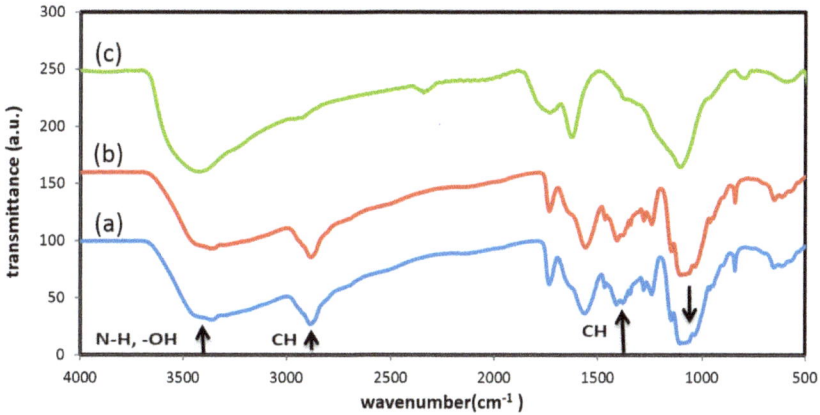

Figure 3. Fourier transform infrared (FT-IR) spectrum of (**a**) CS/BC polymer; (**b**) the nanocomposite fiber containing 3% MND; and (**c**) pristine MND.

2.3. Effect of Nanodiamonds on the Hydrophilicity of Mats

Figure 4 shows changes in the water contact angle of electrospun fibers with the MND concentration. The hydrophilicity at first decreased with the introduction of 1 wt % MND particles, but increased at the higher concentrations. The MND particles with many surface functional groups are hydrophilic but, at the high concentrations, the addition of these nanoparticles increases the hydrophobicity of the mats. It is suggested that changes in the contact angles were more likely due to the morphology/size variations of the fibers. It is known that the surface energy and surface geometric features influence the contact angles of fibrous mats [49,50]. Smaller fibers with agglomerated nanoparticles altered the hydrophilicity due to the roughness issue and surface features [51].

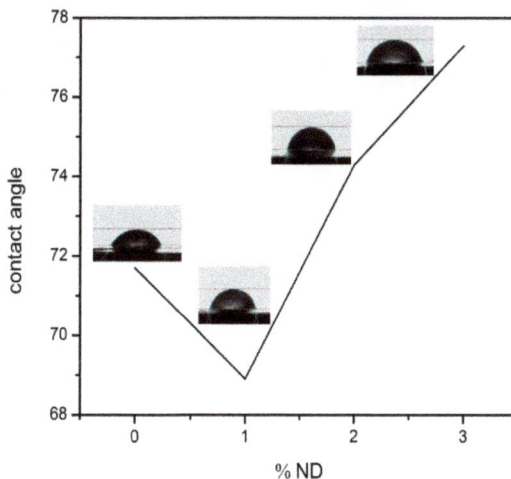

Figure 4. Effect of diamond particles on the hydrophilicity of electrospun CS/BC mats.

2.4. Mechanical Properties of Electrospun Mats

Typical stress-strain curves of the electrospun mats are shown in Figure 5. The effect of MND on the mechanical properties are summarized in Table 2. It was found that the addition of 1 wt % MND particles significantly increased the elastic modulus and yield strength of the fibers along with ductility loss. Tjong et al. [52] related the mechanism of strength enhancement to the effect of nanoparticles on restricted movement of polymer chains. It was noted that the mechanical properties of the mats were close to that of natural skin, as reported in [27]. Meanwhile, the mechanical durability was degraded at high MND concentrations due to severe agglomeration of the nanoparticles. Herein, it should be noted that no chemical interactions occurred between the particles and the polymer matrix, so mechanical interlocking of the polymer chain by the nanoparticles could be the main mechanism of the enhanced durability.

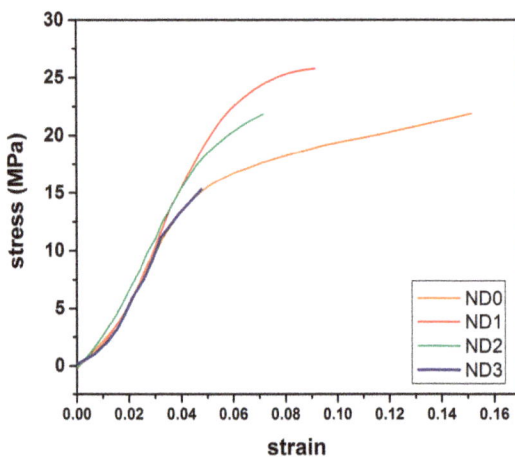

Figure 5. Stress-strain curves of electrospun mats containing different amounts of diamond nanoparticles.

Table 2. Effect of MND on the mechanical properties and permeability of electrospun mats.

Concentration	Elastic Modulus (MPa)	Yield Strength (MPa)	Strain to Failure (%)	Permeability ($\mu g \cdot Pa^{-1} \cdot s^{-1} \cdot m^{-1}$)
0	353	21.7	15.4	423
1	458	25.3	9.9	345
2	393	20.2	7.9	342
3	405	15.9	4.8	359

2.5. Permeability

The water vapor permeability of films was determined by a gravimetric method at room temperature. It is noteworthy that permeability of wound dressings is an important factor in the skin repairing process in order to create the appropriate moisture in wound area and stop over-drying [17]. Figure 6 shows weight change of the mats over time per unit area. The slope of the lines yields the average value of permeability (Table 2). It is seen that the permeability of the electrospun mats decreases with increasing the ND concentration. It is known that the permeability is related to the size and structure of pores in the fibrous mats [53]. As shown in Figure 1, the membranes containing MND exhibited finer fibers with a more closed-packed structure; hence, the permeability was reduced.

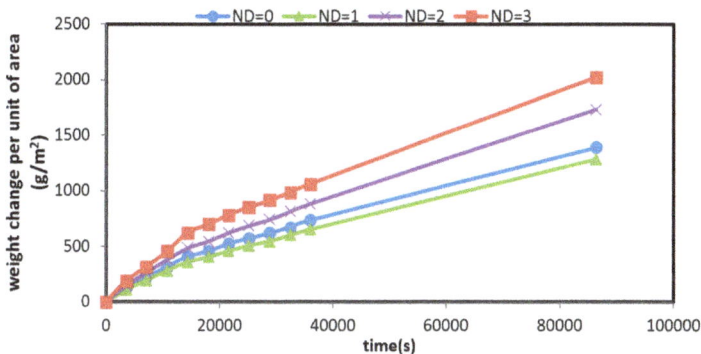

Figure 6. Weight change per unit of area of the mats versus time for CS/BC mats containing different amounts of MND.

2.6. Cell Viability Assessment

Many studies have shown that diamond particles are cytocompatiable [54–56]. To be certain that embedding of these particles in the fibrous structure of CS/BC prepared by electrospinning does not degrade biocompatibility, MTT assay was performed. Figure 7 shows the cell viability of electrospun mats containing different amounts of MND after 24 and 72 h incubation. The viability varied in the range of 75%–90% of the control sample. As compared with previous studies [8], the prepared mats exhibited better cytocompatibility to L929 cells. The cell viability decreased when increasing the amount of MND beyond 2 wt %. This observation might be related to the agglomeration of the nanoparticles as well as refined fibrous structure with different pore sizes.

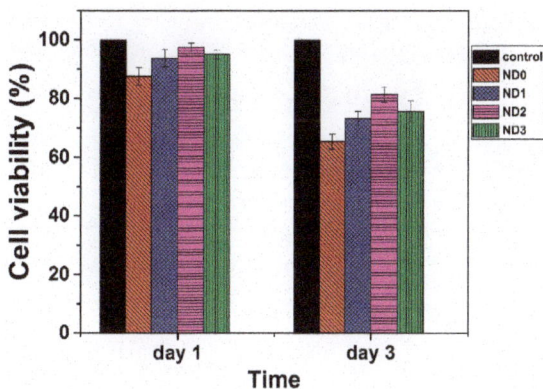

Figure 7. Cell viability of CS/BC mats dependent on the MND content at two incubated times.

3. Experimental Procedure

3.1. Materials

Chitosan, with an average molecular weight of 90–150 kDa and degree of deacetylation of 75%–85%, was supplied by Sigma-Aldrich Co. (St. Louis, MO, USA). Bacterial cellulose nanofibers were purchased from Nano Novin Polymer Co., Sari, Iran. Medical grade diamond nanoparticles with an average particle size of 2–6 nm (Grade PL-D-G, purity > 87%) were supplied by PlasmaChem GmbH (Berlin, Germany). Acetic acid (100%) was obtained from Merck Co., Darmstadt, Germany.

Polyethylene oxide (PEO), with a molecular weight of 900 kDa, was provided by Sigma-Aldrich Co. (St. Louis, MO, USA).

3.2. Preparation of Fibrous Mats

To prepare polymeric solutions for electrospinning, an aqueous solution of chitosan in acetic acid (3 wt %) was prepared. The solution was blended with a bacterial cellulose gel (5 wt %) dissolved in acetic acid (90%). A polyethylene oxide solution in deionized water (5 wt %) was separately prepared and added to the CS/BC suspension. The final composition of the suspension was 45:45:10 CS:BC:PEO. The aim of PEO addition was to reduce the viscosity of the gel and facilitate electrospinning [57].

MND-modified fibrous mats were prepared by electrospinning the polymeric suspension mixed with MND in a concentration of 1, 2, and 3 wt % of the polymer. The diamond nanoparticles were dispersed in deionized water by employing an ultrasonic bath (Wise Clean, Model: WUC-D10h using power of 690 W) for one hour. The dispersion was added to the polymeric suspension and sonicated for one hour.

A single jet electrospinning apparatus (Model HVPS-35/500, ANSTCO, Tehran, Iran) was employed to prepare fibrous mats. The suspension was fed into a horizontally aligned syringe with a needle orifice of 0.55 mm in inner diameter. The distance between syringe and collector was fixed at 10 cm and the applied voltage was 20–22 kV. The electrospinning feeding rate was 0.3 mL/h and the suspensions were spun toward a rotating drum (1000 rpm). The randomly oriented nanofibers were collected on an aluminum foil.

3.3. Materials Characterization

The size and morphology of the fibers were studied by field-emission scanning electron microscopy (FE-SEM; Hitachi Ltd., Tokyo, Japan, F-System 4160) at an acceleration voltage of 20 kV. Gold coating was applied before imaging. Fourier transform infrared (FT-IR) analysis was performed by a Spectrum 400 Perkin Elmer (Waltham, MA, USA) in the range of 450–4000 cm^{-1} with a resolution of 1 cm^{-1}. A universal tensile testing machine (Instron 5566, Norwood, MA, USA) was employed to evaluate the mechanical properties i.e. ultimate Tensile Strength (UTS) and elongation to break, based on ASTM Standard D638. The examined mats had a thickness of 30 $\pm$ 2 μm and a gauge length of 20 mm. The crosshead speed was 5.0 mm/min. Each test was repeated three times and the average values were recorded.

To determine the hydrophilicity of the membranes, water contact measurement was performed by employing an OCA 15 plus video-based optical contact angle meter (Data Physics Instruments GmbH, Filderstadt, Germany). Water vapor permeability (WVP) was gravimetrically determined according to ASTM E96 desiccant method at room temperature. Films with an area of 3.5 cm^2 were prepared and overlaid on cups filled with silica gel. The cups were placed in a desiccator containing saturated salt solution of ammonium nitrate with relative moisture 65%. At several time periods (1–24 h), the weight change was measured. Water vapor transmission (WVT) and permeability (WVP) were determined by [23]:

$$WVT = \frac{G}{t \times A} \ (g/sec.m^2) \tag{1}$$

$$WVP = \frac{WVT}{\Delta P} \times T = \frac{WVT}{S(R_1 - R_2)} \times T \ (g/Pa.sec.m) \tag{2}$$

where G is the weight gain of the cup at time t, A the permeation area, ΔP the vapor pressure difference across the mat—calculated based on the vapor saturation pressure (S) and the relative humidity inside (100%) and outside the cup (49%)—and T the average thickness of the mats.

3.4. Cell Viability

Cell viability was evaluated using the standard 3-(4,5-dimethylthiazol-2-yl)-2,5-diphenyl tetrazolium bromide (MTT) assay protocol. The assay is based on the conversion of MTT into formazan crystals by living cells, which determines mitochondrial activity. Briefly, 5×10^5 mouse skin fibroblast cells (L929) (National Cell Bank, Iran Pasture Institute) were seeded onto the specimens with a 6-well plate and incubated at 37 °C in 5% CO_2 for 24 and 48 h. After each interval, 200 mL of MTT solution (Sigma, St. Louis, MO, USA, 5 mg/mL) in $1\times$ Dulbecco's phosphate-buffered saline (PBS; Sigma, St. Louis, MO, USA) was added to each well and the cells were incubated for another 4 h. Upon removal of the MTT solution, the formed formazan crystals were solubilized with isopropanol for 15 min. Absorbance was read at the wavelength of 570 nm. The data were reported separately for each well by an ELISA reader (BioTek Microplate Reader, BioTek Company, Winooski, VT, USA). An average of triplicate wells was calculated, and the standard deviation for each sample was calculated based on Student's *t*-test ($p < 0.05$). To observe the morphology of the adherent cells, the films were washed by PBS three times and then immersed in 3% glutaraldehyde PBS solution for 30 min for cell fixing. The films were dehydrated in ascending series of ethanol aqueous solutions (50 to 100 percent) at room temperature. The specimens were kept overnight in a desiccator to remove any moisture. The growth of the cells was observed after 24 h incubation.

4. Conclusions

Chitosan/bacterial cellulose nanofibrous membranes modified with diamond nanoparticles were fabricated by electrospinning. It was shown that uniform mats with an average fiber diameter of about 130 nm could be prepared at the spinning distance of 120 mm, applied voltage of 20 kV, and CS/BC ratio of 1:1. The effect of MND particles on the electrospinning of CS/BC blends was also studied. It was shown that MND particles reduced the average fiber diameter. The mechanical properties under tensile loading, the hydrophilicity, and water vapor permeability of the nanocomposites were also examined. An enhancement in the mechanical strength with a decrease in strain to failure was measured due to the addition of MND to the CS/BC nanofibers. Introduction of MND particles was accompanied with a gradual decrease in the hydrophilicity of the nanofibrous membranes as well. The water vapor permeability of the CS/BC nanofibers was also decreased. The cell viability of fibrous membrane after a 1-day incubation was >90% as compared with the control. We concluded that the fibrous mat containing 1% MND could be a promising candidate for wound dress and tissue engineering applications. Meanwhile, in vivo studies and pre-clinical investigations are required to explore the suitability of developed mats for biomedical applications.

Acknowledgments: The authors thank Fatemeh Ostadhossein and Shayan Mousavi. The funding support from the Grant Program of Sharif University of Technology (No. G930305) and Iran Elite Foundation (Grant No. ENL 5418) is highly appreciated.

Author Contributions: M.M. and N.M. helped in design of experiments, analyzing of the results, and manuscript preparation. F.R.A. prepared the specimens and characterized the materials. A.S. designed the experiments, guided the research, and prepared the manuscript.

Conflicts of Interest: The authors declare no conflict of interest.

References

1. Zahedi, P.; Rezaeian, I.; Ranaei-Siadat, S.O.; Jafari, S.H.; Supaphol, P. A review on wound dressings with an emphasis on electrospun nanofibrous polymeric bandages. *Polym. Adv. Technol.* **2010**, *21*, 77–95. [CrossRef]
2. Kokabi, M.; Sirousazar, M.; Hassan, Z.M. Pva-clay nanocomposite hydrogels for wound dressing. *Eur. Polym. J.* **2007**, *43*, 773–781. [CrossRef]
3. Jiang, T.; Carbone, E.J.; Lo, K.W.-H.; Laurencin, C.T. Electrospinning of polymer nanofibers for tissue regeneration. *Prog. Polym. Sci.* **2015**, *46*, 1–24. [CrossRef]
4. Sun, B.; Jiang, X.-J.; Zhang, S.; Zhang, J.-C.; Li, Y.-F.; You, Q.-Z.; Long, Y.-Z. Electrospun anisotropic architectures and porous structures for tissue engineering. *J. Mater. Chem. B* **2015**, *3*, 5389–5410. [CrossRef]

5. Patrulea, V.; Ostafe, V.; Borchard, G.; Jordan, O. Chitosan as a starting material for wound healing applications. *Eur. J. Pharm. Biopharm.* **2015**, *97*, 417–426. [CrossRef] [PubMed]

6. Azuma, K.; Izumi, R.; Osaki, T.; Ifuku, S.; Morimoto, M.; Saimoto, H.; Minami, S.; Okamoto, Y. Chitin, chitosan, and its derivatives for wound healing: Old and new materials. *J. Funct. Biomater.* **2015**, *6*, 104–142. [CrossRef] [PubMed]

7. Mahmoudi, N.; Ostadhossein, F.; Simchi, A. Physicochemical and antibacterial properties of chitosan-polyvinylpyrrolidone films containing self-organized graphene oxide nanolayers. *J. Appl. Polym. Sci.* **2016**, *133*. [CrossRef]

8. Ostadhossein, F.; Mahmoudi, N.; Morales-Cid, G.; Tamjid, E.; Navas-Martos, F.J.; Soriano-Cuadrado, B.; Paniza, J.M.L.; Simchi, A. Development of chitosan/bacterial cellulose composite films containing nanodiamonds as a potential flexible platform for wound dressing. *Materials* **2015**, *8*, 6401–6418. [CrossRef]

9. Zhu, W.; Li, W.; He, Y.; Duan, T. In-situ biopreparation of biocompatible bacterial cellulose/graphene oxide composites pellets. *Appl. Surf. Sci.* **2015**, *338*, 22–26. [CrossRef]

10. Pina, S.; Oliveira, J.M.; Reis, R.L. Natural-based nanocomposites for bone tissue engineering and regenerative medicine: A review. *Adv. Mater.* **2015**, *27*, 1143–1169. [CrossRef] [PubMed]

11. Koosha, M.; Mirzadeh, H. Electrospinning, mechanical properties, and cell behavior study of chitosan/PVA nanofibers. *J. Biomed. Mater. Res. A* **2015**, *103*, 3081–3093. [CrossRef] [PubMed]

12. Jayakumar, R.; Prabaharan, M.; Kumar, P.S.; Nair, S.; Tamura, H. Biomaterials based on chitin and chitosan in wound dressing applications. *Biotechnol. Adv.* **2011**, *29*, 322–337. [CrossRef] [PubMed]

13. Ibrahim, H.; El-Zairy, E. Chitosan as a Biomaterial—Structure, Properties, and Electrospun Nanofibers. *Intech* **2015**, *4*, 7–14. [CrossRef]

14. Jia, Y.; Huang, G.; Dong, F.; Liu, Q.; Nie, W. Preparation and characterization of electrospun poly (ε-caprolactone)/poly (vinyl pyrrolidone) nanofiber composites containing silver particles. *Polym. Compos.* **2015**. [CrossRef]

15. Haider, S.; Al-Masry, W.; Al-Zeghayer, Y.; Al-Hoshan, M.; Ali, F.A. Fabrication chitosan nano fibers membrane via electrospinning. *Une* **2016**, *13*, 15.

16. Millon, L.E.; Guhados, G.; Wan, W. Anisotropic polyvinyl alcohol—Bacterial cellulose nanocomposite for biomedical applications. *J. Biomed. Mater. Res. B Appl. Biomater.* **2008**, *86*, 444–452. [CrossRef] [PubMed]

17. Czaja, W.; Krystynowicz, A.; Bielecki, S.; Brown, R.M. Microbial cellulose—The natural power to heal wounds. *Biomaterials* **2006**, *27*, 145–151. [CrossRef] [PubMed]

18. Millon, L.; Wan, W. The polyvinyl alcohol–bacterial cellulose system as a new nanocomposite for biomedical applications. *J. Biomed. Mater. Res. B Appl. Biomater.* **2006**, *79*, 245–253. [CrossRef] [PubMed]

19. Helenius, G.; Bäckdahl, H.; Bodin, A.; Nannmark, U.; Gatenholm, P.; Risberg, B. In vivo biocompatibility of bacterial cellulose. *J. Biomed. Mater. Res. A* **2006**, *76*, 431–438. [CrossRef] [PubMed]

20. Fu, L.; Zhang, J.; Yang, G. Present status and applications of bacterial cellulose-based materials for skin tissue repair. *Carbohydr. Polym.* **2013**, *92*, 1432–1442. [CrossRef] [PubMed]

21. Jebel, F.S.; Almasi, H. Morphological, physical, antimicrobial and release properties of ZnO nanoparticles-loaded bacterial cellulose films. *Carbohydr. Polym.* **2016**, *149*, 8–19. [CrossRef] [PubMed]

22. Römling, U.; Galperin, M.Y. Bacterial cellulose biosynthesis: Diversity of operons, subunits, products and functions. *Trends Microbiol.* **2015**, *23*, 545–557. [CrossRef] [PubMed]

23. Fernandes, S.C.; Oliveira, L.; Freire, C.S.; Silvestre, A.J.; Neto, C.P.; Gandini, A.; Desbriéres, J. Novel transparent nanocomposite films based on chitosan and bacterial cellulose. *Green Chem.* **2009**, *11*, 2023–2029. [CrossRef]

24. Phisalaphong, M.; Jatupaiboon, N. Biosynthesis and characterization of bacteria cellulose–chitosan film. *Carbohydr. Polym.* **2008**, *74*, 482–488. [CrossRef]

25. Lin, W.-C.; Lien, C.-C.; Yeh, H.-J.; Yu, C.-M.; Hsu, S.-H. Bacterial cellulose and bacterial cellulose–chitosan membranes for wound dressing applications. *Carbohydr. Polym.* **2013**, *94*, 603–611. [CrossRef] [PubMed]

26. Zhang, P.; Chen, L.; Zhang, Q.; Hong, F.F. Using in situ dynamic cultures to rapidly biofabricate fabric-reinforced composites of chitosan/bacterial nanocellulose for antibacterial wound dressings. *Front. Microbiol.* **2016**, *7*. [CrossRef] [PubMed]

27. Azarniya, A.; Eslahi, N.; Mahmoudi, N.; Simchi, A. Effect of graphene oxide nanosheets on the physico-mechanical properties of chitosan/bacterial cellulose nanofibrous composites. *Compos. A Appl. Sci. Manuf.* **2016**, *85*, 113–122. [CrossRef]

28. Ahmed, F.E.; Lalia, B.S.; Hashaikeh, R. A review on electrospinning for membrane fabrication: Challenges and applications. *Desalination* **2015**, *356*, 15–30. [CrossRef]

29. HPS, A.K.; Saurabh, C.K.; Adnan, A.; Fazita, M.N.; Syakir, M.; Davoudpour, Y.; Rafatullah, M.; Abdullah, C.; Haafiz, M.; Dungani, R. A review on chitosan-cellulose blends and nanocellulose reinforced chitosan biocomposites: Properties and their applications. *Carbohydr. Polym.* **2016**, *150*, 216–226.

30. Khalil, H.A.; Davoudpour, Y.; Bhat, A.; Rosamah, E.; Tahir, P.M. Electrospun cellulose composite nanofibers. In *Handbook of Polymer Nanocomposites. Processing, Performance and Application*; Springer: Berlin/Heidelberg, Germany, 2015; pp. 191–227.

31. Liu, Y.; Zhou, J.; Tang, J.; Tang, W. Three-dimensional, chemically bonded polypyrrole/bacterial cellulose/graphene composites for high-performance supercapacitors. *Chem. Mater.* **2015**, *27*, 7034–7041. [CrossRef]

32. Kalashnikova, I.; Das, S.; Seal, S. Nanomaterials for wound healing: Scope and advancement. *Nanomedicine* **2015**, *10*, 2593–2612. [CrossRef] [PubMed]

33. Hsiao, S.-T.; Ma, C.-C.M.; Tien, H.-W.; Liao, W.-H.; Wang, Y.-S.; Li, S.-M.; Chuang, W.-P. Preparation and characterization of silver nanoparticle-reduced graphene oxide decorated electrospun polyurethane fiber composites with an improved electrical property. *Compos. Sci. Technol.* **2015**, *118*, 171–177. [CrossRef]

34. Schrand, A.M.; Dai, L.; Schlager, J.J.; Hussain, S.M.; Osawa, E. Differential biocompatibility of carbon nanotubes and nanodiamonds. *Diam. Relat. Mater.* **2007**, *16*, 2118–2123. [CrossRef]

35. Zhu, Y.; Li, J.; Li, W.; Zhang, Y.; Yang, X.; Chen, N.; Sun, Y.; Zhao, Y.; Fan, C.; Huang, Q. The biocompatibility of nanodiamonds and their application in drug delivery systems. *Theranostics* **2012**, *2*, 302–312. [CrossRef] [PubMed]

36. Kaur, R.; Badea, I. Nanodiamonds as novel nanomaterials for biomedical applications: Drug delivery and imaging systems. *Int. J. Nanomed.* **2013**, *8*, 203.

37. Hsu, C.M.; Shivkumar, S. *N,N*-dimethylformamide additions to the solution for the electrospinning of poly (ε-caprolactone) nanofibers. *Macromol. Mater. Eng.* **2004**, *289*, 334–340. [CrossRef]

38. Li, X.; Bian, F.; Lin, J.; Zeng, Y. Effect of electric field on the morphology and mechanical properties of electrospun fibers. *RSC Adv.* **2016**, *6*, 50666–50672. [CrossRef]

39. Naseri, N.; Mathew, A.P.; Girandon, L.; Fröhlich, M.; Oksman, K. Porous electrospun nanocomposite mats based on chitosan–cellulose nanocrystals for wound dressing: Effect of surface characteristics of nanocrystals. *Cellulose* **2015**, *22*, 521–534. [CrossRef]

40. Rakha, S.A.; Raza, R.; Munir, A. Reinforcement effect of nanodiamond on properties of epoxy matrix. *Polym. Compos.* **2013**, *34*, 811–818. [CrossRef]

41. Kartikowati, C.W.; Suhendi, A.; Zulhijah, R.; Ogi, T.; Iwaki, T.; Okuyama, K. Preparation and evaluation of magnetic nanocomposite fibers containing α''-$Fe_{16}N_2$ and α-Fe nanoparticles in polyvinylpyrrolidone via magneto-electrospinning. *Nanotechnology* **2015**, *27*. [CrossRef]

42. Ul-Islam, M.; Shah, N.; Ha, J.H.; Park, J.K. Effect of chitosan penetration on physico-chemical and mechanical properties of bacterial cellulose. *Korean J. Chem. Eng.* **2011**, *28*, 1736–1743. [CrossRef]

43. Mishra, R.; Rao, K.J. On the formation of poly (ethyleneoxide)-poly (vinylalcohol) blends. *Eur. Polym. J.* **1999**, *35*, 1883–1894. [CrossRef]

44. Duan, B.; Dong, C.; Yuan, X.; Yao, K. Electrospinning of chitosan solutions in acetic acid with poly (ethylene oxide). *J. Biomater. Sci. Polym. Ed.* **2004**, *15*, 797–811. [CrossRef] [PubMed]

45. Osswald, S.; Yushin, G.; Mochalin, V.; Kucheyev, S.O.; Gogotsi, Y. Control of sp^2/sp^3 carbon ratio and surface chemistry of nanodiamond powders by selective oxidation in air. *J. Am. Chem. Soc.* **2006**, *128*, 11635–11642. [CrossRef] [PubMed]

46. Morimune, S.; Kotera, M.; Nishino, T.; Goto, K.; Hata, K. Poly (vinyl alcohol) nanocomposites with nanodiamond. *Macromolecules* **2011**, *44*, 4415–4421. [CrossRef]

47. Zou, Q.; Li, Y.; Zou, L.; Wang, M. Characterization of structures and surface states of the nanodiamond synthesized by detonation. *Mater. Charact.* **2009**, *60*, 1257–1262. [CrossRef]

48. Pan, H.; Xu, D.; Liu, Q.; Ren, H.Q.; Zhou, M. Preparation and Characterization of Corn Starch-Nanodiamond Composite Films. In *Applied Mechanics and Materials*; Trans Tech. Publ.: Zurich, Switzerland, 2014; pp. 156–161.

49. Wang, X.; Yu, J.; Sun, G.; Ding, B. Electrospun nanofibrous materials: A versatile medium for effective oil/water separation. *Mater. Today* **2015**. [CrossRef]

50. Wang, Z.; Macosko, C.W.; Bates, F.S. Fluorine enriched melt blown fibers from polymer blends of poly (butylene terephthalate) and a fluorinated multiblock copolyester. *ACS Appl. Mater. Interfaces* **2016**, *8*, 754–761. [CrossRef] [PubMed]

51. Ma, M.; Mao, Y.; Gupta, M.; Gleason, K.K.; Rutledge, G.C. Superhydrophobic fabrics produced by electrospinning and chemical vapor deposition. *Macromolecules* **2005**, *38*, 9742–9748. [CrossRef]

52. Tjong, S. Structural and mechanical properties of polymer nanocomposites. *Mater. Sci. Eng. R Rep.* **2006**, *53*, 73–197. [CrossRef]

53. Cui, W.; Zhou, Y.; Chang, J. Electrospun nanofibrous materials for tissue engineering and drug delivery. *Sci. Technol. Adv. Mater.* **2016**. [CrossRef]

54. Lee, D.-K.; Kim, S.V.; Limansubroto, A.N.; Yen, A.; Soundia, A.; Wang, C.-Y.; Shi, W.; Hong, C.; Tetradis, S.; Kim, Y. Nanodiamond–gutta percha composite biomaterials for root canal therapy. *ACS Nano* **2015**, *9*, 11490–11501. [CrossRef] [PubMed]

55. Hsiao, W.W.-W.; Hui, Y.Y.; Tsai, P.-C.; Chang, H.-C. Fluorescent nanodiamond: A versatile tool for long-term cell tracking, super-resolution imaging, and nanoscale temperature sensing. *Acc. Chem. Res.* **2016**, *49*, 400–407. [CrossRef] [PubMed]

56. Taylor, A.C.; Vagaska, B.; Edgington, R.; Hébert, C.; Ferretti, P.; Bergonzo, P.; Jackman, R.B. Biocompatibility of nanostructured boron doped diamond for the attachment and proliferation of human neural stem cells. *J. Neural Eng.* **2015**, *12*. [CrossRef] [PubMed]

57. Rieger, K.A.; Birch, N.P.; Schiffman, J.D. Electrospinning chitosan/poly (ethylene oxide) solutions with essential oils: Correlating solution rheology to nanofiber formation. *Carbohydr. Polym.* **2016**, *139*, 131–138. [CrossRef] [PubMed]

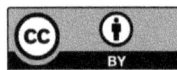

marine drugs

|MDPI|

Article

Effect of Experimental Parameters on Alginate/Chitosan Microparticles for BCG Encapsulation

Liliana A. Caetano [1,2], António J. Almeida [2] and Lídia M.D. Gonçalves [2,*]

[1] ESTeSL-Lisbon School of Health Technology, Polytechnic Institute of Lisbon, 1990-096 Lisbon, Portugal; lacaetano@ff.ulisboa.pt

[2] Research Institute for Medicines (iMed.ULisboa), Faculty of Pharmacy, University of Lisbon, 1649-003 Lisbon, Portugal; aalmeida@ff.ulisboa.pt

* Correspondence: lgoncalves@ff.ulisboa.pt; Tel.: +351-21-7946400

Academic Editor: Paola Laurienzo
Received: 3 February 2016; Accepted: 28 April 2016; Published: 11 May 2016

Abstract: The aim of the present study was to develop novel *Mycobacterium bovis* bacille Calmette-Guérin (BCG)-loaded polymeric microparticles with optimized particle surface characteristics and biocompatibility, so that whole live attenuated bacteria could be further used for pre-exposure vaccination against *Mycobacterium tuberculosis* by the intranasal route. BCG was encapsulated in chitosan and alginate microparticles through three different polyionic complexation methods by high speed stirring. For comparison purposes, similar formulations were prepared with high shear homogenization and sonication. Additional optimization studies were conducted with polymers of different quality specifications in a wide range of pH values, and with three different cryoprotectors. Particle morphology, size distribution, encapsulation efficiency, surface charge, physicochemical properties and biocompatibility were assessed. Particles exhibited a micrometer size and a spherical morphology. Chitosan addition to BCG shifted the bacilli surface charge from negative zeta potential values to strongly positive ones. Chitosan of low molecular weight produced particle suspensions of lower size distribution and higher stability, allowing efficient BCG encapsulation and biocompatibility. Particle formulation consistency was improved when the availability of functional groups from alginate and chitosan was close to stoichiometric proportion. Thus, the herein described microparticulate system constitutes a promising strategy to deliver BCG vaccine by the intranasal route.

Keywords: alginate; chitosan; BCG; microencapsulation; biocompatibility

1. Introduction

Enhanced immunization strategies must be urgently found for tuberculosis control [1,2]. The current available vaccine used for pre-exposure vaccination against tuberculosis is *Mycobacterium bovis* BCG. As with most vaccines nowadays, BCG is parenterally administrated by subcutaneous route. This implies a relatively high production cost, the need for cold chain, and the need for trained personnel for vaccine administration, while it also leads to lower patient compliance. Regarding the resulting immune response, parenterally delivered vaccines usually produce poor mucosal responses, which is critical to preventing tuberculosis, as *Mycobacterium tuberculosis* normally enters the host through mucosal surfaces. The nasal route might therefore be an attractive alternative administration route [3].

Regarding tuberculosis, it is essential for a new vaccine to better target the lungs while improving interaction with antigen presenting cells (APCs) in the lung mucosa, such as alveolar macrophages [4].

It is also well known that the eradication of *Mycobacterium tuberculosis* with pre-exposure vaccination depends on adequate antigen presentation to amplify the elicited immune response, essentially cellular Th1 types [5–8]. As such, whole live attenuated bacteria act as the ideal antigen producers and vectors, as they are multigenic and normally mimic pathogens and surpass natural barriers.

In recent decades, several studies have elucidated the pros and cons of the nasal route for vaccine administration. It is well known that, for soluble antigens, limited absorption occurs at the nasal mucosa due to physiological barriers (*i.e.*, mucosal epithelium, rapid mucociliary clearance, protease degradation) [9]. Many strategies have been proposed in order to surpass these barriers and to increase the immunogenicity of intranasal delivered antigens, namely, the use of permeation enhancers, mucosal adjuvants and nano- and microparticulate delivery systems [10,11]. Some studies refer to a boost in the immune response due to an adjuvant effect of particulate delivery systems, combined with the use of potent immunopotentiators, either present in the formulation or co-delivered with antigens [12–18].

Taking into consideration the aforementioned, it has been hypothesized that BCG bacilli modification through encapsulation in polymeric microparticulate delivery systems could be an alternative to the classical BCG vaccine, suitable for mucosal immunization. Thus, the main goal of this work was to encapsulate whole live BCG into polymers with biocompatible and mucoadhesive properties using only mild conditions, so that BCG viability was maintained and the biocompatibility of the developed microparticulate delivery system was assured. Microencapsulation of BCG in chitosan-alginate microparticles will allow the following to take place *in vivo*, in sequence: bacilli desorption from the particle surface; degradation and erosion of the polymer network; release of bacteria. Moreover, with the entrapment of BCG in polymeric microparticles, it is expected to change the BCG recognition pattern by the immune system and to modulate the mechanism of cellular uptake by APCs cells. The selection of the microsize range was related to the intrinsic length of BCG bacilli rod of approximately 2–4 micrometers, whereas the preference for electropositively charged microparticles depends on their ability to better interact with negatively charged mucin [19–21].

The use of biodegradable polymeric particles has been proposed as a promising approach to elicit adequate immune responses, while protecting antigens from degradation [18]. The preparation of polymeric particles can be achieved through a wide range of preparation methods, each one yielding particle formation within a determined size range. For instance, nanoprecipitation and supercritical fluid technology usually yield nanoparticles, whereas spray-drying and solvent evaporation may produce nano- or microparticles depending on the experimental conditions [22,23]. It is generally stated that, for nasal delivery of antigens, nanoparticles are more favorable than particles in the microsize range, as nanoparticles are better taken up by the M-cells present in the nasal associated lymphoid tissue (NALT), and better transported through the epithelial cells (by paracellular and transcellular transference), thus, leading to increased local and systemic immune responses [24,25]. Nevertheless, microparticles sized up to 40 micron have also been described as successful in eliciting immune responses through nasal administration [11,26–29].

The most commonly described biodegradable polymers are poly(D,L-lactide-co-glycolide) (PLGA) and poly(L-lactide) (PLA); however, particle formation with PLGA and PLA occurs only in the presence of organic solvents. This is a major drawback, for several reasons. Not only the use of organic solvents may lead to relevant toxicological effects, it can also prompt antigen denaturation or hamper cellular vaccine viability, while formulation methods usually require multiple steps and are time consuming. In view of the aim of producing a live vaccine, the longer it takes to carry out the formulation steps, the greater the possibility of losing some of the vaccine or of compromising cell viability, thereby reducing the encapsulation efficiency and potency of the vaccine.

In this context, chitosan (a deacetylated form of chitin extracted from crustaceans), and sodium alginate (a natural product extracted from algae belonging to the Phaeophyceae, mainly species of *Laminaria*) were chosen to prepare polymeric microparticles by ionic cross-linking methods as described elsewhere [30–35]. Both chitosan and alginate have been extensively studied as biomaterials and pharmaceutical excipients due to their biodegradability and low toxicity, and have been included in the composition of several foods and dietary supplements [36,37]. With ionic gelation methods, particles are formed in a single step by a simple mechanism, usually involving two different polymers and one complexation agent, by adding one polymer solution to the other one with stirring. Most commonly described complexation agents used with chitosan and alginate are calcium chloride and tripolyphosphate (TPP) [35,38].

The widespread use of polyionic complexation methods presents many advantages, such as their simplicity, versatility and flexibility, being applicable for virtually all polymers which can be polymerized in the presence of a complexation agent, while being easily adjusted by changing a number of experimental parameters. During optimization studies, the formulation conditions can be changed to obtain desired features, namely, particle size, encapsulation efficiency, surface charge, biocompatibility profile, and production yield. The type of used polymers (*i.e.*, chemical nature, molecular weight, viscosity, purity, pH, and other relevant specifications), the polymer to polymer mass ratio, the type and concentration of complexation agent, the homogenization type (*i.e.*, shear, speed and duration) and the polymer to antigen ratio are some of the variables which significantly influence the particles' characteristics. Furthermore, the mild preparation conditions of these methods allow the encapsulation of antigens without degradation caused by high temperatures, oxidation or hydrolysis, as with other commonly used techniques.

As previously stated, both chitosan and alginate have been extensively used in the preparation of polymeric nano- and micro-particles for immunization purposes. Chitosan and its derivatives are described to increase the absorption of macromolecules through epithelial membranes, and to increase both antigen residence time and uptake at the mucosal site, due to its intrinsic mucoadhesiveness [11,39–44]. Chitosan has been used to prepare nano- and microparticles intended for nasal and oral delivery of vaccines with great results, as chitosan particles were able to elicit strong systemic and local immune responses to different antigens [16,24,25,34,41,45–53].

Alginates are block copolymers polysaccharides, composed of long homopolymeric regions of mannuronate (M) and guluronate (G), as the result of the conversion of mannuronic and guluronic acid through neutralization during extraction from its natural source. The proportion, distribution and length of these blocks determine the chemical and physical properties of the alginate molecules. While G-blocks provide gel-forming capacity, MM and MG units provide flexibility to the uronic acid chains, with flexibility increasing in the order GG < MM < MG.

Alginates constitute a very versatile material, having numerous pharmaceutical applications due to their gelling, film-forming, thickening and stabilizing properties. It is said that the improved stability of chitosan formulations can be assessed by developing chitosan blends with another polymer, namely sodium alginate [36]. Two other valuable properties of alginates are that they are water-soluble, allowing gel formation without heating or cooling, and also that the alginate matrix allows the entrapment of molecules by capillary forces, which remain free to migrate by diffusion, depending on the size. These features make alginates attractive gelling biopolymers for cell encapsulation purposes. Gel formation and gel structure are determined by alginate type and calcium salt (Ca^{2+}), being influenced by pH value, solubility and temperature. For instance, at lower pH values, alginate gel is shrunk and a reduction of the pore size of alginate matrix can be achieved, especially in the case of low G content alginate. As such, these components and factors must be matched in order to optimise the overall formulation of alginate microparticles by ionotropic gelation.

The formulation studies presented in this work aimed the optimization of the preparation conditions of BCG-loaded polymeric particles taking into consideration the final yield of production, encapsulation efficiency, particle size distribution and surface charge. Therefore, variables such as the type of polymer or of polymer blends, polymers solution pH value, the polymer/polymer and BCG/polymers ratio, as well as the type and time of homogenization procedures and order of polymers and counter ions solutions' incorporation were studied. The herein described effects of experimental conditions on critical features of microparticle formulations provide a processing window for manipulating and optimizing particles in the microsize range for intended applications.

The expected advantages of the herein described systems for vaccine delivery include the capacity of polymeric microparticulate systems to increase antigen residence time (due to the differentiated release profile in the presence of alginate and chitosan) and to enhance antigen interaction with the cell surfaces. Moreover, due to chitosan's and alginate's mucoadhesiveness, microparticles would be able to promote mucopenetration, thus increasing antigen delivery.

2. Results and Discussion

2.1. Characterization of Polymeric Microparticles

The purpose of this study was to optimize the experimental parameters to prepare BCG-loaded polymeric microparticles intended for intranasal immunization studies, presenting suitable size distribution or surface charge, critical aspects for vaccine delivery. Therefore, the conditions for microparticle preparation were optimized during preliminary formulation studies. Two polymers—chitosan and sodium alginate—with different quality specifications (molecular weight, viscosity, G-content, deacetylation degree, purity) were used to prepare plain polymeric microparticles, followed by BCG microencapsulation. The prepared polymeric microparticles were characterized considering particle size distribution, surface charge, morphology, and the final yield of production. FT-IR studies were conducted in order to assess the interaction between chitosan and alginate ionic groups. Particle size was the leading assessed property during formulation optimization studies, oriented towards obtaining microparticles with a mean diameter of 5–10 μm, with a narrow and reproducible size distribution. Another key aspect regarding the preparation of vaccine-loaded polymeric particles is encapsulation efficiency, which should be as high as possible. Biocompatibility of the prepared polymeric microparticles was determined in a cell viability MTT assay, using a human monocyte cell line (THP-1) differentiated into macrophage-like cells, as a model for antigen presenting cells [54,55].

2.1.1. Size Distribution and Surface Charge

Previous studies showed that particle size distribution of plain polymeric microparticles prepared by ionic gelation was greatly influenced by the polymers' mass ratio and molecular weight [20,56,57]. Therefore, 14 formulations were initially developed with an alginate to chitosan mass ratio (ALG/CS) ranging from 0.02:1 to 4.23:1 (w/w), according to described Methods I and II, using different combinations of low viscosity (LV) alginate and low molecular weight (LMW) chitosan, medium viscosity (MV) alginate and medium molecular weight (MMW) chitosan, and high viscosity (HV) alginate and high molecular weight (HMW) chitosan. Microparticles were characterised for size distribution (mean diameter and span) and surface charge (zeta potential).

The effect of polymer molecular weight with increasing alginate to chitosan mass ratio on particle size distribution is presented in Table 1. Regarding the use of low molecular weight chitosan, particles ranging from 18 to 34 μm were obtained with a narrow size distribution (span < 2.5) (Table 1). Using chitosan of medium molecular weight yielded a general increase in particle mean diameter, with formulation F13 (0.8:1 alginate to chitosan mass ratio, w/w) being the only exception. Using chitosan of high molecular weight led to an intermediate particle mean diameter, except also for F13 (Table 1). Herein presented formulations were obtained with a relatively narrow size distribution (span ≤ 5), except for formulation F11 prepared with low molecular weight chitosan (span = 9.5). The obtained span values suggest that particles are formed with better consistency when the availability of the functional groups is close to stoichiometric proportion.

Broad particle size distributions can be attributed to the presence of larger single particles, which in turn might prompt aggregate formation [58,59]. By visual inspection, we confirmed the presence of aggregates mainly in formulations obtained with polymers of high MW (Figure 1). Best formulations, defined as suitable to yield turbid solution without aggregation, were obtained with chitosan of medium molecular weight when ALG/CS mass ratio ranged from 0.6:1 to 0.12:1, and with chitosan of low molecular weight when ALG/CS mass ratio ranged from 0.4:1 to 1:1.

Table 1. Particle size distribution (mean diameter and span) and surface charge (zeta potential) of microparticles on the preparation day.

Formulation	ALG:CS Mass Ratio (w/w)	Chitosan MW	Particle Size, d0.5 (µm)	Span	Zeta Potential (mV)	Production Yield (%)
F0	4.23:1	Low	18.5 ± 0.7	1.4 ± 0.0	−20.8 ± 7.9	n.d.
		Medium	260.5 ± 41.3	4.3 ± 0.6	−26.7 ± 4.9	n.d.
		High	68.1 ± 10.6	5.2 ± 2.9	−17.9 ± 6.8	n.d.
F11	0.4:1	Low	37.1 ± 0.7	9.5 ± 0.5	+34.0 ± 0.5	n.d.
		Medium	144.4 ± 5.1	3.0 ± 0.1	+47.1 ± 1.7	n.d.
		High	107.5 ± 10.1	4.1 ± 0.9	+30.4 ± 1.4	n.d.
F12	0.6:1	Low	39.3 ± 2.0	2.6 ± 0.1	+26.7 ± 1.1	n.d.
		Medium	94.7 ± 3.2	3.7 ± 0.2	+30.9 ± 1.1	n.d.
		High	65.9 ± 4.4	4.1 ± 0.7	+25.5 ± 0.5	n.d.
F13	0.8:1	Low	33.8 ± 0.9	2.6 ± 0.1	+22.7 ± 1.6	83.6 ± 0.0
		Medium	23.9 ± 0.6	2.7 ± 0.3	+25.6 ± 1.8	n.d.
		High	51.3 ± 1.8	3.3 ± 0.1	−0.2 ± 0.8	n.d.
F14	1:1	Low	25.9 ± 0.7	1.7 ± 0.1	+16.2 ± 0.6	36.8 ± 0.0
		Medium	139.0 ± 8.5	3.2 ± 0.1	−10.9 ± 1.6	n.d.
		High	80.6 ± 3.8	4.9 ± 0.2	−25.7 ± 3.3	n.d.

F0, microparticles obtained by Method (I) via alginate ionotropic pre-gelation with $CaCl_2$ followed by chitosan addition; F11-F14, microparticles, obtained by Method (II) via chitosan pre-gelation with alginate, followed by TPP (pH 9.0) addition. The pH of alginate and chitosan solutions was initially set to 4.9 and 4.6, respectively. Microparticle size is characterized using the size distribution parameters d0.1, d0.5 and d0.9 (diameter for which 10%, 50% and 90% of the size distribution falls below, respectively) and span (width of particle size distribution, according to the formula (d0.1 − d0.9)/d0.5). Results are expressed as mean and standard deviation ($n \geqslant 3$). n.d., not determined.

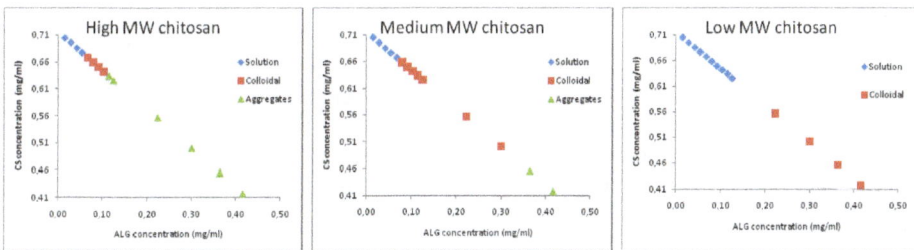

Figure 1. Microparticles domain formation using high, medium and low molecular weight chitosan. The pH of alginate and chitosan solutions was initially set to 4.9 and 4.6, respectively. Three different systems were identified: clear solution (♦), opalescent/colloidal suspension (■), and aggregates (▲).

The obtained results show a greater influence of chitosan molecular weight than alginate to chitosan mass ratio on microparticles size distribution. Overall, the use of chitosan of low molecular weight led to the formation of smaller particles for the majority of ALG/CS mass ratios, resulting in fewer aggregates. This may stem from the ability of chitosan of low molecular weight to diffuse more promptly in the alginate gel matrix to form smaller, more homogeneous particles, whereas, on the contrary, polymers of high molecular weight or viscosity may bind to the surface of such matrices, forming an outer membrane and leading to increment particle size [33,60].

The effect of polymer molecular weight with increasing alginate to chitosan mass ratio on particle surface charge is presented in Figure 2. Alginate to chitosan mass ratios ranging from 0.4:1 to 0.8:1 led to the formation of microparticles with high positive zeta potential values (+22.7 ± 1.6 mV to +47.1 ± 1.7 mV), thus, being positively charged, except for one formulation (F13 prepared with chitosan of high molecular weight) (−0.2 ± 0.8 mV). Higher ALG/CS mass ratios (1:1 and 4.23:1) led to the formation of negatively charged microparticles (−10.9 ± 1.6 mV to −26.7 ± 4.9 mV) with increasing polymer molecular weight. Formulation F14 prepared with chitosan of low molecular weight was the exception (+16.2 ± 0.6 mV).

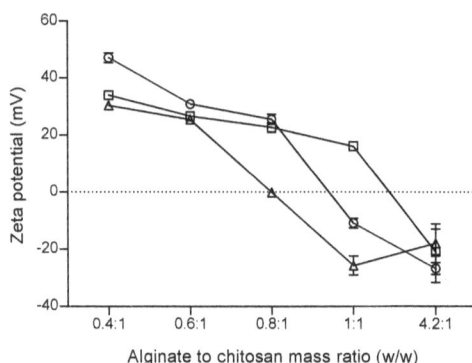

Figure 2. Effect of alginate to chitosan mass ratio on particle surface charge. The pH of alginate and chitosan solutions was initially set to 4.9 and 4.6, respectively. Zeta potential of microparticles prepared with chitosan of low molecular weight (□), medium molecular weight (○), and high molecular weight (Δ). Results are presented as mean ± SD ($n \geqslant 3$).

Zeta potential values provide a quantitative measure of the charge on colloidal particles in liquid suspension. For chitosan-alginate microparticles, surface charge greatly depends on chitosan total protonated amino groups. Zeta potential profiles of ±30 mV are described to prevent aggregation and stabilize particles in suspension [61]. This was also confirmed by visual inspection of the obtained colloidal suspensions, which remained stable without aggregation at room temperature for several days (data not shown).

As for the formulation method, complexation with TPP performed best with 1:1 ALG/CS mass and chitosan of low molecular weight ("F14_Low"), with microparticles presenting a mean diameter of 25.9 ± 0.7 μm, span ≤1.7, and positive surface charge (+22.7 ± 1.6 mV). By using $CaCl_2$ as complexation agent, in alternative to TPP, it was possible to improve particle size distribution with 4.23:1 ALG/CS mass ratio and chitosan of low molecular weight ("F0_Low"), with microparticles presenting a reduced mean diameter of 18.5 ± 0.7 μm (span ≤1.4), and negative surface charge (−20.8 ± 7.9 mV).

These results indicate that the molecular weight of the chitosan used to prepare the microparticles had a major impact in particle size distribution, whereas the alginate to chitosan mass ratio had an important role in modulating particle surface charge. It was also possible to identify the conditions which led to a greater heterogeneity in particle formation, evidenced as a broader particle size distribution revealed in increased span values. Overall, it was possible to observe, for microparticles prepared with a given ALG/CS mass ratio, a higher standard deviation of the span when chitosan of medium and high molecular weight were used (with formulation F11 being the exception), thus, indicating that particle size distribution varied considerably and was not completely reproducible. These results were important to put into evidence how to modulate the microparticles size distribution and surface charge profile according to the selected formulation method.

Particle size is determinant in intranasal delivery and mucosal uptake of particles [29], and in the intracellular traffic of the particles [62,63]. Carriers sizing few microns have shown higher potential as intranasal delivery systems of antigens [64–66]. As size is increased, which can be partially due to the increase in the sample mass by weight of the microparticles, surface area decreases; this in turn might contribute to a slowdown in the antigen release rate as a depot effect. For the purpose of this study, particle size should be at least 5 μm, in order to enable the entrapment of BCG bacilli, which are short to moderate long rods, 0.3–0.6 × 1–4 μm [67,68]. According to some authors, size must not be greater than 10 μm when phagocytosis is required, with 200 nm to 5 μm being the ideal size [69].

Nevertheless, much larger particles ranging from 1 to 40 μm have been successfully used for intranasal immunization, eliciting good systemic and mucosal responses in mice [9].

Concomitantly with particle size distribution, zeta potential determination allows the estimation of particle suspension stability against subsequent aggregation, as ±30 mV can be an indicator of the particulate systems' stability [70,71]. Surface charge is a critical parameter that affects the mucoadhesion of chitosan/alginate microparticles to the lung mucosa, which in turn will prolong the residence time of the vaccine at the site of action. The net positive charge indicates the presence of free surface amino groups in F11–F13 in addition to F14 obtained with chitosan of low molecular weight, which will help in initial adhesion to nasal mucosa. Since mucoadhesive properties of chitosan are mainly explained by the electrostatic interaction and by hydrogen bond of amine groups of this cationic polymer with the negatively charged mucin [36], one can expect positively charged particles to be preferable to negatively charged ones.

Taking into consideration the aforementioned results, it was possible to conclude that the association of 4.23:1 ALG/CS mass ratio (formulation F0) and low molecular weight chitosan provided the formulation's optimal conditions to obtain polymeric microparticles with smaller mean diameter (+18.5 ± 0.7 μm) and narrower particle size distribution (span = 1.4), also with negative surface charge (−20.8 ± 7.9 mV). However, considering that our proposed microparticulate delivery system must be suitable not only to encapsulate whole live BCG bacteria, but also to target the lung mucosa, positively charged particles are expected to be preferable. Therefore, particle size distribution and particle surface charge were considered together, and the 1:1 ALG/CS mass ratio formulation (F14) prepared with chitosan of low molecular weight, with a microparticle size distribution of +25.9 ± 0.7 μm (span = 1.7) and positive surface charge (+16.2 ± 0.6 mV), was chosen to for formulation optimization studies.

Effect of Homogenization Method

Preliminary formulation studies showed that particle size distribution of plain polymeric microparticles prepared with the ionic gelation methods was greatly influenced by the type and time of homogenization. Therefore, different homogenization methods were assessed in four different formulations (F0, F12, F13 and F14), in order to obtain microparticles of desired and consistent size distribution. The effect of high-speed homogenization (ultra-turrax, UT) and ultrasonication (US) used for particle preparation with increasing ALG/CS mass ratios of the final formulation is presented in Table 2.

The homogenization by ultrasonication led to the formation of microparticles within a narrower and smaller size range, with mean diameters between 10.8 μm ("F13_Low") and 14.4 μm ("F14_Low"), and high production yields (>80%) (Table 2). When high-speed homogenization was used, the overall mean diameter of the obtained microparticles greatly increased (Table 2). The use of chitosan of low and high molecular weights resulted in more consistent and reproducible formulation methods, as the size distribution of microparticles with different ALG/CS mass ratios and within the same chitosan molecular weight presented a narrower size distribution, represented by a lower span (Table 2).

Taking into consideration the obtained results, and regarding particle size distribution, method consistency and production yield, we selected formulations "F13_Medium MW chitosan" and "F14_Low MW chitosan" for further optimization studies. In fact, although ultrasonication proved to be effective in the preparation of plain chitosan-alginate microparticles, the ultimate goal was to encapsulate whole live bacilli of BCG. Since both high shear and ultrasonication are said to compromise cell viability, due to the induced cell integrity loss, two alternative homogenization methods were investigated, namely, simple dispersion with a micropipette, or, alternatively, homogenization in an ultrasound water-bath. Increasing homogenization times were evaluated.

Table 2. Size distribution of polymeric microparticles prepared by high-speed homogenization and ultrasonication, and yield of production.

Formulation_Chitosan MW	High-Speed Homogenization			Ultrasonication		
	Particle Size, d0.5 (μm)	Span	Production Yield (%)	Particle Size, d0.5 (μm)	Span	Production Yield (%)
F0_Low	34.5 ± 1.8	6.7 ± 0.5	n.d.	67.8 ± 10.6	5.6 ± 0.9	n.d.
F0_Medium	47.8 ± 2.2	4.1 ± 0.4	n.d.	11.5 ± 3.2	8.8 ± 1.3	n.d.
F0_High	91.8 ± 1.6	3.4 ± 0.1	n.d.	69.5 ± 9.9	6.5 ± 0.8	n.d.
F12_Low	30.2 ± 0.3	3.0 ± 0.0	n.d.	-	-	-
F13_Low	20.4 ± 0.2	2.6 ± 0.0	n.d.	10.8 ± 0.6	6.7 ± 1.9	72.2 ± 0.0
F13_Medium	65.6 ± 1.7	3.5 ± 0.1	n.d.	11.8 ± 0.0	1.6 ± 0.0	97.3 ± 0.9
F13_High	52.9 ± 1.1	2.8 ± 0.0	n.d.	11.2 ± 0.4	4.7 ± 2.4	103.4 ± 2.6
F14_Low	25.2 ± 0.3	3.0 ± 0.0	53.8 ± 0.0	14.4 ± 0.3	1.2 ± 0.0	60.1 ± 10.7

F0, microparticles obtained by Method (I) with modifications, via alginate ionotropic pre-gelation with $CaCl_2$ followed by chitosan addition; F12–F14, microparticles obtained by Method (II) with modifications, via chitosan pre-gelation with alginate followed by precipitation with 2 mg/mL TPP (pH 9.0), with ALG/CS mass ratios ranging from 0.6:1 to 1:1. The pH of alginate and chitosan solutions was initially set to 4.9 and 4.6, respectively. MW, Molecular weight; n.d., not determined.

Particle mean diameter obtained for both formulations was within the 12.5–21.0 μm range (Table 3). The best results were achieved with simple dispersion ("0 min") for formulation "F14_Low" (12.5 ± 0.2 μm; −14.9 ± 0.2 mV) and "20 min" in ultrasound water-bath for formulation "F13_Medium" (12.6 ± 0.1 μm; +12.1 ± 0.9 mV). The use of the ultrasound allowed maintaining particle sizes approximated to the desired particle size (10 μm). Particles were overall negatively charged, as five formulations exhibited negative zeta potential values (−49.8 to −14.1 mV), with formulation "F13_Medium" being the one exception.

Table 3. Size distribution and zeta potential of microparticles prepared by homogenization in an ultrasound water-bath, with increasing homogenization times.

Time (min)	F13_Medium			F14_Low		
	Particle Size, d0.5 (μm)	Span	Zeta Potential (mV)	Particle Size, d0.5 (μm)	Span	Zeta Potential (mV)
0	16.3 ± 0.1	2.0 ± 0.2	−49.8 ± 0.7	12.5 ± 0.2	1.8 ± 0.4	−14.9 ± 0.2
4	19.4 ± 0.6	2.4 ± 0.2	−29.6 ± 1.2	15.7 ± 0.2	1.9 ± 0.2	−19.5 ± 0.7
20	12.6 ± 0.1	2.0 ± 0.2	+12.1 ± 0.9	21.0 ± 0.3	1.6 ± 0.0	−14.1 ± 0.5

F13_Medium, microparticles of 0.8:1 ALG/CS mass ratio prepared with medium molecular weight chitosan and medium viscosity alginate Protanal™; F14_Low, microparticles of 1:1 ALG/CS mass ratio that were prepared with low molecular weight chitosan and low viscosity alginate Protanal™. All microparticles obtained via chitosan precipitation with TPP (pH 9.0) followed by addition of alginate (adapted from *Method III*). The pH of alginate and chitosan solutions was initially set to 4.9 and 4.6, respectively. *Medium* and *Low* refers to chitosan molecular weight and to alginate viscosity.

Particle size increased with increasing homogenization times, as such: from 12.5 to 21.0 μm to "F14_Low" (0 to 20 min); from 16.3 to 19.4 μm to "F13_Medium" (0 to 4 min) (Table 3). Size distribution of microparticles prepared with either 0.8:1 or 1:1 ALG/CS mass ratios, and different chitosan molecular weight, presented with a narrow size distribution (low span) (Table 4), thus indicating a good consistency of the used preparation method. Smaller particle sizes were obtained for F14 formulation at 0 and 4 min, compared to F13, probably due to a more favorable ALG/CS mass ratio, as the stoichiometric proportion of alginate to chitosan of 1:1 might provide a better interaction and nucleation between polymers, leading to smaller sized particles.

Table 4. Effect of pH on particle size distribution, particle surface charge, and yield of production of microparticles prepared with alginate to chitosan mass ratio of 1:1 (F14_Low).

ALG pH	CS pH	F14 pH	Particle Size, d0.5 (μm)		Span	Zeta Potential (mV)		Production Yield * (%)	Aggregates
3.0	3.0	3.3	44.2	±0.9	1.5 ± 0.0	+8.7	±0.1	6.4%	Yes
4.0	3.0	3.6	31.3	±0.3	31.0 ± 16.3	+3.7	±0.0	12.5%	Yes
5.0	3.0	3.9	16.1	±0.1	1.3 ± 0.0	−3.5	±0.0	11.7%	
6.4	3.0	4.0	15.2	±0.2	1.4 ± 0.1	−4.6	±0.0	17.8%	
7.0	3.0	4.0	18.0	±0.4	1.3 ± 0.0	−2.3	±0.0	n.d.	
3.0	4.0	4.1	43.8	±1.0	1.5 ± 0.0	+1.8	±0.0	16.9%	Yes
4.0	4.0	4.3	19.0	±0.8	1.7 ± 0.0	−4.9	±0.0	11.7%	Yes
5.0	4.0	4.5	13.0	±0.3	2.0 ± 0.1	−7.3	±0.1	13.6%	
6.4	4.0	4.6	13.2	±0.7	1.7 ± 0.0	−6.2	±0.1	11.9%	
7.0	4.0	4.6	15.8	±0.4	1.8 ± 0.0	−13.4	±0.1	18.3%	
3.0	5.0	4.9	12.9	±0.5	6.3 ± 1.2	−16.3	±0.0	10.4%	
4.0	5.0	5.0	12.1	±0.4	3.1 ± 0.5	−14.8	±0.0	11.4%	
5.0	5.0	5.3	11.4	±0.3	3.6 ± 0.5	−18.6	±0.1	6.7%	
6.4	5.0	5.4	10.9	±0.4	2.7 ± 0.4	−18.9	±0.1	11.4%	
7.0	5.0	5.4	11.8	±0.3	2.8 ± 0.4	−17.8	±0.1	10.6%	
3.0	6.0	5.7	11.5	±0.2	5.2 ± 0.3	−22.4	±0.1	8.3%	
4.0	6.0	6.3	10.0	±0.7	7.1 ± 0.8	−23.7	±0.2	14.2%	
5.0	6.0	7.2	11.9	±0.3	4.9 ± 0.3	−26.3	±0.1	14.6%	
6.4	6.0	7.5	11.4	±0.2	3.3 ± 0.4	−25.7	±0.1	n.d.	
7.0	6.0	7.6	13.8	±0.3	2.3 ± 0.0	−21.8	±0.2	n.d.	

F14, microparticles obtained using formulation Method (III) with low molecular weight/92% deacetylation degree chitosan (CS), and low viscosity / high-G sodium alginate (ALG) (Protanal™ LF 10/60). Results are expressed as mean and standard deviation ($n \geqslant 3$). *Production yield was determined using gravimetric determination of particles mass following lyophilisation, and it is expressed as mass percentage (w/w), referred to particles theoretical mass; n.d., not determined.

Effect of Alginate Type and Polymers Addition Order

The results obtained during formulation optimization studies led us towards the rejection of Method (I) and the development of a different preparation method—Method (III). In order to evaluate the effect of the polymers' specifications on particle size distribution, three different sets of plain microparticles were prepared using three different commercial brands of low viscosity sodium alginate with distinct G-content, namely: low viscosity sodium alginate of high-G content (65%–75%) Protanal™ LF 10/60; ultra-low viscosity sodium alginate of high-G content (63%) Manugel™ LBA; low viscosity sodium alginate of low-G content (40%) Keltone™ LVCR, all approved as pharmaceutical excipient. Chitosan quality specification was kept constant; low molecular weight chitosan with a deacetylation degree of 92% was used. Microparticles were prepared according to two different formulation methods—Methods (II) and (III)—as described (Materials and Methods section) with modifications. The two methods differ in the addition order of the polymers. By changing the polymers' addition order, it would be possible to modulate the final surface charge of microparticles.

Taking into consideration the aforementioned results obtained for particle size of "F14_Low" prepared by simple dispersion (12.5 ± 0.2 μm), the same homogenization method to prepare these microparticles was used, by simple dispersion with a micropipette for 1 min following additions. In Method (II), chitosan and alginate were allowed to interact prior to TPP addition.

The effect of formulation Methods (II) and (III) with decreasing G-content of the sodium alginate polymers used to prepare microparticles is presented in Figure 3. Regarding particle mean diameter (Figure 3A), microparticles prepared with Method (II) presented a size distribution (d0.5) from 60.9 ± 5.5 μm (Protanal™) to 89.4 ± 6.7 μm (Manugel™). Changing the polymers' addition order by using Method (III) yielded a particle size distribution with a pronounced decrease in d0.5 values, ranging from 14.7 ± 0.6 μm (Manugel™) to 24.0 ± 1.4 μm (Keltone™). No significant differences were observed between alginates of different G-content within the same formulation method ($p = 0.4634$). As for formulation Methods (II) and (III), it was possible to identify a bimodal particle size distribution depending on the used method. The observed differences were not, however, statistically significant ($p = 0.1000$).

Regarding particle surface charge (Figure 3B), microparticles prepared with Method (II) presented zeta potential values from $+14.1 \pm 0.6$ mV (Protanal™) to -16.3 ± 1.3 mV (Keltone™). Particle surface charge decreased for all formulations when Method (III) was used, reaching negative zeta potential values of -29.6 ± 0.9 mV for Keltone™. Differences among the two evaluated methods were not statistically significant ($p = 0.4000$). Nevertheless, the consistent decrease in zeta potential values suggests that a reorganization of the chitosan-alginate matrix occurred when chitosan was allowed to form a pre-gel with TPP, followed by alginate addition.

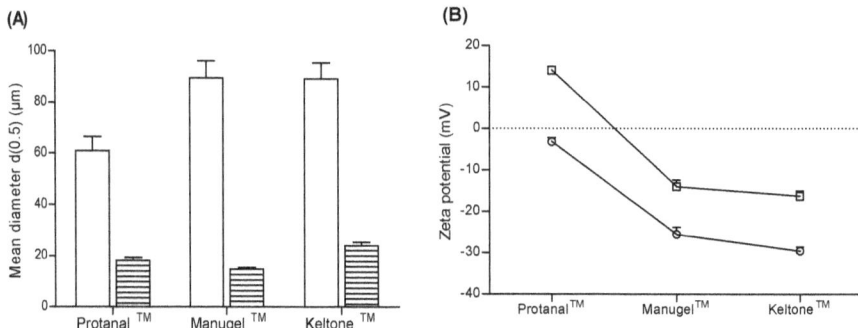

Figure 3. (**A**) Particle size distribution of plain chitosan-alginate microparticles of 1:1 ALG/CS mass ratio, prepared with chitosan of low molecular weight and alginates of decreasing G-content, according to Method (II) (solid) and Method (III) (dashed); (**B**) Zeta potential of plain chitosan-alginate microparticles of 1:1 ALG/CS mass ratio, prepared with chitosan of low molecular weight and alginates of decreasing G-content, according to Method (II) (□) and Method (III) (○).The pH of alginate, chitosan and TPP solutions was initially set to 6.7, 4.1 and 9.0, respectively. Results are presented as mean $\pm$ SD ($n = 3$).

These results were important to evidence how the addition order of the polymers plays an important role in the formation of chitosan-alginate microparticles. So far, it seems that ALG/CS mass ratio, homogenization method, and the addition order of the polymers have greater impact on particle size distribution and surface charge than the herein assessed G-content of sodium alginate. Since Method (III) enabled the formation of microparticles with an inferior mean diameter, within a more stable colloidal suspension, it was chosen as the formulation method for the following optimization studies.

Effect of pH Value

It is well established that an ionic complex between alginate and chitosan is formed due to interactions between the carboxyl groups of alginate with the amino groups of chitosan [35,56,70,71]. The cationic nature of chitosan (pKa $\approx$ 6.5) is conveyed by the positively charged $-NH_3^+$ groups, whereas the anionic nature of alginate (pKa $\approx$ 3.4–3.7) results from the presence of $-COO^-$ groups. The cationic nature of chitosan leads to the amino group protonation in acidic to neutral solution, with charge density depending on pH value and chitosan deacetylation degree. These features contribute to the solubility of chitosan in aqueous acidic solutions. Furthermore, it is key for chitosan bioadhesiveness, since chitosan protonated amino groups readily bind to negatively charged surfaces such as mucosal membranes, and for the enhancement of polar drugs transport across epithelial surfaces.

In order to assess the effect of pH value on microparticle formation, several sets of microparticles from formulation "F14_Low" (ALG/CS mass ratio of 1:1, w/w) were prepared using 1.0 mg/mL solutions of low molecular weight 92% deacetylated chitosan, and low viscosity and high-G content sodium alginate (Protanal™ LF 10/60), with pH value ranging from 3.0 to 7.0. The obtained suspensions were characterized for particle size distribution, surface charge, and yield of production (Table 4).

The use of both alginate and chitosan solutions with a pH value below 5.0 resulted in increased particle size (15 to 44 µm) and particle aggregation (Table 4). Aggregation also occurred when chitosan solution pH was beyond 6.0 (data not shown), due to the loss of chitosan solubility, as chitosan has a pKa value of ≈ 6.5. Considering the desired particle size distribution (*i.e.*, particle mean diameter of approximately 10 µm, and narrow span), the optimal size distributions were obtained when chitosan solution pH value was within 5.0–6.0, and alginate solution pH value within 4.0–6.4, leading to the formation of 10–12 µm sized (d0.5) microparticles. Within this pH range, the carboxyl groups of alginate are ionized, and the amine groups of chitosan are protonated, thus, favouring the optimum interaction for the polyionic complex formation. All these formulations presented a negative particle surface charge (Table 4).

The best system was obtained with formulation final pH value of 5.4, with particle mean diameter of 10.9 ± 0.4 µm, a 2.7 span, and negative surface charge (−18.9 mV) (Table 4). These particles were prepared with chitosan solution at pH = 5.0 and alginate solution pH = 6.4. Although it is well known that the pH-dependent interaction between alginate and chitosan leads to the formation of stronger complexes at a pH value around 4.5–5.0, it is also described that the amine groups of chitosan (pKa ≈ 6.5) have more affinity to alginate mannuronic acid (M) residues (pK$_M$ ≈ 3.38) than to guluronic acid (G) residues (pK$_G$ ≈ 3.65) [36]. Since a high-G content (≈70%) alginate (Protanal LF™ 10/60) was used, overall alginate pKa was closer to 3.65. This might explain why microparticles of lower mean diameter (10.9 ± 0.4 µm) and narrower size distribution (span = 2.7) were obtained with formulation final pH of 5.4. In fact, at this pH range, the high degree of protonation of chitosan amino groups prompts a significant reaction with alginate carboxyl groups, leading to the formation of stable particles. It would be expected that maximum ionic interaction occurs at a slightly lower pH value for high-M content alginates (such as ≈60% M-content Keltone™ alginate).

The production yield was very low (<17%) for all formulations when determined by gravimetry (Table 4). This is probably related to a low responsiveness of the gravimetric method for the determined mass range, as mass variations occurred within the sub-milligram or micro-range. For that reason, the described method in the Materials and Methods section (Section 3.4.2) based on the quantification of chitosan concentration for the determination of the yield of production of microparticles was selected for further studies. The results obtained were analysed by comparing the different pH conditions.

Regarding zeta potential results, microparticles prepared with the majority of pH combinations were negatively charged (Table 4). This is probably due to the contribution of alginate carboxyl groups to the negative net surface charge, therefore suggesting that the Method (III) provides the arrangement of the polymeric matrix in such way that alginate somehow outers the chitosan particulate core.

It can be observed that particle mean diameter is significantly higher for microparticle suspensions with final pH ⩽ 4.3 (Table 4). At this pH value range, alginate approaches its pKa values, and a significant part of alginate starts aggregating and precipitating, which might have contributed to the increased particle mean diameter.

Effect of Cryoprotectants Addition

Table 5 summarizes the different batches of plain "F14_Low" microparticles prepared with two concentrations (5% and 10%, *w/v*) of three different cryoprotectants. Microparticles were prepared according to Method III with addition of cryoprotectant solution, consisting of sucrose, glucose, or trehalose. Samples were prepared in triplicate. Particle size distribution and zeta potential of samples were assessed for samples without cryoprotectant (batch A) and samples with cryoprotectant (batches B to G), both prior to and after freeze-drying.

Table 5. Characterization of plain chitosan-alginate microparticles (formulation "F14_Low") batches without (batch A) and with (batches B to H) cryoprotectants addition (sucrose, glucose, or trehalose), on production day and following freeze-drying.

Batches	Cryoprotectant % (*w/v*)	ALG:CS:Cryoprotectant Mass Ratio (*w/w*)	Before Freeze-Drying			After Freeze-Drying	
			Particle Size (μm)		Zeta Potential (mV)	Particle Size (μm)	
			d0.5	Span		d0.5	Span
A	-	1:1:0	13.3 ± 1.0	3.1 ± 2.3	−19.5 ± 0.7	170.6 ± 50.8	2.6 ± 0.3
B	Sucrose 5%	1:1:120	13.6 ± 0.2	1.8 ± 0.5	+14.9 ± 0.3	93.5 ± 15.6	2.3 ± 0.1
C	Sucrose 10%	1:1:240	13.2 ± 1.1	1.4 ± 0.1	n.d.	65.5 ± 7.3	2.0 ± 0.2
D	Glucose 5%	1:1:120	12.9 ± 0.0	1.8 ± 0.0	n.d.	54.1 ± 9.9	1.9 ± 0.3
E	Glucose 10%	1:1:240	13.5 ± 2.0	2.0 ± 0.7	+11.6 ± 1.2	47.1 ± 8.3	2.4 ± 0.2
F	Trehalose 5%	1:1:120	13.2 ± 0.4	1.8 ± 0.3	+13.3 ± 0.5	81.9 ± 15.5	2.0 ± 0.1
G	Trehalose 10%	1:1:240	12.1 ± 0.6	1.4 ± 0.1	n.d.	63.7 ± 4.5	2.0 ± 0.3

The pH of alginate, chitosan and TPP solutions was initially set to 6.7, 4.1 and 9.0, respectively. Results are expressed as mean and standard deviation ($n \geqslant 3$); n.d., not determined.

The addition of cryoprotectants appears to have contributed to the modification of particle surface charge (Table 5), as microparticles with no cryoprotectant (batch A) presented negative zeta potential values (−19.5 ± 0.7 mV), whereas microparticles prepared with cryoprotectants (batches B, E and F, for 5% sucrose, 10% glucose and 5% trehalose, respectively) presented a positive surface charge, with zeta potential values between +11.6 ± 1.2 mV and +14.9 ± 0.3 mV. This is probably due to the adsorption of the molecules to the surface. It has been described that slightly acidic sucrose and glucose generate a good isotonic medium (in terms of electrostatic stability) for negatively charged particles, but for positively charged particles, as in the case of "F14_Low", these additives reverse zeta potential [72].

Regarding particle mean diameter, it was within micrometer range for all prepared batches (Table 5). With samples analyzed before freeze-drying (on production day), it was possible to observe that there were no significant differences concerning particle size distribution (Table 5). All batches presented similar size distributions, with average d0.5 values of 13.1 ± 0.5 μm, thus, suggesting that addition of cryoprotectants did not influence particle size for batches prepared under thesame conditions.

However, after freeze-drying, particle size distribution profile changed and all batches presented up to 10-fold increased d0.5 values (Table 5), indicating a noteworthy increase of particle mean diameter, probably due to the formation of larger particles or particle aggregates. This could also be seen in the exacerbation of the d0.9 populations for all samples after freeze-drying (data not shown). Nevertheless, the addition of cryoprotectants did prevent some aggregation following freeze-drying, as batch A (particles with no cryoprotectant) presented the highest particle mean diameter, with approximately two-fold higher d0.5 values assigned to batches where cryoprotectant had been added (batches B–G).

As for particle size distribution width, the obtained low span values (2.0 ± 0.5 μm, in average) (Table 5) revealed a high similitude in particle size distribution, thus, suggesting that microparticle preparation was reproducible. Microparticles prepared with 5% and 10% glucose (batches D and E, respectively) performed best, with lower d0.5 values and low span values, thus, corresponding to particles with a smaller, and narrow, particle size distribution.

It can be concluded that microparticle suspensions were affected by the nature and concentration of cryoprotectants, with 10% glucose cryoprotectant (batch E) showing better properties after freeze-drying, with smaller particle size, low span and average zeta potential positive value, compared to microparticles with no cryoprotectant (batch A). Future studies must be conducted with cryoprotectants in order to optimize particle size distribution and surface charge, so that the physicochemical stability of microparticles after freeze-drying can be ensured.

2.1.2. Polymer–Polymer Interaction by FT-IR Analysis

Formation of microparticles of chitosan with alginate is a result of strong interactions by hydrogen bonds between the functional groups of the polymers in which amino and amide groups present in chitosan take part. As a result, there are changes in the FT-IR spectra in the absorption bands of the amino groups, carboxyl groups, and amide bonds [35]. Based on the identification of absorption bands concerned with the vibrations of functional groups present in CS and ALG macromolecules [53], FT-IR analysis was able to illustrate changes in the wave number and absorbance in the region of amino and amide group vibrations with increasing pH of the microparticle suspension (Figure 4).

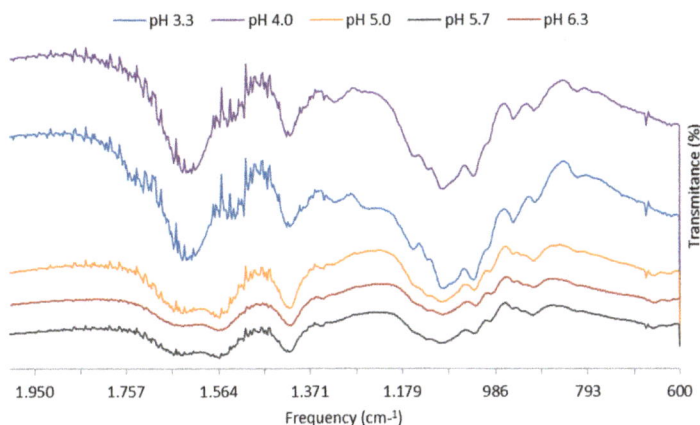

Figure 4. FT-IR spectra of plain chitosan-alginate "F14_Low" microparticles (1:1 ALG/CS mass ratio) with increasing pH of the microparticles suspension. Bands wave numbers (cm^{-1}) are as follows: 1641 (amide bond), 1613 (symmetric COO$^-$ stretching vibration), 1569 (strong protonated amino peak—from partial N-deacetylation of chitin), and 1415 (asymmetric COO$^-$ stretching vibration).

The FT-IR spectrum of microparticles produced with final pH of 4.0 and 5.7 reveals alginate carboxyl peaks slightly shift from 1613 and 1415 cm^{-1} to 1609 and 1414 cm^{-1}, respectively, after complexation with chitosan. Both chitosan peaks were similarly shifted by a few cm^{-1} after complexation with alginate, with the amide peak from 1641 into singlet band at 1609 cm^{-1}, and the amino peak from 1559 to 1533 cm^{-1} or 1560 cm^{-1} at pH 4.0 and 5.7, respectively. The observed changes in the absorption bands of the amino groups, carboxyl groups, and amide bonds can be attributed to an ionic interaction between the carbonyl group of alginate and the amino group of chitosan. The peak absorbance of amino groups of chitosan at 1153 cm^{-1} was also present after complexation, thus, suggesting an effective interaction between polymers at pH 4.0 and 5.7.

2.1.3. Surface Morphology

Microparticle morphology was characterized by microscopy. Both F13 and F14 microparticles presented regular and smooth surfaces related to a generic spherical shape (Figure 5). Additionally, particle size distribution observed in microscopic images was consistent with that obtained by laser diffraction, revealing homogeneous populations of narrow particle size distribution (Figure 6).

Considering the results obtained during formulation optimization studies, F14_Low formulation, produced with 1 mg/mL low MW chitosan (pH = 5.0) and 1 mg/mL Protanal™ sodium alginate (pH = 6.4), the 'simple dispersion' method was chosen for further BCG encapsulation, so that a suitable formulation of BCG-loaded microparticles can be developed and further assessed in immunization studies. This formulation was chosen because it allowed the formation of microparticles of suitable mean diameter and surface charge without aggregation, under mild conditions and only requiring a few steps, critical for future sterile production during vaccine production.

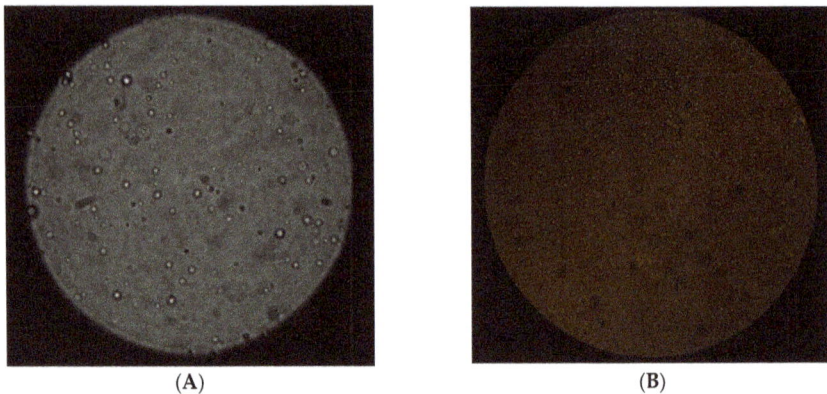

Figure 5. (**A**) Polarized light micrograph (100×) of "F13_Medium" microparticles (0.8:1 ALG/CS) prepared according to Method (III) with chitosan of medium molecular weight; (**B**) Contrast phase micrograph (40×) of "F14_Low" microparticles (1:1 ALG/CS) prepared according to Method (II) with chitosan of low molecular weight.

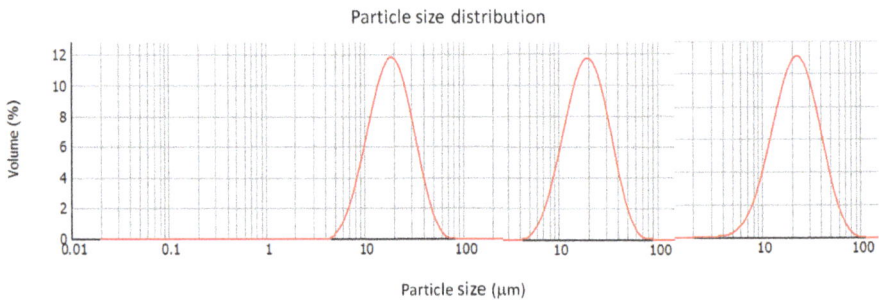

Figure 6. Particle size distribution of microparticles produced with alginate to chitosan ratio of 4.23:1 (F0), 0.8:1 (F13), and 1:1 (F14). F0 microparticles prepared according to Method (I) by alginate ionotropic pre-gelation with $CaCl_2$ followed by chitosan coating; F13-F14 microparticles prepared according to Method (III) by chitosan pre-gelation with TPP followed by alginate coating. LMW, low molecular weight chitosan; MMW, medium molecular weight chitosan; HMW, high molecular weight chitosan.

2.2. Encapsulation Efficiency

The ability of chitosan/alginate microparticles to encapsulate *Mycobacterium bovis* BCG depends to a great extent on bacteria surface charge. Therefore, zeta potential of *Mycobacterium bovis* BCG Pasteur and rBCG-GFP strains was measured at low electrolyte concentration. In order to assess the effect of experimental conditions on BCG bacilli surface charge, BCG strains were suspended in different media, whereas BCG previously suspended in 0.9% NaCl was heat killed as it is described in the Materials and Methods section (Table 6).

Both BCG Pasteur and rBCG-GFP bacilli presented predominantly negative zeta potential values (Table 6). Overall, the surface charge of BCG Pasteur appears to be only slightly more electro-negative than rBCG-GFP for all tested conditions. A different macroscopic behavior of cell suspension was also distinguished—BCG Pasteur suspension formed a fluffy surface layer, which led to partial and ephemeral aggregation; this phenomena was not observed for rBCG-GFP strain.

Table 6. Surface charge of inactivated *Mycobacterium bovis* BCG (strains Pasteur and rBCG-GFP) bacilli suspended in different media. Results are presented as mean $\pm$ SD (n = 3).

Inactivation Method	Medium	Zeta Potential (mV)	
		BCG Pasteur	rBCG-GFP
Temperature (80 °C, 15′)	H$_2$O	−39.3 $\pm$ 1.0	−32.6 $\pm$ 1.0
	Cell culture medium	−27.9 $\pm$ 2.7	−21.2 $\pm$ 2.5
	10 mM PBS	−20.4 $\pm$ 1.5	−13.7 $\pm$ 1.4
	0.9% NaCl	−29.9 $\pm$ 11.5	−23.1 $\pm$ 11.0
	0.025% low MW chitosan	+83.9 $\pm$ 3.5	+90.6 $\pm$ 3.5
	0.1% low MW chitosan	+85.7 $\pm$ 12.1	+92.4 $\pm$ 11.9

The nature of the adsorbing species on the cell surface of the two strains might explain the obtained variations. The negative surface charge for cells of all *Mycobacterium* BCG species arises from the phosphate groups of phosphodiester linkages between the peptidoglycan and the arabinogalactan of the basic cell wall structure which is common to all species of Mycobacteria [73]. Some hydrophobic interaction involving lipid within the surface may also be involved, since the mycobacterial cell envelope is a lipid-rich, complex structure that surrounds the bacillus and is thought to play a critical role in the pathogenicity of *Mycobacterium tuberculosis*. A large number of mycobacterial lipoproteins have been suggested to be important components for the synthesis of the mycobacterial cell envelope, as well as for sensing processes, protection from stressful factors and host–pathogen interactions [74,75].

Zeta potential profiles showed no major differences between bacilli suspension in either 0.9% NaCl, water, 10 mM PBS, or cell culture medium. However, when BCG bacilli from either strains were suspended in low molecular weight chitosan, an inversion of zeta potential values occurred, in a concentration dependent fashion, suggesting that the mechanism of association of the bacteria to chitosan is, at least partially, mediated by ionic interaction between bacilli and chitosan. Other mechanisms, such as hydrophobic interactions, might also be involved in bacteria microencapsulation.

Taking into consideration the abovementioned, it was hypothesised that the greatest encapsulation/association efficiency for *M. bovis* BCG would be obtained by suspending BCG bacteria in chitosan at a pH below its pKa (e.g., pH = 5), so that the polymer is predominantly positively charged. Additionally, we chose to entrap monodisperse bacteria in chitosan microparticles by means of controlled gelation of chitosan with TPP followed by alginate addition. In this way, a good encapsulation efficiency was sought.

Preliminary formulation studies revealed that particle size distribution and surface charge were influenced by the polymer to polymer mass ratio and the formulation method. Whether BCG microencapsulation would have a great impact on microparticles features was uncertain, thus these parameters were investigated. As such, BCG-loaded "F14_Low" microparticles (1:1 ALG/CS mass ratio) were prepared as described in the Materials and Methods section (Section 3.3.1), by Method (II) or Method (III), with modifications. The encapsulation efficiency was also determined. Table 7 summarizes the different batches of BCG-loaded "F14_Low" microparticles that were prepared and the obtained results.

For microparticles prepared according to Method (II), BCG encapsulation led to decreased particle size in comparison with plain microparticles. In opposition, for microparticles prepared according to Method (III), BCG encapsulation led to increased particle size, referred to as plain microparticles (Table 7). Within BCG-loaded microparticles, particle size increased in a concentration dependent fashion, with increasing BCG loads of 8.3×10^6, 1.7×10^7, and 3.3×10^7 CFU/mL for microparticles prepared by Method (II), and with BCG loads of 8.3×10^6 and 1.7×10^7 CFU/mL for microparticles prepared by Method (III) (Table 7).

Table 7. Characterization of batches of BCG-loaded "F14_Low" microparticles prepared with increasing concentrations of BCG.

Batches	Formulation Method	BCG Pasteur Load (CFU/mL)	Particle Size, d(0.5) (μm)	Span	Zeta Potential (mV)	E.E. (%)
A	II	-	60.9 ± 5.5	3.0 ± 5.5	14.1 ± 0.6	–
B	II	1.7×10^6	35.3 ± 2.6	1.8 ± 0.1	10.5 ± 1.5	70.0 ± 1.6
C	II	8.3×10^6	39.3 ± 3.9	2.8 ± 1.8	12.9 ± 2.3	74.0 ± 3.9
D	II	1.7×10^7	41.0 ± 6.3	2.2 ± 0.1	11.8 ± 2.5	85.0 ± 4.8
E	II	3.3×10^7	36.8 ± 2.0	2.0 ± 0.2	13.0 ± 3.9	87.0 ± 3.4
F	III	-	18.2 ± 1.2	3.2 ± 0.7	-3.2 ± 0.9	–
G	III	1.7×10^6	22.2 ± 1.0	6.5 ± 2.6	-16.4 ± 2.1	–
H	III	8.3×10^6	28.3 ± 4.0	25.5 ± 12.3	-12.7 ± 2.4	76.0 ± 1.4
I	III	1.7×10^7	22.5 ± 2.7	4.0 ± 2.8	-13.7 ± 2.0	84.0 ± 3.4
J	III	3.3×10^7	21.4 ± 2.4	2.5 ± 0.4	-12.2 ± 2.6	83.0 ± 10.7

Regarding particle surface charge, two different patterns were obtained, depending on the formulation method (Table 7). Method (II) produced microparticles (both plain and BCG-loaded) that were electropositively charged, with zeta potential values from $+10.5 \pm 1.5$ mV to $+14.1 \pm 0.6$ mV, whereas Method (III) produced electronegatively charged microparticles (both plain and BCG-loaded), with zeta potential values ranging from -3.2 ± 0.9 mV to -16.4 ± 2.1 mV. In comparison to plain microparticles, BCG-loaded microparticles presented lower zeta potential values regardless of the used formulation method (Table 7). These results indicate that negatively charged BCG bacilli is present, thus, indicating that encapsulation occurred.

The encapsulation of BCG Pasteur into microparticles was efficient (70%–87% E.E.) and occred in a concentration dependent fashion, regardless of the formulation method used (Table 7). The encapsulation mechanism, however, was not determined. Due to the extremely high content of complex lipids present in the BCG cell wall, it is extremely difficult and challenging to achieve efficient, uniform and reproducible microencapsulation experiments. Therefore, we accept that BCG bacilli are sometimes microencapsulated and other times just adsorbed due to partial and irregular adsorption onto the microparticle surface.

2.3. BCG Cell Viability

Chitosan is described as having antimicrobial potential [48–50]. Whether BCG suspension in chitosan would compromise BCG cell viability was uncertain. Therefore, BCG cell viability following suspension in chitosan was investigated over time by a colony-forming units (CFUs) assay, as described in the Materials and Methods (Section 3.3.1). Both strains BCG Pasteur and rBCG-GFP were assessed in this cell viability study. Results are presented in Figure 7.

Results showed a significant reduction of BCG cell viability for both BCG strains, with small differences (Figure 7A). For rBCG-GFP, viable cell density decreased 1 log on the 3rd week, and approximately 3 log on the 6th week. Regarding BCG Pasteur, cell viability was further reduced, with a viable cell density decrease of 1–2 log on the third week, and approximately 2.5–4 log on the 6th week. These effects were observed for both strains regardless of the suspension media ($p > 0.05$). Overall, although the suspension of BCG in 0.025% chitosan induced a decrease in BCG cell viability, the same effect was observed in the control groups of 0.9% NaCl-suspended BCG. Therefore, chitosan may not be considered cytotoxic at the tested concentration. Figure 7B confirms that viable cell density decreased approximately 1 log after 3 weeks for BCG-loaded chitosan-alginate microparticles and for BCG suspended in 0.025% chitosan. Overall, the microencapsulation procedures preserved BCG integrity and viability, as there were no statistically significant differences ($P = 0.6314$) in cell viability losses between BCG-loaded microparticles and BCG suspended in 0.025% chitosan or in 0.9% NaCl.

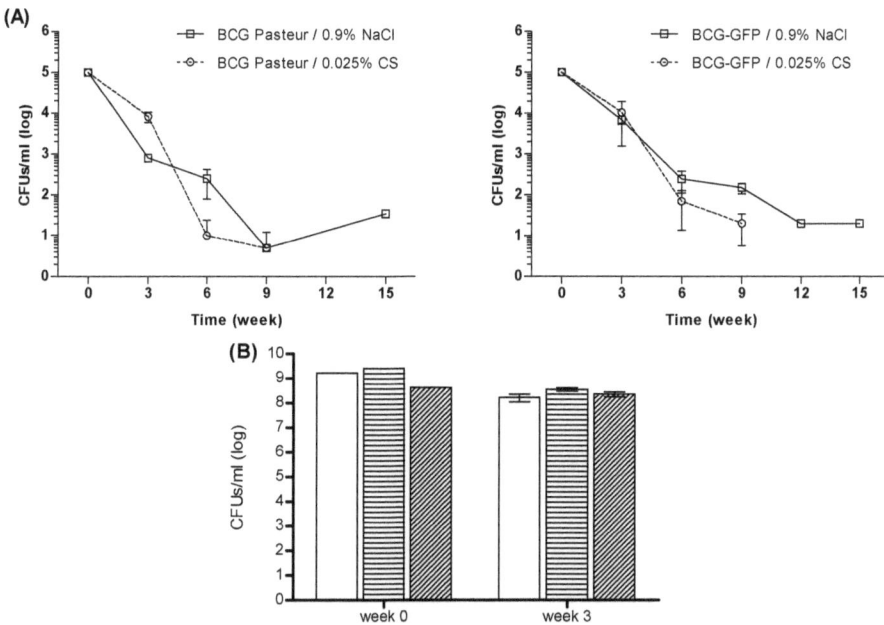

Figure 7. Cell viability of BCG (**A**) After 3 weeks of incubation, agar (Middlebrook 7H10 medium supplemented with OADC) plates inoculated with bacteria of both strains (Pasteur and GFP) that presented a number of colonies of statistical relevance were used to calculate the CFU/mL, by multiplying the colony forming units by the plating factor and the dilution factor. The CFU/mL provides an approximation of the cell density of the original culture. BCG suspension in 0.9% NaCl was used as control; (**B**) BCG Pasteur viability following BCG microencapsulation in "F14_Low" chitosan-alginate microparticles (no fill), BCG suspension in 0.025% low molecular weight chitosan weight (horizontal lines), or BCG suspension in 0.9% NaCl (angled lines). Results are expressed as mean $\pm$ S.D.; *n* = 3.

2.4. In Vitro Cell Viability (MTT Assay)

The *in vitro* biocompatibility of the microparticles was evaluated with the MTT assay using a PMA-differentiated THP-1 cell line (Figure 8), which is recommended as a model for antigen presenting cells [55].

Results showed no significant reduction of cellular viability after 24 h incubation with chitosan-suspended BCG and BCG-loaded microparticles, except for the highest concentrations of chitosan-suspended BCG, namely, 25 µg/mL ($p < 0.00001$), 12.5 µg/mL ($p = 0.0077$) and 6.3 µg/mL ($p < 0.05$), and a high concentration of BCG-loaded microparticles (12.5 µg/mL). These concentrations exceed concentrations intended for vaccination assays (e.g., 25 µg/mL is about five times higher). Overall, although some formulations induced a slight decrease in cell viability (15%–20%), none of the BCG-loaded microparticles may be considered as cytotoxic since the average values were not significantly different from the control group at tested concentrations. The obtained results are in conformity with other studies where chitosan did not interfere with cell viability [31].

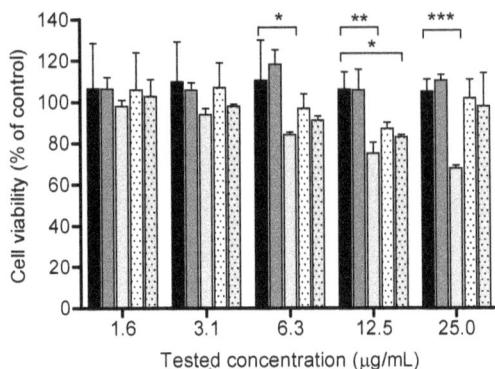

Figure 8. Relative cell viability of THP-1 cell line measured by the MTT reduction. Columns: black—control cells with culture medium; dark grey—BCG-GFP/0.9% NaCl; light grey—BCG-GFP/0.025% LMW chitosan; dotted white—BCG Pasteur/F13_Medium microparticles; dotted grey—BCG Pasteur/F13_High microparticles (1×10^8 CFUs/mL). Results are expressed as mean $\pm$ SD ($n = 3$). Statistical differences between the control group and formulations are reported as: *** $p < 0.001$, ** $p < 0.01$, * $p < 0.05$. Cell viability (% of control) = [A] test/[A] control $\times$ 100.

3. Materials and Methods

3.1. Materials

Sodium alginate polymers of high viscosity (14,000 mPa.s, 20 mg/mL), medium viscosity (3000 mPa.s, 20 mg/mL; M/G ratio of 1.56), and low viscosity (187 mPa.s, 20 mg/mL) (27 mPa.s, 10 mg/mL; M/G ratio of 1.56) were purchased from Sigma-Aldrich (Dorset, UK) (structural viscosity as provided by suppliers). Other tested sodium alginates include: low G-content (40%) Keltone LVCR (218 mPa.s, 20 mg/mL), high G-content (63%) Manugel LBA (773 mPa.s, 100 mg/mL), and high G-content (65%–75%) Protanal LF 10/60 (20–70 mPa.s, 10 mg/mL), which were a gift from FMC BioPolymer A.S. (Sandvika, Norway). Sodium tripolyphosphate (TPP) and calcium chloride ($CaCl_2$) were purchased from Sigma-Aldrich (Dorset, UK). Alginate stock solutions were prepared in ultra-purified water.

Most experiments were performed using solutions containing chitosan of low-molecular weight (<150 kDa) and deacetylation degree of 92%; chitosan of medium molecular weight (<450 kDa) and deacetylation degree of 85%; and chitosan of high molecular weight ($\approx$600 kDa) or high structural viscosity (748 mPas, 1% in acetic acid 1%, 20 °C) and undefined deacetylation degree, all purchased from Sigma–Aldrich (Dorset, UK) (specifications as provided by suppliers). The molecular weights were not verified. Chitosan stock solutions were prepared in 1% acetic acid solution in ultra-purified water.

The BCG strains—*M. bovis* BCG Pasteur strain 1173 (ATCC 35734™) (American Type Culture Collection (ATCC) Manassas, VA, USA)and a recombinant *M. bovis* BCG harboring a pMN437 plasmid for expression of Green Fluorescent Protein (rBCG-GFP) [76], were kindly supplied by Prof Elsa Anes (FFUL). The bacterial cell culture reagents were purchased from Difco, Franklin Lakes, New Jersey, USA. Both *M. bovis* BCG Pasteur and rBCG-GFP cultures were grown on Middlebrook's 7H9 broth Medium supplemented with 5% (v/v) OADC (oleic acid, albumin, dextrose and catalase supplement) at 37 °C/5% CO_2.

The THP1 cells (ATCC TIB-202™) a human monocyte cell line was obtained from (ATCC, USA). All animal cell culture reagents were purchased from Invitrogen (Paisley, UK). Phorbol myristate acetate (PMA), 3-(4,5-dimethyl-2-thiazolyl)-2,5-diphenyl-2*H*-tetrazolium bromide (MTT), dimethylsulfoxide (DMSO) were all from Sigma-Aldrich (Dorset, UK).

3.2. Preparation of Polymeric Microparticles

Polymeric microparticles were initially prepared using modifications of previously described ionic cross-linking methods [30–34], by high speed stirring at room temperature and without organic solvents—Methods (I) and (II). Alginate and chitosan were dissolved in ultra-purified water.

In Method (I), polymeric microparticles were prepared via formation of an alginate ionotropic pre-gel, by allowing sodium alginate solution to react with calcium chloride prior to chitosan addition. (Figure 9). Briefly, a 7.5 mL aliquot of 18 mM calcium chloride solution was added drop wise into a beaker containing 117.5 mL of a 0.6 mg/mL sodium alginate solution, and stirred for 60 min under 600 rpm, to provide an alginate pre-gel. Then, 25.0 mL of a 0.7 mg/mL chitosan solution was added drop wise into the pre-gel and stirred over 90 min, giving a final alginate and chitosan concentration of 0.5 mg/mL and 0.1 mg/mL, respectively (alginate: chitosan mass ratio 4.23:1). A colloidal dispersion formed upon polycationic chitosan addition.

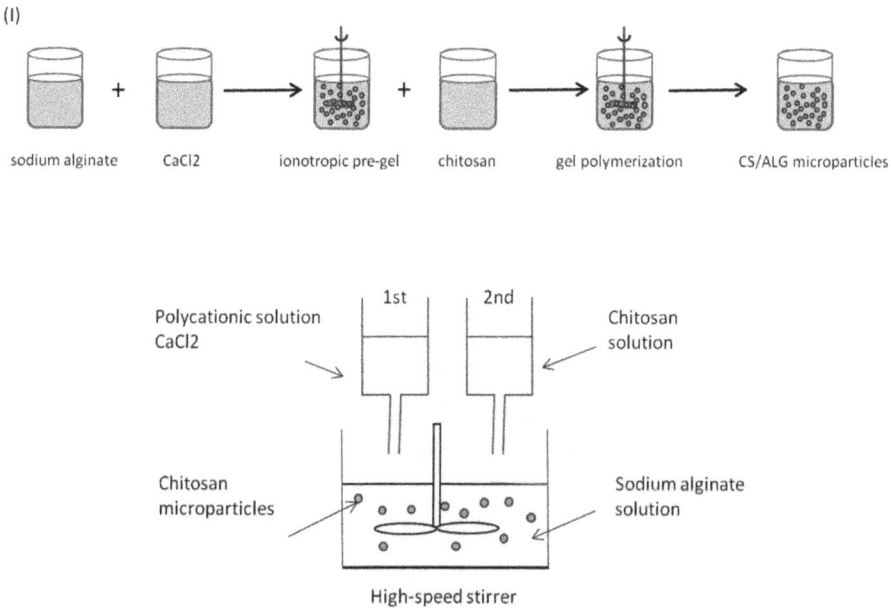

Figure 9. Microparticles formation by alginate ionotropic pre-gelation with CaCl$_2$ followed by chitosan addition (adapted from [33]).

In formulation Method (II), polymeric microparticles were prepared by allowing chitosan and sodium alginate to polymerize, by means of ionic interaction between positively charged amine groups of chitosan and negatively charged carboxyl groups of alginate, prior to TPP addition (Figure 10). Briefly, a 5.0 mL aliquot of 1.0 mg/mL chitosan were added drop wise into a beaker containing volume ranging from 0.1 to 5.0 mL of 1.0 mg/mL of sodium alginate solution, followed by dropwise addition of 1.0 mL of 1.0 mg/mL TPP under high-speed stirring at 600 rpm for 120–150 min. Alginate: chitosan ratios ranged from 0.02:1 to 1:1 (*w:w*).

(II)

sodium alginate   chitosan   gel polymerization   TPP   gel shrinking   CS/ALG microparticles

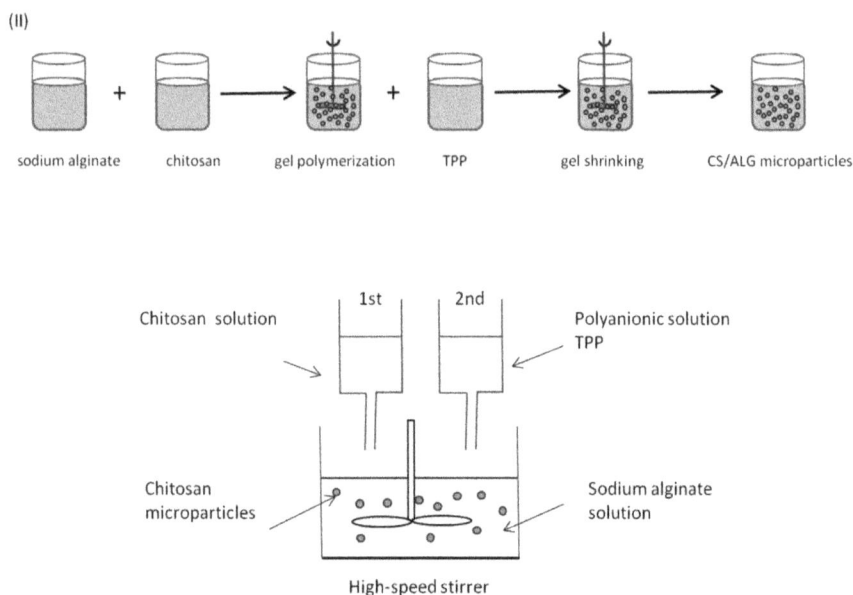

Figure 10. Microparticles formation by chitosan gel matrix formation with sodium alginate followed by TPP addition (adapted from [32,34]).

Preliminary experiments with three replicates were designed in order to investigate the appropriate concentration range for chitosan, alginate and sodium tripolyphosphate, according to a previously described method [32] with modifications (Table 8). The purpose was to identify the impact of the key components of the polyelectrolyte matrix, such as different pH values and polymers mass ratio, on parameters such as particle size and zeta potential. Therefore, high, medium and low molecular weight chitosan, and TPP, were used and their volume was kept constant (5.0 mL and 2.0 mL, respectively), while high, medium and low viscosity alginate was used in increasing volumes.

Table 8. Values for the investigated variables during formulation studies.

Formulation	Chitosan (CS) (% w/v)	Alginate (ALG) (% w/v)	CaCl$_2$* or TPP ** (% w/v)	ALG:CS Mass Ratio (w/w)
F0	0.010	0.050	0.010 *	4.23:1
F1	0.070	0.001	0.028 **	0.02:1
F2	0.069	0.003	0.028 **	0.04:1
F3	0.068	0.004	0.027 **	0.06:1
F4	0.068	0.005	0.027 **	0.08:1
F5	0.067	0.007	0.027 **	0.10:1
F6	0.066	0.008	0.026 **	0.12:1
F7	0.065	0.009	0.026 **	0.14:1
F8	0.064	0.010	0.026 **	0.16:1
F9	0.063	0.011	0.025 **	0.18:1
F10	0.063	0.013	0.025 **	0.20:1
F11	0.056	0.022	0.022 **	0.40:1
F12	0.050	0.030	0.020 **	0.60:1
F13	0.045	0.036	0.018 **	0.80:1
F14	0.042	0.042	0.017 **	1.00:1

F0—ALG/CS microparticles, obtained via alginate ionotropic pre-gelation with CaCl$_2$ followed by chitosan addition—Method (I); F1–F14—CS/ALG microparticles, obtained via chitosan precipitation with TPP followed by gelation with alginate—Method (II). * CaCl$_2$ ** TPP.

High shear homogenization (ultra-turrax T10basic at 11,400 rpm, IKA-Labortechnik, Staufen, Germany) and sonication (Branson Sonifier 250, equipped with a 3 mm microtip probe, BRANSON Ultrasonics Corporation, Danbury, CT, USA) were assessed as potential alternatives to high speed stirring to prepare microparticles. The techniques were evaluated considering physical stability of microparticle suspensions (general aspect, formation of aggregates) and microparticles characteristics, such as size distribution and surface charge. Microparticle preparation was in accordance with above described formulation Method (I) and Method (II), with modifications. Briefly, in accordance with previously described formulation Method (I), 0.75 mL of 18 mM calcium chloride were added to 11.75 mL of 0.6 mg/mL sodium alginate, and either homogenized for 3 min in ultra-turrax or sonicated for 3 min at 20% output intensity, prior to 2.5 mL of 0.7 mg/mL chitosan addition, and subsequent homogenization or sonication as described. As for Method (II), 5.0 mL of 1.0 mg/mL chitosan were added to 0.1–5.0 mL of 1.0 mg/mL of sodium alginate, followed by addition of 1 mL of 2.0 mg/mL TPP, and either homogenized for 3 min in ultra-turrax or sonicated for 3 min at 20% output intensity.

The results obtained during formulation optimization studies led us towards the rejection of Method (I) and the development of a different preparation method—Method (III). In Method (III), polymeric microparticles were prepared by inducing the pre-gelation of chitosan with TPP, followed by alginate coating (Figure 11). Briefly, alginate and chitosan were dissolved in ultra-purified water. Microparticles were formed by the dropwise addition of a 1.0 mL aliquot of 2.0 mg/mL TPP into a beaker containing 5.0 mL of 1.0 mg/mL chitosan solution, followed by polyanionic cross linking with volumes ranging from 0.1 mL to 5.0 mL of 1.0 mg/mL sodium alginate solution, also added drop wise, under high-speed stirring at 600 rpm for 120–150 min.

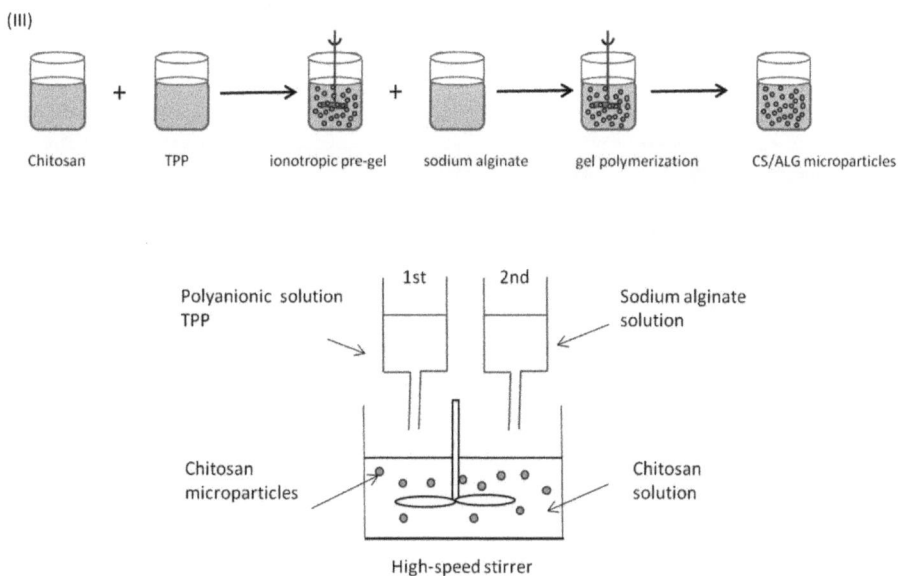

Figure 11. Microparticles formation by chitosan precipitation with TPP followed by alginate addition.

Additional characterization studies were conducted with Methods (II) and (III) to identify the best experimental conditions to obtain microparticles of intended size distribution and surface charge. In these studies, microparticles were prepared with sodium alginate of different quality specifications, namely, viscosity and guluronic acid monomers content (G-content, %), and the influence of pH value variations in microparticle size distribution and surface charge was determined. During pH value studies, a wide range of chitosan- and sodium alginate-solution pH value was assessed (pH from 3.3

to 7.6), while alginate (Protanal™ LF 10/60) concentration was kept constant at 0.1%. Modifications to the formulation methods were introduced along the optimization process accordingly to the conclusions yielded by the obtained results during preliminary studies. Regarding future lyophilisation of microparticles, some preliminary studies using two concentrations (5% and 10% w/v) of three different cryoprotectors (sucrose, glucose, and trehalose) were also conducted.

3.3. BCG Studies

3.3.1. BCG Single Cell Suspension

Bacterial cultures in exponential growth phase (after 7 days) were pelleted at 4000 rpm (1559× g) at 4 °C for 15 min, washed twice in sterile 10 mM PBS pH 7.4 and re-suspended in appropriate medium. The suspension was kept on the bench for 5 min, to allow the decantation of the large clumps of bacteria. Clumps of bacteria were removed by ultrasonic treatment of bacteria suspensions in an ultrasonic water bath for 15 min. For bacteria remaining in clumps, the complete volume of the suspension was collected and pressed through a 21 gauge needle against the syringe tube wall for 10 times, in order to get individualized bacilli.

Single cell suspension was confirmed by phase contrast microscopy or in a fluorescence microscope (for rBCG-GFP). In the absence of clumps, the OD of the suspension at λ = 600 nm was adjusted to 0.1 (we assumed that 0.1 OD_{600} corresponds to 1×10^7 bacteria per mL [76]). This was later confirmed by methylene blue staining and haematocytometer count (for BCG Pasteur) and CFU counts after bacterial suspension plating, in order to more accurately determine the total viable number of bacteria, as this can vary immensely as a function of the growth medium composition of mycobacteria, and also due to a potential growth inhibition effect of chitosan [77–81].

3.3.2. Surface Charge Characterization

In order to modify the physicochemical properties of BCG, monodispersed bacteria were suspended in different concentrations of chitosan and encapsulated or adsorbed into different formulations of microparticles. Then, size distribution and surface charge were determined. These studies were performed for both BCG Pasteur and rBCG-GFP strains. Inactivation studies of both strains were also conducted to assess the effect of viability loss in BCG surface characteristics, and to perform the further characterisation studies in safety. Mycobacteria were submitted to heat inactivation, by submersion of 15 mL falcon containing bacterial suspensions in a water bath preheated and maintained at 80 °C for 15 min [82]. The efficacy of inactivation methods was determined by viability checks, as follows: 100 µL of the heat killed suspension was used to inoculate each of two plates with solid agar Middlebrook 7H10 medium supplemented with 5% OADC and incubated at 37 °C in 5% CO_2 atmosphere for 3 weeks.

3.3.3. Microencapsulation of BCG

BCG-loaded microparticles were prepared by addition of 1.0 mL of whole live attenuated BCG bacillus monodispersed in NaCl 0.9% (range, 1–2 × 10^8 CFUs/mL) to 5.0 mL of 1.0 mg/mL chitosan solution. Next, 1.0 mL of 2.0 mg/mL TPP was added drop wise to chitosan-suspended BCG, followed by drop wise addition of 4.0 to 5.0 mL of 1.0 mg/mL sodium alginate solution to the mixture. Final concentrations of prepared microparticles ranged from 6 to 8 log10 CFUs/mL and from 0.42 to 0.45 mg/mL of chitosan.

3.3.4. BCG Cell Viability

In order to assess BCG viability, a colony-forming units (CFUs) assay was used to count bacteria of both strains (Pasteur and GFP) able to produce colonies in agar Middlebrook 7H10 medium supplemented with OADC (widely used to cultivate and access the CFUs in the case of slow growers such as *M. tuberculosis* and *M. bovis* BCG [77]). Briefly, aliquots of BCG suspended in 0.25 mg/mL chitosan of medium MW and BCG-loaded chitosan-alginate microparticles were seeded in appropriate inoculation medium to determine the effects of processing conditions on cell viability. The samples were maintained at 4 °C for approximately four months (15 weeks), and plates were inoculated with samples for cell count at regular time points. After three weeks of incubation at 37 °C and 5% CO_2, colonies were counted to determine CFUs.

3.4. Characterization of Microparticles

3.4.1. Size Distribution, Surface Charge and Morphology

The microparticles were assessed according to size distribution and surface charge (zeta potential), by laser diffraction and electrophoretic mobility, using a Mastersizer 2000 and a Malvern Zetasizer, respectively (Malvern Instruments, Worcestershire, UK). For particle size analysis, each sample was diluted with filtered purified water to the appropriate concentration to yield 10% obscurity limit. Each analysis was carried out in triplicate at 25 °C. Results were expressed in terms of mean diameter and span (Span = d (0.9) − d (0.1)/d (0.5)). Size distribution is characterized using the d0.5 parameter (diameter for which 50% of the distribution falls below) and the span parameter (width of particle size distribution). For the determination of the electrophoretic mobility, samples were diluted with filtered purified water. The mean values were obtained from the analysis of three different batches, each of them measured three times. Morphological examination of microparticles was performed by microscopy. The ImageJ software, 1.44p version (National Institutes of Health, Bethesda, MA, USA) was used to perform image analysis.

3.4.2. Production Yield

The production yield (YP) (Equation (1)) of the microparticles was determined using an indirect method based on the quantification of the chitosan concentration initially used in the formulation, and that found in the supernatant of the final microparticle suspension as previously published [29]. The method of quantification is based on a colorimetric reaction between amine groups of chitosan and the dye Cibacron brilliant red 3B-A [30].

$$CS \, yield \, (\%) = \frac{[CS] \, total - [CS] \, supernantant}{[CS] \, total} \times 100 \tag{1}$$

3.4.3. Fourier Transform Infrared Spectroscopy (FT-IR) Analysis

Preliminary information on chemical nature of the chitosan-alginate microparticles was collected using FT-IR analysis in an IRAffinity-1 (Shimadzu Corporation, Kyoto, Japan) spectrophotometer. The FT-IR measurements were made directly in the dried microparticles, which were previously lyophilised, and all powder raw materials namely chitosan and alginate, gently mixed with approximately 300 mg of micronized KBr powder and compressed into discs at a force of 10 kN for 1 min using a manual tablet presser (Perkin Elmer, Norwalk, CA, USA). All spectra were recorded at room temperature at the resolution of 4 cm^{-1} and 50-times scanning, between 4000 and 500 cm^{-1} [83].

3.4.4. Encapsulation Efficiency

Encapsulation efficiency (EE, %) was determined by cell count number using a haemocytometer (Neubauer chamber Bürker). The encapsulation efficiency is expressed as the percentage of BCG entrapped/adsorbed in microparticles reported to initial amount of cells in suspension (Equation (2)).

$$Encapsulation \, efficiency \, (\%) = \frac{Total \, cells - Free \, cells}{Total \, cells} \times 100 \tag{2}$$

3.5. In Vitro Cell Viability (MTT Assay)

Animal cell viability was assessed using general cell viability endpoint MTT as previously described with some modification [30,73]. Briefly, THP-1 cells (grown in RPMI 1640 supplemented with 10% FBS, penicillin and streptomycin,) were seeded onto 96 well cultures dishes at a density of 5×10^5 cells/mL and treated for 72 h with 20 nM PMA in order to differentiate into macrophage, and medium exchanged and incubated for one more day. Cells were then incubated for 72 h at 37 °C with different concentrations of CS and ALG solutions and BCG loaded and empty formulations. Controls consisted of cells incubated with only culture medium. Each sample concentration was tested in triplicate in a single experiment, which was repeated at least 3 times.

After the incubation time, culture medium was replaced with culture medium containing 0.5 mg/mL of MTT and incubated for 3 h at 37 °C. The medium was removed after 3 h and the intracellular formazan crystals were solubilised and extracted with dimethylsulfoxide (DMSO). After 15 min at room temperature, the absorbance of the extracted solution was measured at 570 nm in a microplate reader (Infinite M200, Tecan, Männedorf, Switzerland). The percentage of cell viability was determined for each concentration of tested sample according to Equation (3), where *Abs test* is the absorbance value obtained for cells treated with samples, and *Abs control* is the absorbance value obtained for cells incubated with culture medium.

$$\text{Cell viability (\% of Control)} = \frac{Abs\ test}{Abs\ control} \times 100 \tag{3}$$

3.6. Statistical Analysis

Data were subjected to ANOVA for analysis of statistical significance, and a p value of <0.05 was considered to be significant. Unless stated otherwise, results are expressed as mean values $\pm$ standard deviation (SD). The analysis was carried out using GraphPad Prism v. 5.02 (GraphPad Software, La Jolla, CA, USA).

4. Conclusions

During these formulation studies, it was possible to optimize the preparation method for BCG-loaded chitosan-alginate microparticles with reproducible size distribution, encapsulation efficiency and yield of preparation. Particle size and size distribution uniformity were considered to be critical aspects throughout the formulation studies. These parameters are influenced by several experimental conditions, such as the properties of the used polymers, antigen type (whole live bacteria represent additional challenges regarding cell viability maintenance during formulation); type, speed and duration of homogenization, polymer/polymer and polymer/complexation agent mass ratios, and the relationship between the pH values of the different polymers.

In this study, biodegradable and biocompatible polymers (chitosan and sodium alginate), as well as two strains of *Mycobacterium bovis* BCG (BCG Pasteur, clinically available vaccine; and rBCG-GFP), were used. The number of variables that could be optimized was reduced throughout the formulation development. Essentially, the optimization of the preparation method relied on the identification of the best polymeric compositions and identification of the crucial steps in the ionic gelation methods that were determinant for particle size distribution and surface charge.

It was possible to observe that, for chitosan-alginate microparticles, size distribution was mainly influenced by the molecular weight of the used polymers and by the type of polymer blends. On the contrary, particle surface charge was mainly influenced by polymer to polymer mass ratio due to the possibility of particle aggregation. By simply suspending BCG in chitosan, it was possible to tune BCG physicochemical properties, namely surface charge.

Additionally, the encapsulation of monodispersed whole live BCG bacilli into microparticles was of paramount importance since it could directly influence BCG cell viability and particle size and surface charge. It was possible to develop a reproducible method for microencapsulation of whole live bacteria using only mild conditions, through ionic cross-linking, with good production yield and encapsulation efficiency, while maintaining cell viability and assuring the biocompatibility of the developed microparticulate delivery system. The microencapsulation of BCG had no considerable effect on particles key features (*i.e.*, size distribution, surface charge, morphology). However, the formulation method and, to a minor extent, the concentrations of BCG used, proved to be crucial in achieving high encapsulation efficiency values.

Regarding particle surface charge, it was possible to demonstrate that the addition order of the polymers was crucial to obtaining microparticles of either electronegative or electropositive surface charge, as follows: Method (I) produced negatively charged particles, as chitosan droplets were imprisoned in a previously formed, and stoichiometric predominant, alginate matrix); Method (II) allowed the preparation of positively to negatively charged particles, depending on the polymer mass ratio (Figure 2) or polymer specifications such as alginate G-content (Figure 3); and Method (III) allowed the preparation of negatively charged particles, as alginate probably coated previously formed chitosan particles. This was clearly shown with the empty particles (Tables 1, 3 and 4). As expected, due to the negative surface charge of BCG bacilli, BCG encapsulation led to minor modifications of the net charge at the particle surface (as depicted in Table 7), probably due to interference with the polymer arrangement.

In conclusion, a whole, live attenuated, cell-based particulate delivery system was developed for mucosal immunization purposes. Further characterization of these formulations in terms of *in vitro* cellular interaction with macrophages and *in vivo* study following intranasal immunization in mice is ongoing.

Acknowledgments: The authors would like to thanks to Elsa Anes (FFUL) and her team (David Pires, Nuno Carmo) by supplying strains (Pasteur and GFP), for access to the laboratory as well for all advice and practical support. The authors thank iMed.ULisboa for financial support (UID/DTP/04138/2013) from Fundação para a Ciência e Tecnologia (FCT), Portugal and Escola Superior de Tecnologia da Saúde de Lisboa for financial support from merit scholarship for Ph.D. (ESTeSL-IPL/CGD/2012) granted by Caixa Geral de Depósitos, Portugal.

Author Contributions: L.M.D.G. conceived and designed the experiments; L.A.C. and L.M.D.G. performed the experiments; L.A.C., L.M.D.G. and A.J.A. analyzed the data; L.A.C., L.M.D.G. and A.J.A. wrote the paper.

Conflicts of Interest: The authors declare no conflict of interest.

Abbreviations

The following abbreviations are used in this manuscript:

ALG	Alginate
APCs	Antigen presenting cells
BCG	Bacillus Calmette-Guérin
CFU	Colony-forming unit
CS	Chitosan
DMSO	Dimethylsulfoxide
E.E.	Encapsulation efficiency
FT-IR	Fourier transform infrared spectroscopy
G	Guluronate
GFP	Green fluorescence protein
HMW	High molecular weight
HV	High viscosity
LMW	Low molecular weight
LV	Low viscosity
M	Mannuronate

MMW	Medium molecular weight
MV	Medium viscosity
MTT	3-(4,5-dimethyl-2-thiazolyl)-2,5-diphenyl-2H-tetrazolium bromide
NALT	Nasal associated lymphoid tissue
ND	Not determined
OADC	Oleic acid, albumin, dextrose and catalase supplement
OD	Optical density
PBS	Phosphate-buffered saline solution
PLGA	Poly(D,L-lactide-co-glycolide)
PLA	Poly(L-lactide)
PMA	Phorbol myristate acetate
rBCG	Recombinant BCG
THP-1	human monocyte cell line
TPP	Tripolyphosphate
US	Ultrasonication
UT	Ultraturrax
YP	Yield of production

References

1. Kaufmann, S.H.E. Envisioning future strategies for vaccination against tuberculosis. *Nat. Rev. Immunol.* **2006**, *6*, 699–704. [CrossRef] [PubMed]
2. Kaufmann, S.H.E. Future vaccination strategies against tuberculosis: Thinking outside the box. *Immunity* **2010**, *33*, 567–577. [CrossRef] [PubMed]
3. Mohanan, D.; Slütter, B.; Henriksen-Lacey, M.; Jiskoot, W.; Bouwstra, J.A.; Perrie, Y.; Kündig, T.M.; Gander, B.; Johansen, P. Administration routes affect the quality of immune responses: A cross-sectional evaluation of particulate antigen-delivery systems. *J. Control. Release* **2010**, *147*, 342–349. [CrossRef] [PubMed]
4. Cooper, A.M. Cell-mediated immune responses in tuberculosis. *Annu. Rev. Immunol.* **2009**, *27*, 393–422. [CrossRef] [PubMed]
5. Bhatt, K.; Salgame, P. Host innate immune response to *Mycobacterium tuberculosis*. *J. Clin. Immunol.* **2007**, *27*, 347–362. [CrossRef] [PubMed]
6. Ota, M.O.C.; Vekemans, J.; Susanna, E.; Fielding, K.; Sanneh, M.; Kidd, M.; Newport, M.J.; Aaby, P.; Whittle, H.; Lambert, P.H.; *et al.* Influence of *Mycobacterium bovis* bacillus Calmette-Guérin on antibody and cytokine responses to human neonatal vaccination. *J. Immunol.* **2002**, *168*, 919–925. [CrossRef] [PubMed]
7. Dietrich, J.; Billeskov, R.; Doherty, T.M.; Andersen, P. Synergistic effect of bacillus Calmette Guerin and a Tuberculosis subunit vaccine in cationic liposomes: Increased immunogenicity and protection. *J. Immunol.* **2007**, *178*, 3721–3730. [CrossRef] [PubMed]
8. Ajdary, S.; Dobakhti, F.; Taghikhani, M. Oral administration of BCG encapsulated in alginate microspheres induces strong Th1 response in BALB/c mice. *Vaccine* **2007**, *25*, 4595–4601. [CrossRef] [PubMed]
9. Almeida, A.J.; Alpar, H.O. *Antigen Delivery Systems—Imunological and Technical Issues*; Harwood Academic Publishers: Reading, UK, 1997; pp. 207–226.
10. Eyles, J.E.; Sharp, G.J.; Williamson, E.D.; Spiers, I.D.; Alpar, H.O. Intra nasal administration of poly-lactic acid microsphere co-encapsulated Yersinia pestis subunits confers protection from pneumonic plague in the mouse. *Vaccine* **1998**, *16*, 698–707. [CrossRef]
11. Alpar, H.O.; Somavarapu, S.; Atuah, K.N.; Bramwell, V.W. Biodegradable mucoadhesive particulates for nasal and pulmonary antigen and DNA delivery. *Adv. Drug Deliv. Rev.* **2005**, *57*, 411–430. [CrossRef] [PubMed]
12. Tafaghodi, M.; Tabassi, S.A.S.; Jaafari, M.R. Induction of systemic and mucosal immune responses by intranasal administration of alginate microspheres encapsulated with tetanus toxoid and CpG-ODN. *Int. J. Pharm.* **2006**, *319*, 37–43. [CrossRef] [PubMed]
13. Singh, M.; O'Hagan, D.T. Recent advances in vaccine adjuvants. *Pharm. Res.* **2002**, *19*, 715–728. [CrossRef] [PubMed]

14. Slütter, B.; Jiskoot, W. Dual role of CpG as immune modulator and physical crosslinker in ovalbumin loaded *N*-trimethyl chitosan (TMC) nanoparticles for nasal vaccination. *J. Control. Release* **2010**, *148*, 117–121.
15. Pichichero, M.E. Improving vaccine delivery using novel adjuvant systems. *Hum. Vaccin.* **2008**, *4*, 262–270. [CrossRef] [PubMed]
16. Bal, S.M.; Slütter, B.; Verheul, R.; Bouwstra, J.A.; Jiskoot, W. Adjuvanted, antigen loaded *N*-trimethyl chitosan nanoparticles for nasal and intradermal vaccination: Adjuvant- and site-dependent immunogenicity in mice. *Eur. J. Pharm. Sci.* **2012**, *45*, 475–481. [CrossRef] [PubMed]
17. Kazzaz, J.; Singh, M.; Ugozzoli, M.; Chesko, J.; Soenawan, E.; Hagan, D.T.O. Encapsulation of the immune potentiators MPL and RC529 in PLG microparticles enhances their potency. *J. Control. Release* **2006**, *110*, 566–573. [CrossRef] [PubMed]
18. Caetano, L.A.; Almeida, A.J.; Gonçalves, L.M.D. Approaches to tuberculosis mucosal vaccine development using nanoparticles and microparticles: A review. *J. Biomed. Nanotechnol.* **2014**, *10*, 2295–2316. [CrossRef] [PubMed]
19. Thiele, L.; Rothen-Rutishauser, B.; Jilek, S. Evaluation of particle uptake in human blood monocyte-derived cells *in vitro*. Does phagocytosis activity of dendritic cells measure up with macrophages? *J. Control. Release* **2001**, *76*, 59–71. [CrossRef]
20. He, C.; Hu, Y.; Yin, L.; Tang, C.; Yin, C. Effects of particle size and surface charge on cellular uptake and biodistribution of polymeric nanoparticles. *Biomaterials* **2010**, *31*, 3657–3666. [CrossRef] [PubMed]
21. Foged, C.; Brodin, B.; Frokjaer, S.; Sundblad, A. Particle size and surface charge affect particle uptake by human dendritic cells in an *in vitro* model. *Int. J. Pharm.* **2005**, *298*, 315–322. [CrossRef] [PubMed]
22. Douglas, K.L.; Tabrizian, M. Effect of experimental parameters on the formation of alginate-chitosan nanoparticles and evaluation of their potential application as DNA carrier. *J. Biomater. Sci. Polym.* **2005**, *16*, 43–56. [CrossRef]
23. Grabnar, P.A.; Kristl, J. The manufacturing techniques of drug-loaded polymeric nanoparticles from preformed polymers. *J. Microencapsul.* **2011**, *28*, 323–335. [CrossRef] [PubMed]
24. Figueiredo, L.; Cadete, A.; Gonçalves, L.M.D.; Corvo, M.L.; Almeida, A.J. Intranasal immunization of mice against Streptococcus equi using positively charged nanoparticulate carrier systems. *Vaccine* **2012**, *30*, 6551–6558. [CrossRef] [PubMed]
25. Florindo, H.F.; Pandit, S.; Lacerda, L.; Gonçalves, L.M.D.; Alpar, H.O.; Almeida, A.J. The enhancement of the immune response against S. equi antigens through the intranasal administration of poly-epsilon-caprolactone-based nanoparticles. *Biomaterials* **2009**, *30*, 879–891. [CrossRef] [PubMed]
26. Jenkins, P.G.; Coombes, A.G.; Yeh, M.K.; Thomas, N.W.; Davis, S.S. Aspects of the design and delivery of microparticles for vaccine applications. *J. Drug Target.* **1995**, *3*, 79–81. [CrossRef] [PubMed]
27. Davis, S.S. Nasal vaccines. *Adv. Drug Deliv. Rev.* **2001**, *51*, 21–42. [CrossRef]
28. Vajdy, M.; O'Hagan, D.T. Microparticles for intranasal immunization. *Adv. Drug Deliv. Rev.* **2001**, *51*, 127–141. [CrossRef]
29. Almeida, A.J.; Alpar, H.O. Nasal delivery of vaccines. *J. Drug Target.* **1996**, *3*, 455–467. [CrossRef] [PubMed]
30. Cadete, A.; Figueiredo, L.; Lopes, R.; Calado, C.C.R.; Almeida, A.J.; Gonçalves, L.M.D. Development and characterization of a new plasmid delivery system based on chitosan-sodium deoxycholate nanoparticles. *Eur. J. Pharm. Sci.* **2012**, *45*, 451–458. [CrossRef] [PubMed]
31. Figueiredo, L.; Calado, C.C.R.; Almeida, A.J.; Gonçalves, L.M.D. Protein and DNA nanoparticulate multiantigenic vaccines against H. pylori: *In vivo* evaluation. In Proceedings of the 2012 IEEE 2nd Portuguese Meeting in BioEngineering, Coimbra, Portugal, 23–25 February 2012; IEEE EMBS Portuguese Chapter, I.I. p. 1.
32. Calvo, P.; Remuñán-López, C.; Vila-Jato, J.L.; Alonso, M.J. Chitosan and Chitosan-Ethylene Oxide-Propylene oxide block copolymer nanoparticles as novel carriers for proteins and vaccines. *Pharm. Res.* **1997**, *14*, 1431–1436. [CrossRef] [PubMed]
33. Sarmento, B.; Ribeiro, A.J.; Veiga, F.; Ferreira, D.C.; Neufeld, R.J. Insulin-loaded nanoparticles are prepared by alginate ionotropic pre-gelation followed by chitosan polyelectrolyte complexation. *J. Nanosci. Nanotechnol.* **2007**, *7*, 2833–2841. [CrossRef] [PubMed]
34. Calvo, P.; Remuñán-López, C.; Vila-Jato, J.L.; Alonso, M.J. Novel hydrophilic chitosan-polyethylene oxide nanoparticles as protein carriers. *J. Appl. Polym. Sci.* **1997**, *63*, 125–132. [CrossRef]

35. Sarmento, B.; Ferreira, D.; Veiga, F.; Ribeiro, A. Characterization of insulin-loaded alginate nanoparticles produced by ionotropic pre-gelation through DSC and FTIR studies. *Carbohydr. Polym.* **2006**, *66*, 1–7. [CrossRef]

36. Sarmento, B. *Chitosan-Based Systems for Biopharmaceuticals: Delivery, Targeting, and Polymer Therapeutics*; John Wiley & Sons, Ltd.: Hoboken, NJ, USA, 2012.

37. Tønnesen, H.H.; Karlsen, J. Alginate in drug delivery systems. *Drug Dev. Ind. Pharm.* **2002**, *28*, 621–630. [CrossRef] [PubMed]

38. De, S.; Robinson, D. Polymer relationships during preparation of chitosan–alginate and poly-L-lysine–alginate nanospheres. *J. Control. Release* **2003**, *89*, 101–112. [CrossRef]

39. Dodane, V.; Amin Khan, M.; Merwin, J.R. Effect of chitosan on epithelial permeability and structure. *Int. J. Pharm.* **1999**, *182*, 21–32. [CrossRef]

40. Amidi, M.; Mastrobattista, E.; Jiskoot, W.; Hennink, W.E. Chitosan-based delivery systems for protein therapeutics and antigens. *Adv. Drug Deliv. Rev.* **2010**, *62*, 59–82. [CrossRef] [PubMed]

41. Pawar, D.; Goyal, A.K.; Mangal, S.; Mishra, N.; Vaidya, B.; Tiwari, S.; Jain, A.K.; Vyas, S.P. Evaluation of mucoadhesive PLGA microparticles for nasal immunization. *AAPS J.* **2010**, *12*, 130–137. [CrossRef] [PubMed]

42. Lehr, C.; Bouwstra, J.; Schacht, E.; Junginger, H. *In vitro* evaluation of mucoadhesive properties of chitosan and some other natural polymers. *Int. J. Pharm.* **1992**, *78*, 43–48. [CrossRef]

43. Leithner, K.; Bernkop-Schnürch, A. Chitosan and derivatives for biopharmaceutical use: Mucoadhesve properties. In *Chitosan-Based Systems for Biopharmaceuticals: Delivery, Targeting and Polymer Therapeutics*; Sarmento, B., Neves, J., Eds.; John Wiley & Sons, Ltd.: Hoboken, NJ, USA, 2012; pp. 159–180.

44. Van der Lubben, I.M.; Verhoef, J.C.; Borchard, G.; Junginger, H.E. Chitosan and its derivatives in mucosal drug and vaccine delivery. *Eur. J. Pharm. Sci.* **2001**, *14*, 201–207. [CrossRef]

45. Baudner, B.C.; Giuliani, M.M.; Verhoef, J.C.; Rappuoli, R.; Junginger, H.E.; Del, G. The concomitant use of the LTK63 mucosal adjuvant and of chitosan-based delivery system enhances the immunogenicity and efficacy of intranasally administered vaccines. *Vaccine* **2003**, *21*, 3837–3844. [CrossRef]

46. Tafaghodia, M.; Saluja, V.; Kersten, G.F.A.; Kraan, H.; Slütter, B.; Amorij, J.P.; Jiskoot, W. Hepatitis B surface antigen nanoparticles coated with chitosan and trimethyl chitosan: Impact of formulation on physicochemical and immunological characteristics. *Vaccine* **2012**, *30*, 5341–5348. [CrossRef] [PubMed]

47. McNeela, E.A.; Jabbal-Gill, I.; Illum, L.; Pizza, M.; Rappuoli, R.; Podda, A.; Lewis, D.J.M.; Mills, K.H.G. Intranasal immunization with genetically detoxified diphtheria toxin induces T cell responses in humans: Enhancement of Th2 responses and toxin-neutralizing antibodies by formulation with chitosan. *Vaccine* **2004**, *22*, 909–914. [CrossRef] [PubMed]

48. Amidi, M.; Mastrobattista, E.; Jiskoot, W.; Hennink, W.E. *N*-Trimethyl chitosan (TMC) nanoparticles loaded with influenza subunit antigen for intranasal vaccination: Biological properties and immunogenicity in a mouse model. *Vaccine* **2007**, *25*, 144–153. [CrossRef] [PubMed]

49. Jain, R.; Dey, B.; Dhar, N.; Rao, V.; Singh, R.; Gupta, U.D.; Katoch, V.M.; Ramanathan, V.D.; Tyagi, A.K. Enhanced and enduring protection against tuberculosis by recombinant BCG-Ag85C and its association with modulation of cytokine profile in lung. *PLoS ONE* **2008**, *3*, e3869. [CrossRef] [PubMed]

50. Gupta, N.K.; Tomar, P.; Sharma, V.; Dixit, V.K. Development and characterization of chitosan coated poly-(ε-caprolactone) nanoparticulate system for effective immunization against influenza. *Vaccine* **2011**, *29*, 9026–9037. [CrossRef] [PubMed]

51. Vila, A.; Sanchez, A.; Janes, K.; Behrens, I.; Kissel, T.; Jato, J.L.V.; Alonso, M.J. Low molecular weight chitosan nanoparticles as new carriers for nasal vaccine delivery in mice. *Eur. J. Pharm. Biopharm.* **2004**, *57*, 123–131. [CrossRef] [PubMed]

52. Kang, M.L.; Cho, C.S.; Yoo, H.S. Application of chitosan microspheres for nasal delivery of vaccines. *Biotechnol. Adv.* **2009**, *27*, 857–865. [CrossRef] [PubMed]

53. Rodrigues, M.A.; Figueiredo, L.; Padrela, L.; Cadete, A.; Tiago, J.; Matos, H.A.; Azevedo, E.G.; Florindo, H.F.; Goncalves, L.M.; Almeida, A.J. Development of a novel mucosal vaccine against strangles by supercritical enhanced atomization spray-drying of *Streptococcus equi* extracts and evaluation in a mouse model. *Eur. J. Pharm. Biopharm.* **2012**, *82*, 392–400. [CrossRef] [PubMed]

54. Theus, S.A.; Cave, M.D.; Eisenach, K.D. Activated THP-1 cells: An attractive model for the assessment of intracellular growth rates of *Mycobacterium tuberculosis* isolates. *Infect. Immun.* **2004**, *72*, 1169–1173. [CrossRef] [PubMed]

55. Chanput, W.; Mes, J.J.; Wichers, H.J. THP-1 cell line: An *in vitro* cell model for immune modulation approach. *Int. Immunopharmacol.* **2014**, *23*, 1–9. [CrossRef] [PubMed]

56. Makraduli, L.; Crcarevska, M.S.; Geskovski, N.; Dodov, M.G.; Goracinova, K. Factorial design analysis and optimisation of alginate-Ca-chitosan microspheres. *J. Microencapsul.* **2013**, *30*, 81–92. [CrossRef] [PubMed]

57. Takka, S.; Gürel, A. Evaluation of chitosan/alginate beads using experimental design: Formulation and *in vitro* characterization. *AAPS PharmSciTech* **2010**, *11*, 460–466. [CrossRef] [PubMed]

58. Kalkanidis, M.; Pietersz, G.A.; Xiang, S.D.; Mottram, P.L.; Crimeen-Irwin, B.; Ardipradja, K.; Plebanski, M. Methods for nano-particle based vaccine formulation and evaluation of their immunogenicity. *Methods* **2006**, *40*, 20–29. [CrossRef] [PubMed]

59. Ruenraroengsak, P.; Cook, J.M.; Florence, A.T. Nanosystem drug targeting: Facing up to complex realities. *J. Control. Release* **2010**, *141*, 265–276. [CrossRef] [PubMed]

60. Sarmento, B.; Ribeiro, A.; Veiga, F.; Sampaio, P.; Neufeld, R.; Ferreira, D. Alginate/chitosan nanoparticles are effective for oral insulin delivery. *Pharm. Res.* **2007**, *24*, 2198–2206. [CrossRef] [PubMed]

61. Dobakhti, F.; Rahimi, F.; Dehpour, A.R.; Taghikhani, M.; Ajdary, S.; Rafiei, S. Stabilizing effects of calcium alginate microspheres on *Mycobacterium bovis* BCG intended for oral vaccination. *J. Microencapsul.* **2006**, *23*, 844–854. [CrossRef] [PubMed]

62. Bramwell, V.W.; Perrie, Y. Particulate delivery systems for vaccines: What can we expect? *J. Pharm. Pharmacol.* **2006**, *58*, 717–728. [CrossRef] [PubMed]

63. Griffiths, G.; Nyström, B.; Sable, S.B.; Khuller, G.K. Nanobead-based interventions for the treatment and prevention of tuberculosis. *Nat. Rev. Microbiol.* **2010**, *8*, 827–834. [CrossRef] [PubMed]

64. Storni, T.; Kündig, T.M.; Senti, G.; Johansen, P. Immunity in response to particulate antigen-delivery systems. *Adv. Drug Deliv. Rev.* **2005**, *57*, 333–355. [CrossRef] [PubMed]

65. Hagan, D.T.O. Microparticles and polymers for the mucosal delivery of vaccines. *Adv. Drug Deliv. Rev.* **1998**, *34*, 305–320. [CrossRef]

66. Van der Lubben, I.M.; Kersten, G.; Fretz, M.M.; Beuvery, C.; Verhoef, J.C.; Junginger, H.E. Chitosan microparticles for mucosal vaccination against diphtheria: Oral and nasal efficacy studies in mice. *Vaccine* **2003**, *21*, 1400–1408. [CrossRef]

67. Garrity, G.M.; Bell, J.A.; Lilburn, T.G.; Lansing, E. Taxonomic outline of the prokaryotes. In *Bergey's Manual of Systematic Bacteriology*; Springer-Verlag: New York, NY, USA, 2004.

68. Zhang, A.; Groves, M.J. Size characterization of *Mycobacterium bovic* BCG (Bacillus Calmette Guérin) Vaccine, Tice Substrain. *Pharm. Res.* **1988**, *5*, 607–610. [CrossRef] [PubMed]

69. Desjardins, M.; Griffiths, G. Phagocytosis: Latex leads the way. *Curr. Opin. Cell Biol.* **2003**, *15*, 498–503. [CrossRef]

70. Simsek-Ege, F.A.; Bond, G.M.; Stringer, J. Polyelectrolye complex formation between alginate and Chitosan as a function of pH. *J. Appl. Polym. Sci.* **2003**, *88*, 346–351. [CrossRef]

71. Chen, S.; Wu, Y.; Mi, F.; Lin, Y.; Yu, L.; Sung, H. A novel pH-sensitive hydrogel composed of *N,O*-carboxymethyl chitosan and alginate cross-linked by genipin for protein drug delivery. *J. Control. Release* **2004**, *96*, 285–300. [CrossRef] [PubMed]

72. Kaasalainen, M.; Mäkilä, E.; Riikonen, J.; Kovalainen, M.; Järvinen, K.; Herzig, K.-H.; Lehto, V.-P.; Salonen, J. Effect of isotonic solutions and peptide adsorption on zeta potential of porous silicon nanoparticle drug delivery formulations. *Int. J. Pharm.* **2012**, *431*, 230–236. [CrossRef] [PubMed]

73. Mosmann, T. Rapid colorimetric assay for cellular growth and survival: Application to proliferation and cytotoxicity assays. *J. Immunol. Methods* **1983**, *65*, 55–63. [CrossRef]

74. Zhang, A.; Groves, M.J.; Klegerman, M.E. The surface charge of cells of *Mycobacterium bovis* BCG vaccine, Tice substrain. *Microbios* **1988**, *53*, 191–195. [PubMed]

75. Jordao, L.; Bleck, C.K.E.; Mayorga, L.; Griffiths, G.; Anes, E. On the killing of mycobacteria by macrophages. *Cell. Microbiol.* **2008**, *10*, 529–548. [CrossRef] [PubMed]

76. Bettencourt, P.; Pires, D.; Carmo, N.; Anes, E. *Microscopy: Science, Technology, Applications and Education*; Méndez-Vilas, A., Díaz, J., Eds.; FORMATEX: Badajoz, Spain, 2010; pp. 614–621.

77. Zheng, L.Y.; Zhu, J.F. Study on antimicrobial activity of chitosan with different molecular weights. *Carbohydr. Polym.* **2003**, *54*, 527–530. [CrossRef]

78. Devlieghere, F.; Vermeulen, A.; Debevere, J. Chitosan: Antimicrobial activity, interactions with food components and applicability as a coating on fruit and vegetables. *Food Microbiol.* **2004**, *21*, 703–714. [CrossRef]

79. Liu, N.; Chen, X.; Park, H.; Liu, C.; Liu, C.; Meng, X.; Yu, L. Effect of MW and concentration of chitosan on antibacterial activity of *Escherichia coli*. *Carbohydr. Polym.* **2006**, *64*, 60–65. [CrossRef]

80. Raafat, D.; Sahl, H.-G. Chitosan and its antimicrobial potential—A critical literature survey. *Microb. Biotechnol.* **2009**, *2*, 186–201. [CrossRef] [PubMed]

81. Goy, R.C.; De Britto, D.; Assis, O.B.G. A review of the antimicrobial activity of chitosan. *Polím. Ciênc. Tecnol.* **2009**, *19*, 241–247. [CrossRef]

82. Doig, C.; Seagar, A.L.; Watt, B.; Forbes, K.J. The efficacy of the heat killing of *Mycobacterium tuberculosis*. *J. Clin. Pathol.* **2002**, *55*, 778–779. [CrossRef] [PubMed]

83. Pawlak, A.; Mucha, M. Thermogravimetric and FTIR studies of chitosan blends. *Thermochim. Acta* **2003**, *396*, 153–166. [CrossRef]

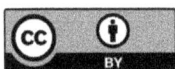

marine drugs

MDPI

Article

The Mucus of *Actinia equina* (Anthozoa, Cnidaria): An Unexplored Resource for Potential Applicative Purposes

Loredana Stabili [1,2,*], Roberto Schirosi [3], Maria Giovanna Parisi [4], Stefano Piraino [2,5] and Matteo Cammarata [4]

[1] Institute for Marine Coastal Environment (Unit of Taranto), National Research Council (IAMC-CNR) Via Roma 3, 74100 Taranto, Italy
[2] Department of Biological and Environmental Sciences and Technologies (DiSTeBA), Università del Salento, Via Prov.le Lecce-Monteroni, 73100 Lecce, Italy; stefano.piraino@unisalento.it
[3] Lachifarma s.r.l., S.S.16 Zona Industriale, Zollino (Le) 73010, Italy; robertoschirosi@libero.it
[4] Department of Biological, Chemical and Pharmaceutical Sciences and Technologies (STEBICEF), Università di Palermo, Via Archirafi, 18, 90123 Palermo, Italy; mariagiovanna.parisi@unipa.it (M.G.P.); matteo.cammarata@unipa.it (M.C.)
[5] National Interuniversity Consortium for Marine Sciences (CoNISMa), Local Research Unit Lecce, Lecce 73100, Italy
* Author to whom correspondence should be addressed; loredana.stabili@iamc.cnr.it; Tel.: +39-0832-298-971.

Academic Editor: Paola Laurienzo
Received: 16 June 2015; Accepted: 6 August 2015; Published: 19 August 2015

Abstract: The mucus produced by many marine organisms is a complex mixture of proteins and polysaccharides forming a weak watery gel. It is essential for vital processes including locomotion, navigation, structural support, heterotrophic feeding and defence against a multitude of environmental stresses, predators, parasites, and pathogens. In the present study we focused on mucus produced by a benthic cnidarian, the sea anemone *Actinia equina* (Linnaeus, 1758) for preventing burial by excess sedimentation and for protection. We investigated some of the physico-chemical properties of this matrix such as viscosity, osmolarity, electrical conductivity, protein, carbohydrate, and total lipid contents. Some biological activities such as hemolytic, cytotoxic, and antibacterial lysozyme-like activities were also studied. The *A. equina* mucus is mainly composed by water (96.2% ± 0.3%), whereas its dry weight is made of 24.2% ± 1.3% proteins and 7.8% ± 0.2% carbohydrates, with the smallest and largest components referable to lipids (0.9%) and inorganic matter (67.1%). The *A. equina* mucus matrix exhibited hemolytic activity on rabbit erythrocytes, cytotoxic activity against the tumor cell line K562 (human erythromyeloblastoid leukemia) and antibacterial lysozyme-like activity. The findings from this study improve the available information on the mucus composition in invertebrates and have implications for future investigations related to exploitation of *A. equina* and other sea anemones' mucus as a source of bioactive compounds of high pharmaceutical and biotechnological interest.

Keywords: mucus; *Actinia equina*; antibacterial activity; hemolytic activity; cytotoxicity; tumor cell line K562

1. Introduction

To adhere on immersed substrata in their aquatic habitats, many marine organisms, including invertebrates, secrete viscoelastic adhesive gels such as mucus consisting primarily of a network of polysaccharides and proteins entangled to form a weak gel containing more than 95% water [1–4]. Different from synthetic glue polymers, these bio-molecules are produced in an aqueous environment, therefore including water as a key constituent [5]. This represents a major difference between natural adhesive and synthetic polymers. Mucus is essential to several aquatic organisms for various reasons, e.g., to reduce drag forces, prevent sedimentation, enhance adhesion, limit water loss, and facilitate locomotion [6]. In addition mucus can serve as a "scaffolding" that provides anchorage and protection for egg-laying and a barrier against infection [3]. A mucus layer indeed provides a physical shield [7] and a slippery coating that prevents bacteria and debris from accumulating on the body surface [8], with a number of defence mechanisms [9–13]. Many marine invertebrates are sessile, *i.e.*, steadily attached to the sea bottom or with low locomotion ability, thus vulnerable either to predation and threat from a rich surrounding microbiota with pathogenic potential. Besides mechanical protection, the mucus of many invertebrates contains specific compounds to make the animal poisonous, distasteful or irritating, or a combination of these features [14]. Also, it is not surprising that these invertebrates developed an innate immune system producing a considerable number of defence molecules such as lytic compounds [15], bioactive antimicrobials [16–18], toxins, and carbohydrate antiadhesives [19]. Lectin-like molecules able to agglutinate red blood cells were characterized from mucus of the gastropod snail *Helix aspersa*, whose agglutinating activity was inhibited by D-GalNAc [20]. In addition, the potential to reduce the bacterial adhesion was demonstrated from mucus glycoproteins of the starfish *Marthasterias glacialis* [21], together with an antibacterial lysozyme-like activity [22], also observed in the annelid polychaetes *Sabella spallanzanii* [10,23] and *Myxicola infundibulum* [12].

As suggested by Calow [24], mucus could be made more or less susceptible to microbial attack. Some invertebrates could lace their mucus with antibiotic molecules when it is more advantageous for them to inhibit bacterial attack; in those cases, the mucus contains less proteins and does not promote bacterial growth. By contrast, some invertebrates, including corals [25], may release mucus with high content of proteins rapidly used by microbes. Due to their high turnover rates and their physiological diversity, microbes are likely to react quickly to released protein-rich mucus. Bacteria indeed possess a wide range of exo-enzymes potentially capable of degrading mucoid polymers, boosting the development of a mucus-specific microbiome. These microbes may transform mucus-derived (dissolved and particulate) organic matter into living biomass, *i.e.*, forming the so-called "microbial loop" trophic pathway [26], where mucus can be the scaffolding matrix eventually supporting a mucus-based food web [27–29].

Most cnidarians, including both medusozoans and anthozoans, are capable of secreting a mucus-based surface layer essential for a number of processes such as feeding, protection against pathogens, desiccation, and a number of environmental stresses. Mucus production may account for as much as 40% of the net daily fixed carbon in the coral *Acropora acuminata* [30]. Other uses that should be considered are protection from aggression and as an offensive weapon. The coral *Lobactis* (*Fungia*) *scutaria* in response to contact with other corals or rough human handling secretes mucus containing cytotoxic molecules to other corals. A highly active cytolysin as well as aliphatic-antibiotic compounds have been isolated from the mucus secretion of the sea anemone *Heteractis magnica* [31]. In spite of the multitude of ecological and physiological roles played by the cnidarian mucus, relatively little is known about the link between biochemical structures and functions. In the present study we focused on the mucus of the intertidal sea anemone *Actinia equina* produced as mechanical protection against excess sedimentation or desiccation as well as barrier against microbial attacks. Tissue extracts of *A.equina* has been long investigated for their peptide and protein toxins. Besides at least five isoforms of pore-forming cytolysins (equinatoxins) of proteinic nature, tissues of *A. equina* also contain several peptide toxins (Ae I, Ae K, acrorhagin I and II) isolated from different body portions [32,33]. Here, we investigated some of the physico-chemical properties of the secreted mucus of *A. equina* such as viscosity, osmolarity, electrical conductivity, protein, carbohydrate, and total lipid contents. Some biological activities, such as the hemolytic, cytotoxic, and antibacterial lysozyme-like activities were also investigated to highlight the potential of sea anemone mucus as a source of bioactive compounds of interest for biotechnological applications.

2. Results

2.1. Mucus Viscosity, Osmolarity, and Electrical Conductivity

Adult specimens of *A. equina* were employed for both the study of the physical and chemical properties of the mucus and the determination of its biological activities. The mean viscosity of *A. equina* mucus was 2.1 ± 0.02 cPs in respect to the 1 cPs viscosity of water measured at 20 °C (Table 1). The mean osmolarity value of the cnidarian mucus was 1205 ± 10 mOsmol/L, similar to seawater (1152 ± 25 mOsmol/L). The mean electrical conductivity of mucus was 124 ± 4 mS·cm^{-1} whilst the electrical conductivity of the seawater is 35 mS·cm^{-1}.

Table 1. Main physico-chemical characteristics of *Actinia equina* mucus.

Physico-Chemical Feature	Mean ± SD
Inorganic matter (%)	67.1 ± 2.3
Organic matter (%)	32.9 ± 0.2
Viscosity 20 °C (cps)	2.1 ± 0.02
Osmolarity (mOsmol/L)	1205 ± 10
Conductivity (mS·cm^{-1})	124 ± 4.0

2.2. Water and Inorganic Content

The water content of *A. equina* mucus was 96.1% ± 0.5% (Figure 1A). After dehydration, inorganic salts represented the main part (67.1% ± 2.3%) of the mucus dry weight (DW) (Figure 1B). Mean percentages of the elements are listed in Table 2: In all samples, Cl and Na were abundant whereas C, Mg and K represented only 2.8%–2.1% of the inorganic content.

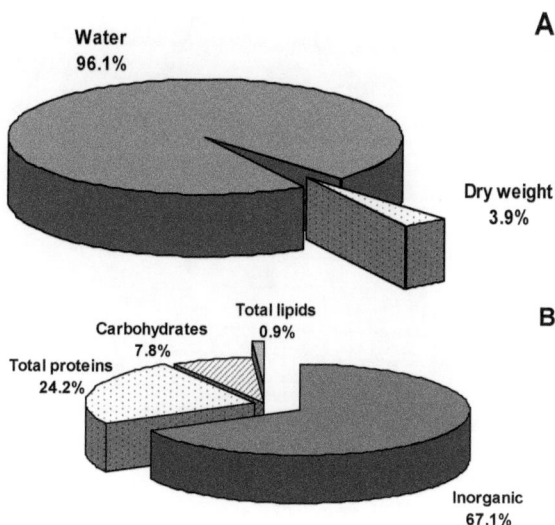

Figure 1. *Actinia equina* mucus composition: (**A**) water content and dried weight; (**B**) organic and inorganic residuals.

Table 2. Elements detected in mucus sample of *Actinia equine*.

Element	Content (%)
Cl	44.48 ± 0.12
Na	13.38 ± 0.11
Mg	2.41 ± 0.03
H	1.53 ± 0.10
K	2.11 ± 0.02
Ca	0.71 ± 0.02
C	2.13 ± 0.02
N	0.45 ± 0.02
Zn	0.06 ± 0.005
Cu	absent
Fe	absent
P	absent
Se	absent
Sn	absent

2.3. Protein, Carbohydrate, and Lipids Concentration

The organic residual of *A. equina* mucus DW was composed of proteins (24.2% ± 1.3%), carbohydrates (7.8% ± 0.2%) and lipids (0.9% ± 0.02%) (Figure 1B) with protein/glucose ratio equals to 3.2. The electrophoretic analysis revealed at least fourteen major protein bands, ranging from 12 to 200 kDa (Figure 2B).

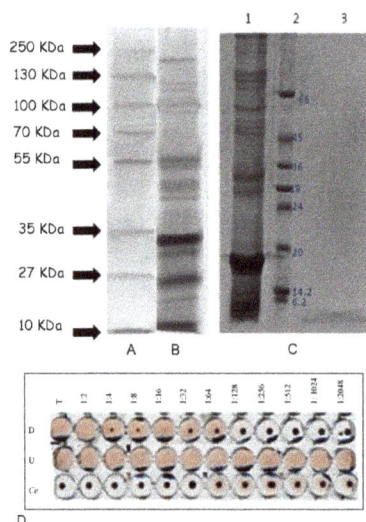

Figure 2. SDS-PAGE analysis of *Actinia equina* mucus. Panel **A**: Molecular weight standards furnished by Fermentas. Molecular weights (kDa) of standard proteins are on left; Panel **B**: *A. equina* total mucus; (**C**) *Actinia equina* different molecular weight fractions from total mucus extract obtained by membrane filtration system (pore size: 10 kDa). SDS-PAGE 15% acrylamide gel stained with Coomassie Blue R-250. Lane 1: Fraction >10 kDa named "U" (Upper), Lane 2: Standard Low sigma, Lane 3: Fraction <10 kDa. Named "D" (Lower); (**D**) Micro plate lysis assay carried out against Rabbit erythrocytes (RRBCs) in TBS buffer. Hemolysis is evidenced by free hemoglobin, when the erythrocytes are not lysed a central pellet of erythrocytes is visible on the well center. Lower fraction (**D**) showing lysis until dilution of 1:64, Upper fraction (U) showing lysis until dilution of 1:2048, Control experiment (Ce) with RRBCs and buffer.

2.4. Lysozyme Like Activity

Mucus of *A. equina* showed a natural lysozyme like activity (Figure 3A). This activity was strictly affected by pH (Figure 3B) and ionic strength (I) (Figure 3C) of the sample and of the reaction medium. The maximum diameter of lysis was reported at pH 6.0. The lytic activity increased after dialysis of the mucus at pH 6.0 and I = 0.175. The largest diameters of lysis were recorded at 37 °C (Figure 3D). By the standard assay on Petri dishes the maximum diameter of lysis (16.2 $\pm$ 0.5 mm corresponding to 2.21 mg/mL of hen egg-white lysozyme) was reported at I = 0.175, pH 6.0 and incubation temperature of 37 °C.

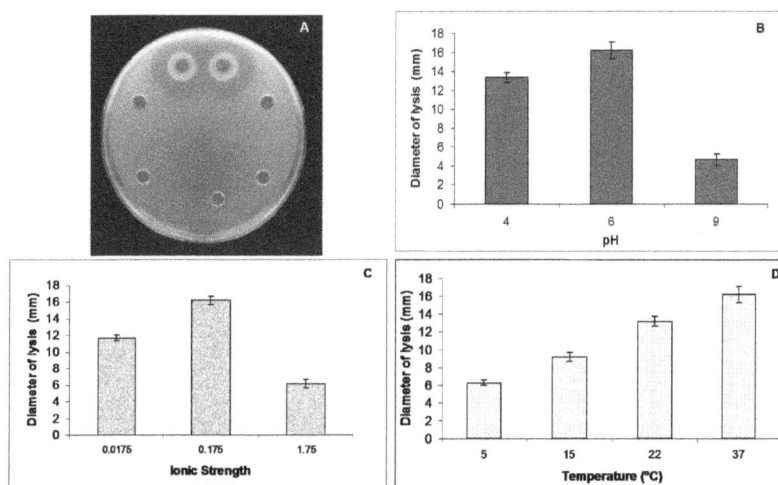

Figure 3. Lysozyme-like activity of *Actinia equina* mucus. (**A**) Standard assay on Petri dish inoculated with *Micrococcus lysodeikticus* cell walls to detect the lysozyme-like activity of *A. equina* mucus; (**B**) Effect of the pH on the lysozyme-like activity of *A. equina* mucus. Columns are mean values (n = 20) (vertical bars $\pm$ Standard Deviation); (**C**) Effect of the ionic strength on the lysozyme-like activity of mucus. Columns are mean values (n = 20) (vertical bars $\pm$ Standard Deviation); (**D**) Effect of the incubation temperature on the lysozyme-like activity of mucus. Columns are mean values (n = 20) (vertical bars $\pm$ Standard Deviation).

2.5. Hemolytic Activity

Mucus of *A. equina* with a protein concentration of 0.8 mg/mL exerted a hemolytic effect after incubation at 37 °C against rabbit and sheep erythrocytes with a lysis titer of 1:526 and 1:1048, respectively.

2.6. Cytotoxic Activity

The trypan blue dye exclusion test was used to determine the number of viable cells present in a cell suspension incubated with *A. equina* mucus sample. Human erythromyeloid leukemia-derived (K562) treated cells were damaged by mucus compounds (Figure 4A). Control cells (without mucus incubation) show intact cell membranes and do not incorporate trypan blue (Figure 4B).

The mucus of *A. equina* exhibits direct cytotoxic activity on K562 target cells (Figure 4C). Lactate dehydrogenase release into the supernatant of cells was used to calculate the percentage of target cell lysis. At the mucus protein concentration of 0.8 mg/mL and 0.4 mg/mL, the percentage of lysis was found significantly higher than control cells and quantified respectively equal to 62% and 58% of total target cells in suspension.

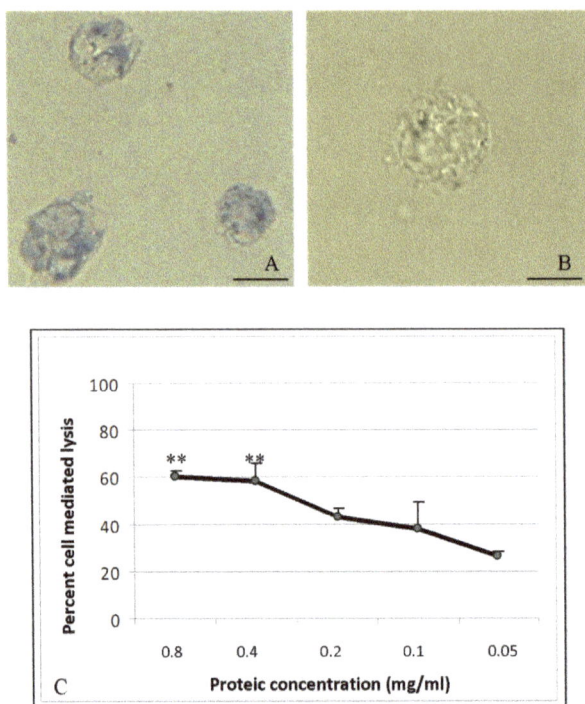

Figure 4. (**A**) Light Microscopic observation of Human erythromyeloblastoid leukemia (K562) cells treated with *A. equine* mucus crude extract. The target cell lysis was also determined by trypan blue exclusion test. Bar: 25 μm; (**B**) Control cell observed in the absence of mucus Bar. 25 μm; (**C**) Colorimetric assay of *A. equina* mucus extract on human chronic myelogenous leukemia cells K562 (Cytotoxic detection Kit. Boehringer Mannheim, Mannheim, Germany). Lactate dehydrogenase release into the supernatant was used to calculate the percentage of target cell lysis.

2.7. Fractionation of Actinia Equina Mucus

The system of separation by centrifugation through Nanosep devices membrane has allowed to obtain two fractions starting from the sample of mucus (1.2 ± 0.3 mg/mL). Molecules larger than the membrane pores of 10 kDa were retained at the surface of the membrane and concentrated during the ultrafiltration process. This component was defined "U" (upper) with a concentration of 1.5 ± 0.2 mg/mL, while the fraction with molecular weight below 10 kDa was named "D" (lower) (0.256 ± 0.022 mg/mL). The SDS electrophoresis analysis of the two mucus components showed a major component to occur in the D fraction, with an apparent mass less than 6 kDa (Figure 2C).

In microplate the isolated fractions showed a different lytic activity toward rabbit erythrocytes (Figure 2D). The lysis capacity was identified until 1:2048 dilution of the sample in the U fraction, and till dilution of 1:64 in the D fraction.

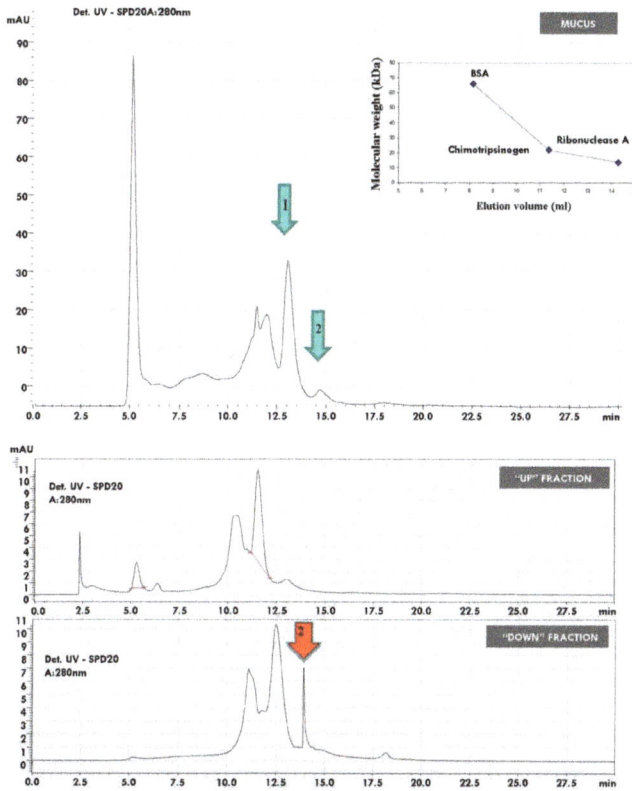

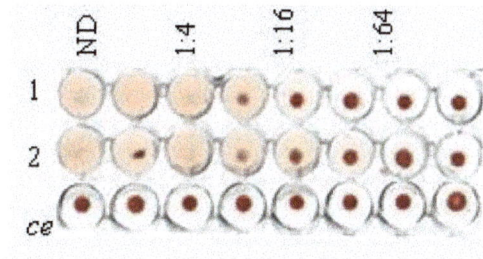

Figure 5. (**A**) High performance liquid chromatography separation of *A. equina* mucus components. The first plot shows profile of HPLC analysis of the crude mucus extract. Green arrows 1 and 2 indicate the isolated peaks at 12.5 and 14.5 min. Insert shows HPLC profiles of bovine serum albumin (BSA-66 kDa), chimotrypsinogen (25 kDa) and ribonuclease (13.7 kDa) used as standards separated on a molecular weight exclusion column BioSuite 250 (10 microns; Waters, Milford, CT, USA). The second plot shows the purification profiles of the high molecular weight fraction (u = upper) and low molecular weight fraction (d = lower) previously separated via centrifugation system on 10 kDa membrane. Red arrow indicate peak 2 detected at 14.5 min post HPLC start running; (**B**) Lytic activity detected in microplate toward rabbit erythrocytes of peaks 1 and 2 (Ce: Control experiment).

2.8. HPLC Separation of Mucus Components

Profiles of high pressure liquid chromatography (HPLC) on a column of size exclusion chromatography (BioSuite 250, 10 μm SEC, 7.5 mm × 300 mm) revealed the separation plot obtained from the mucus sample and the U fraction to be similar (Figure 5A). Two peaks are detected at 12.5 min (1) and 14.5 min (2). The first one contains proteins with a high molecular weight while the second peak includes molecules of lower dimensions. The profile of purification of the D fraction resulted enriched in the second component of low molecular weight. All the HPLC fractions of 1 mL/min were collected and subsequently analyzed to assess the hemolytic activity. The results of the assays (Figure 5B) showed the presence of hemolytic activity toward rabbit erythrocytes up to 1:16 for the peak 1 and 1:32 for the peak 2. Thus, different components within the sample showed similar hemolytic activity. Comparing the elution volume of standards used before purification of samples, the fraction 1 contains mainly a 20 kDa electrophoretic band while the peak 2 includes the 6 kDa component. The nature of equinatoxins-related activity of the 20 kDa fraction was suggested by inhibition experiments using bovine sphingomyelin (data not shown). One of the hallmarks of actinoporins is they efficiently make pores in lipid membranes containing this lipid. Thus, the interaction between erythrocytes membrane lipids and lysins was evaluated by inhibition experiments carried out using rabbit erythrocytes.

3. Discussion

Underwater attachment will undoubtedly have many technological applications including the design of water-resistant adhesives, sealants, and biomedical coatings and the development of new antifouling strategies [34]. Nonetheless a considerable dearth of information still remains regarding the biochemical composition of marine adhesives and the link between biochemical structure and function. Hitherto, studies on adhesives from invertebrates mainly concerned the characterization of permanent secretions from mussels and barnacles [5,35]. In comparison, non-permanent adhesives, (more hydrated than permanent ones and consisting of a mixture of proteins and polysaccharides) received so far much less attention [4,36–39]. The present paper represents a preliminary contribution on this topic since we provide novel data on the physico-chemical and biological properties of the sea anemone *A. equina* mucus. We analyzed some rheological properties of mucus such as osmolarity and viscosity since they are believed to be critical in fulfilling specific biological functions and are intimately related to the chemical composition [23]. Compared to mucus from typical marine sources [40] with a water content ranging 96%–98% of the wet weight, the mucus of *A. equina* has water content up of 96.2% ± 0.3%. The high percentage of inorganic material (about 67.1%) presumably results from dried salts left over when the seawater in a gel evaporates as already suggested for limpets and periwinkles mucus by Smith *et al.* [4] and Smith and Morin [40] which observed a similar proportion of inorganic material. The mucus of the studied cnidarian is mostly composed of proteins, representing the most conspicuous organic component (24% of total mucus dry matter, 73% of dry organic matter residual), and carbohydrates (7.8% of total mucus dry matter, near 24% of dry organic matter residual). Similar values were recorded for the mucus of limpets [4] as well as for the mucus of the annelid polychaete *Sabella spallanzanii* [10]. From studies on the biochemical composition of adhesive footprints of the sea star *Asterias rubens* [41,42] the amount of protein and carbohydrate (20% and 8% respectively) resulted similar to those recorded in *A. equina* mucus. As observed in the mucus of *A. equina*, the co-occurrence of proteins and carbohydrates seems to be a common trait among non-permanent adhesives of marine invertebrates, from cnidarians to deuterostomes [37] and protostomes [40,43]. These protein-carbohydrate complexes typically form highly hydrated adhesives with viscoelastic properties [42,43]. The mucus of *A. equina* corresponds to this kind of adhesives also on account of the obtained values of viscosity and osmolarity. This matrix indeed exhibits a low viscosity (2.1 ± 0.02 cps) and its osmolarity is of the same order of magnitude as the seawater such that mucus achieves near ionic equilibrium with the surrounding medium.

A noteworthy result of the present paper is the protein pattern of the *A. equina* mucus: from the electrophoretic analysis a complex of at least fourteen major proteins ranging from 12 to 200 kDa was highlighted. This is in agreement with the general multi-protein nature of other marine invertebrate adhesives. Indeed, in the sea urchin *Paracentrotus lividus* footprint material SDS-PAGE analysis revealed that the soluble fraction contains about 13 protein bands with molecular masses ranging from 10 to 200 kDa [39]. Moreover, in the mucus of the polychaete *Sabella spallanzanii* the electrophoretic analysis revealed at least 10 major protein bands, with molecular weights ranging from 16 to 90 kDa, and six minor components, with molecular weights ranging from 14 to 116 kDa [23]. In non-permanent adhesives, multi-protein complexes have been also evidenced in sea cucumbers and limpets [34,43]. The lysozyme activity recorded in mucus of *A. equina* mucus can be ascribed to one the fourteen major protein bands evidenced by electrophoretic analysis. Interestingly, one of the "known proteins in the databases" described in a marine adhesive is a homolog of lysozyme in barnacle cement [44]. Lysozyme represents the best characterized enzyme involved in self-defence from bacteria [45]. This enzyme is a glycoside hydrolase and dissolves certain bacteria by hydrolyzing the glycosidic β1-4 bonds between *N*-acetylglucosamine and *N*-acetylmuramic acid of bacterial cell walls. A bacterial cell devoid of a wall usually bursts because of the high osmotic pressure inside the cell. The constitutive levels of lysozyme protect the organism from bacteria living in the same environment and control its natural symbiotic flora. Lysozyme-like proteins have also already been found in other cnidarians, including some species of sea anemones [46,47]. In the present work it a lysozyme-like activity was also highlighted in the mucus of *A. equina*. This lysozyme had a maximum of activity when the pH of the reaction medium and sample was 6 and the ionic strength 0.175, as previously reported for other lysozymes [48–52].

We also showed hemolytic activity of *A. equina* mucus extract toward RRBC target cells. After purification by membrane separation system and HPLC, different components exhibiting hemolytic activity have been found. Among the mucus components of high molecular weight, fraction "up", the hemolytic activity resides in a 20 kDa protein corresponding to Equinatoxin, as demonstrated by the experiment of hemolysis carried out on peaks isolated by HPLC. Results of hemolytic assays showed also an active fraction with a lowest molecular weight, of approximately 6 kDa in SDS. Both these lytic fractions are inhibited by sphingomyelin. This suggests that the mucus of *A. equina* could contain actinoporin-like molecules, known to be specifically inhibited by sphingomyelin [53] which may have an interaction with erythrocyte membrane permeability, leading to lysis. Actinoporins belong to the unique family of the α-pore-forming toxins (PFTs) due to their ability to hold the membrane phospholipids domains of the host organism forming cation selective pores [54]. Interestingly, the mucus of *Heteractis magnifica* showed a strong hemolytic activity toward fish erythrocytes, and exerted an antibacterial activity towards pathogenic bacterial strains. The presence in *A. equina* mucus of a hemolytic, cytotoxic activity and an antibacterial activity suggests that this matrix may provide a defensive tool for the cnidarian from microbial attacks serving as substrate into which the humoral substances are released. The role of mucus as a defence against potentially pathogenic microorganisms has been already demonstrated for the mucus of other marine invertebrates including corals [3,9]. The antibacterial functions of coral mucus are particularly well documented in the soft corals. Slattery *et al.* [55] demonstrated anti-microbial and anti-fouling activity in Antarctic soft corals also and suggested that, although mucus secretion in these species was low, it was likely to be important in preventing bacterial attachment to the coral surface.

The results obtained in the present study not only improve the available information on the mucus composition in invertebrates, but also have implications for future studies aimed to the employment of *A. equina* mucus as source of compounds with antimicrobial lysozyme-like and antitumor activity of pharmaceutical and biotechnological interest. As regards pharmaceuticals, the ongoing explosion of antibiotic-resistant infections due to new opportunistic pathogen multidrug-resistant microbes continues to plague global health care. This clearly highlights the need for new antibacterial agents with fundamentally different modes of action than that of traditional antibiotics. The enormous demand has triggered worldwide efforts in developing novel antibacterial alternatives. Bacterial cell wall hydrolases (BCWH) are among the most promising candidates and lysozyme was recently chosen as a model protein. For the first time, this led a great opportunity for potential use of lysozyme in drug systems as a new antimicrobial agent [56,57]. A possible application of lysozyme, which is attracting considerable interest, is the use of this molecule in veterinary work and in aquaculture facilities in particular. The emergence of microbial diseases in aquaculture industries is of major concern implying serious financial loss. Therefore, *A. equina* mucus appears as a promising and valuable alternative source of lysozyme for drug development and the marine origin of this lysozyme represents an added value. Last but not least, indeed, the lysozyme produced by *A. equina* mucus is salt-stable and this feature makes it more suitable to be used to control fish or shellfish pathogens in mariculture in the case of antibiotic efficacy reduction due to high-salt conditions.

The utilization of *A. equina* mucus to extract bioactive substances of pharmaceutical interest is encouraged also with the evidence of the cytotoxic activity against the tumor cell line K562. In *A. equina* the first indication about cytotoxicity of its venom due to equinatoxin action was elucidated by dye exclusion test on Ehrlich carcinoma and L1210 leukemia inoculated in mice [58]. In another study, crude extracts from nematocyst and surrounding tissues of the sea-anemone *A. equina* were tested on V79 fibroblasts [59]. Moreover Isoform II of Equinatoxin (Eq. II) *showed* cytotoxic capability against human glioblastoma U87 and A172 cell lines [60]. Eq. II was found to affect the survival of U87 glioblastoma cells by a necrosis-like action and increasing lactate dehydrogenase (LDH) release [61]. On account of our results it seems that in addition to Eq. II a low molecular component, responsible for the toxicity to K562 tumor cells, is present in the mucus. This finding demonstrates that not only nematocysts or the granulocytes of *A equina* produce and release cytotoxins [62] but also the matrix outside of the body which, releasing toxic substances, is involved in defense mechanisms.

Finally, the antibacterial and cytotoxic activity of *A. equina* mucus could be employed to avoid the settlement of bacteria, which is the primary colonizing process in marine biofouling development. Alternative marine technologies employing biogenic compounds that function as natural anti-settlement agents are sought taking into account that some compounds such as TBT, copper [63], and organic biocides [64] used as antifouling agents in paints have been banned after 2008 [65–67]. Recently we have also purified new thermo-stable proteases and antimicrobial peptides from the body and tentacle of *A. equina* and *Anemonia sulcata* which were applied for biocleaning or controlling microbial growth on heritage objects [68]. In particular, the protease-containing fraction was tested for the hydrolysis of protein layers on old paintings. The cleaning protocol including sea anemone proteases offered a novel selective procedure preventing damage to the original materials constituting the heritage object. The fraction containing the antimicrobial peptide was used to control fungal growth during the restoration of the painting [68]. Bioactive molecules extracted from sea anemones' mucus are currently under investigation.

4. Experimental Section

4.1. Animals and Samples Preparation

Adult specimens of *Actinia equina* were collected at Porto Cesareo (Lecce, Italy, 40.25 N, 17.9 E) using SCUBA equipment.

About 100 adult specimens of *A. equina* were collected and transferred to the laboratory. Here the sea anemones were washed with filtered (0.2 μm) sterile sea water and kept for 30 min in a Petri dish in order to stimulate the secretion of the mucus for both the study of its physico-chemical properties and the determination of its biological activities such as hemolytic, cytotoxic and antibacterial, lysozyme-like activities. Within the secreted mucus, we checked for trapped material by microscopic observations, whilst we excluded any contamination of other excretion products by pH measurements. Secreted mucus was collected and centrifuged at $12,000 \times g$ for 30 min at 4 °C. A previous work [10] showed that the protein content of the mucus varies between individuals. To avoid the introduction of this variable, in the present work the mucus of the whole group of 100 individuals was pooled into five samples (each pool collected from 20 sea anemones) which were stored at −80 °C until use.

4.2. Mucus Viscosity, Osmolarity, Electrical Conductivity and Water Content

Mucus viscosity was measured at 200 rpm in 1 mL aliquots with a cone-plate viscometer (cone angle of 1.565°, model LVT-C/P 42, Brookfield Engineering Laboratories, Middleboro, MA, USA) connected to a circulating water bath (Thermoline, Wetherill Park, Sydney, Australia) set at 17 ± 0.1 °C. Due to differences in temperature and equipment used between studies, comparison of viscosity data can be difficult without reference to a common, known viscosity. Thus, we documented the relative viscosity of mucus with respect to the viscosity of water, similar to Rosen and Cornford [69] and Cone [70]. The viscosity of water is 1 cP at 20 °C and it is only slightly dependent on temperature [71].

Osmolarity was measured using a VAPRO vapour pressure osmometer (model 5520, WESCOR, Logan, UT, USA), all measurements being carried out in triplicate. Electrical conductivity was measured using a GLP 31 conductimeter (Crison, Barcelona, Spain).

For water content measurement, the wet weights of mucus of 15 samples (three replicates for each of the five groups of 20 individuals each) were measured on an analytical balance. They were then dehydrated in a SpeedVac, and their dry weight (DW) was measured.

4.3. Determination of the Inorganic Composition

The inorganic composition was determined for each sample after lyophilization of sample solution at 52 °C and 0.061 mbar using a LIO 5P CINQUEPASCAL freeze-dryer.

C, H, and N analyses were performed using a 1106 Carlo Erba elemental analyzer, while an AA-6200 Shimadzu atomic absorption flame emission spectrophotometer was used for the determination of Fe, Ca, Mg, Zn, Cu, K, Na. A P/N 206-17143 Shimadzu hydride vapor generator was coupled to the atomic absorption spectrophotometer in order to analyze the Sn and Se content. In general, each sample was mineralized to oxidize the organic fraction. To this end a weighted sample of the mucus (*ca.* 10 mg) was treated with HNO_3 (1 mL) and H_2SO_4 96% w/w (2.5 mL) at high temperature until no more fumes were released. The residue was treated again with the acids two more times. The final liquid residue was dissolved in water to give a 100 mL solution. For each element a calibration curve was obtained by using standard solutions. The quantitative analysis of phosphorous was performed using an UV-1601 Shimadzu spectrophotometer according to the method reported in the literature [72,73]. A 785 DMP Metrohm Titrino was used for the quantitative determination of the inorganic chloride using a potentiometric determination.

4.4. Lipid, Protein, and Carbohydrate Concentration

Total lipids from each mucus sample were extracted according to the method of Folch *et al.* [74]. The mucus was homogenized with chloroform/methanol (2:1) to a final volume 20 times the volume of the mucus sample. After centrifugation and siphoning of the upper phase, the lower chloroform phase contained the lipids. Total lipid content was determined by the colorimetric enzymatic method [75] using commercial kit (FAR, Verona, Italy).

The protein concentration of each mucus sample was measured using the Bradford assay [76] with bovine serum albumin (BIO-RAD, Hercules, CA, USA) as standard.

The carbohydrate concentration of the mucus was assayed using the method described by Dubois *et al.* [77] and Kennedy and Pagliuca [78]. The assay was calibrated with known amounts of D-glucose.

4.5. Electrophoresis

Mucus samples were analyzed by SDS-polyacrylamide gel electrophoresis (SDS-PAGE). They were run on discontinuous gels, based on the method of Laemmli [79] and the detailed protocols of Hames [80]. The gels contained 10% of acrylamide, and were 8 cm × 9 cm by 1.0 mm thick. The migration buffer consisted of 25 mM Tris, 192 mM glycine, pH 8.5. After migration, gels were stained using Silver Stain kit (Sigma, Saint Louis, MO, USA). Molecular standards (PageRuler™ Prestained

Protein Ladder range 10–250 kDa, Fermentas, Waltham, Massachusetts, USA) consisted in a mixture of eight recombinant, highly purified, coloured proteins with apparent molecular weights of 10 to 250 kDa.

4.6. Lysozyme-Like Activity

To detect lysozyme activity, inoculated Petri dishes were used as standard assay, 700 µL of 5 mg/mL of dried *Micrococcus luteus* cell walls (Sigma, Saint Louis, MO, USA) were diluted in 7 mL of 0.05 M PB-agarose (1.2%, pH 5.0) then spread on a Petri dish. Four wells of 6.3 mm diameters were sunk in agarose gel and each filled with 30 µL of mucus. The diameter of the cleared zone of the four replicates was recorded after overnight incubation at 37 °C and compared with those of reference samples containing known amounts of standard hen-egg-white lysozyme (Merck, Darmstadt, Germany). The effects of pH, ionic strength (I), and temperature were examined. The pH effect was tested by dialyzing the mucus in PB 0.05 M, ionic strength, I = 0.175, adjusted at pH 4, 5, 6, 7, 8 and by dissolving agarose in PB at the same I- and pH-values. The ionic strength effect was tested in PB 0.05 M (pH 6.0), adjusted at I = 0.0175, 0.175, 1.75. Agarose was dissolved in PB at the same I-values. The temperature effect was tested with incubations of samples (in PB, at pH 6.0, and I = 0.175) at 5, 15, 22, and 37 °C.

4.7. Hemolytic Activity

The rabbit erythrocytes (RRBCs) obtained by Istituto Zooprofilattico della Sicilia in Alsever solution (0.42% NaCl; 0.08% sodium citrate dihydrate, citric acid monohydrate 0.045%, 2.05% D-glucose pH 7.2) were washed three times with erythrocytes-Phosphate-buffered saline (PBSE) (KH_2PO_4 6 mM; Na_2HPO_4 0.11 M; NaCl 30 mM; pH 7.4) and centrifuged at 1800 rpm for 10 min at 4 °C. Suspensions of RRBCs (2.5% in Tris buffer: Tris HCl 0.05 M, 0.15 M NaCl pH 8) were used to test the lysis of RRBCs by mucus. For the microplate assay 25 µL of mucus or serial (two-fold) dilution were mixed with an equal volume of the RRBCs suspension.in 96-well round-bottom microtiter plates (Nunc, Roskilde, Denmark). After 1 h incubation at 37 °C the lytic activity was recorded as the reciprocal of the highest dilution showing complete RRBCs lysis.

For the quantitative hemoglobin release evaluation, one hundred microlitres of mucus in triplicate were mixed with 100 µL RRBCs suspension in glass tubes with U bottom, incubated for 60 min at 37 °C and then centrifuged for 5 min at 1500× *g*. One mL of Tris buffer was added to the supernatant in order to obtain an adequate amount of sample for spectrophotometric evaluation (541 nm) of the hemoglobin content. The degree of hemolysis was calculated by: [(absorbance of sample − absorbance of control)/absorbance of total hemolysis] × 100. Total hemolysis (100%) was achieved by adding 100 µL of distilled water to the same volume of RRBCs suspension.

Control erythrocyte suspensions were also prepared in the same medium and incubated as reaction mixtures: spontaneous hemoglobin release never exceeded 5% of the total release. For each experiment three samples were assayed.

4.8. Cytoxicity Assay against the Tumor Cell Line K562

The human erythromyeloid leukemia-derived cell line K562 were kindly provided by Dr. Domenico Schillaci (STEBICEF, University of Palermo) and was maintained for short time in RPMI 1640 medium (Gibco, Grand Island, NY, USA) supplemented with 10% heat inactivated fetal calf serum (Flow Laboratories, Irvine, Scotland), gentamycin, streptomycin, and Hepes buffer (Boehringer Mannheim, Mannheim, Germany).

Cytotoxicity effect of mucus against tumor cell lines was performed using a cytotoxic detection Kit (Boehringer Mannheim, Mannheim, Germany) based on determination of lactate dehydrogenase (LDH) activity released from lysed target cells [81]. The target cells were washed and suspended in PBS supplemented with 1% bovine serum albumin (PBS-BSA, 370 mOsm kg^{-1}) at a concentration of 10^5 cells mL^{-1}. All tests were performed in triplicate with 10^4 target cells $well^{-1}$ in V-shaped microplates

(Nunc, Roskilde, Denmark) in a total volume of 200 μL. Plates were centrifuged for 1 min at 100× *g* and incubated for 2 h at 18 °C. The plates were then centrifuged for 5 min at 400× *g*, and the release of LDH from lysed cells in 100 μL of supernatant from each well was determined by reading the absorbance at 490 nm in a microplate reader (Uniskan I, Labsystems, Helsinki, Finland). Spontaneous and maximum release were measured in 100 μL of supernatant from wells containing target cells only or target cells with 1% Triton X-100 (Sigma, Saint Louis, MO, USA).

Spontaneous baseline LDH release from target (10^4 cells well^{-1}) was used as controls. The values of the controls were subtracted from the degree of target cell lysis determined according to the equation:

Percent lysis = (measured release − spontaneous target release)/(complete release − spontaneous target release) × 100.

The living cells were observed through Nomarski differential interference contrast optics (DIC). Unless otherwise specified the cytotoxic reactions against tumour cells were carried out at 18 °C for 2 h. This is the optimal temperature for the molecule activity, for this short time the cells neither show any modifications nor do they die.

In addition trypan blue exclusion test was used for dead cells determination by addition of 0.01% trypan blue to the medium. This test was also used to evaluate the cytotoxic activity against tumor cell lines, the dye was added into the reaction mixture after 2 h incubation. To show target cell death following an *in vitro* cytotoxic reaction, the trypan blue was added to the medium 20 min after the mucus were mixed with target cells. Samples of the reaction mixture were smeared on slides and examined under the microscope.

4.9. Fractionation of Actinia Equina Mucus

Although ultrafiltration is primarily a separation technique, under some conditions it can be used for the gross fractionation of proteins that differ significantly in size. Briefly, the 10 kDa Nanosep device has been inserted into one of the provided microcentrifuge tubes and 500 μL of mucus sample was added. The filter device was positioned into the centrifuge rotor with a counterbalance with a similar device. After 20 min of centrifugation at 6000× *g* the filtrate was transferred from the bottom receiver to a new tube for storage. The sample with low molecular mass was filtered through the membrane (10 kDa size pores) and collected as down fraction, while the component with higher molecular mass remained above the membrane and was collected as up and stored at −20 °C until the proteic concentration evaluation and the use for the assays.

4.10. HPLC Size Exclusion Chromatography

Mucus extract were subjected to size exclusion chromatography using BioSuite 250, 10 μm SEC, 7.5 mm × 300 mm column (Waters, Milford, USA) on a HPLC system (Shimadzu Scientific Instruments, Columbia, MD, USA). The column was washed with Tris buffered saline (TBS) (150 mM NaCl, 10 mM Tris, pH 7.4). 200 μL of each sample were injected into the column which was eluted with TBS at a flow rate of 1 mL/min for 30 min. The chromatogram was recorded with a UV detector at 280 nm (mAU). The collected fractions were concentrated by centrifugation at 500× *g* with micro-concentrators (3 K Omega Centrifugal Devices Nanosep, Pall Corporation, Port Washington, NY, USA), and the final concentrated samples were stored at −80 °C until use.

5. Conclusions

Compared with terrestrial ecosystem and organisms, marine ecosystems and biodiversity are largely unexplored and underexploited in terms of potential provision for biomaterials, food, energy, and beneficial services for humans. Here we showed the mucus of the cnidarian sea anemone *A. equina* might represent a novel source of bioactive molecules with potential applicative purposes in drug discovery and biotechnological processes. Further investigations will be required in order to isolate and better characterize the molecular effectors responsible for the observed biological activities of the sea anemone mucus. The search for novel biomolecules deserves the development of appropriate measures to strengthen the focus on untapped source organisms from marine environments.

Acknowledgments: This work was financially supported by (a) the ENPI CBCMED project MED-JELLYRISK (Integrated monitoring of jellyfish outbreaks under anthropogenic and climatic impacts in the Mediterranean Sea coastal zones: Trophic and socio-economic risks—Project registration number I-A/1.3/098); (b) the PRIN Project "Genes and molecules of invertebrate immunity. Structures, functions, evolutionary precursors and transferability to applied research" (2010–2011); (c) RITMARE Flagship Project (Italian Ministry of University and Research) and (d) MC FFR project "Conoscenza di base e prospettive applicative di molecole bioattive da molluschi bivalvi di interesse commerciale: caratterizzazione di lectine, fattori antimicrobici e citotossici" (University of Palermo).

Author Contributions: Loredana Stabili, Stefano Piraino and Roberto Schirosi carried out the experiments on the physico-chemical mucus composition. Loredana Stabili, Maria Giovanna Parisi and Matteo Cammarata carried out the assays on the mucus biological activites. Loredana Stabili, Stefano Piraino, Maria Giovanna Parisi and Matteo Cammarata designed the experiment and wrote the manuscript.

Conflicts of Interest: The authors declare no conflict of interest.

References

1. Connor, V.M. The use of mucous trails by intertidal limpets to enhance food resources. *Biol. Bull.* **1986**, *171*, 548–564. [CrossRef]

2. Davies, M.S.; Jones, H.D.; Hawkins, S.J. Seasonal variation in the composition of pedal mucus from *Patella vulgata* L. *J. Exp. Mar. Biol. Ecol.* **1990**, *144*, 101–112. [CrossRef]

3. Davis, J.M.; Viney, C. Water-mucin phases: Conditions for mucus liquid crystallinity. *Thermochim. Acta* **1998**, *315*, 39–49. [CrossRef]

4. Smith, A.M.; Quick, T.J.; Peter, S.T.R.L. Differences in the Composition of Adhesive and Non-Adhesive Mucus from the Limpet *Lottia limatula*. *Biol. Bull.* **1999**, *196*, 34–44. [CrossRef] [PubMed]

5. Kamino, K. Underwater adhesive of marine organisms as the vital link between biological science and material science. *Mar. Biotechnol.* **2008**, *10*, 111–121. [CrossRef] [PubMed]

6. Branch, G.M. The biology of limpets: Physical factors, energy flow and ecological interactions. *Oceanogr. Mar. Biol. Ann. Rev.* **1981**, *19*, 235–380.

7. Martin, R.; Walther, P. Protective mechanisms against the action of nematocysts in the epidermis of *Cratena peregrina* and *Flabellina affinis* (Gastropoda, Nudibranchia). *Zoomorphology* **2003**, *122*, 25–35.

8. Baier, R.E.; Gucinski, H.; Meenaghan, M.A.; Wirth, J.; Glantz, P.Q. Biophysical studies of mucosal surfaces. In *Oral Interfacial Reactions of Bone, Soft Tissue and Saliva*; Glantz, P.Q., Leach, S.A., Ericson, T., Eds.; IRL Press: Oxford, UK, 1985; pp. 83–95.

9. Clare, A.S. Marine natural product antifoulants: Status and potential. *Biofouling* **1995**, *9*, 211–229. [CrossRef]

10. Stabili, L.; Schirosi, R.; Licciano, M.; Giangrande, A. The mucus of *Sabella spallanzanii* (Annelida, Polychaeta): Its involvement in chemical defence and fertilization success. *J. Exp. Mar. Biol. Ecol.* **2009**, *374*, 144–149. [CrossRef]

11. Iori, D.; Forti, L.; Massamba-N'Siala, G.; Prevedelli, D.; Simonini, R. Toxicity of the purple mucus of the polychaete *Halla parthenopeia* (Oenonidae) revealed by a battery of ecotoxicological bioassays. *Sci. Mar.* **2014**, *78*, 589–595.

12. Stabili, L.; Schirosi, R.; Licciano, M.; Giangrande, A. Role of *Myxicola infundibulum* (Polychaeta, Annelida) mucus: From bacterial control to nutritional home site. *J. Exp. Mar. Biol. Ecol.* **2014**, *461*, 344–349. [CrossRef]

13. Waite, J.H. Nature's underwater adhesive specialist. *Int. J. Adhes. Adhes.* **1987**, *7*, 9–14. [CrossRef]

14. Derby, C.D. Escape by inking and secreting: Marine molluscs avoid predators through a rich array of chemicals and mechanisms. *Biol. Bull.* **2007**, *213*, 274–289. [CrossRef] [PubMed]

15. Mayer, A.M.; Rodriguez, A.D.; Taglialatela-Scafati, O.; Fusetani, N. Marine Pharmacology in 2009–2011: Marine Compounds with Antibacterial, Antidiabetic, Antifungal, Anti-Inflammatory, Antiprotozoal, Antituberculosis, and Antiviral Activities; Affecting the Immune and Nervous Systems, and other Miscellaneous Mechanisms of Action. *Mar. Drugs* **2013**, *11*, 2510–2573. [PubMed]

16. Aneiros, A.; Garateix, A. Bioactive peptides from marine sources: Pharmacological properties and isolation procedures. *J. Chromatogr. B Anal. Technol. Biomed. Life Sci.* **2004**, *803*, 41–53. [CrossRef] [PubMed]

17. Otero Gonzalez, A.J.; Magalhaes, B.S.; Garcia Villarino, M.; Lopez Abarrategui, C.; Sousa, D.A.; Dias, S.C.; Franco, O.L. Antimicrobial peptides from marine invertebrates as a new frontier for microbial infection control. *FASEB J.* **2010**, *24*, 1320–1334. [CrossRef] [PubMed]

18. Smith, V.J.; Desbois, A.P.; Dyrynda, E.A. Conventional and unconventional antimicrobials from fish, marine invertebrates and micro-algae. *Mar. Drugs* **2010**, *8*, 1213–1262. [CrossRef] [PubMed]

19. Bavington, C.D.; Lever, R.; Mulloy, B.; Grundy, M.M.; Page, C.P.; Richardson, N.V.; McKenzie, J.D. Anti-adhesive glycoproteins in echinoderm mucus secretions. *Comp. Biochem. Physiol. B Biochem. Mol. Biol.* **2004**, *139*, 607–617. [CrossRef] [PubMed]

20. Fountain, D.W.; Campbell, B.A. A lectin isolated from mucus of *Helix aspersa*. *Comp. Biochem. Physiol.* **1984**, *77*, 419–425.

21. McKenzie, J.D.; Grigovala, I.V. The echinoderm surface and its role in preventing microfouling. *Biofouling* **1996**, *10*, 261–272. [CrossRef] [PubMed]

22. Canicatti, C.; D'Ancona, G. Biological protective substances in *Marthasterias glacialis* (Asteroidea) epidermal secretion. *J. Zool.* **1990**, *222*, 445–454. [CrossRef]

23. Stabili, L.; Schirosi, R.; Di Benedetto, A.; Merendino, A.; Villanova, L.; Giangrande, A. First insights into the biochemistry of *Sabella spallanzanii* (Annelida: Polychaeta) Mucus: A potentially unexplored resource for applicative purposes. *J. Mar. Biol. Assoc. UK* **2011**, *91*, 199–208. [CrossRef]

24. Calow, P. Why some metazoan mucus secretions are more susceptible to microbial attack than others. *Am. Nat.* **1979**, *114*, 149–152. [CrossRef]

25. Azam, F. Microbial control of oceanic carbon flux: The plot thickens. *Science* **1998**, *280*, 694–696. [CrossRef]

26. Azam, F.; Smith, D.C.; Steward, G.F.; Hagström, A. Bacteria-organic matter coupling and its significance for oceanic carbon cycling. *Microbial Ecol.* **1993**, *28*, 167–179. [CrossRef] [PubMed]

27. Peduzzi, P.; Herndl, G.J. Mucus trails in the rocky intertidal: A highly active microenvironment. *Mar. Ecol. Prog. Ser.* **1991**, *75*, 267–274. [CrossRef]

28. Davies, M.S.; Hawkins, S.J.; Jones, H.D. Pedal mucus and its influence on the microbial food supply of two intertidal gastropods, *Patella vulgata* L. and *Littorina littorea* (L.). *J. Exp. Mar. Biol. Ecol.* **1992**, *161*, 57–77. [CrossRef]

29. Imrie, D.W. The role of pedal mucus in the feeding behaviour of *Littorina littorea* (L.). In Proceedings of the 3rd International Symposium on Littorinid Biology, Dale Fort Field Centre, Wales, UK, 5–12 September 1990; Grahame, J., Mill, P.J., Reid, D.G., Eds.; The Malacological Society of London: London, UK, 1992; p. 221.

30. Wild, C.; Woyt, H.; Markus Huettel, M. Influence of coral mucus on nutrient fluxes in carbonate sand. *Mar. Ecol. Progr. Ser.* **2005**, *287*, 87–98. [CrossRef]

31. Gunasundari, V.; Ajith Kumar, T.T.; Kumaresan, S.; Balagurunathan, R.; Balasubramanian, T. Isolation of aliphatic-antibiotic compounds from marine invertebrate, *Heteractis magnifica* "Quoy & Gaimard1833" against captive marine ornamental fish pathogens. *Indian J. Geomar. Sci.* **2013**, *42*, 807–811.

32. Lin, X.Y.; Ishida, M.; Nagashima, Y.; Shiomi, K. A polypeptide toxin in the sea anemone *Actinia equina* homologous with other sea anemone sodium channel toxins: Isolation and amino acid sequence. *Toxicon* **1996**, *34*, 57–65. [CrossRef]

33. Frazão, B.; Vasconcelos, V.; Antunes, A. Sea Anemone (Cnidaria, Anthozoa, Actiniaria) Toxins: An Overview. *Mar. Drugs* **2012**, *10*, 1812–1851. [CrossRef] [PubMed]

34. Flammang, P.; Santos, R.; Haesaerts, D. Echinoderm adhesive secretions: From experimental characterization to Evidence-Based Complementary and Alternative Medicine biotechnological applications. In *Progress in Molecular and Subcellular Biology, Marine Molecular Biotechnology, Echinodermata*; Matranga, V., Ed.; Springer: Berlin, Germany, 2005; pp. 201–220.

35. Taylor, S.W.; Waite, J.H. Marine adhesives: From molecular dissection to application. In *Protein-Based Materials*; McGrath, K., Kaplan, D., Eds.; Birkhauser: Boston, MA, USA, 1997; pp. 217–248.

36. Hamwood, T.E.; Cribb, B.W.; Halliday, J.A.; Kearn, G.C.; Whittington, I.D. Preliminary characterization and extraction of anterior adhesive secretion in monogean (plathyelminth) parasites. *Folia Parasitol.* **2002**, *49*, 39–49. [CrossRef] [PubMed]

37. DeMoor, S.; Waite, H.; Jangoux, M.; Patrick, P. Characterization of the adhesive from Cuvierian tubules of the sea cucumber *Holothuria forskali* (Echinodermata, Holothuroidea). *Mar. Biotechnol.* **2003**, *5*, 45–57. [CrossRef] [PubMed]

38. Pawlicki, J.M.; Pease, L.B.; Pierce, C.M.; Startz, T.P.; Zhang, Y.; Smith, A.M. The effect of molluscan glue proteins on gel mechanics. *J. Exp. Biol.* **2004**, *207*, 1127–1135. [CrossRef] [PubMed]

39. Santos, R.; da Costa, G.; Franco, C.; Gomes-Alves, P.; Flammang, P.; Coelho, A.V. First insights into the biochemistry of tube foot adhesive from the sea urchin *Paracentrotus lividus* (Echinoidea, Echinodermata). *Mar. Biotechnol.* **2009**, *11*, 686–698. [CrossRef] [PubMed]

40. Smith, A.M.; Morin, M.C. Biochemical differences between trail mucus and adhesive mucus from marsh periwinkles. *Biol. Bull.* **2002**, *203*, 338–346. [CrossRef] [PubMed]

41. Flammang, P.; Walker, G. Measurement of the adhesion of the podia in the asteroid *Asterias rubens* (Echinodermata). *J. Mar. Biol. Assoc. UK* **1997**, *77*, 1251–1254. [CrossRef]

42. Flammang, P.A.; van Cauwenberge, M.A.; Alexandre, H.; Jangoux, M. A study of temporary adhesion of the podia in the sea star *Asterias rubens* (Echinodermata, Asteroidea) through their footprints. *J. Exp. Biol.* **1998**, *201*, 2383–2395. [PubMed]

43. Smith, A.M. The biochemistry and mechanics of gastropod adhesive gels. In *Biological Adhesives*; Smith, A.M., Callow, J.A., Eds.; Springer-Verlag: Berlin, Germany, 2006; pp. 167–182.

44. Kamino, K. Barnacle underwater attachment. In *Biological Adhesives*; Smith, A.M., Callow, J.A., Eds.; Springer-Verlag: Berlin, Germany, 2006; pp. 145–166.

45. Jolles, P.; Jolles, J. What's new in lysozyme research? *Mol. Cell. Biochem.* **1984**, *63*, 165–189. [CrossRef] [PubMed]

46. Lesser, M.P.; Stochaj, W.R.; Tapley, D.W.; Shick, J.M. Bleaching in coral reef anthozoans: Effects of irradiance, ultraviolet radiation, and temperature on the activities of protective enzymes against active oxygen. *Coral Reefs* **1995**, *8*, 225–232. [CrossRef]

47. Leclerc, M. Humoral factors in marine invertebrates. In *Molecular and Subcellular Biology: Invertebrate Immunology*; Rinkevich, B., Muller, W.E.G., Eds.; Springer-Verlag: Berlin, Germany, 1996; pp. 1–9.

48. Cheng, T.C.; Rodrick, G.E. Identification and characterization of lysozyme from the hemolymph of the soft-shelled clam, *Mya arenaria*. *Biol. Bull.* **1974**, *147*, 311–320. [CrossRef] [PubMed]

49. Maginot, N.; Samain, J.F.; Daniel, J.Y.; Le Coz, J.R.; Moal, J. Kinetic properties of lysozyme from the digestive glands of *Ruditapes philippinarum*. *Oceanis* **1989**, *15*, 451–464.

50. Sotelo-Mundo, R.R.; Islas-Osuna, M.A.; de-la-Re-Vega, E.; Hernandez-Lopez, J.; Vargas-Albores, F.; Yepiz-Plascencia, G. cDNA cloning of the lysozyme of the white shrimp *Penaeus vannamei*. *Fish Shellfish Immunol.* **2003**, *15*, 325–333. [CrossRef]

51. Huag, K.; Olsen, Ø.M.; Sandsdalen, E.; Styrvold, O.B. Antibacterial activities in various tissues of the horse mussel *Modiolus modiolus*. *J. Invertebr. Pathol.* **2004**, *85*, 112–119. [CrossRef] [PubMed]

52. Xue, O.G.; Schey, K.L.; Volety, A.K.; Chu, F.L.E.; La Peyre, J.F. Purification and characterization of lysozyme from plasma of the eastern oyster *Crassostrea virginica*. *Comp. Biochem. Physiol. B Biochem. Mol. Biol.* **2004**, *139*, 1–25. [CrossRef] [PubMed]

53. Kristan, K.; Viero, G.; Dalla Serra, M.; Macek, P.; Anderluh, G. Molecular mechanism of pore formation by actinoporins. *Toxicon* **2009**, *54*, 1125–1134. [CrossRef] [PubMed]

54. Monastyrnaya, M.I.; Leychenko, E.; Isaeva, M.; Likhatskaya, G.; Zelepuga, E.; Kostina, E.; Trifonov, E.; Nurminski, E.; Kozlovskaya, E. Actinoporins from the sea anemones, tropical *Radianthus macrodactylus* and northern *Oulactis orientalis*: Comparative analysis of structure-function relationships. *Toxicon* **2010**, *56*, 1299–1314. [CrossRef] [PubMed]

55. Slattery, M.; McClintock, J.B.; Heine, J.N. Chemical defences in Antarctic soft corals: Evidence for anti-fouling compounds. *J. Exp. Mar. Biol. Ecol.* **1995**, *190*, 61–77. [CrossRef]

56. Ibrahim, H.R.; Aoki, T.; Pellegrini, A. Strategies for new antimicrobial proteins and peptides: Lysozyme and aprotinin as model molecules. *Curr. Pharm. Des.* **2002**, *8*, 671–693. [CrossRef] [PubMed]

57. Niyonsaba, F.; Ogawa, H. Protective roles of the skin against infection: Implication of naturally occurring human antimicrobial agents β-defensins, cathelicidin LL-37 and lysozyme. *J. Dermatol. Sci.* **2005**, *40*, 157–168. [CrossRef] [PubMed]

58. Giraldi, T.; Ferlan, I.; Romeo, D. Antitumor activity of equinatoxin. *Chem. Biol. Interact.* **1976**, *13*, 199–203. [CrossRef]

59. Mariottini, G.L.; Robbiano, L.; Carli, A. Toxicity of *Actinia equina* (Cnidaria: Anthozoa) crude venom on cultured cells. *Boll. Soc. Ital. Biol. Sper.* **1998**, *74*, 103–110. [PubMed]

60. Soletti, R.C.; de Faria, G.P.; Vernal, J.; Terenzi, H.; Anderluh, G.; Borges, H.L.; Moura-Neto, V.; Gabilan, N.H. Potentiation of anticancer-drug cytotoxicity by sea anemone pore-forming proteins in human glioblastoma cells. *Anticancer Drugs* **2008**, *19*, 517–525. [CrossRef] [PubMed]

61. Soletti, R.C.; Alves, T.; Vernal, J.; Terenzi, H.; Anderluh, G.; Borges, H.L.; Gabilan, N.H.; Moura-Neto, V. Inhibition of MAPK/ERK, PKC and CaMKII signaling blocks cytolysin-induced human glioma cell death. *Anticancer Res.* **2010**, *30*, 1209–1215. [PubMed]

62. Parisi, M.G.; Trapani, M.R.; Cammarata, M. Granulocytes of sea anemone *Actinia equina* (Linnaeus, 1758) body fluid contain and release cytolysins forming plaques of lysis. *ISJ* **2014**, *11*, 39–46.

63. Jelic-Mrcelic, G.; Sliskovic, M.; Antolic, B. Biofouling communities on test panels coated with TBT and TBT-free copper-based antifouling paints. *Biofouling* **2006**, *22*, 293–230. [CrossRef] [PubMed]

64. Turley, P.A.; Fenn, R.J.; Ritter, J.C.; Callow, M.E. Pyrithiones as antifoulants: Environmental fate and loss of toxicity. *Biofouling* **2005**, *21*, 31–40. [CrossRef] [PubMed]

65. Stupak, M.E.; Garcia, M.T.; Perez, M.C. Non-toxic alternative compounds for marine antifouling paints. *Int. Biodeter. Biodegr.* **2003**, *52*, 49–52. [CrossRef]

66. Konstantinou, I.K.; Albanis, T.A. Worldwide occurrence and effects of antifouling paint booster biocides in the aquatic environment: A review. *Environ. Int.* **2004**, *30*, 235–248. [CrossRef]

67. Ostroumov, S.A. On the concepts of biochemical ecology and hydrobiology: Ecological chemomediators. *Contemp. Probl. Ecol.* **2008**, *1*, 238–244. [CrossRef]

68. Barresi, G.; di Carlo, E.; Trapani, M.R.; Parisi, M.G.; Chille, C.; Mule, M.F.; Cammarata, M.; Palla, F. Marine organisms as source of bioactive molecules applied in restoration projects. *Herit. Sci.* **2015**, *3*. [CrossRef]

69. Rosen, M.W.; Cornford, N.E. Fluid friction of fish slimes. *Nature* **1971**, *234*, 49–51. [CrossRef]

70. Cone, R.A. Mucus. In *Mucosal Immunology*; Ogra, P.L., Mestecky, J., Lamm, M.E., Strober, W., Bienenstock, J., McGhee, J.R., Eds.; Academic Press: San Diego, CA, USA, 1999; pp. 43–64.

71. Withers, P.C. *Comparative Animal Physiology*; Saunders College Publishing: Ft. Worth, TX, USA, 1992; p. 669.

72. Kitson, R.E.; Mellon, M.G. Colorimetric determination of phosphorus as molybdivanadophosphoric acid. *Ind. Eng. Chem. Anal.* **1944**, *16*, 379–383. [CrossRef]

73. Quinlan, K.P.; Desesa, M.A. Spectrophotometric determination of phosphorus as molybdovanadophosphoric acid. *Anal. Chem.* **1955**, *27*, 1626–1629. [CrossRef]

74. Folch, J.; Less, M.; Stone Stanley, G.H. A simple method for the isolation and purification of total lipids from animal tissues. *J. Biol. Chem.* **1957**, *226*, 497–508. [PubMed]

75. Zöllner, N.; Kirsch, K. Determination of the total lipid concentration in serum. *Z. Gesamte Exp. Med.* **1962**, *135*, 545–549. [CrossRef]

76. Bradford, M. A rapid and sensitive method for the quantification of microgram quantities of protein utilizing the principle of proteins dye binding. *Anal. Biochem.* **1976**, *72*, 248–254. [CrossRef]

77. Dubois, M.; Gilles, K.A.; Hamilton, J.K.; Rebers, P.A.; Smith, F. Colorimetric method for determination of sugars and related substances. *Anal. Chem.* **1956**, *28*, 350–356. [CrossRef]

78. Kennedy, J.F.; Pagliuca, G. Chapter 2. Oligosaccharides. In *Carbohydrate Analysis A Practical Approach*, 2nd ed.; Chapling, M.F., Kennedy, J.F., Eds.; Oxford University Press: New York, NY, USA, 1994; pp. 43–72.

79. Laemmli, V.H. Cleavage of structural proteins during the assembly of the head of bacteriophage T4. *Nat. Lond.* **1970**, *227*, 680–682. [CrossRef]

80. Hames, B.D. One-dimensional polyacrylamide gel electrophoresis. In *IRL Gel Electrophoresis of Proteins. A Practical Approach*; Hames, B.D., Rickwood, D., Eds.; Press Oxford: Oxford, UK, 1990; pp. 1–147.

81. Korzeniewski, C.; Callewaert, D.M. An enzyme-release assay for natural cytotoxicity. *J. Immunol. Methods* **1983**, *64*, 313–320. [CrossRef]

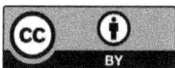

marine drugs

MDPI

Article

Alginate Hydrogels Coated with Chitosan for Wound Dressing

Maria Cristina Straccia [1], Giovanna Gomez d'Ayala [1], Ida Romano [2], Adriana Oliva [3] and Paola Laurienzo [1,*]

[1] Institute for Polymers, Composites and Biomaterials (IPCB), CNR, via Campi Flegrei 34, Pozzuoli 80078, Italy; mariacristina.straccia@ictp.cnr.it (M.C.S.); giovanna.gomez@ictp.cnr.it (G.G.A.)

[2] Institute of Biomolecular Chemistry, CNR, via Campi Flegrei 34, Pozzuoli 80078, Italy; iromano@icb.cnr.it

[3] Department of Biochemistry, Biophysics and General Pathology, Second University of Naples, via L. De Crecchio 7, Naples 80138, Italy; adriana.oliva@unina2.it

* Author to whom correspondence should be addressed; paola.laurienzo@ictp.cnr.it; Tel.: +39-81-867-5215; Fax: +39-81-867-5230.

Academic Editor: Alejandro M. Mayer

Received: 24 February 2015; Accepted: 29 April 2015; Published: 11 May 2015

Abstract: In this work, a coating of chitosan onto alginate hydrogels was realized using the water-soluble hydrochloride form of chitosan (CH-Cl), with the dual purpose of imparting antibacterial activity and delaying the release of hydrophilic molecules from the alginate matrix. Alginate hydrogels with different calcium contents were prepared by the internal setting method and coated by immersion in a CH-Cl solution. Structural analysis by cryo-scanning electron microscopy was carried out to highlight morphological alterations due to the coating layer. Tests *in vitro* with human mesenchymal stromal cells (MSC) were assessed to check the absence of toxicity of CH-Cl. Swelling, stability in physiological solution and release characteristics using rhodamine B as the hydrophilic model drug were compared to those of relative uncoated hydrogels. Finally, antibacterial activity against *Escherichia coli* was tested. Results show that alginate hydrogels coated with chitosan hydrochloride described here can be proposed as a novel medicated dressing by associating intrinsic antimicrobial activity with improved sustained release characteristics.

Keywords: chitosan hydrochloride; alginate; hydrogels; antibacterial activity; sustained release; wound dressing

1. Introduction

The local treatment of wounds is crucial to prevent infections, to control the removal of exudates and to create a moist environment to allow for skin healing [1]. Research is nowadays increasingly oriented towards "bioactive dressings". These dressings are made of materials that can play an active role in wound protection and healing. The first strategy consists of the application of skin substitutes, following a cell therapy approach [2]. A second strategy is the realization of "medicated dressings", able to release biomolecules in a sustained manner and to perform functions other than passive protection [3].

Due to their characteristics, hydrogels find application in wound dressing, especially in cases where a conventional dressing can be difficult to apply, as deep and irregular lesions. Hydrogels based on natural polysaccharides are highly hydrophilic and sometimes sensitive to enzymatic degradation [4–6]. In particular, alginates (Alg) are known for their ability to crosslink under mild conditions through a series of divalent cations. Alginates are a family of popular biocompatible polysaccharides extracted from brown algae [7]. Their hydrogels, in combination with other biopolymers or active agents, are used as dressing for wounds and burns, as they help to maintain an optimum moisture environment and cool temperature [8–10]. Alginate is approved for healthcare and present on the market with several trademarks. Another merit of alginate hydrogels is that they can be easily and quickly prepared at the time of need starting from sterilized solutions in a sterile area, making them appealing from a galenic, as well as an industrial point of view.

Alginate beads and hydrogels are stable in acidic media, whereas they easily swell and disintegrate in alkaline media and normal saline solution [11], conditions similar to those found in wound exudates. As calcium ions are being released by the ion exchange with sodium in the medium, electrostatic repulsion between the carboxylate anions further accelerates the swelling and erosion of alginate gels [12]. Moreover, on account of short time release in alkaline and neutral media, alginate is not an ideal material for sustained release. There were many attempts to control the disintegration of alginate-based drug delivery systems (DDS) and extend drug release characteristics through coating with polycationic polymers, such as poly(L-lysine) [13] or chitosan [14]. In contrast to alginate, which is polyanionic in nature, chitosan is a polycationic polysaccharide, derived from chitin [15,16]. Due to its gel-forming properties, it has been also employed in the design of DDS [17,18]. Complexation of alginate with chitosan reduces the porosity of the alginate gel and decreases the leakage of the encapsulated drugs [19–24]. In the case of wound dressing, encapsulated drugs are mainly antibiotics able to prevent or combat infections or growth factors to accelerate the healing process.

Nowadays, there are many concerns about the prolonged use of antibiotics, as required in the case of chronic wounds. The rise of bacterial resistance to antibiotics is well documented, both in the scientific literature and in the popular press. The World Health Organization recently described antimicrobial resistance as "a problem so serious that it threatens the achievements of modern medicine" [25]. Another concern is the safety of silver and titanium nanoparticles, often used in wound dressing for their antimicrobial activity [26,27]. Due to the small size, nanoparticles are easily absorbed into biological tissues and may interact with mitochondria, inducing structural damages, specifically in the liver cells [28]. In this regard, the use of materials with intrinsic antibacterial activity, avoiding the release of nanoscopic particles, may represent a valid alternative. As the antibacterial properties of chitosan are well documented in the literature [29,30], coating of alginate hydrogels with chitosan looks to be a possible strategy to realize intrinsic antimicrobial dressings with sustained release characteristics. Anyway, the difficulty in realizing alginate-chitosan hydrogels derives from their different pH-dependent water solubilities. To overcome these drawbacks, several examples of the use of water-soluble chitosan derivatives are found in literature [31,32]. Nevertheless, chemical modification usually involves amines, with the loss of antibacterial activity.

In the present work, a coating of chitosan onto alginate hydrogels was realized using chitosan hydrochloride (CH-Cl), a protonated form of chitosan, with the dual purpose of imparting antibacterial activity and delaying the release of hydrophilic molecules from the alginate matrix. Chitosan hydrochloride was characterized by FTIR analysis. Alginate hydrogels with different calcium contents were prepared by the internal setting method and coated by immersion in a CH-Cl solution. Structural analysis by cryo-scanning electron microscopy permits highlighting the morphological alterations due to the coating layer. Tests *in vitro* with human mesenchymal stromal cells (MSC) were assessed to check the absence of toxicity of CH-Cl. Swelling, stability in physiological solution and release characteristics using rhodamine B as the hydrophilic model drug were compared to those of relative uncoated hydrogels. Finally, the antibacterial activity against *Escherichia coli* was tested.

2. Results and Discussion

2.1. Preparation of CH-Cl

CH-Cl is a charged form of chitosan, completely soluble in acid-free water [33]. It is known from the literature that the methodology employed here results in highly pure samples, which preserve an identical degree of deacetylation [34]. FTIR spectra of chitosan and CH-Cl are shown in Figure 1.

The appearance in the CH-Cl spectrum of typical bands of symmetric and asymmetric stretching of ammonium N-H (1624 and 1518 cm^{-1}, respectively) is evidence of the protonation of free amines.

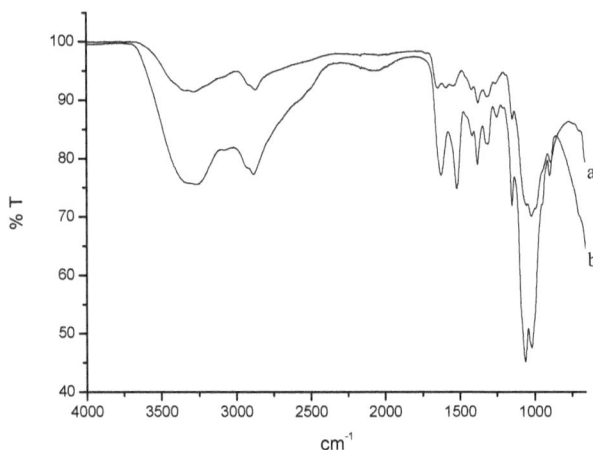

Figure 1. (a) FTIR spectrum of chitosan; (b) FTIR spectrum of chitosan hydrochloride (CH-Cl).

2.2. Preparation and Preliminary Characterization of Hydrogels

Alginate hydrogels were prepared via internal gelation, using CaCO$_3$ as the calcium source. This methodology allows one to obtain highly regular and homogeneous gels through a slow release of calcium ions. Different CaCO$_3$ and D-(+)-gluconate-δ-lactone (GDL) amounts were used, as reported in Table 1.

Table 1. Composition and codes of hydrogels. GDL, D-(+)-gluconate-δ-lactone; Alg, alginate.

CaCO$_3$ (mmol)	GDL (mmol)	GDL (mL)	Alg/Ca^{2+} * (mol/mol)	GDL/CaCO$_3$ (mol/mol)	Code
0.999	0.999	17.8	5.155	1	Alg1
0.999	1.998	35.6	5.155	2	Alg2
1.998	1.998	35.6	2.577	1	Alg3
1.998	3.997	71.2	2.577	2	Alg4

* The reported data refer to 1 g of alginate = 0.0051 mol of repeating units.

The intrinsic features of hydrogels are strictly dependent on the relative concentrations of calcium carbonate and GDL. In particular, the molar ratio between GDL and calcium carbonate is crucial to obtain a complete salt dissolution and to determine the final gel pH (acid or neutral) [35,36], whereas the molar ratio between alginate repeating units and calcium ions regulates the number of carboxylates engaged in ionic interactions and, therefore, the crosslinking density of the resulting gel. Such characteristics are important for the final properties of the gel and for the interactions of alginate with chitosan hydrochloride, as will be discussed. Two GDL/CaCO$_3$ molar ratios were chosen, in order to obtain neutral or acid gels (1/1 and 2/1, respectively). Concerning the Alg/Ca^{2+} ratio, a value close to the stoichiometric one or its half (2.5/1 and 5/1) was investigated.

Coating of alginate hydrogels was achieved simply by immersion in a 1% (*w/w*) CH-Cl water solution. The dipping time (1 h) and CH-Cl concentration were established after several attempts. During immersion, shrinkage is observed for all hydrogels to a different extent. All coated hydrogels (c-Alg) retain transparency, a desirable feature for wound dressing to allow inspection of the injury bed. Furthermore, the hydrogels are harder and easier to handle upon coating.

Gelation time, bulk pH value and water content are reported in Table 2. Gelation time is mainly influenced by the calcium ion concentration, passing from a slow (around half an hour) to a fast (a few minutes) gelation when the amount of calcium carbonate is doubled. Of course, an excess of GDL (GDL/$CaCO_3$ equal to two) further accelerates gelation as a consequence of two effects: faster calcium carbonate dissolution and partial acidification of carboxylate groups, which contribute to gelation via hydrogen bonding.

pH measurements evidence that hydrogels with a GDL/Ca^{2+} molar ratio equal to one (Alg1 and Alg3) are basic, suggesting that calcium carbonate is not completely neutralized. When an excess of GDL is used (Alg2 and Alg4), the pH is lowered until neutral. After coating, a decrease of bulk pH values is generally observed, likely due to diffusion of CH-Cl within the hydrogel during immersion. In particular, c-Alg2 and c-Alg4 show an acid pH value.

Table 2. Gelation times, pH values and water content. c, coated.

Sample	Gelation Time (min)	pH	Water Content (wt %)
Alg1	40 ± 4	8.34 ± 0.14	69.37 ± 1.32
Alg2	28 ± 3	6.49 ± 0.70	68.61 ± 1.15
Alg3	8 ± 1	7.24 ± 0.83	69.63 ± 0.32
Alg4	5 ± 1	7.12 ± 0.01	68.76 ± 0.84
c-Alg1	*	7.53 ± 0.54	69.42 ± 0.96
c-Alg2	*	5.19 ± 0.36	67.70 ± 0.82
c-Alg3	*	7.34 ± 0.81	65.94 ± 1.02
c-Alg4	*	5.10 ± 0.40	53.51 ± 0.64

* Gelation times are the same as the corresponding uncoated hydrogels.

The water content of Alg hydrogels is in line with what is reported in the literature for calcium alginate spray formulations [37]. Upon coating, a slight decrease is generally observed, likely due to the release of water associated with shrinking. This behavior is more pronounced in the case of c-Alg4, which visually shows greater shrinkage associated with volume reduction.

Figure 2 displays the gel homogeneity, estimated according to the literature [38]. The results show that, despite shrinking, the coating does not substantially influence the homogeneity of the gels.

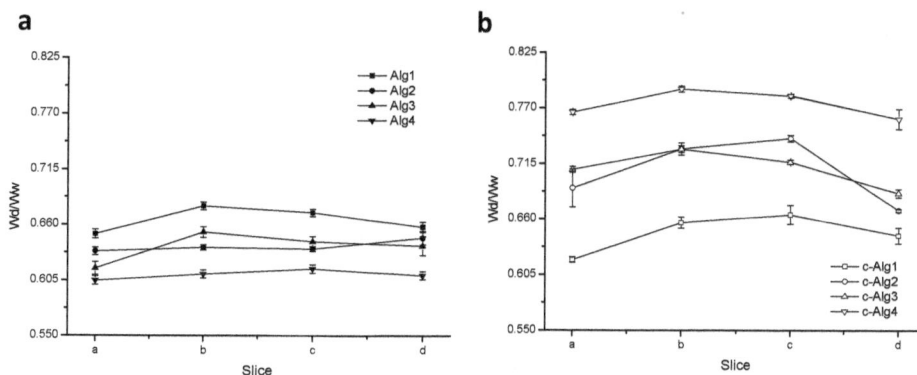

Figure 2. (a) Homogeneity profiles of Alg hydrogels; (b) homogeneity profiles of c-Alg hydrogels.

2.3. Swelling

The water uptake ability of hydrogels was monitored with time by weight determinations. Swelling kinetics curves are reported in Figure 3a,b. Alg hydrogels (Figure 3a) show a fast water uptake in the first two hours followed by a short plateau and a second phase in which swelling rapidly increases, perhaps due to incoming gel disintegration, until achievement of the equilibrium water content after around 8 h. Swelling is generally related to crosslinking degree: hydrogels with a low crosslinking density are expected to have a large pore size and greater ability to swell, but ultimately may tend to dissolve. On the contrary, an increase of Ca^{2+} concentration or a pH decrease would limit swelling ability. Accordingly, swelling regularly decreases going from Alg1 to Alg4. Alg1 and Alg2 (low calcium content) reach over 400% swelling, whereas Alg3 and Alg4 swell less (below 200%).

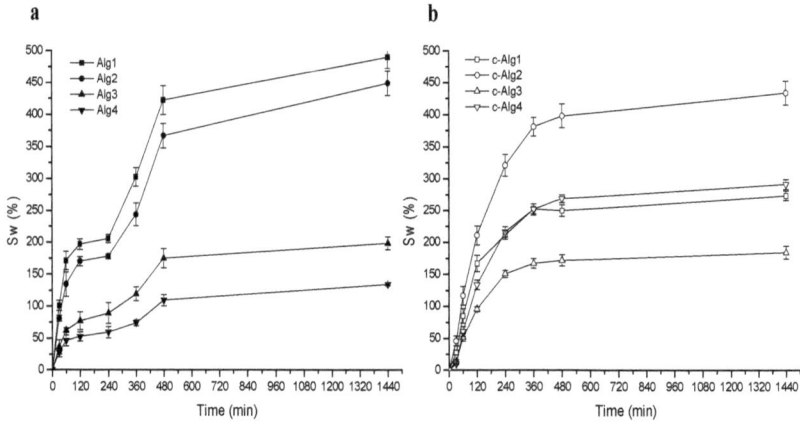

Figure 3. (**a**) Swelling curves of Alg hydrogels; (**b**) swelling curves of c-Alg hydrogels.

Swelling of c-Alg hydrogels increases regularly for all samples (Figure 3b), but the trend is not regular any more: whereas c-Alg2 preserves a high swelling percentage, close to that of Alg2, in the case of c-Alg1, swelling falls from ~460% to ~200% upon coating. This suggests that an alginate hydrogel with a low calcium concentration and besides being characterized by a basic pH, such as Alg1, holds a greater amount of CH-Cl, due to the high number of free carboxylate groups available for ionic interactions with ammonium groups of CH-Cl, thus creating a tight coating layer in which ion pairs are uniformly distributed. It is known from the literature that ionic aggregates represent a barrier to water diffusion [39]; the strong swelling decrease of c-Alg1 is likely a consequence of the reduced water diffusion throughout the coating. Concerning c-Alg2, instead, the partial protonation of carboxylates, as evidenced by the pH value of Alg2, reduces the ionic interactions between alginate and chitosan hydrochloride; thus, CH-Cl is just physically absorbed, and no significant variations of swelling properties are detected. Similarly, in the case of c-Alg3, carboxylate groups are saturated, due to the large excess of calcium ions, and no change of swelling occurs. On the opposite end, c-Alg4 shows higher swelling with respect to Alg4. This result is reasonably related to the re-uptake of water expelled during the coating process as a consequence of shrinkage (see Table 1 and the Discussion Section).

2.4. Stability in Normal Saline Solution

In order to verify the resistance of hydrogels to degradation in a medium close to the environment of the wound bed, a stability test was performed by immersion in normal saline solution for 24 h. Curves relative to weight change percentage with time are shown in Figure 4a,b. It is important to underline that weight loss due to alginate chain dissolution is partially hidden by simultaneous swelling.

From a comparison, it is evident that coating induces an increase of stability: after initial swelling, Alg hydrogels undergo around a 10% weight loss in eight hours, whereas c-Alg does not lose weight during the whole range of time. As can be seen, c-Alg has just a low weight loss of about 5% at first, attributed to the loss of CH-Cl slightly absorbed onto the surface. Interactions between alginate and chitosan hydrochloride are not sensitive to sodium exchange, so the coating is stable, and disintegration of the hydrogel is delayed. It is also worth noticing that the Alg1 and Alg2 samples appear broken into several pieces just after two hours, while all other hydrogels preserve their physical integrity during 24 h.

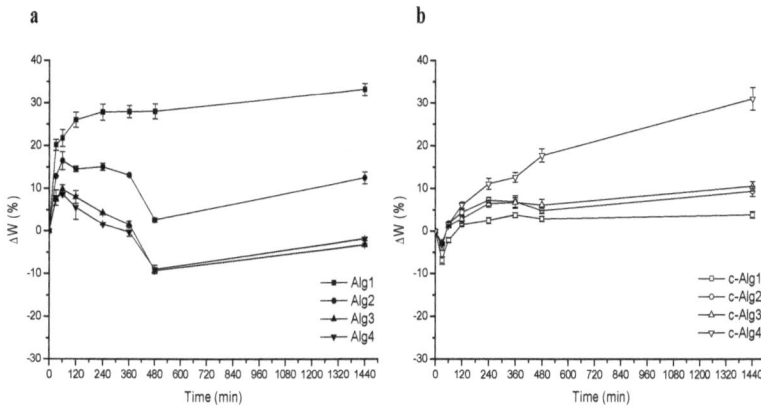

Figure 4. (**a**) Stability test in normal saline solution of Alg hydrogels; (**b**) stability test in normal saline solution of c-Alg hydrogels.

2.5. Cryo-SEM Analysis

Coated and uncoated hydrogels have been observed by cryo-SEM. Micrographs of Alg1 and c-Alg1 are reported in Figure 5a–f as an example. From a comparison between the outer surfaces of Alg1 (Figure 5a,b) and c-Alg1 (Figure 5d,e), it seems that in the last case, the surface is more regular and compact, whereas Alg1 shows an irregular surface, with the presence of numerous depressions, likely due to water evaporation. This evidence suggests a reduction in water loss from the coated hydrogel. Low-temperature fracture allows the exposure of the internal structure; the pore dimension can be roughly estimated in the range of 10–20 µm (Figure 5c,f). The morphology of the internal structure is not altered by the presence of the coating layer.

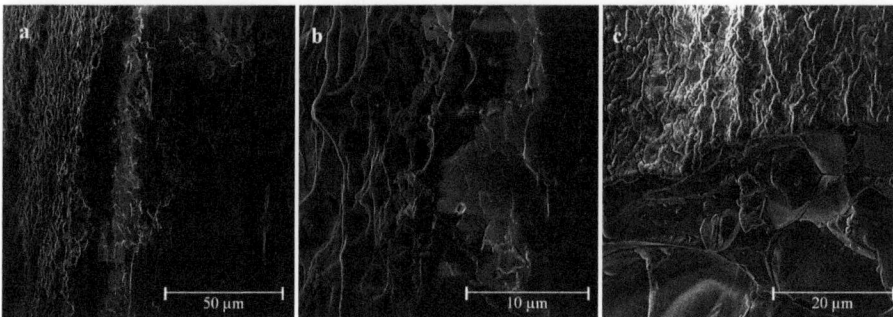

Figure 5. *Cont.*

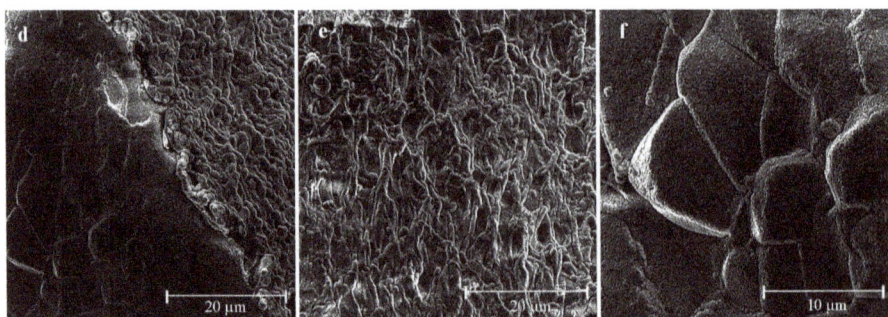

Figure 5. (a–c) Cryo-SEM images of Alg1; (d–f) cryo-SEM images of c-Alg1.

2.6. Release Study

In order to verify the effect of coating on the release properties, rhodamine B (RhB) was chosen as a model of a low molecular weight hydrophilic drug and encapsulated within the hydrogel. To evaluate the release kinetics in physiological conditions, hydrogels were placed on a porous glass set in order to be in contact with PBS medium (pH 7.4) only by the lower surface (Figure 6). This equipment was designed to mimic exudate penetration into the hydrogel from the wound bed. The release profiles of Alg hydrogels compared to coated hydrogels are reported in Figure 7. As can be seen, c-Alg always exhibits a lower release rate with respect to the relative uncoated hydrogels. After eight hours, Alg hydrogels released about 70%–80% of their content, whereas c-Alg hydrogels released only about 60%–50%. The different rate of release can be easily related to the presence of a coating layer on the hydrogel surface. Release from hydrogels is dependent on the diffusion of drug molecules throughout the alginate matrix; the presence of a coating layer acts as a barrier that delays diffusion and, hence, slows down release.

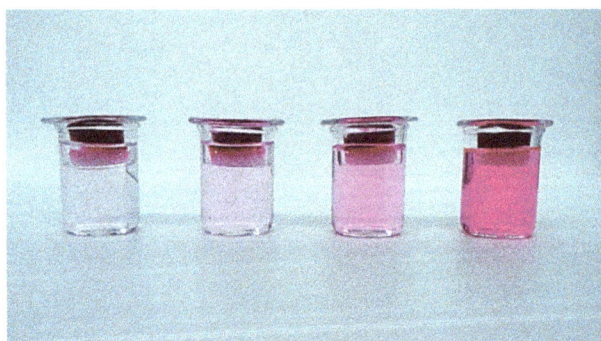

Figure 6. Equipment employed to study the release of rhodamine B in physiological conditions. The photo refers to different release times.

a

b

c

d

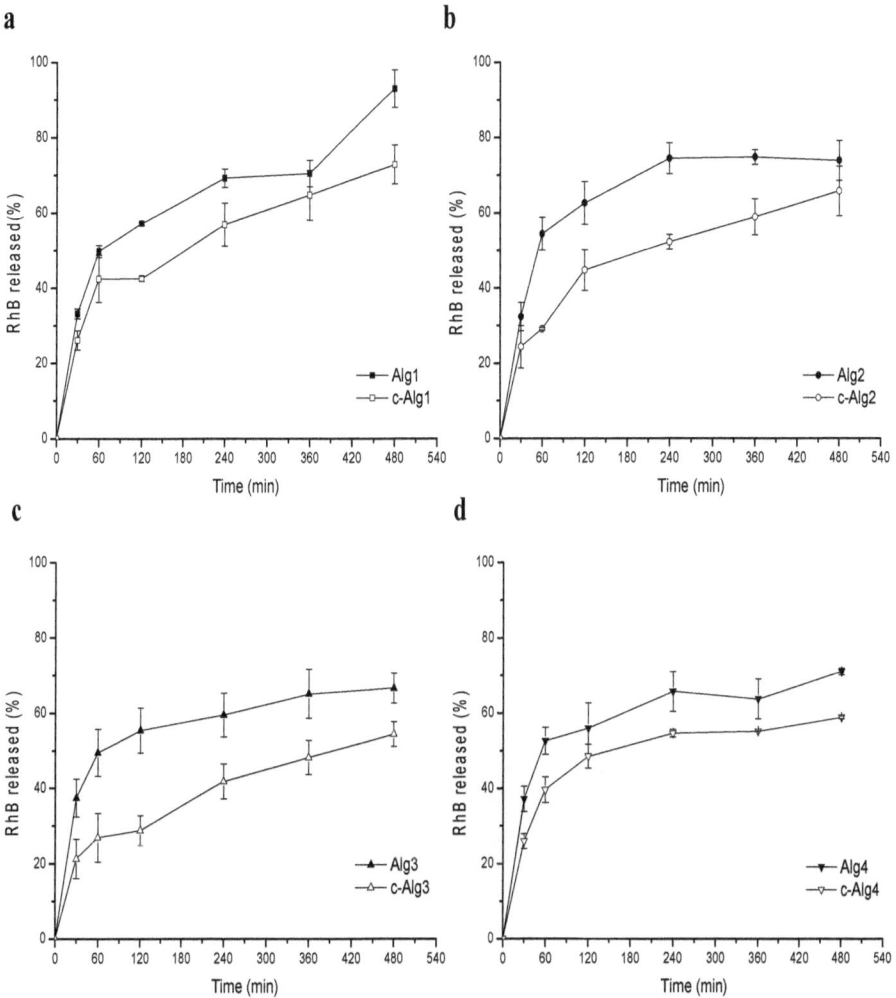

Figure 7. Release profiles of RhB from: (**a**) Alg1 and c-Alg1; (**b**) Alg2 and c-Alg2; (**c**) Alg3 and c-Alg3; (**d**) Alg4 and c-Alg4.

2.7. Cytotoxicity Test

A cytotoxicity test to analyze the effects of CH-Cl solution on mesenchymal stromal cells (MSC) was performed. Cells were treated for seven days with culture medium (control) or with culture medium added with 0.1% (w/v) solution of CH-Cl. MSC were examined every day for one week to observe any possible appearance of cytotoxicity signs, such as morphologic changes, cellular lysis areas or cell death. Figure 8 shows the microscopic images of cells cultured for one week in control medium (a,b) and in 0.1% CH-Cl medium (c,d) after crystal violet staining. It appears evident that in both cases (control and treated MSC), the morphology was substantially unmodified; most important, growth was not inhibited, and cells were able to reach confluence to the same extent as the controls. Anyway, it has to be underlined that this test represents only the first, pivotal approach in the evaluation of biocompatibility, which allows one to exclude an acute cytotoxicity. Other tests, namely sensitization and irritation tests, will be necessary to confirm the absence of adverse effects on living tissues.

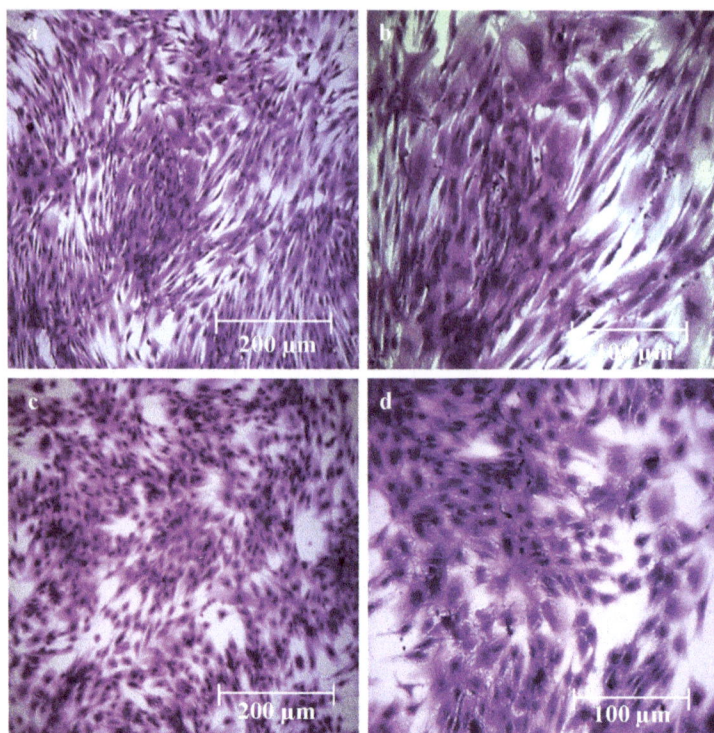

Figure 8. (**a,b**) Microscopic images of MSC cultured for seven days in control culture medium after crystal violet staining; (**c,d**) microscopic images of MSC cultured for seven days in 0.1% CH-Cl culture medium after crystal violet staining.

2.8. Antibacterial Activity

The antibacterial activity of CH-Cl and c-Alg was tested against the *Escherichia coli* wild-type strain, the second most common single pathogen involved in postoperative wound infections [40]. To test the activity of CH-Cl as an antimicrobial agent, MIC and minimum bactericidal concentration (MBC) were determined. MIC and MBC define the antibacterial efficiency of an antimicrobial agent in terms of the concentration at which it will inhibit growth (MIC) or completely kill (MBC) 1×10^6 challenge microorganisms during 24 h of incubation. Both MIC and MBC were found to fall at a 1:32 dilution, corresponding to 0.31 mg/mL of CH-Cl.

Preliminary tests based on the solid agar medium contact method carried out on hydrogels evidenced the presence of an inhibition zone around the contact area in the case of coated hydrogels, completely absent in uncoated hydrogels. Figure 9a,b shows photos of *Escherichia coli* growing on agar plates in contact with Alg1 and c-Alg1 hydrogels as an example. No significant differences were noted among the coated hydrogels (c-Alg1, c-Alg2, c-Alg3 and c-Alg4).

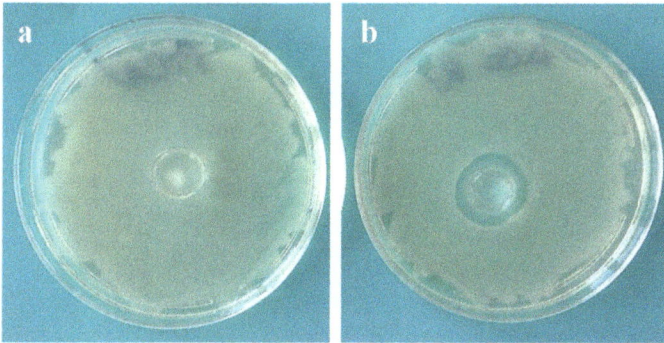

Figure 9. (a) Optical photo of *E. coli* growing on agar in contact with Alg1; (b) optical photo of *E. coli* growing on agar in contact with c-Alg1.

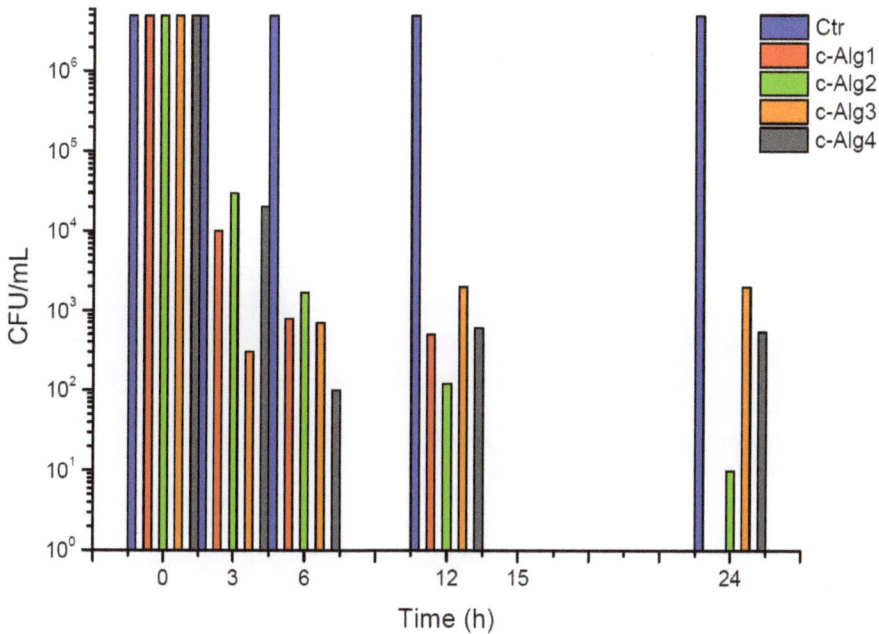

Figure 10. Antimicrobial activity kinetics of c-Alg hydrogels against *E. coli*.

The kinetics of antimicrobial activity against *Escherichia coli* of coated hydrogels is reported in Figure 10. Uncoated hydrogels were tested as the negative control (Ctr). Results show that all c-Alg cause a bacterial inactivation higher than 99% already after 3 h of contact, and a complete killing of bacteria was reached after 24 h in the case of c-Alg1. The concentration of CH-Cl is likely equal or higher than the MIC and MBC values in all coated hydrogels. The slight difference in bactericidal activity among hydrogels is attributed to the different degree of interaction between CH-Cl and alginate in the various hydrogels, as previously discussed (e.g., swelling behavior, see Section 2.2). Alginate hydrogel with the highest concentration of free carboxylate groups (Alg1) binds more CH-Cl via ionic interactions with ammonium groups, forming a denser layer coating on the surface. As a consequence, bacterial killing is complete, whereas surviving bacterial cells (less than 1%) are found with the other hydrogels. Furthermore, in the case of c-Alg3 and c-Alg4, the activity stops after 6 h, as no further reduction is detected after this time. Once again, the occurrence of antibacterial activity can be related to the interaction of alginate with CH-Cl. In fact, in the case of hydrogels with high calcium content (c-Alg3 and c-Alg4), most of the carboxylates groups of alginate are engaged in calcium ion chelation and not available for interactions with ammonium groups, reducing the coating layer.

3. Experimental Section

3.1. Materials

Pharmaceutical-grade alginic acid sodium salt (Alg), extracted from *Laminaria hyperborean* (viscosity 360 mPa·s, 1% *w/v* water solution; mannuronic and guluronic acids: ratio 1.8:2.2), was supplied by Farmalabor (Canosa di Puglia, Brindisi, Italy). Chitosan (CH) extracted from crab shells (high molecular weight; viscosity 400 mPa·s, 1% acetic acid (20 °C); 80% deacetylation degree), calcium carbonate, D-(+)-glucono-δ-lactone (GDL), rhodamine B (RhB) and sodium phosphate monobasic monohydrate ($Na_2HPO_4 \cdot H_2O$) were purchased from Sigma Aldrich (Milan, Italy). Streptomycin sulfate was supplied by Applichem (Darmstadt, Germany). Potassium chloride, sodium bicarbonate, calcium chloride hexahydrate and sodium chloride were purchased from J.T. Baker (Avantor Performance Materials, Milan, Italy). Yeast extract, tryptone and agar, used as the culture medium, were purchased from Oxoid, England. Opti-MEM was purchased from Life technologies Italia (Monza, Italy).

3.2. Preparation of Chitosan Hydrochloride

Water-soluble chitosan hydrochloride (CH-Cl) was prepared following literature reports [34]. Briefly, a solution of chitosan (1 g/100 mL, 1% acetic acid) was filtered and dialyzed against NaCl 0.4 mol/L for eight days. NaCl solution was then replaced by freshly-distilled water, and the dialysis continued for another two days. CH-Cl was finally recovered by freeze-drying in the form of white powder.

3.3. Preparation of Alginate Hydrogels by Internal Setting Method

Alginate hydrogels were prepared using the internal setting method [35,36]. Fine suspensions of calcium carbonate in distilled water (0.1% or 0.2% *w/v*) were obtained by sonication (Vibracell VC 505, Sonics, Newton, CT, USA; 500 Hz, 50% amplitude, 10 min). One gram of sodium alginate was dissolved in 100 mL of suspension under stirring, then a chosen amount of 1% *w/v* GDL solution was added. Five milliliters of each final alginate solution were immediately poured into a petri dish (3.6 cm diameter) and left for 24 h in air at room temperature to complete gelation. Hydrogels were washed in water by quick immersion and briefly blotted on paper before characterization.

3.4. Preparation of Coated Hydrogels

Samples coated with CH-Cl were prepared by immersion in CH-Cl solution. Freshly-prepared alginate hydrogels (1.9 cm diameter, corresponding to 1 mL of alginate solution) were embedded in 10 mL of CH-Cl solution (1 g/100 mL, water) for 60 min under mild stirring. The coated hydrogels were carefully recovered with a strainer and withdrawn by briefly blotting on paper.

3.5. FTIR Analysis

FTIR spectra were obtained in the attenuated total reflection mode (ATR) using a Perkin-Elmer spectrometer (Norwalk, CT, USA) equipped with universal-ATR accessory, fitted with a diamond optical element and ZnSe focusing elements. The apparatus operates with a single reflection at an incident angle of 45°. The analysis was carried out on powders at room temperature and ambient humidity. Spectra were acquired between 4000 and 400 cm^{-1} with a spectral resolution of 4 cm^{-1} and 32 scans collected.

3.6. Gelation Time

Gelation time, defined as the time between the addition of GDL and the formation of a fixed gel, was assessed using a method adapted from the literature [38]. The petri dish containing the gelling solution was periodically tilted during the gelation process. Gel was said to be formed when there was no longer flowing when the dish was kept at an angle of 45° for more than 30 s.

3.7. pH Measurements

Bulk pH determinations were carried out by a CRISON 507 pH-meter (CRISON, Barcelona, Spain) equipped with type 52-00 electrodes and a probe tip 52-32 for penetration analysis.

3.8. Water Content

Water content (W) of hydrogels was calculated as a percentage by the ratio between the wet gel weight and the dry gel weight (after drying at 40 °C in air until constant weight). Measurements were performed in triplicate.

3.9. Homogeneity

The homogeneity of alginate gels was estimated according to the literature [38]. Hydrogels were cut into four slices of equal dimension (a–d). Each slice was weighed, then dried to constant weight and reweighed. The dry to wet weight ratio (W_d/W_w) of slices provides an indication of the homogeneity. A homogeneous gel will have a consistent dry to wet weight ratio across its constituent slices. Data are the mean of three measurements for each sample.

3.10. Swelling

Swelling was determined gravimetrically by monitoring the water up-take with time. Hydrogels were immersed in distilled water, withdrawn at different times and weighed after blotting on paper. For each sample, the measurements were performed in triplicate, and average data were used for the calculations.

3.11. Stability Test

A degradation test in normal saline solution (NaCl 0.9%, w/v) was achieved in order to get information about the stability of hydrogels when in contact with physiological fluids. Hydrogels were weighed and immersed in 100 mL of saline solution at room temperature. At set time intervals, the samples were withdrawn, briefly blotted on filter paper and weighed. Stability was expressed as weight variation percentage ($\Delta W\%$). All measurements were performed in triplicate, and average data were reported.

3.12. Cryo-SEM Analysis

The morphology of coated hydrogels was examined through cryo-scanning electron microscopy (cryo-SEM) using a cryo-system Gatan Alto 1000E (Gatan, Pleasanton, CA, USA) installed on a FEI Quanta 200 FEG SEM (FEI, Eindhoven, The Netherlands). The sample was placed on the holder, mounted on the cryo-transfer rod, slam-frozen in nitrogen slush and transferred to the cryo-chamber, where it was cryo-fractured and sputter coated with gold/palladium. The sample was finally moved to the SEM chamber where either fracture or top surfaces were observed at −140 °C, using an acceleration voltage of 5–10 kV.

3.13. Release Study

Alg and c-Alg hydrogels (1.9 cm diameter), prepared as previously described (Section 2.3), were loaded with RhB by dissolving 10 mg of alginate in 1 mL of RhB aqueous solution of different concentrations, in order to obtain in each gel a final RhB concentration of 13.05 µM. Release studies were performed using a modified Enslin apparatus, designed to mimic the wound bed [41]. Twelve milliliters of phosphate buffer saline solution (PBS; NaCl 120 mM, KCl 2.7 mM, Na$_2$HPO$_4$ 10 mM, pH 7.4) were in contact with the hydrogels only by their lower surface. At set times, 1.0 mL of buffer medium was withdrawn, replaced by the same amount of fresh PBS and analyzed by UV spectroscopic analysis. Release was followed for 8 h. The RhB% released was calculated using a 10-point calibration curve ($R^2 = 0.9993$) in the concentration range 13.05–1.30 μM. Experiments were performed in triplicate.

3.14. Cytotoxicity Test

In order to exclude the cytotoxic effects of chitosan hydrochloride, an assay was performed on mesenchymal stromal cells (MSC) obtained from normal human bone marrow, as previously described [42]. Cells were seeded in multi-well plates at a density of 20,000/cm^2 and treated with culture medium (control) or with culture medium added with 0.1% (*w/v*) solution of CH-Cl. The test was performed in triplicate. MSC were grown for one week renewing the medium every second day and observed daily by optical microscopy. Finally, control and treated MSC were stained with crystal violet and observed with a Workstation Leica DMI6000 microscope (Leica Microsystems GmbH, Wetzlar, Germany). Images were acquired using a digital camera Leica DFC 340FX (Leica Microsystems GmbH, Wetzlar, Germany) and analyzed by LAS AF 2.2.0 software.

3.15. Antibacterial Activity

Antibacterial activity of CH-Cl and c-Alg hydrogels was tested against *Escherichia coli* (DSM 498), purchased from Deutsche Samlug von Mikroorganismen und Zellkulturen GmbH (DSMZ, Braunschweig, Germany). Growth of bacterial strain occurs on sterile Luria-Bertani (LB) medium (10 g/L tryptone, 5 g/L yeast extract, 10 g/L NaCl distilled water) in an aerated incubator at 37 °C, 120 rpm, for 18–24 h. Bacterial growth was verified measuring the optical density of bacteria at 600 nm (OD$_{600}$) by means of a spectrophotometer. After growth and harvesting, bacterial cells were washed twice with sterile Ringer solution (RS), a neutral buffer saline solution (0.150 g KCl, 2.25 g NaCl, 0.05 g NaHCO$_3$ and 0.12 g CaCl$_2$ per liter of distilled water, pH 7.0) and then re-suspended in RS up to an absorbance of 0.250 ± 0.01, which corresponds to a concentration of approximately 1.5–3.0 × 10^8 colony-forming units per milliliter (CFU/mL). A second dilution was carried out to obtain working bacterial suspensions of about 10^6 CFU/mL.

The minimum inhibitory concentration (MIC) of CH-Cl, defined as the lowest concentration of the antimicrobial agent that inhibits the visible growth of the test microorganism, was determined using the broth dilution methods [43,44]. CH-Cl solution (10 mg/mL, water) was serially diluted with LB medium: 10 mL of CH-Cl solution were added to 10 mL of LB and mixed by vortexing for 1 min; successive dilutions were repeated in order to obtain a concentration range spanning from 0.078 to 10 mg/mL. Ten milliliters of each diluted CH-Cl solution were inoculated with 100 μL of 10^8 CFU/mL microbial suspension of *Escherichia coli*. The inoculum assay and streptomycin sulfate (15 μg/mL) were evaluated as negative and positive controls, respectively; the optical density of bacteria after 24 h was assessed.

The minimum bactericidal concentration (MBC) was measured following MIC determination. One hundred microliters of each of the two dilution suspensions preceding the MIC dilution were plated onto LB medium agar 1.8% and incubated at 37 °C overnight. The highest dilution (and conversely, the lowest concentration) that resulted in a 99.9% reduction in bacterial cells number was recorded as the MBC.

Each measurement was replicated three times.

Preliminary screening of the antimicrobial properties of c-Alg hydrogels (1.9 cm diameter) was carried out by the solid phase contact method on an LB agar medium plate (1.5% agar) in petri dishes. Hydrogels were prepared in sterile conditions. Working bacterial suspensions (0.1 mL) were spread onto the solid surface of the medium agar plate, then hydrogels were put on it, and the plates were incubated at 37 °C for 24 h. After incubation, the inhibition areas were evaluated. Alg hydrogels were tested as the negative control.

The kinetics of killing of c-Alg1, c-Alg2, c-Alg3 and c-Alg4 (1.9 cm diameter) was determined by measuring bacteria logarithmic reduction as a function of time. Hydrogels were kept in contact with 10 mL of working bacterial suspension at room temperature on a wrist-action shaker (ASTM standard Test Method E 2149-01). Then, 0.1 mL of working solution were used to prepare decimal dilutions, which were plated onto the LB solid medium agar plate. Plates were incubated at 37 °C for 24 h. After 0 h (t_0), 3 h (t_3), 6 h (t_6), 12h (t_{12}) and 24 h (t_{24}) of contact time, surviving cells were evaluated by the standard plate count method, and inactivation tests were performed in duplicate. The inoculum assay and Alg hydrogels were used as the negative control, while streptomycin sulfate (15 μg/mL) was tested as the positive control. The average colony count of duplicate plates was used to calculate the CFU/mL. Tests were performed three times.

The percentage reduction was calculated by the following equation:

$$\text{Reduction \%} \left(\text{CFU mL}^{-1} \right) = \left(\frac{B - A}{B} \right) \times 100 \tag{1}$$

where A = bacterial concentration after a specific contact time and B = bacterial concentration at t_0 contact time.

4. Conclusions

Alginate chitosan-coated hydrogels were prepared by using water-soluble chitosan hydrochloride. The internal gelation setting method was used for the realization of hydrogels. Coated hydrogels retain good homogeneity and high water content, whereas a decrease of bulk pH was detected. Overall, hydrogels were found to have a water uptake weight percentage ranging from 450 to 200, which would prevent the wound bed from accumulating exudates and, at the same time, protect it from excessive dehydration. Stability in normal saline solution increases upon coating. Cryo-SEM analysis highlighted a more regular and compact surface on coated hydrogels, while the internal morphology was not altered. Coated hydrogels exhibit antibacterial activity against *Escherichia Coli*, and cytotoxicity tests demonstrate that chitosan hydrochloride does not elicit any acute toxic effects on mesenchymal stromal cells. Release studies using rhodamine B as a model of a low molecular weight hydrophilic drug show that the coating induces a decrease in the release kinetics.

To summarize, in this work, novel hydrogels based on alginate and chitosan hydrochloride have been investigated in order to explore their potential application as novel medicated dressings by associating intrinsic antimicrobial activity with improved sustained release characteristics.

Acknowledgments: The authors gratefully acknowledge the project "High-tech devices for biomedical applications" (acronym: DIATEME) in the frame of the National Operative Program (PON 2007–2013), for financial support. The authors wish to thank Cristina Del Barone from Laboratory of Electron Microscopy "LaMEST" of IPCB, CNR for technical assistance with the cryo-SEM analysis. The authors are also indebted to Roberta Imperatore (Institute of Applied Sciences and Intelligent Systems, CNR) for assistance with the optical microscopy.

Author Contributions: Conceived and designed the experiments: GGA AO PL. Performed the experiments: MCS, IR. Analyzed the data: MCS, GGA, IR, AO, PL. Wrote the paper: PL.

Conflicts of Interest: The authors declare no conflict of interest.

References

1. Eming, S.A.; Krieg, T.; Davidson, J.M. Inflammation in wound repair: Molecular and cellular mechanisms. *J. Investig. Dermatol.* **2007**, *127*, 514–525. [CrossRef] [PubMed]

2. Moura, L.I.; Dias, M.A.; Carvalho, E.; de Sousa, H.C. Recent advances on the development of wound dressings for diabetic foot ulcer treatment—A review. *Acta Biomater.* **2013**, *9*, 7093–7114. [CrossRef] [PubMed]

3.   Boateng, J.S.; Matthews, K.H.; Stevens, H.N.; Eccleston, G.M. Wound healing dressings and drug delivery systems: A review. *J. Pharm. Sci.* **2008**, *97*, 2892–2923. [CrossRef] [PubMed]

4.   Altinisik, A.; Yurdacoc, K. Synthesis, characterization, and enzymatic degradation of chitosan/PEG hydrogel films. *J. Appl. Polym. Sci.* **2011**, *122*, 1556–1563. [CrossRef]

5.   Gorgieva, S.; Kokol, V. Preparation, characterization, and *in vitro* enzymatic degradation of chitosan-gelatine hydrogel scaffolds as potential biomaterials. *J. Biomed. Mater. Res. A* **2012**, *100*, 1655–1667. [CrossRef] [PubMed]

6.   Tan, H.; Rubin, J.P.; Marra, K.G. Injectable *in situ* forming biodegradable chitosan-hyaluronic acid based hydrogels for adipose tissue regeneration. *Organogenesis* **2010**, *6*, 173–180. [CrossRef] [PubMed]

7.   Laurienzo, P. Marine polysaccharides in pharmaceutical applications: An overview. *Mar. Drugs* **2010**, *8*, 2435–2465. [CrossRef] [PubMed]

8.   Brachkova, M.I.; Marques, P.; Rocha, J.; Sepodes, B.; Duarte, M.A.; Pinto, J.F. Alginate films containing *Lactobacillus plantarum* as wound dressing for prevention of burn infection. *J. Hosp. Infect.* **2011**, *79*, 375–377. [CrossRef] [PubMed]

9.   Dantas, M.D.; Cavalcante, D.R.; Araujo, F.E.; Barretto, S.R.; Aciole, G.T.; Pinheiro, A.L.; Ribeiro, M.A.; Lima-Verde, I.B.; Melo, C.M.; Cardoso, J.C.; *et al.* Improvement of dermal burn healing by combining sodium alginate/chitosan-based films and low level laser therapy. *J. Photochem. Photobiol. B* **2011**, *105*, 51–59. [CrossRef] [PubMed]

10.   Peng, C.W.; Lin, H.Y.; Wang, H.W.; Wu, W.W. The influence of operating parameters on the drug release and anti-bacterial performances of alginate wound dressings prepared by three-dimensional plotting. *Mater. Sci. Eng. C* **2012**, *32*, 2491–2500. [CrossRef]

11.   Acarturk, F.; Takka, S. Calcium alginate microparticles for oral administration: II. Effect of formulation factors on drug release and drug entrapment efficiency. *J. Microencapsul.* **1999**, *16*, 291–301. [CrossRef] [PubMed]

12.   Kikuchi, A.; Kawabuchi, M.; Sugihara, M.; Sakurai, Y. Pulsed dextran release from calcium-alginate gel vedas. *J. Control. Release* **1997**, *47*, 21–29. [CrossRef]

13.   Lemoine, D.; Wauters, F.; Bouchend'homme, S.; Préat, V. Preparation and characterization of alginate microspheres coating a model antigen. *Int. J. Pharm.* **1998**, *176*, 9–19. [CrossRef]

14.   Murata, Y.; Meada, T.; Miyamoto, E.; Kawashima, S. Preparation of chitosan-reinforced alginate gel beads—effects of chitosan on gel matrix erosion. *Int. J. Pharm.* **1993**, *96*, 139–145. [CrossRef]

15.   Ravi Kumar, M.N.V.; Muzzarelli, R.A.A.; Muzzarelli, C.; Sashiwa, H.; Domb, A.J. Chitosan chemistry and pharmaceutical perspectives. *Chem. Rev.* **2004**, *104*, 6017–6084. [CrossRef] [PubMed]

16.   Dash, M.; Chiellini, F.; Ottenbrite, R.M.; Chiellini, E. Chitosan-A versatile semi-synthetyic polymer for biomedical applications. *Prog. Polym. Sci.* **2011**, *36*, 981–1014. [CrossRef]

17.   Hu, L.; Sun, Y.; Wu, Y. Advances in chitosan-based drug delivery vehicles. *Nanoscale* **2013**, *5*, 3103–3111. [CrossRef] [PubMed]

18.   Patel, M.P.; Patel, R.R.; Patel, J.K. Chitosan mediated targeted drug delivery system: A review. *J. Pharm. Sci.* **2010**, *13*, 536–557.

19.   Polk, A.; Amsden, B.; de Yao, K.; Peng, T.; Goosen, M.F.A. Controlled release of albumin from chitosan—Alginate microcapsules. *J. Pharm. Sci.* **1994**, *83*, 178–185. [CrossRef] [PubMed]

20.   Sezer, A.D.; Akbuga, J. Release characteristics of chitosan treated alginate beads: II. Sustained release of a low molecular drug from chitosan treated alginate beads. *J. Microencapsul.* **1999**, *16*, 678–696. [CrossRef]

21.   Sarmento, B.; Ribeiro, A.; Veiga, P.F.; Sampaio, P.; Neufeld, R.; Ferreira, D. Alginate/chitosan nanoparticles are effective for oral insulin delivery. *Pharm. Res.* **2007**, *24*, 2198–2206. [CrossRef] [PubMed]

22.   González-Rodríguez, M.L.; Holgado, M.A.; Sánchez-Lafuente, C.; Rabasco, A.M.; Fini, A. Alginate/chitosan particulate systems for sodium diclofenac release. *Int. J. Pharm.* **2002**, *232*, 225–234. [CrossRef] [PubMed]

23.   Xu, Y.; Zhan, C.; Fan, L.; Wang, L.; Zheng, H. Preparation of dual crosslinked alginate-chitosan blend gel beads and *in vitro* controlled release in oral site-specific drug delivery system. *Int. J. Pharm.* **2007**, *336*, 329–337. [CrossRef] [PubMed]

24.   Lucinda-Silva, R.M.; Evangelista, M.C. Microspheres of alginate-chitosan containing isoziadin. *J. Microencapsul.* **2003**, *20*, 145–152. [CrossRef]

25.   World Health Organisation. *Antimicrobial Resistance: Global Report on Surveillance*; WHO Press: Geneva, Switzerland, 2014.

26. Cortivo, R.; Vindigni, V.; Iacobellis, L.; Abatangelo, G.; Pinton, P.; Zavan, B. Nanoscale particle therapies for wounds and ulcers. *Nanomedicine* **2010**, *5*, 641–656. [CrossRef] [PubMed]

27. Goh, Y.F.; Shakir, I.; Hussain, R. Electrospun fibers for tissue engineering, drug delivery, and wound dressing. *J. Mater. Sci.* **2013**, *48*, 3027–3054. [CrossRef]

28. Hussain, S.M.; Hess, K.L.; Gearhart, J.M.; Geiss, K.T.; Schlager, J.J. In vitro toxicity of nanoparticles in BRL 3A rat liver cells. *Toxicol. In Vitro* **2005**, *19*, 975–983. [CrossRef] [PubMed]

29. Muzzarelli, R.A.A. Chitins and chitosans for the repair of wounded skin, nerve cartilage and bone. *Carbohydr. Polym.* **2009**, *76*, 167–182. [CrossRef]

30. Kong, M.; Chen, X.G.; Xing, K.; Park, H.J. Antimicrobial properties of chitosan and mode of action: A state of the art review. *Int. J. Food Microbiol.* **2010**, *144*, 51–63. [CrossRef] [PubMed]

31. Chung, Y.C.; Yeh, J.Y.; Tsai, C.F. Antibacterial characteristics and activity of water-soluble chitosan derivatives prepared by the Maillard reaction. *Molecules* **2011**, *16*, 8504–8514. [CrossRef] [PubMed]

32. Kyzas, G.Z.; Bikiaris, D.N. Recent modifications of chitosan for adsorption applications: A critical and systematic review. *Mar. Drugs* **2015**, *13*, 312–337. [CrossRef] [PubMed]

33. Signini, R.; Desbrières, J.; Campana Filho, S.P. On the stiffness of chitosan hydrochloride in acid-free aqueous solutions. *Carbohydr. Polym.* **2000**, *43*, 351–357. [CrossRef]

34. Signini, R.; Campana Filho, S.P. On the preparation and characterization of chitosan hydrochloride. *Polym. Bull.* **1999**, *42*, 159–166. [CrossRef]

35. Draget, K.I.; Oestgaard, K.; Smidsrod, O. Homogeneous alginate gels: A technical approach. *Carbohydr. Polym.* **1990**, *14*, 159–178. [CrossRef]

36. Draget, K.I.; Skjak-Braek, G.; Smidsrod, O. Alginate based new materials. *Int. J. Biol. Macromol.* **1997**, *21*, 47–55. [CrossRef] [PubMed]

37. Catanzano, O.; Straccia, M.C.; Miro, A.; Ungaro, F.; Romano, I.; Mazzarella, G.; Santagata, G.; Quaglia, F.; Laurienzo, P.; Malinconico, M.; *et al. Spray-by-Spray in situ* cross-linking alginate hydrogels delivering a tea tree oil microemulsion. *Eur. J. Pharm. Sci.* **2015**, *66*, 20–28. [CrossRef]

38. Alexander, B.R.; Murphy, K.E.; Gallagher, J.; Farrell, G.F.; Taggart, G. Gelation time, homogeneity, and rupture testing of alginate-calcium carbonate-hydrogen peroxide gels for use as wound dressings. *J. Biomed. Mater. Res. B* **2012**, *100B*, 425–431. [CrossRef]

39. Del Nobile, M.A.; Laurienzo, P.; Malinconico, M.; Mensitieri, G.; Nicolais, L. New functionalized ethylene/vinyl alcohol co-polymers: Synthesis and water vapour transport properties. *Packag. Technol. Sci.* **1997**, *10*, 95–108. [CrossRef]

40. Insan, N.G.; Payal, N.; Singh, M.; Yadav, A.; Chaudhary, B.; Srivastava, A. Post operative wound infection: Bacteriology and antibiotic sensitivity pattern. *Int. J. Cur. Res. Rev.* **2013**, *5*, 74–79.

41. Rossi, S.; Marciello, M.; Sandri, G.; Ferrari, F.; Bonferoni, M.C.; Papetti, A.; Caramella, C.; Dacarro, C.; Grisoli, P. Wound dressings based on chitosan and hyaluronic acid for the release of chlorhexidine diacetate in skin ulcer therapy. *Pharm. Dev. Technol.* **2007**, *12*, 415–422. [CrossRef] [PubMed]

42. Oliva, A.; Passaro, I.; di Pasquale, A.; di Feo, A.; Criscuolo, M.; Zappia, V.; Della Ragione, F.; D'Amato, S.; Annunziata, M.; Guida, L. *Ex vivo* expansion of bone marrow stromal cells by platelet-rich plasma: A promising strategy in maxillo facial surgery. *Int. J. Immunopathol. Pharmacol.* **2006**, *19*, 47–53.

43. Amsterdam, D. Susceptibility testing of antimicrobials in liquid media. In *Antibiotics in Laboratory Medicine*, 4th ed.; Loman, V., Ed.; Williams & Wilkins: Baltimore, MD, USA, 1996; pp. 52–111.

44. Wiegand, I.; Hilpert, K.; Hancock, R.E. Agar and broth dilution methods to determine the minimal inhibitory concentration (MIC) of antimicrobial substances. *Nat. Protoc.* **2008**, *3*, 163–175. [CrossRef] [PubMed]

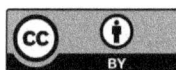

![marine drugs logo] *marine drugs*

MDPI

Article

Chitin-Lignin Material as a Novel Matrix for Enzyme Immobilization

Jakub Zdarta [1], Łukasz Klapiszewski [1], Marcin Wysokowski [1], Małgorzata Norman [1], Agnieszka Kołodziejczak-Radzimska [1], Dariusz Moszyński [2], Hermann Ehrlich [3], Hieronim Maciejewski [4,5], Allison L. Stelling [6] and Teofil Jesionowski [1,*]

[1] Institute of Chemical Technology and Engineering, Faculty of Chemical Technology, Poznan University of Technology, Berdychowo 4, 60965 Poznan, Poland; jakub_zdarta@wp.pl (J.Z.); lukasz.klapiszewski@put.poznan.pl (L.K.); wysokowski@wp.pl (M.W.); malgorzata.norman@hotmail.com (M.N.); agnieszka.kolodziejczak-radzimska@put.poznan.pl (A.K.-R.)
[2] Institute of Inorganic Chemical Technology and Environmental Engineering, West Pomeranian University of Technology, Pulaskiego 10, 70322 Szczecin, Poland; dmoszynski@zut.edu.pl
[3] Institute of Experimental Physics, TU Bergakademie Freiberg, Leipziger Str. 23, 09599 Freiberg, Germany; Hermann.Ehrlich@physik.tu-freiberg.de
[4] Adam Mickiewicz University in Poznan, Faculty of Chemistry, Umultowska 89b, 61614 Poznan, Poland; maciejm@amu.edu.pl
[5] Poznan Science and Technology Park, Adam Mickiewicz University Fundation, Rubież 46, 61612 Poznan, Poland
[6] Duke University, Center for Materials Genomics, Department of Mechanical Engineering and Materials Science,144 Hudson Hall, Durham, NC 27708, USA; antistokes@gmail.com
* Author to whom correspondence should be addressed; teofil.jesionowski@put.poznan.pl; Tel.: +48-61-665-37-20; Fax: +48-61-665-36-49.

Academic Editor: Paola Laurienzo
Received: 19 February 2015; Accepted: 27 March 2015; Published: 20 April 2015

Abstract: Innovative materials were made via the combination of chitin and lignin, and the immobilization of lipase from *Aspergillus niger*. Analysis by techniques including FTIR, XPS and ^{13}C CP MAS NMR confirmed the effective immobilization of the enzyme on the surface of the composite support. The electrokinetic properties of the resulting systems were also determined. Results obtained from elemental analysis and by the Bradford method enabled the determination of optimum parameters for the immobilization process. Based on the hydrolysis reaction of para-nitrophenyl palmitate, a determination was made of the catalytic activity, thermal and pH stability, and reusability. The systems with immobilized enzymes were found to have a hydrolytic activity of 5.72 mU, and increased thermal and pH stability compared with the native lipase. The products were also shown to retain approximately 80% of their initial catalytic activity, even after 20 reaction cycles. The immobilization process, using a cheap, non-toxic matrix of natural origin, leads to systems with potential applications in wastewater remediation processes and in biosensors.

Keywords: chitin-lignin matrix; enzyme immobilization; hydrolytic activity; lipase; immobilized lipase stability

1. Introduction

Continuing technological progress means that scientists are constantly finding new solutions that make use of lignin and its derivatives. When suitably modified, lignin is a polarographically active material [1] capable of undergoing a variety of electrochemical reactions, in the course of both oxidation and reduction [2]. Consequently, in recent years it has found interesting applications in electrochemistry. One of these was the creation of a cheap and fully environmentally friendly cathode, developed by Milczarek and Inganäs [3]. The valuable properties of lignin and its particular structure had previously been exploited by Milczarek in the construction of electrochemical sensors and detectors, as described in [4–7]. Interesting work using lignin-based material to create an innovative, cheap battery was reported by Gnedenkov *et al.* [8–10]. Literature reports also indicate the possibility of using lignocellulose materials, including pure lignin, as a filler in a wide range of polymers, both in strongly polar (poly(ethylene terephthalate)—PET; poly(ethylene oxide)—PEO) [11,12] and in hydrophobic (polypropylene—PP) [13,14] polymer matrices. Studies have also been carried out using poly(vinyl chloride) [15]. The biopolymer may also serve as a potential cheap and easily available biosorbent for environmentally harmful metal ions [16–20]. As a sorbent, lignin may be obtained chiefly as a waste product of the paper industry, and subjected to chemical modification to increase the number of functional groups [21,22]. It has also been reported that lignin has multifunctional barrier properties, protecting against harmful UV radiation, as well as antibacterial properties [23]. There are also promising possibilities for the use of lignin in the pharmaceutical industry and in medicine.

Chitin is an aminopolysaccharide, built of a long polymer chain consisting of *N*-acetylglucosamine units connected by β-1,4-glycoside bonds [24]. Chitin is a natural polymer, obtained chiefly from the shells of marine invertebrates, including the marine sponges [25–28]. It is friendly to the natural environment, and it exhibits high chemical stability and high reactivity, and is also non-toxic, bioactive, biodegradable and biocompatible [29]. Because of these features it is used in many areas of biomedicine and biotechnology [30,31]. One of these fields is the immobilization of enzymes [32–34]. Krajewska [35] presents a wide-ranging review of the literature concerning the use of chitin as a support for many catalytic proteins. Enzymes were immobilized by cross-linking with chitin by glutaraldehyde to reduce the viscosity of fruit and vegetable juices [36]. Outside the food industry, mention might be made of the use of enzymes immobilized on chitin via physisorption [37] or with the formation of covalent bonds [38] to detect and remove phenols. One of the most industrially useful groups of enzymes are the lipases, which are hydrophobic enzymes. To take full advantage of their technical and economic possibilities, they are used in a form immobilized on chitin [39]. An important factor in the widespread use of chitin as a support is the universality of the forms in which it can be used. Available morphological forms include powder, flakes, beads, nanoscale whiskers and fibers [40].

The creation of a stable material with defined properties provides the possibility of combining the undoubted advantages of both precursors, such as the aforementioned biocompatibility and non-toxicity, in the process of enzyme immobilization. The presence of multiple reactive functional groups in the structure of both materials increases their affinity to biomolecules [41]. It should be noted that the fact that the matrix is made using relatively cheap waste materials has a positive impact with regard to the economic aspects of the immobilization process [42]. The systems so produced may have potential uses in many fields where there is a need for highly pure and non-toxic catalysts.

The aim of the present study was to use a chitin-lignin material as a novel matrix for immobilization by adsorption of the lipase from *Aspergillus niger*. This is work of an innovative aspect, because there are no reports in the literature concerning the use of this system in enzyme immobilization. The systems produced may find uses in the transesterification and hydrolysis of a wide range of compounds, as well as in the production of biosensors. The results of the analysis confirmed the effective immobilization of the lipase on the chitin-lignin support. A detailed analysis was also made of the effect of process parameters on the properties of the resulting systems, and it was shown that lipase immobilized on the composite offers greater thermal and chemical stability than the native enzyme.

2. Results and Discussion

2.1. Physicochemical Evaluation

2.1.1. FTIR Spectroscopy

Figure 1 shows the FTIR spectra of the chitin–lignin material, lipase from *Aspergillus niger* (Figure 1a), and the products following enzyme immobilization (Figure 1b). The major bands are summarized in Table 1.

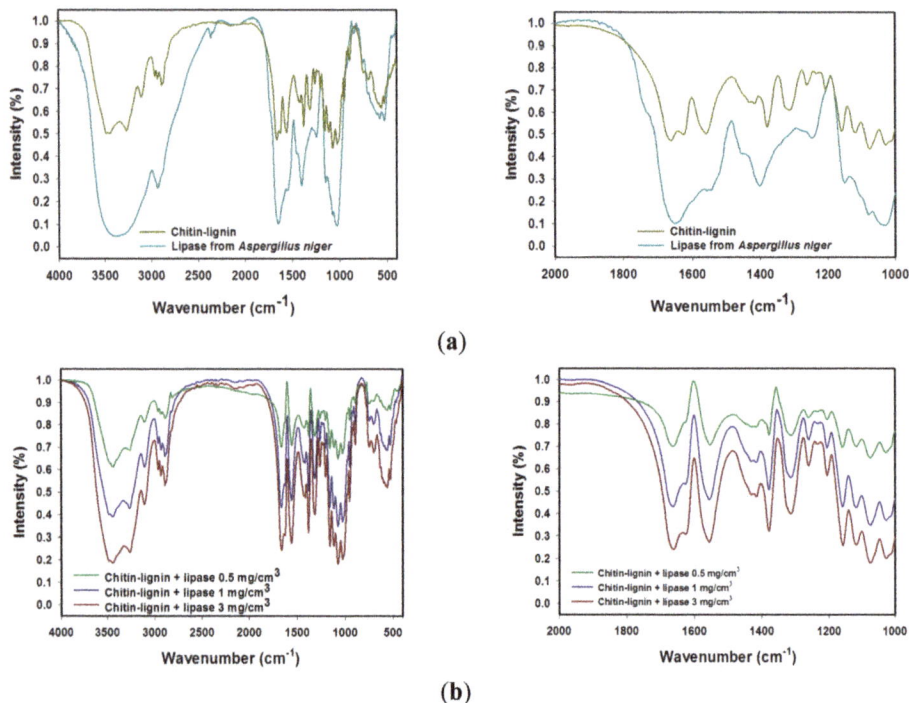

Figure 1. FTIR spectra of chitin-lignin composite and lipase (**a**) and selected products following 24 h of enzyme immobilization (**b**), in two different spectral range.

Table 1. Maximal vibrational wavenumbers (cm^{-1}) attributed to lipase from *Aspergillus niger*, chitin-lignin material, and products following immobilization.

Lipase from *Aspergillus niger*	Chitin-Lignin Material	Products after Immobilization	Vibrational Assignment
3460	3444	3457	O-H stretching
3242	3257	3264	N-H stretching
-	3111	3112	C_{Ar}-H stretching
2931	2965, 2930, 2877	2966, 2935, 2879	CH_x stretching
-	1674	1676	C=O stretching
1647	1625	1639	amide I stretching
1546	1556	1552	amide II bending
1448	1432	1438	CH_2 bending
-	1420	1417	C_{Ar}-C_{Ar} stretching
1402	1388	1401	O-H stretching
-	1323	1329	C-O (syringyl unit) streching
1257	1268	1261	amide III bending
1151, 1073, 1037	1158, 1116, 1077, 1022	1162, 1113, 1081, 1027	C-O-C (ring), C-O stretching
-	953	957	CH_3 bending
-	903	905	β-1,4-glycosidic bonds
-	745	745	aromatic C-H(guaiacyl unit), bending
576	558	571	N-H bending
531	527	530	C-C scissoring

Analysis of the FTIR spectrum of the enzyme prior to immobilization shows the presence of a band in the range 3550–3200 cm^{-1} associated with stretching vibrations of O-H and N-H groups, and one at wavenumber 2931 cm^{-1} from stretching vibrations of C-H (CH_3 and CH_2). The most important signals in the spectrum of the native lipase are peaks at wavenumbers 1647 cm^{-1}, 1546 cm^{-1} and 1257 cm^{-1}, whose presence is characteristic of stretching vibrations of amide I, II and III bonds [43,44]. The FTIR spectrum of the enzyme also features a peak at wavenumber 1402 cm^{-1}, generated by stretching vibrations of O-H groups, and a low-intensity signal at 1448 cm^{-1} confirming the presence of bending vibrations of CH_2. The group of signals at 1151 cm^{-1}, 1073 cm^{-1} and 1037 cm^{-1} are associated with the presence of C-O-C bonds in the protein structure [45]. In addition, of note are two signals below 1000 cm^{-1}: at 576 cm^{-1} a band of N-H stretching vibrations, and at 531 cm^{-1} a band of scissor vibrations of the C-C bonds forming the skeleton of the enzyme structure [46].

Analysis of the spectrum of the chitin–lignin matrix confirms that the expected product was obtained. It also features a large number of bands, this being a result of the complex structure of the system. Attention is drawn to the bands with maxima at 3444 cm^{-1} and 3257 cm^{-1}, attributed to stretching vibrations of O-H and N-H groups. A peak with a maximum at 3111 cm^{-1} is associated with stretching vibrations of C_{Ar}-H groups present in the lignin structure [47]. A series of signals in the range 2970–2870 cm^{-1} confirms the presence of CH_2 and CH_3 groups in the structure of the composite, while the distinct band with a maximum at 1674 cm^{-1} comes from stretching vibrations of C=O bonds. Four signals between 1160 cm^{-1} and 1020 cm^{-1} can be attributed to stretching vibrations of C-O-C bonds in the glucose ring in chitin, as well as other C-O bonds in the material [48]. The interpretation of the carbon–oxygen bonds present in the system is supplemented by a peak at wavenumber 905 cm^{-1}, which is a consequence of the β-1,4-glycosidic bonds in chitin [49]. Note should also be taken of the signals originating from vibrations of amide I, II and III bonds. These are bands analogous to those present in the enzyme structure, but appearing at slightly different wavenumbers, respectively 1639 cm^{-1}, 1552 cm^{-1} and 1261 cm^{-1}, as a result of the different chemical environment of the bonds. Very significant bands, confirming the production of a chitin–lignin material, are present at 1420 cm^{-1},

1329 cm^{-1} and 745 cm^{-1}, and originate from the stretching and bending vibrations of the aromatic structures present in lignin [50].

The FTIR spectra of the systems following immobilization carried out for 24 h using solutions of the enzyme in various concentrations are shown in Figure 1b. Analysis of the data obtained shows that the lipase was effectively immobilized on the matrix surface. In spite of the similarity of the bands present on the spectra of the support and the enzyme, an indication is provided by the presence of signals associated with vibrations of amide I, II and III bonds contained in the protein structure, at wavenumbers 1639 cm^{-1}, 1552 cm^{-1} and 1261 cm^{-1} respectively [51]. The intensity of these bands increases, and their absorption maxima are shifted, compared with the spectrum of the support. Analogous observations apply to the signals from stretching vibrations of O-H groups at wavenumber 3457 cm^{-1}, and from stretching vibrations of C=O bonds at 1676 cm^{-1}. The changes provide additional evidence confirming the immobilization, as well as indicating hydrogen bonding between the matrix and enzyme [52]. It is also interesting that as the concentration of the enzyme solution used for immobilization increases, particular bands in the product spectra become more intense. This provides indirect evidence that there is also an increase in the quantity of the enzyme deposited on the matrix surface.

2.1.2. ^{13}C CP MAS NMR Spectroscopy

Figure 2 shows the ^{13}C CP MAS NMR spectra of the obtained chitin–lignin material, the native lipase, and the product following 24 h of immobilization of the enzyme from solution at a concentration of 3 mg/cm^3.

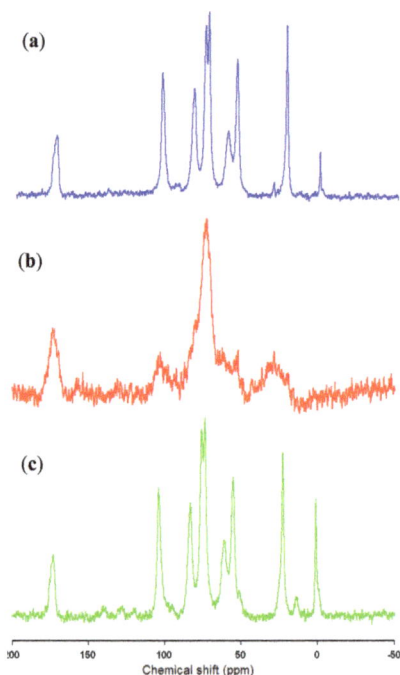

Figure 2. ^{13}C CP MAS NMR spectra of chitin-lignin (**a**); lipase (**b**) and chitin-lignin matrix with immobilized enzyme (**c**).

The ^{13}C CP MAS NMR spectrum of the chitin-lignin material shows the presence of signals characteristic of the precursors, which provides confirmation of the effective formation of the expected material. The signal at 22 ppm originates from the carbon in CH$_3$ in acetamide groups from chitin, while the entire group of peaks in the range 55–105 ppm is generated by carbon atoms in N-acetylglucosamine mers [53]. The distinct signal at 175 ppm originates from the carbonyl carbons in acetamide groups in the chitin structure [54]. The spectrum of the immobilized enzyme provides confirmation of the previous findings concerning the great similarity in structure of the lipase and the chitin; which is the chief component of the composite. The spectrum of the protein contains two clear signals, with maxima at 76 and 177 ppm, as well as several bands of much smaller intensity and wider range. The spectrum of the product formed after immobilization, in view of the similarity of the spectra of the precursors, does not show many changes. There is a different shape, particularly at the base, in the signals at 56 and 107 ppm. There is also a characteristic area between 115 and 145 ppm, where there appear signals which were not observed in the spectrum of the support, but which appear with low intensity in the spectrum of the native enzyme. Analysis of the ^{13}C CP MAS NMR spectra confirms the effectiveness of the immobilization process and the immobilization of the enzyme on the surface of the chitin-lignin matrix. In addition, in the case of the signals on the spectrum of the system after immobilization, there is seen to be a small shift in their maxima, which may suggest that the protein is attached to the support by way of the formation of hydrogen bonds.

2.1.3. Elemental Analysis

Table 2 contains the results of elemental analysis, describing the change in the content of such elements as nitrogen, carbon, hydrogen and sulfur in the immobilized enzyme preparations and in the matrix used.

Table 2. Elemental content of examined elements in the chitin-lignin matrix and in products following immobilization.

Enzyme Solution Concentration (mg/cm³)	Immobilization Time	Elemental Content (%)			
		N	C	H	S
Chitin-lignin matrix		5.07	33.86	4.93	0.03
0.5	1 min	5.23	35.42	5.40	0.02
	2 h	5.58	37.17	5.67	0.01
	24 h	6.41	37.77	5.73	0.03
1.0	1 min	5.75	38.31	5.54	0.01
	2 h	5.96	38.77	5.78	0.03
	24 h	6.66	39.81	5.95	0.02
3.0	1 min	5.96	39.01	5.91	0.03
	2 h	6.03	39.30	6.05	0.02
	24 h	6.77	39.92	6.07	0.02

The initial matrix, prior to enzyme immobilization, has a carbon content of 33.86% and a hydrogen content of 4.93%. These elements are present in the structure of both lignin and chitin. Nitrogen, found in the elemental composition of the hybrid material with a content of 5.07%, is associated with the presence of N-acetylglucosamine groups in chitin. The presence of sulfur in the composite is explained by the use of sulfuric acid in the kraft process used to produce the lignin precursor.

The elemental analysis of systems resulting from the immobilization of lipase on the surface of the chitin-lignin matrix showed an increase in the contents of carbon, nitrogen and hydrogen, compared with the initial material. These changes are a result of the presence of those three elements in the structure of the enzyme, and confirm the effective immobilization of the protein on the surface of the support. The increase in the content of the analyzed components with higher initial concentration of protein solution and longer time of immobilization indicates that both of these parameters have a significant effect on the quantity of enzyme immobilized. The most distinct changes compared with the chitin–lignin material were observed for the system produced following a process lasting 24 h using a solution of concentration 3 mg/cm^3, which may be taken as confirmation that the greatest quantity of protein was immobilized under such conditions.

2.1.4. XPS Analysis

The surface composition for samples of lipase, chitin–lignin material and the product following enzyme immobilization was examined with X-ray photoelectron spectroscopy. The surface of all samples is composed of carbon, oxygen and nitrogen. Some traces of calcium, potassium and sulfur were detected, but these are not considered in the quantitative calculations. The elemental surface compositions calculated from XPS data are given in Table 3.

Table 3. Elemental composition of the surface of samples.

Sample Name	Atomic %			N/C Ratio	O/C Ratio
	C	O	N	H	S
Lipase	58.2	30.7	11.1	0.19	0.53
Chitin-lignin matrix	61.4	32.6	6.0	0.10	0.53
Chitin-lignin + lipase	62.5	30.0	7.5	0.12	0.48

The elemental composition of the lipase as reported by Tomizuka *et al.* and expressed as a C:O:N molar ratio is 61:25:14 [55]. These values are in good agreement with the ratio obtained in the present study for the surface of lipase, namely 58:31:11. Similar good agreement is obtained for the surface composition of the chitin-lignin matrix, which was reported previously [53]. The oxygen-carbon ratio close to 0.5 obtained for chitin-lignin, as well as the surface composition of the matrix, are very close to the values observed for nanocrystalline chitin [56]. Since the elemental composition of lignin differs significantly from the ratio observed here, it is concluded that the surface of the support matrix is composed mainly of chitin. The nitrogen-carbon ratio is almost twice as high for the lipase as for the chitin-lignin material. Therefore an increase in this parameter can be used as an indicator for successful enzyme immobilization, as reported previously [57]. Indeed the N/C ratio increases from 0.10 for the pure chitin-lignin matrix to 0.12 for the sample after immobilization. The elemental analysis of samples before and after immobilization, as described in Section 2.1.3., indicates an increase of approximately 20% in the nitrogen content after enzyme immobilization. This is corroborated by XPS data. This increase in nitrogen concentration following the immobilization process is taken as indirect evidence of successful lipase immobilization.

Evaluation of the chemical composition of the surface of the examined materials is based mainly on analysis of the XPS C 1s peak. The spectra have a relatively complex profile (Figure 3). Deconvolution of the experimental data was performed using a model consisting of four basic components of the C 1s transition: C_1–C_4. Component C_1, with a binding energy of 284.4 ± 0.1 eV, corresponds essentially to non-functionalized carbon atoms located in the aromatic rings expected to be in the lignin structure. Component C_2, with a binding energy of 284.8 eV, is attributed to all other non-functionalized sp^2 and sp^3 carbon atoms, bonded either to other carbon or to hydrogen atoms. Component C_3, shifted by 1.4 ± 0.2 eV from component C_2 in the direction of increasing binding energies, is attributed to a set of groups with a carbon atom bonded to one atom of oxygen or nitrogen. These include the following functional groups which are presumed to be present in the studied materials: C-O-C, C-OH, C-N-C, C-NH$_2$. Component C_4, shifted by 2.9 ± 0.2 eV from component C_2 in the direction of increasing binding energies, also corresponds to a set of functional groups: C=O, O-C-O, N-C-O and N-C=O. The binding energy interpretations given above are based on the energy shifts given in Appendix E [58]. A relative surface functional group composition obtained from decomposition of the C 1s signal is given in Table 4. The total C 1s peak intensity is taken as 100.

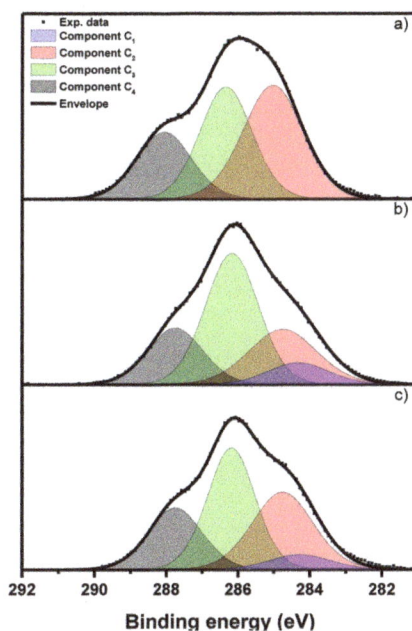

Figure 3. The XPS C 1s spectra for chitin-lignin (**a**); lipase (**b**); and the chitin-lignin + lipase product (**c**).

Table 4. Distribution of functional groups calculated on the basis of the deconvolution model of the XPS C 1s peak.

Sample Name	Total C 1s Peak Intensity (%)			
	C_1	C_2	C_3	C_4
Lipase	-	42	36	22
Chitin-lignin	9	25	46	20
Chitin-lignin + lipase	6	32	39	23

Since lipase contains a relatively small number of aromatic rings, originating from amino acids such as phenylalanine or tyrosine [55], the component C_1 is not considered in the deconvolution of the C 1s spectrum for that substance. Component C_2 prevails in the XPS signal, followed by C_3. The support material is a mixture of chitin and lignin. The expected component ratio for pure chitin is $C_2:C_3:C_4 = 25:50:25$ [59], while the ratio $(C_1 + C_2):C_3:C_4$ observed for lignin is 65:29:3 [60]. On the surface of the chitin–lignin matrix observed here, the contributions of components C_1 and C_2 are lower than would be given by a simple average for the mixture of chitin and lignin. Therefore, as suggested earlier, it is concluded that chitin prevails on the surface of the support. Comparison of the spectra of the chitin-lignin material and the product following enzyme immobilization indicates that C_1 diminishes slightly, while C_2 increases. Since C_2 is dominant in the XPS spectrum of lipase, we believe this to be an indication of successful enzyme immobilization.

Some additional evidence of the successful immobilization of lipase on the chitin-lignin matrix can be observed in the XPS O 1s spectra shown in Figure 4. The XPS O 1s transition observed for lipase is symmetric, with a maximum at binding energy 531.8 eV (dotted curve). In the case of the chitin-lignin matrix and the product of enzyme immobilization, the maximum of the O 1s peak is shifted in the direction of high binding energy to 532.4 eV. The structure of both chitin and lignin is dominated by C-OH groups, while in the case of the lipase a more equal ratio between hydroxyl and carboxyl groups is expected. The characteristic position of the O 1s peak for C-OH groups is approximately 532.5 eV, while its position for C=O groups is reported to be about 531.3 eV [61]. Accordingly, a shift in the XPS O 1s spectra is observed between the lipase and chitin-lignin. A small difference is also observed between the profile of the O 1s peak for chitin-lignin and for the chitin-lignin + lipase product. On the high-energy side of the spectrum the intensity of the O 1s peak obtained for the product following enzyme immobilization is slightly higher than the intensity of the peak obtained for the chitin-lignin support. The difference is small, but considering the relatively low quantity of immobilized lipase, it can be taken as confirmation of the increased concentration of C=O groups, which is an expected result of lipase being attached to the support.

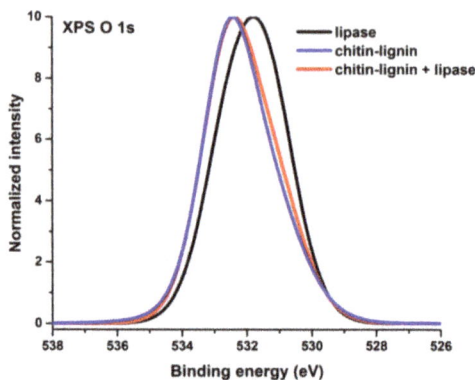

Figure 4. XPS O 1s spectra for lipase, chitin-lignin matrix and the product following enzyme immobilization.

XPS analysis provides no direct confirmation of lipase immobilization, since there is no apparent evidence of the formation of a new chemical environment. However, the formation of hydrogen bonds is not excluded. Moreover, the increase in the nitrogen-carbon ratio in combination with the subtle changes in the C 1s and O 1s component ratios can be considered an indication of successful immobilization of the enzyme.

2.1.5. Electrokinetic Characteristic

Studies of zeta potential and the effect of pH provide very valuable data about the electrokinetic properties of dispersed systems. Figure 5 shows the results obtained. Determination of the zeta potential of the biocomposite with and without immobilized enzyme provides indirect confirmation of the effectiveness of the suggested method of immobilization. The graph shows the values of the zeta potential obtained for selected samples following immobilization for 24 h.

The zeta potential of the chitin–lignin system is negative over the whole of the investigated pH range, and the isoelectric point is not attained. This results from the presence of specific functional groups (-COOH and -OH) on the surface of the component biopolymers. The electrokinetic potential of pure kraft lignin is even more negative; its value increased when the lignin was combined with chitin (due to the presence of surface NH_2 functional groups, which in an acidic environment can undergo protonation to NH_3^+) [53]. Lipase consists of several amino acids. The high percentage of acidic amino acids (Asp and Glu) gives the molecule a net negative charge, which is higher than the total for the positively charged residues (Arg, Lys, and His) [62]. That is why the isoelectric point of this protein is about 4 [63,64]. This value indicates that only at pH values below it will the surface charge (and indirectly zeta potential) be positive. The absolute value of zeta potential of chitin-lignin + lipase is smaller than this for matrix, especially in acidic condition, which can be explained by adsorption of lipase.

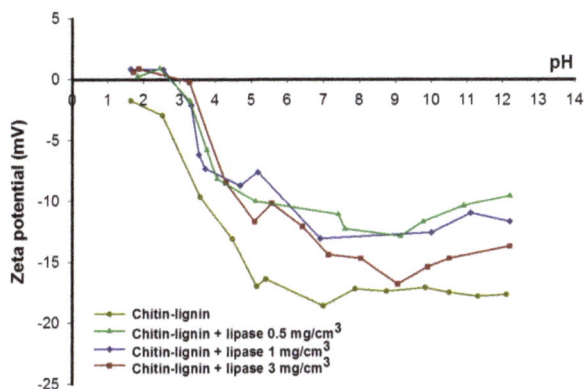

Figure 5. The zeta potential, as a function of pH, of the chitin-lignin material and selected products following immobilization.

Following immobilization of the enzyme on the surface of the support, as a result of interactions between the surface groups of the support and of the enzyme, the absolute values of the zeta potential decreased. This provides indirect evidence of the adsorptive nature of the attachment of the enzyme to the chitin–lignin support [65–67]. There was a decrease in the number of the free functional groups which are responsible for generating the charge. In addition, the chitin-lignin products upon addition of enzyme attain their isoelectric point (the pH at which the zeta potential is zero), which had previously not been observed. From the measured values of zeta potential it can be concluded that the quantity of immobilized enzyme influences its electrokinetic properties [68]. Nevertheless, irrespective of the quantity of adsorbed enzyme, the value of the isoelectric point is 2.7.

2.1.6. Quantity of Immobilized Enzyme

Based on the Bradford method [69] it was determined how the quantity of enzyme immobilized on the surface of the chitin-lignin support is affected by the concentration of the solution used in the immobilization process, and by the duration of the process. Table 5 contains detailed data on the quantity of biocatalyst adsorbed, depending on the concentration of the protein solution and the time of the process. The results are presented in terms of milligrams of enzyme per 1 gram of used matrix.

The results show that increasing the time of the immobilization process causes greater quantities of enzyme to be adsorbed. It should nonetheless be noted that the greatest increase in adsorbed protein occurs in the initial stages of the process. After the process time exceeds 4 h, the quantity of immobilized biocatalyst does not increase significantly, and the maximum change, depending on the concentration of the enzyme solution, is approximately 2 mg/g.

Table 5. Content of investigated elements in the chitin-lignin matrix and in the products following immobilization.

Immobilization Time	Concentration of Enzyme Solution (mg/cm^3)		
	0.5	1	3
	Amount of Immobilized Enzyme (mg/g)		
1 min	1.45	5.13	6.19
1 h	6.23	9.76	14.97
2 h	8.17	10.84	18.46
4 h	8.58	11.37	18.72
24 h	9.22	11.84	19.31
96 h	9.94	12.57	20.28

Another parameter having a significant effect on the quantity of protein in the products following immobilization is the concentration of the solution used. The results show that the greatest quantity of protein is adsorbed from the solution with a concentration of 3 mg/cm^3. When identical times of immobilization are compared, this solution enables the adsorption of more than twice as much protein as when a solution of concentration 0.5 mg/cm^3 is used.

The greatest quantity of the enzyme was adsorbed from the solution with a concentration of 3 mg/cm^3 following a process lasting 96 h. However, the optimum time of the immobilization process is 4 h, enabling comparable quantities of protein to be immobilized in a much shorter time, which has a positive impact on the economics of the studied process.

2.2. Hydrolytic Activity

2.2.1. Determination of Hydrolytic Activity

The hydrolytic activity of the free and immobilized enzyme was assessed spectrophotometrically based on the hydrolysis reaction of para-nitrophenyl palmitate. Figure 6 shows the results for catalytic activity of preparations with immobilized lipase obtained using enzyme solutions with concentrations of 0.5, 1 and 3 mg/cm^3, subjected to immobilization over different time intervals. The measurements were performed at 30 °C.

The systems with immobilized enzymes have lower catalytic activity than the native lipase, for which the activity is measured at 7.46 mU. Irrespective of the concentration of the protein solution, the greatest activity is found for the products formed after 4 h of immobilization. The results showed the enzyme solution with a concentration of 3 mg/cm^3 to be optimum for immobilization on a chitin–lignin support. The resulting immobilized lipase has the highest activity of all of the systems investigated, equal to 5.76 mU. This sample was selected for further analysis to determine the stability of the resulting system depending on the conditions of the catalyzed reaction.

The results show unambiguously that a greater quantity of immobilized enzyme does not lead directly to an increase in the system's catalytic activity. The products obtained following 96 h of immobilization, which have the greatest quantities of immobilized protein, exhibit a lower activity. This is caused by the accumulation of too great a quantity of the enzyme on the matrix surface, blocking the active sites on the biocatalyst and thus reducing its activity [70].

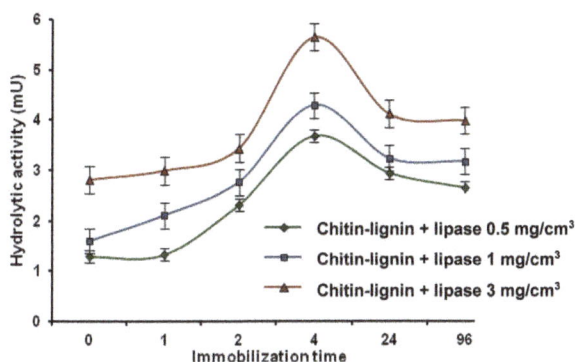

Figure 6. Graph showing changes in the catalytic activity of products depending on the time of immobilization and the concentration of the enzyme solution.

2.2.2. Thermal Stability

Thermal stability is one of the most important properties of immobilized enzymes. The thermal stability of the immobilized lipase was studied, in comparison with the native enzyme, over a temperature range of 10–80 °C. For this analysis, the system selected was one that underwent 4 h immobilization in the enzyme solution at a concentration of 3 mg/cm^3 in phosphate buffer at pH = 7. Figure 7 shows a comparison of the thermal stability of the native lipase with that of the lipase immobilized on a chitin-lignin matrix.

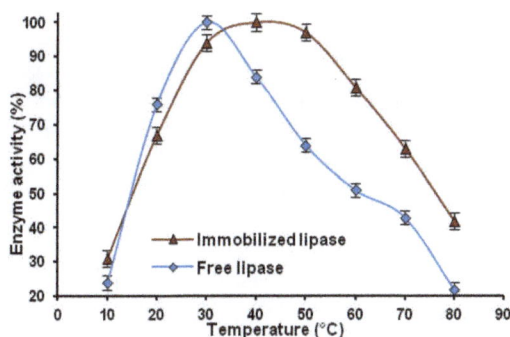

Figure 7. Graph of thermal stability of immobilized and native lipase in the temperature range 10–80 °C.

The native lipase attains its maximum hydrolytic activity at 30 °C, while that of the immobilized enzyme occurs at 40 °C. It should be noted, however, that the immobilized lipase retains more than 90% of its initial activity even at 50 °C, where the properties of the free enzyme are lost to a significant degree. These results show clearly that attaching the biocatalyst to a solid support has a positive effect on its resistance to denaturation at high temperature. This has been shown to be a result of an increase in the rigidity of the protein structure [71]. The thermal stability increased because the immobilization process could protect the tertiary structure of the peptide from conformational changes caused by the higher temperature [72].

2.2.3. pH Stability

The pH stability is an important characteristic of systems resulting from immobilization. The pH stability of the immobilized lipase, compared with that of the native enzyme, was studied over a pH range of 3 to 11 at 30 °C. Figure 8 shows a comparison of the pH stability of the native lipase with that of the lipase immobilized on a chitin-lignin matrix.

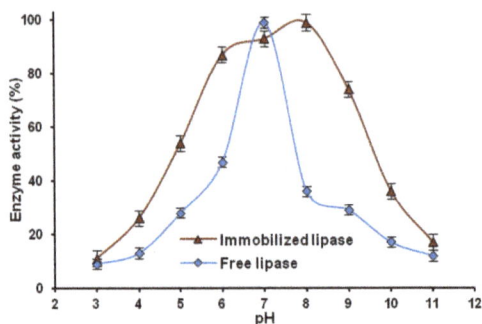

Figure 8. Graph showing changes in the catalytic active of immobilized and native lipase over the pH range 3–11.

The data above show that the pH has a large effect on the activity of the lipase in an aqueous environment. The activity of native lipase reaches a maximum at pH = 7, and small changes in pH cause a large decrease in hydrolytic activity, by as much as 50%. The immobilized lipase has its highest activity at pH = 8, which is characteristic of immobilized enzymes in this catalytic group [73]. The attachment of the enzyme to a solid support also causes it to retain more than 70% of its activity in the pH range 6–9. The improved stability of the immobilized enzyme compared with the native protein is probably a result of conformational changes taking place in the protein tertiary and quaternary structure following immobilization [74]. An increase in pH stability of the immobilized lipase is also connected with the changes in spatial orientation of secondary structure of the protein backbone, caused by the formation of hydrogen bonds between the enzyme and matrix [75].

2.2.4. Reusability

Figure 9 shows the reusability of the lipase immobilized on the chitin-lignin matrix over 20 cycles. In each cycle, the immobilized lipase was separated and washed with phosphate buffer, and the activity was calculated for p-NPP hydrolysis.

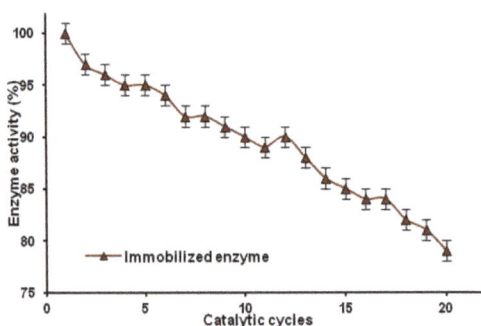

Figure 9. Changes in catalytic activity of immobilized lipase over 20 catalytic cycles.

The immobilized lipase was tested over 20 catalytic cycles, and was found to retain approximately 80% of its initial activity. The high reusability of products based on a chitin-lignin matrix may also lead to widespread use of this support in the immobilization of enzymes of other catalytic groups. Prolongation of the catalytic activity of these products may also lead to a significant reduction in the costs of carrying out reactions in real-life applications.

3. Experimental Section

3.1. Materials

The precursors, α-chitin powder from crab shells (technical grade) and kraft lignin (reagent grade), and 15% hydrogen peroxide as an oxidizing agent, were obtained from Sigma-Aldrich (Munich, Germany). Immobilization was carried out using commercial lipase from *Aspergillus niger* (Sigma-Aldrich, Munich, Germany) and phosphate buffer at pH = 7 (Amresco, Solon, OH, USA). The 85% phosphoric acid and 96% ethyl alcohol used in the Bradford method were obtained from Chempur (Piekary Śląskie, Poland). Coomassie Brilliant Blue G-250 (CBB G-250) was obtained from Sigma-Aldrich (Munich, Germany). The catalytic activity tests used para-nitrophenyl palmitate, Triton X-100 and gum arabic from Sigma-Aldrich (Munich, Germany) and 2-propanol from Chempur (Piekary Śląskie, Poland).

3.2. Preparation of Chitin-Lignin Material

The process of obtaining the chitin–lignin material (precursors ratio 1:1, *m/m*) began with the addition of 15 cm^3 of 15% hydrogen peroxide to the lignin, according to the procedure reported in previously published work [53]. The mixture was subjected to intensive mixing at approximately 800 rpm for about 30 min using a high-speed stirrer (Eurostar Digital, IKA Werke GmbH, Staufen, Germany). Chitin was then added to the reactor, and mixing continued for 60 min. The resulting chitin-lignin material was filtered under reduced pressure and washed with distilled water. The product was then dried in a convectional dryer (Memmert, Munich, Germany) at approximately 105 °C for about 24 h.

3.3. Enzyme Immobilization

The process of immobilization of lipase from *Aspergillus niger* on the surface of the chitin-lignin composite was carried out using solutions of the enzyme at concentrations of 0.5, 1 and 3 mg/cm^3 in a phosphate buffer at pH = 7, for times of 1 min and 1, 2, 4, 24 and 96 h. Quantities of 250 mg of the previously obtained matrix were placed in conical flasks, and 15 cm^3 of the solution of the enzyme in the required concentration was added. The mixture was placed in a KS260 BASIC shaker (IKA Werke GmbH, Staufen, Germany), and shaken for the required length of time. Afterwards the precipitate was filtered under reduced pressure and left to dry at room temperature for 24 h.

3.4. Physicochemical Evaluation

The presence of the expected functional groups was confirmed by Fourier transform infrared (FTIR) spectroscopy, using a Vertex 70 spectrophotometer (Bruker, Karlsruhe, Germany). The materials were analyzed in the form of tablets, made by placing a mixture of anhydrous KBr (*ca.* 0.25 g) and 1.5 mg of the tested substance in a steel ring under a pressure of 10 MPa. The tests were performed at a resolution of 0.5 cm^{-1} in the wavenumber range 4000–400 cm^{-1}.

^{13}C CP MAS NMR measurement was carried out on a DSX spectrometer (Bruker, Karlsruhe, Germany). For the determination of NMR spectra, a sample of approximately 100 mg was placed in a ZrO_2 rotator with diameter 4 mm, which enabled spinning of the sample. Centrifugation at the magic angle was performed at a spinning frequency of 8 kHz. The ^{13}C CP MAS NMR spectra were recorded at 100.63 MHz in a standard 4 mm MAS probe using single pulse excitation with high power proton decoupling (pulse repetition 10 s, spinning speed 8 kHz).

The elemental contents of the chitin-lignin hybrid material and the immobilized enzyme were determined using a Vario EL Cube instrument (Elementar Analysensysteme GmbH, Hanau, Germany), which is capable of registering the percentage content of carbon, hydrogen, nitrogen and sulfur in samples after high-temperature combustion. A properly weighed sample was placed in an 80-position autosampler and subjected to combustion. The decomposed sample was transferred in a stream of inert gas into an adsorption column. The results are given to ±0.01%, and each is obtained by averaging three measurements.

The X-ray photoelectron spectra were obtained using Al $K\alpha$ (hv = 1486.6 eV) radiation with a Prevac system equipped with a Scienta SES 2002 (VG Scienta, Uppsala, Sweden) electron energy analyzer operating at constant transmission energy (E_p = 50 eV). The spectrometer was calibrated using the following photoemission lines (with reference to the Fermi level): EB Cu $2p_{3/2}$ = 932.8 eV, EB Ag $3d_{5/2}$ = 368.3 eV, EB Au $4f_{7/2}$ = 84.0 eV. The instrumental resolution, as evaluated by the full width at half maximum (FWHM) of the Ag $3d_{5/2}$ peak, was 1.0 eV. The samples were placed loose in a grooved molybdenum sample holder. The analysis chamber was evacuated during the experiments to better than $1 \cdot 10^{-9}$ mbar. Data processing involved background subtraction by means of an "S-type" integral profile and a curve-fitting procedure (a mixed Gaussian–Lorentzian function was employed) based on a least-squares method (CasaXPS software). The experimental errors were estimated to be ±0.1 eV for the photoelectron peaks of carbon and oxygen. Charging effects were corrected using the C 1s component attributed after deconvolution to aliphatic carbon bonds (component C_2) and determined at 284.8 eV. The reproducibility of the peak position thus obtained was ±0.1 eV. The surface composition of the samples was obtained on the basis of the peak area intensities of the C 1s, O 1s, and N 1s transitions using the sensitivity factor approach and assuming homogeneous distribution of elements in the surface layer.

The electrokinetic stability of the materials with immobilized enzyme was determined on the basis of zeta potential dependence on pH, using a Zetasizer Nano ZS (Malvern Instruments Ltd., Worcestershire, UK) equipped with an autotitrator. Measurements were made in a 0.001 M NaCl solution over the pH range 2–12, using 0.001 M NaCl solution.

The quantity of immobilized enzyme was determined by the Bradford method [69]. A solution of the Bradford reagent was prepared by dissolving 10 mg of Coomassie Brilliant Blue G-250 in 5 cm^3 of 96% ethyl alcohol, 15 cm^3 of 85% phosphoric acid and 80 cm^3 of water. In a quartz cuvette, 4 cm^3 of the Bradford reagent was mixed with 800 μL of the analyzed protein solution and 100 μL water, and the analysis was performed 10 min after the preparation of the mixture. Measurements were made at wavelength 595 nm, using a JASCO 650 spectrophotometer (Jasco, Tokyo, Japan).

3.5. Evaluation of Hydrolytic Activity

The activity of the immobilized lipase was measured by the method used in our previous work [76], with slight modifications. Spectrophotometric measurements were made for 2 min at wavelength 410 nm at 30 °C, based on the transesterification reaction of para-nitrophenyl palmitate (p-NPP) to para-nitrophenyl (p-NP). Hydrolytic activity was measured in 1 cm^3 quartz cuvettes containing 5 mg of immobilized lipase with 2.7 cm^3 of substrate solution containing 10 mM phosphate buffer, 10 mM of p-NPP solution in 2-propanol, 0.44% mass fraction of Triton X-100 and 0.11% mass fraction of gum arabic. One mUnit of immobilized enzyme activity was defined as the release of 1 μmoL of p-NP per minute.

3.5.1. Thermal Stability

The thermal stability of the immobilized and native lipase was determined over a temperature range of 10–80 °C. Hydrolytic activity was calculated as described in Section 3.5.

3.5.2. pH Stability

The pH stability of the immobilized and native lipase was determined by incubating the substrate solution at different pH values (3, 5, 7, 9, 11) to compare the activity of the free and immobilized lipase. Catalytic activity was calculated as described in Section 3.5.

3.5.3. Reusability

The reusability of the immobilized lipase was determined by testing over 20 cycles. Between each reaction step, the chitin-lignin matrix with the immobilized enzyme was separated from the substrate solution by centrifugation and washed with phosphate buffer. The hydrolytic activity was calculated as described in Section 3.5.

4. Conclusions

In this study, a chitin-lignin system was used as an innovative matrix in the process of immobilizing lipase from *Aspergillus niger*. Detailed characteristics of the obtained matrix, and confirmation of the effective immobilization of the enzyme, were obtained using such techniques as FTIR, XPS, ^{13}C CP MAS NMR and elemental analysis. It was shown that both the time of the process and the initial concentration of the protein solution have a significant effect on the properties of the products obtained. A determination was also made of the quantity of enzyme immobilized on the surface of the system, and of the catalytic activity of the system following lipase immobilization. It was found that the immobilized lipase exhibits lower activity than the free enzyme, but retains its catalytic properties for a greater number of reaction cycles. The enzyme bound to the chitin-lignin matrix also has greater thermal and chemical stability than the native protein. Measurement of the zeta potential enabled determination of the electrokinetic properties of the systems obtained. Detailed analysis of the FTIR spectra of the products of the immobilization process, and changes in the zeta potential and shifts in signal maxima on ^{13}C CP MAS NMR spectra, indicate that the enzyme is attached by way of physical adsorption, probably through the formation of hydrogen bonds.

Acknowledgments: The study was financed within the Polish National Center of Science funds according to decision No. DEC-2013/09/B/ST8/00159.

Author Contributions: J.Z.: Planning studies. Preparation of functional chitin-lignin biosorbent. Evaluation of enzyme immobilization efficiency. Results development. Ł.K.: Analysis of physicochemical properties of the materials obtained. Results development. M.W.: Analysis of structural properties of the materials obtained. Results development. D.M.: Implementation and description of the XPS analysis. M.N.: Implementation and description of the zeta potential analysis. A.K.-R.: Evaluation of enzyme immobilization efficiency. Results development. H.E.: Supervising manuscript with data interpretation. H.M.: Supervising manuscript with data interpretation. A.L.S.: Supervising manuscript with data interpretation. T.J.: Coordination of all tasks in the paper. Planning studies. Results development.

Conflicts of Interest: The authors declare no conflict of interest.

References

1. Evstigneyev, E.; Shevchenko, S.; Mayorova, H.; Platonow, A. Polarographically active structural fragments of lignin. II. Dimeric model compounds and lignins. *J. Wood Chem. Technol.* **2004**, *24*, 263–278. [CrossRef]
2. Lund, H.; Baizer, M.M. *Organic Electrochemistry—An Introduction and Guide*; Marcel Dekker: New York, NY, USA, 1991.
3. Milczarek, G.; Inganäs, O. Renewable cathode materials from biopolymer/conjugated polymer interpenetrating networks. *Science* **2012**, *335*, 1468–1471. [CrossRef] [PubMed]
4. Milczarek, G. Preparation and characterization of a lignin modified electrode. *Electroanalsia* **2007**, *19*, 1411–1414. [CrossRef]
5. Milczarek, G. Preparation, characterization and electrocatalytic properties of an iodine/lignin modified gold electrode. *Electrochim. Acta* **2009**, *54*, 3199–3205. [CrossRef]
6. Milczarek, G. Lignosulfonate-modified electrodes: Electrochemical properties and electrocatalysis of NADH oxidation. *Langmuir* **2009**, *25*, 10345–10353. [CrossRef] [PubMed]

7.   Milczarek, G.; Rębiś, T. Synthesis and electroanalytical performance of a composite material based on poly(3,4-ethylenedioxythiophene) doped with lignosulfonate. *Int. J. Electrochem.* **2012**, *130980*, 1–7. [CrossRef]

8.   Gnedenkov, S.V.; Opra, D.P.; Sinebryukhov, S.L.; Tsvetnikov, A.K.; Ustinov, A.Y.; Sergienko, V.I. Hydrolysis lignin-based organic electrode material for primary lithium batteries. *J. Solid State Electrochem.* **2014**, *17*, 2611–2621. [CrossRef]

9.   Gnedenkov, S.V.; Opra, D.P.; Sinebryukhov, S.L.; Tsvetnikov, A.K.; Ustinov, A.Y.; Sergienko, V.I. Hydrolysis lignin: Electrochemical properties of the organic cathode material for primary lithium battery. *J. Ind. Eng. Chem.* **2014**, *20*, 903–910. [CrossRef]

10. Opra, D.P.; Gnedenkov, S.V.; Sinebryukhov, S.L.; Tsvetnikov, A.K.; Sergienko, V.I. Fabrication of battery cathode material based on hydrolytic lignin. *Solid State Phenom.* **2014**, *213*, 154–159. [CrossRef]

11. Kadla, J.F.; Kubo, S. Lignin-based polymer blends: Analysis of intermolecular interactions in lignin-synthetic polymer blends. *Compos. A Appl. Sci. manuf.* **2004**, *35*, 395–400. [CrossRef]

12. Canetti, M.; Bertini, F. Supermolecular structure and thermal properties of poly(ethylene terephthalate)/lignin composites. *Compos. Sci. Technol.* **2007**, *67*, 3151–3157. [CrossRef]

13. Chen, F.; Dai, H.; Dong, X.; Yang, J.; Zhong, M. Physical properties of lignin-based polypropylene blends. *Polym. Compos.* **2011**, *32*, 1019–1025. [CrossRef]

14. Borysiak, S. Fundamental studies on lignocellulose/polypropylene composites: Effects of wood treatment on the transcrystalline morphology and mechanical properties. *J. Appl. Polym. Sci.* **2013**, *127*, 1309–1322. [CrossRef]

15. Gozdecki, C.; Wilczyński, A.; Kociszewski, M.; Zajchowski, S. Mechanical properties of wood-polypropylene composites with industrial wood particles of different sizes. *Wood Fiber. Sci.* **2012**, *44*, 14–21.

16. Guo, X.; Zhang, S.; Shan, X. Adsorption of metal ions on lignin. *J. Hazard. Mater.* **2008**, *151*, 134–142. [CrossRef] [PubMed]

17. Betancur, M.; Bonelli, P.R.; Velásquez, J.A.; Cukierman, A.L. Potentiality of lignin from the Kraft pulping process for removal of trace nickel from wastewater: Effect of demineralization. *Bioresour. Technol.* **2009**, *100*, 1130–1137. [CrossRef] [PubMed]

18. Bulgariu, L.; Bulgariu, D.; Malutan, T.; Macoveanu, M. Adsorption of lead(II) ions from aqueous solution onto lignin. *Adsorp. Sci. Technol.* **2009**, *27*, 435–445. [CrossRef]

19. Harmita, H.; Karthikeyan, K.G.; Pan, X.J. Copper and cadmium sorption onto kraft and organosolv lignins. *Bioresour. Technol.* **2009**, *100*, 6183–6191. [CrossRef] [PubMed]

20. Ahmaruzzaman, M. Industrial wastes as low-cost potential adsorbents for the treatment of wastewater laden with heavy metals. *Adv. Colloid Interface Sci.* **2011**, *166*, 36–59. [PubMed]

21. Lei, Y.; Huizhen, Y. Modification of reed alkali lignin to adsorption of heavy metals. *Adv. Mater. Res.* **2013**, *622*, 1646–1650.

22. Ge, Y.; Li, Z.; Kong, Y.; Song, Q.; Wang, K. Heavy metal ions retention by bi-functionalized lignin: Synthesis, applications, and adsorption mechanisms. *J. Ind. Eng. Chem.* **2014**, *20*, 4429–4436. [CrossRef]

23. Toh, K.; Yokoyama, H.; Takahashi, C.; Watanabe, T.; Noda, H. Effect of herb lignin on the growth of enterobacteria. *J. Gen. Appl. Microbiol.* **2007**, *53*, 201–205. [CrossRef] [PubMed]

24. Ehrlich, H. Chitin and collagen as universal and alternative templates in biomineralization. *Int. Geol. Rev.* **2010**, *52*, 661–699. [CrossRef]

25. Ehrlich, H.; Krautter, M.; Hanke, T.; Simon, P.; Knieb, C.; Heinemann, S.; Worch, H. First evidence of the presence of chitin in skeleton of marine sponges. Part II. Glass sponges. (Hexactinellida: Porifera). *J. Exp. Zool. B* **2007**, *308*, 473–478. [CrossRef]

26. Ehrlich, H.; Maldonado, M.; Spindler, K.D.; Eckert, C.; Hanke, T.; Born, R.; Goebel, C.; Simon, P.; Heinemann, S.; Worch, H. First evidence of chitin as a component of the skeletal fibers of marine sponges. Part I. Verongidae (Demospongia: Porifera). *J. Exp. Zool. B* **2007**, *308*, 347–356. [CrossRef]

27. Brunner, E.; Ehrlich, H.; Schupp, P.; Hedrich, R.; Hunoldt, S.; Kammer, M.; Machill, S.; Paasch, S.; Bazhenov, V.V.; Kurek, D.V.; *et al.* Chitin-based scaffolds are an integral part of the skeleton of the marine demosponge *Ianthella basta*. *J. Struct. Biol.* **2009**, *168*, 539–547. [CrossRef] [PubMed]

28. Ehrlich, H.; Ilan, M.; Maldonado, M.; Muricy, G.; Bavestrello, G.; Kljajic, Z.; Carballo, J.L.; Schiaparelli, S.; Ereskovsky, A.; Schupp, P.; *et al.* Three-dimensional chitin-based scaffolds from Verongida sponges

(Demospongiae: Porifera). Part I. Isolation and identification of chitin. *Int. J. Biol. Macromol.* **2010**, *47*, 132–140. [CrossRef] [PubMed]

29. Yang, T.C.; Zall, R.R. Absorption of metals by natural polymers generated from seafood processing wastes. *Ind. Eng. Chem. Prod. Res. Dev.* **1984**, *23*, 168–172. [CrossRef]

30. Muzzarelli, R.A.A. Chitins and chitosans for the repair of wounded skin, nerve, cartilage and bone. *Carbohydr. Polym.* **2009**, *76*, 167–182. [CrossRef]

31. Jayakumar, R.; Nair, A.; Sanoj Rejinold, N.; Maya, S.; Nair, S.V. Doxorubicin-loaded pH-responsive chitin nanogels for drug delivery to cancer cells. *Carbohydr. Polym.* **2012**, *87*, 2352–2356. [CrossRef]

32. Liu, H.S.; Chen, W.H.; Lai, J.T. Immobilization of isoamylase on carboxymethyl-cellulose and chitin. *Appl. Biochem. Biotechnol.* **1997**, *66*, 57–67. [CrossRef]

33. Chang, R.C.; Shaw, J.F. The immobilization of *Candida cylindracea* lipase on PVC, chitin and agarose. *Bot. Bull. Acad. Sin.* **1987**, *28*, 33–42.

34. Romo-Sanchez, S.; Arevalo-Villena, M.; Garcia Romero, E.; Ramirez, H.L.; Briones Perez, A. Immobilization of β-glucosidase and its application for enhancement of aroma precursors in muscat wine. *Food Bioprocess Technol.* **2014**, *7*, 1381–1392. [CrossRef]

35. Krajewska, B. Application of chitin- and chitosan-based materials for enzyme immobilizations: A review. *Enzyme Microb. Technol.* **2004**, *35*, 126–139. [CrossRef]

36. Vaillant, F.; Millan, A.; Millan, P.; Dormier, M.; Decloux, M.; Reynes, M. Co-immobilized pectinlyase and endocellulase on chitin and nylon supports. *Process Biochem.* **2000**, *35*, 989–996. [CrossRef]

37. Batra, R.; Gupta, M.N. Non-covalent immobilization of potato (*Solanum tuberosum*) polyphenol oxidase on chitin. *Biotechnol. Appl. Biochem.* **1994**, *19*, 209–215.

38. Wang, G.; Xu, J.J.; Ye, L.H.; Zhu, J.J.; Chen, H.Y. Highly sensitive sensors based on the immobilization of tyrosinase in chitosan. *Bioelectrochemistry* **2002**, *57*, 33–38. [CrossRef] [PubMed]

39. Gomes, F.M.; Pereira, E.B.; de Castro, H.F. Immobilization of lipase on chitin and its use in nonconventional biocatalysis. *Biomacromolecules* **2004**, *5*, 17–23. [CrossRef] [PubMed]

40. Zeng, J.B.; He, Y.S.; Li, S.L.; Wang, Y.Z. Chitin whiskers: An overwiev. *Biomacromolecules* **2012**, *13*, 1–11. [CrossRef] [PubMed]

41. Filipkowska, U. Desorption of reactive dyes from modified chitin. *Environ. Technol.* **2008**, *29*, 681–690. [CrossRef] [PubMed]

42. Jesionowski, T.; Zdarta, J.; Krajewska, B. Enzymes immobilization by adsorption: A review. *Adsorption* **2014**, *20*, 801–821. [CrossRef]

43. Wong, P.T.T.; Nong, R.K.; Caputo, T.A.; Godwin, T.A.; Rigas, B. Infrared spectroscopy of exfoliated human cervical cells: Evidence of extensive structural changes during carcinogenesis. *Proc. Natl. Acad. Sci. USA* **1991**, *88*, 10988–10992. [CrossRef] [PubMed]

44. Dousseau, F.; Pezolet, M. Determination of the secondary structure content of proteins in aqueous solutions from their amide I and amide II infrared bands. Comparison between classical and partial least-squares methods. *Biochemistry* **1990**, *29*, 8771–8779. [CrossRef] [PubMed]

45. Dong, L.; Ge, C.; Qin, P.; Chen, Y.; Xu, Q. Immobilization and catalytic properties of candida lipolytic lipase on surface of organic intercalated and modified MgAl-LDHs. *Sol. Sci.* **2014**, *31*, 8–15. [CrossRef]

46. Cabrera-Padilla, R.Y.; Lisboa, M.C.; Pereira, M.M.; Figueiredo, R.T.; Franceschi, E.; Fricks, A.T.; Lima, A.S.; Silva, D.P.; Soares, C.M.F. Immobilization of *Candida rugosa* lipase onto an eco-friendly support in the presence of ionic liquid. *Bioprocess Biosyst. Eng.* **2014**. [CrossRef]

47. Klapiszewski, Ł.; Zdarta, J.; Szatkowski, T.; Wysokowski, M.; Nowacka, M.; Szwarc-Rzepka, K.; Bartczak, P.; Siwińska-Stefańska, K.; Ehrlich, H.; Jesionowski, T. Silica/lignosulfonate hybrid materials: Preparation and characterization. *Cent. Eur. J. Chem.* **2014**, *12*, 719–735. [CrossRef]

48. Lavall, R.L.; Assis, O.B.G.; Campana-Filho, S.P. β-Chitin from the pens of *Loligo* sp.: Extraction and characterization. *Bioresource Technol.* **2007**, *98*, 2465–2472. [CrossRef]

49. Jang, M.K.; Kong, B.G.; Jeong, Y.I.; Lee, C.H.; Nah, J.W. Physicochemical characterization of α-chitin, β-chitin, and γ-chitin separated from natural resources. *J. Polym. Sci. A* **2004**, *42*, 3423–3432. [CrossRef]

50. Klapiszewski, Ł.; Wysokowski, M.; Majchrzak, I.; Szatkowski, T.; Nowacka, M.; Siwińska-Stefańska, K.; Szwarc-Rzepka, K.; Bartczak, P.; Ehrlich, H.; Jesionowski, T. Preparation and characterization of multifunctional chitin/lignin materials. *J. Nanomater.* **2013**, 1–13. [CrossRef]

51. Naidja, A.; Liu, C.; Huang, P.M. Formation of protein-birnessite complex: XRD, FTIR, and AFM analysis. *J. Colloid Interface Sci.* **2002**, *251*, 46–56. [CrossRef] [PubMed]

52. Portaccio, M.; Della Ventura, B.; Mita, D.G.; Manolova, N.; Stoilova, O.; Rashkov, I.; Lepore, M. FT-IR microscopy characterization of sol–gel layers prior and after glucose oxidase immobilization for biosensing applications. *J. Sol-Gel Sci. Technol.* **2011**, *57*, 204–211. [CrossRef]

53. Wysokowski, M.; Klapiszewski, Ł.; Moszyński, D.; Bartczak, P.; Majchrzak, I.; Siwińska-Stefańska, K.; Bazhenov, V.V.; Jesionowski, T. Modification of chitin with kraft lignin and development of new biosorbents for removal of cadmium(II) and nickel(II) ions. *Mar. Drugs* **2014**, *12*, 2245–2268. [CrossRef] [PubMed]

54. Cardenas, G.; Cabrera, G.; Taboada, E.; Miranda, S.P. Chitin characterization by SEM, FTIR, XRD, and ^{13}C cross polarization/mass angle spinning NMR. *J. Appl. Polym. Sci.* **2004**, *93*, 1876–1885. [CrossRef]

55. Tomizuka, N.; Ota, Y.; Yamada, K. Lipase from *Candida cylindracea II*. Amino acid composition, carbohydrate component, and some physical properties. *Agric. Biol. Chem.* **1966**, *30*, 1090–1096. [CrossRef]

56. Wang, B.; Li, J.; Zhang, J.; Li, H.; Chen, P.; Gu, Q.; Wang, Z. Thermo-mechanical properties of the composite made of poly (3-hydroxybutyrate-co-3-hydroxyvalerate) and acetylated chitin nanocrystals. *Carbohydr. Polym.* **2013**, *95*, 100–106. [CrossRef] [PubMed]

57. Song, J.; Kahveci, D.; Chen, M.; Guo, Z.; Xie, E.; Xu, X.; Besenbacher, F.; Dong, M. Enhanced catalytic activity of lipase encapsulated in PCL nanofibers. *Langmuir* **2012**, *28*, 6157–6162. [CrossRef] [PubMed]

58. Briggs, D.; Grant, J.T. *Surface Analysis by Auger and X-ray Photoelectron Spectroscopy*; IM Publications and SurfaceSpectra Limited: Charlton, UK, 2003.

59. Wang, J.; Wang, Z.; Li, J.; Wang, B.; Liu, J.; Chen, P.; Miao, M.; Gu, Q. Chitin nanocrystals grafted with poly(3-hydroxybutyrate-co-3-hydroxyvalerate) and their effects on thermal behavior of PHBV. *Carbohydr. Polym.* **2012**, *87*, 784–789. [CrossRef]

60. De Lange, P.J.; Mahy, J.W.G. ToF-SIMS and XPS investigations of fibers, coatings and biomedical materials. *Fresenius' J. Anal. Chem.* **1995**, *353*, 487–493. [CrossRef]

61. Rouxhet, P.G.; Genet, M.J. XPS analysis of bio-organic systems. *Surf. Interface Anal.* **2011**, *43*, 1453–1470. [CrossRef]

62. Namboodiri, V.M.H.; Chattaopadhyaya, R. Purification and biochemical characterization of a novel thermostable lipase from *Aspergillus niger*. *Lipids* **2000**, *35*, 495–502. [CrossRef] [PubMed]

63. Pokorny, D.; Cimerman, A.; Steiner, W. *Aspergillus niger* lipases: Induction, isolation and characterization of two lipases from a MZKI Al 16 strain. *J. Mol. Cat. B Enzym.* **1997**, *2*, 215–222. [CrossRef]

64. Xiaoming, L.; Breddam, K. A novel carboxylesterase from *Aspergillus niger* and its hydrolysis of succinimide esters. *Carlsberg Res. Commun.* **1989**, *54*, 241–249. [CrossRef]

65. Rezwan, K.; Studart, A.R.; Vo1ro1s, J.; Gauckler, L.J. Change of ζ potential of biocompatible colloidal oxide particles upon adsorption of bovine serum albumin and lysozyme. *J. Phys. Chem. B* **2005**, *109*, 14469–14474. [CrossRef] [PubMed]

66. Rezwan, K.; Meier, L.P.; Rezwan, M.; Voros, J.; Textor, M.; Gauckler, L.J. Bovine serum albumin adsorption onto colloidal Al_2O_3 particles: A new model based on zeta potential and UV-Vis measurements. *Langmuir* **2004**, *20*, 10055–10061. [CrossRef] [PubMed]

67. Bernsmann, F.; Frisch, B.; Ringwald, C.; Ball, V. Protein adsorption on dopamine–melanin films: Role of electrostatic interactions inferred from ζ-potential measurements *versus* chemisorption. *J. Colloid Interface Sci.* **2010**, *344*, 54–60. [CrossRef] [PubMed]

68. Li, S.; Hu, J.; Liu, B. A study on the adsorption behavior of protein onto functional microspheres. *Chem. Technol. Biotechnol.* **2005**, *80*, 531–536. [CrossRef]

69. Bradford, M.M. Rapid and sensitive method for the quantitation of microgram quantities of protein utilizing the principle of protein-dye binding. *Anal. Biochem.* **1976**, *72*, 248–254. [CrossRef] [PubMed]

70. Sheldon, R.A.; van Pelt, S. Enzyme immobilisation: Why, what and how? *Chem. Soc. Rev.* **2013**, *42*, 6223–6235. [CrossRef] [PubMed]

71. Abdel-Naby, M.A. Immobilization of Aspergillus niger NRC 107 xylanase and beta-xylosidase, and properties of the immobilzed enzymes. *Appl. Biochem. Biotechnol.* **1993**, *38*, 69–81. [CrossRef] [PubMed]

72. Jia, J.; Hu, Y.; Liu, L.; Jiang, L.; Zou, B.; Huang, H. Enhancing catalytic performance of porcine pancreatic lipase by covalent modification using functional ionic liquids. *ACS Catal.* **2013**, *3*, 1976–1983. [CrossRef]

73. Emregul, E.; Sungur, S.; Akbulut, U. Polyacrylamide-gelatine carrier system used for invertase immobilization. *Food Chem.* **2006**, *97*, 591–597. [CrossRef]

74. Zhu, Y.T.; Ren, X.Y.; Liu, Y.M.; Wei, Y.; Qing, L.S.; Liao, X. Covalent immobilization of porcine pancreatic lipase on carboxyl-activated magnetic nanoparticles: Characterization and application for enzymatic inhibition assays. *Mater. Sci. Eng. C Mater Boil. Appl.* **2014**, *38*, 278–285. [CrossRef]
75. Melgosa, R.; Sanz, M.T.; Solaesa, A.G.; Bucio, S.L.; Beltran, S. Enzymatic activity and conformational and morphological studies of four commercial lipases treated with supercritical carbon dioxide. *J. Supercrit. Fluids* **2015**, *97*, 51–62. [CrossRef]
76. Zdarta, J.; Sałek, K.; Kołodziejczak-Radzimska, A.; Siwińska-Stefańska, K.; Szwarc-Rzepka, K.; Norman, M.; Klapiszewski, Ł.; Bartczak, P.; Kaczorek, E.; Jesionowski, T. Immobilization of *Amano Lipase A* onto Stöber silica surface: Process characterization and kinetic studies. *Open Chem.* **2015**, *13*, 138–148.

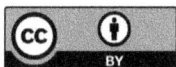

marine drugs

MDPI

Article

Effect of Fucoidan Extracted from Mozuku on Experimental Cartilaginous Tissue Injury

Tomohiro Osaki [1],*, Koudai Kitahara [1], Yoshiharu Okamoto [1], Tomohiro Imagawa [1], Takeshi Tsuka [1], Yasunari Miki [2], Hitoshi Kawamoto [2], Hiroyuki Saimoto [3] and Saburo Minami [1]

[1] Department of Veterinary Clinical Medicine, School of Veterinary Medicine, Tottori University, 4-101 Koyama Minami, Tottori 680-8553, Japan; sakurayama@ninus.ocn.ne.jp (K.K.); yokamoto@muses.tottori-u.ac.jp (Y.O.); imagawat@muses.tottori-u.ac.jp (T.I.); tsuka@muses.tottori-u.ac.jp (T.T.); minami@muses.tottori-u.ac.jp (S.M.)

[2] Marine Products Kimuraya, 3307 Watari, Sakaiminato, Tottori 684-0072, Japan; miki@mozuku-1ban.jp (Y.M.); kawamoto@mozuku-1ban.jp (H.K.)

[3] Graduate School of Engineering, Tottori University, 4-101 Koyama Minami, Tottori 680-8553, Japan; saimoto@chem.tottori-u.ac.jp

* Author to whom correspondence should be addressed; tosaki@muses.tottori-u.ac.jp; Tel./Fax: +81-857-31-5434.

Received: 20 August 2012; in revised form: 25 October 2012; Accepted: 6 November 2012; Published: 13 November 2012

Abstract: We investigated the effect of fucoidan, a sulfated polysaccharide, on acceleration of healing of experimental cartilage injury in a rabbit model. An injured cartilage model was surgically created by introduction of three holes, one in the articular cartilage of the medial trochlea and two in the trochlear sulcus of the distal femur. Rabbits in three experimental groups (F groups) were orally administered fucoidan of seven different molecular weights (8, 50, 146, 239, 330, 400, or 1000 kD) for 3 weeks by screening. Control (C group) rabbits were provided water *ad libitum*. After the experimental period, macroscopic examination showed that the degree of filling in the fucoidan group was higher than that in the C group. Histologically, the holes were filled by collagen fiber and fibroblasts in the C group, and by chondroblasts and fibroblasts in the F groups. Image analysis of Alcian blue- and safranin O-stained F-group specimens showed increased production of glycosaminoglycans (GAGs) and proteoglycans (PGs), respectively. Some injured holes were well repaired both macroscopically and microscopically and were filled with cartilage tissues; cartilage matrices such as PGs and GAGs were produced in groups F 50, F 146, and F 239. Thus, fucoidan administration enhanced morphologically healing of cartilage injury.

Keywords: articular cartilage; fucoidan; rabbit

1. Introduction

Our joints make complex movements easily because articular cartilage and subchondral bone absorb exercise-induced physical impact. Normal hyaline cartilage consists of chondrocytes ($\leq 5\%$ total volume) and extracellular matrix ($\geq 95\%$ total volume). Matrix consists of 70%–80% water, 20%–25% collagen, and 5%–10% proteoglycans (PGs) [1]. The collagen triple-helix consists of a repeating (Gly-X-Y)n sequence, and cartilage contains mixed fibrils of collagen type II, IV, IX, and XI. Proteoglycans act to pump water inside dense fiber networks and have the function of expanding pressure [2]. Aggrecan, the large species of PGs found in cartilage, has a crucial function in distributing the load in weight-bearing joints [3]. Degenerative joint disease (DJD) in humans results from excessive exercise combined with the natural aging processes [4].

In recent years, various combinations of non-steroid anti-inflammatory drugs, steroids, surgical treatment, oral administration of glucosamine and/or collagen supplements, weight control, and restriction of physical activity have been used for supportive treatment of patients with DJD. The glucosamine and/or collagen supplements have low toxicity and are suitable for long-term administration, although they have low analgesic effects [5,6]. In the 1980s, glucosamine (GlcN) in particular was used in the management of DJD (primarily in Europe) and had a reputation for providing clinical symptom relief [7]. We have reported accelerated healing of experimental cartilage damage by GlcN [8]. Chondroitin sulfate (CS) is also thought to heal cartilage damage, and oral CS at a dose of 800 mg per day was reported to be a pain relieving agent for the treatment of DJD. In addition, CS might stabilize the joint space width and modulate bone and joint metabolism [9].

Degenerative joint disease is primarily characterized by areas of destruction of articular cartilage and synovitis. Articular damage and synovitis are secondary to local increases of pro-inflammatory cytokines (interleukin-1b and tumor necrosis factor-α), enzymes with proteolytic activity (matrix metalloproteinases), and enzymes with pro-inflammatory activity (cyclooxygenase-2 and nitric oxide synthase-2). Enhanced expression of these proteins in chondrocytes and synovial membrane appears to be associated with the activation and nuclear translocation of nuclear factor-κB (NF-κB). CS reduces NF-κB nuclear translocation, probably by diminishing extracellular levels of signal-regulated kinase 1/2, p38 mitogen-activated protein kinase, and c-Jun *N*-terminal kinase activity [10]. The sulfate salt of GlcN stimulates *in vitro* production of aggrecan core protein mRNA and protein, and at the same time inhibits production and enzymatic activity of matrix-degrading MMP-3 in chondrocytes cultured from osteoarthritic articular cartilage [11]. These observations suggest that materials containing the sulfate group are prominently involved in the prevention and treatment of DJD.

Fucoidan, which is extracted from brown algae such as kelp, wakame, and mozuku, is a sulfated polysaccharide with L-fucose building blocks and predominantly α1–2 and α1–4 linkages. Fucoidan extracted from Okinawa mozuku contains fucose (30.9%), glucose (2.2%), xylose (0.7%), uronic acid (23.4%), and sulfate groups (15.1%). Differences in composition influence the anti-inflammatory effects, anti-angiogenic effects, and anti-adhesive action [12]. Differences in the absorption and bioavailability of the various CS formulations are strongly influenced by the structure and characteristics, such as molecular mass, charge density, and clusters of disulfated disaccharides [13]. These reports suggest that differences in the molecular weight of various fucoidan preparations influence their bioactivity.

The objective of the present study was to investigate the morphological effects of orally administered fucoidans of various molecular weights on cartilage repair by screening.

2. Results

2.1. General Condition

In the C group, one rabbit presented with swelling of a stifle joint. In the F groups, 19% of the rabbits presented with swelling of stifle joints (F 8 group, $n = 2$; F 239 group, $n = 1$; F 330 group, $n = 1$). Nineteen percent of the rabbits also presented with diarrhea (F 400 group, $n = 2$; F 1000 group, $n = 2$).

2.2. Changes in Muscle Weight

The weights of the lateral great muscle and biceps muscle were not significantly different between the C group and the F groups.

2.3. Macroscopic Findings

In the C group, the surgically created holes were incompletely healed. In the F groups, the holes were filled with regenerated tissue, though there was variability in the degree of healing. The average scores for restoration of the defective pores in the C group, F 8 group, F 50 group, F 146 group, F 239 group, F 330 group, F 400 group, and F 1000 group were 1.10, 1.67, 2.22, 2.44, 2.00, 1.78, 2.22, and 2.00, respectively. The surgically created holes in the F 50 group, F 146 group, and F 400 group exhibited significantly more healing than was found in the C group specimens ($p < 0.05$) (Figure 1).

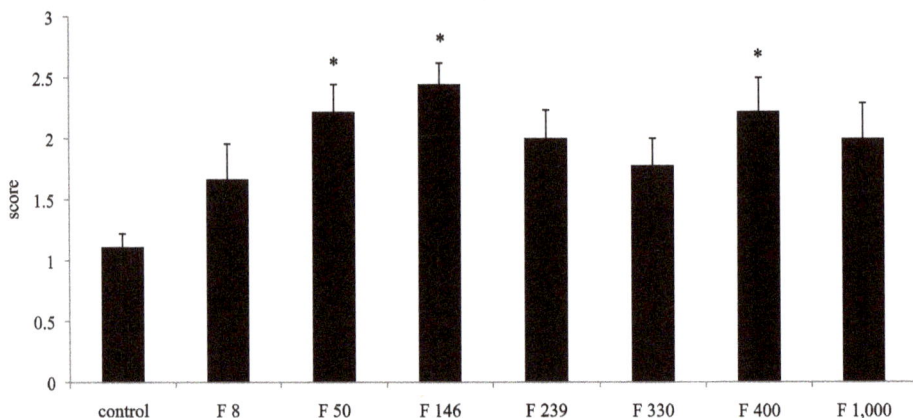

Figure 1. Average defect restoration scores. Data are expressed as the average $\pm$ standard deviation. * $p < 0.05$.

2.4. Histological Findings

In the control group, cartilage tissues were not observed in the deeper layer (Figure 2A), and bone trabeculae were lacking.

In the fucoidan group, regenerated cartilage tissues were observed in the deeper layer of cancellous bone (Figures 3F and 4F), and bone trabeculae were regenerated in the F 50 and F 146 groups (Figure 4D). The greatest degree of regeneration of cartilage tissues was observed in the F 146 group.

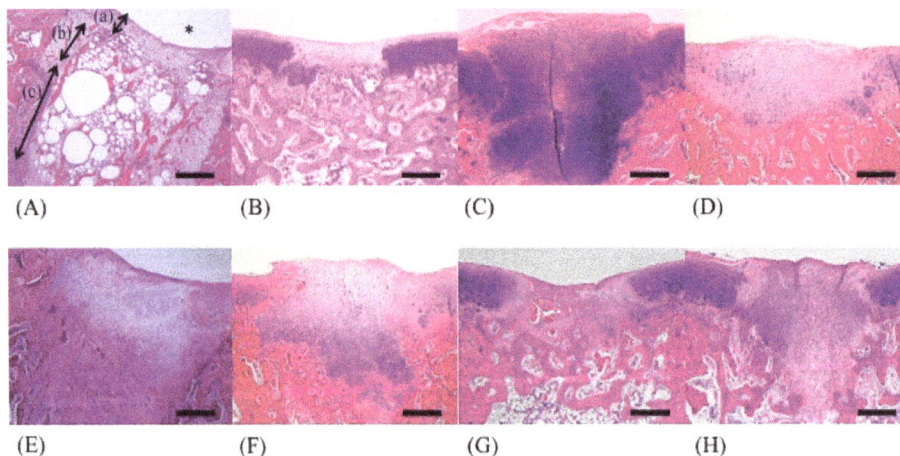

Figure 2. Light microscopy of tissues from each group (HE stain; 40×). (**A**) C group; (**B**) F 8 group; (**C**) F 50 group; (**D**) F 146 group; (**E**) F 239 group; (**F**) F 330 group; (**G**) F 400 group; (**H**) F 1000 group. (a) cartilage layer; (b) superficial layer of cancellous bone; (c) deeper layer of cancellous bone. * joint cavity.

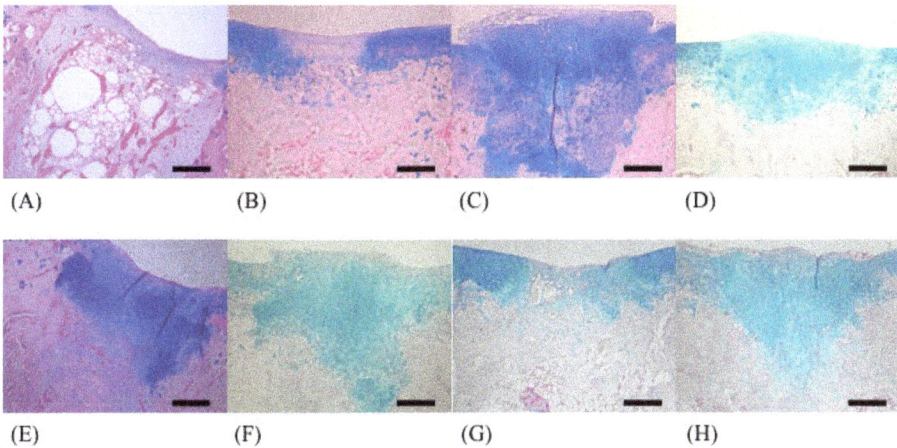

Figure 3. Light microscopy of tissues from each group (Alcian blue stain; ×40). (**A**) C group; (**B**) F 8 group; (**C**) F 50 group; (**D**) F 146 group; (**E**) F 239 group; (**F**) F 330 group; (**G**) F 400 group; (**H**) F 1000 group.

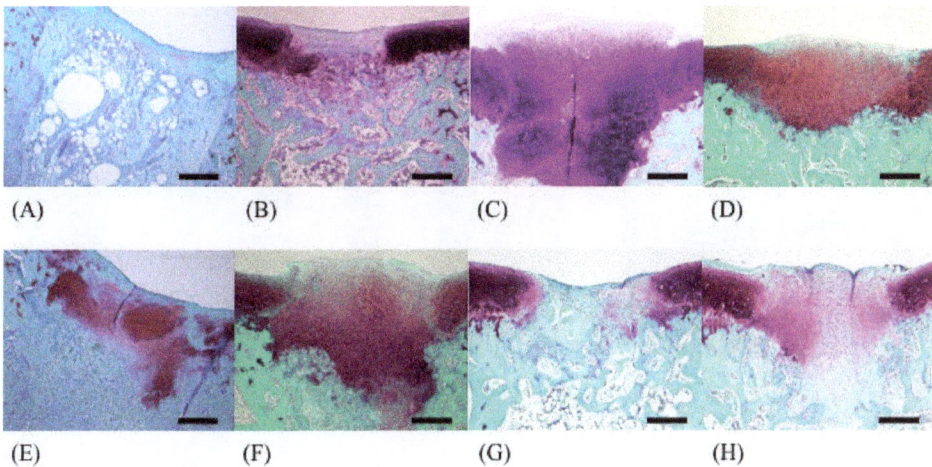

Figure 4. Light microscopy of tissues from each group (safranin O stain; 40×). (**A**) C group; (**B**) F 8 group; (**C**) F 50 group; (**D**) F 146 group; (**E**) F 239 group, (**F**) F 330 group; (**G**) F 400 group; (**H**) F 1000 group.

2.5. Image Analysis for Safranin O- and Alcian Blue-Stained Specimens

In Alcian blue-stained specimens, the number of pixels in the C group, F8 group, F 50 group, F 146 group, F 239 group, F 330 group, F 400 group, and F 1000 group were 5989, 22,087, 46,617, 50,580, 41,392, 27,175, 28,967, and 29,146, respectively. The number of pixels in the F 50 and F 146 groups was significantly greater than that in the C group ($p < 0.05$) (Figure 5).

In safranin O-stained specimens, the number of pixels in the C group, F 8 group, F 50 group, F 146 group, F 239 group, F 330 group, F 400 group, and F 1000 group were 2018, 29,686, 47,083, 56,788, 34,085, 29,474, 31,163, and 31,096, respectively. The number of pixels in the F 50 group and F 146 group were significantly higher than that in the C group ($p < 0.05$) (Figure 6).

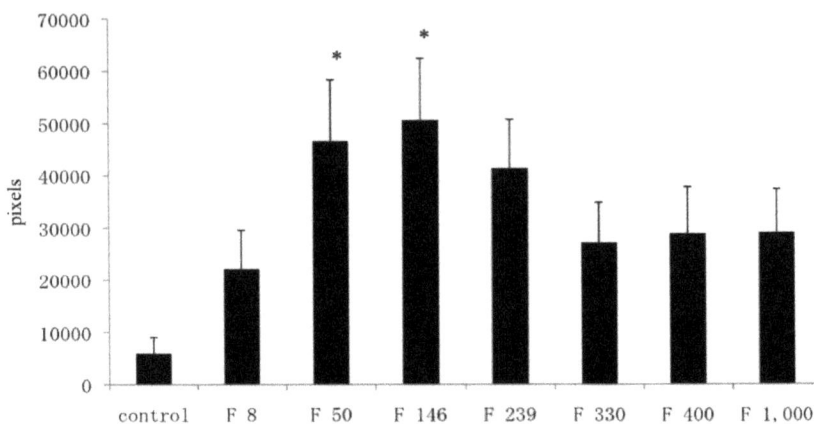

Figure 5. Image analysis of Alcian blue-stained specimens. Data are expressed as the average ± standard deviation. *$p < 0.05$.

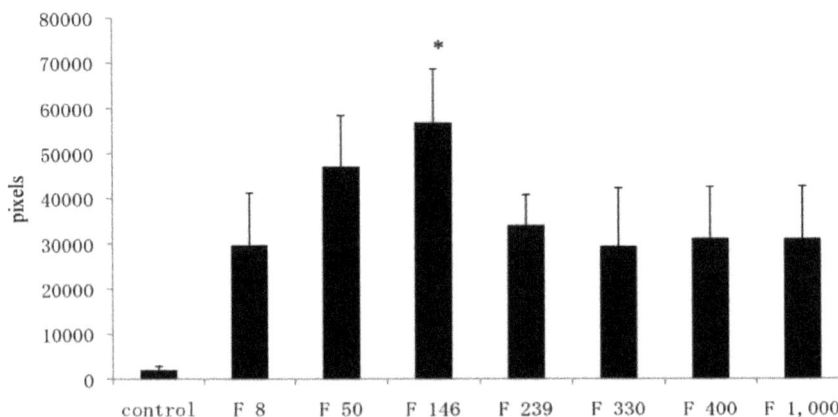

Figure 6. Image analysis of safranin O-stained specimens. The data are expressed as the average ± standard deviation. * $p < 0.05$.

3. Discussion

Oral administration of GlcN at a dose of 1.5 g/day is effective for DJD in humans at a dose of 30 mg per kilogram of body weight [14,15]. In this study, 1 g/head of fucoidan was administered to rabbits. The dose was 500 mg/kg, which is a high dose. Nineteen rabbits developed mild diarrhea during the experiment. Although it is still unclear whether fucoidan is absorbed in the digestive tract, Becker *et al.* reported that fucoidan inhibits the absorption of trace elements [16]. In this study, diarrhea may have been caused because the high dose of fucoidan was not absorbed and was eliminated with unabsorbed foods.

Repair of cartilage injury involves fibrous tissue, fibrocartilaginous tissue, or hyaline cartilage tissue [17]. In many cases, osteochondral defects heal by formation of fibrous tissue or fibrocartilaginous tissue. Eventual deterioration of these tissues is the usual sequel to this imperfect healing. One study on cartilage injury reported that the regenerated tissue at the injured area after 12 months was fibrous rather than cartilage tissue [18]. In healed cartilage injury, the late morphological changes to a more fibrous texture might result from a loss of PGs rather than from an overt transition of all tissues to fibrocartilage [19]. In our previous study using GlcN, the holes were completely filled by proliferating chondroblasts; remodeling of bony trabeculae was also observed [20]. Therefore, our present study design was based on the period 3 weeks after surgery to enable comparison between our studies. In addition, regenerated tissue analyzed more than 3 weeks after cartilage injury has been reported to be non-functional fibrous tissue instead of hyaline cartilage [8,20]. Osteochondral defects may not heal with cartilage tissues because of the slow transition of fibrin clots into undifferentiated mesenchyme and insufficient amounts of fundamentally important regulatory factors [21].

Both chondroblasts and osteoblasts are derived from primitive mesenchymal cells of the bone marrow [22], and the undifferentiated cells that migrate to the injury site secrete primarily type I collagen, along with smaller amounts of other extracellular matrix components [17]. Furthermore, differentiated cartilage cells secrete type II collagen and PGs, and macrophages activated by these factors produce chondrocyte-stimulating factor [23]. Because direct quantification of collagen was not possible in our study, bone morphogenetic proteins (BMPs) in plasma, which are members of the TGF-β superfamily of molecules, were measured. BMPs showed a marked tendency to increase (data not shown) in the F 146.

In this study, well-repaired injuries were observed in the F 8, F 330, F 400, and F 1000 groups. However, individual variability was considerable, and many of the injured holes were filled with fibrous tissues, as in the C group. On the other hand, some injured holes were well repaired both macroscopically and microscopically and were filled with cartilage tissues; cartilage matrices such as PGs and GAGs were produced in the F 50, F 146, and F 239 groups. In a previous study using an injured cartilage model, the main collagen found in the repaired tissue after 3 weeks was type I. By 6 to 8 weeks, type II had become predominant and continued to be enriched for up to 1 year. However, type I still persisted as a significant constituent of the repair tissue even after 1 year, so the repaired cartilage never fully resembled normal articular cartilage [19]. In contrast, the present study found that the injury holes leading to cancellous bone were completely filled by proliferating chondroblasts, and remodeling of bony trabeculae was observed in the F 146 group.

The difference between the mechanism of action of GlcN and that of fucoidans is unclear. GlcN is a monomer and is absorbed in the gut. Maximam plasma GlcN concentrations are reached at 0.5 hr after oral administration of GlcN [24]. Absorbed GlcN influences the metabolism of amino acids associated with collagen synthesis [25]. In contrast, fucoidan is a polymer composed of fucose, and an increase in plasma fucose was not observed in this study (data not shown). Because fucoidan is a sulfated polysaccharide, it was considered to be not directly associated with the synthesis of collagen. Although PGs and GAGs were evaluated in the present study, it might need to estimate the synthesis of collagen in future. We therefore suspect that the mechanism of hole repair may differ between GlcN and fucoidan. We also noted that the individual variability seen in this study was more marked than that in studies using glucosamine. Further investigation is required to evaluate the relationship between the molecular weight of fucoidans and their bioactive effects, such as collagen synthesis.

4. Experimental Section

4.1. Preparation of Fucoidan

Fucoidans with varying average molecular weight (330, 400, and 1000 KD) were extracted from Okinawa mozuku with hot water. Extracted fucoidans (molecular weight: 330 KD) were further treated under hydrothermal conditions for conversion to low-molecular weight fucoidans (8, 50, 146, and 239 KD). Fucoidans with seven different molecular weights were used for the experiment.

4.2. Animals

An injured cartilage model was made in the same manner as our previous report [21]. Twenty-four clinically healthy rabbits (female Japanese albino; average age, 12 weeks) with a body weight of 2.0–2.5 kg were used. The animals were used in the experiment after 1-week acclimatization to the laboratory environment. All experimental procedures were approved by the animal care and use committees of Tottori University and were conducted in accordance with The American Physiological Society's guiding principles for the care and use of animals.

4.3. Fucoidans

The experimental rabbits were divided into eight groups (*n* = 3), namely the control group (C group), the group receiving 8 KD fucoidan (F 8 group), the group receiving 50 KD fucoidan (F 50 group), the group receiving 146 KD fucoidan (F 146 group), the group receiving 239 KD fucoidan (F 239 group), the group receiving 330 KD fucoidan (F 330 group), the group receiving 400 KD fucoidan (F 400 group), and the group receiving 1000 KD fucoidan (F 1000 group). The fucoidan groups were administered a solution of fucoidan dissolved in tap water that was administered at a rate of 1 g/head/day for three weeks.

4.4. Preparation of the Model of Articular Cartilage Injury

An analgesic (xylazine hydrochloride, 10 mg/kg) was administered as premedication. After sedation, induction of anesthesia was performed in a box with a mixture of 5% isoflurane in oxygen. Anesthesia was maintained by inhalation of a mixture of 3% isoflurane in oxygen using a mask. The fur at the left knee joint was clipped and the area disinfected with chlorhexidine solution (Hibiscrub, Zeneka, Osaka) and 70% alcohol. Approaching from the lateral portion of the knee joint, an incision was made vertically on the skin from the central part of the femur toward the tibial tuberosity. The articular capsule was incised, and the patella of the stifle joint was exposed completely by artificially dislocating the patella toward the medial side. Three holes measuring 2 mm in diameter and 4 mm in depth were made using a hand drill (Micro-engine D-2, Osada medical, Tokyo) at the articular cartilage of the medial trochlea (one hole) and the trochlear sulcus (two holes) of the distal femur. Afterwards, the wound was rinsed with saline solution, and the articular capsule was sutured and closed with a synthetic absorbent thread (3-0 PDSII, Johnson & Johnson, Tokyo). The subcutaneous tissues and skin were sutured with nylon (USP 3-0 suture, Suprylon, Vomel, Germany). During the 1-week period after the operation, the wound surface was disinfected by povidone-iodine (Isodine, Meiji confectionery, Tokyo) once a day, and 10 mg/kg of oxytetracycline (Terramycin, Pfizer, Tokyo) was subcutaneously administered twice a day to prevent infection.

4.5. Postmortem Examination

At three weeks after the operation, the rabbits were euthanized by overdose (80 mg/kg) of pentobarbital (Nembutal, Dainippon Pharmaceutical Co., Osaka) through intravenous injection. The stifle joints were opened and were macroscopically observed at the operated site for assessment of injured cartilage. The lateral great muscle and the biceps muscle in the left and right hind legs were then collected for weight comparison. The muscle weight ratio (%) was calculated by comparing the operation side with the non-operation side.

4.6. Evaluation of Healing at Injured Sites

For the macroscopic findings, the proportion of restoration of the defective pores was scored according to previous our report [20]: less than 50% repair of defect depth, score 0; less than 60% repair of defect depth, score 1; less than 80% repair of defect depth, score 2; and more than 80% repair of defect depth, score 3.

4.7. Histological Examination

The recovered left femur was fixed in a 10% neutral buffered formaldehyde solution. After fixation, the operated stifle joint was trimmed to a thickness of 5 mm and decalcified for 1 day by shaking in 5% formic acid solution. After decalcification, the tissue was soaked for neutralization in a

Mar. Drugs **2012**, *10*, 2560–2570

5% sodium sulfate solution for 1 day, and was then washed for approximately 10 h under running water. After using the usual method of paraffin embedding, the tissue was sliced by a microtome into 5-μm sections. Staining was carried out using the hematoxylin/eosin double staining method; safranin O and Alcian blue stains were used for staining PGs and GAGs, respectively. We recorded the difference between restored substances at the injured parts in all groups using a microscope (BX51-FL, Olympus, Tokyo). The 200× magnified images of restored parts, articular cartilage, and growing zone stained with safranin stains and Alcian blue stains were captured by a computer using Photograb ab-300 version 1.0 (Macintosh software, Fujifilm, Tokyo), and the images were digitized using Adobe Photoshop 3.0 (Macintosh software, Adobe System, Tokyo). In safranin stains, the red colored pixels that indicated PGs were counted in order not to include non-specific colored pixels. In Alcian blue stains, the indigo colored pixels that indicated GAGs were also counted. The proportion of each colored pixels out of a total of 120,000 pixels accounted for the observed hue (random sampling of 20,000 pixels at 6 locations) was then calculated through the image processing technique.

4.8. Statistical Analysis

Statistical analysis was performed using the Turkey-Kramer method. A p value of less than 0.05 was considered significant.

5. Conclusion

The administration of fucoidan effectively promoted the healing and restoration of cartilage injury. The degree of healing promoted by fucoidan may be associated with the steric structure and composition of the fucoidan as well as the size and molecular weight. Further investigations are necessary to evaluate the relationship between the molecular weight of fucoidans and their bioactive effects, such as collagen synthesis.

References

1. Maroudas, A.; Bayliss, M.T.; Venn, M.F. Further studies on the composition of human femoral head cartilage. *Ann. Rheum. Dis.* **1980**, *39*, 514–523. [CrossRef]
2. Heinegard, D. Proteoglycans and more from molecules to biology. *Int. J. Exp. Pathol.* **2009**, *90*, 575–586. [CrossRef]
3. Hardingham, T.E.; Fosang, A.J. Proteoglycans: Many forms and many functions. *FASEB J.* **1992**, *6*, 861–870.
4. Barclay, T.S.; Tsourounis, C.; McCart, G.M. Glucosamine. *Ann. Pharmacother.* **1998**, *32*, 574–579. [CrossRef]
5. Qiu, G.X.; Gao, S.N.; Giacolli, G.; Rovati, L.; Setnikar, I. Efficacy and safety of glucosamine sulfate *versus* ibuprofen in patients with knee osteoarthritis. *Arzneimittelforschung* **1998**, *48*, 469–474.
6. Setnikar, I.; Giacchti, C.; Zanolo, G. Pharmacokinetics of glucosamine in the dog and in man. *Arzneimittelforschung* **1991**, *36*, 729–735.
7. Deal, C.L.; Moskowitz, R.W. Nutraceuticals as therapeutic agents in osteoarthritis: The role of glucosamine, chondroitin sulfate, and collagen hydrolysate. *Rheum. Dis. Clin. North. Am.* **1999**, *25*, 379–395. [CrossRef]
8. Tamai, Y; Miyatake, K.; Okamoto, Y.; Takamori, Y.; Sakamoto, K.; Minami, S. Enhanced healing of cartilaginous injuries by N-acetyl-D-glucosamine and blucuronic acid. *Carbohydr. Polym.* **2003**, *54*, 251–262. [CrossRef]
9. Uebelhart, D.; Thonar, E.J.; Delmas, P.D.; Chantraine, A.; Vignon, E. Effects of oral chondroitin sulfate on the progression of knee osteoarthritis. *Osteoarthr. Cartil.* **1998**, *6*, 39–46. [CrossRef]
10. Iovu, M.; Dumais, G.; Souich, P.D. Anti-inflammatory activity of chondroitin sulfate. *Osteoarthr. Cartil.* **2008**, *16*, S14–S18.
11. Dodge, G.R.; Jimenez, S.A. Glucosamine sulfate modulates the levels of aggrecan and matrix metalloproteinase-3 synthesized by cultured human osteoarthritis articular chondrocytes. *Osteoarthr. Cartil.* **2003**, *11*, 424–432. [CrossRef]

12. Cumashi, A.; Ushakova, A.N.; Preobrazhenskaya, E.M.; Incecco, D.A.; Piccoli, A.; Totani, L.; Tinari, N.; Morozevich, E.G.; Berman, E.A.; Bilan, I.M.; *et al.* A comparative study of the anti-inflammatory, anticoagulant, antiangiogenic, and antiadhesive activities of nine different fucoidans from brown seaweeds. *Glycobiology* **2007**, *17*, 541–552.

13. Volpi, N. Oral absorption and bioavailability of ichthyic origin chondroitin sulfate in healthy male volunteers. *Osteoarthr. Cartil.* **2003**, *11*, 433–441. [CrossRef]

14. Dovanti, A.; Bignamini, A.A.; Rovati, A.L. Therapeutic activity of oral glucosamine sulfate in osteoarthritis: A placebo-controlled double-blind investigation. *Clin. Ther.* **1980**, *3*, 260–272.

15. Reichelt, A.; Förster, K.K.; Fischer, M.; Rovati, L.C.; Setnikar, I. Efficacy and safety of intramuscular glucosamine sulfate in osteoarthritis of the knee. A randomised placebo-controlled, double-blind study. *Arzneim. Forsch.* **1994**, *44*, 75–80.

16. Becker, G.; Osterloh, K.; Schafer, S.; Forth, W.; Paskins-Hurlburt, A.J.; Tanaka, G.; Skoryna, S.C. Influence of fucoidan on the intestinal absorption of iron, cobalt, manganese and zinc in rats. *Digestion* **1981**, *21*, 6–12. [CrossRef]

17. Suh, J.K.; Scherping, S.; Mardi, T.; Steadman, J.R.; Woo, S.L.Y. Basic science of articular cartilage injury and repair. *Oper. Tech. Sports Med.* **1995**, *3*, 78–86. [CrossRef]

18. Mitchell, N.; Shepard, N. The resurfacing of adult rabbit articular cartilage by multiple perforations through the subchondral bone. *J. Bone Joint Surg. Am.* **1976**, *58A*, 230–233.

19. Furukawa, T.; Eyre, D.R.; Kiode, S.; Glimcher, M.J. Biochemical studies on repair cartilage resurfacing experimental defects in the rabbit knee. *J. Bone Joint Surg. Am.* **1980**, *62A*, 79–89.

20. Hashida, M.; Miyatake, K.; Okamoto, Y.; Fujita, K.; Matsumoto, T.; Morimatsu, F.; Sakamoto, K.; Minami, S. Synergistic effects of D-glucosamine and collagen peptides on healing experimental cartilage injury. *Macromol. Biosci.* **2003**, *3*, 596–603. [CrossRef]

21. Metsaranta, M.; Kujala, U.M.; Pelliniemi, L.; Osterman, H.; Aho, H.; Vuorio, E. Evidence for insufficient chondrocytic differentiation during repair of full-thickness defects of articular cartilage. *Matrix Biol.* **1996**, *15*, 39–47. [CrossRef]

22. Shapiro, F.; Koide, S.; Glimcher, M.J. Cell origin and differentiation in the repair of full-thickness defects of articular cartilage. *J. Bone Joint Surg. Am.* **1993**, *75*, 532–553.

23. Phadke, K.; Nanda, S. Secretion of chondrocyte stimulating factor by macrophages as a result of activation with collagen and proteoglycans. *Clin. Exp. Immunol.* **1983**, *51*, 494–500.

24. Azuma, K.; Osaki, T.; Tsuka, T.; Imagawa, T.; Okamoto, Y.; Takamori, Y.; Minami, S. Effects of oral glucosamine hydrochloride administration on plasma free amino acid concentrations in dogs. *Mar. Drugs* **2011**, *9*, 712–718. [CrossRef]

25. Osaki, T.; Azuma, K.; Kurozumi, S.; Takamori, Y.; Tsuka, T.; Imagawa, T.; Okamoto, Y.; Minami, S. Metabolomic analyses of blood plasma after oral administration of D-glucosamine hydrochloride to dogs. *Mar. Drugs* **2012**, *10*, 1873–1882. [CrossRef]

Samples Availability: Available from the authors.

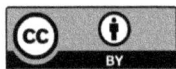

MDPI

Review

Marine Polysaccharides in Microencapsulation and Application to Aquaculture: "From Sea to Sea"

Massimiliano Borgogna, Barbara Bellich and Attilio Cesàro *

Department of Life Sciences, University of Trieste, Via L. Giorgieri, 1-I-34127 Trieste, Italy;
mborgogna@units.it (M.B.); bbellich@units.it (B.B.)

* Author to whom correspondence should be addressed; cesaro@units.it; Tel.: +39-040-558-3684;
Fax: +39-040-558-3691.

Received: 10 October 2011; in revised form: 18 November 2011; Accepted: 22 November 2011;
Published: 8 December 2011

Abstract: This review's main objective is to discuss some physico-chemical features of polysaccharides as intrinsic determinants for the supramolecular structures that can efficiently provide encapsulation of drugs and other biological entities. Thus, the general characteristics of some basic polysaccharides are outlined in terms of their conformational, dynamic and thermodynamic properties. The analysis of some polysaccharide gelling properties is also provided, including the peculiarity of the charged polysaccharides. Then, the way the basic physical chemistry of polymer self-assembly is made in practice through the laboratory methods is highlighted. A description of the several literature procedures used to influence molecular interactions into the macroscopic goal of the encapsulation is given with an attempt at classification. Finally, a practical case study of specific interest, the use of marine polysaccharide matrices for encapsulation of vaccines in aquaculture, is reported.

Keywords: polysaccharide properties; conformation and dynamics; hydrogels; encapsulation; fish vaccination

---

1. Introduction

The polymer science viewpoint has been extended in the last two decades to many other fields of research, from food science and technology to pharmaceutical and biomedicine application.

It is a first principle in the general polymer textbook that, when specific interactions are weak or absent, most polymers are by definition incompatible and show a tendency to undergo liquid-liquid phase separation. In addition to the phase behavior enhanced either by a decrease or an increase in temperature, some polymers may also have further elements of topological complexity in their ordering processes which make the event of phase separation more complex. Thus, understanding solution phase behavior and associative phenomena of mixed polymers, and biopolymers in particular, is important from many viewpoints. The thermodynamic phase boundary location and the dynamic aspects of phase separation are related to the non-equilibrium relaxation processes that follow the perturbation of the system from a thermodynamically stable to a thermodynamically unstable state. Indeed, these processes are usually induced not only by changes in temperature, but also solvent (concentration or composition) or pressure. Polymer compatibility, in the sense of thermodynamic stability, depends in a subtle way on molecular parameters, both intrinsically conformational and energetic. As a general principle, two high molecular weight polymers are mutually incompatible in the absence of favorable interaction. Of a great practical interest is the situation when one or both polymers are weakly charged and modulation of the solution compatibility can be achieved by tuning the ionic strength or pH [1]. Some aspects of these phenomena are briefly described in the following sections, reporting in particular on the phenomenon of polymer complexation and gelation of weakly charged polysaccharides and their self-assembly in forms of beads (from nano to micro) for several practical applications, including the delivery of vaccines in aquaculture.

The intent of this review is to examine a progressive field of research through the authors experience and interests; therefore it is not necessarily exhaustive or comprehensive. The paper is organized in part in a semi-tutorial way, from the description of some basic blocks of polysaccharides (glycans) to form chain topologies and supramolecular structures that can usefully provide encapsulation of drugs, for application in vaccines. Thus, the following section reports on several molecular aspects involved in the construction of polymeric self-assembled structures, aiming at the basic phenomena behind the bench work. Then, by introducing the requirement of biocompatibility and, moreover, of biodegradation and safety of the polymeric matrices, an analysis of some polymeric categories generally regarded as safe (or GRAS) is provided, illustrating in particular those polymers that are largely used, both from the historical and from the economical viewpoint. The third section illustrates the way the basic physical chemistry of polymer self-assembly is made in practice through laboratory methods, by coarsening the fine tuning of the molecular interactions into the macroscopic goal of encapsulation of a macromolecular drug. Finally, the last section is devoted to a case study of specific interest, the use of polysaccharidic matrix for encapsulation of vaccines for aquaculture, by exploring the formulation and the characterization of several systems.

2. Polysaccharides

2.1. Structure and Shape Determinants for Aggregation and Gelation

This work points out the biophysical rules in the construction of nanostructures with application in food, cosmeceutical and pharmaceutical fields. Attention is mainly given to the polysaccharide conformational and solution properties which are at the basis of the self-interaction processes generating nano- and micro-structures. The main reason for focusing attention on polysaccharides is certainly due to their versatility accompanied by the fully biocompatibility and biodegradability. A description of the topological and dynamical parameters characterizing the conformational properties of polysaccharides has been presented elsewhere [2] and is summarized in Section 2.3. The relevance of spatial and temporal concepts has been clearly pointed out in a recent paper dealing with the statistical conformational analysis of glycans. This problem was summarized in the question "What conformational states does the glycan adopt and what are their population?" as opposed to the other simpler one "What is the shape of my glycan?" [3].

The solution properties of biopolymers, and polysaccharides in particular, have always been of considerable interest for many commercial applications, such as thickening, suspending and gelling agents [4,5]. The wide range of rheological behavior shown by polysaccharides in aqueous solution is due to the variety of conformations and chain flexibility, spanning from the more or less expanded coil (like dextran or guar) to the rigid rod limit (like xanthan) which is peculiar for this class of polymers. Still lacking is, however, the direct correlation of the chemical structure and the conformational features of the chains with the rheological behavior displayed, although experimental and simulation studies have been addressed more recently to understanding the process of elasticity and dissipation at nanoscale level by means of atomic force microscopy and conformational analysis [6,7]. The main reason to refer to rheological properties is due to the clear definition that the ratio of the elastic modulus to the dissipative viscous one gives for the identification of the presence of a gel phase, often called "soft condensed matter". A gel phase occurs as an irreversible phenomenon for chemically cross-linked polymer chains, while it is a consequence of solvent or temperature perturbation in many other cases, classified as "reversible gels".

The formation of thermoreversible (physical) gels has been observed in many dilute polymer solutions and has previously provoked an enormous interest because of both the fundamental aspects of the morphology and of the gelation kinetics of these systems [8–10]. Polymer physical gels are also formed by crystallization from quiescent solutions, while for a time the belief persisted that, apart from the biopolymer gel networks [8], shearing was required. As a notable example, the crystals formed during gelation of many synthetic polymers are of lamella type, like those formed from dilute solution [11].

According to experimental findings in gel formation, many variables are involved to control the resulting structures, in particular, cooling rate, gelation temperature, and solvent properties, which are all important for the crystallization process. As the solution is cooled, chains can form crystalline domains that serve as reversible cross-links if the chain entanglement in the solution is sufficiently developed. This scheme is in line with Flory's concept of the minimum functionality which can generate cross-linking gelation [12] and with the statistical model of Tanaka and Stochmayer [13].

Recent results reported in the literature [14–16] provide the basis for a better understanding of the gel structure and gelation mechanism for many systems, either synthetic or natural polymers. The mechanism of thermoreversible gelation of polysaccharides in solution is investigated through the study of the temperature-concentration relations, the thermodynamic behavior of the solvent and the gel melting, the change in molecular conformation by several spectroscopic methods and structural and dynamic analysis by light scattering. In particular, the time dependence of structural and dynamic parameters can be measured after a rapid quenching of the polysaccharide solution at a given concentration (above the critical threshold), providing a picture such as schematically reported in Figure 1. The mechanism consists of different steps: a coil to (double) helix transition followed by an intermolecular association that finally leads to a macroscopic network like a crystal lattice.

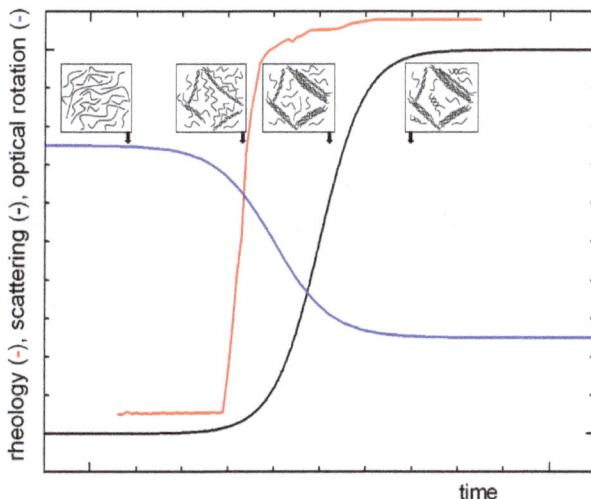

Figure 1. General mechanism (nucleation and growth) of gel formation as macroscopically measured by viscoelastic, optical and chiroptical properties. The insets show sketch of the polymer solution microstructure at the various stages.

Models for fibrillar aggregation arise especially from the polysaccharide field and have also been pictured by several microscopy methods in the case of gellan, agarose, carrageenan, and other relatively stiff chains [14,17,18]. Many of these biopolymers have low flexibility (e.g., worm-like polysaccharides with persistence length Lp > 60 nm) and show a remarkable deviation from the solution behavior described for flexible molecules. They often undergo gelation in a cooperative process triggered by small changes in temperature, ionic strength, pH [8,19]. A similar suggestion has also been put forward for polystyrene gels [20], in which the complexation with the solvent is the crucial factor affecting the chain stiffening. However, neither the solution features nor the gel morphology and behavior exhibited by many biopolymers can support the molecular mechanism or the conformational motifs as those ascribed to stiff polysaccharides and solvent-complexed polystyrene.

2.2. Thermodynamic Considerations

As chain dimension and stiffness not only depend on structural characteristics but also on the solvent quality, the other point to discuss is the more general thermodynamic aspect of the gel. In physical gelation processes, the important driving force is the conformational ordering of segments of chains which reach a critical size for the Gibbs free energy stability. The dimensionality of the gel nucleus is again governed by the stiffness of the chain. On this basis, it does not seem appropriate to assume that very flexible chains which are known to form gels in dilute solutions are organized with the same mechanism proposed for rigid polymers. Therefore, both in biopolymers and synthetic polymers the process of local crystallization and gelation can occur either in the lamella-like (e.g., starches) or fibrillar-like (e.g., gelatin) organization.

Independent of the structure of crystalline junctions, the size of the ordered gel phase is a relevant aspect which determines the thermodynamic stability and therefore the changes in the melting temperature Tm of the gel phase. The other is the presence of a component (solvent or plasticizer) which acts as a solvent for the amorphous/liquid phase in equilibrium at Tm with the solid crystalline phase. The first development of a theoretical formulation was given by Flory and Mandelkern [21] and uses the Flory-Huggins model for the thermodynamic properties of the polymer solution. However, this is not sufficient for many cases, where the crystalline phase is formed by crystals whose dimension and morphology are dependent upon the experimental conditions [22]. In a schematic representation of the Gibbs free-energy diagram *vs.* temperature, the energy surface is described by a family of curves for the liquid phase (*i.e.*, the Gibbs free-energy curve of the liquid polymer and those of the pure liquid polymer with increasing concentration of the other component) and also by a family of curves for the solid phase (*i.e.*, the Gibbs free-energy curve of the perfect crystal of infinite size and those of the crystals with an increasing number of defects and decreasing size). Melting temperatures, such as those in Figure 2, are then a function of both the composition of the system and the dimensional features of the crystal (*i.e.* by the Gibbs-Thomson-Tamman equation), as recently "rediscovered" in the field of nanomaterials. Many literature results confirm this general interpretation, although they are not always reported in this form.

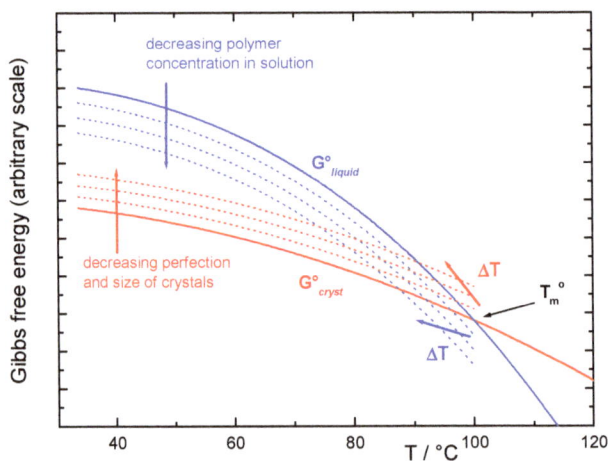

Figure 2. Schematic representation of the Gibbs free-energy curve *vs.* temperature for the liquid phase (as a function of composition, blue lines); and for the crystalline phase as a function of decreasing crystal size (red lines). The practical effect is a decrease in the measured melting temperature.

Mar. Drugs **2011**, *9*, 2572–2604

Having discussed how the overall process of chain-chain interaction is governed by chemical and physical parameters, it is also worth pointing out the principles that shape the polymer aggregates for specific functions. Indeed, the most important feature for spherical gel particles is not only the diameter (from millimeters to nanometers) but also the distribution of polymer aggregates as the actual texture may change from the interior to the surface. To make this clear with one single example, it is sufficient to mention the relevance of survival of a cell encapsulated within a gel particle in terms of dimension of the confined cavity and of the extent of diffusion of metabolites and catabolytes, in addition to the proper environmental chemical properties. For the above reasons, gel systems in the biological fields (especially for applications in foods and pharmaceutics) are mainly based on biopolymers and polysaccharides in particular.

Finally, in several less stringent applications, other kinds of gels are prepared from synthesis of natural polymers through chemical cross-linkers or by the free radical polymerization of monomers in the presence of a bifunctional cross-linking agent. New classes of gels with two levels of structural hierarchy have also been engineered by first making gel nanoparticles and then covalently bonding them together. In this way the primary network is made by cross-linked polymer chains in each individual particle, while the secondary network is a system of cross-linked nanoparticles. Such nanostructured gels have appealing properties that conventional gels do not have, including a high surface area, a bright color at room temperature, and temperature-tunable heterogeneity on the nanometer scale [23].

2.3. How Do Polysaccharide Chain Solution Properties Depend on Sugar Monomer Composition?

It is now well known that linear glycans, differing from one another only in glycosidic linkage position and stereochemistry, can display a wide range of equilibrium conformational features [24,25]. The variability of chain flexibility arises from the large number of naturally available sugar residues with several linkage patterns and from the possible occurrence of intra- and intermolecular interactions. The former controls the overall chain geometry and the latter governs the pattern of shapes and dimensions characterizing the polymer in solution. Under given conditions the above constraints may induce regular helical conformations to some extent. A "portfolio" sketch of how the main structural blocks of polysaccharides prefigure the local conformational features and therefore the chain topology is given in Figure 3.

Commonly, some of these well known equilibrium conformational differences are schematically illustrated by the typical stiff and extended $(1{\rightarrow}4)$-β-linked chain of cellulose [26,27] and similar "cellulosic" chains, like chitosan [28]. Other features are exhibited by the "pseudo-helical" $(1{\rightarrow}4)$-α-linked random coil chain of amylose [29] or by the more disordered open helical-like that of the $(1{\rightarrow}3)$-β-linked chain of curdlan [25,30]. Additional examples of chain topology are provided by industrially important polysaccharides, like hyaluronan [31,32], schizophyllan [6] and scleroglucan [7], which have been modeled with a reasonable level of accuracy.

Although schematically simple in the statements given above, it is more complicated in practice to experimentally develop structural (molecular) understanding of the conformational mobility and dynamics of oligo- and polysaccharides in solution. While modern Molecular Dynamics investigations provide a huge amount of numerical simulations, the underlying physical rules are hidden behind the "beauty" of the molecular figures the computation productions.

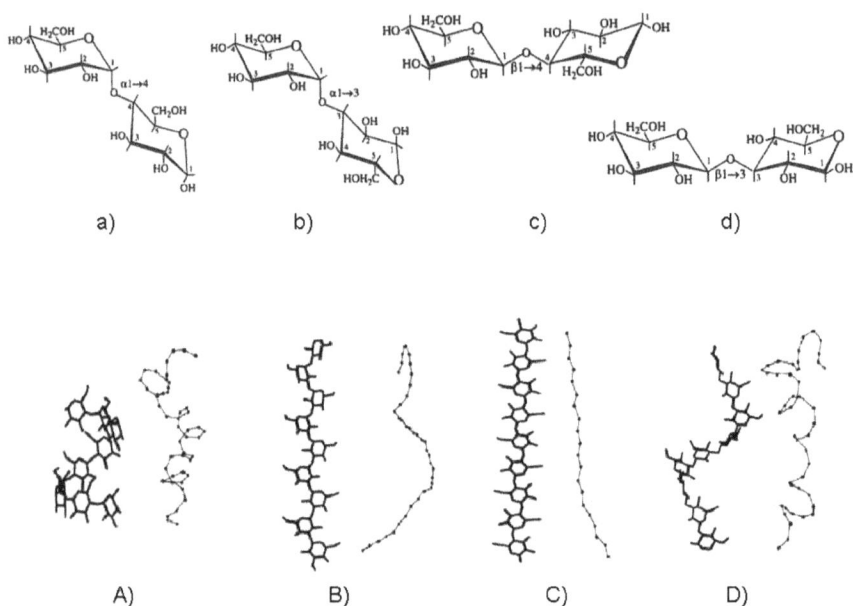

Figure 3. Structural representation of four disaccharides from glucose: (**a**) maltose (α-(1-4)-linked); (**b**) nigerose (α-(1-3)-linked); (**c**) cellobiose (β-(1-4)-linked); (**d**) laminarabiose (β-(1-3)-linked). The related polysaccharide structures of amylose (**A**), nigeran (**B**), cellulose (**C**) and laminaran (**D**) are shown in the ordered helical conformations as measured by X-ray fiber diffraction studies (left) and as snapshots of random chains modeled by Monte Carlo calculation (right).

For an implementation of these pictorial views, the time dependence of the conformational changes in solution has to be considered as this is likely also to be dependent on the features of the glycosidic linkages [7,31,33]. The full physical description of all these local motions are conveniently given by the spectral density of $^{13}C-^{1}H$ bond motions in the nanosecond frequency range [34–36]. Thus, some correlations between the conformational dynamics and the structural details have been sought, although systematic theoretical investigation of the structure dynamics relationships for naturally occurring sugar sequences is still in progress [37].

In an attempt to scrutinize the above features, the very preliminaries for a correct setting of knowledge about the shape of polysaccharides in solution are essentially given by the correlation between three contributions: the primary structure (*i.e.*, the chemical identity of the carbohydrates polymerized in the chain), the intrinsic conformational features dictated by the rotational equilibrium (often the major contributions are due to the rotation about the glycosidic linkages) and the interaction with the other molecular species in the system, *i.e.*, solvent and cosolutes [38].

As already mentioned, the primary structure of polysaccharides is complicated by different kinds of linkages in homopolymers and different kinds of monomer units, facts which give rise to a huge number of different polymers. Glucans (see a general formula in Figure 3) are those composed exclusively of glucose, while glucuronans are polymers of glucuronic acid. Similarly mannans and galactans as well as mannuronans and galacturonans, are homopolymers of mannose, galactose, mannuronic acid and galacturonic acid, respectively. Although the listed polysaccharides have a structural regularity (homopolymers), many other glycans are not homopolymers and their chemical structure can often be fairly complicated, as in the case of microbial and plant polysaccharides [39–41].

From the experimental point of view, several omo- and co-polysaccharides with different chain linkage and anomeric configurations have been studied to determine to what extent the polymeric linkage structure and the nature of the monomeric unit are responsible for the preferred solvation and for the chain topology and dimensions [42]. Conversely, since it is generally understood that the structure and topology of many macromolecules are affected by solvation, theoretical models must include these solvent effects in addition to the internal flexibility, in order to estimate changes in the accessible conformations as a result of the presence of the solvent molecules. The practical problem is to what extent do solvents and co-solutes contribute to stabilizing some conformational states rather than others. Since solution properties reflect the distribution of conformations of the chain molecules, the experimental data are the unique solution to the statistical thermodynamic average over all the accessible conformational states of the molecule. This aspect has been illustrated by taking into consideration the accessible conformational states of a simple sugar unit *"in vacuo"* and the conformational perturbation arising from a solvent medium [43–50]. Therefore, in most realistic situations, account must be taken of the conformational perturbations given by specific molecular interactions. These interactions often modulate the conformation to a local minimum and impose some structural constraints giving long range pseudo-order. The naïve response to these questions, which requires a complete knowledge of the time-space dependence of the chain topology, is often "rounded-off" by the use of empirical terms like "flexibility".

Passing from monomer units to oligomers (disaccharides and higher oligosaccharides), the dominant features of molecular flexibility become those due to rotations about the glycosidic linkages. Although all other conformational fluctuations contribute to the local dynamics of the atoms or group of atoms, only the glycosidic linkage rotations are able to dramatically change the conformational topology of oligomers at ambient temperature. The aim of a conformational analysis of oligosaccharides is thus to evaluate the probability (that is the energy) of all mutual orientations of the two monosaccharide units, as a function of rotations about the glycosidic linkages, defined by the dihedral angles φ and ψ. The important regions of φ and ψ rotations are those with energy variations in the order of kT, the thermal motion energy, because this may produce a large ensemble of accessible conformational states for the oligosaccharide. There are some contrasting interpretations as to whether the presence of water contributes to the increase or decrease of the glycosidic conformational freedom. This is sometimes due to the possibility of contribution of water molecules bridging two adjacent sugar rings, an event which is more probable in stiff disaccharides than in the more flexible $1{\rightarrow}6$ linked disaccharides.

Even when the rotational motion is restricted to only a few angles, the fluctuations of many such glycosidic bonds is amplified along the chain backbone, as the molecular weight increases. The accumulation of even limited local rotations may produce very large topological variations in the case of polymeric chains and consequently relevant changes in thermodynamic, hydrodynamic and rheological properties of these systems. Other internal motions often make only small contributions to the observable properties on the macromolecular scale [26]. Attempts to take into account the full range of conformations have been made in the past in order to predict some suitable set of experimental data, like hydrodynamic volume and radius of gyration, and, more recently, Small-Angle X-ray Scattering results [47,51].

2.4. Solutions of Ionic Polysaccharides

The solution behavior of ionic macromolecules (polyelectrolytes) is by far more complicated. Based on the experimental evidence of polyelectrolyte solutions, all high molecular weight ionic macromolecules are characterized by a peculiar behavior which sets them apart from all other ionic low molecular weight molecules as well as from non-ionic macromolecules. A general consequence of the presence of charged groups on the chain is a favorable contribution to the solubility of polymer in water. Also, a strongly attractive potential is generated between the charge density on the polymer and the opposite charges in solution. As a consequence, the value of the activity coefficient of the counterions is strongly reduced with respect to that of the same ions in the presence of the univalent opposite charged species. When the ionizable groups are rather weak (e.g., carboxylic groups), the behavior of the polymer is a function of pH (*i.e.*, of the degree of ionization α). For these reasons, the study of the protonation-deprotonation process of a carboxylic polymer is an efficient tool for understanding the various contributions and for revealing, through the change of charge density, variations occurring in the intramolecular and intermolecular interactions. However, because the flexibility of conformation alters the distances between charged groups on the polymeric chain, a new equilibrium is statistically defined by the total Gibbs energy minimum of the system [52]. As an important consequence of this energy balance, changes in temperature, ionic strength, pH, *etc.*, can provoke changes in polyelectrolyte conformation and dimension, often cooperatively in many biopolymers, between states with different values of the charge density. These states may be characterized by different structural orders (e.g., helix→extended chain transition), by different degrees of flexibility of the chain (globular coil→expanded chain) or by different extents of aggregation (monomeric→dimeric or multimeric chains).

For the interpretation of the experimental data and for the understanding of the correlation between properties and structure, a theoretical approach based on a molecular model is necessary. The central problem is that of quantifying the interactions among charges on the polymer and among these and their respective counterions. The most common approaches are those which describe the linear polyelectrolyte using a model with local cylindrical geometry. Although no derivation is given here of the thermodynamic functions associated with the process of "ion binding" [53,54], let us briefly state that a polyelectrolyte approach, based on the counterion condensation theory developed for dilute solutions by Manning [55], predicts a positive enthalpy change on mixing the polymer with a simple salt. Under the same circumstances, a positive volume change and a negative entropy change are also predicted for the merely electrostatic interaction of the point charges with the linear polyelectrolyte.

The measured enthalpy of binding evaluated by direct calorimetric experiments has been published for different cations and polysaccharides and nicely confirms the predicted behavior, when other conformational changes or aggregative processes are absent. In other cases, scrutiny of the dependence of the experimental enthalpy changes as a function of the degree of complexation (or of the ion-to-polymer molar ratio) discloses cooperativity (binding and/or state transition), that easily monitor the occurrence of a chain conformational transition [56], in particular if the dependence is contrasted to the theoretical trend of the purely polyelectrolytic binding. Furthermore, the analysis can detect the actual charge density of the ionic polysaccharides (either single chains or multiple chain aggregates), since the free mono- or di-valent cation effectively acts as a "thermodynamic probe" of the true chemical potential associated to the structural characteristics of the charged species. Figure 4 illustrates this concept of the ion as a thermodynamic probe by comparing the structural information obtained by scattering experiments with that achievable by molecular thermodynamic experiments, both using suitable theories.

EXPERIMENT   OUTPUT – DATA ANALYSIS

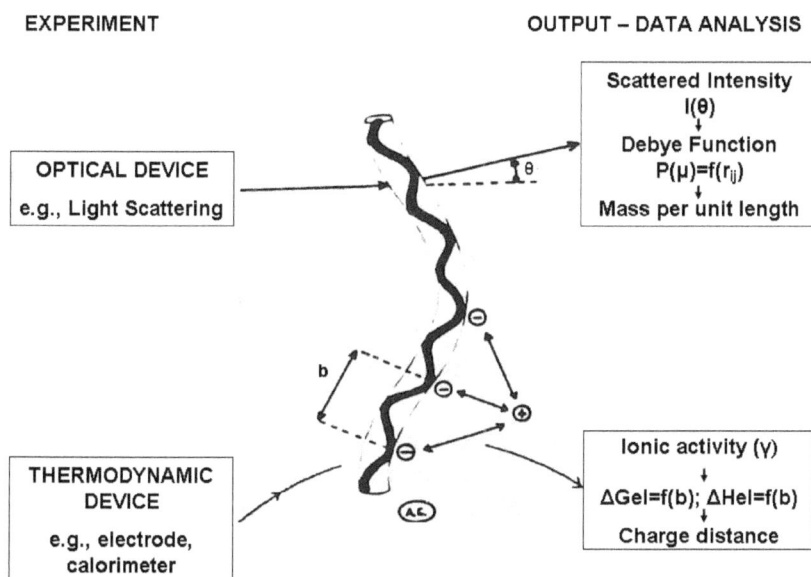

Figure 4. Correlation between structural conformational data obtained by scattering experiments (top) and structural data obtained by molecular thermodynamic theories (bottom). The example refers to the chain mass-per-unit length (from light scattering) and to the average distance between charged groups (from potentiometry or calorimetry).

Within this perspective, the theoretical derivation of the Gibbs energy, enthalpy and volume change on mixing a polyelectrolyte with monovalent and divalent ions has been explored for many cases, e.g., for carrageenans with Cs^+ [54,57], always compared with experimentally measured values of the same properties. It is also clear that the volume change, as experimentally observed, may be larger than that which would be calculated on the basis of theory alone, since no provision is made in the theory for the volume change upon ion desolvation.

As far as it concerns the short-range interactions in the absence of aggregates or gel formation, the introduction of charged groups modifies the equilibrium geometry of the monomeric units and the contribution of the electrostatic nature on the nearest-neighbor conformational energy. There are at least two approaches that are relevant for this review; one is that described by Haug and Smidsrød [58] for the rationalization of the dimensional properties of polyelectrolytes as a function of salt concentration, the other is the already mentioned formulation of a statistical thermodynamic theory for the "physical" framing of the ion-polyelectrolyte interactions. Both these theoretical formulations deal with the conformation of the polymer and predict that the conformational features must be a function of ionic strength (see for example [53,59]). More recent developments in the exploitations of structure-property-applications of ionic polysaccharides [60–63] make indirect use of the above concepts.

2.5. Marine Polysaccharides: Alginate and Chitosan Solutions

Some aspects of the main phenomena that describe the conformational properties, and their perturbation, of carbohydrate polymers have been covered in this section. One of the major concerns has been to describe these "effects" starting with the complex conformational equilibria generated in the simple chains. In fact, only recently has the quantitative relationship between conformational population and physical properties been fully appreciated. This section, however, does not give extensive references to the experimental determination of the polysaccharide shape and size in different experimental conditions, but rather it attempts to focus on the molecular reasons for these perturbations. A digression is also made to include the electrostatic charges in polyelectrolytic polysaccharides, because of their diffusion and use and because of interesting variations occurring in these systems, including the marine polysaccharides discussed in the following section. In particular, since alginate and chitosan will be used for the application given in Section 4, the relation between the structural features of these compounds and their use in gelation systems are focused on here.

Alginate is a polysaccharide of algal or bacterial origin. It is composed of units of D-mannuronic acid (M) and L-guluronic acid (G) which form homopolymeric block structures along the chains, namely M-blocks and G-blocks interspaced by alternate MG sequences [64]. The original work on elucidation of alginate binding properties goes back to the seventies, pointing out the important relation between the cooperative sequence of guluronan residues [65–67] and the egg-box model proposed by Rees and coworkers [68,69]. This model has been central for the phenomenological description of alginate gelation, although more recently both a refinement and an extension of the original model shed some more light on the structural features of the "dimeric forms" of guluronan sequences involved in the chelation with calcium ions and responsible for the gel strength [70–72]. A recent review on alginate as a "biomaterial" [73] describes the role of several features of comonomer fraction and sequence in the ion-binding properties of alginate towards divalent ions and includes the extended description of the thermodynamic aspects of "egg-box" model and of the mechanism of hydrogel formation [74–76]. The concluding remarks on the gelation features of alginate attribute to calcium ions the right size and charge to fit into the distorted egg-box structure, including a non-negligible effect of the secondary junctions due to the alternating sequences of MG-type [77].

Chitosan derives from the chitin (extracted from crustacean and insect exoskeleton or from some algae and fungi) and is essentially a polyglucosamine varying in the degree of acetylation (DA) and molecular weight. The presence of a variable number of free amino groups and substitutions is responsible for the tunable interaction with anionic and polyanionic systems [78]. Although less modeled, chitosan conformational properties are mainly ascribed to the two-fold cellulose-like helix [79]. These features largely explain the intrinsic conformational stiffness as measured by several hydrodynamic and scattering experiments, sometimes affected in the past by uncertainties due to the microgel formation for samples at high DA [80]. Recent experimental results converge toward assigning to random acetyl substitution the relevant key-factor in controlling the changes in the chain stiffness, with a significant flexibility achieved at moderate to medium DA (<50%). This result is at least in part due to the common "co-monomer" effect, but must contain other contributing factors, such as short-range nearest-neighbor interactions [28] and long range excluded volume effect [81]. More recently, enhancement of chain flexibility and solubility properties has been reached by controlled chemical-etching of the glucosidic ring with periodate oxidation [82], as well as by introducing several types of pendant groups at the amino functionality [83].

3. Encapsulation in Polysaccharide Hydrogels

3.1. Polysaccharide-Based Hydrogels for Technological Applications

In biomaterial science, hydrogels are defined as "three-dimensional, hydrophilic, polymeric networks capable of imbibing large amounts of water or biological fluids" [84]. Such networks can be chemically (covalently) or physically cross-linked (by reversible molecular entanglements, ionic and hydrophobic interactions, H-bonds, *etc.*). Due to their high water content and soft consistency, hydrogels are very similar to natural living tissues, with performances that overcome the other classes of biomaterials. Generally, hydrogels are classified as natural polymer hydrogels, synthetic polymer hydrogels and combination of the two types. Several polymeric materials are employed as biomaterials, each one with specific properties which influence the hydrogel design parameters [84–87]. Among the natural polymers, polysaccharides have a wide application due to their peculiarities: they are abundant and obtained from renewable sources (such as plants, algae, bacteria); they present a large variety of composition and properties, not easily reproducible by synthetic routes; their production is generally easier and cheaper than for synthetic polymers. Thus, the number of polysaccharides investigated for technological applications of hydrogels is extremely extensive [88]. Polysaccharides are also employed as derivatives obtained by chemical or physical modification, to tailor the final properties of interest; moreover, biotechnology can enable the *in vitro* production of high levels of polysaccharides from micro-organisms [89–91].

In bio-oriented applications, polysaccharide hydrogels are exploited as immobilization matrices and protective structures (as scaffolds and capsules) for sensible materials, such as living cells and active compounds. The application to relevant technological fields (pharmaceutical, food, and biomedical) of hydrogels based on two representative marine polysaccharides, alginate and chitosan, will be reviewed.

3.2. Pharmaceutical Applications

Pharmaceutical applications of hydrogels are based on their capability to act as exceptional drug delivery vehicles. Drugs and bioactive compounds are incorporated into the matrices and can be released according to various release profiles depending on the hydrogel properties [84,92]. It is generally accepted that the drug release from the matrix follows two main mechanisms, that is diffusion of the protein through the pores of the polymer network and degradation of the polymer network [93]. In addition, water diffusion and swelling through the hydrogel are two of the major factors affecting drug release rate [94]. Thus, drug release from a hydrogel is governed by several parameters: pore volume fraction; pore sizes; extent of interconnections; size and physico-chemical nature of the drug molecule, and in general type and strength of interactions between drugs and polymeric chains [86]. When alginate and chitosan are used for the preparation of hydrogel matrices for drug release, the fine control of the polymer structure and molecular weight [95–98], and of the conditions employed for the formulations (such as type and concentration of gelling ions, polymer concentration, procedures, *etc.*) [99–101], enable tailoring the functional properties of the drug delivery system. At a molecular level, the alginate hydrogel structure is strictly related to the composition and sequence of the polymer, and thus to the origin of the sample. Chitosan properties are also determined by the acetylation degree. All these factors deeply influence the characteristics of the hydrogel, and thus the capability to entrap, protect and release the drug payload.

Some peculiar properties of hydrogels are shown in physiological conditions: for example, they can swell depending on the external environment, behaving as physiologically-responsive hydrogels. Some hydrogels show significant changes in the swelling ratio, and thus in release capability, in relation to pH, ionic strength, temperature or electromagnetic radiation. Moreover, hydrogels are used as muco-adhesive drug carriers able to interact with the mucosal surface (for example in the gastrointestinal tract or the respiratory epithelium) prolonging their residence time at the site of delivery. The interaction between carriers and mucosal glycoproteins occurs primarily via hydrogen bonding, and materials containing a high density of carboxyl and hydroxyl groups are chosen for these applications [84,102,103]. Hydrogel-based systems have been exploited for protection and delivery of low-molecular weight drugs and macromolecular payloads [104,105], such as peptide and protein drugs (insulin, melatonin, heparin, haemoglobin, parathyroid hormone, calcitonin, *etc.*) [106–108], nucleic acids (DNA, siRNA) [109,110] and antigens (from pathogens responsible of influenza, pertussis, diphtheria, tetanus, *etc.*) [107,111–113]. In addition to antigens, also vaccines have been encapsulated (attenuated or inactivated pathogens) in both medical and veterinary fields, combining the cell immobilization to a drug delivery system. Such technology is gaining great attention, due to the possibility to protect the vaccine during the administration (also for the oral route) and hopefully to control the targeting and delivery rate [114,115]. A detailed example of the application of biopolymer encapsulation of fish vaccinations will be presented in Section 4.2.

3.3. Other Applications

The oldest application of polysaccharide hydrogels is in food technology: in foodstuff, they are naturally responsible of the texture, so they have been used as thickening or gelling agents (for example in juices and chocolate). Nowadays, the use of microencapsulation with biopolymers has gained great importance in the development of food enriched with bioactive components (lipids, vitamins, peptides, fatty acids, antioxidants, minerals and also living cells, such as probiotics) and nutraceuticals (ingredients with potential health benefits [116–118]), for the protection of the compounds against inactivation or degradation, and also for their controlled delivery. The addition of such substances to food matrices is pursued to produce physiological benefits or reduce the risk of specific diseases. This implies a huge challenge, in common with pharmaceutical applications, since only a reduced amount of molecules remains available after oral administration, due to several factors, such as low permeability or solubility within the gut, and instability in the gastro-intestinal tract (due to pH, enzymes, presence of other nutrients) [117], or under food processing conditions (temperature, oxygen, light). Microencapsulation is used to stabilize reactive, sensitive, or volatile ingredients, and can be considered the source of totally new ingredients with exceptional properties, thanks to the tailored controlled-release properties: targeted and controlled release enhances the effectiveness of food additives, ensuring the optimal dosage, and (not marginally at all) improves the cost effectiveness [119]. Many encapsulation procedures have also been developed in the food industry: each technology suits different systems in order to meet the physico-chemical and molecular requirements of a specific bioactive component.

A lot of GRAS biopolymers are compatible with many food components and are already used in the food industry (such as alginate, pectins, dextran, starch, cellulose and derivatives) and can combine a proper protection of the product and a targeted delivery. Often these polymers are modified to optimize the compatibility with the food matrices [118,120]. In principle, no real distinction exists between procedures used in food and in pharmaceutical technology, but of the entrapped molecules.

In the biomedical technology (tissue engineering and regenerative medicine) hydrogels are the most relevant materials, thanks to their peculiarities, such as biocompatibility, physical properties, flexibility in the synthesis, and variety of constituents [121]. Hydrogels are currently used in several applications: as scaffolds, as tissue barriers and bioadhesives, as drug depots, as delivery systems for bioactive agents (that enhance the natural reparative process), as matrices to encapsulate and deliver cells [121]. Thus tissue engineering represents a great potential for the regeneration of tissues and organs, as an alternative to the traditional approaches to tissue or organ failure, mainly based on the replacement of the tissue with a synthetic implant, on the transplantation of the organ, and also on extracorporeal treatments (passive membrane exchange, experimental biohybrid systems, *etc.*). Among several strategies, the most appealing is based on the combination of cells and polymer scaffolds [86]. The 3D-scaffolds are used as substrates for supporting and guiding tissue regeneration in several *in vitro* and *in vivo* systems which mimic the extracellular matrix (ECM), a structure made of protein and sugar-based macromolecules, that provides the physical and biological support for cell and tissue growth. The preparation of ECM-mimicking biomaterials with defined shape and complex porous architecture represents still a technical challenge [122]. Hydrogels designed as 3D-scaffolds should present pores with an ideal size to accommodate living cells; moreover, they can be designed to dissolve, releasing active molecules [85,86]. Nowadays a variety of tissues has been engineered, with systems at the stage of clinical trial or application, including artery, bladder, skin, cartilage, bone, ligament, and tendon [85,123].

The cell immobilization and encapsulation systems have a broad range of applications: one of the most studied and described is the transplantation of microencapsulated cells, proposed as a therapy for the treatment of a wide variety of diseases. This technology is based on the principle that foreign cells (xenogeneic or allogeneic) are physically segregated and protected from the host immune system by an artificial membrane [124–126]. Thus hydrogel microcapsules can provide immunoisolation, without interfering with the diffusion of oxygen, nutrients, and metabolic products [121]. Various cell types including primary cells, stem cells [127] or bioengineered cells have been investigated for the treatment of the different diseases [128]. Some relevant examples are the treatment of cardiovascular diseases, kidney and liver failure, and diabetes mellitus (by the microencapsulation of islets of Langerhans) [123,129,130].

3.4. Methods for Microencapsulation

As previously reported, the encapsulation in polymeric hydrogels is employed to protect a wide range of materials of biological interest, from small molecules to cells (of bacterial, yeast, plant and animal origin). As a general definition, microencapsulation is "the technology of packaging solid, liquid and gaseous materials in small capsules that release their contents at controlled rates over prolonged periods of time" [116]. A variety of methods of encapsulation has been developed, and the best choice is based on the final requirements, such as mean particle size, physical/chemical properties, payload application, desired release mechanisms, industrial manufacturing scale and the acceptable processing cost [123].

Among all the existing methods, here the attention will be primarily given to the microencapsulation by ionotropic gelation which is one of the most employed, by exploiting the capability of some marine polymers to form hydrogels in the presence of proper multivalent counterions (such as calcium ions for alginate [124] or triphosphate for chitosan [131]). The protection is based on the embedding effect of the polymeric matrix, which controls interactions between the internal and external parts. Although such versatile technology is widely used in the technological fields of food industry, pharmaceutics and biomedicine, the variety of procedures requires some systematization that necessarily includes the other methods.

In the literature definition [93,116], gel particle technology mainly includes three different methods to prepare microspheres by ionotropic gelation (as schematically represented in Figure 5): (a) dropping the polyelectrolyte solution into a solution of small ions; (b) via a water in oil emulsification technique; and (c) complexation of oppositely charged polyelectrolytes by mixing, with additional coating procedures. These original classifications merged over the years into other approaches that use, indeed, several different techniques and procedures, often generating a confusion of terms.

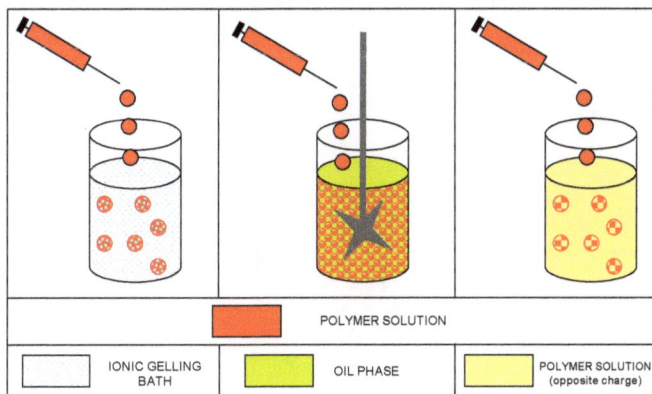

Figure 5. Schematic representation of the methods described for gel particle technology.

In the attempt to rationalize the several approaches into the frame outlined in the previous sections, a graphical classification of the procedures and techniques to encapsulate in polysaccharide hydrogels is proposed in Figure 6. The microparticle production is regarded as a preliminary step for the physical generation of spherical microdomains, independently of the final stage of preparation. Thereafter, whichever production method of microparticles is used, the use of an appropriate gelation mechanism is foreseen to stabilize the microdomains.

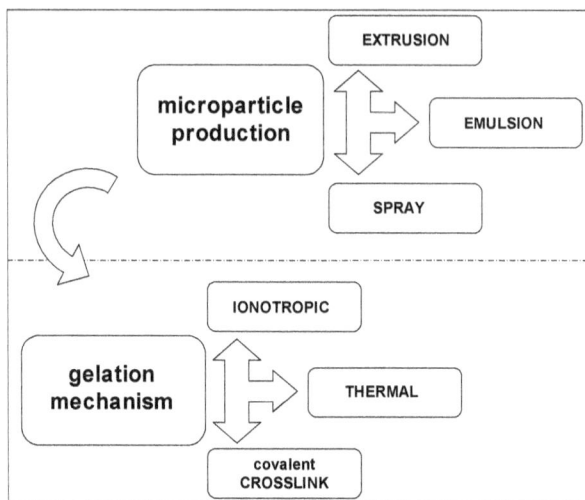

Figure 6. Graphical classification of the encapsulation procedures and techniques in polysaccharide hydrogels.

Thus, in the following part, the methods to obtain microscale droplets/particles and those to transform them in hydrogels will be separately described by reviewing some recent literature classifications [116,123,132,133]. The focus will be on the encapsulation in hydrogels of biological entities (biomolecules, drugs, *etc.*), taking into account that the literature nomenclature for the procedures could vary in different application fields [118].

3.5. Microparticle Production

The first step in the preparation of hydrogel microcapsules is to obtain micro-droplets which will then be gelled in different ways. Three procedures will be presented: extrusion, emulsion and spray-technologies.

The "extrusion" technique is widely exploited and, in the simplest case, can be performed by using a syringe with a needle. As a general principle, the polymer solution is extruded through an orifice and dripped into a hardening (gelling) bath. The size of the droplets determines the final dimensions of the gel particles, and can be controlled through several system parameters: the diameter of the orifice, the flow rate, the viscosity of the solution, the distance between the hardening solution and the orifice, the polymer concentration and the temperature [123]. The reduction of the droplet (and gel particle size) is a fundamental technical problem, which has been handled by developing several devices based on different physical mechanisms. The most used are the coaxial laminar air-flow, the air atomization, the electrostatic potential, the vibrating nozzle, the jet cutting and the spinning disk atomization [134–136]. The resulting particle size is not the only factor to be considered since other aspects are relevant, such as reproducibility, size tunability and distribution, time and yield of production.

Emulsification is the process of dispersing a liquid in a second liquid that is immiscible [118]. The resulting emulsion can be defined basically as a system of two phases (dispersed and dispersing) in which droplets of one liquid are dispersed in another: when the emulsion is made of oil droplets in an aqueous phase it is called "oil-in-water" (O/W), while the opposite system is called "water-in-oil" (W/O). The stability of an emulsion can be regulated by the addition of a surfactant. By working on the composition of the two phases, the type of polymer and surfactant, this technique has been employed also for the production of nanometric droplets and particles. Advances in this technology have been obtained also by the application of microfluidic principles [137,138].

Among the spray-technologies, spray-drying is based on the formation of dried particulate starting from a fluid material (a solution, an emulsion or a suspension), by the atomization in heated gas (air or nitrogen), and the fast removal of the solvent (water). The powder particles are then separated from the drying air. This continuous process is influenced by the temperatures of the system (feed, air inlet and air outlet temperatures), the viscosity and concentration of the feed solution, the morphology of the polymer. Hydrogel particles can thereafter be produced by re-hydrating the powders under gelling conditions. Other methods, such as spray-cooling and spray-chilling, are based on a different principle and in the absence of solvent: the dispersion of a bioactive product in a polymeric matrix is cooled (or chilled) to allow solidification and immobilization [118,123,139]. Finally, the spray-coating technology is often reported in association with gel particle production. It is an efficient coating technique, based on devices such as the fluidized bed, to be used with virtually any polymer. The core particles are suspended by an air flow and then coated with the polymer solution sprayed from different directions (top, bottom and using a tangential spray). This technique can be used on hydrogel microcapsules after the gelation step [116,123].

3.6. Gelation Methods

The step that follows the preparation of micro-droplets of the desired dimension is the gelation, which can occur in different ways through physical and chemical mechanisms.

Physical gelation is mainly done by ionotropic and thermal gelation. The ionotropic gelation is in turn carried out by two main techniques, diffusion and internal setting. The first one is based on the introduction (mainly a dripping) of the polymer solution into an ionic solution: gelation occurs when the ions diffuse into the polymer solution droplets. The second is based on the addition of gelling ions in inactive form (such as calcium carbonate for calcium alginate gels). The gelation is triggered by changes in some system properties, generally pH changes [123]. The ionotropic gelation is suitable for marine biopolymers such as alginate, chitosan, carrageenan and also for materials of different origin (for example pectins). Microencapsulation in alginate hydrogels is probably the most exploited [140–143].

Also polyelectrolyte complexation (PEC), between polymers of opposite charges, is associated to the hydrogel formation, either as method to form the gel structure, or as technique to improve the quality (mechanical strength and permeability barrier) of hydrogel beads already prepared. In the latter case, the complexation can be concurrent with the ion-based gelation, or subsequent (coating step). PEC formation between chitosan and alginate (or other biopolymers) has been exploited for a long time, mainly for pharmaceutical applications for the production of micro- and nano-particles based systems [144–148].

Thermal gelation is applied to agarose, as marine polysaccharide, but also to gelatin, maltodextrin and several synthetic polymers, such as polymethylmethacrylate, polystyrene, poly(*N*-isopropyl-acrylamide), *etc.* Some hints for understanding the theory of this phenomenon have been given in Section 1. Concerning cell encapsulation, the agarose-based hydrogels have been widely studied for several biological applications [149,150].

Chemical gelation is based on the covalent cross-linking of the polymer chains, which results in the formation of the 3D-matrix. Several examples have been reported in literature, the oldest being the reticulation of dextrans to prepare gel beads for size-exclusion chromatography. The formation of chitosan microcapsules was initially based on the glutaraldehyde cross-linking. However, its use is avoided in cell and human applications because of the toxicity of such a reactant. Covalent cross-link can be obtained also by enzymatic routes, among which the safe cross-linker genipine has been employed for the preparation of hydrogels and beads of chitosan [88]. There is also a long list of covalent cross-linking reactions induced by the exposure to UV or visible light (photo-crosslinked hydrogels) [151].

In addition, several strategies of combinations of physical and chemical hydrogel formation techniques have been proposed, leading to "in tandem" mechanisms, in order to tailor and enhance the properties of the microcapsules produced [152–154].

It is also mandatory to mention the application of the natural biopolymers at the nanoscale level. Biopolymeric nanocapsules, nanogels and nanoparticles have been developed since the early nineties (in parallel to the liposome and the other lipid-based nanosystems) with the logical application to the encapsulation of biological entities of smaller dimensions (mainly drugs, therapeutic proteins, nucleic acids) [155–158]. Drug delivery systems based on polysaccharide nanoparticles present several advantages: the capability to penetrate cells and tissues; the possibility to improve the bioavailability of drugs, reducing toxic side effects; the ability to control release properties due to the biodegradability and the stimuli (pH, ion and temperature), and sensibility of materials [146]. The rationalization of the assembly mechanisms and the capability to tailor the properties (size, charge, and loading capability) to desirable levels are essential goals to advance biodegradable polysaccharidic nanoparticles as efficient drug delivery vehicles. Nowadays the results obtained by the researchers in this field have generated a huge number of patents [159,160] and remarkable scientific production [138,161–165].

4. Microencapsulation for Fish Vaccination in Aquaculture: A Case Study

4.1. Fish Vaccination in Aquaculture

Aquaculture represents a fast growing sector of the food industry, providing one half of the fish consumed by humans [166]. Over the past three decades, aquaculture has expanded, intensified, and diversified. However, the intensive production of fish farming results in stress for fish and health problems, such as increased vulnerability to disease outbreaks. This situation influences dramatically the economic and socio-economic development of many countries [166,167].

The prevention of diseases, by using optimal husbandry practice and biological control methods (such as vaccination and the use of immunostimulants) is mandatory, due to the concerns regarding the environmental pollution associated with chemical treatments, the emergence of multiple resistance to antibiotics, and the resulting consumer unsafe products [168]. At an international level, the urgent requirement of pro-active and reactive programs has been expressed, to solve health questions in order to sustain the growth of aquatic animal food production [166].

Currently, the applied research is oriented towards the development of new preventive strategies based on fish vaccinations. This practice has a great relevance in large-scale commercial fish farming and, for example, has been responsible for successful salmon cultivation. In general, commercial vaccines are based on inactivated bacterial pathogens, but at the moment few viral and no parasite vaccines are commercially available [169]. In this context, oral vaccinations are appealing since the first contact with pathogens occurs through the mucosal surfaces of the gut at the level of the gut-associated lymphoid tissue (GALT). Fish intestine indeed does not present Peyer's patches and antigen-transporting M cells: however lymphoid cells and macrophages are present between the epithelial cells and in the lamina propria, and enterocytes show an antigen-transporting capacity [170]. Compared to intra-peritoneal injection, oral administration of vaccines is simple, cost-effective, stress free and easy to administer to large numbers of fish at one time, thus being suitable for mass fish immunization. Oral vaccines are generally produced in two ways: by top coating the feed with the antigen or by preparing a mix with the feed during the production. Oral vaccination at the moment presents also relevant disadvantages, such as the generally high amount of antigen required to provoke an immune response; the lack of an adequate duration of the immunoprotection; the damages from digestive hydrolysis; the necessity to enhance the uptake by the hind gut, in order to induce an effective protective immune response; the physiological and anatomical differences among the species (gastric or agastric fish) [115,167]. These limitations led researchers to develop methods of protecting the vaccine, and thus new fish vaccines and advanced technology have been implemented. For a systematic overview on the most diffuse fish diseases, the vaccines already available, the species that are treated and the developments in the delivery strategies, the reader is addressed to some relevant review publications [115,169,171].

4.2. Case Study

Part of the work here summarized as a case study has been set up in the frame of a Research Project [172] in which a network of scientific institutions and fish farming plants shared their competences to develop an oral vaccination protocol for lactococcosis in trout, exploiting the administration of the inactivated bacteria microencapsulated in biodegradable biopolymeric matrices. Lactococcosis by *Lactococcus garvieae*, is one of the most relevant fish diseases in intensive aquaculture, causing substantial economic losses to rainbow trout (*Oncorhynchus mykiss*) farming [173]. Microencapsulation has been employed since the late nineties as a way to protect the vaccine to be delivered in aquaculture. Three polymers (alginate, chitosan and PLGA) have been mainly used to encapsulate various pathogens (such as *Vibrio anguillarum*, *Lactococcus garvieae*, *Aeromonas hydrophila*) or nucleic acids (for example DNA plasmids containing genes coding for antigens), in order to treat several fish species (carp, Japanese flounder, trout, Nile tilapia, *etc.*) [115]. The results so far obtained for the specific case of alginate encapsulation of the lactococcosis pathogen show that the system is still not optimal: at the moment it resulted mainly in a successful boost, in association with the traditional injection [173,174].

The set up of a microencapsulation system for large scale production of vaccine loaded microcarriers is technologically very challenging. The system developed in our study [175] is an upgrade of a previous one, produced on a laboratory scale, that has been successfully tested in preliminary trials, both on fish (sea bass) and mammal (mice) models [176,177]. It is based on a mixture of biopolymers that have been chosen among other candidate biomaterials. In particular, alginate, chitosan and a cellulose derivative (hydroxypropyl methyl cellulose, HPMC) have been used in a procedure, based on an ionotropic gelation combined with a polyelectrolyte complexation. Lysozyme has been also added as adjuvant and co-encapsulated with the vaccine, due to its immunomodulating properties [178]. The system has been fully characterized and has been tested in two seasonal trials; the evaluation of the results is not the object of this paper.

The preparation of the microcapsules on a large scale [179] has been paralleled by the set-up of a model system (polymer beads), obtained at bench scale by a simple extrusion technique [180]. The feeding solutions and the beads have been characterized for properties [181,182] derived from the combination of different materials (alginate, chitosan, HPMC and lysozyme). The compositional effect on the encapsulation process and formulation is detected also from bead shape, transparency and morphology. The rationale for the employment of a simple model system comes up from the necessity to collect information regarding the role of each component and their mutual interactions within the system. Moreover, the effects of the polymer nature (such as type and origin of alginate samples, or chitosan characteristics) on the resulting hydrogels have been studied and optimized.

The composite biopolymeric beads can be used as a general model of drug delivery system, and thus have been tested in a variety of "environmental" conditions (pH, temperature, ionic strength, *etc.*) which correspond to different physiological conditions (mimicking, for example, gastric or intestinal release, stomach-less or stomach-containing fish, *etc.*), thus enabling the investigation of both human and veterinary applications.

The application presented here, typically follows the understanding of the concepts exposed in the previous sections of this review; in that sense it is not only a case study, but also a real "proof of concept" in the field. As reported in Section 3.2, drug release is influenced by several parameters, which are dependent on the matrix structure (pore size, pore volume fractions, extent of the interconnections, *etc.*) and from the surrounding environment (such as pH, ionic strength, temperature, chemical composition, *etc.*). For this reason, the effect of the composition of the buffer medium on the release of the encapsulated protein has been also evaluated. Release studies have been carried out in buffer medium to guarantee the maintenance of the pH (phosphate buffer and Tris buffer with the addition of NaCl at pH = 7.4).

Figure 7a reports the release profiles of lysozyme from alginate beads in phosphate buffer and in Tris/NaCl. In phosphate buffer, release occurs very rapidly and it is completed during the first hour. The rapid release kinetics is not due to the pH value, but rather to a fast erosion of the alginate matrix in the presence of phosphate ions, which subtract calcium ions from the guluronate sites of the gel (see egg-box model illustrated in Section 2.5). In fact, a different behavior is observed in Tris/NaCl buffer. The use of Tris prevents the matrix from erosion and the release of lysozyme is partially hampered.

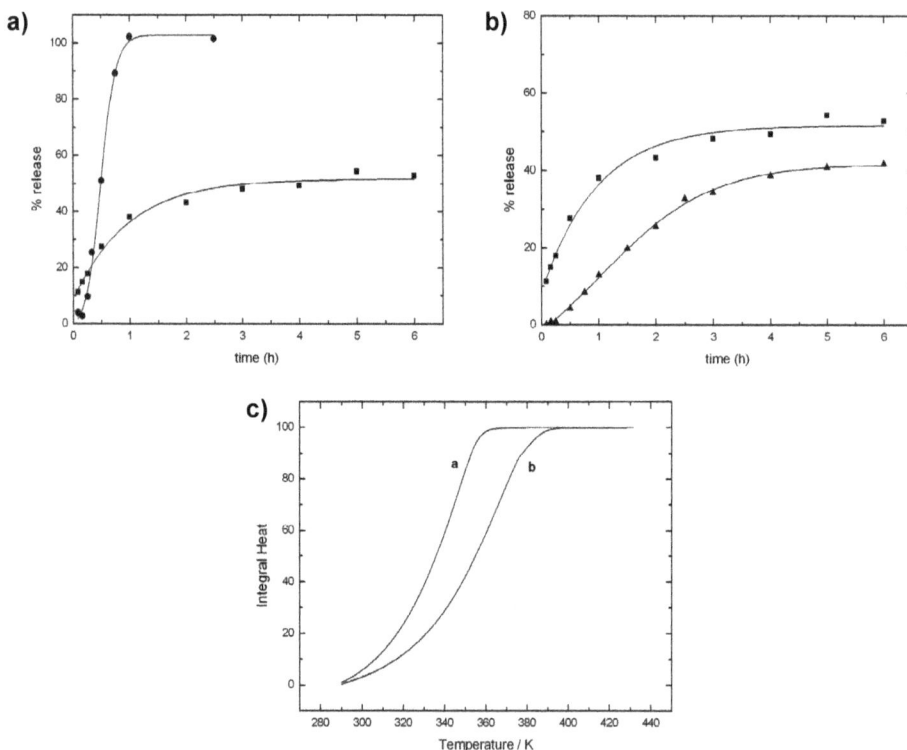

Figure 7. (a) Comparison of lysozyme release from alginate beads in phosphate buffer (●) and in Tris/NaCl (■) at pH = 7.4; (b) Comparison of lysozyme release in Tris/NaCl from alginate beads (■) and from alginate/chitosan beads (▲); (c) Experimental integral heat of water evaporation from alginate beads (curve a); and from alginate/chitosan beads (curve b). Polymer samples: alginate (F_G = 0.4; Mv = 86 kDa); chitosan (Mv = 492 kDa; DA = 11%). Other experimental details in refs [182,183].

The alginate gel matrix can be reinforced by employing other polysaccharides able to interact with alginate either with electrostatic and/or dipolar interactions. This structurization is an effective hampering factor to the rapid release of proteins. The two polymers here exploited have been already largely used in the past, one is chitosan [97,184], and the other is the cellulose derivative HPMC. Both polymers have been employed in order to modify the barrier properties of the matrix. Cellulose derivatives, like HPMC, are also commonly used as a polymer generating swellable matrix, since in solid tablets it undergoes a glassy-rubbery transition as water penetrates [185,186]. Figure 7b reports the release profiles of lysozyme in Tris/NaCl from the alginate beads and the chitosan-reinforced alginate beads. In Tris buffer, the main process occurring is diffusion. The effect of the addition of chitosan is clear from the release profile, which is lower than that of the sole alginate.

The idea that the addition of other polysaccharide to the basic alginate matrix produces a more intricate matrix has been already modeled in the literature and it is referred as "obstruction effect" [187]. In a previous study [183], a calorimetric approach has been proposed to measure this effect. Indeed, differential scanning calorimetry has proven to be a powerful tool to study the barrier properties of the different systems. In particular, water evaporation rate from beads of different compositions, obtained by adding HPMC and/or chitosan, has been investigated to evaluate the effect of additional carbohydrate polymers on the alginate matrix [182]. The rationale of this approach is that the study of water evaporation can be helpful in understanding the structural arrangement of the polymer chains in the beads. It is claimed that the shift of the thermograms, arising from the addition of other components, reflects the "obstructive" character of the polymer network in the bead. Therefore, it is expected that a delay of water evaporation is paralleled by a decrease in protein release as it is shown in Figure 7c which reports the experimental integral heat of water evaporation from alginate and alginate/chitosan gel beads.

The addition of chitosan produces a delay of water evaporation, thus confirming the effect of chitosan, as demonstrated also by release data. The results of several experiments carried out to compare water evaporation and protein release from gel beads with different compositions are very helpful in predicting the release properties of new formulations by a rapid analysis. Besides the above reported tests and the positive response of this system to the "*in vitro*" analyses, trials in the field have shown remarkable but, as yet, not fully analyzed results; this is also due to some unavoidable variability in the trial conditions when compared to a laboratory set-up.

The superior properties of the mixed alginate/chitosan with a proper addition of a little amount of an extra-marine polysaccharide (HPMC) is the reason for stating that the systems made with polymers from the sea, contribute to solve a problem in the sea.

5. Conclusions

The overview provided in this paper has been mainly devoted to the elucidation at the molecular level of the main polysaccharide properties and of the processes on which the encapsulation in polysaccharides is based. This methodological approach to the comprehension of the physico-chemical properties of the systems being developed enables their efficient exploitation and provides a solution to technical and experimental problems, often encountered, but not always reported in literature.

The superior properties of the polysaccharide-based systems described here and reviewed provide the reasons for stating that systems made with biopolymers from the sea may contribute to solve a problem in the sea, although limited to the aquaculture environment.

Acknowledgments: The acknowledge their colleagues and coworkers Sergio Paoletti, Ivan Donati, Gianni Sava and Moreno Cocchietto, for fruitful discussion and long standing collaboration. The encapsulation work has been carried out in the frame of projects "Oral vaccine carrier for fish farming of Friuli Venezia Giulia" and NanoBioPharmaceutics (FP6 EU Project no. 026723-2) with support of the University of Trieste. MB is recipient of a grant from MIUR (Rome).

References and Notes

1. Donati, I.; Borgogna, M.; Turello, E.; Cesàro, A.; Paoletti, S. Tuning Supramolecular Structuring at the Nanoscale Level: Nonstoichiometric Soluble Complexes in Dilute Mixed Solutions of Alginate and Lactose-Modified Chitosan (Chitlac). *Biomacromolecules* **2007**, *8*, 1471–1479.
2. Cesàro, A.; Bellich, B.; Borgogna, M. Biophysical functionality in polysaccharides: from Lego-blocks to nano-particles. *Eur. Biophys. J.* **2011**, in press.
3. Woods, R.J.; Tessier, M.B. Computational glycoscience: characterizing the spatial and temporal properties of glycans and glycan-protein complexes. *Curr. Opin. Struct. Biol.* **2010**, *20*, 575–583.

4. Yalpani, M.; Sandford, P.A. *Industrial Polysaccharides*; Yalpani, M., Ed.; Elsevier: Amsterdam, The Netherlands, 1987; p. 31.

5. Ross-Murphy, S.B.; Tobitani, A. *Hydrocolloids: Physical Chemistry and Industrial Application of Gels, Polysaccharides, and Proteins*; Nishinari, K., Ed.; Elsevier: Amsterdam, The Netherlands, 2000; p. 379.

6. Kawakami, M.; Byrne, K.; Khatri, B.; McLeish, T.C.B.; Radford, S.E.; Smith, D.A. Viscoelastic properties of single polysaccharide molecules determined by analysis of thermally driven oscillations of an atomic force microscope cantilever. *Langmuir* **2004**, *20*, 9299–9303.

7. Khatri, B.S.; Kawakami, M.; Byrne, K.; Smith, D.A.; McLeish, T.C.B. Entropy and barrier-controlled fluctuations determine conformational viscoelasticity of single biomolecules. *Biophys. J.* **2007**, *92*, 1825–1835.

8. Clark, A.; Ross-Murphy, S. Structural and mechanical properties of biopolymer gels. *Adv. Polym. Sci.* **1987**, *83*, 57–192.

9. *Makromolekulare Chemie. Macromolecular Symposia*; Eichinger, B.E. (Ed.) Wiley-VCH: Weinheim, Germany, 1993; Volume 76, pp. 1–290.

10. te Nijenhuis, K. *Thermoreversible Networks*; Springer: Berlin-Heidelberg, Germany, 1997; Volume 130, p. 1.

11. Mandelken, L.; Edwards, C.O.; Domszy, R.C.; Davidson, M.W. *Microdomains in Polymer Solutions*; Dubin, P., Ed.; Plenum Press: New York, NY, USA, 1985; p. 121.

12. Flory, P.J. Introductory lecture. *Faraday Discuss. Chem. Society* **1974**, *57*, 7–18.

13. Tanaka, F.; Stockmayer, W.H. Thermoreversible gelation with junctions of variable multiplicity. *Macromol. Symposia* **1994**, *81*, 171–175.

14. Xiong, J.Y.; Narayanan, J.; Liu, X.Y.; Chong, T.K.; Chen, S.B.; Chung, T.S. Topology evolution and gelation mechanism of agarose gel. *J. Phys. Chem. B* **2005**, *109*, 5638–5643.

15. Clark, A.; Ross-Murphy, S.B. Biopolymer network assembly: measurement and theory. In *Modern Biopolymer Science*; Kasapis, S., Norton, I.T., Ubbink, J.B., Eds.; Elsevier: London, UK, 2009; p. 1.

16. Nordqvist, D.; Vilgis, T. Rheological study of the gelation process of agarose-based solutions. *Food Biophys.* **2011**, *6*, 450–460.

17. Nishinari, K.; Takahashi, R. Interaction in polysaccharide solutions and gels. *Curr. Opin. Colloid Interface Sci.* **2003**, *8*, 396–400.

18. Dai, B.; Matsukawa, S. NMR studies of the gelation mechanism and molecular dynamics in agar solutions. *Food Hydrocoll.* **2012**, *26*, 181–186.

19. Miles, M.J. *Developments in Crystalline Polymers*; Bassett, D.C., Ed.; Elsevier Applied Science: London, UK, 1988; p. 233.

20. Guenet, M.J. Factors influencing gelation versus crystallization in cooling polymer solutions. *Trends Polym. Sci.* **1996**, *4*, 6–11.

21. Mandelkern, L. Polymer-diluent mixtures. In *Crystallization of Polymers*; McGraw-Hill: New York, NY, USA, 1964; Chapter 3.

22. Keller, A.; Rastogi, S.; Hikosaka, M.H. Polymer crystallisation: Role of metastability and the confluence of thermodynamic and kinetic factors. *Macromol. Symposia* **1997**, *124*, 67–81.

23. Hu, Z.; Lu, X.; Gao, J.; Wang, C. Polymer Gel Nanoparticle Networks. *Adv. Mater.* **2000**, *12*, 1173–1176.

24. Rees, D.A. *Polysaccharide Shapes*; Chapman and Hall: London, UK, 1977.

25. Burton, B.A.; Brant, D.A. Comparative flexibility, extension, and conformation of some simple polysaccharide chains. *Biopolymers* **1983**, *22*, 1769–1792.

26. Brant, D.A.; Christ, M.D. Realistic Conformational Modeling of Carbohydrates. In *Computer Modeling of Carbohydrate Molecules*; French, A.D., Brady, J.W., Eds.; American Chemical Society: Washington, DC, USA, 1990; p. 42.

27. Kroon-Batenburg, L.M.J.; Kruiskamp, P.H.; Vliegenthart, J.F.G.; Kroon, J. Estimation of the persistence length of polymers by MD simulations on small fragments in solution. Application to cellulose. *J. Phys. Chem. B* **1997**, *101*, 8454–8459.

28. Skovstrup, S.; Hansen, S.G.; Skrydstrup, T.; Schiøtt, B. Conformational flexibility of chitosan: A molecular modeling study. *Biomacromolecules* **2010**, *11*, 3196–3207.

29. Jordan, R.C.; Brant, D.A.; Cesàro, A. A Monte Carlo study of the amylosic chain conformation. *Biopolymers* **1978**, *17*, 2617–2632.

30. Kitamura, S.; Minami, T.; Nakamura, Y.; Isuda, H.; Kobayashi, H.; Mimura, M.; Urakawa, H.; Kajiwara, K.; Ohno, S. Chain dimensions and scattering function of (1→3)-β-D-glucan simulated by the Monte Carlo method. *J. Mol. Struct. Theochem* **1997**, *395-396*, 425–435.

31. Furlan, S.; La Penna, G.; Perico, A.; Cesàro, A. Hyaluronan chain conformation and dynamics. *Carbohydr. Res.* **2005**, *340*, 959–970.

32. Hargittai, I.; Hargittai, M. Molecular structure of hyaluronan: An introduction. *Struct. Chem.* **2008**, *19*, 697–717.

33. Brant, D.A. Shapes and motions of polysaccharide chains. *Pure Appl. Chem.* **1997**, *69*, 1885–1892.

34. Kadkhodaei, M.; Wu, H.; Brant, D.A. Comparison of the conformational dynamics of the (1→4)- and (1→6)-linked a-D-glucans using ^{13}C-NMR relaxation. *Biopolymers* **1991**, *31*, 1581–1592.

35. Brant, D.A.; Liu, H.-S.; Zhu, Z.S. The dependence of glucan conformational dynamics on linkage position and stereochemistry. *Carbohydr. Res.* **1995**, *278*, 11–26.

36. Perico, A.; Mormino, M.; Urbani, R.; Cesàro, A.; Tylianakis, E.; Dais, P.; Brant, D.A. Local dynamics of carbohydrates. 1. dynamics of simple glycans with different chain linkages. *J. Phys. Chem. B* **1999**, *103*, 8162–8171.

37. Landström, J.; Widmalm, G. Glycan flexibility: insights into nanosecond dynamics from a microsecond molecular dynamics simulation explaining an unusual nuclear Overhauser effect. *Carbohydr. Res.* **2010**, *345*, 330–333.

38. Urbani, R.; Cesàro, A. Solvent effects on the unperturbed chain conformation of polysaccharides. *Polymer* **1991**, *32*, 3013–3020.

39. Bertocchi, C.; Navarini, L.; Cesàro, A.; Anastasio, M. Polysaccharides from cyanobacteria. *Carbohydr. Polym.* **1990**, *12*, 127–153.

40. Li, P.; Harding, S.E.; Liu, Z. Cyanobacterial exopolysaccharides: their nature and potential biotechnological applications. *Biotechnol. Genet. Eng. Rev.* **2001**, *18*, 375–404.

41. Sutherland, I.W. Polysaccharides from Microorganisms, Plants and Animals. In *Biopolymers*; Vandamme, E.J., De Baets, S., Steinbüchel, A., Eds.; Wiley-VCH: Weinheim, Germay, 2002; Volume 5, p. 1.

42. Straub, P.R.; Brant, D.A. Measurement of preferential solvation of some glucans in mixed solvent systems by gel-permeation chromatography. *Biopolymers* **1980**, *19*, 639–653.

43. Kirschner, K.N.; Woods, R.J. Solvent interactions determine carbohydrate conformation. *Proc. Natl. Acad. Sci. USA* **2001**, *98*, 10541–10545.

44. Almond, A.; Sheenan, J.K. Predicting the molecular shape of polysaccharides from dynamic interactions with water. *Glycobiology* **2003**, *13*, 255–264.

45. Kuttel, M.M.; Naidoo, K.J. Free energy surfaces for the α(1→4)-glycosidic linkage: Implications for polysaccharide solution structure and dynamics. *J. Phys. Chem. B* **2005**, *109*, 7468–7474.

46. Pereira, C.S.; Kony, D.; Baron, R.; Müller, M.; Van Gunsteren, W.F.; Hünenberger, P.H. Conformational and dynamical properties of disaccharides in water: A molecular dynamics study. *Biophys. J.* **2006**, *90*, 4337–4344.

47. Antoniou, E.; Buitrago, C.F.; Tsianou, M.; Alexandridis, P. Solvent effects on polysaccharide conformation. *Carbohydr. Polym.* **2010**, *79*, 380–390.

48. Perić-Hassler, L.; Hansen, H.S.; Baron, R.; Hünenberger, P.H. Conformational properties of glucose-based disaccharides investigated using molecular dynamics simulations with local elevation umbrella sampling. *Carbohydr. Res.* **2010**, *345*, 1781–1801.

49. Brady, J.W.; Schmidt, R.K. The role of hydrogen bonding in carbohydrates: Molecular dynamics simulations of maltose in aqueous solution. *J. Phys. Chem.* **1993**, *97*, 958–966.

50. Ueda, K.; Ueda, T.; Sato, T.; Nakayama, H.; Brady, J.W. The conformational free-energy map for solvated neocarrabiose. *Carbohydr. Res.* **2004**, *339*, 1953–1960.

51. Dogsa, I.; Štrancar, J.; Laggner, P.; Stopar, D. Efficient modeling of polysaccharide conformations based on Small-Angle X-ray Scattering experimental data. *Polymer* **2008**, *49*, 1398–1406.

52. Cesàro, A.; Paoletti, S.; Urbani, R.; Benegas, J. Polyelectrolytic effects in semi-flexible carboxylate polysaccharides. Part 2. *Int. J. Biol. Macromol.* **1989**, *11*, 66–72.

53. Paoletti, S.; Cesàro, A.; Delben, F.; Crescenzi, V.; Rizzo, R. *Microdomains in Polymer Solutions*; Dubin, P., Ed.; Plenum Press: New York, NY, USA, 1985; p. 159.

54. Paoletti, S.; Benegas, J.; Cesàro, A.; Manzini, G.; Fogolari, F.; Crescenzi, V. Limiting-laws of polyelectrolyte solutions. Ionic distribution in mixed-valency counterions systems. I: The model. *Biophys. Chem.* **1991**, *41*, 73–80.

55. Manning, G.S. Counterion binding in polyelectrolyte theory. *Acc. Chem. Res.* **1979**, *12*, 443–449.

56. Cesàro, A.; Delben, F.; Paoletti, S. Interaction of divalent cations with polyuronates. *J. Chem. Soc. Faraday Trans. 1* **1988**, *84*, 2573–2584.

57. Paoletti, S.; Delben, F.; Cesàro, A.; Grasdalen, H. Conformational transition of κ-carrageenan in aqueous solution. *Macromolecules* **1985**, *18*, 1834–1841.

58. Smidsrød, O.; Haug, A. Estimation of the relative stiffness of the molecular chain in polyelectrolytes from measurements of viscosity at different ionic strengths. *Biopolymers* **1971**, *10*, 1213–1227.

59. Manning, G.S.; Paoletti, S. *Industrial Polysaccharides*; Crescenzi, V., Dea, I.C.M., Stivala, S.S., Eds.; Gordon & Breach: New York, NY, USA, 1987; p. 305.

60. Rotureau, E.; Van Leeuwen, H.P. Kinetics of metal ion binding by polysaccharide colloids. *J. Phys. Chem. A* **2008**, *112*, 7177–7184.

61. Sriamornsak, P.; Kennedy, R.A. Swelling and diffusion studies of calcium polysaccharide gels intended for film coating. *Int. J. Pharm.* **2008**, *358*, 205–213.

62. Kristiansen, K.A.; Schirmer, B.C.; Aachmann, F.L.; Skjåk-Bræk, G.; Draget, K.I.; Christensen, B.E. Novel alginates prepared by independent control of chain stiffness and distribution of G-residues: Structure and gelling properties. *Carbohydr. Polym.* **2009**, *77*, 725–735.

63. Haidara, H.; Vonna, L.; Vidal, L. Unrevealed self-assembly and crystallization structures of Na-alginate, induced by the drying dynamics of wetting films of the aqueous polymer solution. *Macromolecules* **2010**, *43*, 2421–2429.

64. Draget, K.I.; Smidsrød, O.; Skjåk-Bræk, G. Alginates from Algae. In *Polysaccharides and Polyamides in the Food Industry. Properties, Production, and Patents*; Steinbüchel, A., Rhee, S.K., Eds.; WILEY-VCH: Weinheim, Germany, 2005; p. 1.

65. Smidsrød, O.; Haug, A. Dependence upon gel-sol state of ionexchange properties of alginates. *Acta Chem. Scand.* **1972**, *26*, 2063–2074.

66. Smidsrød, O. Molecular basis for some physical properties of alginates in the gel state. *Faraday Discuss. Chem. Soc.* **1974**, *57*, 263–274.

67. Kohn, R. Ion binding on polyuronates-alginate and pectin. *Pure Appl. Chem.* **1975**, *42*, 371–397.

68. Grant, G.T.; Morris, E.R.; Rees, D.A.; Smith, P.J.C.; Thom, D. Biological interactions between polysaccharides and divalent cations: The egg-box model. *FEBS Lett.* **1973**, *32*, 195–198.

69. Morris, E.R.; Rees, D.A.; Thom, D.; Boyd, J. Chiroptical and stoichiometric evidence of a specific, primary dimerisation process in alginate gelation. *Carbohydr. Res.* **1978**, *66*, 145–154.

70. Braccini, I.; Pérez, S. Molecular basis of Ca^{2+}-induced gelation in alginates and pectins: The egg-box model revisited. *Biomacromolecules* **2001**, *2*, 1089–1096.

71. Li, L.; Fang, Y.; Vreeker, R.; Appelqvist, I.; Mendes, E. Reexamining the egg-box model in calcium-alginate gels with X-ray diffraction. *Biomacromolecules* **2007**, *8*, 464–468.

72. Sikorski, P.; Mo, F.; Skjåk-Bræk, G.; Stokke, B.T. Evidence for egg-box-compatible interactions in calcium-alginate gels from fiber X-ray diffraction. *Biomacromolecules* **2007**, *8*, 2098–2103.

73. Donati, I.; Paoletti, S. Material properties of alginates. In *Alginates: Biology and Applications*; Rehm, B.H.A., Ed.; Springer-Verlag: Berlin Heidelberg, Germany, 2009; p. 1.

74. Donati, I.; Cesàro, A.; Paoletti, S. Specific Interactions *versus* counterion condensation. 1. Nongelling ions/polyuronate systems. *Biomacromolecules* **2005**, *7*, 281–287.

75. Donati, I.; Benegas, J.C.; Cesàro, A.; Paoletti, S. Specific Interactions *versus* counterion condensation. 2. Theoretical treatment within the counterion condensation theory. *Biomacromolecules* **2006**, *7*, 1587–1596.

76. Donati, I.; Benegas, J.C.; Paoletti, S. Polyelectrolyte study of the calcium-induced chain association of pectate. *Biomacromolecules* **2006**, *7*, 3439–3447.

77. Donati, I.; Holtan, S.; Mørch, Y.A.; Borgogna, M.; Dentini, M.; Skjåk-Bræk, G. New hypothesis on the role of alternating sequences in calcium-alginate gels. *Biomacromolecules* **2005**, *6*, 1031–1040.

78. Vårum, K.M.; Smidsrød, O. Structure-Property Relationship in Chitosans. In *Polysaccharides. Structural Diversity and Functional Versatility*; Dumitriu, S., Ed.; Marcel Dekker: New York, NY, USA, 2004; p. 625.

79. Ogawa, K.; Yui, T.; Okuyama, K. Three D structures of chitosan. *Int. J. Biol. Macromol.* **2004**, *34*, 1–8.

80. Signini, R.; Desbrières, J.; Campana Filho, S.P. On the stiffness of chitosan hydrochloride in acid-free aqueous solutions. *Carbohydr. Polym.* **2000**, *43*, 351–357.

81. Lamarque, G.; Lucas, J.-M.; Viton, C.; Domard, A. Physicochemical behavior of homogeneous series of acetylated chitosans in aqueous solution: Role of various structural parameters. *Biomacromolecules* **2004**, *6*, 131–142.

82. Christensen, B.E.; Vold, I.M.N.; Vårum, K.M. Chain stiffness and extension of chitosans and periodate oxidised chitosans studied by size-exclusion chromatography combined with light scattering and viscosity detectors. *Carbohydr. Polym.* **2008**, *74*, 559–565.

83. Ravi Kumar, M.N.V.; Muzzarelli, R.A.A.; Muzzarelli, C.; Sashiwa, H.; Domb, A.J. Chitosan chemistry and pharmaceutical perspectives. *Chem. Rev.* **2004**, *104*, 6017–6084.

84. Peppas, N.A.; Bures, P.; Leobandung, W.; Ichikawa, H. Hydrogels in pharmaceutical formulations. *Eur. J. Pharm. Biopharm.* **2000**, *50*, 27–46.

85. Lee, K.Y.; Mooney, D.J. Hydrogels for tissue engineering. *Chem. Rev.* **2001**, *101*, 1869–1879.

86. Hoffman, A.S. Hydrogels for biomedical applications. *Adv. Drug Deliv. Rev.* **2002**, *54*, 3–12.

87. Lee, K.Y.; Yuk, S.H. Polymeric protein delivery systems. *Prog. Polym. Sci.* **2007**, *32*, 669–697.

88. Coviello, T.; Matricardi, P.; Marianecci, C.; Alhaique, F. Polysaccharide hydrogels for modified release formulations. *J. Control. Release* **2007**, *119*, 5–24.

89. D'Ayala, G.; Malinconico, M.; Laurienzo, P. Marine derived polysaccharides for biomedical applications: Chemical modification approaches. *Molecules* **2008**, *13*, 2069–2106.

90. Rinaudo, M. Main properties and current applications of some polysaccharides as biomaterials. *Polym. Int.* **2008**, *57*, 397–430.

91. Laurienzo, P. Marine polysaccharides in pharmaceutical applications: An overview. *Mar. Drugs* **2010**, *8*, 2435–2465.

92. Van Vlierberghe, S.; Dubruel, P.; Schacht, E. Biopolymer-based hydrogels as scaffolds for tissue engineering applications: a review. *Biomacromolecules* **2011**, *12*, 1387–1408.

93. Gombotz, W.R.; Wee, S. Protein release from alginate matrices. *Adv. Drug Deliv. Rev.* **1998**, *31*, 267–285.

94. Faroongsarng, D.; Sukonrat, P. Thermal behavior of water in the selected starch- and cellulose-based polymeric hydrogels. *Int. J. Pharm.* **2008**, *352*, 152–158.

95. Martinsen, A.; Skjåk-Bræk, G.; Smidsrød, O. Alginate as immobilization material: I. Correlation between chemical and physical properties of alginate gel beads. *Biotechnol. Bioeng.* **1989**, *33*, 79–89.

96. Thu, B.; Bruheim, P.; Espevik, T.; Smidsrød, O.; Soon-Shiong, P.; Skjåk-Bræk, G. Alginate polycation microcapsules: II. Some functional properties. *Biomaterials* **1996**, *17*, 1069–1079.

97. Gåserød, O.; Sannes, A.; Skjåk-Bræk, G. Microcapsules of alginate-chitosan. II. A study of capsule stability and permeability. *Biomaterials* **1999**, *20*, 773–783.

98. Takka, F.; Acarturk, S. Calcium alginate microparticles for oral administration: II effect of form ulation factors on drug release and drug entrapment efficiency. *J. Microencapsul.* **1999**, *16*, 291–301.

99. Acarturk, S.; Takka, F. Calcium alginate microparticles for oral administration: I: effect of sodium alginate type on drug release and drug entrapment efficiency. *J. Microencapsul.* **1999**, *16*, 275–290.

100. Vandenberg, G.W.; Drolet, C.; Scott, S.L.; de la Noüe, J. Factors affecting protein release from alginate–chitosan coacervate microcapsules during production and gastric/intestinal simulation. *J. Control. Release* **2001**, *77*, 297–307.

101. Bhattarai, N.; Gunn, J.; Zhang, M. Chitosan-based hydrogels for controlled, localized drug delivery. *Adv. Drug Deliv. Rev.* **2010**, *62*, 83–99.

102. Serra, L.; Doménech, J.; Peppas, N.A. Engineering design and molecular dynamics of mucoadhesive drug delivery systems as targeting agents. *Eur. J. Pharm. Biopharm.* **2009**, *71*, 519–528.

103. Bonferoni, M.C.; Sandri, G.; Rossi, S.; Ferrari, F.; Caramella, C. Chitosan and its salts for mucosal and transmucosal delivery. *Expert Opin. Drug Deliv.* **2009**, *6*, 923–939.

104. Agnihotri, S.A.; Mallikarjuna, N.N.; Aminabhavi, T.M. Recent advances on chitosan-based micro- and nanoparticles in drug delivery. *J. Control. Release* **2004**, *100*, 5–28.

105. Oh, J.K.; Lee, D.I.; Park, J.M. Biopolymer-based microgels/nanogels for drug delivery applications. *Prog. Polym. Sci.* **2009**, *34*, 1261–1282.

106. He, P.; Davis, S.S.; Illum, L. Chitosan microspheres prepared by spray drying. *Int. J. Pharm.* **1999**, *187*, 53–65.

107. Illum, L.; Jabbal-Gill, I.; Hinchcliffe, M.; Fisher, A.N.; Davis, S.S. Chitosan as a novel nasal delivery system for vaccines. *Adv. Drug Deliv. Rev.* **2001**, *51*, 81–96.

108. George, M.; Abraham, T.E. Polyionic hydrocolloids for the intestinal delivery of protein drugs: Alginate and chitosan—A review. *J. Control. Release* **2006**, *114*, 1–14.

109. Borchard, G. Chitosans for gene delivery. *Adv. Drug Deliv. Rev.* **2001**, *52*, 145–150.

110. Mao, S.; Sun, W.; Kissel, T. Chitosan-based formulations for delivery of DNA and siRNA. *Adv. Drug Deliv. Rev.* **2010**, *62*, 12–27.

111. Tafaghodi, M.; Sajadi Tabassi, S.A.; Jaafari, M.R. Induction of systemic and mucosal immune responses by intranasal administration of alginate microspheres encapsulated with tetanus toxoid and CpG-ODN. *Int. J. Pharm.* **2006**, *319*, 37–43.

112. Amidi, M.; Mastrobattista, E.; Jiskoot, W.; Hennink, W.E. Chitosan-based delivery systems for protein therapeutics and antigens. *Adv. Drug Deliv. Rev.* **2010**, *62*, 59–82.

113. Wen, Z.-S.; Xu, Y.-L.; Zou, X.-T.; Xu, Z.-R. Chitosan Nanoparticles Act as an Adjuvant to Promote both Th1 and Th2 Immune Responses Induced by Ovalbumin in Mice. *Mar. Drugs* **2011**, *9*, 1038–1055.

114. Año, G.; Esquisabel, A.; Pastor, M.; Talavera, A.; Cedré, B.; Fernández, S.; Sifontes, S.; Aranguren, Y.; Falero, G.; García, L.; *et al.* A new oral vaccine candidate based on the microencapsulation by spray-drying of inactivated Vibrio cholerae. *Vaccine* **2011**, *29*, 5758–5764.

115. Plant, K.P.; Lapatra, S.E. Advances in fish vaccine delivery. *Develop. Comp. Immunol.* **2011**, in press.

116. Champagne, C.P.; Fustier, P. Microencapsulation for the improved delivery of bioactive compounds into foods. *Curr. Opin. Biotechnol.* **2007**, *18*, 184–190.

117. Chen, L.; Remondetto, G.E.; Subirade, M. Food protein-based materials as nutraceutical delivery systems. *Trends Food Sci. Technol.* **2006**, *17*, 272–283.

118. de Vos, P.; Faas, M.M.; Spasojevic, M.; Sikkema, J. Encapsulation for preservation of functionality and targeted delivery of bioactive food components. *Int. Dairy J.* **2010**, *20*, 292–302.

119. Desai, K.G.H.; Park, H.J. Recent developments in microencapsulation of food ingredients. *Dry. Technol.* **2005**, *23*, 1361–1394.

120. Wandrey, C.; Bartkowiak, A.; Harding, S.E. Materials for Encapsulation. In *Encapsulation Technologies for Active Food Ingredients and Food Processing*; Zuidam, N.J., Nedović, V., Eds.; Springer: New York, NY, USA, 2009.

121. Slaughter, B.V.; Khurshid, S.S.; Fisher, O.Z.; Khademhosseini, A.; Peppas, N.A. Hydrogels in regenerative medicine. *Adv. Mater.* **2009**, *21*, 3307–3329.

122. Luo, Y.; Engelmayr, G.; Auguste, D.T.; Ferreira, L.; Karp, J.M.; Saigal, R.; Langer, R. Three Dimensional Scaffolds. In *Principles of Tissue Engineering*; Lanza, R., Langer, R., Vacanti, J.P., Eds.; Elsevier Academic Press: San Diego, CA, USA, 2007; p. 359.

123. Brun-Graeppi, A.K.A.S.; Richard, C.; Bessodes, M.; Scherman, D.; Merten, O.-W. Cell microcarriers and microcapsules of stimuli-responsive polymers. *J. Control. Release* **2011**, *149*, 209–224.

124. Smidsrød, O.; Skjåk-Bræk, G. Alginate as immobilization matrix for cells. *Trends Biotechnol.* **1990**, *8*, 71–78.

125. Dulieu, C.; Poncelet, D.; Neufeld, R.J. Encapsulation and Immobilization Techniques. In *Cell Encapsulation Technology and Therapeutics*; Kühtreiber, W.M., Lanza, R.P., Chick, W.L., Eds.; Birkhäuser: Boston, MA, USA, 1999.

126. de Vos, P.; Faas, M.M.; Strand, B.; Calafiore, R. Alginate-based microcapsules for immunoisolation of pancreatic islets. *Biomaterials* **2006**, *27*, 5603–5617.

127. Lutolf, M.P.; Gilbert, P.M.; Blau, H.M. Designing materials to direct stem-cell fate. *Nature* **2009**, *462*, 433–441.

128. Hernandez, R.M.; Orive, G.; Murua, A.; Pedraz, J.L. Microcapsules and microcarriers for *in situ* cell delivery. *Adv. Drug Deliv. Rev.* **2010**, *62*, 711–730.

129. Murua, A.; Portero, A.; Orive, G.; Hernandez, R.M.; de Castro, M.; Pedraz, J.L. Cell microencapsulation technology: Towards clinical application. *J. Control. Release* **2008**, *132*, 76–83.

130. Hunt, N.C.; Grover, L.M. Cell encapsulation using biopolymer gels for regenerative medicine. *Biotechnol. Lett.* **2010**, *32*, 733–742.

131. Janes, K.A.; Calvo, P.; Alonso, M.J. Polysaccharide colloidal particles as delivery systems for macromolecules. *Adv. Drug Deliv. Rev.* **2001**, *47*, 83–97.

132. Gouin, S. Microencapsulation. *Trends Food Sci. Technol.* **2004**, *15*, 330–347.

133. Gharsallaoui, A.; Roudaut, G.; Chambin, O.; Voilley, A.; Saurel, R. Applications of spray-drying in microencapsulation of food ingredients: An overview. *Food Res. Int.* **2007**, *40*, 1107–1121.

134. Cui, J.H.; Goh, J.S.; Park, S.Y.; Kim, P.H.; Lee, B.J. Preparation and physical characterization of alginate microparticles using air atomization method. *Drug Develop. Ind. Pharm.* **2001**, *27*, 309–319.

135. Teunou, E.; Poncelet, D. Rotary disc atomisation for microencapsulation applications-prediction of the particle trajectories. *J. Food Eng.* **2005**, *71*, 345–353.

136. Prüsse, U.; Bilancetti, L.; Bučko, M.; Bugarski, B.; Bukowski, J.; Gemeiner, P.; Massart, B.; Nastruzzi, C.; Nedovic, V.; Poncelet, D.; *et al.* Comparison of different technologies for alginate beads production. *Chem. Pap.* **2008**, *62*, 364–374.

137. Pinto Reis, C.; Neufeld, R.J.; Ribeiro, A.J.; Veiga, F. Nanoencapsulation I. Methods for preparation of drug-loaded polymeric nanoparticles. *Nanomed. Nanotechnol. Biol. Med.* **2006**, *2*, 8–21.

138. Anton, N.; Benoit, J.P.; Saulnier, P. Design and production of nanoparticles formulated from nano-emulsion templates—A review. *J. Control. Release* **2008**, *128*, 185–199.

139. Barbosa-Cánovas, G.V.; Ortega-Rivas, E.; Juliano, P.; Yan, H. *Food Powders: Physical Properties, Processing, and Functionality*; Kluwer Academic/Plenum Publishers: New York, NY, USA, 2005.

140. Tønnesen, H.H.; Karlsen, J. Alginate in drug delivery systems. *Drug Develop. Ind. Pharm.* **2002**, *28*, 621–630.

141. Zimmermann, H.; Shirley, S.G.; Zimmermann, U. Alginate-based encapsulation of cells: Past, present, and future. *Curr. Diabetes Rep.* **2007**, *7*, 314–320.

142. de Vos, P.; Bučko, M.; Gemeiner, P.; Navrátil, M.; Švitel, J.; Faas, M.; Strand, B.L.; Skjåk-Bræk, G.; Morch, Y.A.; Vikartovská, A.; *et al.* Multiscale requirements for bioencapsulation in medicine and biotechnology. *Biomaterials* **2009**, *30*, 2559–2570.

143. Lee, K.Y.; Mooney, D.J. Alginate: Properties and biomedical applications. *Prog. Polym. Sci.* **2011**.

144. Gåserød, O.; Smidsrød, O.; Skjåk-Bræk, G. Microcapsules of alginate-chitosan—I: A quantitative study of the interaction between alginate and chitosan. *Biomaterials* **1998**, *19*, 1815–1825.

145. Ribeiro, A.J.; Silva, C.; Ferreira, D.; Veiga, F. Chitosan-reinforced alginate microspheres obtained through the emulsification/internal gelation technique. *Eur. J. Pharm. Sci.* **2005**, *25*, 31–40.

146. Liu, Z.; Jiao, Y.; Wang, Y.; Zhou, C.; Zhang, Z. Polysaccharides-based nanoparticles as drug delivery systems. *Adv. Drug Deliv. Rev.* **2008**, *60*, 1650–1662.

147. Hamman, J.H. Chitosan based polyelectrolyte complexes as potential carrier materials in drug delivery systems. *Mar. Drugs* **2010**, *8*, 1305–1322.

148. Patil, J.S.; Kamalapur, M.V.; Marapur, S.C.; Kadam, D.V. Ionotropic gelation and polyelectrolyte complexation: The novel techniques to design hydrogel particulate sustained, modulated drug delivery system: A review. *Digest J. Nanomater. Biostruct.* **2010**, *5*, 241–248.

149. Batorsky, A.; Liao, J.; Lund, A.W.; Plopper, G.E.; Stegemann, J.P. Encapsulation of adult human mesenchymal stem cells within collagen-agarose microenvironments. *Biotechnol. Bioeng.* **2005**, *92*, 492–500.

150. Kumachev, A.; Greener, J.; Tumarkin, E.; Eiser, E.; Zandstra, P.W.; Kumacheva, E. High-throughput generation of hydrogel microbeads with varying elasticity for cell encapsulation. *Biomaterials* **2011**, *32*, 1477–1483.

151. Jeon, O.; Bouhadir, K.H.; Mansour, J.M.; Alsberg, E. Photocrosslinked alginate hydrogels with tunable biodegradation rates and mechanical properties. *Biomaterials* **2009**, *30*, 2724–2734.

152. Cellesi, F.; Tirelli, N. A new process for cell microencapsulation and other biomaterial applications: Thermal gelation and chemical cross-linking in "tandem". *J. Mater. Sci.: Mater. Med.* **2005**, *16*, 559–565.

153. Shen, F.; Li, A.A.; Cornelius, R.M.; Cirone, P.; Childs, R.F.; Brash, J.L.; Chang, P.L. Biological properties of photocrosslinked alginate microcapsules. *J. Biomed. Mater. Res. Part B* **2005**, *75*, 425–434.

154. Rokstad, A.M.; Donati, I.; Borgogna, M.; Oberholzer, J.; Strand, B.L.; Espevik, T.; Skjåk-Bræk, G. Cell-compatible covalently reinforced beads obtained from a chemoenzymatically engineered alginate. *Biomaterials* **2006**, *27*, 4726–4737.

155. Rajaonarivony, M.; Vauthier, C.; Couarraze, G.; Puisieux, F.; Couvreur, P. Development of a new drug carrier made from alginate. *J. Pharm. Sci.* **1993**, *82*, 912–917.

156. Skiba, M.; Morvan, C.; Duchene, D.; Puisieux, F.; Wouessidjewe, D. Evaluation of gastrointestinal behaviour in the rat of amphiphilic β-cyclodextrin nanocapsules, loaded with indomethacin. *Int. J. Pharm.* **1995**, *126*, 275–279.

157. Calvo, P.; Remuñan-López, C.; Vila-Jato, J.L.; Alonso, M.J. Chitosan and chitosan/ethylene oxide-propylene oxide block copolymer nanoparticles as novel carriers for proteins and vaccines. *Pharm. Res.* **1997**, *14*, 1431–1436.

158. Riley, T.; Govender, T.; Stolnik, S.; Xiong, C.D.; Garnett, M.C.; Illum, L.; Davis, S.S. Colloidal stability and drug incorporation aspects of micellar-like PLA-PEG nanoparticles. *Colloid. Surf. B* **1999**, *16*, 147–159.

159. Bhavna, M.A.; Sanjula, B.; Javed, A. Patents on nanoparticulate drug delivery systems—A review. *Recent Pat. Drug Deliv. Formul.* **2008**, *2*, 83–89.

160. Wong, T.W. Chitosan and its use in design of insulin delivery system. *Recent Pat. Drug Deliv. Formul.* **2009**, *3*, 8–25.

161. Bawarski, W.E.; Chidlowsky, E.; Bharali, D.J.; Mousa, S.A. Emerging nanopharmaceuticals. *Nanomed. Nanotechnol. Biol. Med.* **2008**, *4*, 273–282.

162. Millotti, G.; Bernkop-Schnürch, A. Nano- and Microparticles in Oral Delivery of Macromolecular Drugs. In *Oral Delivery of Macromolecular Drugs*; Bernkop-Schnürch, A., Ed.; Springer: New York, NY, USA, 2009; p. 153.

163. Mishra, B.; Patel, B.B.; Tiwari, S. Colloidal nanocarriers: a review on formulation technology, types and applications toward targeted drug delivery. *Nanomed. Nanotechnol. Biol. Med.* **2010**, *6*, 9–24.

164. Mora-Huertas, C.E.; Fessi, H.; Elaissari, A. Polymer-based nanocapsules for drug delivery. *Int. J. Pharm.* **2010**, *385*, 113–142.

165. Phillips, M.A.; Gran, M.L.; Peppas, N.A. Targeted nanodelivery of drugs and diagnostics. *Nano Today* **2010**, *5*, 143–159.

166. *Fish Health Management in Aquaculture*; Fisheries and Aquaculture Department, Food and Agriculture Organization of the United Nations: Rome, Italy. Available online: www.fao.org/fishery/en (accessed on 27 May 2005).

167. Vandenberg, G.W. Oral vaccines for finfish: academic theory or commercial reality? *Anim. Health Res. Rev.* **2004**, *5*, 301–304.

168. Adams, A.; Thompson, K.D. Biotechnology offers revolution to fish health management. *Trends Biotechnol.* **2006**, *24*, 201–205.

169. Sommerset, I.; Krossøy, B.; Biering, E.; Frost, P. Vaccines for fish in aquaculture. *Expert Rev. Vaccines* **2005**, *4*, 89–101.

170. Joosten, P.H.M.; Tiemersma, E.; Threels, A.; Caumartin-Dhieux, C.; Rombout, J.H.W.M. Oral vaccination offish against Vibrio anguillarum using alginate microparticles. *Fish Shellfish Immunol.* **1997**, *7*, 471–485.

171. Toranzo, A.E.; Magariños, B.; Romalde, J.L. A review of the main bacterial fish diseases in mariculture systems. *Aquaculture* **2005**, *246*, 37–61.

172. Research project "Oral vaccine carrier for fish farming of Friuli Venezia Giulia"-Region Friuli Venezia Giulia, Italy.

173. Romalde, J.L.; Luzardo-Alvárez, A.; Ravelo, C.; Toranzo, A.E.; Blanco-Méndez, J. Oral immunization using alginate microparticles as a useful strategy for booster vaccination against fish lactoccocosis. *Aquaculture* **2004**, *236*, 119–129.

174. Altun, S.; Kubilay, A.; Ekici, S.; Didinen, B.I.; Diler, O. Oral vaccination against lactococcosis in rainbow trout (*Oncorhynchus mykiss*) using sodium alginate and poly (lactide-co-glycolide) carrier. *Kafkas Univ. Vet. Fak. Derg.* **2010**, *16*, S211–S217.

175. Bellich, B.; Borgogna, M.; Zorzin, L.; Cocchietto, M.; Blasi, P.; Lapasin, R.; Sava, G.; Cesàro, A. Oral vaccines for aquaculture: development of a vaccine microencapsulation system based on biodegradable polymers. In *Third Biotech Workshop—"Drug Delivery Systems For Biotech Products"*, Pavia, Italy, 24–25 March 2010; University of Pavia.

176. Paolini, A.; Ridolfi, V.; Zezza, D.; Cocchietto, M.; Musa, M.; Pavone, A.; Conte, A.; Giorgetti, G. Vaccination trials of sea bass (*Dicentrarchus labrax*) against pasteurellosis using oral, intraperitoneal and immersion methods. *Vet. Ital.* **2005**, *41*, 137–144.

177. Zorzin, L.; Cocchietto, M.; Voinovich, D.; Marcuzzi, A.; Filipović-Grčić, J.; Mulloni, C.; Crembiale, G.; Casarsa, C.; Bulla, R.; Sava, G. Lysozyme-containing chitosan-coated alginate microspheres for oral immunisation. *J. Drug Deliv. Sci. Technol.* **2006**, *16*, 413–420.

178. Sava, G. Pharmacological aspects and therapeutic applications of lysozymes. In *Lysozyme: Model Enzymes in Biochemistry and Biology*; Jolles, P., Ed.; Birkhäuser Verlag: Basel, Switzerland, 1996; p. 433.

179. Zorzin, L.; Cocchietto, M.; Voinovich, D.; Blasi, P.; Bellich, B.; Borgogna, M.; Sava, G. Production of microparticles by a novel pneumatic -assisted technology: preliminary results. In Proceeding of 17th International Symposium on Microencapsulation, Nagoya, Japan, 29 September–1 October 2009.

180. Bellich, B.; Borgogna, M.; Carnio, D.; Cesàro, A. Thermal behavior of water in micro-particles based on alginate gel. *J. Therm. Anal. Calorim.* **2009**, *97*, 871–878.

181. Borgogna, M.; Bellich, B.; Zorzin, L.; Lapasin, R.; Cesàro, A. Food microencapsulation of bioactive compounds: Rheological and thermal characterisation of non-conventional gelling system. *Food Chem.* **2010**, *122*, 416–423.

182. Bellich, B.; Borgogna, M.; Cok, M.; Cesàro, A. Release Properties of Hydrogels: Water Evaporation from Alginate Gel Beads. *Food Biophys.* **2011**, *6*, 259–266.

183. Bellich, B.; Borgogna, M.; Cok, M.; Cesàro, A. Water evaporation from gel beads: A calorimetric approach to hydrogel matrix release properties. *J. Therm. Anal. Calorim.* **2011**, *103*, 81–88.

184. Martins, S.; Sarmento, B.; Souto, E.B.; Ferreira, D.C. Insulin-loaded alginate microspheres for oral delivery—Effect of polysaccharide reinforcement on physicochemical properties and release profile. *Carbohydr. Polym.* **2007**, *69*, 725–731.

185. Lee, D.W.; Hwang, S.J.; Park, J.B.; Park, H.J. Preparation and release characteristics of polymer-coated and blended alginate microspheres. *J. Microencapsul.* **2003**, *20*, 179–192.

186. Joshi, S.C.; Chen, B. Swelling, Dissolution and Disintegration of HPMC in Aqueous Media. In Proceeding of 13th International Conference on Biomedical Engineering; Lim, C.T., Goh, J.C.H., Eds.; Springer: Berlin Heidelberg, Germany, 2009; 23, p. 1244.

187. Lin, N.; Huang, J.; Chang, P.R.; Feng, L.; Yu, J. Effect of polysaccharide nanocrystals on structure, properties, and drug release kinetics of alginate-based microspheres. *Colloid. Surf. B* **2011**, *85*, 270–279.

Samples Availability: Available from the authors.

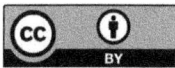

marine drugs

MDPI

Article

Employment of Marine Polysaccharides to Manufacture Functional Biocomposites for Aquaculture Feeding Applications

Marina Paolucci [1,2], **Gabriella Fasulo** [1] and **Maria Grazia Volpe** [1,*]

[1] Istituto di Scienze dell'Alimentazione—CNR Via Roma 52, 83100 Avellino, Italy;
paolucci@unisannio.it (M.P.); gabriella.fasulo@isa.cnr.it (G.F.)

[2] Department of Science and Technologies, University of Sannio, Via Port'Arsa, 11, 82100 Benevento, Italy

* Author to whom correspondence should be addressed; mgvolpe@isa.cnr.it; Tel.: +39-0825-299-513;
Fax: +39-0825-781-585.

Academic Editor: Paola Laurienzo

Received: 3 March 2015; Accepted: 17 April 2015; Published: 29 April 2015

Abstract: In this study, polysaccharides of marine origin (agar, alginate and κ-carrageenan) were used to embed nutrients to fabricate biocomposites to be employed in animal feeding. The consistency of biocomposites in water has been evaluated up to 14 days, by several methods: swelling, nutrient release and granulometric analysis. Biocomposites were produced with varying percentages of nutrients (5%–25%) and polysaccharides (1%–2%–3%). All possible biopolymer combinations were tested in order to select those with the best network strength. The best performing biocomposites were those manufactured with agar 2% and nutrients 10%, showing the lowest percentage of water absorption and nutrient release. Biocomposites made of agar 2% and nutrients 10% were the most stable in water and were therefore used to analyze their behavior in water with respect to the release of quercetin, a phenolic compound with demonstrated high antibacterial and antioxidant activities. The leaching of such molecules in water was therefore employed as a further indicator of biocomposite water stability. Altogether, our results confirm the suitability of agar as a binder for biocomposites and provide a positive contribution to aquaculture.

Keywords: functional biocomposites; quercetin release; aquaculture applications; welfare fish

1. Introduction

Marine organisms synthesize a considerable variety of biopolymers, which can begrouped into three main classes: polysaccharides, proteins and nucleic acids. The exploitation of marine biopolymers for industrial and medical purposes is a fast-growing sector of enormous interest, not only in research, but also in the progress of society, as demonstrated by the increasing number of different types of compounds isolated fromaquatic organisms and transformed into profitable products for health applications and food/feed industry [1–3]. Differently from feed for livestock, feed for aquaculture requires an adequate level of processing to guarantee good stability in water, long enough for animals to consume it. Indeed, some species are grazers and need time to eat the feed offered. Thus, in order to facilitate rearing management, the addition of binders to the feed has been considered [4]. Binders are essential for the manufacturing of formulated feed, and research is always on the look-out for new solutions based on eco-friendly, sustainable and cost-effective materials. Carbohydrates are natural biopolymers whose molecular diversity includes structures and characteristics with a large array of functions of great significance, making them suitable candidates as binders. Carbohydrates create three-dimensional networks or hydrogels that entrap nutrients and are sustainable and biodegradable [5]. Carbohydrate binders, mainly polysaccharides, in animal

Mar. Drugs **2015**, 13, 2680–2693

feed have been tested for water stability and growth performance in aquatic species with conflicting results [4]. Consistent results have been obtained regarding improved growth rates in crayfish fed on manufactured pellets [6–8].

Agar is an unbranched polysaccharide obtained from the cell walls of some species of red algae, primarily the genera belonging *Gelidium* and *Gracilaria*. Its structure consists of a gelling fraction, agarose and other non-gelling portions, agaropectins [9]. To allow the solubilization of agar, the water solution is heated up to 80–85 °C; at this temperature, agar macromolecules are statistically distributed in predominant random coil arrangements. As the sol cools down close to gelling temperature (32–43 °C), macromolecular chains start to organize in a left-handed dual helix structure due to hydrogen bond formation; the macro-grid thus obtained is stable up to 85 °C, the temperature at which it become a sol. Sodium alginate is the sodium salt of alginic acid, the structural component of the intercellular walls of *Phaeophyceae* brown seaweeds. In water solution and in the presence of divalent cations, such as calcium ion, sodium alginate yields water-insoluble gels. The divalent ions strongly interact with the-COO^- groups of the base residual of guluronic blocks forming ionic bridges between different chains [10]. Carrageenan is the hydrocolloid obtained from some red seaweeds [11,12]. Its structure consists principally of sodium, potassium, calcium, magnesium and ammonium sulfate esters of galactose and 3,6-anhydrogalactose copolymers. These hexoses are alternately linked α-1,3 and β-1,4 in the polymer. The content of sulfate groups varies 18%–40%, and according to the number and position of these groups in the units of galactose, it is possible to distinguish different types of carrageenans: kappa-carrageenan (κ-carrageenan), iota-carrageenan (ι-carrageenan) and lambda-carrageenan (λ-carrageenan). κ-Carrageenan contains residues of β-D-galactose-4-sulfate with 1,3 bonds with residues of 3,6-anhydro-α-D-galactose with 1,4 bonds. ι-Carrageenan has a similar structure to κ-carrageenan, with a difference in the degree of sulfation on Carbon 2. λ-Carrageenan contains residues of β-D-galactose-2-sulfate and 1,3 bonds with residues of β-D-galactose-2,6-disulfate bonds with 1,4. κ-Carrageenan is the most suitable to form resistant gels, because the mechanism of gelation is based on the formation of a double helix structure [13]. Quercetins are phenolic compounds (flavonoids) with several hydroxyl groups on aromatic rings [14] with demonstrated high antioxidant activities and also potential antiviral [15], antibacterial [16–18] and antiparasitic effects [19–21].

In this study, a number of polysaccharide binders of marine origin were mixed with various percentages of nutrients to manufacture biocomposites with prolonged firmness that were then tested for water retention and nutrient release up to two weeks' immersion in water. Moreover, quercetin, an active compound with antimicrobial and antifungal action, was employed to generate functional biocomposites. In particular, we focused on the application of sodium alginate, κ-carrageenan and agar as binders to manufacture feed for aquatic species.

2. Results and Discussion

2.1. Biocomposites Manufacturing and Selection

In this paper, functional biocomposites manufactured with different percentages of marine polysaccharides as binders, nutrients and quercetin were analyzed to determine the binder's capability to improve the biocomposites' stability in water.

To investigate the water stability, biocomposites manufactured with percentages ranging from 1% to 3% of each one of the following polysaccharides, agar, κ-carrageenan and sodium alginate made with percentages of nutrients ranging from 5% to 25%,were compared according to the network strength graduation used by Pearce *et al.* (2002) [22]. Figure 1 reports pictures of samples of biocomposites cast in small Petri capsules.

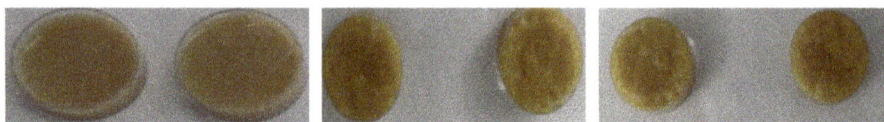

Figure 1. Pictures of biocomposites made with 2% polymer and 10% nutrients. (Right) agar; (center) alginate; (left) κ-carrageenan.

Agar-based biocomposites at any percentage had a smooth and glossy surface, while both sodium alginate- and κ-carrageenan-based biocomposites appeared bumpy and dull. In Table 1, the complete list of manufactured biocomposites is reported, along with their consistency. Biocomposites made with agar 2% and 3% and nutrients 5%–10% gave the best results in terms of consistency, followed by agar 1% with all percentages of nutrients tested and agar 2% and 3% with nutrients 15%, 20%–25%. Sodium alginate and κ-carrageenan performed less well at all percentages of polysaccharide and nutrients tested. This is probably due to the different supermolecular structure of the gels. Alginate forms the so-called "egg-box" structure, where the contact points of the polymeric chainsare formed by ionic bonds by means of divalent ions (Ca^{2+}). In gels made with κ-carrageenan, the molecules assume a helical shape due to the effects of torsional movements. The association of many chains leads to the formation of multiple helices, whose anionic nature requires the presence of cations, such as Ca^{2+}. Thus, with both alginate and κ-carrageenan, the gels formed are rigid, even at low concentrations. Thus, although alginate and κ-carrageenan are well known by their good gel-forming capability, lowconsistent systems of alginate and κ-carrageenan are probably due to interference of the molecules of nutrients with the crosslinking process thatoccurs with calcium ions.The mechanism of agar gel formation is instead temperature dependendant reversible. At the beginning, single and double helices are formed, then individual helices aggregate into multiple helices [23]. Although speculative, we may hypothesize that the slower gelation process occurring in agar gel allowed the nutrients to embed in the network, thus leading to biocomposites with good and very good consistency with respect to gels made of sodium alginate and κ-carrageenan.

Only biocomposites with very good and good consistency were further tested for water uptake and nutrients release being. Thus, agar-based biocomposites made with percentages of nutrients ranging from 5% to 25% were manufactured and further analyzed for water behavior. The proximate composition is shown in Table 2.

Table 1. Consistency evaluation according to the terminology used by Pearce *et al.* [22]: 1, very good consistency; 2, good consistency; 3, weak consistency; 4, inconsistent.

No.	Biocomposites	Biopolymer %	Nutrients %	Consistency
1	Sodium Alginate	1	15–20–25	4
2	Sodium Alginate	1	5–10	3
3	Sodium Alginate	2	15–20–25	4
4	Sodium Alginate	2	5–10	3
5	Sodium Alginate	3	15–20–25	4
6	Sodium Alginate	3	5–10	3
7	κ-Carrageenan	1	15–20–25	4
8	κ-Carrageenan	1	5–10	3
9	κ-Carrageenan	2	15–20–25	4
10	κ-Carrageenan	2	5–10	3
11	κ-Carrageenan	3	15–20–25	4
12	κ-Carrageenan	3	5–10	3
13	Agar	1	15–20–25	2
14	Agar	1	5–10	2
15	Agar	2	15–20–25	2
16	Agar	2	5–10	1
17	Agar	3	15–20–25	2
18	Agar	3	5–10	1

2.2. Biocomposites Water Stability

Water stability of feed is of primary importance in the processing of aquaculture diets; it is greatly influenced by the properties of the binders, although the ingredients themselves have an influence on the characteristics of the binders [24]. Despite the water stability representing a major concern of the aquaculture industry, there is no standard method to determine feed water stability. It is usually estimated by the method of dry matter weight loss, according to which a certain amount of feed, usually in the form of pellets, is placed in a water-containing beaker and allowed to stay for a variable length of time [4]. In the present study, the stability in water of biocomposites was evaluated through the degree of water absorption (swelling test), dry matter loss (nutrients release) and granulometric analysis.

Table 2. Proximate analysis of agar (1%–2%–3%)-based biocomposites and nutrients ranging from 5% to 25%.

Agar (%)	Nutrients (%)	Total Lipids (%)	Protein (%)	Carbohydrates (%)	Water (%)
1	5	0.240 ± 1.04	2.56 ± 0.44	7.9 ± 1.12	89.3 ± 0.98
1	10	0.420 ± 1.08	3.06 ± 0.60	14.7± 0.98	81.2 ± 1.01
1	15	0.740 ± 0.98	4.47 ± 0.38	21.7 ± 1.02	73.09± 1.15
1	20	0.975 ± 0.79	5.96 ± 1.02	30.5 ± 0.76	62.6 ± 1.30
1	25	1.58 ± 0.08	7.39 ± 0.79	38.4 ± 0.54	52.6 ± 0.94
2	5	0.257 ± 0.16	2.32 ± 1.12	7.7 ± 0.38	88.3 ± 0.84
2	10	0.432 ± 0.21	3.46 ± 0.74	13.7 ± 0.44	82.2 ± 0.79
2	15	0.750 ± 0.38	4.50 ± 0.67	21.0 ± 0.67	72.8 ± 0.78
2	20	0.946 ± 0.20	5.89 ± 0.21	30.3 ± 1.23	62.1 ± 1.05
2	25	1.64 ± 0.24	7.25 ± 1.02	38.0 ± 1.21	51.9 ± 1.16
3	5	0.235 ± 0.19	2.32 ± 0.14	7.5 ± 1.34	89.1 ± 0.60
3	10	0.453 ± 0.32	3.38 ± 0.23	14.3 ± 0.98	81.7 ± 0.59
3	15	0.736 ± 0.48	4.86 ± 0.36	21.9 ± 0.87	73.32 ± 0.54
3	20	0.967 ± 0.21	6.02 ± 0.16	31.1 ± 1.37	62.3 ± 0.54
3	25	1.59 ± 0.38	7.63 ± 0.76	38.2 ± 0.97	52.1 ± 0.38

2.2.1. Swelling

In general, the percentage of water absorbed by biocomposites increased with the time of immersion and the percentage of nutrients employed. Figure 2a,c,e,g,i shows how agar 2%-based biocomposites show the best behavior in water, in terms of swelling, with respect to agar 1% and 3%. Indeed, biocomposites made of agar 2% absorbed less water with respect to biocomposites made of agar 1% and 3%, at any nutrient concentration. The amount of absorbed water increased according to the increase in the percentage of nutrients present in the biocomposites. In any case, water absorption was quite limited. In both 1% and 2% agar-based biocomposites, the percentage of absorbed water reached a maximum value of 10% after 14 days of immersion, while in the 3% agar-based biocomposites, it reached a value of 15% after 14 days of immersion. The agarose molecules that constitute the highly gelling fraction of agar have a high molecular weight due to the presence of left-handed triple helices that enable the polymer to generate a strong and stable gel, which can accommodate and firmly bind water molecules in thefree inter- and intra-molecular interstices [25], a phenomenon that could explain the greater degree of absorption of water in the biocomposites based on 3% agar.

2.2.2. Nutrient Release

In spite of the importance of assessing nutrient release, there is still no standard method to determine it. In this study, we evaluated the dry matter loss after water immersion and indicate it as nutrient release. Nutrient release Figure 2b,d,f,h,j appeared to be proportional to the nutrient percentage in the biocomposites, with the exception of biocomposites based on agar1%,whichreleased less nutrients at 25% than nutrients at 15% and 20%. Moreover, nutrient release appeared to be proportional to the percentage of agar in the biocomposites. This outcome is in disagreement with observations made by Partridge and Southgate (1999) [26], who reported that nutrient release increased with decreasing binder concentration. However, it is possible that such a discrepancy may be attributed to the ample variability in feed ingredients and manufacturing technologies employed. It can be hypothesized that the greater degree of nutrient release from biocomposites based on agar 3% could be attributed to the ability held a higher amount of water that consequently determines thelower stability of the nutrients inside the three-dimensional networks of the gel. In 1% agar-based biocomposites, the lower amount of water held could conversely explain the higher stability of nutrients and, therefore, the lower nutrient release with respect to the 3% agar.Only in one case, that is biocomposites made of agar 1% with nutrients 10%, was the amount of water held higher than biocomposites made of agar 3%. Unfortunately, we do not have an explanation for such a discrepancy. Nevertheless, we cannot rule out the possibility that agar could undergo degradation during water incubation, thus altering the amount of nutrients released.

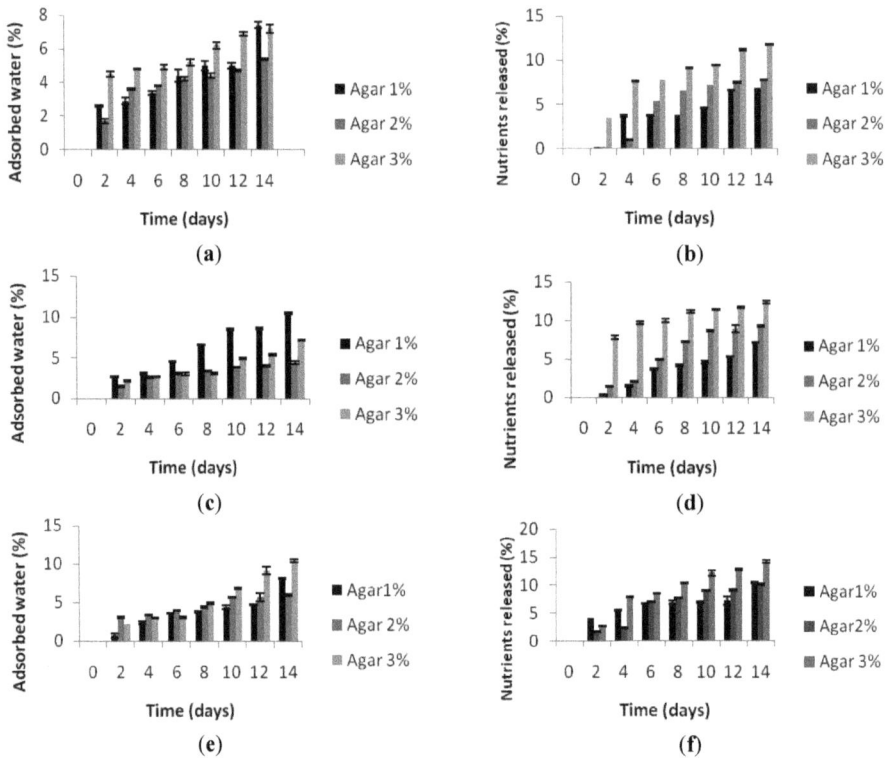

Figure 2. *Cont.*

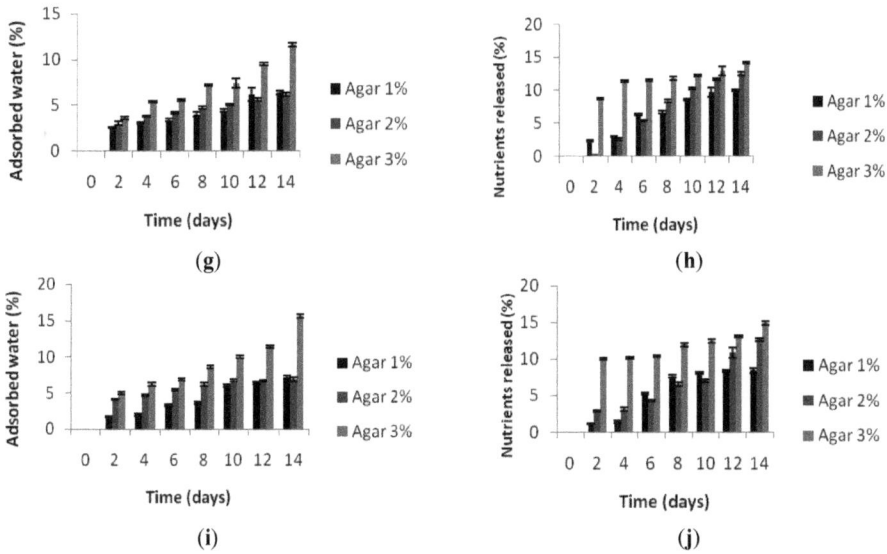

Figure 2. (**a,c,e,g,i**) percentage of water adsorbed by biocomposites made with agar 1%–2%–3% and containing nutrients 5%–10%–15%–20%–25%; (**b,d,f,h,j**) percentage of nutrients released by biocomposites with agar 1%–2%–3% and containing nutrients 5%–10%–15%–20%–25%.

2.2.3. Granulometric Analysis

Granulometric analysis allows the monitoring of particles released by the biocomposites in water and the measurement of the diameter of the particles expressed as derived diameter. The low angle laser light scattering technique has been long employed in our laboratory to determine the water stability of feed for aquatic species [4,6–8,27]. The diameters of particles released by the biocomposites are continuously monitored over time, providing a time-course indication about the water stability as a function of the released particle diameter inasmuch as biocomposites that disaggregate into small particles are less stable in water than biocomposites that disaggregate into particles of a larger diameter. In Table 3 are reported the derived diameter of agar-based biocomposites at different percentages of nutrients.

The diameter of the released particles was quite constant throughout the experiment, ranging from about 10 to about 400 μm. All agar percentages behave well with all of the percentages of nutrients employed. The outcome is in agreement with previous observations carried out using the low angle laser light scattering technique to determine the diameter of particles released by agar-based biocomposites specifically designed for sea urchin feeding, which proved to have good water stability at least up to seven days [27].

Table 3. (a) Derived diameters (μm) of particles released in water at time intervals up to 14 days of biocomposites manufactured with percentages of nutrients of 5% and 10%; (b) derived diameters (μm) of particles released in water at time intervals up to 14 days of biocomposites manufactured with percentages of nutrients of 15% and 20%.

	(a)					
	Derived Diameters (μm) Nutrients 5%			Derived Diameters (μm) Nutrients 10%		
Days	Agar 1%	Agar 2%	Agar 3%	Agar 1%	Agar 2%	Agar 3%
2	46.24 ± 0.02	13.82 ± 0.03	44.50 ± 0.22	54.41 ± 0.02	269.71 ± 0.41	108.35 ± 0.04
4	284.28 ± 0.11	57.44 ± 0.02	56.91 ± 0.23	304.51 ± 0.32	223.34 ± 0.32	171.62 ± 0.12
6	272.58 ± 0.04	160.62 ± 0.14	121.64 ± 0.02	251.39 ± 0.44	326.05 ± 0.19	206.51 ± 0.22
8	260.88 ± 0.04	162.90 ± 0.22	141.17 ± 0.02	204.66 ± 0.34	356.84 ± 0.24	142.19 ± 0.32
10	245.33 ± 0.12	176.49 ± 0.03	181.60 ± 0.02	287.82 ± 0.27	242.10 ± 0.12	64.83 ± 0.28
12	239.62 ± 0.02	286.53 ± 0.05	310.29 ± 0.02	324.26 ± 0.78	248.48 ± 0.52	67.62 ± 0.34
14	233.92 ± 0.12	255.93 ± 0.11	333.36 ± 0.02	339.68 ± 0.05	140.13 ± 0.62	70.42 ± 0.25

	(b)					
	Derived diameters (μm) Nutrients 15%			Derived diameters (μm) Nutrients 20%		
Days	Agar 1%	Agar 2%	Agar 3%	Agar 1%	Agar 2%	Agar 3%
2	317.48 ± 0.32	121.37 ± 0.04	109.40 ± 0.08	277.23 ± 0.04	258.04 ± 0.14	245.63 ± 0.18
4	335.00 ± 0.22	224.71 ± 0.24	327.59 ± 0.18	323.17 ± 0.11	218.70 ± 0.29	211.55 ± 0.21
6	303.12 ± 0.12	242.44 ± 0.14	218.19 ± 0.13	349.98 ± 0.12	295.13 ± 0.30	227.21 ± 0.24
8	217.69 ± 0.02	271.51 ± 0.12	114.81 ± 0.10	375.91 ± 0.12	265.84 ± 0.34	258.74 ± 0.34
10	306.61 ± 0.23	119.16 ± 0.05	153.46 ± 0.12	364.81 ± 0.09	236.55 ± 0.27	290.28 ± 0.27
12	280.82 ± 0.11	186.35 ± 0.11	192.12 ± 0.09	273.88 ± 0.09	330.72 ± 0.24	286.87 ± 0.38
14	238.41 ± 0.11	254.70 ± 0.12	356.19 ± 0.08	231.23 ± 0.22	188.70 ± 0.38	106.41 ± 0.44

2.2.4. Quercetin Release

Release of nutrients is an important feature of feed, since they can function as attractant molecules. Indeed, a certain degree of leaching should always be allowed. In this study, we used quercetin to monitor the amount of small molecule leaching and chose quercetin due to its characteristics. Akroum *et al.* (2010) [28] tested the antibacterial activity of 11 flavonoids extracted from some medicinal plants and concluded that quercetin was the most interesting compound for all of the tested activities. Thus, quercetin could be usefully employed to improve both biocomposites' shelf-life and the health performances of the farmed species due to its antioxidant and anti-microbial activities. The concentration of quercetin released by biocomposites in water is reported in Figure 3.

The trend of quercetin release was similar in all agar-based biocomposites. Quercetin release in water increased sharply during the first four days in 1% and 3% agar-based biocomposites, reaching values of respectively 87.01 ± 0.33 mg/100 g fresh tissue (quercetin 0.25%) and 73.75 ± 0.85 mg/100 g fresh tissue (quercetin 0.50%) in 1% agar-based biocomposites and 64.58 ± 0.02 mg/100 g fresh tissue (quercetin 0.25%) and 47.45 ± 0.03 mg/100 g fresh tissue (quercetin 0.50%) in 3% agar-based biocomposites. Slightly different was the behavior of 2% agar-based biocomposites that released a lower concentration of quercetin (27.80 ± 0.02 and 29.28 ± 0.02 mg/100 g fresh tissue for respectively quercetin 0.25% and 0.50%) up to the sixth day. From the eight day on, the quercetin concentrations released in water increased, but never as much as the values showed by 1% and 3% agar-based biocomposites. Again 2% agar-based biocomposites showed the best performances in terms of water behavior. As expected, the release of quercetin follows the same trends of nutrients.

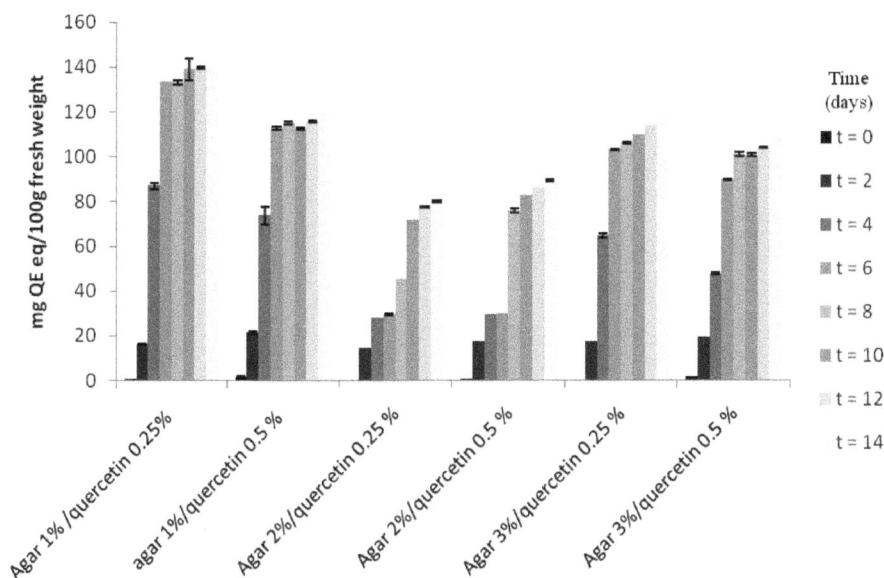

Figure 3. Quantity of quercetin (mg QE eq/100 g fresh weight) released by biocomposites made with agar 1%–2%–3% and containing nutrients 5%. Fresh weight refers to biocomposites formulated without any treatment before analysis.

3. Materials and Methods

3.1. Biocomposites Formulation and Preparation

The following biopolymers were employed: agar, sodium alginate and κ-carrageenan, supplied by Sigma (St. Louis, MO, USA). Biocomposites were first produced with varying percentages of nutrients (5%–25%) and polymers (1%–2%–3%), adding $CaCl_2$ either alone or as a solution (0.5%–1%) to sodium alginate and κ-carrageenan as a networking agent.The best results were obtained with 0.5%of powdered $CaCl_2$; therefore, the following descriptions refer to such parameters. All possible biopolymer combinations were tested in order to select those with the best network strength. The feed used for the nutrients was formulated on the basis of the current literature on aquatic species (Table 4).

Quercetin (Sigma-Aldrich Co., St. Louis, MO, USA) (0.25%–0.5%) was added to all biocomposites for its antimycotic and antioxidant properties. Biocomposites were manufactured by the following procedure: each biopolymer in powder form was dissolved to the desired percentage in tap water and heated to the boiling point on a magnetic plate, stirring constantly. The solution was allowed to boil for a few minutes and was then cooled at RT to a temperature of 45 ± 5 °C. Nutrients in powder form and $CaCl_2$ (only in the presence of alginate and carrageenan) were then added to the mixture while stirring vigorously. The biocomposite was then poured into Petri capsules and allowed to cool at RT for 12 h. The round biocomposites (1-cm high, 4-cm diameter) were then removed from the Petri capsules and used for the further analyses. Network strength was subjectively evaluated in accordance with the terminology used by Pearce *et al.*, (2002) [22]: 1, very good consistency; 2, good consistency; 3, weak consistency; 4, inconsistent. Samples with "weak consistency" and "inconsistent" were discarded and were not considered for further trials. A complete list of manufactured biocomposites is provided in Table 4.

Table 4. Feed ingredients used in biocomposites.

Ingredient	Dry Weight (%)
Fish meal	19.00
Legume meal	27.00
Corn meal [a]	24.00–25.00
Algae meal	25.00
Fish oil	1.80
Mineral mix	0.10
Vitamin mix	0.10

[a] Percentage adjusted depending on the percentage of binder employed.

3.2. Behavior in Water of Biocomposites

3.2.1. Swelling

Samples of round biocomposites listed in Table 4 among those selected for further trials were soaked at 20°C in water for up to 14 days. A round biocomposite was placed in a beaker and submerged with 200 mL of tap water. Only biocomposites with a network strength of 2 or less according to the terminology used by Pearce *et al.* (2002) [22], were tested for swelling. The swelling degree was expressed as a percentage of the increase in weight against the initial weight of the biocomposites and was calculated using the following equation:

$$\text{water uptake (\%)} = [(W_f - W_0)/W_0] \times 100$$

where W_0 and W_f are the initial and final weight, respectively. Samples were recovered every two days and re-weighed in order to assess weight gain. All tests were carried out in triplicate.

3.2.2. Nutrients Release

To evaluate nutrients release, quantitative analysis was performed at 20 °C by evaporating the water in which the biocomposites were immersed. At time intervals of 2 days, up to 14 days, the amount of nutrients deposited on the bottom was determined by ponderal analysis according to A.O.A.C 2007 (Association of Official Agricultural Chemists) [29]. For each analysis, three samples for each type of biocomposites were employed.

3.2.3. Granulometric Analysis

The diameter of nutrients released in water was measured by immersing samples of each biocompositi up to 14 days. For each analysis, three samples for each type of biocomposites were employed. After the required immersion time, samples were recovered, freeze-dried for 24 h and re-weighed. The recovered liquid was analyzed by monitoring the released particles in water during immersion. Particle size distributions were measured by LALLS (low angle laser light scattering technique) using Master Sizer Model S equipped with Malvern Application Software Version 1.1.a (Malvern Instruments, Malvern, UK) and fitted with a Small Volume Presentation Unit, as described in Volpe *et al.* (2008) [6]. The refractive index of samples and of dispersants was measured using an Optech Model RM Abbe refractometer at a temperature of 20 °C and white light. Specifically, LALLS and laser diffraction are based on the interaction of light-particle, called diffraction, which, as a physical principle, produces a dispersion of light on the ends of the particles with an angle inversely proportional to the size of the particle invested. After having focused on the center of a light-multi element detector, the effect of dispersion leading to signals on the elements is not central to the detector. Among the technical characteristics of the laser granulometer, there is an optics-unique and fixed measuring range: 0.02 to 2000 μM.

3.2.4. Quercetin Release

To evaluate quercetin leaching in water, biocomposites were submerged in water at 20 °C. For each analysis, three samples for each type of biocomposite were employed. At different time intervals (2 days up to 14 days), an aliquot of water (1 mL) was taken and employed to determine the quercetin concentration by spectrophotometric analysis. After the quercetin measurement, the water aliquot was returned to the beaker to keep thewater volume constant throughout the experiment. Quercetin absorbance was measured at 515 nm using a Beckman Coulter model. DU 730 Spectrophotometer (Indianapolis, IN, USA). The results were expressed as mg of quercetin equivalents/100 g fresh weight.

3.3. Statistical Analysis

Data were analyzed by one-way ANOVA, and the significant difference was determined at the 0.05 level by Duncan's multiple range test. All analyses were performed with the StatSoft, Inc., STATISTICA data analysis software system, Version 8.0.

4. Conclusions

The feeding of aquatic animals stimulates the interest of researchers towards improving feed formulation. The feed must first be able to meet the different nutritional requirements in such a way as to ensure a degree of optimal growth; secondly, the critical issues related to the management of aquaculture systems must be considered, so as to minimize waste and pollution. In this experimental work, attention was focused on a particular aspect of the preparation of feed with structural characteristics, so as to prevent or at least minimize the release of nutrients in the water. To achieve these objectives, biopolymer-based feeds have been formulated, using macromolecules found in large quantities from natural renewable sources that, thanks to the peculiarity of forming hydrogels, are able to incorporate the nutrients in the three-dimensional network conferring firmness and stability to the feed. This study showed that the use of the agar-based biocomposites has a great degree of stability in water; this is in full agreement with the gelling characteristics of the polymer, which also in low percentages allows one to obtain three-dimensional networks that are strongly interpenetrated and resistant, so as to minimize the absorption of water and the release of nutrients.

Our results confirm the suitability of agar as a binder for biocomposites and provide a positive contribution to aquaculture.

Acknowledgments: This research was supported by the European Fund for Fisheries 2007–2013 (Regulation (CE) N. 1198/2006) Tool 3.5 "Pilot Projects" to Marina Paolucci.

Author Contributions: Marina Paolucci and Maria Grazia Volpe designed the experiments and wrote the manuscript. Gabriella Fasulo carried out the experiments.

Conflicts of Interest: The authors declare no conflict of interest.

References

1. Silva, T.H.; Alves, A.; Ferreira, B.M.; Oliveira, J.M.; Reys, L.L.; Ferreira, R.J.F.; Sousa, R.A.; Silva, S.S.; Mano, J.F.; Reis, R.L. Materials of marine origin: A review on polymers and ceramics of biomedical interest. *Int. Mater. Rev.* **2012**, *57*, 276–306. [CrossRef]
2. Farris, S.; Schaich, K.M.; Liu, L.; Piergiovanni, L.; Yam, K.L. Development of polyion-complex hydrogels as an alternative approach for the production of bio-based polymers for food packaging applications: A review. *Trends Food Sci. Technol.* **2009**, *20*, 316–332. [CrossRef]
3. Volpe, M.G.; Malinconico, M.; Varricchio, E.; Paolucci, M. Polysaccharides as biopolymers for food shelf-life extention. *Rec. Pat. Food Nutr. Agric.* **2010**, *2*, 129–139. [CrossRef]
4. Paolucci, M.; Fabbrocini, A.; Volpe, M.G.; Varricchio, E.; Coccia, E. Development of biopolymers as binders for feed for farmed aquatic organisms. In *Aquaculture*; Muchlisin, Z.A., Ed.; InTech Publishers: New York, NY, USA, 2012; pp. 3–34.

5. Volpe, M.G.; Santagata, G.; Coccia, E.; di Stasio, M.; Malinconico, M.; Paolucci, M. Pectin based pellets for crayfish aquaculture: Structural and functional characteristics and effects on redclaw *Cherax quadricarinatus* performances. *Aquac. Nutr.* **2014**, in press.

6. Volpe, M.G.; Monetta, M.; di Stasio, M.; Paolucci, M. Rheological behavior of polysaccharide based pellets for crayfish feeding tested on growth in the crayfish *Cherax albidus*. *Aquaculture* **2008**, *274*, 339–346. [CrossRef]

7. Volpe, M.G.; Varricchio, E.; Coccia, E.; Santagata, G.; di Stasio, M.; Malinconico, M.; Paolucci, M. Manufacturing pellets with different binders: Effect on water stability and feeding response in juvenile *Cherax albidus*. *Aquaculture* **2012**, *324–325*, 104–110. [CrossRef]

8. Coccia, E.; Santagata, G.; Malinconico, M.; Volpe, M.G.; di Stasio, M.; Paolucci, M. *Cherax albidus* juveniles fed polysaccharide-based pellets: Rheological behavior and effect on growth. *Freshw. Crayfish* **2010**, *17*, 13–18.

9. Usov, A.I. Structure analysis of red seaweed galactan of agar and carrageenan groups. *Food Hydrocoll.* **1998**, *12*, 301–308. [CrossRef]

10. Draget, K.I.; Skjak-Bræk, G.; TorgerStokke, B. Similarities and differences between alginic acid gels and ionically crosslinked alginate gels. *Food Hydrocoll.* **2006**, *20*, 170–175. [CrossRef]

11. Murano, E.; Toffanin, R.; Zanetti, F.; Knutsen, S.H.; Paoletti, S.; Rizzo, R. Chemical and macromolecular characterisation of agar polymers from *Gracilaria dura* (C. Agardh) J. agardh (Gracilariaceae, Rhodophyta). *Carbohydr. Polym.* **1992**, *18*, 171–178. [CrossRef]

12. Kalia, A.N. *Textbook of Industrial Pharmacognosy*; CBS Publishers and Distributors: New Delhi, India, 2005; ISBN 8123912099.

13. Anderson, N.S.; Campbell, J.W.; Harding, M.M.; Rees, D.A.; Samuel, J.W.B. X-ray diffraction studies of polysaccharide sulphates: Double helix models of κ-and ι-carrageenans. *J. Mol. Biol.* **1969**, *45*, 85–88. [CrossRef] [PubMed]

14. Manach, C.; Scalbert, A.; Morand, C.; Rémésy, C.; Jiménez, L. Polyphenols, food sources and bioavailability. *Am. J. Clin. Nut.* **2004**, *79*, 727–747.

15. Zandi, K.; Teoh, B.T.; Sam, S.S.; Wong, P.F.; Mustafa, M.R.; AbuBakar, S. Antiviral activity of four types of bioflavonoid against dengue virus type-2. *Virol. J.* **2011**, *8*, 560. [CrossRef]

16. Funatogawa, K.; Hayashi, S.; Shimomura, H.; Yoshida, T.; Hatano, T.; Ito, H.; Iría, Y. Antibacterial activity of hydrolysable tannins derived from medicinal plants against *Helicobacter pylori*. *Microbiol. Immunol.* **2004**, *48*, 251–261. [CrossRef] [PubMed]

17. Karou, D.; Dicko, M.H.; Simpore, J.; Traore, A.S. Antioxidant and antibacterial activities of polyphenols from ethnomedicinal plants of Burkina Faso. *Afr. J. Biotechnol.* **2005**, *4*, 823–828.

18. Tavassoli, S.; Djomeh, Z.E. Total phenols, antioxidant potential and antimicrobial activity of methanol extract of rosemary (*Rosmarinus officinalis* L.). *Glob. Vet.* **2011**, *7*, 337–341.

19. Yang, C.Y.L.; Yen, K.Y. Induction of apoptosis by hydrolysable tannins from *Eugenia jambos* L. on human leukemia cells. *Cancer Lett.* **2000**, *157*, 65–75. [CrossRef] [PubMed]

20. Tanimura, S.; Kadomoto, R.; Tanaka, T.; Zhang, Y.J.; Kouno, I.; Kohno, M. Suppression of tumor cell invasiveness by hydrolyzable tannins (plant polyphenols) via the inhibition of matrix metalloproteinase-2/-9 activity. *Biochem. Biophys. Res. Commun.* **2005**, *330*, 1306–1313.

21. Molan, A.L.; Faraj, A.M. The effects of condensed tannins extracted from different plant species on egg hatching and larval development of *Teladorsagia circumcincta* (Nematoda: Trichostrongylidae). *Folia Parasitol.* **2010**, *57*, 62–68. [CrossRef] [PubMed]

22. Pearce, C.M.; Daggett, T.L.; Robinson, S.M.C. Effect of binder type and concentration of prepared feed stability and gonad yield and quality of the green sea urchin, *Strongylocentrotus droebachiensis*. *Aquaculture* **2002**, *205*, 301–323. [CrossRef]

23. Armisen, R.; Galactas, F. Production, properties and uses of agar. In *Production and Utilisation of Products from Commercial Seaweeds*; McHugh, D.J., Ed.; FAO Fisheries Technical Paper Publisher: Roma, Italy, 1987; pp. 1–57.

24. Dominy, W.G.; Lim, C. Performance of binder in pelleted shrimp diets. In Proceedings of the Aquaculture Fee Processing and Nutrition Workshop, Thailand and Indonesia, 19–25 September 1991; pp. 149–157.

25. Araki, C. Some recent studies on the polysaccharides of agarophytes. *Proc. Int. Seaweed Symp.* **1966**, *5*, 3–19.

26. Partridge, G.J.; Southgate, P.C. The effect ofbinder composition on ingestion and assimilation of microbound diets (MBD) by barramundi *Lates calcarifer* Bloch larvae. *Aquac. Res.* **1999**, *30*, 879–886. [CrossRef]

27. Fabbrocini, A.; Volpe, M.G.; di Stasio, M.; D'Adamo, R.; Maurizio, D.; Coccia, E.; Paolucci, M. Agar-based pellet as feed for sea urchins (*Paracentrotus lividus*): Rheological behaviour, digestive enzymes and gonad growth. *Aquac. Res.* **2012**, *43*, 321–331. [CrossRef]

28. Akroum, S.; Bendjeddou, D.; Satta, D.; Lalaoui, K. Antibacterial, antioxidant and acute toxicity tests on flavonoids extracted from some medicinal plants. *Int. J. Green Pharm.* **2010**, *4*, 165–169. [CrossRef]

29. AOAC Official Method International. Available online: http://www.aoac.org (accessed on 8 October 2007).

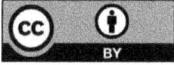

MDPI

Article

Sulfated-Polysaccharide Fraction from Red Algae *Gracilaria caudata* Protects Mice Gut Against Ethanol-Induced Damage

Renan Oliveira Silva [1], Geice Maria Pereira dos Santos [1], Lucas Antonio Duarte Nicolau [1], Larisse Tavares Lucetti [2], Ana Paula Macedo Santana [2], Luciano de Souza Chaves [3], Francisco Clark Nogueira Barros [3], Ana Lúcia Ponte Freitas [3], Marcellus Henrique Loiola Ponte Souza [2] and Jand-Venes Rolim Medeiros [1,*]

[1] LAFFEX—Laboratory of Experimental Physiopharmacology, Biotechnology and Biodiversity Center Research (BIOTEC), Federal University of Piauí-CMRV, 64202-020, Parnaíba, PI, Brazil; renan.oliveira25@yahoo.com.br (R.O.S.); geicysantos2009@hotmail.com (G.M.P.d.S.); lucasnicolau5@hotmail.com (L.A.D.N.)

[2] LAFICA—Laboratory of Pharmacology of Inflammation and Cancer, Department of Physiology and Pharmacology, Federal University of Ceará, 60430-270, Fortaleza, CE, Brazil; larisselucetti@hotmail.com (L.T.L.); apmacedo1@hotmail.com (A.P.M.S.); souzamar@ufc.br (M.H.L.P.S.)

[3] Laboratory of Proteins and Carbohydrates of Marine Algae, Department of Biochemistry and Molecular Biology, Federal University of Ceará, 60455-760, Fortaleza, CE, Brazil; lucianoscsep@hotmail.com (L.d.S.C.); clarkfc@gmail.com (F.C.N.B.); pfreitas@ufc.br (A.L.P.F.)

* Author to whom correspondence should be addressed; jandvenes@ufpi.edu.br; Tel.: +55-86-99862374 or +55-86-33234750; Fax: +55-86-33235406.

Received: 14 September 2011; in revised form: 17 October 2011; Accepted: 24 October 2011; Published: 2 November 2011

Abstract: The aim of the present study was to investigate the gastroprotective activity of a sulfated-polysaccharide (PLS) fraction extracted from the marine red algae *Gracilaria caudata* and the mechanism underlying the gastroprotective activity. Male Swiss mice were treated with PLS (3, 10, 30 and 90 mg·kg^{-1}, *p.o.*), and after 30 min, they were administered 50% ethanol (0.5 mL/25 g^{-1}, *p.o.*). One hour later, gastric damage was measured using a planimeter. Samples of the stomach tissue were also obtained for histopathological assessment and for assays of glutathione (GSH) and malondialdehyde (MDA). Other groups were pretreated with L-NAME (10 mg·kg^{-1}, *i.p.*), DL-propargylglycine (PAG, 50 mg·kg^{-1}, *p.o.*) or glibenclamide (5 mg·kg^{-1}, *i.p.*). After 1 h, PLS (30 mg·kg^{-1}, *p.o.*) was administered. After 30 min, ethanol 50% was administered (0.5 mL/25g^{-1}, *p.o.*), followed by sacrifice after 60 min. PLS prevented-ethanol-induced macroscopic and microscopic gastric injury in a dose-dependent manner. However, treatment with L-NAME or glibenclamide reversed this gastroprotective effect. Administration of propargylglycine did not influence the effect of PLS. Our results suggest that PLS has a protective effect against ethanol-induced gastric damage in mice via activation of the NO/K$_{ATP}$ pathway.

Keywords: polysaccharide; gastric damage; ethanol; nitric oxide; hydrogen sulfide

1. Introduction

Marine organisms are sources of numerous new compounds with multiple pharmacological properties [1]. At present, the number of substances being isolated from such sources is growing. Most of their chemical structures have been elucidated, and they are being investigated for their potential to meet various biological objectives, as well as to expand the scientific knowledge base in the area of naturally bioactive compounds [2]. Currently, about 25–30% of all active agents used in treatments are extracted from natural products [3]. In the last 50 years, sulfated-polysaccharide has drawn the attention of researchers, since it has become clear that it is involved in several cellular processes [4] and therefore, may present many pharmacological opportunities [5,8].

In algae, these sulfated-polysaccharides are complex macromolecular constituents of the extracellular matrix, and they evidently play an important role in the mechanical, osmotic, and ionic regulation of these beings [9,10]. Investigation of these biomolecules has been steadily increasing in recent years owing to their broad potential development as antithrombotic, anti-viral, anticoagulant, antioxidant, anti-inflammatory, and anti-proliferative agents [11,14]. However, studies of sulfated-polysaccharide extracted from sea algae (hereafter referred to as "PLS" throughout this manuscript) in ethanol-induced gastric damage models are scarce.

In the gastrointestinal tract, ethanol can produce acute hemorrhagic gastric damage, and excessive ingestion can result in gastritis characterized by mucosal edema, subepithelial hemorrhages, cellular exfoliation, and inflammatory cell infiltration [15,16]. Multiple mechanisms are likely to be involved in this pathogenic process, including depletion of non-protein sulfhydryl groups (thereby increasing reactive oxygen species (ROS) that have ulcerogenic activity), modulation of the nitric oxide system, and reduction of gastric mucosal blood flow. It has also been suggested that oxidative stress and depletion of anti-oxidants may be a crucial step in ethanol-induced mucosal damage [17]. In recent years, algal sulfated-polysaccharides have been demonstrated to play an important role as free-radical scavengers and antioxidants in the prevention of oxidative damage in living organisms [13,18].

Nitric oxide (NO) and hydrogen sulfide (H_2S) are crucial mediators of gastrointestinal mucosal defense [19,22]. Studies have demonstrated that these gases are responsible for the modulation of some general components of mucosal defense such as increase of the gastric mucosal blood flow, mucus and bicarbonate secretion, and inhibition of neutrophil adherence to endothelial cells [19,23,25]. Thus, considering that the sea algae are important sources of new chemical substances with potential therapeutic effects, this study sought to evaluate the gastroprotective effect of a sulfated-polysaccharide fraction extracted from the sea algae *Gracilaria caudata* (PLS) against ethanol-induced gastric damage in mice, and the possible mechanisms involved.

2. Results and Discussion

Alcohol-related diseases of the gastrointestinal tract play an important role in clinical gastroenterology. However, the mechanisms and pathophysiology underlying the effects of ethanol on the organs of the digestive tract are not yet completely understood. The gastroprotective activity of PLS was evaluated using the ethanol-induced gastric damage model, the most commonly employed model in the evaluation of anti-ulcer/cytoprotective activity. Ethanol administration evidently resulted in severe macroscopic and microscopic gastric mucosal damage through an increase in reactive oxygen species generation and a decrease in the endogenous anti-oxidant defense mechanisms [26]. In the present study, we confirmed that ethanol induced gastrophathy (61.3 ± 18.9 mm^2) and that PLS treatment reduced the macroscopic and microscopic ethanol-induced gastric damage. Figure 1 shows that the PLS prevented ethanol-gastropathy in a dose-dependent manner, reaching maximal effect at a dose of 30 mg·kg^{-1} (4.9 ± 3.7 mm^2). Because a PLS dose of 30 mg·kg^{-1} afforded the most protection against gastric lesions induced by ethanol, this dose was selected for the study of the possible mechanisms of action involved in PLS-mediated gastroprotective effects.

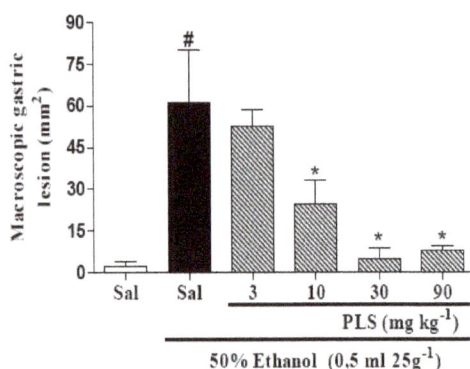

Figure 1. The effect of PLS on ethanol-induced gastric damage. Mice were treated by gavage with either saline or PLS (3, 10, 30 and 90·mg·kg^{-1}). Thirty minutes later, mice in experimental groups were administered 50% ethanol (0.5 mL/25 g^{-1}); the negative control group was administered saline. The total area of macroscopic gastric lesions was determined after 1 h. The results are expressed as mean ± SEM of a minimum of 5 animals per group. $^{#}$ $p < 0.05$ *vs.* saline group; * $p < 0.05$ *vs.* ethanol group; ANOVA and Newman-Keuls test.

Figure 2 shows that ethanol administration induced a gastric superficial region disruption with epithelial cell loss and intense hemorrhage. Conversely, these afflictions were not observed in mice treated with ethanol and 30·mg·kg^{-1} of PLS. These data suggest that PLS has a gastroprotective effect in this context. Table 1 shows that PLS treatment (30 mg·kg^{-1}) resulted in less ethanol-induced hemorrhagic damage, edema, and epithelial cell loss. Notably, these data indicate that ethanol did not increase inflammatory cell infiltration in the gastric mucosa compared with controls; however, this is probably due to mice being sacrificed just 1 h after ethanol administration (Figure 2 and Table 1).

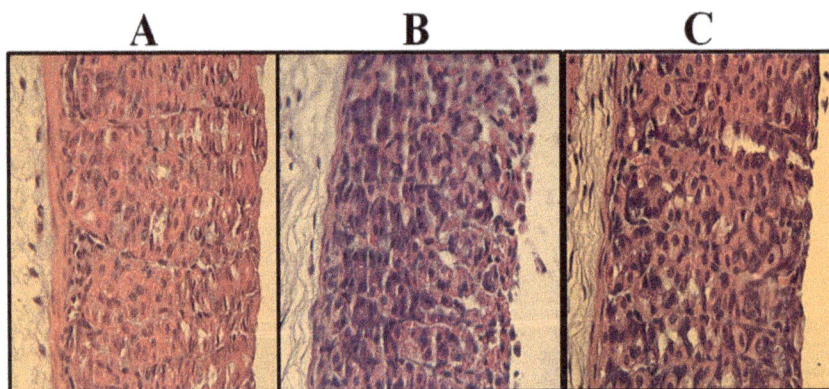

Figure 2. Photomicrographs of gastric mucosa (Magnification, 100×): (**A**) saline control; (**B**) animals treated with 50% ethanol, showing disruption of the superficial region of the gastric gland with epithelial cell loss and intense hemorrhage; (**C**) animals treated with 50% ethanol + polysaccharide (30 mg·kg^{-1}), showing preservation of the gastric mucosa. Quantitative results from these assessments are shown in Table 1.

Table 1. The effect of PLS (30 mg·kg^{-1}) on ethanol-induced microscopic gastric damage.

Experimental group (n = 5)	Hemorrhagic damage (score, 0–4)	Edema (score, 0–4)	Epithelial cell loss (score, 0–3)	Inflammatory cells (score, 0–3)	Total (score, 0–14)
Saline	0	0 (0–1)	0	0	0
Ethanol	3 (3–4)	3 (3–4)	2 (2–3)	0 (0–1)	8 (6–10)
Ethanol + PLS 30 mg·kg^{-1}	1 (0–2) *	1 (0–1) *	1 (0–1) *	0	3 (0–3) *

Data shown are medians with minimal and maximal scores shown in parentheses. The Kruskal-Wallis nonparametric test, followed by Dunn's test was used for multiple comparisons of histological analyses. * $p < 0.05$ *vs.* control (ethanol) group.

It has been suggested that oxygen-derived free radicals (ROS) may contribute to ethanol-induced gastric mucosal lesions [27,28] and deplete the reduced glutathione (GSH) content in stomach tissues [21,27,29]. Our results are in accordance with these reports; ethanol induced a decrease in gastric GSH (298.3 ± 18.2 μg/g tissue) as compared to the saline group (415.0 ± 28.7 μg/g tissue) (Figure 3). Thus, PLS may function by decreasing the redox state in ethanol-induced gastropathy. Our results showed that administration of PLS (30 mg·kg^{-1}; 369.7 ± 19.4 μg/g tissue) reversed the decrease in the gastric GSH levels after ethanol administration. Therefore, we inferred that the protective effect of PLS administration might be explained by a resultant increase in the gastric GSH concentration. Another possibility is that an increase in GSH levels could be secondary to a decrease in the free radical production. Superoxide produced by peroxidase in the stomach tissues might damage cell membranes and cause ulcers by increasing malondialdehyde (MDA) level, the most widely used index of lipid peroxidation [30]. Our results suggest that administration of 30 mg·kg^{-1} (20.0 ± 11.9 nmol·g^{-1} of tissue) of PLS resulted in a significant decrease in the MDA concentrations in ethanol-induced gastropathy (115.1 ± 7.4 nmol·g^{-1} of tissue) (Figure 4). Several authors evaluated the effect of different gastroprotective and antioxidants extracts, also had similar results [29,31]. Thus, the mechanism through which PLS exerts gastroprotective effects seems to involve an indirect antioxidant activities and a reduction of the lipid peroxidation induced by ethanol.

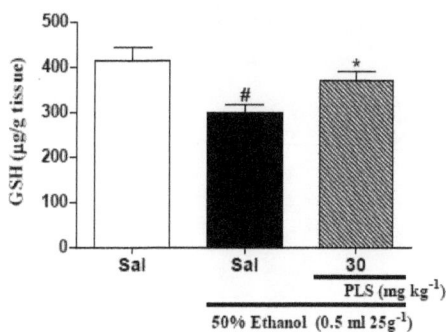

Figure 3. The effect of PLS on glutathione (GSH) levels in the gastric mucosa of mice treated with ethanol. Mice were treated by gavage with saline or PLS (30 mg·kg^{-1}). Thirty minutes later, 50% ethanol (0.5 mL 25 g^{-1}) was administered to the experimental groups, while the control group was administered saline. Ethanol administration promoted a reduction in the GSH gastric levels. This effect was partially reverted when the animals were treated with PLS. The results are expressed as mean ± SEM of 5 animals per group. $^{\#}$ $p < 0.05$ *vs.* saline group; * $p < 0.05$ *vs.* ethanol group; ANOVA and Newman-Keuls test.

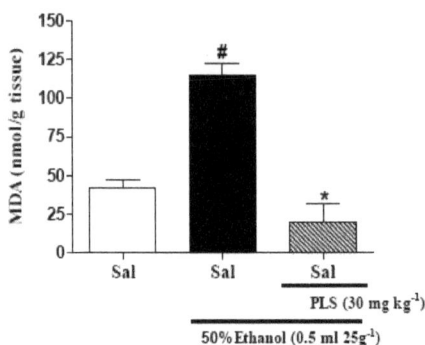

Figure 4. The effect of PLS on malondialdehyde (MDA) concentration in the gastric mucosa of mice treated with ethanol. Mice were treated by gavage with PLS (30 mg·kg^{-1}). Thirty minutes later, mice in the experimental group were administered 50% ethanol (0.5 mL 25 g^{-1}), and the control group was administered saline. The ethanol evidently promoted an increase in MDA gastric levels. When the animals were pre-treated with PLS, this effect was reverted. The results are expressed as the Means ± SEM of 5 animals per group. [#] $p < 0.05$ *vs.* saline group; * $p < 0.05$ *vs.* ethanol group; ANOVA and Newman-Keuls test.

Using a pharmacological approach it was demonstrated that PLS provides a protective effect against ethanol-induced gastric damage via the NO/K$_{ATP}$ pathway. As shown in Figure 5, in animals treated with L-NAME (74.9 ± 22.9 mm^2, a non selective inhibitor of nitric oxide synthase) or with glibenclamide (41.6 ± 6.5 mm^2, a drug that blocks K$_{ATP}$-dependent channels), the gastroprotective effect of PLS 30 mg·kg^{-1} (12.5 ± 8.3 mm^2) was abrogated. This attests to the involvement of the NO/K$_{ATP}$ pathway in the protection conferred by PLS. However, when the animals were pretreated with DL-propargylglycine (9.8 ± 3.5 mm^2, an H$_2$S synthesis inhibitor that blocks CSE activity), it did not alter the protective effect of PLS.

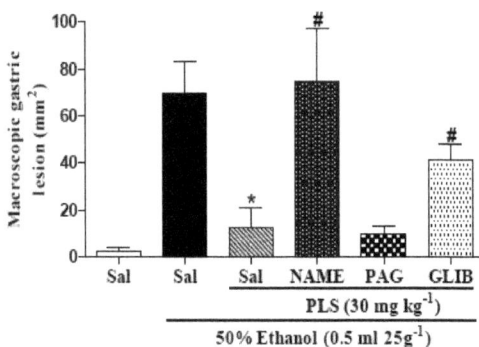

Figure 5. The effect of L-NAME, PAG, and glibenclamide on PLS-mediated protection against macroscopically visible ethanol-induced gastric damage. Mice were initially treated with L-NAME (10 mg·kg^{-1}, *i.p.*), DL-propargylglycine (PAG, 50 mg·kg^{-1}, *p.o.*), or glibenclamide (5 mg·kg^{-1}, *i.p.*). After 1 h, PLS (30 mg·kg^{-1}, *p.o.*) was administered. Thirty minutes later, 50% ethanol was administered to the experimental groups, and the control group was administered saline. The total area of the macroscopic gastric lesions was determined after 1 h. The results are expressed as mean ± SEM of a minimum of 5 animals per group. * $p < 0.05$ *vs.* ethanol group; [#] $p < 0.05$ *vs.* PLS + ethanol group; ANOVA and Newman-Keuls test.

Nitric oxide (NO) modulates several elements of gastric mucosal defense, including blood flow [32], neutrophil adhesion [33,34], and mucus secretion [25,35]. NO and cyclic GMP can both activate various types of K^+ channels [36,37]. Recently, it was demonstrated that the activation of ATP-sensitive potassium channels (K_{ATP}) is involved in gastric defense [38,39]. Our findings suggest that the PLS defensive effect is a NO-dependent process and that blockage of the NO/K_{ATP} pathway with L-NAME/glibenclamide abrogated the protective effect of PLS against ethanol-induced gastric damage.

It has been demonstrated that the development of stress-induced gastric mucosal injury, including an increase in the gastric acid secretion, is involved in the pathogenesis of ethanol-induced gastric mucosal injury [40]. Several studies suggest that hypersecretion of gastric acid is associated with ethanol-induced gastric damage, and the anti-ulcer activity of many compounds may be related to the inhibition of gastric acid secretion [41,42]. However, in our study, PLS did not alter gastric acid secretion. As shown in Table 2, administration of PLS did not change the volume of gastric juice, the pH or the total acidity as compared to similarly derived values observed in the saline group. In contrast, histamine treatment increased the volume and total acidity, while ranitidine (an H_2 antagonist) decreased the volume and total acidity, as compared to corresponding values in the saline group (Table 2).

Table 2. The effects of PLS on gastric secretion in 4-h pylorus-ligated mice.

Experimental Group ($n = 5$)	Volume (μL)	pH	Total Acid (mEq[H^+]/L/4 h)
Saline	504 ± 39.2	1.6 ± 0.4	5.0 ± 0.3
PLS (30 mg·kg^{-1})	550 ± 89.1	1.8 ± 0.8	5.4 ± 0.6
Histamine	993 ± 90.8 *	1.5 ± 0.5	10 ± 0.6 *
Ranitidine	295 ± 78.3 #	2.7 ± 0.5	2.4 ± 0.5 #

Data shown are expressed as mean $\pm$ SEM ($n = 5$). * $p < 0.05$; # $p < 0.05$, *vs.* saline group; ANOVA and Newman-Keuls test.

In summary, our results indicate that PLS prevents ethanol-induced gastric damage. While there are many mechanisms through which this effect could potentially occur, our data supports the hypothesis that the reduction of lipid peroxidation and the activation of the NO/K_{ATP} pathway are of primary importance. These observations also raise the possibility of polysaccharides being used to improve resistance to gastric mucosal injury.

3. Experimental Section

3.1. Extraction of Soluble Polysaccharide

Specimens of the red algae *Gracilaria caudata* were collected in August 2008 from the Atlantic coast northeast of Brazil (Fleixeira Beach, Trairi-Ceará). After collection, the algae were cleaned of epiphytes, washed with distilled water, and stored at -20 °C. In order to enable extraction of polysaccharide, 5 g of dried *G. caudata* tissue was ground into a fine powder and incubated in stirring distilled water (1.5% w/v) for 2 h at 100 °C. After filtration and concentration of the solution, the polysaccharide was precipitated with ethanol (1:3 v/v) followed by washing with acetone and dried with hot air flow. The polysaccharide fraction was then re-dissolved in distilled water (1.5% w/v) and subjected to the same process to achieve precipitation, washing, and drying. The polysaccharide fraction thus derived constitutes what is referred to throughout this manuscript as "PLS".

3.2. Animals

Male Swiss mice (25–30 g) were fasted for 18 to 24 h before the experiments. Animals were housed in cages in temperature-controlled rooms, and food and water were available *ad libitum*. All animal treatments and surgical procedures were performed in accordance with the Guide for Care and Use of Laboratory Animals (National Institute of Health, Bethesda, MD, USA) and were approved by the appropriate ethics committee (protocol No. 0066/10).

3.3. The Effect of PLS on Ethanol-Induced Gastric Damage

Male Swiss mice were initially treated with PLS (3, 10, 30 and 90 mg·kg^{-1}) by gavage. After 30 min, gastric damage was induced in the experimental groups by ethanol administration (0.5 mL/25 g^{-1} *p.o.*), while the control group received saline. One hour later, the animals were sacrificed and their stomachs rapidly removed—opened via an incision along the greater curvature and pinned out on a wax block. Gastric damage (hemorrhagic or ulcerative lesions) was measured using a computer planimetry program (Image J®). A sample of the corpus region of each stomach was fixed in 10% formalin immediately after removal for subsequent histopathological assessment. Further gastric corpus samples were then weighed, frozen, and stored at -70 °C until they were assayed for GSH [43] and MDA [44].

3.4. The Roles of NO and H₂S in the Protective Effect of PLS

Animals were pre-treated with a non-selective NO-synthase inhibitor, N-nitro-L-arginine methyl ester hydrochloride (L-NAME, 10 mg kg^{-1}, *i.p.*), or with DL-propargylglycine (PAG, 50 mg·kg^{-1}, *p.o.*), an inhibitor of H₂S synthesis. After 1 h, the mice were administered PLS (30 mg·kg^{-1} *p.o.*). Thirty minutes later, gastric damage was induced in the experimental mice by intragastric instillation of ethanol 50% (0.5 mL/25 g^{-1} *p.o.*), while the control group received saline. One hour later, gastric damage was analyzed as described above.

3.5. The Role of K$_{ATP}$ in PLS-Mediated Gastric Protection

To study the role of K$_{ATP}$ in PLS-mediated gastric protection, animals were pre-treated with glibenclamide (5 mg·kg^{-1}, *i.p.*), a drug that blocks K$_{ATP}$-dependent channels. After 1 h, the mice received PLS (30 mg·kg^{-1} *p.o.*). Thirty minutes later, gastric damage was induced in experimental mice by intragastric instillation of ethanol 50% (0.5 mL/25 g^{-1} *p.o.*), while the control group received saline. One hour later, gastric damage was determined as described above.

3.6. Histological Assessment

For histological assessment, stomach samples were fixed in 10% formalin solution, sectioned, and embedded in paraffin. Four-micrometer-thick sections were deparaffinized, stained with hematoxylin and eosin, and then examined under a microscope. The specimens were assessed according to the criteria described in Laine and Weinstein (1988) [45]. In brief, 1 cm lengths of each histological section were assessed for epithelial cell loss (a score of 0–3), edema in the upper mucosa (a score of 0–4), hemorrhagic damage (a score of 0–4) and the presence of inflammatory cells (a score of 0–3). Subsequently, the sections were assessed as "blind" (without knowledge of the prior treatments) by an experienced pathologist.

3.7. GSH Assay

The reduced GSH content of the stomach tissues was estimated according to the method described in Sedlak and Lindsay (1968) [43]. A segment from each stomach was homogenized in 5 mL of cold 0.02 M EDTA solution (1 mL 100 mg^{-1} tissue). Aliquots (400 μL) of tissue homogenate were mixed with 320 μL of distilled water and 80 μL of 50% (w/v) trichloroacetic acid in glass tubes and centrifuged at 3000 rpm for 15 min. Next, 400 μL of each supernatant was mixed with 800 μL of Tris buffer (0.4 M, pH 8.9), and 20 μL of 0.01 M 5,5-dithio-bis (2-nitrobenzoic acid). After shaking the preparation, absorbance was measured at 412 nm on a spectrophotometer. GSH concentration was ascertained via

Mar. Drugs **2011**, *9*, 2188–2200

a reduced GSH standard curve, generated in parallel. The results are expressed as micrograms of GSH per gram of tissue.

3.8. MDA Assay

The level of MDA in the homogenate from each group was measured using the method described in Mihara and Uchiyama (1978) [44], which is based on a thiobarbituric acid reaction. Fragments of the gastric mucosa weighing between 100 and 150 mg were homogenized with cold 1.15% KCl to prepare 10% homogenates. In brief, 250 μL of each homogenate was added to 1.5 mL of 1% H_3PO_4 and 0.5 mL of 0.6% *tert*-butyl alcohol (aqueous solution). Then, this mixture was stirred and heated in a boiling water bath for 45 min. The preparation was then cooled immediately in an ice water bath, followed by the addition of 4 mL of *n*-butanol. This mixture was shaken and the butanol layer was separated by centrifugation at 1200 g for 10 min. Optical density was determined to be 535 and 520 nm, and the optical density difference between the 2 determinations was calculated as the *tert*-butyl alcohol value. MDA concentrations are expressed as millimoles per gram of tissue.

3.9. Gastric Acid Secretion

The technique described in Shay *et al.* (1945) [46] was utilized in the current study. Firstly, pylorus ligature was performed under inhalation anesthesia. Then saline and PLS (30 mg·kg^{-1}) were injected intraperitoneally. In another group, gastric acid secretion in pylorus-ligated mice induced by histamine (5 mg·kg^{-1}) or ranitidine (5 mg·kg^{-1}) via *i.p.* injection was tested. After 4 h, the animals were sacrificed by deep inhalatory anesthesia, their stomachs were opened, and the gastric content collected. The final volume and pH were directly determined after washing the mucosal side of the stomach with 2 mL of distilled water. Total acidity of the gastric juice was titrated with NaOH 0.01 N, using 2% phenolphthalein as an indicator.

3.10. Statistical Analysis

All values are expressed as mean ± SEM. ANOVA and the Student-Newman-Keuls test were used to determine the statistical significance of the differences between the groups. For histological assessment, the Kruskal-Wallis nonparametric test was used, followed by Dunn's test for multiple comparisons. Differences were considered to be significant when $p < 0.05$.

4. Conclusions

In conclusion, our results indicate that PLS has a potential gastroprotective effect against ethanol-induced gastrophathy. In addition, the mechanism of PLS-mediated protection may be related to decreases in free radical production and lipid peroxidation.

Although there are many mechanisms through which this gastroprotective effect could occur, our data support the hypothesis that NO and the activation of K_{ATP} channels are of primary importance. These observations also raise the possibility of PLS being used to improve resistance to gastric mucosal injury.

Acknowledgments: The authors gratefully acknowledge the technical assistance of Maria Silvandira Freire França, and we thank UFPI/CNPq for fellowship support.

References

1.   Arif, J.M.; Al-Hazzani, A.A.; Kunhi, M.; Al-Khodairy, F. Marine compounds: Anticancer or genotoxic? *J. Biomed. Biotechnol* **2004**, *2*, 93–98.
2.   Blunt, J.W.; Copp, B.R.; Munro, M.H.G.; Northcote, P.T.; Prinsep, M.R. Marine natural products. *Nat. Prod. Rep* **2006**, *23*, 26–78.
3.   Silva, J.S.E.; Moura, M.D.; Oliveira, R.A.G.; Diniz, M.F.F.M.; Barbosa-Filho, J.M. Natural products inhibitors of ovarian neoplasia. *Phytomedicine* **2003**, *10*, 221–232.

4. Han, F.; Yao, W.; Yang, X.; Liu, X.; Gao, X. Experimental study on anticoagulant and antiplatelet aggregation activity of a chemically sulfated marine polysaccharide YCP. *Int. J. Biol. Macromol* **2005**, *36*, 201–207.

5. Toida, T.; Sakai, S.; Akiyama, H.; Linhardt, R.J. Immunological activity of chondroitin sulfate. *Adv. Pharmacol* **2006**, *53*, 403–415.

6. Toida, T.; Chaidedgumjorn, A.; Linhardt, R. Structure and bioactivity of sulfated polysaccharides. *J. Trends Glycosci. Glycotechnol* **2003**, *15*, 29–46.

7. Lee, J.B.; Hayashi, K.; Maeda, M.; Hayashi, T. Antiherpetic activities of sulfated polysaccharides from green algae. *Planta Med* **2004**, *70*, 813–817.

8. Athukorala, Y.; Lee, K.W.; Kim, S.K.; Jeon, Y.J. Anticoagulant activity of marine green and brown algae collected from Jeju Island in Korea. *Bioresour. Technol* **2007**, *98*, 1711–1716.

9. Kloareg, B.; Quatrano, R.S. Structure of cell wall of marine algae and ecophysiological function of matrix polysaccharides. *Oceanogr. Mar. Biol. Ann. Rev* **1988**, *26*, 259–315.

10. Rocha, H.A.O.; Leite, E.L.; Medeiros, V.P.; Lopes, C.C.; Nascimento, F.D.; Tersariol, I.L.S.; Sampaio, L.O.; Nader, H.B. Natural Sulfated Polysaccharides as Antithrombotic Compounds. Structural Characteristics and Effects on the Coagulation Cascade. In *Insight into Carbohydrate Structure and Biological Function*; Verli, H., Guimarães, J.A., Eds.; Transworld Research Network: Kerala, India, 2006; pp. 51–67.

11. Almeida-Lima, J.; Costa, L.S.; Silva, N.B.; melo-Silveira, R.F.; Silva, F.V.; Felipe, M.B.M.C.; Medeiros, S.R.B.M.; Leite, E.L.; Rocha, H.A.O. Evaluating the possible genotoxic, mutagenic and tumor cell proliferation-inhibition effects of a non-anticoagulant, but antithrombotic algal heterofucan. *J. Appl. Toxicol* **2010**, *30*, 708–715.

12. Barroso, E.M.; Costa, L.S.; Medeiros, V.P.; Cordeiro, S.L.; Costa, M.S.; Franco, C.R.; Nader, H.B.; Leite, E.L.; Rocha, H.A.O. A non-anticoagulant heterofucan has antithrombotic activity *in vivo*. *Planta Med* **2008**, *74*, 712–718.

13. Costa, L.S.; Fidelis, G.P.; Cordeiro, S.L.; Oliveira, R.M.; Sabry, D.A; Câmara, R.B.G.; Nobre, L.T.D.B.; Costa, M.S.S.P.; Almeida-Lima, J.; Farias, E.H.C.; *et al.* Biological activities of sulfated polysaccharides from tropical seaweeds. *Biomed. Pharmacother* **2010**, *64*, 21–28.

14. Cumashi, A.; Ushakova, N.A.; Preobrazhenskaya, M.E.; D'incecco, A.; Picooli, A.; Totani, L.; Tinari, N.; Morozevich, G.E.; Berman, A.E.; Bilan, M.I.; *et al.* A comparative study of the anti-inflammatory, anticoagulant, antiangiogenic, and antiadhesive activities of nine different fucoidans from brown seaweeds. *Glycobiology* **2007**, *17*, 541–552.

15. Guslandi, M. Effect of ethanol on the gastric mucosa. *Dig. Dis* **1987**, *5*, 21–32.

16. Ko, J.K.; Cho, C.H.; Lam, S.K. Adaptive cytoprotection through modulation of nitric oxide in ethanol-evoked gastritis. *World J. Gastroenterol* **2004**, *1*, 2503–2508.

17. La Casa, C.; Villegas, I.; De La Lastra, C.A.; Motilva, V.; Martin Calero, M.J. Evidence for protective and antioxidant properties of rutin, a natural flavone, against ethanol induced gastric lesions. *J. Ethnopharmacol* **2000**, *71*, 45–53.

18. Zhang, Z.; Wang, F.; Wang, X.; Liu, X.; Hou, Y.; Zhang, Q. Extraction of the polysaccharides from five algae and their potential antioxidant activity *in vitro*. *Carbohydr. Polym* **2010**, *82*, 118–121.

19. Muscara, M.N.; Wallace, J.L. Nitric oxide. V. Therapeutic potential of nitric oxide donors and inhibitors. *Am. J. Physiol* **1999**, *276*, 1313–1316.

20. Fiorucci, S.; Antonelli, E.; Distrutti, E.; Rizzo, G.; Mencarelli, A.; Orlandi, S.; Zanardo, R.; Renga, B.; Di Sante, M.; Morelli, A.; *et al.* Inhibition of hydrogen sulfide generation contributes to gastric injury caused by anti-inflammatory nonsteroidal drugs. *Gastroenterology* **2005**, *129*, 1210–1224.

21. Medeiros, J.V.; Gadelha, G.G.; Lima, S.J.; Garcia, J.A.; Soares, P.M.; Santos, A.A.; Brito, G.A.; Ribeiro, R.A.; Souza, M.H. Role of the NO/cGMP/K_{ATP} pathway in the protective effects of sildenafil against ethanol-induced gastric damage in rats. *Br. J. Pharmacol* **2008**, *153*, 721–727.

22. Medeiros, J.V.; Bezerra, V.H.; Gomes, A.S.; Barbosa, A.L.; Lima-Júnior, R.C.; Soares, P.M.; Brito, G.A.; Ribeiro, R.A.; Cunha, F.Q.; Souza, M.H. Hydrogen sulfide prevents ethanol-induced gastric damage in mice: Role of ATP-sensitive potassium channels and capsaicin-sensitive primary afferent neurons. *J. Pharmacol. Exp. Ther* **2009**, *330*, 764–770.

23. Coruzzi, G.; Adami, M.; Morini, G.; Pozzoli, C.; Cena, C.; Bertinaria, M.; Gasco, A. Antisecretory and gastroprotective activities of compounds endowed with H$_2$ antagonistic and nitric oxide (NO) donor properties. *J. Physiol. Paris* **2000**, *94*, 5–10.

24. Fiorucci, S.; Distrutti, E.; Cirino, G.; Wallace, J.L. The emerging roles of hydrogen sulfide in the gastrointestinal tract and liver. *Gastroenterology* **2006**, *131*, 259–271.

25. Wallace, J.L.; Miller, M.J. Nitric oxide in mucosal defense: A little goes a long way. *Gastroenterology* **2000**, *119*, 512–520.

26. Jonsson, I.M.; Verdrengh, M.; Brissler, T.M.; Lindblad, S.; Bokarewa, M.; Islander, U.; Carlsten, H.; Ohlsson, C.; Nandakumar, K.S.; Holmdahl, R.; Tarkowski, A. Ethanol prevents development of destructive arthritis. *Proc. Natl. Acad. Sci. USA* **2007**, *104*, 258–263.

27. Trier, J.S.; Szabo, S.; Allan, C.H. Ethanol-induced damage to mucosal capillaries of rat stomach. Ultrastructural features and effects of prostaglandin E_2 and cysteamine. *Gastroenterology* **1987**, *92*, 13–22.

28. Matsumoto, T.; Moriguchi, R.; Yamada, H. Role of polymorphonuclearleucocytes and oxygen-derived free radicals in the formation of gastric lesions induced by HCl/ethanol, and a possible mechanism of rotection by antiulcer polysaccharide. *J. Pharm. Pharmacol* **1992**, *45*, 535–539.

29. Gomes, A.S.; Gadelha, G.G.; Lima, S.J.; Garcia, J.A.; Medeiros, J.V.R.; Havt, A.; Lima, A.A.; Ribeiro, R.A.; Brito, G.A.; Cunha, F.Q.; *et al.* Gastroprotective effect of heme-oxygenase 1/ biliverdin/CO pathway in ethanol-induced gastric damage in mice. *Eur. J. Pharmacol* **2010**, *642*, 140–145.

30. Alimi, H.; Hfaiedh, N.; Bouoni, Z.; Hfaiedh, M.; Sakly, M.; Zourgui, L.; Rhouma, K.B. Antioxidant and antiulcerogenic activities of Opuntia ficus indica f. inermis root extract in rats. *Phytomedicine* **2010**, *17*, 1120–1126.

31. Alvarez-Suarez, J.M.; Dekanski, D.; Ristić, S.; Radonjić, N.V.; Petronijević, N.D.; Giampieri, F.; Astolfi, P.; González-Paramás, A.M.; Santos-Buelga, C.; Tulipani, S.; *et al.* Strawberry polyphenols attenuate ethanol-induced gastric lesions in rats by activation of antioxidant enzymes and attenuation of MDA increase. *PLoS One* **2011**, *6*, e25878.

32. Whittle, B.J.; Kauffman, G.L.; Moncada, S. Vasoconstriction with thromboxane A2 induces ulceration of the gastric mucosa. *Nature* **1981**, *292*, 472–474.

33. Kubes, P.; Suzuki, M.; Granger, D.N. Nitric oxide: An endogenous modulator of leukocyte adhesion. *Proc. Natl. Acad. Sci. USA* **1991**, *88*, 4651–4655.

34. May, G.R.; Crook, P.; Moore, P.K.; Page, C.P. The role of nitric oxide as an endogenous regulator of platelet and neutrophil activation within the pulmonary circulation of the rabbit. *Br. J. Pharmacol* **1991**, *102*, 759–763.

35. Allen, A.; Flemstrom, G.; Garner, A.; Kivilaakso, E. Gastroduodenal mucosal protection. *Physiol. Rev* **1993**, *73*, 823–857.

36. Archer, S.L.; Huang, J.M.; Hampl, V.; Nelson, D.P.; Shultz, P.J.; Weir, E.K. Nitric oxide and cGMP cause vasorelaxation by activation of a charybdotoxin-sensitive K channel by cGMP-dependent protein kinase. *Proc. Natl. Acad. Sci. USA* **1994**, *91*, 7583–7587.

37. Bolotina, V.M.; Najibi, S.; Palacino, J.J.; Pagano, P.J.; Cohen, R.A. Nitric oxide directly activates calcium-dependent potassium channels in vascular smooth muscle. *Nature* **1994**, *368*, 850–853.

38. Peskar, B.M.; Ehrlich, K.; Peskar, B.A. Role of ATP-sensitive potassium channels in prostaglandin-mediated gastroprotection in the rat. *J. Pharmacol. Exp. Ther* **2002**, *301*, 969–974.

39. Gomes, A.S.; Lima, L.M.; Santos, C.L.; Cunha, F.Q.; Ribeiro, R.A.; Souza, M.H. LPS from Escherichia coli protects against indomethacin-induced gastropathy in rats: Role of ATP-sensitive potassium channels. *Eur. J. Pharmacol* **2006**, *547*, 136–142.

40. Moody, F.G.; Cheung, L.Y.; Simons, M.A.; Zalewsky, C. Stress and acute gastric mucosal lesion. *Am. J. Dig. Dis* **1976**, *21*, 148–154.

41. Oates, P.J.; Hakkinen, J.P. Studies on the mechanism of ethanol-induced gastric damage in rats. *Gastroenterology* **1988**, *94*, 10–21.

42. Vela, S.M.; Souccar, C.; Lima-Landman, M.T.; Lapa, A.J. Inhibition of gastric acid secretion by the aqueous extract and purified extracts of *Stachytarpheta cayennensis*. *Planta Med* **1997**, *63*, 36–39.

43. Sedlak, J.; Lindsay, R.H. Estimation of total, protein-bound, and nonprotein sulfhydryl groups in tissue with Ellman's reagent. *Anal. Biochem* **1968**, *25*, 1192–1205.

44. Mihara, M.; Uchiyama, M. Determination of malonaldehyde precursor in tissues by thiobarbituric acid test. *Anal. Biochem* **1978**, *86*, 271–278.

45. Laine, L.; Weinstein, W.M. Histology of alcoholic hemorrhagic gastritis: A prospective evaluation. *Gastroenterology* **1988**, *94*, 1254–1262.
46. Shay, M.; Kamarov, S.A.; Fels, D.; Meranze, D.; Gruenstein, H.; Siplet, H. A simple method for the uniform production of gastric ulceration in the rats. *Gastroenterology* **1945**, *5*, 43–61.

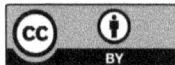

marine drugs

MDPI

Review

Prebiotics from Marine Macroalgae for Human and Animal Health Applications

Laurie O'Sullivan [1], Brian Murphy [1], Peter McLoughlin [1], Patrick Duggan [1], Peadar G. Lawlor [2], Helen Hughes [1,*] and Gillian E. Gardiner [1]

[1] Eco-Innovation Research Centre, Department of Chemical and Life Sciences, Waterford Institute of Technology, Waterford, Ireland; losullivan@wit.ie (L.O.S.); bmurphy@wit.ie (B.M.); pmcloughlin@wit.ie (P.M.); pduggan@wit.ie (P.D.); ggardiner@wit.ie (G.E.G.)

[2] Teagasc, Pig Development Unit, Moorepark Research Centre, Fermoy, County Cork, Ireland; peadar.lawlor@teagasc.ie

* Author to whom correspondence should be addressed; hhughes@wit.ie; Tel.: +353-51-834047; Fax: +353-51-302679.

Received: 13 May 2010; in revised form: 11 June 2010; Accepted: 28 June 2010; Published: 1 July 2010

Abstract: The marine environment is an untapped source of bioactive compounds. Specifically, marine macroalgae (seaweeds) are rich in polysaccharides that could potentially be exploited as prebiotic functional ingredients for both human and animal health applications. Prebiotics are non-digestible, selectively fermented compounds that stimulate the growth and/or activity of beneficial gut microbiota which, in turn, confer health benefits on the host. This review will introduce the concept and potential applications of prebiotics, followed by an outline of the chemistry of seaweed polysaccharides. Their potential for use as prebiotics for both humans and animals will be highlighted by reviewing data from both *in vitro* and *in vivo* studies conducted to date.

Keywords: marine macroalgae; polysaccharides; prebiotics; human and animal health

---

1. Introduction

Marine macroalgae, or seaweeds as they are more commonly known, are one of nature's most biologically active resources, as they possess a wealth of bioactive compounds. For example, compounds isolated from marine macroalgae have demonstrated various biological activities, such as antibacterial activity [1], antioxidant potential [2,3], anti-inflammatory properties [4], anti-coagulant activity [5], anti-viral activity [6] and apoptotic activity [7]. As a result, seaweed-derived compounds have important applications in a range of products in food, pharmaceuticals and cosmetics [8,10]. In addition to bioactive components, macroalgae are a rich source of dietary fiber (25–75% dry weight), of which water-soluble fiber constitutes approximately 50–85% [11]. Seaweeds are commonly classified into three main groups based on their pigmentation. Phaeophyta, or brown seaweeds, are predominantly brown due to the presence of the carotenoid fucoxanthin and the primary polysaccharides present include alginates, laminarins, fucans and cellulose [12,13]. Chlorophyta, or green seaweeds, are dominated by chlorophyll a and b, with ulvan being the major polysaccharide component [14]. The principal pigments found in rhodophyta, or red seaweeds, are phycoerythrin and phycocyanin and the primary polysaccharides are agars and carrageenans [15].

In the past decade, considerable research has been conducted on dietary modulation of intestinal microbiota. One particular area of research has focused on the concept of dietary "prebiotics" as functional ingredients for gut health, both for humans and animals. This review will examine evidence that polysaccharides from marine macroalgae, such as fucoidan, laminarin, alginate and their derivatives, may offer potential for use as prebiotics, with particular emphasis on their use in human and animal health applications. First the concept of prebiotics will be introduced, followed by a summary of the chemistry of seaweed polysaccharides, and a discussion of data from both *in vitro* and *in vivo* studies that have examined the prebiotic potential of seaweed polysaccharides.

2. The Prebiotic Concept

The gastrointestinal tract (GIT) of both humans and animals is a complex, diverse, microbial ecosystem. The colon is the most heavily colonized region of the GIT with up to 10^{12} bacteria per gram of intestinal contents. The dominant genera include *Bacteroides, Prevotella, Eubacterium, Clostridium* and *Bifidobacterium*, with *Lactobacillus, Staphylococcus, Enterococcus, Streptococcus, Enterobacter* and *Escherichia* part of the sub-dominant flora (Figure 1) [16]. Potentially pathogenic and beneficial bacteria co-exist (Figure 1); however, strategies are being sought to influence this composition towards a more favorable balance, by reducing the amount of potentially harmful or pathogenic species and promoting the growth of species thought to have beneficial effects on host health [17]. Dietary modulation of the intestinal microflora can either be achieved via oral administration of probiotic micro-organisms or prebiotic compounds. The prebiotic concept was first proposed by Gibson and Roberfroid in 1995 [17] and the most recent definition of a prebiotic is "a selectively fermented ingredient that allows specific changes, both in the composition and/or activity of the gastrointestinal microflora that confers benefits upon the host wellbeing and health" [18]. To be considered prebiotic, a compound must satisfy a number of criteria; firstly it must be resistant to digestion in the upper GIT and therefore resistant to acid and enzymatic hydrolysis; secondly, it must be a selective substrate for the growth of beneficial bacteria and therefore result in a shift in the profile of the microflora and finally, it must induce luminal or systemic effects that are beneficial to host health [18]. In theory, any carbohydrate that enters the colon can potentially be considered prebiotic. However, while many naturally occurring carbohydrates from sources such as fruits and vegetables (*i.e.*, chicory, artichoke, garlic, bananas) and milk have been investigated both *in vitro* and *in vivo* [19]; evidence that the compound satisfies the prebiotic criteria outlined above must ultimately be obtained in well-controlled human/animal studies. To date, only three carbohydrates types are accepted as true prebiotics; inulin and oligofructose, galactooligosaccharides and lactulose [20]. Many polysaccharides from various sources have displayed prebiotic activity both *in vitro* and *in vivo*. As seaweeds are rich in polysaccharides, they are an obvious choice for investigation as a source of prebiotics.

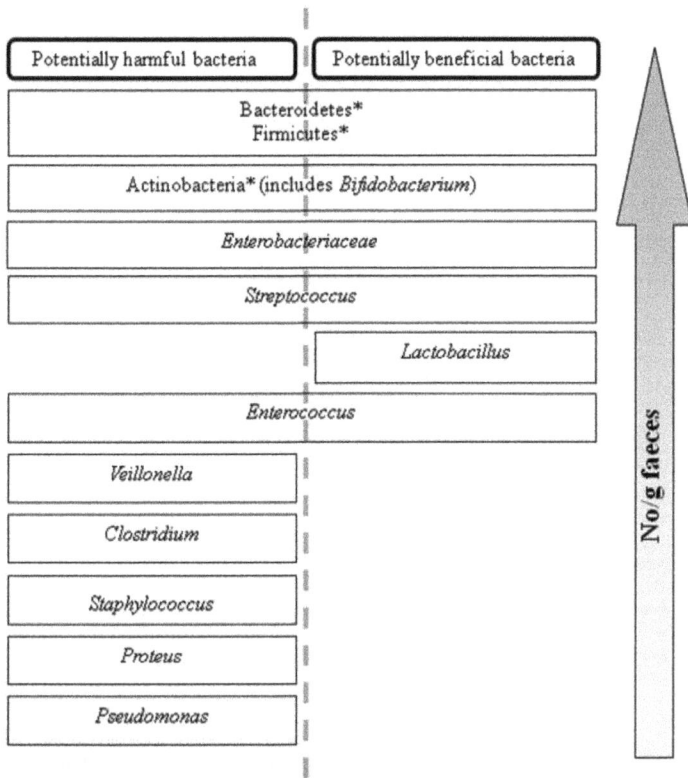

Figure 1. Distribution of the dominant, sub-dominant and minor components of human fecal microflora. Major dominant phyla are denoted. *: Other components are at the family or genus level (adapted from reference [16]).

Applications of prebiotics

There are numerous purported health benefits attributed to the consumption of prebiotics by both humans and animals (Figure 2). The most notable and direct effects of prebiotics *in vivo* are mediated via modulation of intestinal microbiota (Figure 2) populations. A number of health effects in humans can be attributed to modulation of gut microflora and these have been extensively studied and reviewed [21,26]. Prebiotics can be consumed as dietary supplements or in functional foods. A functional food is defined as a food which provides a health benefit beyond basic nutrition [27]. At present, there are a number of functional foods on the market which contain prebiotic compounds; for example, infant formula, soy milk, breakfast cereals and yogurts [28].

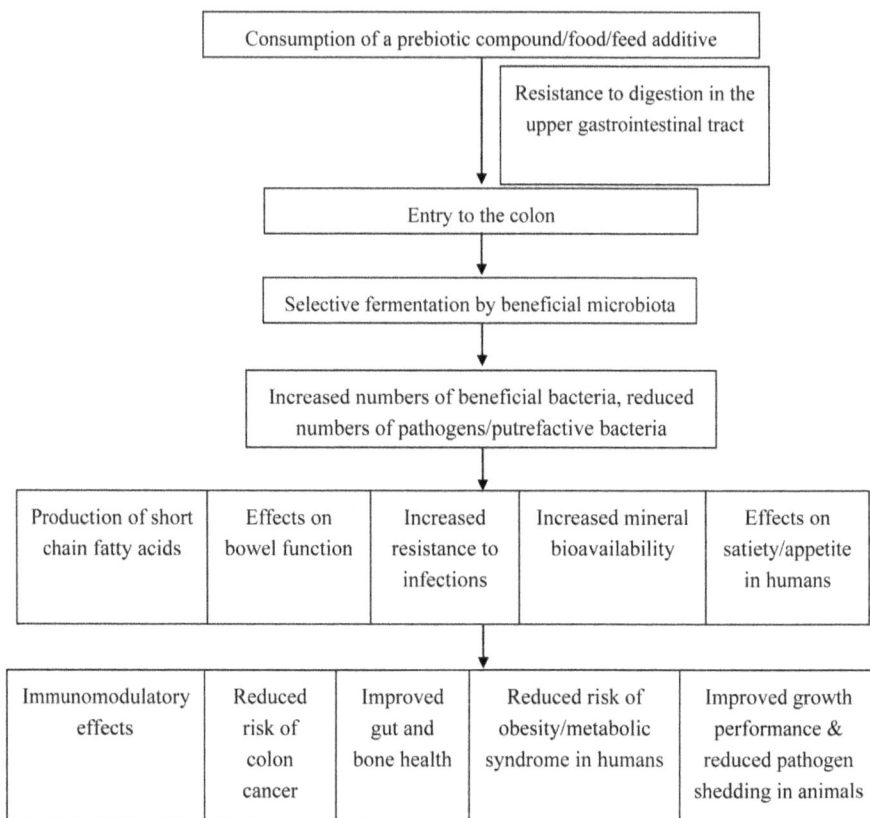

Figure 2. Mode of action of prebiotics and purported health benefits in humans and animals.

Prebiotic compounds may also be added to animal feed, as an alternative to antibiotics. Sub-therapeutic doses of antibiotics were used in-feed in Europe and continue to be used in the US as a management tool to promote growth and maintain health in farm animals, in particular pigs and poultry. However, due to concerns over increasing bacterial antibiotic resistance, in-feed antibiotics are no longer permitted for use as growth promoters in the EU since 2006. Consequences, including increased enteric infections, reduced pig performance and increased mortality have been seen in Nordic countries where the antibiotic ban has been in place since the late 1990s [29]. Therefore, one of the challenges facing the livestock industry is maintaining the growth performance targets required for Consumption of a prebiotic compound/food/feed additive Resistance to digestion in the upper gastrointestinal tract Entry to the colon Selective fermentation by beneficial microbiota Increased numbers of beneficial bacteria, reduced numbers of pathogens/putrefactive bacteria Production of short chain fatty acids Effects on bowel function Increased resistance to infections Effects on satiety/appetite in humans Increased mineral bioavailability Immunomodulatory effects Reduced risk of colon cancer Improved gut and bone health Reduced risk of obesity/metabolic syndrome in humans Improved growth performance & reduced pathogen shedding in animals cost-effective animal production without the use of antibiotic growth promoters. Although the exact mode of action of antibiotic growth promoters is unknown, they most likely act via modulation of intestinal microbial populations, including reduction of pathogenic microorganisms. Prebiotic compounds therefore offer potential as an alternative to in-feed antibiotic growth promoters [30]. Apart from improving animal performance and health, prebiotics may also reduce carriage of enteric pathogens, thereby preventing transmission to humans (Figure 2) [30].

Dietary prebiotics sourced from seaweeds may provide a means to modulate the intestinal microbiota thereby improving the overall health of animals and humans. In particular, seaweeds contain a high concentration of polysaccharides of varying structure and functionality which could potentially be exploited as prebiotics.

3. Chemistry of Seaweed Polysaccharides

The chemical structures of seaweed polysaccharides have been described extensively [31,35]. Contained primarily in the cell walls, key functions of these relatively high molecular weight polysaccharides include, acting as a food reserve, provision of strength and flexibility to withstand wave action, maintenance of ionic equilibrium in the cell and prevention of cell desiccation. The composition varies according to season, age, species, and geographic location [36]. They are found with a wide variety of chemical structures, but some general characteristics have been identified [34]. They are rich in hydroxyl (-OH) groups, making them hydrophilic and often water soluble, and are known to establish intra-chain H-bond networks, making them stiff and rigid and suitable as thickeners. The regularity of their structures also promotes interaction with external ions and inter-chain H-bonding (e.g., gelation). Key polysaccharides found in chlorophyta, phaeophyta and rhodophyta are described in the following sections.

3.1. Polysaccharides from chlorophyta

Complex sulfated hetero-polysaccharides

The cell wall matrix of chlorophyta contains highly complex sulfated hetero-polysaccharides [37]. The extracted polysaccharides from *Ulva* spp. (12% of the algal dry weight) have been reported to contain 16% sulfate and 15–19% uronic acids [38,39]. Each molecule of these heteropolysaccharides is made up of several different residues, with the major sugars being glucuronic acid, rhamnose, arabinose and galactose, in a variety of combinations [31]. Figure 3 shows the structures of rhamnose and glucuronic acid, two of the constituent sugars of green seaweed polysaccharides.

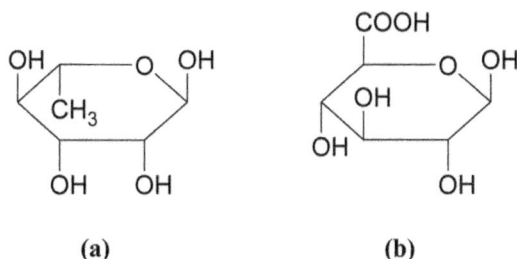

(a)   **(b)**

Figure 3. Green seaweed constituents: **(a)** α-L-rhamnose and **(b)** glucuronic acid [31].

The polysaccharide ulvan is easily extracted from *Ulva rigida* [40,41]. It is composed of β-(1,4)-xyloglucan, glucuronan and cellulose in a linear arrangement [31,41]. It corresponds to a water-soluble dietary fiber and is resistant to both human digestive tract enzymes and degradation by colonic bacteria. This polysaccharide cannot therefore be considered prebiotic; however, it could potentially be hydrolysed to bioactive oligosaccharides [42].

3.2. Polysaccharides from phaeophyta

3.2.1. Alginates (also called alginic acid or algin)

Alginic acid is an anionic polysaccharide that occurs in all brown algae. It is the most abundant cell wall polysaccharide in brown algae [43]. For example, the alginate content of a number of seaweeds, based on dry weight, is as follows: *Ascophylum nodosum*, 22–30%; *Laminaria digitata* fronds, 25–44%; *L. digitata* stipes, 35–47%; *L. hyperborea* fronds, 17–33%; *L. hyperborea* stipes, 25–38% [34]. Alginate contents of between 17 and 45% have been reported in *Sargassum* spp. [44,45]. The industrial process for the extraction of alginates from brown seaweeds is as follows [35]:

- The seaweed is washed, macerated, extracted with sodium carbonate and filtered
- Sodium/calcium chloride is added to the filtrate and a fibrous precipitate of sodium/calcium alginate is formed
- The alginate salt is transformed to alginic acid by treatment with hydrochloric acid
- The alginate is purified, dried and powdered

Alginic acid is a linear polysaccharide containing 1,4-linked β-D-mannuronic acid (M) and α-L-guluronic acid (G) residues, arranged in a non-regular block-wise order along the chain [46]. The residues typically occur as $(-M-)_n$, $(-G-)_n$ and $(-MG-)_n$ sequences or blocks [43]. The carboxylic acid dissociation constants have been determined as $pK_a = 3.38$ and $pK_a = 3.65$ for M and G, respectively, with similar values obtained for the polymers [47]. Figure 4 illustrates the structure of β-D-mannuronic acid and α-L-guluronic acid.

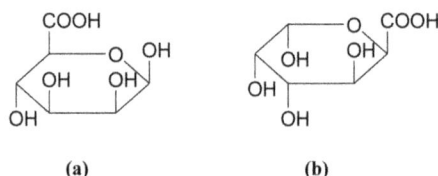

Figure 4. Constituent acids of alginic acid, where **(a)** is β-D-mannuronic acid and **(b)** is α-L-guluronic acid [43].

Mannuronic and guluronic acids are classed as uronic acids. The uronic acids are simple monosaccharides in which the primary hydroxyl group at C_6 has been oxidized to the corresponding carboxylic acid. Their names retain the root of the monosaccharides, but the *-ose* sugar suffix is changed to *-uronic acid*. For example, galacturonic acid has the same configuration as galactose, and the structure of glucuronic acid corresponds to that of glucose. Uronic acids are present in all three algal divisions [31].

3.2.2. Fucans/Fucoidans

Fucoidans are a complex series of sulfated polysaccharides found both intercellularly and in the cell wall of brown algae, with molecular weights typically of the magnitude 1,000,000. They play a role in cell organization and may be involved in the cross-linkage of alginate and cellulose [34]. Fucoidan is a water-soluble branched matrix polysaccharide sulfate ester, with L-fucose building blocks as the major component with predominantly α-(1,2) linkages [48]. Brown algae contain 5–20% fucoidan [44], about 40% of which is sulfate esters. The basic structure of fucoidan is shown in Figure 5.

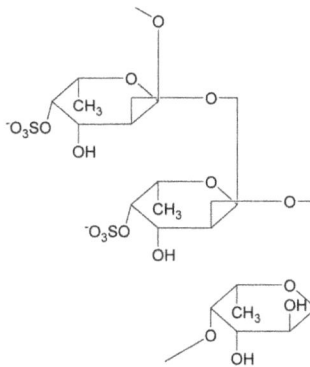

Figure 5. Fucoidan: Branched polysaccharide sulfate ester with L-fucose building blocks as the major component with predominantly α-(1,2) linkages [43].

Fucoidans are reported to display physiological and biological activities, including anticoagulant, antithrombotic, antiviral, antitumor, immunomodulatory, antioxidant, and anti-inflammatory [49], with therapeutic potential increasing with the degree of sulfation [34]. In addition, they protect gastric mucosa against the proteolytic activity of gastric juice. Furthermore, studies have demonstrated that fucoidan may prevent *Helicobacter pylori* infection in the stomach, thereby reducing the risk of associated gastric cancers [50].

3.2.3. Laminarin

Laminarin is a relatively low molecular weight storage polysaccharide found commonly in brown algae. It may constitute up to 35% of the dried weight of the seaweed [34]. A member of the 1–3-β-D-glucan family, laminarin, consists of a linear structure with a small degree of side branching [51]. It is composed of (1,3)-β-D-glucopyranose residues, in which some 6-O-branching in the main chain and some β-(1,6) intrachain links are present (Figure 6 and Table 1) [52]. Laminarins from different algal species may vary in structural features; for example the degree of branching, the degree of polymerization (up to 50 carbohydrate residues, commonly about 25), and the ratio of (1,3)- and (1,6)-glycosidic bonds [52]. Most laminarins form complex structures that are stabilized by inter-chain hydrogen bonds and are therefore resistant to hydrolysis in the upper GIT and are considered as dietary fibers [53].

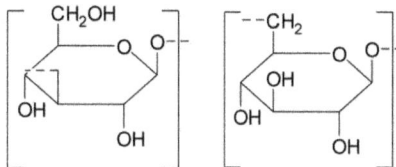

Figure 6. Basic chemical units of laminarin, made up of β-(1,3) and β-(1,6) linked glucose.

Table 1. Chemical structure of laminarins from various seaweeds [34].

Seaweed	Structure of Laminarin
Several species of *Laminaria*	Linear β-(1,3) linked D-glucose
Laminaria digitata	Linear backbone of β-(1,3) linked D-glucose, with β-(1,6) linked side chains
Eisenia bicyclis	Linear chain of (1–3) and (1–6) links, in the ratio of 2:1

Laminarin has been identified as a modulator of intestinal metabolism through its effects on mucus composition, intestinal pH and short chain fatty acid (SCFA) production, especially butyrate [54,55] (see Section 4.3).

3.3. Polysaccharides from rhodophyta

Most red algal polysaccharides are galactans in which α-(1,3) and β-(1,4) links alternate [31]. Variety in the polysaccharides comes from sulfation, pyruvation and methylation of some of the hydroxyl groups and from the formation of an anhydride bridge between C_3 and C_6.

3.3.1. Agar

Agars, the gel-forming polysaccharides extracted from certain families of rhodophyta, mainly Gracilariaceae and Gelidiaceae [56], are linear polymers with a sugar skeleton consisting of alternating 3-linked β-D-galactopyranosl and 4-linked 3,6-anhydro-α-L-galactopyranosyl units [57]. The basic structure of the constituent galactose residues is shown in Figure 7. Agar may be fractionated into two components [58]:

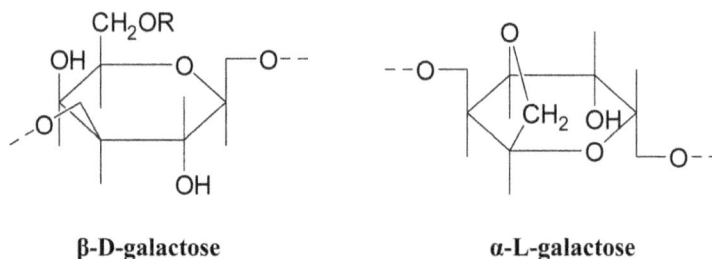

β-D-galactose   α-L-galactose

Figure 7. Agar constituents [31] (R=H or CH$_3$).

- Agarose (the gelling fraction)—A neutral linear molecule, free of sulfates
- Agaropectin (the non-gelling fraction)—Contains all the charged polysaccharide components, with some galactose residues substituted with pyruvic acid ketal, 4,6-O-(1-carboxyethylidene)D-galactopyranose, or methylated or sulfated sugar units [58]. Agaropectin is a slightly branched heterogeneous mixture of smaller molecules.

The ratio of the two fractions varies according to seaweed species and environmental conditions, and will affect the physiochemical, mechanical and rheological properties of agar. The molecular weight of agarose is about 120,000. Due to the substitutions in agaropectin, the molecular weight of agar is typically higher (up to 250,000), with a wide distribution [58].

Agarose is widely used as a gelling agent in microbiological media and for biotechnological applications [34]. Hu *et al.* [59] found that neoagaro-oligosaccharides (NAOS), obtained from the enzymatic hydrolysis of agarose, demonstrated prebiotic activity which was dependant on the degree of polymerization (see Section 4.2).

3.3.2. Carrageenans (sulfated polysaccharides)

In carrageenans, β-D-galactose alternates with α-D-galactose, not α-L-galactose as in agars. The degree of sulfation in carrageenans is generally much greater than that in agars. Based on physical properties, carrageenans are commonly classified into three types; kappa (strong rigid gels), iota (soft elastic gels) and lambda (thickening polymer) [34]. The basic structures of the three classes are shown in Figure 8.

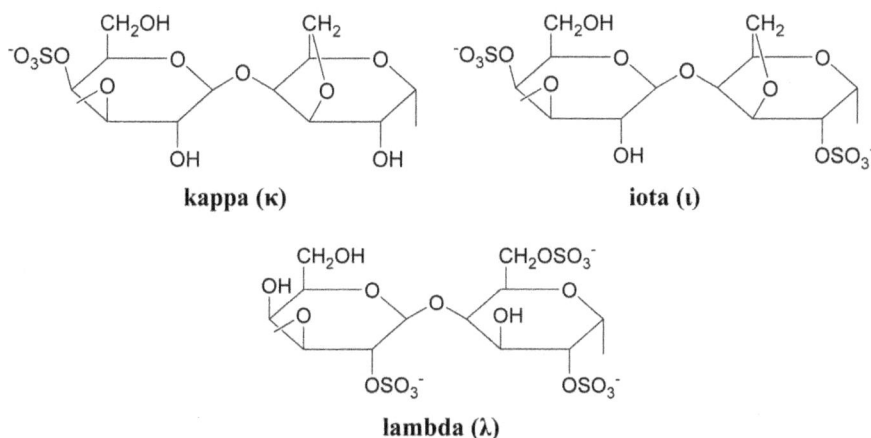

Figure 8. Basic structure of kappa-, iota-, and lambda-carrageenan [60].

Carrageenans are used in a wide variety of applications; for example, as thickening, stabilizing and encapsulation agents. It has been reported that degraded carrageenans may cause ulcerations in the GIT and gastrointestinal cancer [34].

3.3.3. Other polysaccharides and polysaccharide derivatives

The presence of uronic acids in red seaweed polysaccharides has been reported. For example, a neutral xylan and a xylogalactan, with 4.8% uronic acids, were obtained from *Palmaria decipiens* [32]. Errea *et al.* [61] reported unusual structures in polysaccharides from the red seaweed *Pterocladiella capillacea*. Structural analysis indicated the presence of xylogalactans, with a low content of 3,6-anhydrogalactose and low molecular weight. The polysaccharides varied in the degree of xylopranosyl and sulfate substitution. The presence of 3-substituted, 4-linked D-galactopyranosyl residues was also reported.

A number of potentially useful sulfated polysaccharides from lesser-known red seaweed species have been reported [34]:

- Hypneans are extracted from the *Hypnea* spp. Structurally, hypneans are similar to agar and carrageenan, but with a higher percentage of 3,6-anhydrogalactose. They are primarily used as gelling agents in food applications and as fertilizers in dry arid soils.
- Porphyran is a highly substituted polysaccharide extracted from the *Porphyra* genus. It is used as a gelling agent, a nutritional supplement (e.g., to help cope with stress) and an antioxidant.
- Funorans, extracted from species such as *Gloiopeltis complanata*, are composed of a heterogeneous series of polysaccharides and sulfated galactans. Funoran has been shown to inhibit the adherence and colonization of oral bacteria, reducing dental caries in rat studies [62]. It is also reported to reduce blood pressure, lower cholesterol and exhibit anti-tumor properties.

Oligosaccharides are commonly defined as carbohydrate molecules with a low degree of polymerization (between 2 and 25) [19]. These molecules may be found naturally or derived from larger polysaccharides. Examples of depolymerization methods for algal polysaccharides include; free radical depolymerization for fucoidan, thermal degradation and enzymatic hydrolysis for alginate and chemical degradation for ulvan. While numerous studies have reported prebiotic activity for plant-derived oligosaccharides [19], few studies have specifically examined the effects of algal-derived oligosaccharides (see Section 5.1).

4. *In Vitro* Studies Examining the Prebiotic Potential of Seaweed Polysaccharides and Oligosaccharide Derivatives

While prebiotic activity must ultimately be determined *in vivo, in vitro* studies are useful for preliminary screening of candidate compounds and can generate information on functional mechanisms. The three main criteria that are tested *in vitro* are; non-digestibility, fermentability and selectivity [20]. Studies that have evaluated seaweeds and/or seaweed polysaccharides *in vitro* will be reviewed here.

4.1. Resistance to digestive enzymes

As discussed in Section 2, a prebiotic compound must be resistant to digestion in the upper GIT so that it can reach the lower intestine intact [18]. This can be investigated *in vitro* by testing resistance to acidic and enzymatic hydrolysis. Hu *et al.* [59] showed that agarose-derived NAOS were resistant to amylolytic enzymes by demonstrating via electrophoretic analysis that the compounds remained intact after 24 h incubation with an enzyme mixture. Similarly, glycerol galactoside, determined to be the fermentable component of the red alga *Porphyra yezoensis*, was not digested by salivary, gastric, pancreatic or intestinal enzymes [63]. Neither was it absorbed across excised segments of rat small intestine. A study by Deville *et al.* [55] showed that laminarin remained intact following incubation *in vitro* with HCl, human saliva and human gastric, pancreatic, small intestinal and colonic homogenates.

4.2. Selective fermentation by pure cultures

One of the criteria that a compound must meet in order to be classified as a prebiotic is "fermentation by intestinal microbiota" [18]. Compounds should be selectively fermented, *i.e.,* fermentable by beneficial species but not pathogens (Figure 1). This can be determined *in vitro* by incubating pure cultures of representative beneficial bacteria (usually *Lactobacillus* and *Bifidobacterium* spp.) as well as potentially pathogenic species (e.g., *E. coli, Enterococcus*) with the compound and investigating bacterial growth [18]. The usual procedure is to inoculate a range of bacterial strains into a microbiological medium in which the carbon source has been replaced by the test compound and measure growth in comparison to a glucose control. While many studies have evaluated potential prebiotics in this way [16], few have evaluated seaweed-derived compounds. However, studies conducted more than three decades ago showed that laminarin and alginate could be degraded by human colonic bacteria [64,65]. Hu *et al.* [59] showed that NAOS obtained from agarose were fermented by *Lactobacillus* and *Bifidobacterium* but not *E. coli* or *Enterococcus*. Increased growth rates, as determined by plate counts and pH decrease, were observed in comparison to fructo-oligosaccharides (FOS) but glucose was not included as a control. Nori, a dried form of the red seaweed *Porphyra yezoensis,* was fermented by all but one of five intestinal *Bifidobacterium* strains, but only when it had a high protein content [63]. In a subsequent experiment with 17 bacterial strains, glycerol galactoside, which was determined to be the fermentable component, was comparable with glucose as a substrate for *Bifidobacterium*. It was also fermented by *Bacteroides, Clostridium* and *E. coli,* albeit not as well as glucose but failed to stimulate the growth of *Enterococcus, Eubacterium* or *Lactobacillus* spp.

These results, while useful, should be interpreted with caution, as the test strains and conditions used may not be representative of those found within the intestinal tract. Therefore, these types of assays are recommended only as a screening tool in preliminary investigations [18].

4.3. Fermenter studies to determine effects on intestinal microbiota

A more meaningful way to assay potential prebiotic compounds is to test them in anaerobic fermenter systems inoculated with fecal/intestinal material [66]. This not only tests the ability of the intestinal microflora to ferment the compound but also evaluates stimulatory effects on microbial growth and/or activity. Effects on microbial growth can be monitored by culturing fermenter samples on selective media; however, culture-independent approaches employing molecular methods such as fluorescece *in situ* hybridization (FISH), polymerase chain reaction (PCR), denaturing gradient gel electrophoresis (DGGE) and 16S rRNA gene sequencing provide a more complete representation of microbial diversity [18]. Microbial activity is usually evaluated by measuring metabolic end products, such as SCFA and gases.

Total algal fibers extracted from whole *Himanthalia elongata*, *L. digitata* and *Undaria pinnatifida* were fermented by human fecal microflora after 24 h in a batch system, as determined by substrate disappearance, but were not completely metabolized to SCFA compared with sugarbeet fiber [67]. In a subsequent experiment, purified laminarins were highly fermented after an initial lag period (explained by the time required for induction of bacterial enzymes), alginates were fermented but not completely degraded to SCFA and fucans were not fermented at all. However, effects on microbial counts were not evaluated, so no conclusions on prebiotic activity can be made.

Deville *et al.* [54] showed that laminarin (either extracted from *L. saccharina* or *L. digitata*) was almost completely fermented in a human fecal batch fermenter system after an initial lag period, as measured by its disappearance over 48 h. Turbidity increases and pH decreases (both indicative of bacterial growth) were comparable in vessels containing laminarin, FOS or glucose after 24–48 h. Total SCFA concentrations were higher for *L. digitata* laminarin in comparison to glucose with higher amounts of propionate and butyrate observed. SCFA were, however, not measured for the *L. saccharina*-derived laminarin or FOS treatments. Furthermore, while FOS increased culturable *Lactobacillus* and decreased *Bacteroides*, laminarin had no effects on bacterial counts. Although PCR was used to confirm counts, no culture-independent analyses were performed. Similarly, SCFA concentrations increased in a human fecal batch culture on addition of laminarin or alginate compared to a control [68]. Reduced concentrations of potentially harmful microbial end products (ammonia, indole compounds, phenol compounds) were also observed. Taken together, this data was interpreted as an indication of fermentation of the seaweed polysaccharides by intestinal bacteria but, as is the case in many studies, no microbiological analyses were performed. However, Dierick *et al.* [69] demonstrated that dried whole *Ascophyllum nodosum* decreased potential pathogens (*E. coli*, streptococci) and total anaerobes in batch systems inoculated with either porcine small intestinal or cecal suspensions. This inhibitory activity may have been due to the reduction in pH, as the pH was not controlled during fermentation. However, a decrease in beneficial bacteria (*i.e.*, *Lactobacillus*) was also observed. The authors concluded that this intact brown seaweed is not a suitable fermentation substrate, however, further experiments were not conducted to evaluate this and only culturable microflora was investigated. Furthermore, the control vessel contained a synthetic diet which would have supplied all of the nutrients necessary for microbial growth, while the experimental vessels contained seaweed only. In practice, diets would be supplemented with *A. nodosum*, rather than consisting entirely of seaweed.

Michel *et al.* [70] evaluated alginate- and laminarin-derived oligosaccharides in continuous as well as batch human fecal fermentations compared with FOS. While total concentrations of SFCA did not differ between treatments, propionate production was increased by all of the test compounds relative to FOS. These and additional data reported in the study indicated that the oligosaccharides tested were fermented by the fecal microflora [70]. However, oligosaccharides from either source did not alter counts of *Bacteroides*, *Lactobacillus*, total anaerobes or aerobes and, in fact, *Bifidobacterium* counts were reduced ~1000-fold. The latter is in keeping with the reductions in *Lactobacillus* observed by Dierick *et al.* [69].

The most promising evidence of prebiotic activity of algal polysaccharides comes from a recent study that evaluated the effects of a dietary supplement containing a mixture of plant polysaccharides including *Undaria pinnatifida* fucoidans on human fecal microflora in a three-vessel colon model [71]. No control vessels were used; instead there was a control period before supplement addition and a washout period after. The product tested was predominantly fermented in the distal colon vessel. Although no effects on total SCFA were observed before, during or after supplement addition, lactate and butyrate were decreased in the ascending and descending colon vessels, respectively during the treatment period. Although some increases in individual SCFA were observed during the washout period (most notably butyrate in the distal colon), a concomitant increase in ammonium, a potentially toxic metabolite, was observed in the descending colon during treatment. It is encouraging to note that increases in *Bifidobacterium* were seen, both via plate counts and quantitative PCR (qPCR). Furthermore, DGGE revealed compositional changes within bifidobacterial populations. Cultivable *Lactobacillus* were increased but qPCR failed to show such an effect, although it did reveal increases in the *Bacteroides-Prevotella* group. Taken together, these data demonstrate that the product tested appears promising as a prebiotic; however, as it was a mixture of plant-derived polysaccharides, no conclusions can be made regarding prebiotic activity of the seaweed fucoidan component.

Overall, a number of studies mainly conducted in batch fermentation systems have demonstrated that seaweed polysaccharides are fermented by the intestinal microflora but few demonstrate selective stimulation of beneficial intestinal microbial populations. Additional studies in multi-chamber continuous culture systems are needed, as these replicate different gastrointestinal regions more closely. Even these systems suffer limitations, as an increase in a limited number of bacterial genera within a complex mixture is not definitive proof of a prebiotic effect. Further studies utilizing detailed molecular methods, such as metagenomics, are required in order to fully elucidate the impact of algal polysaccharides on the entire intestinal microbiome.

5. *In Vivo* Studies Examining the Prebiotic Potential of Macroalgal Polysaccharides and Oligosaccharide Derivatives

In vitro studies give an indication of the prebiotic potential of algal polysaccharides. However, *in vivo* studies are necessary to demonstrate prebiotic activity before worthwhile conclusions may be drawn. While there is substantial evidence in the literature to suggest that certain polysaccharides such as inulin and FOS have modulatory effects on the gut microflora in humans, to date no human trials have been conducted on polysaccharides from seaweeds. Studies have, however, been conducted in laboratory animals to determine prebiotic properties of seaweed polysaccharides with a view to establishing suitability for applications in other animals and humans. Feeding trials have also been performed in farm animals to investigate effects on animal health and growth performance.

5.1. Studies in laboratory animals

Wang *et al.* [72] demonstrated that rats fed test diets supplemented with 2.5% alginate oligosaccharides displayed a selective increase in the numbers of *Bifidobacterium* and *Lactobacillus* in both the cecum and feces. The prebiotic effect was greater than that observed in the control group which was fed a diet containing FOS, a well-established prebiotic. A study conducted by Hu *et al.* [59] demonstrated similar increases in fecal *Lactobacillus* and *Bifidobacterium* populations after feeding mice diets supplemented with either 2.5% or 5% agarose hydrolysate (NAOS) compared with a control diet or a diet containing FOS. The authors also demonstrated that the NAOS-fed group had increased *Lactobacillus* counts in the cecum seven days post-administration compared to the control group; however, cecal *Lactobacillus* counts in the test group were similar to those in the group fed FOS. In addition, the NAOS-fed group had lower numbers of *Bacteroides* compared to the control group.

Overall, the NAOS-fed groups demonstrated large increases in populations of beneficial bacteria, with no adverse effects on animal health, suggesting that NAOS could be a potential algal prebiotic. Kuda *et al.* [68] reported that dietary supplementation with 1% laminarin resulted in an increase in *Bifidobacterium* counts in the cecum of rats compared to a control diet, but there was no significant difference in *Lactobacillus* counts. In the same study, laminarin was shown to suppress indole, cresol and sulfide, which are putrefactive compounds considered risk markers for colon cancer. Further evidence that laminarin is fermented by the intestinal microbiota was found in a study which showed that laminarin was not detected in the feces of rats fed laminarin [55]. A study by Gudiel-Urbano and Goni [73] demonstrated that rats fed *Undaria pinnatifida* and *Porphyra ternera* extracts had lower bacterial enzyme activity in the cecum. This provides additional indirect evidence of the effects of seaweed extracts on the intestinal microflora. Furthermore, the enzymatic activities that were reduced are implicated in the conversion of procarcinogens to carcinogens, suggesting a possible link between seaweed extract intake and reduced risk of colon cancer (also implied from data generated by Kuda *et al.* [68], as outlined above). Neyrinck *et al.* [53] demonstrated that dietary supplementation with laminarin also has systemic effects, as it protected against lipopolysaccharide-induced liver toxicity in a rodent model of systemic inflammation. Dietary laminarin had immunomodulatory effects, which the authors suggest are due either to a direct effect of laminarin on immune cells or to an indirect effect via modulation of the intestinal microbiota. However, intestinal microbial populations were not measured so no conclusions can be made regarding the latter. Overall, from the studies conducted to date, it is evident that seaweed polysaccharides and oligosaccharide derivatives demonstrate prebiotic effects in rodents.

5.2. Studies in farm animals

Prebiotics have a role to play in animal health; they are assumed to stimulate the growth of beneficial bacteria, thereby improving intestinal health and stimulating growth performance, particularly following weaning. The post-weaning period in pigs is stressful due to factors such as separation from the sow and littermates, digestive disruption as a result of the sudden shift from milk to a cereal-based diet and exposure to a new environment [74]. These stressors can cause a microbial imbalance in the gut, leading to undesirable effects such as reduced feed intake, a consequential reduction in growth rate and increased susceptibility to post-weaning diarrhea and pathogenic infections [75]. Modulation of the gut microbiota by prebiotics may prove to be a useful strategy in promoting growth and may alleviate some of the undesirable effects observed in weanling pigs. Many studies have evaluated the effects of seaweed extracts and seaweed polysaccharides, such as laminarin in feeding experiments, mainly in pigs but also in lambs and cattle. Such experiments have been conducted as seaweed extracts and seaweed polysaccharides are considered good prebiotic candidates as they are resistant to digestion in the small intestine and are fermented by colonic microbiota, as outlined in section 4 [54,55]. However, the differences in digestive physiology and anatomy must be borne in mind when attempting to extrapolate data from ruminants (cattle and sheep) to pigs, which are monogastric. Effects on parameters, such as growth performance, nutrient digestibility, volatile fatty acids and intestinal microbiota have been studied in detail, particularly in relation to swine health and nutrition and will be reviewed below. Only statistically significant results (cut-off of $P < 0.05$) are discussed.

5.2.1. Effects of marine polysaccharides on growth performance

Reilly *et al.* [76] found that dietary inclusion of seaweed extracts containing both laminarin and fucoidan had no effect on feed intake, weight gain, feed conversion ratio or nutrient digestibility in weanling pigs (Table 2). A lack of improvement in weight gain, feed intake and feed efficiency has also been reported in finishing lambs fed diets supplemented with Tasco 14™ (sun-dried whole *A. nodosum*) [77]. Furthermore, Gardiner *et al.* [78] found no effects on feed intake or feed conversion ratio but reported a decrease in weight gain when an *A. nodosum* extract was fed to grower-finisher pigs (Table 2). The authors suggested that the presence of anti-nutritional phyto-chemicals and a high level of chelated metals in the crude seaweed extract may have been responsible for the decreased growth performance. As a consequence, Gahan *et al.* [79] supplemented diets with a more refined seaweed extract containing only laminarin and fucoidan with a view to replacing lactose in the diet of weaned pigs. The authors extract increased feed intake and weight gain and improved feed conversion ratio in a manner similar to lactose (Table 2).

High health status of animals is often cited as a reason for lack of effects on growth performance. For this reason, McDonnell *et al.* [80] fed pigs a nutritionally challenged diet supplemented with laminarin and found increased weight gain and increased gain to feed ratio (equivalent to reduced feed conversion ratio). However, fucoidan had no effect on pig growth or daily feed intake. A more recent study conducted by O'Doherty *et al.* [81] reported that dietary inclusion of a laminarin-fucoidan extract increased average daily weight and gain to feed ratio in pigs fed diets formulated to create a nutritional challenge, similar to those fed by McDonnell *et al.* [80] (Table 2). Similarly, Turner *et al.* [82] observed a positive linear effect on feed intake and a quadratic effect on weight in young pigs challenged with *Salmonella* and fed an *A. nodosum* extract.

Table 2. Effects of algal prebiotics on pig health.

Algal supplement	Age and heath status of pigs	Dose	Effect on gut microbiota	Effect on growth performance and health	Ref
A. nodosum extract (ANE)	Healthy grower-finisher pigs	0, 3, 6 or 9 g/kg basal feed	Animals supplemented with 6 or 9 g ANE/kg had lower (P < 0.05) ileal coliform counts than animals that received 3 g/kg. Linear reduction (P < 0.05) in coliform counts in the ileal contents as ANE increased. Reduction (P < 0.05) in cecal Bifidobacterium counts with increasing ANE supplementation	Linear decrease (P < 0.05) in weight gain with increasing levels of extract	[78]
A. nodosum meal (ANM)	Healthy, weanling piglets	10 or 20 g/kg basal feed	Reduced (P < 0.05)E. coli in the small intestine and increased (P < 0.05) Lactobacillus/E. coli ratio in animals fed 10 g/kg	No effects on final weight. No effects on intestinal histology or intestinal immune cells	[69]
Laminaria spp. extract containing a combination of laminarin & fucoidan (ranging from 0.112–0.446 and 0.890–0.356 g/kg, respectively)	Healthy, weanling piglets	0, 1, 2, 4 g/kg basal feed containing increasing levels of lactose (60–250 g/kg)	Effects on gut microbiota were not determined	Weight gain and feed intake increased (P < 0.05) as the level of seaweed extract increased; however, this was only observed when fed in combination with low and medium levels of lactose	[79]
Laminaria spp. extract containing either laminarin or fucoidan or a combination of both (0.3 and 0.24 g/kg, respectively)	Healthy, weanling piglets fed a nutritionally-challenged diet (high protein, low lactose)	Basal feed + 0.3 g/kg laminarin; basal feed + 0.24 g/kg fucoidan; basal feed + 0.3 g/kg laminarin and 0.24 g/kg fucoidan	Laminarin supplementation resulted in lower (P < 0.05) fecal E. coli populations compared to control group. Interaction (P < 0.01) between laminarin and fucoidan with respect to fecal lactobacilli populations	Laminarin supplementation resulted in increased (P < 0.01) daily weight gain. Pigs offered combination of laminarin and fucoidan had reduced (P < 0.05) diarrhoea	[80]
Alginate	Healthy, weanling piglets	1 g/kg starter feed	Higher enterococci counts in distal small intestine, cecum and proximal colon (P < 0.001) compared with inulin or control group. Reduced (P < 0.05) lactobacilli in all intestinal segments but only after 6 days of alginate supplementation, and not before or thereafter. Increased microbial diversity	Animals were in good health throughout the study	[84]
Exp 1: L. hyperborea extract (112 g/kg laminarin & 89 g/kg fucoidan). Exp 2: Purified laminarin (0.30 g/kg), fucoidan (0.24 g/kg) and a combination of both laminarin and fucoidan (0.30 and 0.24 g/kg, respectively)	Healthy finishing boars	Exp 1:0.7, 1.4, 2.8, 5.6 g/kg extract. Exp 2: Basal diet + 0.30 g/kg laminarin; basal diet + 0.24 g/kg fucoidan; basal diet + 0.30 g/kg laminarin and 0.24 g/kg fucoidan	Exp 1: Quadratic response (P < 0.05) to seaweed extract on cecal (P < 0.05) Enterobacterium spp., colonic (P < 0.05) Enterobacterium spp. and (P < 0.001) Bifidobacterium spp. Linear decrease in cecal Bifidobacterium spp and colonic Lactobacillus spp. with increasing seaweed extract (P < 0.01, P < 0.05, respectively). Exp 2: Fucoidan diet resulted in increases in colonic Lactobacillus spp. Combination diet resulted in increase in Enterobacterium spp. (P < 0.05).	Growth performance was not evaluated	[83]
L. hyperborea extract (LHE), containing laminarin and fucoidan (0.17 and 0.13 g/kg, respectively). L. digitata extract (LDE), containing laminarin and fucoidan (0.17 and 0.14 g/kg, respectively). Combination of LHE and LDE containing laminarin and fucoidan (0.17 and 0.13 g/kg, respectively)	Healthy, weanling piglets	Basal feed + 1.5 g/kg LHE. Basal feed + 1.5 g/kg LDE. Basal feed + 1.5 g/kg LHE & LDE	Animals offered LHE diet had lower (P < 0.05) numbers of colonic Bifidobacterium and lower populations of cecal and colonic (P < 0.05, P < 0.001, respectively) lactobacilli compared to control diet. Supplementation with LDE resulted in lower populations of cecal and colonic (P < 0.05) Enterobacterium, cecal (P < 0.05) Bifidobacterium and cecal and colonic (P < 0.05, P < 0.001, respectively) Lactobacillus compared to control diet. Animals offered combination diet had lower (P < 0.05) populations of colonic and cecal Enterobacterium and Lactobacillus (P < 0.01) compared to control diet	No effects on animal performance Marginal differences in systemic immune response reported in animals fed combination diet	[76]
L. digitata extract containing laminarin (0.11 g/kg), and fucoidan (0.89 g/kg)	Healthy, weanling piglets fed a nutritionally-challenged diet	Diet 1: 150g lactose (L)/kg. Diet 2: 150 g/kg lactose + 2.8 g/kg seaweed extract (SE). Diet 3: 250g lactose/kg. Diet 4: 250g lactose/kg + 2.8 g/kg SE	The inclusion of SE decreased (P < 0.05) fecal E. coli counts compared to non-SWE diets. Dietary inclusion of SE increased (P < 0.001) Lactobacillus counts in pigs fed high L diets	Animals offered seaweed diets had higher (P < 0.01) average daily gain and gain to feed ratio (P < 0.05) Fecal score not affected by dietary inclusion of SE	[81]

Overall, the evidence examining the effect of seaweed extracts on growth performance in farm animals is equivocal, a trend which is also observed in studies examining the effects of established prebiotics in animals [30]. Reasons for the differences in responses observed between studies may be due to factors such as, differences in dietary inclusion levels, variations in the types and purity of seaweed extracts evaluated and differences in the species, age and health status of animals used (Table 2). Additional studies examining the effects of purified polysaccharides from seaweeds are needed.

5.2.2. Effects on intestinal microflora

In addition to the studies conducted in rodents (see Section 5.1), a number of research groups have examined the effect of feeding seaweed extracts on the gut microflora of farm animals. Dierick *et al.* [69] reported that inclusion of *A. nodosum* meal in the diets of weanling pigs resulted in lower numbers of *E. coli* in the small intestine. Furthermore, the authors reported that the small intestinal *Lactobacillus/E. coli* ratio was increased in the test group indicating a potentially beneficial shift in the microbial ecosystem. However, Gardiner *et al.* [78] reported that dietary supplementation with a crude *A. nodosum* extract in finisher pigs resulted in reduced ileal coliform counts but also reduced cecal bifidobacteria, which are considered beneficial (Table 2). Similarly Reilly *et al.* [76] reported reductions in enterobacteria but also bifidobacteria and lactobacilli in the cecum and/or colon of weaned pigs fed *L. digitata* containing laminarin and fucoidan. Similar effects were seen in a group fed *L. hyperborea* (also containing laminarin and fucoidan), but there were no reductions in enterobacteria. However, a combination of both extracts resulted in a reduction of enterobacteria and lactobacilli in the cecum and colon but no effects on bifidobacteria were observed (Table 2). Lynch *et al.* [83] found that finisher pigs offered diets supplemented with increasing amounts of an intact *L. hyperborea* extract had reduced cecal *Bifidobacterium* and colonic *Lactobacillus* counts [76]. In a subsequent experiment also in finisher pigs, dietary supplementation with a purer fucoidan extract increased *Lactobacillus* counts in the proximal and distal colon (Table 2). On the other hand, McDonnell *et al.* [70] demonstrated that weanling pigs offered diets supplemented with laminarin alone or laminarin in combination with fucoidan had reduced fecal *E. coli* counts compared to pigs fed diets without laminarin. However, laminarin alone or in combination with fucoidan did not affect fecal lactobacilli but fucoidan alone resulted in higher counts of fecal lactobacilli compared to control animals (Table 2). The authors suggest that fucoidan has antimicrobial activity, while laminarin exerts prebiotic activity. In another study, O'Doherty *et al.* [81] hypothesized that a laminarin-fucoidan seaweed extract might prevent any negative effects of lactose removal from weanling pig diets. Inclusion of seaweed extract in either high or low lactose diets resulted in decreased fecal *E. coli* counts compared to non-seaweed diets. Decreases were similar to those observed in pigs fed high lactose diets alone. Increased lactobacilli numbers were also observed in pigs fed diets supplemented with seaweed extract but only in combination with high lactose levels. Janczyk *et al.* [84] reported that dietary supplementation with alginate resulted in higher enterococci counts in the distal small intestine, cecum and proximal colon of weanling pigs after an 11-day administration period compared with inulin or a control diet. However, reductions in lactobacilli were also observed in all intestinal segments but only after 6 days of alginate supplementation, and not prior to or after this timepoint. Molecular analysis of the intestinal microbiota by DGGE also demonstrated higher microbial diversity in the distal small intestine of alginate-supplemented pigs compared to animals fed a control diet. To our knowledge this is the only study to date that has examined effects of a seaweed polysaccharide on the intestinal microflora at a molecular level. Dietary supplementation with prebiotic compounds is also promising as a means of reducing pathogen shedding in farm animals as a strategy to improve food safety. Braden *et al.* [85] examined the effects of dietary supplementation with 2% dried *A. nodosum* (Tasco 14™), on fecal enterohemorrhagic *E. coli* O157:H7 populations on cattle hides and in feces. The authors reported reductions in the prevalence of fecal *E. coli* O157 and O157:H7 in hide swabs and fecal samples of *A. nodosum*-supplemented animals compared to animals offered a control diet. Bach *et al.* [77] also examined the effect of feeding Tasco 14™ on *E. coli* O157:H7 shedding but in cattle deliberately challenged with the pathogen. *E. coli* O157:H7 detection was less frequent in fecal samples of animals fed diets supplemented with either 10 g/kg of Tasco 14™ for 14 days or 20 g/kg for seven days compared to animals fed the control diets or diets supplemented with 20 g/kg for 14 days. The exact mode of action of the seaweed extract was not identified in either study but inhibitory effects against *E. coli* were attributed to direct antimicrobial activity rather than a prebiotic effect. This was concluded due to a lack of effects on microbial metabolites in the feces, indicating that the seaweed extract did not alter intestinal microbial populations and was therefore not fermented; however, only fecal metabolites were measured and further studies are warranted to explore effects on colonic microflora.

Overall, while increases in beneficial intestinal microbial populations are seen in some experiments where animals were fed seaweed-extracts, there is evidence to show that feeding purer extracts containing known amounts of characterized polysaccharides may be more effective in achieving a prebiotic effect. On the other hand, some extracts result in decreases in Gram negative intestinal populations but are not selective, as concomitant decreases in populations considered beneficial are sometimes also observed. This is most likely due to a direct antimicrobial effect rather than prebiotic activity. It has been suggested that certain seaweed polysaccharides may exert inhibitory effects while others might stimulate microbial populations and for this reason polysaccharides should perhaps be fed in combination.

In addition to examining the effects of potential prebiotic compounds on gut microbial ecology, microbial activity can be elucidated by examination of fermentation end products such as SCFA. These are predominantly produced in the hindgut which is where they exert the majority of their effects. For example, within the colon, SCFA are a source of energy for the host but also have important effects on host epithelial physiology [86]. SCFA also stimulate gut integrity and lower intestinal pH, which is associated with a reduction in pathogen growth [87]. Lynch *et al.* [83] observed that a crude *L. hyperborea* extract resulted in changes in the concentration of total fatty acids and molar proportions of individual fatty acids in the cecum but not the proximal colon of finisher pigs. However, Reilly *et al.* [76] demonstrated that supplementation with a crude *L. hyperborea* extract increased the concentration of colonic volatile fatty acids, whilst an extract derived from *L. digitata* increased volatile fatty acids in the cecum of weanling pigs. Therefore, extracts from different seaweeds, although similar in laminarin and fucoidan content, are fermented in different areas of the GIT and this may be due to differences in the purity of these extracts. It is also apparent that results can also vary between studies even when the same seaweed is fed; this was perhaps due to the differing age of the animals used. In a subsequent experiment, Lynch *et al.* [83] examined the effects of purified laminarin, fucoidan and a combination of both on the concentration of fatty acids in the proximal and distal colon (but not the cecum) of finishing pigs. Interestingly, the fucoidan-supplemented diet increased total fatty acid concentrations in the proximal and distal colon; there were however, no changes in fatty acid concentrations in the proximal colon of pigs fed the crude seaweed extract, as outlined above. This indicates that the purified polysaccharides were broken down to a greater extent than the crude extract. McDonnell *et al.* [80] reported increases in fecal lactobacilli populations in weanling animals offered a laminarin-fucoidan extract, however, no changes in fecal fatty acids in this group were observed. Similarly, O'Doherty *et al.* [81] reported increases in *Lactobacillus* spp. in weanling pigs fed a laminarin-fucoidan extract in combination with a high lactose diet but reported no effects on total fecal volatile fatty acid concentrations or the fatty acid profile. However, measurement of fecal volatile fatty acids in pigs may not be indicative of the degree of fermentation in the large intestine, as the fatty acids produced in the cecum and colon will most likely have been absorbed there and hence will not be excreted in the feces.

5.2.3. Additional benefits of prebiotics in swine husbandry

Dietary prebiotic supplementation in pigs may reduce nitrogen excretion, which may have positive environmental implications. Prebiotics, such as inulin have yielded a reduction in fecal ammonia concentrations in pigs [86]. While limited studies have examined this effect using polysaccharides from algal sources, Reilly *et al.* [76] reported a significant reduction in ammonia concentrations in the colon of pigs offered diets containing either a *L. hyperborea* extract or an *L. digitata* extract.

Boar taint is an undesirable taste or odor which can be evident when cooking or eating pork from non-castrated male pigs once they reach puberty. It is mainly caused by an accumulation of skatole and androstenone in adipose tissues. Skatole is produced by bacterial fermentation of tryptophan in the hindgut of animals [87]. Where slaughter weight is high and consequentially pigs are older at slaughter, as is the case in North America and continental Europe, boar taint is usually controlled by castration. Countries like Ireland and the UK still produce entire male pigs since slaughter weight/age has traditionally been low in these countries. However, as slaughter weight and hence age at slaughter is increasing in Ireland and the UK and there is European pressure to ban the practice of castration, alternative nutritional means of mitigating against boar taint are being investigated. Lanthier *et al.* [88] demonstrated that animals offered a diet containing inulin had significantly reduced plasma, cecal and fat skatole concentrations compared to animals offered a control diet. The authors suggest that this is possibly due to a reduction in hindgut proteolytic bacteria in favor of carbohydrate-fermenting bacteria. In addition, Byrne *et al.* [89] demonstrated that feeding pigs chicory root, a rich source of inulin, resulted in a significant reduction in boar taint sensory characteristics and reduced blood and back fat concentrations to below detectable levels. To the best of our knowledge, no studies have been conducted to date to assess the effects of marine polysaccharides on skatole or adrostenone levels in pigs.

6. Conclusions

Seaweed grows in abundance in coastal areas and may be a source of compounds which could be exploited for novel functional ingredients for human and animal health applications. This review has examined the evidence from both *in vitro* and *in vivo* experiments and found that seaweed-derived polysaccharides may have prebiotic activity. While a substantial amount of research has been conducted to date on animals, no studies have been conducted in human subjects to date. Results from *in vivo* studies using laboratory animals and domestic pigs are promising. However, it is difficult to reach consensus on the benefits because of the conflicting results obtained in different studies. This is most likely due to a number of factors such as, experimental conditions, intra-laboratory variations in age and physiology of the animals studied, variations in the type, purity and dose of seaweed extracts fed, differences in the concentration of active compounds within seaweed extracts and differences in dietary inclusion of other feed ingredients. In addition to these factors, seasonal variations in the composition of seaweed polysaccharides also require consideration when feeding intact seaweed meal. Future work in the area of seaweed-derived prebiotics should aim to examine the effects of purified seaweed polysaccharides on gut morphology and intestinal microbiota in parallel with well-established prebiotics, such as FOS or inulin. Furthermore, the role of seaweed prebiotics in animal husbandry may go beyond that of health applications with potential for improvement of environmental pollution and meat quality.

Abbreviations

GIT	Gastrointestinal tract
SCFA	short-chain fatty acids
NAOS	Neoagaro-oligosaccharides
FOS	Fructo-oligosaccharides
FISH	Fluorescence in situ hybridization
PCR	Polymerase chain reaction
DGGE	Denaturing gradient gel electrophoresis
qPCR	Quantitative PCR

References

1. Gonzalez del Val, A; Platas, G; Basilio, A; Cabello, A; Gorrochategui, J; Suay, I; Vicente, F; Portillo, E; Jimenez del Rio, M; Reina, GG; Pelaez, F. Screening of antimicrobial activities in red, green and brown macroalgae from Gran Canaria (Canary Islands, Spain). *Int. Microbiol* **2001**, *4*, 35–40.

2. Yuan, YV; Walsh, NA. Antioxidant and antiproliferative activities of extracts from a variety of edible seaweeds. *Food Chem. Toxicol* **2006**, *44*, 1144–1150.

3. Chandini, SK; Ganesan, P; Bhaskar, N. *In vitro* antioxidant activities of three selected brown seaweeds of India. *Food Chem* **2008**, *107*, 707–713.

4. Kang, JY; Khan, MNA; Park, NH; Cho, JY; Lee, MC; Fujii, H; Hong, YK. Antipyretic, analgesic, and anti-inflammatory activities of the seaweed *Sargassum fulvellum* and *Sargassum thunbergii* in mice. *J. Ethnopharmacol* **2008**, *116*, 187–190.

5. Pushpamali, WA; Nikapitiya, C; De Zoysa, M; Whang, I; Kim, SJ; Lee, J. Isolation and purification of an anticoagulant from fermented red seaweed Lomentaria catenata. *Carbohydr. Polym* **2008**, *73*, 274–279.

6. Sinha, S; Astani, A; Ghosh, T; Schnitzler, P; Ray, B. Polysaccharides from *Sargassum tenerrimum*: structural features, chemical modification and anti-viral activity. *Phytochemistry* **2009**, *71*, 235–242.

7. Kwon, MJ; Nam, TJ. Porphyran induces apoptosis related signal pathway in AGS gastric cancer cell lines. *Life Sci* **2006**, *79*, 1956–1962.

8. d'Ayala, GG; Malinconico, M; Laurienzo, P. Marine derived polysaccharides for biomedical applications: Chemical modification approaches. *Molecules* **2008**, *13*, 2069–2106.

9. Guo, JH; Skinner, GW; Harcum, WW; Barnum, PE. Pharmaceutical applications of naturally occurring water-soluble polymers. *Pharm. Sci. Technol. Today* **1998**, *1*, 254–261.

10. Dhargalkar, VK; Verlecar, XN. Southern Ocean seaweeds: A resource for exploration in food and drugs. *Aquaculture* **2009**, *287*, 229–242.

11. Jimenez-Escrig, A; Sanchez-Muniz, FJ. Dietary fiber from edible seaweeds: chemical structure, physicochemical properties and effects on cholesterol metabolism. *Nut. Res* **2000**, *20*, 585–598.

12. Goni, I; Valdivieso, L; Gudiel-Urbano, M. Capacity of edible seaweeds to modify *in vitro* starch digestibility of wheat bread. *Nahrung* **2002**, *46*, 18–20.

13. Haugan, JA; Liaaenjensen, S. Algal Carotenoids 54. Carotenoids of Brown-Algae (Phaeophyceae). *Biochem. Syst. Ecol* **1994**, *22*, 31–41.

14. Robic, A; Gaillard, C; Sassi, JF; Lerat, Y; Lahaye, M. Ultrastructure of Ulvan: A Polysaccharide from Green Seaweeds. *Biopolymers* **2009**, *91*, 652–664.

15. McHugh, DJ. A guide to seaweed industry. *FAO Fish. Tech. Pap.* **2003**, *T441*, 118.

16. Roberfroid, MB. Gibson, GR, Roberfroid, MB, Eds.; Prebiotics in Nutrition. In *Handbook of Prebiotics*, 1st ed; CRC Group: Boca Raton, FL, USA, 2008; pp. 1–11.

17. Gibson, GR; Roberfroid, MB. Dietary Modulation of the Human Colonic Microbiota: Introducing the Concept of Prebiotics. *J. Nutr* **1995**, *125*, 1401–1412.

18. Roberfroid, M. Gibson, GR, Roberfroid, M, Eds.; Prebiotics: Concept, definition, criteria, methodologies, and products. In *Handbook of Prebiotics*; CRC Press: Boca Raton, FL, USA, 2008; pp. 39–69.

19. Courtois, J. Oligosaccharides from land plants and algae: production and applications in therapeutics and biotechnology. *Curr. Opin. Microbiol* **2009**, *12*, 261–273.

20. Kolida, S; Gibson, GR. Gibson, GR, Roberfroid, M, Eds.; The prebiotic effect: Review of experimental and human data. In *Handbook of Prebiotics*; CRC Press: Boca Raton, FL, USA, 2008; pp. 69–93.

21. Manning, TS; Gibson, GR. Prebiotics. *Best Pract. Res. Clin. Gastroenterol* **2004**, *18*, 287–298.

22. Kelly, G. Inulin-Type Prebiotics: A Review (Part 2). *Altern. Med. Rev* **2009**, *14*, 36–55.

23. Spiller, R. Review article: probiotics and prebiotics in irritable bowel syndrome. *Aliment. Pharm. Therap* **2008**, *28*, 385–396.

24. Davis, CD; Milner, JA. Gastrointestinal microflora, food components and colon cancer prevention. *J. Nut. Biochem* **2009**, *20*, 743–752.

25. Lomax, AR; Calder, PC. Prebiotics, immune function, infection and inflammation: a review of the evidence. *Br. J. Nutr* **2009**, *101*, 633–658.

26. Tuohy, KM; Probert, HM; Smejkal, CW; Gibson, GR. Using probiotics and prebiotics to improve gut health. *Drug Discov. Today* **2003**, *8*, 692–700.

27. Sanders, ME. Overview of Functional Foods: Emphasis on Probiotic Bacteria. *Int. Dairy J* **1998**, *8*, 341–347.
28. Saulnier, DMA; Spinler, JK; Gibson, GR; Versalovic, J. Mechanisms of probiosis and prebiosis: considerations for enhanced functional foods. *Curr. Opin. Biotechnol* **2009**, *20*, 135–141.
29. Wierup, M. The Swedish experience of the 1986 year ban of antimicrobial growth promoters, with special reference to animal health, disease prevention, productivity, and usage of antimicrobials. *Microb. Drug Res* **2001**, *7*, 183–190.
30. Gaggia, F; Mattarelli, P; Biavati, B. Probiotics and prebiotics in animal feeding for safe foods production. *Int. J. Food Microbiol* **2010**. [CrossRef]
31. Percival, E; McDowell, RH. *Chemistry and Enzymology of Marine Algal Polysaccharides*; Academic Press: New York, NY, USA, 1967.
32. Percival, E. Polysaccharides of Green, Red and Brown Seaweeds: Their Basic Structure, Biosynthesis and Function. *Br. Phycol. J* **1979**, *14*, 103–117.
33. Rioux, LE; Turgeon, SL; Beaulieu, M. Characterization of polysaccharides extracted from brown seaweeds. *Carbohydr. Polym* **2007**, *69*, 530–537.
34. Rinaudo, M. Kamerling, JP, Ed.; Comprehensive Glycoscience. In *Seaweed Polysaccharides*; Elsevier: Amsterdam, The Netherland, 2007; Volume 2.
35. Pereira, L; Amado, AM; Critchley, AT; van de Velde, F; Ribeiro-Claro, PJA. Identification of selected seaweed polysaccharides (phycocolloids) by vibrational spectroscopy (FTIR-ATR and FT-Raman). *Food Hydrocolloid* **2009**, *23*, 1903–1909.
36. Graham, LE; Wilcox, LW. *Algae*, 1st ed; Prentice Hall: Upper Saddle River, NJ, USA, 2000.
37. Murphy, V. An investigation into the mechanisms of heavy metal binding by selected seaweed species. Ph.D. Thesis, Waterford Institute of Technology, Waterford, Ireland, 2007.
38. Mckinnell, JP; Percival, E. Acid polysaccharide from green seaweed. *Ulva-lactuca. J. Chem. Soc* **1962**, 2082–2083.
39. Lahaye, M; Axelos, MAV. Gelling properties of water-soluble polysaccharides from proliferating marine green seaweeds (*Ulva* Spp). *Carbohydr. Polym* **1993**, *22*, 261–265.
40. Paradossi, G; Cavalieri, F; Chiessi, E. A conformational study on the algal polysaccharide ulvan. *Macromolecules* **2002**, *35*, 6404–6411.
41. Ray, B; Lahaye, M. Cell-wall polysaccharides from the marine green-alga *Ulva-rigida* (Ulvales, Chlorophyta) - chemical-structure of ulvan. *Carbohydr. Res* **1995**, *274*, 313–318.
42. Andrieux, C; Hibert, A; Houari, AM; Bensaada, M; Popot, F; Szylit, O. *Ulva lactuca* is poorly fermented but alters bacterial metabolism in rats inoculated with human fecal flora from methane and non-methane producers. *J. Sci. Food Agric* **1998**, *77*, 25–30.
43. Davis, TA; Volesky, B; Mucci, A. A review of the biochemistry of heavy metal biosorption by brown algae. *Water Res* **2003**, *37*, 4311–4330.
44. Chapman, VJ; Chapman, DJ. *Seaweeds and Their Uses*; Chapman & Hall: London, UK, 1980.
45. Fourest, E; Volesky, B. Contribution of sulfonate groups and alginate to heavy metal biosorption by the dry biomass of *Sargassum fluitans*. *Environ. Sci. Technol* **1996**, *30*, 277–282.
46. Haug, A; Larsen, B; Smidsrod, O. Studies on sequence of uronic acid residues in alginic acid. *Acta Chem. Scand* **1967**, *21*, 691–704.
47. Haug, A. Affinity of some divalent metals to different types of alginates. *Acta Chem. Scand* **1961**, *15*, 1794–1795.
48. Mackie, W; Preston, RD. Stewart, WDP, Ed.; Algal physiology and biochemistry. In *Cell Wall and Intercellular Region Polysaccharides*; Blackwell Scientific Publications: Oxford, UK, 1974.
49. Li, B; Lu, F; Wei, XJ; Zhao, RX. Fucoidan: Structure and bioactivity. *Molecules* **2008**, *13*, 1671–1695.
50. Shibata, H; Iimuro, M; Uchiya, N; Kawamori, T; Nagaoka, M; Ueyama, S; Hashimoto, S; Yokokura, T; Sugimura, T; Wakabayashi, K. Preventive effects of Cladosiphon fucoidan against *Helicobacter pylori* infection in Mongolian gerbils. *Helicobacter* **2003**, *8*, 59–65.
51. Dunstan, DE; Goodall, DG. Terraced self assembled nano-structures from laminarin. *Int. J. Biol. Macromol* **2007**, *40*, 362–366.
52. Chizhov, AO; Dell, A; Morris, HR; Reason, AJ; Haslam, SM; McDowell, RA; Chizhov, OS; Usov, AI. Structural analysis of laminarans by MALDI and FAB mass spectrometry. *Carbohydr. Res* **1998**, *310*, 203–210.

53. Neyrinck, AM; Mouson, A; Delzenne, NM. Dietary supplementation with laminarin, a fermentable marine beta (1–3) glucan, protects against hepatotoxicity induced by LPS in rat by modulating immune response in the hepatic tissue. *Int. Immunopharmacol* **2007**, *7*, 1497–1506.
54. Deville, C; Gharbi, M; Dandrifosse, G; Peulen, O. Study on the effects of laminarin, a polysaccharide from seaweed, on gut characteristics. *J. Sci. Food Agric* **2007**, *87*, 1717–1725.
55. Deville, C; Damas, J; Forget, P; Dandrifosse, G; Peulen, O. Laminarin in the dietary fiber concept. *J. Sci. Food Agric* **2004**, *84*, 1030–1038.
56. Marinho-Soriano, E. Agar polysaccharides from *Gracilaria* species (Rhodophyta, Gracilariaceae). *J. Biotech* **2001**, *89*, 81–84.
57. Falshaw, R; Furneaux, RH; Stevenson, DE. Agars from nine species of red seaweed in the genus Curdiea (Gracilariaceae, Rhodophyta). *Carbohydr. Res* **1998**, *308*, 107–115.
58. Labropoulos, KC; Niesz, DE; Danforth, SC; Kevrekidis, PG. Dynamic rheology of agar gels: theory and experiments. Part I. Development of a rheological model. *Carbohydr. Polym* **2002**, *50*, 393–406.
59. Hu, B; Gong, QH; Wang, Y; Ma, YM; Li, JB; Yu, WG. Prebiotic effects of neoagaro-oligosaccharides prepared by enzymatic hydrolysis of agarose. *Anaerobe* **2006**, *12*, 260–266.
60. Falshaw, R; Bixler, HJ; Johndro, K. Structure and performance of commercial kappa-2 carrageenan extracts I. Structure analysis. *Food Hydrocollid* **2001**, *15*, 441–452.
61. Errea, MI; Matulewicz, MC. Unusual structures in the polysaccharides from the red seaweed *Pterocladiella capillacea* (Gelidiaceae, Gelidiales). *Carbohydr. Res* **2003**, *338*, 943–953.
62. Saeki, Y; Kato, T; Naito, Y; Takazoe, I; Okuda, K. Inhibitory effects of funoran on the adherence and colonization of mutans streptococci. *Caries Res* **1996**, *30*, 119–125.
63. Muraoka, T; Ishihara, K; Oyamada, C; Kunitake, H; Hirayama, I; Kimura, T. Fermentation properties of low-quality red alga susabinori *Porphyra yezoensis* by intestinal bacteria. *Biosci. Biotechnol. Biochem* **2008**, *72*, 1731–1739.
64. Salyers, AA; Vercellotti, JR; West, SEH; Wilkins, TD. Fermentation of mucin and plant polysaccharides by strains of *bacteroides* from the human colon. *Appl. Environ. Microbiol* **1977**, *33*, 319–322.
65. Salyers, AA; West, SEH; Vercellotti, JR; Wilkins, TD. Fermentation of mucins and plant polysaccharides by anaerobic bacteria from the human colon. *Appl. Environ. Microbiol* **1977**, *34*, 529–533.
66. Coles, LT; Moughan, PJ; Darragh, AJ. *In vitro* digestion and fermentation methods, including gas production techniques, as applied to nutritive evaluation of foods in the hindgut of humans and other simple-stomached animals. *Anim. Feed Sci. Tech* **2005**, *123*, 421–444.
67. Michel, C; Macfarlane, GT. Digestive fates of soluble polysaccharides from marine macroalgae: Involvement of the colonic microflora and physiological consequences for the host. *J. Appl. Bacteriol* **1996**, *80*, 349–369.
68. Kuda, T; Yano, T; Matsuda, N; Nishizawa, M. Inhibitory effects of laminaran and low molecular alginate against the putrefactive compounds produced by intestinal microflora *in vitro* and in rats. *Food Chem* **2005**, *91*, 745–749.
69. Dierick, N; Ovyn, A; De Smet, S. Effect of feeding intact brown seaweed *Ascophyllum nodosum* on some digestive parameters and on iodine content in edible tissues in pigs. *J. Sci. Food Agric* **2009**, *89*, 584–594.
70. Michel, C; Benard, C; Lahaye, M; Formaglio, D; Kaeffer, B; Quemener, B; Berot, S; Yvin, JC; Blottiere, HM; Cherbut, C. Algal oligosaccharides as functional foods: *in vitro* study of their cellular and fermentative effects. *Food Sci* **1999**, *19*, 311–332.
71. Marzorati, M; Verhelst, A; Luta, G; Sinnott, R; Verstraete, W; Van de Wiele, T; Possemiers, S. *In vitro* modulation of the human gastrointestinal microbial community by plant-derived polysaccharide-rich dietary supplements. *Int. J. Food Microbiol* **2010**, *139*, 168–176.
72. Wang, Y; Han, F; Hu, B; Li, JB; Yu, WG. *In vivo* prebiotic properties of alginate oligosaccharides prepared through enzymatic hydrolysis of alginate. *Nut. Res* **2006**, *26*, 597–603.
73. Gudiel-Urbano, M; Goni, I. Effect of edible seaweeds (*Undaria pinnatifida* and *Porphyra ternera*) on the metabolic activities of intestinal microflora in rats. *Nut. Res* **2002**, *22*, 323–331.
74. Pluske, JR; Hampson, DJ; Williams, IH. Factors influencing the structure and function of the small intestine in the weaned pig: a review. *Livestock Prod. Sci* **1997**, *51*, 215–236.
75. Estrada, A; Drew, MD; Van Kessel, A. Effect of the dietary supplementation of fructooligosaccharides and *Bifidobacterium longum* to early-weaned pigs on performance and fecal bacterial populations. *Can. J. Anim. Sci* **2001**, *81*, 141–148.

76. Reilly, P; O'Doherty, JV; Pierce, KM; Callan, JJ; O'Sullivan, JT; Sweeney, T. The effects of seaweed extract inclusion on gut morphology, selected intestinal microbiota, nutrient digestibility, volatile fatty acid concentrations and the immune status of the weaned pig. *Animal* **2008**, *2*, 1465–1473.

77. Bach, SJ; Wang, Y; McAllister, TA. Effect of feeding sun-dried seaweed (*Ascophyllum nodosum*) on fecal shedding of *Escherichia coli* O157: H7 by feedlot cattle and on growth performance of lambs. *Anim. Feed Sci. Tech* **2008**, *142*, 17–32.

78. Gardiner, GE; Campbell, AJ; O'Doherty, JV; Pierce, E; Lynch, PB; Leonard, FC; Stanton, C; Ross, RP; Lawlor, PG. Effect of *Ascophyllum nodosum* extract on growth performance, digestibility, carcass characteristics and selected intestinal microflora populations of grower-finisher pigs. *Anim. Feed Sci. Tech* **2008**, *141*, 259–273.

79. Gahan, DA; Lynch, MB; Callan, JJ; O'Sullivan, JT; O'Doherty, JV. Performance of weanling piglets offered low-, medium- or high-lactose diets supplemented with a seaweed extract from *Laminaria* spp. *Animal* **2009**, *3*, 24–31.

80. McDonnell, P; Figat, S; O'Doherty, JV. The effect of dietary laminarin and fucoidan in the diet of the weanling piglet on performance, selected fecal microbial populations and volatile fatty acid concentrations. *Animal* **2010**, *4*, 579–585.

81. O'Doherty, JV; Dillon, S; Figat, S; Callan, JJ; Sweeney, T. The effects of lactose inclusion and seaweed extract derived from *Laminaria* spp. on performance, digestibility of diet components and microbial populations in newly weaned pigs. *Anim. Feed Sci. Tech* **2010**, *157*, 173–180.

82. Turner, JL; Dritz, SS; Higgins, JJ; Minton, JE. Effects of *Ascophyllum nodosum* extract on growth performance and immune function of young pigs challenged with *Salmonella* typhimurium. *J. Anim. Sci* **2002**, *80*, 1947–1953.

83. Lynch, MB; Sweeney, T; Callan, JJ; O'Sullivan, JT; O'Doherty, JV. The effect of dietary *Laminaria*-derived laminarin and fucoidan on nutrient digestibility, nitrogen utilization, intestinal microflora and volatile fatty acid concentration in pigs. *J. Sci. Food Agric* **2010**, *90*, 430–437.

84. Janczyk, P; Pieper, R; Smidt, H; Souffrant, WB. Effect of alginate and inulin on intestinal microbial ecology of weanling pigs reared under different husbandry conditions. *FEMS Microbiol. Ecol* **2010**, *72*, 132–142.

85. Braden, KW; Blanton, JR; Allen, VG; Pond, KR; Miller, MF. *Ascophyllum nodosum* supplementation: A preharvest intervention for reducing *Escherichia coli* O157:H7 and *Salmonella* spp. in feedlot stears. *J. Food Prot* **2004**, *67*, 1824–1828.

86. Awati, A; Williams, BA; Bosch, MW; Gerrits, WJJ; Verstegen, MWA. Effect of inclusion of fermentable carbohydrates in the diet on fermentation end-product profile in feces of weanling piglets. *J. Anim. Sci* **2006**, *84*, 2133–2140.

87. Yokoyama, MT; Carlson, JR. Microbial metabolites of tryptophan in the intestinal-tract with special reference to skatole. *Am. J. Clin. Nutr* **1979**, *32*, 173–178.

88. Lanthier, F; Lou, Y; Terner, MA; Squires, EJ. Characterizing developmental changes in plasma and tissue skatole concentrations in the prepubescent intact male pig. *J. Anim. Sci* **2006**, *84*, 1699–1708.

89. Byrne, DV; Thamsborg, SM; Hansen, LL. A sensory description of boar taint and the effects of crude and dried chicory roots (*Cichorium intybus* L.) and inulin feeding in male and female pork. *Meat Sci* **2008**, *79*, 252–269.

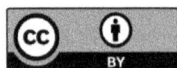

marine drugs

MDPI

Article

Nature and Lability of Northern Adriatic Macroaggregates

Jadran Faganeli [1],*, Bojana Mohar [1], Romina Kofol [1], Vesna Pavlica [1], Tjaša Marinšek [1], Ajda Rozman [1], Nives Kovač [1] and Angela Šurca Vuk [2]

[1] Marine Biological Station, National Institute of Biology, 6330 Piran, Slovenia; moharbojana@yahoo.co.uk (B.M.); rkofol@gmail.com (R.K.); vesna.pavlica@gmail.com (V.P.); tjasa.marinsek@gmail.com (T.M.); ajdaroz@yahoo.co.uk (A.R.); kovac@mbss.org (N.K.)

[2] National Institute of Chemistry, Hajdrihova 19, 1000 Ljubljana, Slovenia; angela.surca.vuk@ki.si

* *Author to whom correspondence should be addressed; Jadran.Faganeli@mbss.org; Tel.: +386-5-923-2911; Fax: +386-5-671-2902.

Received: 22 July 2010; in revised form: 30 August 2010; Accepted: 3 September 2010; Published: 6 September 2010

Abstract: The key organic constituents of marine macroaggregates (macrogels) of prevalently phytoplankton origin, periodically occurring in the northern Adriatic Sea, are proteins, lipids and especially polysaccharides. In this article, the reactivity of various macroaggregate fractions in relation to their composition in order to decode the potentially »bioavailable« fractions is summarized and discussed. The enzymatic hydrolysis of the macroaggregate matrix, using α-amylase, β-glucosidase, protease, proteinase and lipase, revealed the simultaneous degradation of polysaccharides and proteins, while lipids seem largely preserved. In the fresh surface macroaggregate samples, a pronounced degradation of the α-glycosidic bond compared to β-linkages. Degradation of the colloidal fraction proceeded faster in the higher molecular weight (MW) fractions. N-containing polysaccharides can be important constituents of the higher MW fraction while the lower MW constituents can mostly be composed of poly- and oligosaccharides. Since the polysaccharide component in the higher MW fraction is more degradable compared to N-containing polysaccharides, the higher MW fraction represents a possible path of organic nitrogen preservation. Enzymatic hydrolysis, using α-amylase and β-glucosidase, revealed the presence of α- and β-glycosidic linkages in all fractions with similar decomposition kinetics. Our results indicate that different fractions of macroaggregates are subjected to compositional selective reactivity with important implications for macroaggregate persistence in the seawater column and deposition.

Keywords: marine macroaggregates; lability; northern Adriatic

1. Introduction

The northern Adriatic "mucilage phenomena", or mucous macroaggregates, usually develop in late spring or early summer. Although their formation is not yet completely understood, these events seems to be significantly linked to preceding changes of the seawater inorganic N/P ratio [1,2] which can influence the rate of phytoplankton growth and phytoplankton metabolism inducing the production of mucilaginous material [3,5]. The phytoplankton origin is also indicated by mucilage composition, mostly composed of heteropolysaccharides produced by phytoplankton exudation [6] and cell lysis [7]. Microscopic observations [7,11] indicate diatoms as their crucial producers although other phytoplankton species and bacteria are also present in macroaggregates. Concentrations of nutrients present during the marked retention of freshened waters and water column stratification in the northern Adriatic [12] seem to be less critical for mucous formation. Specific oceanographic conditions, including the formation of a gyre, higher seawater residence time, and development of a marked pycnocline during stable summer conditions with low turbulent shear [13], significantly contribute to the subsequent concentration and agglomeration of macromolecular organic matter, phytoplankton cells and other organics and minerals. The aggregation process can be explained by polymer gel theory [14] through the formation of nanogels, later microgels which continue to aggregate into macrogels and POM [15,16]. Macroaggregates represent basically the transition from colloidal organic matter (COM, macromolecules) into macrogels and particulate organic matter (POM). Their gel-like nature is manifested by a high content of water, sometimes exceeding 95%, and organic matter which represents about 35–57% of dry mass. The organic component is mostly composed of carbohydrates (12–34%), proteins (1–12%) and lipids (0.1–8%)[17] and the inorganic fraction is predominantly composed of quartz, calcite and clays. The latter generally results from the scavenging and inclusion of autochthonous and allochthonous particles [11] from the ambient seawater. The association of inorganic and organic particles [18] and that of colloids with cations [15] probably contributes to the stabilization and persistence of those macrogels in the aquatic environment.

Mucous macroaggregates can be observed in various forms, in the surface layer, in the water column and on the seabed. Their different color, size and shape depends on their biological and chemical composition, maturation stage, *i.e.*, age, basic water-column characteristics and environmental conditions, as well as local hydrodynamics [9,10,19,21]. Macroaggregates are continuously subjected to microbial and various chemical and photochemical transformations [17]. However, the bacteria are believed to be a principal decomposer of the macroaggregate biopolymers [21,22] leading to low molecular weight products finally released to marine dissolved matter. Complete disappearance of macroaggregates, mostly in the late summer, usually coincides with rain storm events, changes in the water column stratification and circulation pattern [23].

The principal aim of this article was to present our recent investigations on the reactivity of various macroaggregate fractions, namely matrix and interstitial water colloids, in relation to their composition as well as the linkage of macroaggregate structural units using laboratory based enzymatic and natural degradation approaches.

2. Results and Discussion

2.1. Macroaggregate composition: matrix

The matrix can be viewed as the water-insoluble fraction of macroaggregates. Major spectrum bands (Figure 1) could be assigned: 3000–3600 cm^{-1} (O-H, N-H stretching band region), 3000–2800 cm^{-1} (aliphatic groups), 1730 cm^{-1} (C=O stretching of COOH, ketones or aldehides), 1650–1640 cm^{-1} (C=O stretching of amide I; C=N stretch; stretching of COO$^-$; C=C signals of aromatic ring and/or olefins C=C, water deformational modes), 1430 cm^{-1} (aliphatic C-H deformation of CH$_2$ and CH$_3$ groups; symmetric stretching of COO$^-$), 1150–1000 cm^{-1} (carbohydrates, Si-O stretch). Spectra of surface matrix display also main calcite peaks situated at 2516, 1420–1450, 876 and 713 cm^{-1} and that of silicates (527–535 and 472 cm^{-1}). The elemental composition of surface and water column samples revealed higher values for surface macroaggregates, averaging 16.4% of C$_{org.}$, 0.7% of N$_{tot.}$ and 254 ppm of P$_{tot.}$, with a mean C:N:P ratio (molar) of 772:26:1. Accordingly, higher contents of total carbohydrates and proteins, averaging 13.5% and 4.7%, respectively, were determined in surface samples compared to deeper seawater layer samples. This statement is supported also by FTIR analyses (Figure 1) showing the presence of carbohydrates, evidenced by bands at ~1150–900 cm^{-1} and proteins, evidenced by bands at 1654–1635 cm^{-1}, in both samples. The lipid contents, clearly indicated by bands at 2950–2850 cm^{-1} in FTIR spectra (Figure 1), are lower, averaging 2.2%.

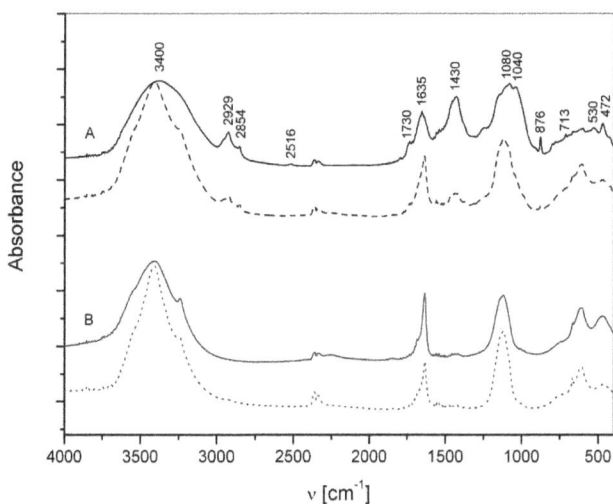

Figure 1. FT-IR spectra of (**A**) macroaggregate matrix, surface sample (black bold line) and water column sample (black dotted line); and (**B**) macroaggregate interstitial water colloids, surface sample (blue bold line) and water column sample (blue dotted line).

2.2. Macroaggregate composition: interstitial water colloids

FTIR spectra of interstitial water colloids (the "water-soluble" fraction) show the presence of both basic constituents, *i.e.*, carbohydrates and proteins (Figure 1). In FT-IR spectra of all colloidal fractions (not shown), the presence of a band at 2240 cm^{-1} probably indicates the cyanogenic glycosides [24] represents the greatest part of organic nitrilated compounds [25]. Their existence was previously confirmed also by monosaccharide analyses in bulk macroaggregates [26]. Their source is most probably linked to amino acids [25]. The bands assigned to lipids, *i.e.*, aliphatic components, at 2800–3000 cm^{-1} are less evident. The important contribution of carbohydrates in all colloid fractions was supported by higher UV absorption at $\lambda = 250$ nm, more typical of polysaccharides, compared to $\lambda = 205$ nm, being more typical of proteins [27] and humics [28]. The highest carbohydrate content and the lower C/N and C/P ratios (Figure 2) were found in the higher molecular weight (MW) colloidal fraction indicating the important presence of N and P containing [29] carbohydrates as well as their important role in mucilage composition. The δ^{15}N data exhibiting low values, especially in the >30 kDa fraction [30] and previous reports on non-protein nitrogen compounds [31], also sustain the presence of non-protein N compounds, *i.e.*, amino sugars, chlorophyll and nucleic acids, in the colloidal fraction. In contrast, the lower MW fractions seem mostly composed of oligo- and polysaccharides.

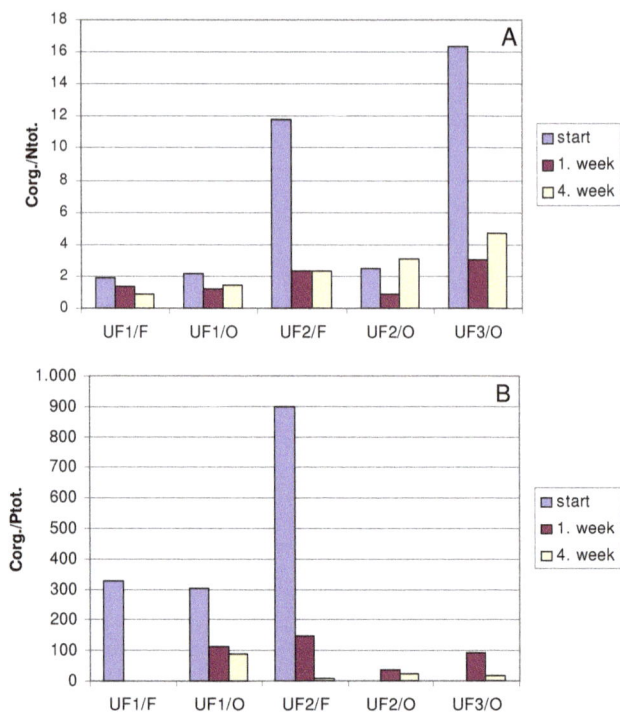

Figure 2. $C_{org.}/N_{tot.}$ (**A**) and $C_{org.}/P_{tot.}$ (**B**) molar ratios ultrafiltrate retentates (UF/0) and permeates (UF/F) using a nominal molecular weight cutoff of 30–10 (UF1), 10–5 (UF2) and <5 kDa (UF3) at the start, after 1 week and after 4 weeks of the degradation experiment.

3. Macroaggregate Lability

3.1. Matrix

According to macroaggregate enzymatic hydrolysis with α-amylase and β-glucosidase, the α (1–4) reserve polysaccharides, abundantly present in dinofllagelates in surface bulk macroaggregate samples taken in July 2004, are the most susceptible for enzymatic hydrolysis. In contrast, in the water column macroaggregates, containing prevalently diatoms, the impact of α-amylase is lower (Figure 3).

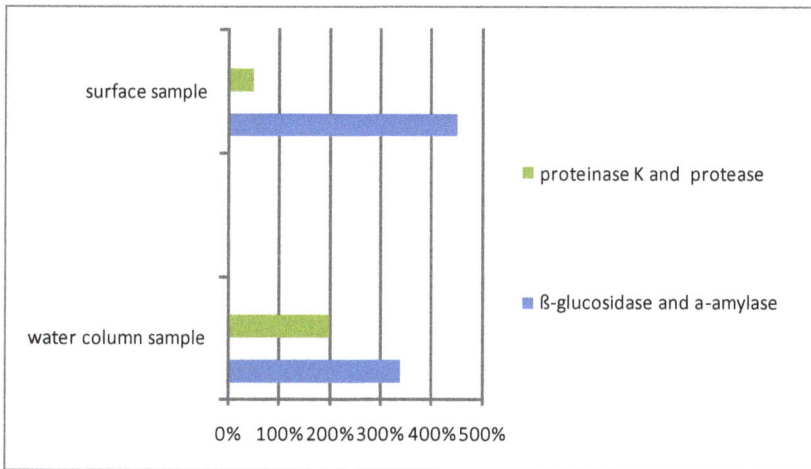

Figure 3. Concentration changes of carbohydrates and proteins during various enzyme hydrolyses (6 hours at 26 °C).

The presence of α- and β-glycosidic linkages in macroaggregates was previously confirmed by ^{1}H-NMR spectroscopy [32] and a shift from α- to the more refractory β-glycosidic linkage was described in aged macroaggregates dominated by diatoms containing storage β-glucans [19,22]. These findings are in accordance with the observations of Herndl *et al.* [33] and Zaccone *et al.* [34] who found that the activities of α- and β-glucosidase in macroaggregates were opposite due to microbial response to the composition of substrates, *i.e.*, macroaggregate components, where β-glycosidic linkage seems more refractory. The compositional difference between "fresher" surface and aged water column macroaggregate samples is also indicated by results of enzymatic hydrolysis (Figure 4). The addition of α-amylase and β-glucosidase produces high carbohydrate release in both samples (Figure 4). Protease and proteinase K, the most active ectoenzymes found in particles [35] and macroaggregates [22], produce, in addition to proteins, higher carbohydrate release in the water column sample which is clearly evident from FTIR spectra (Figure 4) showing a greater decrease in the carbohydrate band at ~1150–1000 cm^{-1}.

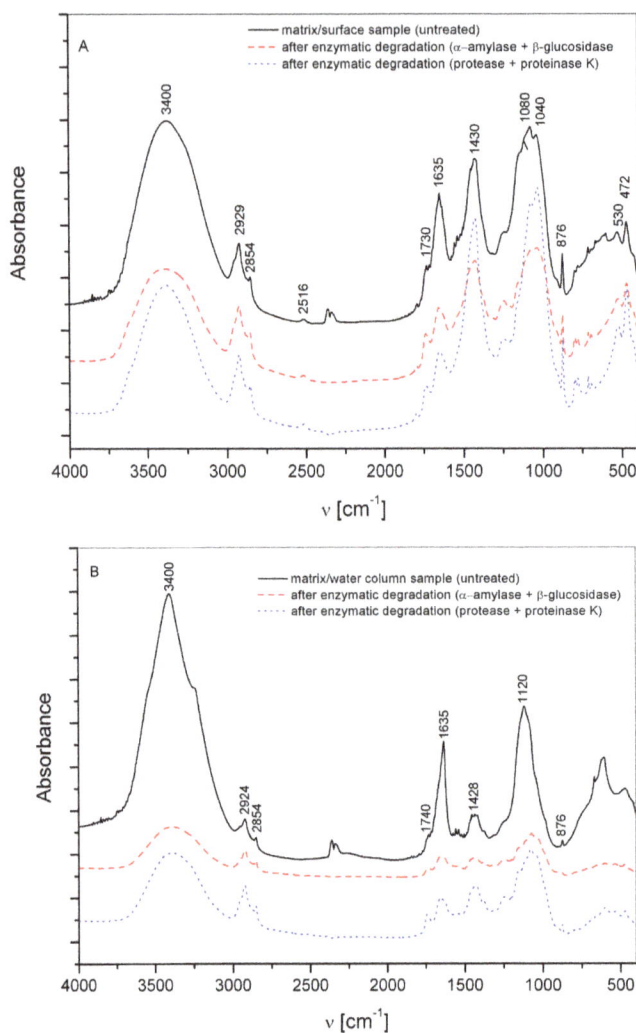

Figure 4. FT-IR spectra of the (**A**) surface and (**B**) water column macroaggregate matrices, and after (i) α-amylase + β-glucosidase, (ii) protease + proteinase K hydrolysis: carbohydrate bands (region ~1150–900 cm^{-1}), protein bands (region 1654–1635 cm^{-1}), lipid bands (region 2950–2850 cm^{-1}) and inorganic (mineral) components (region <1000 cm^{-1}).

FTIR spectra of the water phase from macroaggregate matrix slurries, obtained after hydrolysis with α-amylase + β-glucosidase, indicate the presence of minerals (Figure 5) such as calcite (signals at 2516, 1430, 876 cm^{-1}) and silicates (530 and 472 cm^{-1}). These results confirm the importance of associations between carbohydrates and minerals (inorganic species) for mucilage events. The release of minerals was not observed in the case of the same treatment of more mature water column sample, probably due to more intense interactions between organic and inorganic components; the latter acting as a stabilizing agent.

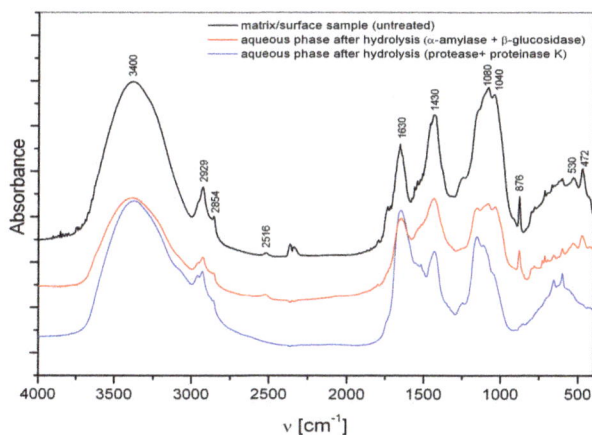

Figure 5. FT-IR spectra of the surface macroaggregate matrix and aqueous phase of experimental slurries after α-amylase + β-glucosidase and protease + proteinase K hydrolysis.

In aged macroaggregates, the carbohydrates can be linked to proteins, probably in the form of glycoproteins, and thus the organic N can be preserved in these probably more crosslinked samples [36]. The rapid hydrolysis of organophosphorus in the macroaggregate matrix by phosphatase, a nearly 300% increase of phosphate concentrations in the first ten minutes, suggests faster cycling of P with respect to N. Phosphatase can also be involved in the hydrolysis and release of organic constituents [37].

The hydrolysis of surface (fresher) macroaggregates with lipase showed primarily the degradation of lipids and polysaccharides, suggesting an association of lipids with polysaccharides possibly in the form of glycolipids. Using lipase (Figure 6) the macroagregate degradation is slower, ranging from days to weeks, compared to proteinase K and protease, ranging from hours to days. In the three week long degradation experiment, the relative intensities of absorptions indicating the lipidic component ($2800–3000 \ cm^{-1}$, $1730–1740 \ cm^{-1}$, $1430–1450 \ cm^{-1}$), revealed a large decrease in lipids, only at the end of the experiment due to their lower degradability.

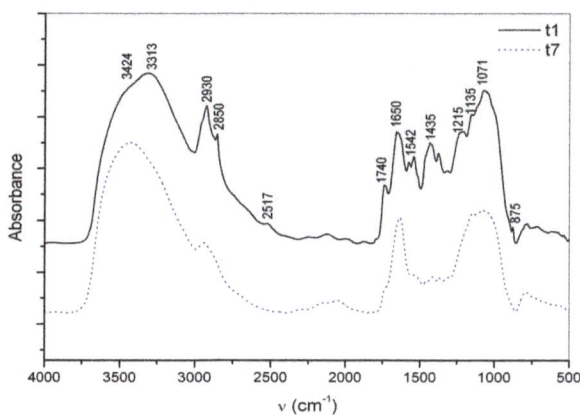

Figure 6. FT-IR spectra of the surface macroaggregate matrix (sampled at the beginning of the degradation experiment; t_1—black line), and after lipase (after 3 weeks at 26 °C, t_1—blue line) hydrolysis: carbohydrate bands (region ~1150–900 cm^{-1}), protein bands (region 1654–1635 cm^{-1}), lipid bands (region 2950–2850 cm^{-1}) and inorganic (mineral) components (region <1000 cm^{-1}).

The previous studies [18,36] of temporal compositional changes of the northern Adriatic bulk macroaggregates in the summer stratified seawater column, using ^{1}H- and ^{13}C-NMR and FTIR spectroscopy, also revealed the preferential degradation of carbohydrates in comparison to the aliphatic components—lipids. Similar results were obtained in the spectroscopic ^{1}H-NMR study of the bulk macroaggregates, showing much faster degradation of carbohydrates compared to lipids during the mucilage event [31]. All these findings seem to contradict the reported observations of the high hydrolytic activity of lipases, one of the most active ectoenzymes in aquatic systems [38] and in macroaggregates [39].

Regardless of bacterial enzymatic activity, the macroaggregate hydrogel structure can slow microbial degradation [40]. The gel microhabitat can represent an important site of organic matter degradation (microbial functioning) but, on the other hand, the gel polymers can be preserved due to their sterical hindrance [40] and the presence of organic-inorganic associations.

3.2. Interstitial water colloids

The enzymatic hydrolysis of all colloidal fractions using α-amylase and β-glucosidase indicates the presence of α- and β-gycosidic linkages in nearly equimolar proportions. Similar kinetics of hydrolysis appears in the >30 kDa and 10–30 kDa fractions. In the 5–10 kDa fraction, the increase of carbohydrate content after seven days is probably due to the prevalently polysaccharidic nature of this fraction making it more suitable for enzymatic hydrolisis. Contents of $C_{org.}$, $N_{tot.}$ and $P_{tot.}$ and the results of HPSEC analyses [41] from the »natural« degradation of macroaggregate colloidal fractions, indicate faster degradation in the >30 kDa and 30–10 kDa fractions compared to the 10–5 kDa fraction. This could be due to the higher contents of N-containing polysaccharides in the higher MW fractions. The microbial degradation of the carbohydrate component of glycoproteins is reported to proceed up to 3-fold faster compared to the proteinaceous components [42,43] explaining the preservation of organic nitrogen and the decreasing C/N ratio in aged degraded mature macroaggregates.

4. Experimental Section

4.1. Samples

Macroaggregate samples were collected on 1 July, 2004, in the southern part of the Gulf of Trieste at a fixed sampling site (45° 31.46′ N, 13° 33.72′ E) at the sea surface and at a depth of 10 m above the pycnocline. The sea water temperature was 25 °C. Both macroaggregate samples were in macrogel form; hence it was possible to collect them by hand by SCUBA divers, using polyethylene bottles with a minimal amount of surrounding water. The macroaggregate interstitial water was isolated by filtration through a 50 μm mesh size plankton net and centrifuged at 4000 g. The supernatant was successively filtered through preignited 0.7 μm pore size Whatman GF/F filters. The sediment (water-insoluble fraction) experiments and filtered supernatant (water-soluble fraction) were freeze-dried and used for subsequent degradation and fractionation, and degradation experiments, respectively.

4.2. Degradation experiments and separations

4.2.1. Matrix

The dry macroaggregate matrix was diluted with distilled water (aqueous phase) to obtain aqueous slurries of water-insoluble macroaggregate matrix. It was further enzymatically hydrolyzed for 0, 5, 10, 30, 60, 120, 240 and 360 min at 26 °C using 0.5 mL of α-amylase, β-glucosidase, protease or 1 mL proteinase K (all Sigma). The concentrations of all used aqueous enzyme stock solutions were 1 mg/mL. Enzymatic hydrolisis with 0.2 mL of lipase (Sigma) at 26 °C lasted for 0, 20, 60 min, and 1, 7, 14 and 21 days. The concentration of the used lipase stock solution was 6 mg/mL. The hydrolyzates were successively centrifuged at 3000 g, and the supernatant and sediment used for determination of total carbohydrates, proteins and lipids, and FTIR analyses. The blanks, consisting of samples without the addition of enzymes, represented substrates in a »natural« degradation experiment. All experiments were performed in triplicate.

4.2.2. Interstitial water colloids

In the natural degradation study, the filtrate was incubated for four weeks at 26 °C in the dark and subsamples were taken at the start (t = 0), after one (t = 1), two (t = 2), three (t = 3) and four weeks (t = 4). The subsamples were subsequently filtered through 0.22 μm pore size Nucleopore filters and separated by ultrafiltration. Ultrafiltration in a "cascade fashion" through membranes with nominal molecular weight cutoff (MWCO) values of 30, 10 and 5 kDa was performed using a Vivascience VivaFlow 200 unit (Sartorius) with a MasterFlex L/S membrane pump (Cole-Palmer) at a flow rate of 300 mL min^{-1} at 2.5 bar. The permeates (F) and retentates (O) were freeze-dried and analyzed for $C_{org.}$, $N_{tot.}$, $P_{tot.}$ and carbohydrate contents, and used for FTIR analyses.

For enzymatic study, the macroaggregate interstitial water used as a substrate was firstly filtered through 0.7 μm pore size Whatman GF/F filters and then filtered through a 0.22 μm pore size Nucleopore filter and, finally, separated by ultrafiltration as described above. The obtained retentates were subsequently hydrolyzed using α-amylase and β-glucosidase at 26 °C, the mean summer surface temperature in the Gulf of Trieste, for 14 days, and the products freeze-dried and analyzed for $C_{org.}$, $N_{tot.}$ and total carbohydrate content, and characterized using FTIR analyses. Concentration of both enzyme stock solutions was 1 mg/mL. All experiments were performed in triplicate.

4.3. Analyses

$C_{org.}$ and $N_{tot.}$ in freeze-dried samples were analyzed using a Carlo Erba mod. EA 1108 C, H, N, S analyzer and $P_{tot.}$ colorimetrically [44] after sample digestion with $K_2S_2O_8$. Total proteins, carbohydrates and lipids were assayed colorimetrically using the Coomassie Brilliant Blue method of Setchell *et al.* [45], the phenol-sulphuric acid method of Dubois *et al.* [46] and the Folch [47] method, respectively. Standards comprised solutions of D-glucose (Sigma) for carbohydrates and BSA (Sigma) for proteins in Milli-Q water. All colorimetric analyses were performed in triplicate. FTIR spectra were obtained from homogenized samples using a Perkin-Elmer Spectrum One spectrometer with a diffuse reflectance sampling accessory. The micro-cup of the accessory was filled with the sample diluted by anhydrous KBr to give up to a 5% mixture. Spectra were collected at room temperature with a resolution of 4 cm^{-1} and 4–10 scans were accumulated for each spectrum in a frequency range of 4000–450 cm^{-1}.

5. Conclusions

Results obtained from the enzymatically hydrolyzed macroaggregate matrix, prevalently of phytoplankton origin, by amylase, glucosidase, protease, proteinase and lipase, reveal fast, almost simultaneous, decomposition of polysaccharides and proteins, but slower decomposition of lipids probably in the form of glycolipids. Hence, the majority of carbohydrate and protein pools are potentially degradable, while the great majority of lipids can be preserved in the water column and transported away and finally deposited on the seabed. A pronounced degradation of the α-glycosidic bond compared to β-linkages was observed, probably due to the presence of α-reserve algal polysaccharides. The rapid hydrolysis of the organophosphorus component suggests fast cycling of macroaggregate phosphorus.

Hydrolysis of the macroaggregate matrix with α-amylase + β-glucosidase resulted in a release of inorganic particles, indicating an important interaction between carbohydrates and minerals. Minerals act as an important aggregation nucleus in mucilage formation and stabilization.

N-containing polysaccharides seem to be important constituents of the higher MW colloidal fractions, whereas poly- and oligosaccharides prevailed in the lower MW fractions. Degradation of the polysaccharide component proceeded faster in the higher MW fractions contributing to the preservation of organic nitrogen in the form of less degradable N-containing polysaccharides.

Our present knowledge indicates that various macroaggregate fractions and components are subjected to compositionally selective lability with important implications for macroaggregate persistence.

The compositional and degradation studies of marine mucous macroaggregates can contribute to the general knowledge of gels, gelation and aggregation (sol-gel transition) processes, binding capacity and other adsorbing properties, ion-exchange processes and inter- and intra-associations of such substrates, and the outcomes can potentially be used for technological purposes. To our knowledge, there are no reports on technological and pharmaceutical use of marine macroaggregates.

References

1. Cozzi, S; Ivančić, I; Catalano, G; Djakovac, T; Degobbis, D. Dynamics of the oceanographic properties during mucilage appearance in the Northern Adriatic Sea: Analysis of the 1997 event in comparison to earlier events. *J. Mar. Syst* **2004**, *50*, 223–241.
2. Penna, N; Kovac, N; Ricci, F; Penna, A; Capellacci, S; Faganeli, J. The role of dissolved carbohydrates in the northern Adriatic macroaggregate formation. *Acta Chim. Slov* **2009**, *56*, 305–314.
3. Myklestad, SM. Production of carbohydrates by marine planktonic diatoms. Influence of N/P ratio in the growth medium on the assimilation ratios, growth rate and production of cellular and extracellular carbohydrates by *Chaetoceros affinis* var, *willei* (Gran) Husted and *Skeletonema costatum* (Grev) Cleve. *J. Exp. Mar. Biol. Ecol* **1977**, *29*, 161–179.
4. Penna, N; Rinaldi, A; Montanari, G; Di Paolo, A; Penna, A. Mucilaginous masses in the Adriatic Sea in the summer of 1989. *Water Res* **1993**, *27*, 1767–1771.
5. Maestrini, SY; Breret, M; Bechim, C; Berland, BR; Poletti, R; Rinaldi, A. Nutrients limiting the algal growth potential (AGP) in the Po River Plume and an adjacent area, northwest Adriatic Sea: Enrichment bioassays with the test algae *Nitzschia closterium* and *Thalassiosira pseudonana*. *Estuaries* **1997**, *20*, 416–429.
6. Myklestad, SM. Release of extracellular products by phytoplankton with special emphasis on polysaccharides. *Sci. Total Environ* **1995**, *165*, 155–164.
7. Baldi, F; Minacci, A; Saliot, A; Mejanelle, L; Mozetic, P; Turk, V; Malej, A. Cell lysis and release of particulate polysaccharides in extensive marine mucilage assessed by lipid biomarkers and molecular probes. *Mar. Ecol. Prog. Ser* **1997**, *153*, 45–58.
8. Fanuko, N; Rode, J; Drašlar, K. Microflora from the Adriatic mucous aggregations. *Biol. Vestn* **1989**, *37*, 27–34.
9. Stachowitsch, M; Funuko, N; Richter, M. Mucus aggregates in the Adriatic Sea: An overview of stages and occurrences. *Mar. Ecol* **1990**, *11*, 327–350.
10. Degobbis, D; Fonda-Umani, S; Franco, P; Malej, A; Precali, R; Smodlaka, N. Changes in the northern Adriatic ecosystem and the hypertrophic appearance of gelatinous aggregates. *Sci. Total Environ* **1995**, *165*, 43–58.
11. Kovač, N; Mozetič, P; Trichet, J; Défarge, C. Phytoplankton composition and organic matter organization of mucous aggregates by means of light and cryo-scanning electron microscopy. *Mar. Biol* **2005**, *147*, 261–271.
12. Degobbis, D; Precali, R; Ferrari, CR; Djakovac, T; Rinaldi, A; Ivančić, I; Gismondi, M; Smodlaka, N. Change in nutrient concentrations and ratios during mucilage event in the period 1999–2002. *Sci. Total Environ* **2005**, *353*, 103–114.
13. Supić, N; Orlić, M. Seasonal and interannual variability of the northern Adriatic surface fluxes. *J. Mar. Syst* **2000**, *20*, 205–229.
14. Chin, WC; Orellana, MV; Verdugo, P. Spontaneous assembly of marine dissolved organic matter in polymer gels. *Nature* **1998**, *391*, 568–572.
15. Verdugo, P; Alldredge, AL; Azam, F; Kirchman, DL; Passow, U; Santschi, PH. The oceanic gel phase: A bridge in the DOM-POM continuum. *Mar. Chem* **2004**, *92*, 67–85.
16. Svetličić, V; Žutić, V; Zimmermann, AH. Biophysical scenario of giant gel formation in the Northern Adriatic Sea. *Ann. N. Y. Acad. Sci* **2005**, *1048*, 524–527.
17. Kovač, N; Faganeli, J; Bajt, O. Stefansson, O, Ed.; Mucous macroaggregates in the Northern Adriatic. In *Geochemistry Research Advances*; Nova Science: New York, NY, USA, 2008; pp. 119–141.
18. Kovac, N; Faganeli, J; Bajt, O; Sket, B; Orel, B; Penna, N. Chemical composition of macroaggregates in the northern Adriatic Sea. *Org. Geochem* **2004**, *35*, 1095–1104.

19. Herndl, GJ. Marine snow in the Northern Adriatic Sea: Possible couses and consequences for a shallow ecosystem. *Mar. Microb. Food Webs* **1992**, *6*, 149–172.

20. Rinaldi, A; Montanari, G; Ferrari, CR; Ghetti, A; Vollenweider, AR. Evoluzione dello stato trofico nelle acque costiere Emiliano-Romagnole nel periodo 1982–1994. Proceedings of Evoluzione dello stato trofico in Adriatico: Analisi degli interventi attuati e future linee di intervento, Bologna, Italy, 28–29 September 1995; pp. 33–49.

21. Mingazzini, M; Thake, B. Summary and conclusions of the workshop on marine mucilages in the Adriatic Sea and elsewhere. *Sci. Total Environ* **1995**, *165*, 9–14.

22. Müller-Niklas, S; Schuster, S; Kaltenböck, E; Herndl, GJ. Organic content and bacterial metabolism in amorphous aggregations of the Northern Adriatic Sea. *Limnol. Oceanogr* **1994**, *39*, 58–68.

23. Grilli, F; Marini, M; Degobbis, D; Ferrari, CR; Fornasiero, P; Russo, A; Gismondi, M; Djakovac, T; Precali, R; Simonetti, R. Circulation and horizontal fluxes in the northern Adriatic Sea in the period June 1999–July 2002. Part II: Nutrients transport. *Sci. Total Environ* **2005**, *353*, 115–125.

24. Nishikida, K; Hannah, RW. *Selected Applications of Modern FT-IR Techniques*; CRC: Boca Raton, FL, USA, 1996; p. 279.

25. Legras, JI; Chuzel, G; Arnaud, A; Galzy, P. Natural nitriles and their metabolism. *World J. Microbiol. Biotechnol* **1990**, *6*, 83–108.

26. Leskovšek, H; Perko, S; Žigon, D; Faganeli, J. Analysis of carbohydrates in marine particulates by gas chromatography and tandem mass spectrometry. *Analyst* **1994**, *119*, 1125–1128.

27. Binkley, ER; Binkley, RW. *Carbohydrate Photochemistry*; American Chemical Society: Washington DC, USA, 1999; p. 448.

28. Chin, Y-P; Aiken, GR; O'Loughlin, E. Molecular weight, polydispersity, and spectroscopic properties of aquatic humic substances. *Environ. Sci. Technol* **1994**, *28*, 1853–1858.

29. Sannigrahi, P; Ingall, ED; Benner, R. Nature and dynamics of phosphorous-containing components of marine dissolved and particulate organic matter. *Geochim. Cosmochim. Acta* **2006**, *70*, 5868–5882.

30. Faganeli, J; Ogrinc, N; Kovac, N; Kukovec, K; Falnoga, I; Mozetic, P; Bajt, O. Carbon and nitrogen isotope composition of particulate organic matter in relation to mucilage formation in the northern Adriatic Sea. *Mar. Chem* **2009**, *114*, 102–109.

31. Smucker, RA; Dawson, R. Products and photosynthesis by marine phytoplankton: Chitin in TCA "protein" precipitates. *J. Exp. Mar. Biol. Ecol* **1986**, *104*, 143–152.

32. Kovac, N; Bajt, O; Faganeli, J; Sket, B; Orel, B. Study of macroaggregate composition using FT-IR and ^{1}H-NMR spectroscopy. *Mar. Chem* **2002**, *78*, 205–215.

33. Herndl, GJ; Arrieta, JM; Stoderegger, K. Interaction between specific hydrological and microbial activity leading to extensive mucilage formation in the northern Adriatic Sea. *Ann. Ist. Super. Sanità* **1999**, *35*, 405–409.

34. Zaccone, R; Carus, G; Cal, C. Heterotrophic bacteria in the northern Adriatic Sea: Seasonal changes and ectoenzyme profile. *Mar. Environ. Res* **2002**, *54*, 1–19.

35. Grossart, HP; Ploug, H. Microbial degradation of organic carbon and nitrogen on diatom aggregates. *Limnol. Oceanogr* **2001**, *46*, 267–277.

36. Kovac, N; Faganeli, J; Bajt, O; Sket, B; Surca Vuk, A; Orel, B; Mozetič, P. Degradation and preservation of organic matter in marine macroaggregates. *Acta Chim. Slov* **2006**, *53*, 81–87.

37. Hoppe, HG; Ullrich, S. Profile of ectoenzymes in the Indian Ocean: Phenomena of phosphatase activity in the mesopelagic zone. *Aquat. Microb. Ecol* **1999**, *19*, 139–148.

38. Chrost, RJ; Gajewski, AJ. Microbial utilization of lipids in lake water. *FEMS Microbiol. Ecol* **1995**, *18*, 45–50.

39. Zoppini, A; Puddu, A; Fazi, S; Rosati, M; Sist, P. Extracellular enzyme activity and dynamics of bacterial community in mucilaginous aggregates of the northern Adriatic Sea. *Sci. Total Environ* **2005**, *353*, 270–286.

40. Aldrkamp, A-C; Buma, AGJ; Rijssel, M. The carbohydrates of *Phaeocystis* and their degradation in the microbial food web. *Biogeochemistry* **2007**, *83*, 99–118.

41. Koron, N; Faganeli, J; Falnoga, I; Kovac, N. Interaction and recativity of macroaggregates and Hg in coastal waters (Gulf of Trieste, northern Adriatic Sea). *Geomicrobiol. J* **2010**. submitted.

42. Ogawa, H; Amagai, Y; Koike, I; Kaiser, K; Benner, R. Production and refractory dissolved organic matter by bacteria. *Science* **2001**, *292*, 917–920.

43. Nagata, T; Meon, B; Kirchman, DL. Microbial degradation of peptidoglycan in seawater. *Limnol. Oceanogr* **2003**, *48*, 745–754.

44. Murphy, J; Riley, JP. A modified single solution method for the determination of phosphate in natural waters. *Anal. Chim. Acta* **1962**, *27*, 31–36.

45. Setchell, FW. Particulate protein measurements in oceanographic samples by dye binding. *Mar. Chem* **1981**, *10*, 301–313.

46. Dubois, M; Gilles, KA; Hamilton, JK; Rebers, PA; Smith, F. Colorimetric method for determination of sugars and related substances. *Anal. Chem* **1956**, *28*, 350–356.

47. Folch, J; Lees, M; Sloane-Stanley, GH. A simple method for the isolation and purification of total lipids from animal tissues. *J. Biol. Chem* **1957**, *226*, 497–502.

Samples Availability: Available from the authors.

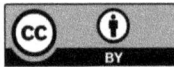

marine drugs

MDPI

Article

Degradation of Marine Algae-Derived Carbohydrates by Bacteroidetes Isolated from Human Gut Microbiota

Miaomiao Li [1,2], Qingsen Shang [1], Guangsheng Li [3], Xin Wang [4,*] and Guangli Yu [1,2,*]

[1] Shandong Provincial Key Laboratory of Glycoscience and Glycoengineering,
School of Medicine and Pharmacy, Ocean University of China, Qingdao 266003, China;
liaa99@163.com (M.L.); shangqingsen@163.com (Q.S.)

[2] Laboratory for Marine Drugs and Bioproducts of Qingdao National Laboratory for Marine Science and Technology, Qingdao 266237, China

[3] DiSha Pharmaceutical Group, Weihai 264205, China; gsli-87@163.com

[4] State Key Laboratory of Breeding Base for Zhejiang Sustainable Pest and Disease Control and Zhejiang Key Laboratory of Food Microbiology, Academy of Agricultural Sciences, Hangzhou 310021, China

* Correspondence: xxww101@sina.com (X.W.); glyu@ouc.edu.cn (G.Y.);
Tel.: +86-571-8641-5216 (X.W.); +86-532-8203-1609 (G.Y.)

Academic Editor: Paola Laurienzo
Received: 2 January 2017; Accepted: 20 March 2017; Published: 24 March 2017

Abstract: Carrageenan, agarose, and alginate are algae-derived undigested polysaccharides that have been used as food additives for hundreds of years. Fermentation of dietary carbohydrates of our food in the lower gut of humans is a critical process for the function and integrity of both the bacterial community and host cells. However, little is known about the fermentation of these three kinds of seaweed carbohydrates by human gut microbiota. Here, the degradation characteristics of carrageenan, agarose, alginate, and their oligosaccharides, by *Bacteroides xylanisolvens*, *Bacteroides ovatus*, and *Bacteroides uniforms*, isolated from human gut microbiota, are studied.

Keywords: carrageenan; agarose; alginate; oligosaccharides; *Bacteroides xylanisolvens*; *Bacteroides ovatus*; *Bacteroides uniforms*

1. Introduction

Marine carbohydrates contain a great deal of polysaccharides and oligosaccharides, some of them have been used as food additives for a long time, such as carrageenan, agarose, and alginate; all play an important role in Asian food, however, these marine carbohydrates cannot be digested by the enzymes encoded by the human genome. By now, most of the reported enzymes responsible for digesting marine carbohydrates are from ocean bacteria [1–3]; however, recent studies showed that the genes encoding porphyranase and agarase, which, respectively, cleave the algal polysaccharides porphyran and agarose, were found in *Bacteroides plebeius*, isolated from the microbiota of Japanese individuals [4,5]. This means that the human gut microbiota assist humans in utilizing marine carbohydrates that could not be digested by humans.

Genome analysis showed that human gut microbiota contained abundant and a variety of carbohydrate-active enzymes, which endow us with metabolic abilities that compensate for the paucity of glycoside hydrolases and polysaccharide lyases encoded by our genome [6]. However, the human gut microbiota is a massive colony, with 10^{14} microbes, including 1000 to 1150 phylotypes [7]; it is hard to assign the degradation of carbohydrates to specific bacterium. Notably, for marine carbohydrates, despite the fact that they have been used as food additives for a long time, little is known regarding their degradation and utilization by specific bacterium from human gut microbiota.

Our previous results showed the degradation of agarooligosaccharides [8], alginate, and alginate oligosaccharides [9] by Chinese gut microbiota. Here, we report the degradation of several kinds of marine carbohydrates (carrageenan oligosaccharides, agarose, alginate, and alginate oligosaccharides) by several Bacteroidetes isolated from Chinese individuals' feces, and analyze the structure of degradation products and the enzymes responsible for degrading marine carbohydrates. The results showed that *Bacteroides uniforms* L8 could degrade agarose (AP) completely, and the major enzyme secreted was β-agarase. The enzyme produced by isolate 38F6 (*Bacteroides xylanisolvens* and *Escherichia coli*), which degrades κ-carrageenan oligosaccharides, is β-carrageenase; for *Bacteroides ovatus* G19, based on its digestion pattern of alginate (Alg), guluronic acid oligosaccharides (GO), and mannuronic acid oligosaccharides (MO); the enzymes contain both α-1,4-guluronanlyase and β-1,4-mannuronanlyase.

2. Results and Discussion

2.1. Chemical Structures of the Products Generated by the Degradation of κ-Carrageenan Oligosaccharides by B. xylanisolvens and E. coli

Isolate 38F6 that degraded κ-carrageenan oligosaccharides was identified as two kinds of bacterium: *B. xylanisolvens* and *E. coli*. We attempted to purify *B. xylanisolvens* from the complex isolate, but the degrading ability of the single *B. xylanisolvens* is much weaker than that of the complex [10]. Then, 38F6 was used to inoculate neocarratetraose (NK-DP4), neocarrahexaose (NK-DP6), and carraheptadecaose (K-DP17). κ-carrageenan is a linear polysaccharide composed of repeating disaccharides of (1→3)-4-SO$_4$-β-D-galactose (G4S) and (1→4)-3,6-anhydro-α-D-galactose (A). The sequence of NK-DP4, NK-DP6 and K-DP17 are A-G4S-A-G4S, A-G4S-A-G4S-A-G4S, and (-G4S-(A-G4S)$_n$-, n = 8).

In order to analyze the enzyme hydrolyzing κ-carrageenan oligosaccharides in 38F6, the products generated by K-DP17 degradation after 144 h were separated using gel filtration and determined with electrospray ionization mass spectrometry (ESI-MS). The degradation products were identified mainly as 4-O-sulfate-D-galactose, κ-carratriose, κ-carrapentaose, κ-carraheptaose, and also a minor part was disaccharides and tetrasaccharides of κ-carrageenan (Table 1). The sequence of odd oligosaccharides can be easily verified based only on the results of ESI-MS for the different molecular weight of G4S and A (Table 1); however, for even oligosaccharides, there are two kinds of sequences, carraoligosaccharides (G4S-A-(G4S-A)$_n$) and neocarraoligosaccharides (A-G4S-(A-G4S)$_n$), and their molecular weights are the same. ESI-MS could not distinguish the difference between them according to mass spectrometry (MS); however, MS^2 plus with oligosaccharide reduction could help to solve this problem. The m/z of ions generated from the reducing terminal fragments will increase after reduction, but there will be no change for fragments from non-reducing terminals [11]. Using neocarrabiose (A-G4S) as an example, m/z 259 (Y1) and 241 (Z1) (Figure 1a), which are from the reducing terminal, will become m/z 261 (Y1) and 243 (Z1) after reduction (Figure 1b); and based on the molecular weights, ions of m/z 259 and 241 should be from G4S, but not A, thus, G4S is at the reducing terminal. The electrospray ionization collision-induced-dissociation mass spectrometry (ESI-CID-MS^2) spectrums of disaccharides (Figure 2a) and tetrasaccharides (Figure 2c) of κ-carrageenan from the degradation of K-DP17 showed that m/z 259 and 241 became m/z 261 and m/z 243 after reduction (Figure 2b,d). For tetrasaccharides, there is an additional ion, m/z 322 (double charged) (Figure 2c) became m/z 323 (double charged) (Figure 2d). All of the results indicated that the even-numbered oligosaccharides in the degradation production of K-DP17 are neocarrabiose (A-G4S) and neocarratetraose (A-G4S-A-G4S).

Table 1. Negative-ion electrospray ionization mass spectrometry (ESI-MS) analysis of the fragments generated from K-DP17 degradation by 38F6 at 144 h.

Fractions	Found Ions (Charge)	Calculated Mol Mass (Na Form)	Assignment	
			DP	Sequences
A 1	403.06 (−1)	426.05	2	A-G4S
A 2	322.03 (−2)	690.05	3	G4S-A-G4S
A 3	394.05 (−2)	834.10	4	A-G4S-A-G4S
A 4	343.03 (−3)	1098.09	5	G4S-A-G4S-A-G4S
A 5	391.06 (−3)	1245.18	6	A-G4S-A-G4S-A-G4S

G4S: (1→3)-4-SO$_4$-β-D-galactose; A: (1→4)-3,6-anhydro-α-D-galactose.

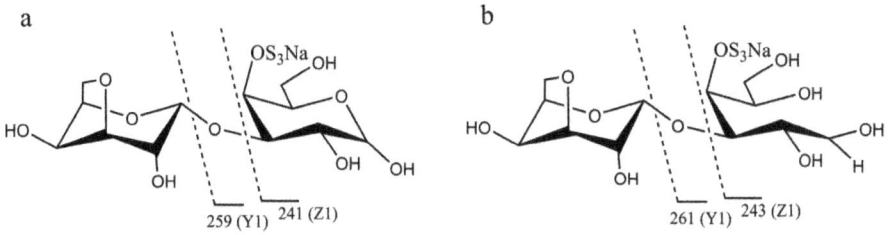

Figure 1. Diagram of fragments generated from electrospray ionization collision-induced-dissociation mass spectrometry (ESI-CID-MS^2) of neocarrabiose and neocarradiitol. (**a**) neocarrabiose; (**b**) neocarradiitol.

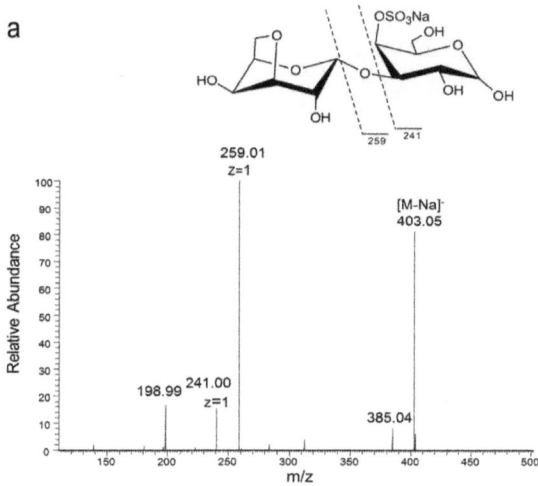

Figure 2. *Cont.*

537

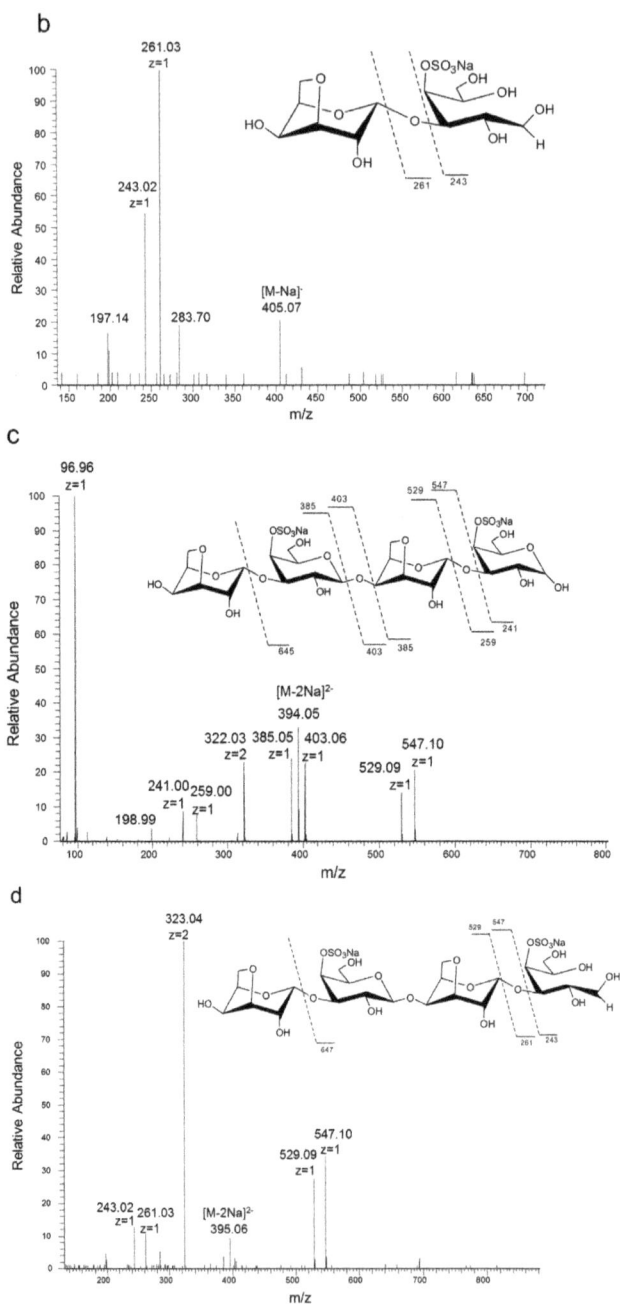

Figure 2. Electrospray ionization collision-induced-dissociation mass spectrometry (ESI-CID-MS^2) spectrums of products of K-DP17 degraded by 38F6. (**a**) ESI-CID-MS^2 spectrum of disaccharides generated from K-DP17 degradation by 38F6, (**b**) ESI-CID-MS^2 spectrums of reduced disaccharides generated from K-DP17 degradation by 38F6, (**c**) ESI-CID-MS^2 spectrums of tetrasaccharides generated from K-DP17 degradation by 38F6, (**d**) ESI-CID-MS^2 spectrums of reduced tetrasaccharides generated from K-DP17 degradation by 38F6.

The degradation pattern of NK-DP4 and NK-DP6 also confirmed our inference. Thin-layer chromatography (TLC) results showed that the product of NK-DP4 is neocarrabiose (Figure 3), and of NK-DP6 are neocarrabiose and neocarratetraose (Figure 3), which further demonstrate that the enzyme secreted by 38F6 is β-carrageenase, specifically cleaving β-1,4-glycoside (Figure 6a).

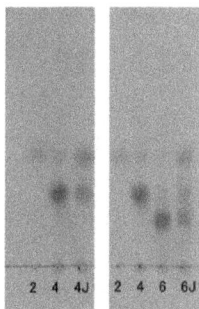

Figure 3. Thin-layer chromatography (TLC) analysis of degradation of neocarratetraose (NK-DP4) and neocarrahexaose (NK-DP6) by 38F6; 2: neocarrabiose (NK-DP2), 4: NK-DP4, 6: NK-DP6, 4J: NK-DP4 fermentation by 38F6, 6J: NK-DP6 fermentation by 38F6.

2.2. Chemical Structures of the Intermediates Produced by the Degradation of AP by B. uniformis L8

TLC patterns showed that the intermediates produced from the degradation of AP by *B. uniformis* L8 contained a range of fragments with different molecular weights after 48 h of incubation (Figure 4a). However, the product generated after 96 h of incubation consisted of only a single spot (Figure 4a), which was identified as D-galactose by HPLC, using the 1-phenyl-3-methyl-5-pyrazolone (PMP)-derivatization method (Figure 4b). The chemical structures of the intermediates at 48 h were determined using ESI-MS analyses and NMR. The ESI-MS results showed that the composition of the intermediates from AP degradation by *B. uniformis* L8, after 48 h, mainly included disaccharides, tetrasaccharides, hexasaccharides, and octasaccharides of agarose (Table 2). Agarose is made up of 3, 6-anhydro-L-galactose (A) and D-galactose (G) units, alternately linked by α-(1, 3) and β-(1, 4) glycosidic bonds. Like κ-carrageenan oligosaccharides, there are still two different sequences for the oligosaccharides of agarose: Agaroligosaccharides (G-A-(G-A)$_n$) and neoagaroligosaccharides (A-G-(A-G)$_n$); ESI-MS could not tell the difference between these two sequences, thus, part of the degradation products at 48 h was taken for NMR analysis to determine the sequence. Compared to the standard spectrums of agaroligosaccharides and neoagaroligosaccharides, the signals, 92.8 ppm, 96.8 ppm, and 98.3 ppm, were, respectively, ascribed to the $G_r1(\alpha)$, $G_r1(\beta)$, and $A_{nr}1$ residues, which were exactly in accord with the typical anomeric carbon signals of neoagaroligosaccharides [12] (Figure 5 and Table 3).

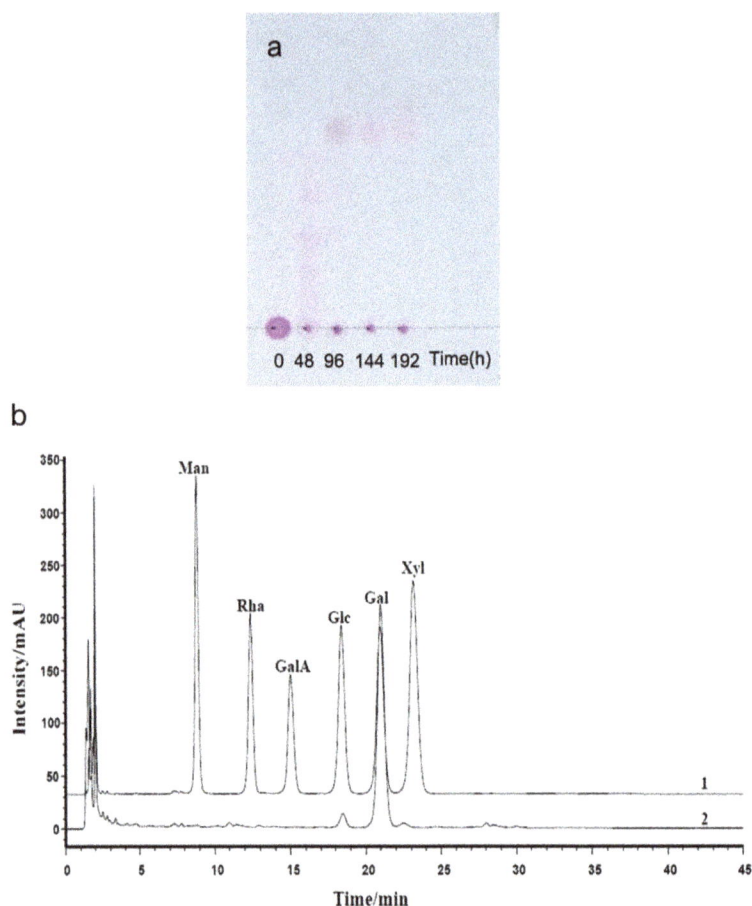

Figure 4. Analysis of the products of agarose (AP) degraded by *B. uniformis* L8 (**a**) TLC analysis of degradation of AP by *B. uniformis* L8 at 0, 48, 96, 144 and 192 h; (**b**) HPLC chromatography of final products of AP degraded by *B. uniformis* L8 at 96 h; 1. monosaccharide standard (Man: mannose, Rha: rhamnose, GalA: galacturonic acid, Glc: glucose, Gal: Galactose, Xyl: xylose); 2. final products of AP degraded by *B. uniformis* L8 at 96 h.

Table 2. Positive-ion electrospray ionization mass spectrometry (ESI-MS) analysis of the fragments generated from agarose (AP) degradation by *B. uniformis* L8 at 48 h.

Fraction	Found Ions (Charge)	Calculated Mol Mass (H Form)	Assignment	
			DP	Sequences
B1	325.11 * (+1)	324.11	2	A-G
B2	653.19 ** (+1)	630.20	4	A-G-A-G
B3	959.29 ** (+1)	936.30	6	A-G-A-G-A-G
B4	1265.38 ** (+1)	1242.39	8	A-G-A-G-A-G- A-G

G: (1→3)-β-D-galactose; A: (1→4)-3,6-anhydro-α-L-galactose; * the found ion is H form; ** the found ion is Na form.

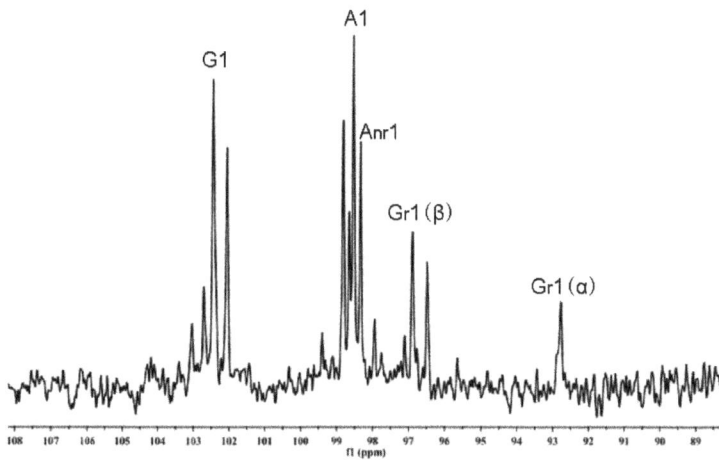

Figure 5. NMR ^{13}C spectrum of the oligosaccharides generated from agarose (AP) degradation by *B. uniformis* L8 at 48 h.

Table 3. NMR ^{13}C spectrum ascription of standard agarose oligosaccharides and products generated from agarose (AP) degraded by *B. uniformis* L8 at 48 h.

Compound	G1	G$_r$1	G$_{nr}$1	A1	A$_r$1	A$_{nr}$1
neoagaroligosaccharides [a]	102.4	92.8(α) 96.8(β)	-	98.5	-	98.3
neoagarotetraose [a] A$_{nr}$-G$_{nr}$-A$_r$-G$_r$	102.4	92.8(α) 96.8(β)	-	98.5	-	98.3
agaroligosaccharides [b]	102.6	-	102.6	98.4	90.4	
agarotetraose [b] G$_{nr}$-A$_{nr}$-G$_r$-A$_r$	102.6	-	102.5	98.5	63.3	
AP-L8	102.44	92.77(α) 96.88(β)		98.53	-	98.33

G: (1→3)-β-D-galactose; A: (1→4)-3,6-anhydro-α-L-galactose; r: reducing end; nr: non-reducing end; a: agarose oligosaccharides generated from agarose hydrolyzed by β-agarase; b: agarose oligosaccharides generated from agarose hydrolyzed by α-agarase.

There are two types of agarase: α-agarase and β-agarase. α-agarase cleaved α-1,3-glycosidic bonds, releasing agaroligosaccharides (G-A-(G-A)$_n$), on the other hand, β-agarase cleaved β-1,4-glycosidic bonds and the degradation products are neoagaroligosaccharides (A-G-(A-G)$_n$). Considering the results of ESI-MS and NMR, the major secreted enzyme of *B. uniforms* L8 should be β-agarase, which specifically cleaves the β-1,4-glycosidic bonds between G and A (Figure 6b). However, the end product of AP degradation by *B. uniforms* L8 is D-galactose, so it is possible that during the later period of hydrolysis, *B. uniforms* L8 secreted another glycoside hydrolase, which could help to hydrolyze neoagarobiose to D and A. The reason that 3,6-anhydro-galactose was not detected during the PMP-derivatization method is that it was further degraded to 5-hydroxymethyl-furfural due to its instability [13].

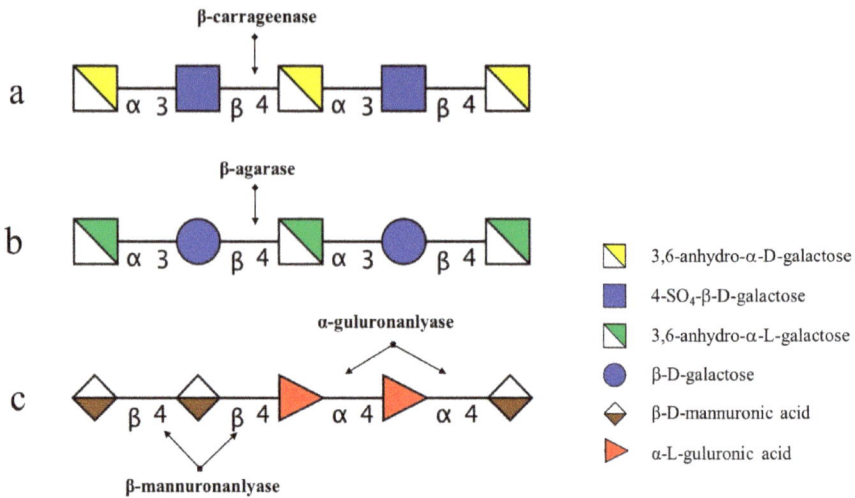

Figure 6. Profile of degradation position and mode of action of enzymes on marine carbohydrates. (**a**) degradation position of carrageenan oligosaccharides by enzymes secreted by 38F6 (*B. xylanisolvens* and *E. coli*); (**b**) degradation position of agarose (AP) by enzymes from *B. uniformis* L8; (**c**) degradation position of alginate by enzymes from *B. ovatus* G19.

2.3. Chemical Structures of the Intermediates Produced by the Degradation of Alg, MO and GO by B. ovatus G19

Alginate consists of hexuronic acid residues, β-D-mannuronic acid (M), and α-L-guluronic acid (G) with only 1→4 glycosidic linkages. MO and GO used for digestion were obtained from acid hydrolysis; controlled acid hydrolysis results in random cleavage along the polysaccharide chains and produces oligosaccharide fragments with unmodified hexuronic acid residues at both termini, and there are no unsaturated hexuronic acid residues in the products from acid hydrolysis. Alginate lyase are classified as α-1,4-guluronanlyase and β-1,4-mannuronanlyase; some bacteria can only secrete one kind of alginate lyase [14,15], and there are also bacteria that can secrete both [16]. All of the oligosaccharides generated from the digested enzyme had the 4,5-unsaturated hexuronic acid residue (Δ) at the non-reducing terminus.

The degradation productions of Alg, MO, and GO were prepared following the above-mentioned method. Fractions of C1, C2, C3, and C4 were obtained from degradation products of Alg and the procedure was performed on a LTQ Orbitrap XL instrument in order to determine molecular weight. Based on the molecular weight from the ESI-MS results (Table 4), C1 to C4 were assigned as unsaturated alginate disaccharides, trisaccharides, tetrasccharide, and pentasaccharides. MO and GO could also be digested by *B. ovatus* G19; the products contained saturated and unsaturated disaccharides, trisaccharides, and tetrasccharide (data not shown). According to *B. ovatus* G19's degrading ability of Alg, MO, and GO, the enzymes from *B. ovatus* G19 contain both α-1,4-guluronanlyase and β-1,4-mannuronanlyase, resulting in unsaturated alginate oligosaccharides (Figure 6c). For MO and GO, because the original substrate was prepared using acid hydrolysis, the saturated oligosaccharides are from the hexuronic acid residues at the non-reducing end.

Table 4. Negative-ion electrospray ionization mass spectrometry (ESI-MS) analysis of the fragments generated from alginate (Alg) degradation by *B. ovatus* G19 at 144 h.

Fraction	Found Ions (Charge)	Calculated Mol Mass (H Form)	Assignment DP	Assignment Sequences
C1	351.05 (−1)	351.06	2	ΔNN
C2	527.08 (−1)	527.09	3	ΔNNN
C3	351.05 (−2), 703.11 (−1)	704.13	4	ΔNNNN
C4	439.06 (−2), 879.13 (−1)	880.16	5	ΔNNNNN

N = β-D-mannuronic acid (M) or α-L-guluronic acid (G).

3. Experimental Section

3.1. Polysaccharide and Oligosaccharide Materials

AP was obtained from Qingdao Judayang Seaweed Co. Ltd., Qingdao, China. Other marine oligosaccharides used in the current study, including several kinds of κ-carrageenan oligosaccharides: NK-DP4, NK-DP6, and K-DP17, were kindly provided by Glycoscience and Glycoengineering Laboratory, Ocean University of China. GO and MO were obtained from Qingdao Haida Science and Technology Pharmaceutical Company (Qingdao, China). The purity of MO (with a molecular weight of 2.5 kD) and GO (with a molecular weight of 4.0 kD) were at least 90%, based on monosaccharide analyses using pre-column derivation with PMP by HPLC.

3.2. Bacteroidetes Material

Bacteroidetes responsible for degrading these marine carbohydrates were all isolated from human fecal samples and identified by sequencing their 16S rRNA gene. *Bacteroides uniforms* L8 could degrade agaro-oligosaccharides [8]; *Bacteroides xylanisolvens* and *E. coli* (38F6) were identified for degrading κ-carrageenan oligosaccharides mixture [10]; and *Bacteroides ovatus* G19 was reported to degrade alginate and alginate oligosaccharides [9].

3.3. Degradation of Marine Carbohydrates by Human Gut Bacteria Isolates

Batch culture fermentations were conducted using the procedure described by Lei et al. [17]. Briefly, the basic growth medium VI contained the following (g/L): Yeast extract, 4.5; tryptone, 3.0; peptone, 3.0; bile salts No. 3, 0.4; L-cysteine hydrochloride, 0.8; NaCl, 4.5; KCl, 2.5; $MgCl_2·6H_2O$, 0.45; $CaCl_2·6H_2O$, 0.2; KH_2PO_4, 0.4; Tween 80, 1 mL; and 2 mL of a solution of trace elements. Different marine carbohydrates were added to VI separately at different concentrations for their own properties: NK-DP4, NK-DP6, K-DP17, MO, GO, 8 g/L; AP, 1 g/L; Alg, 5 g/L. Medium with κ-carrageenan oligosaccharides (NK-DP4, NK-DP6 and K-DP17), AP, and alginate type (Alg, GO, MO) were autoclaved and inoculated with 38F6, *B. uniforms* L8, and *Bacteroides ovatus* G19 separately, then incubated at 37 °C in an anaerobic chamber. Samples were removed at different times for analyses of degradation.

3.4. General Experimental Procedures

The derivatives generated from NK-DP4, NK-DP6, and AP were confirmed using TLC analysis. Samples (0.2 μL) were loaded on a pre-coated silica gel-60 TLC aluminum plates (Merck, Darmstadt, Germany). After development with a solvent system consisting of formic acid/n-butanol/water (6:4:1, $v/v/v$), the plate was soaked in orcinol reagent and visualized by heating at 120 °C for 3 min.

The derivatives generated from K-DP17, AP, Alg, MO, and GO with Bacteroidetes were determined by gel filtration chromatography and analyzed using negative-ion ESI-MS for K-DP17, Alg, MO and GO; positive-ion ESI-MS for AP. In brief, after removing the bacteria by centrifugation, the supernatant was separated on a Superdex Peptide 10/300 column [18] and the sequence of each fraction was determined on a Thermo LTQ Orbitrap XL instrument (Thermo Fisher Scientific, Waltham, MA, USA) [13,19,20]. Samples were dissolved in CH_3CN/H_2O (1:1, v/v) at a concentration of 10 pmol/µL and 5 µL was injected. Solvent volatilization temperature and capillary temperatures were 275 °C and the sheath flow gas flow rate was 8 arb. The flow rate was 8 µL/min in the ESI-MS analysis and 3–5 µL/min in the ESI-CID-MS^2 analysis. Helium was used as the collision gas with a collision energy of 20–25 eV.

Because TLC analyses showed only one spot of AP after 96 h of incubation with *B. uniformis* L8, monosaccharide analysis was performed using pre-column derivation with PMP [21]. Briefly, the end products of AP were derivatized with PMP and then analyzed using HPLC system (Agilent 1260, Santa Clara, CA, USA) on a XDB-C18 column with acetonitrile/phosphate buffer solution (18:82, pH 6.7) at a flow rate of 1.0 mL/min at 30 °C; the detection wavelength was set to 254 nm. The composition of the end products was determined by retention time, in comparison with monosaccharide standards (mannose, rhamnose, xylose, galactose, glucose, and glucuronic acid; Sigma-Aldrich Company, Shanghai, China).

Part of the AP degradation solution after centrifugation was precipitated with 2 volumes of ethanol, twice, and then dried. Thirty milligrams of dried sample were co-evaporated by lyophilization, twice, with 1 mL of D_2O (99.96%), to remove exchangeable protons before a final dissolution in 0.5 mL of D_2O for NMR analysis. ^{13}C-NMR spectra were acquired at 25 °C with a JEOL ECP 600 MHz spectrometer (JEOL, Tokyo, Japan). Chemical shift values were calibrated using acetone-d66 as an internal standard.

3.5. Oligosaccharide Reduction

In order to analyze the sequence of products generated from K-DP17 degradation, disaccharides and tetrasaccharides of carrageenan (20–50 µg) were added 20 µL of NaBD$_4$ reagent (0.05 M NaBD$_4$ in 0.01 M NaOH) and the reduction was carried out at 4 °C overnight, as previously described [22]. The reaction solution was then neutralized to pH 7 with a solution of AcOH/H$_2$O (1:1) to damage borodeuterides before passing through a mini-column of cation exchange (AG50W-X8, Bio-Rad, Hercules, CA, USA). Boric acid was removed by repeated co-evaporation with MeOH.

4. Conclusions

Our study showed that marine carbohydrates (carrageenan, agarose, alginate, and their oligosaccharide derivatives), which could not be digested by humans, can be degraded by specific Bacteroidetes isolated from human gut microbiota; we also analyzed the enzymes responsible for hydrolysis, secreted by these Bacteroidetes. It was reported that all of the oligosaccharides of carrageenan, agarose, and alginate showed many potential activities with respect to antiviral [23], anticancer [24], and hypolipidemic effects [25]. Thus, the oligosaccharides generated from the degradation have the potential to affect the structure of human gut microbiota, and also gut health. Further animal studies are required to evaluate the effects of these marine carbohydrates, combined with degrading Bacteroidetes in organisms.

Acknowledgments: This work was supported in part by the National Natural Science Foundation of China (31670811, 31370156), the NSFC-Shandong Joint Fund for Marine Science Research Centers (U1406402 and U1606403), the National Science & Technology Support Program of China (2013BAB01B02), Taishan Scholar Project special funds (G. Yu) and Major Science and Technology projects in Shandong province (2015ZDJS04002), National High Technology Research and Development Program of China (2015AA020701), and the Scientific and Technological Innovation Project Financially Supported by Qingdao National Laboratory for Marine Science and Technology (2015ASKJ02).

Author Contributions: G.Y., M.L. and X.W. conceived and designed the experiments; M.L. and Q.S. performed the experiments; G.Y. and M.L. analyzed the data; G.L. contributed to materials, analytical methods and data interpretation; M.L. and G.Y. wrote the paper.

Conflicts of Interest: The authors declare no conflict of interest.

References

1. Yagi, H.; Fujise, A.; Itabashi, N.; Ohshiro, T. Purification and characterization of a novel alginate lyase from the marine bacterium Cobetia sp. NAP1 isolated from brown algae. *Biosci. Biotechnol. Biochem.* **2016**, *80*, 2338–2346. [CrossRef] [PubMed]

2. Shan, D.; Ying, J.; Li, X.; Gao, Z.; Wei, G.; Shao, Z. Draft genome sequence of the carrageenan-degrading bacterium Cellulophaga sp. strain KL-A, isolated from decaying marine algae. *Genome Announc.* **2014**, *2*. [CrossRef] [PubMed]

3. Hu, Z.; Lin, B.K.; Xu, Y.; Zhong, M.Q.; Liu, G.M. Production and purification of agarase from a marine agarolytic bacterium Agarivorans sp. HZ105. *J. Appl. Microbiol.* **2009**, *106*, 181–190. [CrossRef] [PubMed]

4. Hehemann, J.-H.; Kelly, A.G.; Pudlo, N.A.; Martens, E.C.; Boraston, A.B. Bacteria of the human gut microbiome catabolize red seaweed glycans with carbohydrate-active enzyme updates from extrinsic microbes. *Proc. Natl. Acad. Sci. USA* **2012**, *109*, 19786–19791. [CrossRef] [PubMed]

5. Hehemann, J.-H.; Correc, G.; Barbeyron, T.; Helbert, W.; Czjzek, M.; Michel, G. Transfer of carbohydrate-active enzymes from marine bacteria to Japanese gut microbiota. *Nature* **2010**, *464*, 908–912. [CrossRef] [PubMed]

6. Kaoutari, A.E.; Armougom, F.; Gordon, J.I.; Raoult, D.; Henrissat, B. The abundance and variety of carbohydrate-active enzymes in the human gut microbiota. *Nat. Rev. Microbiol.* **2013**, *11*, 497–504. [CrossRef] [PubMed]

7. Qin, J.; Li, R.; Raes, J.; Arumugam, M.; Burgdorf, K.S.; Manichanh, C.; Nielsen, T.; Pons, N.; Levenez, F.; Yamada, T.; et al. A human gut microbial gene catalogue established by metagenomic sequencing. *Nature* **2010**, *464*, 59–65. [CrossRef] [PubMed]

8. Li, M.; Li, G.; Zhu, L.; Yin, Y.; Zhao, X.; Xiang, C.; Yu, G.; Wang, X. Isolation and characterization of an agaro-oligosaccharide (AO)-hydrolyzing bacterium from the gut microflora of Chinese individuals. *PLoS ONE* **2014**, *9*, e91106. [CrossRef] [PubMed]

9. Li, M.; Li, G.; Shang, Q.; Chen, X.; Liu, W.; Pi, X.; Zhu, L.; Yin, Y.; Yu, G.; Wang, X. In vitro fermentation of alginate and its derivatives by human gut microbiota. *Anaerobe* **2016**, *39*, 19–25. [CrossRef] [PubMed]

10. Li, M. The Degradation and Utilization Study of Agarose,κ-carrageenan and Their Oligosaccharides by Human Gut Microbiota. Ph.D. Thesis, Ocean University of China, Qingdao, China, 2014.

11. Yang, B. Preparation and Sequence Analysis of Oligosaccharides and Neoglycolipids Probes from Marine-Derived Sulfated Galactan & Construction of Oligosaccharide-Chips. Ph.D. Thesis, Ocean University of China, Qingdao, China, 2009.

12. Ji, M. *Seaweed Chemistry*; Science Press: Beijing, China, 1997.

13. Yang, B.; Yu, G.; Zhao, X.; Jiao, G.; Ren, S.; Chai, W. Mechanism of mild acid hydrolysis of galactan polysaccharides with highly ordered disaccharide repeats leading to a complete series of exclusively odd-numbered oligosaccharides. *FEBS J.* **2009**, *276*, 2125–2137. [CrossRef] [PubMed]

14. Ostgaard, K.; Knutsen, S.H.; Dyrset, N.; Aasen, I.M. Production and characterization of guluronate lyase from Klebsiella pneumoniae for applications in seaweed biotechnology. *Enzyme Microb. Technol.* **1993**, *15*, 756–763. [CrossRef]

15. Linker, A.; Evans, L.R. Isolation and characterization of an alginase from mucoid strains of Pseudomonas aeruginosa. *J. Bacteriol.* **1984**, *159*, 958–964. [PubMed]

16. Sawabe, T.; Ohtsuka, M.; Ezura, Y. Novel alginate lyases from marine bacterium Alteromonas sp. strain H-4. *Carbohydr. Res.* **1997**, *304*, 69–76. [CrossRef]

17. Lei, F.; Yin, Y.; Wang, Y.; Deng, B.; Yu, H.D.; Li, L.; Xiang, C.; Wang, S.; Zhu, B.; Wang, X. Higher-level production of volatile fatty acids in vitro by chicken gut microbiotas than by human gut microbiotas as determined by functional analyses. *Appl. Environ. Microbiol.* **2012**, *78*, 5763–5772. [CrossRef] [PubMed]

18. Wang, P.; Zhao, X.; Lv, Y.; Li, M.; Liu, X.; Li, G.; Yu, G. Structural and compositional characteristics of hybrid carrageenans from red algae Chondracanthus chamissoi. *Carbohydr. Polym.* **2012**, *89*, 914–919. [CrossRef] [PubMed]

19. Zhang, Z.; Yu, G.; Zhao, X.; Liu, H.; Guan, H.; Lawson, A.M.; Chai, W. Sequence analysis of alginate-derived oligosaccharides by negative-ion electrospray tandem mass spectrometry. *J. Am. Soc. Mass Spectrom.* **2006**, *17*, 621–630. [CrossRef] [PubMed]

20. Yu, G.; Zhao, X.; Yang, B.; Ren, S.; Guan, H.; Zhang, Y.; Lawson, A.M.; Chai, W. Sequence determination of sulfated carrageenan-derived oligosaccharides by high-sensitivity negative-ion electrospray tandem mass spectrometry. *Anal. Chem.* **2006**, *78*, 8499–8505. [CrossRef] [PubMed]
21. Jiao, G.; Yu, G.; Wang, W.; Zhao, X.; Zhang, J.; Ewart, S.H. Properties of polysaccharides in several seaweeds from Atlantic Canada and their potential anti-influenza viral activities. *J. Ocean Univ. China* **2012**, *11*, 205–212. [CrossRef]
22. Chai, W.; Luo, J.; Lim, C.K.; Lawson, A.M. Characterization of heparin oligosaccharide mixtures as ammonium salts using electrospray mass spectrometry. *Anal. Chem.* **1998**, *70*, 2060–2066. [CrossRef] [PubMed]
23. Wang, W.; Zhang, P.; Hao, C.; Zhang, X.-E.; Cui, Z.-Q.; Guan, H.-S. In vitro inhibitory effect of carrageenan oligosaccharide on influenza A H1N1 virus. *Antivir. Res.* **2011**, *92*, 237–246. [CrossRef] [PubMed]
24. Zhou, G.; Sun, Y.; Xin, H.; Zhang, Y.; Li, Z.; Xu, Z. In vivo antitumor and immunomodulation activities of different molecular weight lambda-carrageenans from Chondrus ocellatus. *Pharmacol. Res.* **2004**, *50*, 47–53. [CrossRef] [PubMed]
25. Liu, X.; Hao, J.; Zhang, L.; Zhao, X.; He, X.; Li, M.; Zhao, X.; Wu, J.; Qiu, P.; Yu, G. Activated AMPK explains hypolipidemic effects of sulfated low molecular weight guluronate on HepG2 cells. *Eur. J. Med. Chem.* **2014**, *85*, 304–310. [CrossRef] [PubMed]

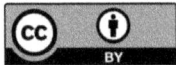

marine drugs

MDPI

Article

Seaweed Polysaccharides (Laminarin and Fucoidan) as Functional Ingredients in Pork Meat: An Evaluation of Anti-Oxidative Potential, Thermal Stability and Bioaccessibility

Natasha C. Moroney [1], Michael N. O'Grady [1], Sinéad Lordan [2], Catherine Stanton [2] and Joseph P. Kerry [1,*]

[1] Food Packaging Group, School of Food and Nutritional Sciences, College of Science, Engineering and Food Science, University College, Cork, Ireland; natasha.moroney@gmail.com (N.C.M.); Michael.OGrady@ucc.ie (M.N.G.)

[2] Teagasc Food Research Centre, Moorepark, Fermoy, Co. Cork, Ireland; s.lordan@ucc.ie (S.L.); Catherine.Stanton@teagasc.ie (C.S.)

* Author to whom correspondence should be addressed; joe.kerry@ucc.ie; Tel.: +353-21-4903798; Fax: +353-21-4270001.

Academic Editor: Paola Laurienzo
Received: 5 February 2015; Accepted: 30 March 2015; Published: 20 April 2015

Abstract: The anti-oxidative potential of laminarin (L), fucoidan (F) and an L/F seaweed extract was measured using the DPPH free radical scavenging assay, in 25% pork (*longissimus thoracis et lumborum* (LTL)) homogenates (TBARS) (3 and 6 mg/mL) and in horse heart oxymyoglobin (OxyMb) (0.1 and 1 mg/mL). The DPPH activity of fresh and cooked minced LTL containing L (100 mg/g; L_{100}), F_{100} and L/$F_{100,300}$, and bioaccessibility post *in vitro* digestion (L/F_{300}), was assessed. Theoretical cellular uptake of antioxidant compounds was measured in a transwell Caco-2 cell model. Laminarin displayed no activity and fucoidan reduced lipid oxidation but catalysed OxyMb oxidation. Fucoidan activity was lowered by cooking while the L/F extract displayed moderate thermal stability. A decrease in DPPH antioxidant activity of 44.15% and 36.63%, after 4 and 20 h respectively, indicated theoretical uptake of L/F antioxidant compounds. Results highlight the potential use of seaweed extracts as functional ingredients in pork.

Keywords: laminarin; fucoidan; seaweed extract; *in vitro* digestion; bioaccessibility; pork

1. Introduction

Seaweed polysaccharides (laminarin and fucoidan) isolated from the cell walls of brown seaweed (*Laminaria digitata*) possess immunomodulatory, anti-inflammatory, antiviral, antitumor, antithrombotic anticoagulant and antioxidant bioactivities [1,2]. Structurally, laminarin is composed of β-(1,3)-linked glucose containing large amounts of sugars and a low fraction of uronic acids. Two types of polymeric chains are present in laminarin, G-chains with glucose at the end and M-chains with mannitol as the terminal reducing end [3]. The antioxidant activity of laminarin has been linked to molecular structure, degree and length of branching and the monosaccharide constituents [4]. The structure of fucoidan consists mainly of α(1,3)-linked L-fucopyranose residues with sulphates at the C-2 position [5]. Distinct conclusions regarding chemical structures of fucoidans are often difficult to formulate due to structural heterogeneity and lack of regularity in fucoidan molecules [6]. Sulphate content, degree of sulphation and molecular weight are often attributed as factors influencing the antioxidant activity of fucoidan [7].

A wide range of analytical techniques (e.g., HPLC, ATR-FTIR and NMR spectroscopy) may be used to characterise and quantify structurally complex polysaccharides, such as laminarin and fucoidan, present in seaweeds [8]. Such techniques can involve detailed and time consuming extraction, preparation and sample clean-up procedures, depending on the parent seaweed material or the matrix in which the compounds of interest (polysaccharides) are contained [9]. *In vitro* antioxidant assays (e.g., FRAP, ABTS, ORAC and DPPH free radical scavenging activities) are frequently used to assess the antioxidant activity and potency of plant extracts [10]. The DPPH assay (based on a quick electron transfer reaction, followed by a slower hydrogen transfer reaction) is a simple, rapid, sensitive and reproducible index of antioxidant activity [11]. DPPH free radical scavenging activity of seaweed extracts, including laminarin and fucoidan, has been reported for a number of seaweed species [11,12].

The addition of antioxidant compounds to muscle foods (via the animals' diet or direct addition) in order to enhance meat quality and shelf-life has attracted much research attention in recent years. Previous research indicated that functional ingredients, such as laminarin and fucoidan, have beneficial effects pre-(animal health) [13] and post-slaughter (meat quality) [14]. Moroney *et al.* [15] reported that the addition of seaweed extracts, containing laminarin and fucoidan, to pig diets, resulted in lower levels of lipid oxidation in fresh pork steaks. However, direct addition of the same seaweed extract, promoted lipid oxidation and decreased the surface redness of fresh pork patties [16]. Catalysis of lipid oxidation was linked to the presence of salt and minerals in the seaweed extract. Increased discolouration (oxymyoglobin oxidation) was attributed to the effect of oxidising lipids and potential interactions between seaweed polysaccharides and oxymyoglobin. The anti- and pro-oxidative activity of laminarin and fucoidan on lipid and oxymyoglobin oxidation processes will be further examined in the present study.

The chemical structure of plant cell wall polysaccharides (e.g., cellulose, pectin substances, inulin and gums) and other associated non-carbohydrate components (*i.e.*, resistant protein) can be sensitive to chemical, mechanical, thermal and enzymatic processing [17]. Therefore the consequence of cooking on the potential bioactivity of laminarin and fucoidan in a meat matrix should be considered when formulating a functional meat product [18]. Cooking may sometimes improve the antioxidant activity of plant based materials due to the formation of other antioxidant components such as Maillard reaction products (MRPs) [19]. MRPs have been reported to possess antiradical activity including inhibition of the DPPH, oxygen peroxyl and hydroxyl radicals as well as copper and Fe^{2+} chelators [20]. In a previous study, Moroney *et al.* [16] reported a reduction in lipid oxidation of cooked minced pork patties containing laminarin and fucoidan which was attributed partially to the cooking process and the formation of MRPs which were not present in the fresh pork patties.

The digestion process may influence the bioactivity and bioaccessibility of laminarin and fucoidan. Bioaccessibility is defined as the fraction of a compound transferred from the food matrix during digestion, and thus made accessible for intestinal absorption and cellular uptake [21]. *In vitro* digestion models provide a useful alternative to animal and human models and simulate the digestion process of the human gastrointestinal tract (GIT). Cell culture models, in particular the Caco-2 cell culture model, have been widely utilised as part of *in vitro* digestion models as a predictive tool for the absorption of bioactive compounds from foods [22].

Studies on the anti-oxidative potential of seaweed polysaccharides in meat products are limited and merit investigation. Furthermore, the literature lacks information regarding the bioaccessibility of seaweed polysaccharides in meat products after cooking and post digestion. The initial objective of this study was to profile the antioxidant activity of laminarin (L), fucoidan (F) and a seaweed extract containing L and F, using the DPPH free radical scavenging assay. The antioxidative potential of L, F and L/F was further examined in fresh pork *longissimus thoracis et lumborum* (LTL) homogenates and in commercial horse heart oxymyoglobin. The DPPH radical scavenging and thermal stability of L, F and L/F in cooked pork patties was assessed. Finally cooked pork patties were subjected to an *in vitro* digestion procedure to determine the effects of digestion on the antioxidant potential of L, F and L/F and L/F digestates were examined in a transwell Caco-2 cell model to assess theoretical cellular uptake of antioxidant components of L/F.

2. Results and Discussion

2.1. Free Radical Scavenging Activity of Seaweed Polysaccharides (L, F and L/F)

In general, the DPPH free radical scavenging activity of seaweed polysaccharides increased over 20 h and followed the order: Trolox > F_1 > L/F_3 > L/F_1 > L_{10} ≈ L_1 (Table 1). DPPH free radical scavenging activity of L/F increased as a function of concentration. The DPPH free radical scavenging activities reported for L_1 and L_{10} were comparable to previously reported values (1.4%–5.3%) for laminarin extracted from *Laminaria digitata* at concentrations ranging from 0.125 to 1.0 mg/mL [12]. The DPPH free radical scavenging activity of F_1 (66.13%) after 1 h in the present study was similar to the inhibition of the DPPH radical (55.22%) after 30 min by fucoidan (1 mg/mL) from Sigma reported by Mak *et al.* [7].

Limited research suggests that carbohydrate polymers such as β-glucans (laminarin) possess free radical scavenging activity, however the addition of high levels of β-glucans is often necessary before radical scavenging activity is observed [23,24]. At concentrations of 20–200 mg/mL (higher than those used in the present study) a 1,3 β-D-glucan enriched extract from cereal grains demonstrated 25%–80% inhibition of the DPPH radical [23]. The mechanism of antioxidant action of β-D-glucans against free radicals is still not well understood, but a number of theories exist [25]. Tsiapali *et al.* [24] reported enhanced antioxidant activity of laminarin polymers over monomeric units due to greater ease of abstraction of anomeric hydrogen from one of the internal monosaccharide units rather than from the reducing end. In the present study, laminarin exhibited weak radical scavenging activity which may be due to the level examined.

Table 1. Free radical scavenging activity (DPPH) of L, F and L/F for up to 20 h at ~20 °C.

Incubate	Time, h		
	1	4	20
L_1 *	1.09 ± 0.92 [ab]	1.39 ± 0.96 [ab]	1.64 ± 1.30 [ab]
L_{10}	1.55 ± 1.21 [b]	2.72 ± 1.77 [b]	3.16 ± 2.72 [b]
F_1	66.13 ± 0.32 [c]	76.48 ± 0.30 [c]	90.68 ± 0.55 [c]
L/F_1	35.43 ± 2.04 [d]	47.35 ± 1.79 [d]	69.51 ± 1.37 [d]
L/F_3	56.18 ± 1.01 [e]	68.40 ± 0.89 [e]	78.41 ± 0.21 [e]
Trolox	95.89 ± 0.08 [f]	95.92 ± 0.14 [f]	95.76 ± 0.48 [f]

* Subscripts 1, 3 and 10 denote concentrations in mg/mL; [a–f] Within each storage time, mean values (± standard deviation) in the same column bearing different superscripts are significantly different, $p < 0.05$.

For some antioxidants, such as Trolox, the reaction with DPPH is rapid while other compounds may react more slowly [26]. The ability of seaweed extracts to quench free radicals is known to take place over longer periods of time compared to rapid acting synthetic antioxidants such as butylated hydroxyanisole (BHA) [27,28]. Slower reacting compounds are hypothesised to have a more complex reaction mechanism involving one or more secondary reactions in quenching the DPPH radical [10]. In the present study, after 20 h, the DPPH free radical scavenging activity of F_1 was equivalent (although statistically lower) to the positive control (Trolox), and significantly ($p < 0.05$) higher than both L_1 and L_{10}. Therefore the ability of an antioxidant to reduce and quench free radicals over a longer period of time may have benefits for extending the shelf-life of processed foods [28].

2.2. Effect of Seaweed Polysaccharides on Lipid Oxidation in Pork Muscle Model Systems

In vitro antioxidant assays (e.g., the DPPH assay) highlight the potential antioxidant activities of compounds but may not accurately predict activity in complex test systems such as muscle foods. To further investigate antioxidant activities of L, F and L/F, pork meat homogenates were subjected to iron/ascorbate (FeCl$_3$/sodium ascorbate)-induced lipid oxidation. Compared to the control, after 4 h at 4 °C, lipid oxidation significantly increased ($p < 0.05$) in the pork meat homogenates with the addition of pro-oxidants (Figure 1). No difference was observed for L_3 and L_6 compared to the control. Similarly no inhibition of lipid oxidation by laminarin, at levels comparable to those in the present study (3 mg/mL), was observed in a linoleic acid emulsion system [25]. F_3 and F_6 significantly decreased ($p < 0.05$) levels of lipid oxidation in pork meat homogenates. Trends indicated that levels of lipid oxidation in L/F_3 and L/F_6 were lower than the control (with pro-oxidants) although results were not statistically significant. In a previous study, Moroney *et al.* [16] reported that salt and minerals, present in the L/F extract, may have promoted lipid oxidation in fresh pork patties. Minerals and salt present in L/F_3 and L/F_6 may have counteracted the antioxidant activity of other constituents in the extract, thus impeding ability to significantly enhance lipid stability in the pork meat homogentates (Figure 1).

Structurally laminarin does not contain sulphate groups, which reportedly increases the antioxidant activity of fucoidan [29]. Sulphate groups can enhance the steric hindrance between polymer chains in polysaccharides leading to a more ordered and expanded conformation thus improving homogeneity in aqueous solution [30]. Lower molecular weight polysaccharides are often linked to increased free radical scavenging ability, presumably due to a non-compact structure which may allow more available sulphate and hydroxyl groups react with free radicals [9]. However, this was not observed for L in the present study indicating that even at low molecular weight, the structure in the presence of pork meat was unable to inhibit lipid oxidation, similar to the lack of DPPH free radical scavenging activity observed in Section 2.1 (Table 1).

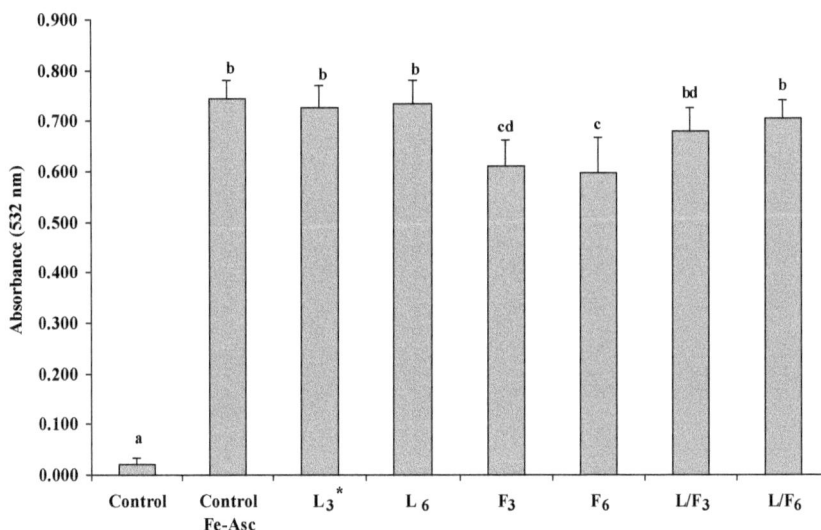

Figure 1. Lipid oxidation in 25% *longissimus thoracis et lumborum* (LTL) pork muscle homogenates following the addition of L, F or L/F and storage for up to 4 h at 4 °C. * Subscripts 3 and 6 denote concentrations in mg/mL. abcd Mean values (± standard deviation error bars) bearing different superscripts are significantly different, $p < 0.05$.

In general, it is accepted that natural antioxidants scavenge free oxygen-centered radicals via two major mechanisms, hydrogen atom transfer (HAT) reactions and electron transfer (ET) reactions. Yan *et al.* [30] suggested the HAT reaction is more likely to occur in neutral polysaccharides, such as laminarin, while the ET is the probable mechanism in acidic polysaccharides, like fucoidan where the negative charge of the sulphate groups plays a large part in the radical scavenging activity. In the present study, fucoidan is most likely responsible for the antioxidant activity observed by the L/F extract in the pork meat homogenates presumably due to ET reactions between the sulphate groups and the free radicals in the pork meat homogenates.

2.3. Effect of Seaweed Polysaccharides on Oxymyoglobin Oxidation

Oxymyoglobin oxidation (represented by a reduction in OxyMb, %) increased during storage for up to 8 days at 4 °C (Table 2). $L_{0.1}$ and L_1 had no influence on OxyMb oxidation, however $F_{0.1}$ and F_1 significantly ($p < 0.05$) enhanced OxyMb oxidation compared to the control in a dose dependant manner on days 4 and 8 of storage. Similarly, a significant increase ($p < 0.05$) in OxyMb oxidation was observed for $L/F_{0.1}$ and L/F_1. The presence of metmyoglobin is characterised by an increased absorption at ~628 nm [31] which is evident in the spectral scan for OxyMb alone and OxyMb + F_1 (Figure 2). At the wavelengths examined, no spectral shift in the presence of F_1 was observed.

Table 2. Oxymyoglobin (OxyMb) oxidation (represented by a reduction in OxyMb) following the addition of L, F or L/F and storage for up to 8 d at 4 °C.

Incubate	time, d		
	0	**4**	**8**
Control	76.53 ± 2.28 [a]	59.92 ± 2.30 [a]	54.46 ± 2.02 [a]
$L_{0.1}$ *	76.57 ± 2.31 [a]	59.68 ± 2.14 [ab]	54.00 ± 2.50 [a]
L_1	76.59 ± 2.73 [a]	58.11 ± 3.12 [abc]	52.51 ± 2.75 [a]
$F_{0.1}$	74.73 ± 2.54 [ac]	53.44 ± 2.44 [bd]	45.42 ± 2.56 [b]
F_1	67.55 ± 2.50 [b]	32.95 ± 2.00 [e]	21.71 ± 1.34 [c]
$L/F_{0.1}$	74.93 ± 2.06 [ad]	52.91 ± 2.44 [cd]	44.95 ± 2.82 [b]
L/F_1	69.03 ± 2.78 [bcd]	39.01 ± 1.90 [e]	28.78 ± 2.25 [d]

* Subscripts 0.1 and 1 denote concentrations in mg/mL; [abcde] Within each storage time, mean values ($\pm$ standard deviation) in the same column bearing different superscripts are significantly different $p < 0.05$.

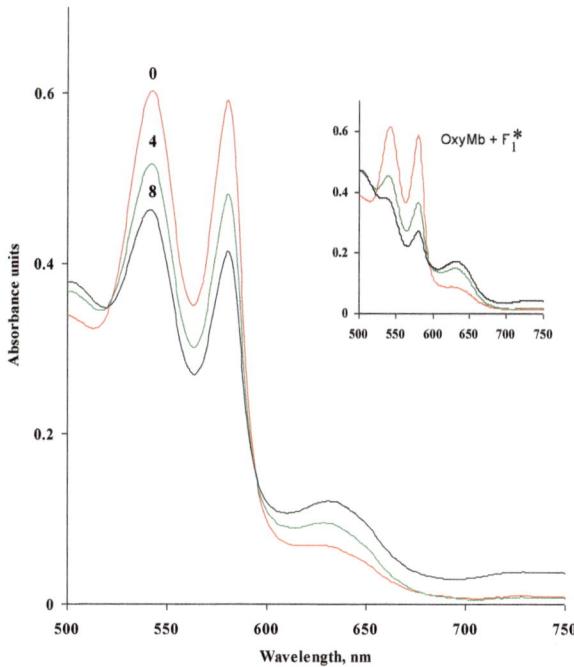

Figure 2. Absorbance spectra of oxymyoglobin (OxyMb) alone and following the addition of F_1 (* Subscript 1 denotes concentration in mg/mL) and storage for up to 8 days at 4 °C.

The exact mechanism by which fucoidan promotes OxyMb oxidation is unclear. The ability of fucoidan to bind to proteins such as antithrombin (a glycoprotein) and bovine serum albumin (a globular protein) has previously been linked to molecular weight as well as the sulphation patterns of the polysaccharide [32–34]. Generally, interactions between anionic polysaccharides and positively charged OxyMb have been reported to be electrostatic in nature due to opposing charges [35].

Similarly, Satoh *et al.* [36] demonstrated that oxidation of OxyMb was initiated via nucleophilic attack at the iron (II) centre of OxyMb by a water molecule with strong proton assistance from the distal histidine, or a hydroxide anion (OH^-). These reactions can cause irreversible displacement of bound dioxygen from OxyMb resulting in the formation of ferric metmyoglobin and generation of the superoxide anion. In the present study, the anionic sulphate groups of fucoidan potentially enhanced the oxidation of OxyMb through the nucleophilic displacement mechanism described above.

2.4. Effect of Cooking on the DPPH Free Radical Scavenging Activity of Seaweed Polysaccharides in Pork Meat

Statistical analysis indicated that the DPPH free radical scavenging of L, F and L/F in the presence of fresh minced LTL ($F_{100} > L/F_{300} \approx L/F_{100} \approx L_{100}$) followed a similar pattern to the DPPH free radical scavenging activities of seaweed polysaccharides reported in Section 2.1. L_{100} DPPH free radical scavenging was similar to the control before and after cooking (Figure 3). The DPPH free radical scavenging activity of F_{100} significantly ($p < 0.05$) decreased after cooking. Thermal processing is known to modify the physicochemical properties of plant cell wall polysaccharides [17]. The DPPH free radical scavenging activities of fresh and cooked L/F_{100} and L/F_{300} were similar indicating moderate thermal stability of the L/F extract. Similarly, Moroney *et al.* [14] reported low to moderate thermal stability of L/F in cooked minced pork patties from pigs fed the L/F extract for 3 weeks pre-slaughter.

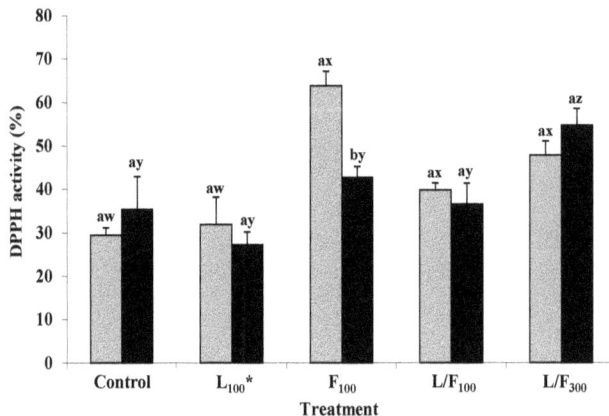

Figure 3. Free radical scavenging activity (DPPH) of L, F or L/F in fresh and cooked minced *longissimus thoracis et lumborum* (LTL) pork muscle stored for 20 h at ~20 °C. * Subscripts 100 and 300 denote concentrations in mg/g. [ab] Within each treatment, mean values (± standard deviation error bars) bearing different superscripts are significantly different, $p < 0.05$. Comparing [wx] fresh and [yz] cooked LTL pork muscle treatments to their respective controls, mean values bearing different superscripts are significantly different, $p < 0.05$. (▢), fresh; (■), cooked.

L/F_{300} significantly ($p < 0.05$) enhanced the DPPH free radical scavenging activity of cooked minced LTL compared to the control (Figure 3). Similarly, Prabhasankar *et al.* [37] reported an increase in DPPH free radical scavenging activity of cooked pasta with the addition of a brown seaweed (*Undaria pinnatifida*) to uncooked pasta. The formation of Maillard reaction products (MRP) and other novel antioxidant compounds such as mycosporine-like amino acids during heat treatment of seaweed extracts has been reported [38–40]. Additionally, MRP have proven effective inhibitors of lipid oxidation in cooked minced pork patties [41]. In the present study, MRP formed during heating of L/F_{300} most likely enhanced the DPPH free radical scavenging of cooked minced LTL.

2.5. DPPH Free Radical Scavenging Activity of Seaweed Polysaccharides in Pork Meat Following in Vitro Digestion

During the digestion procedure, cooked minced LTL from each treatment was subjected to pH changes and enzymatic reactions which resulted in increased (~30%–44%) DPPH free radical scavenging activities in digestates compared to undigested aqueous fractions (data not shown). The DPPH free radical scavenging activity of the control post digestion increased from 14.4% to 44.8% and was attributed to the presence of compounds such as peptides released from the pork meat during the *in vitro* digestion procedure. Escudero *et al.* [42] reported 51 different peptides were released from pork meat (*longissimus dorsi*) following *in vitro* digestion. Additionally, peptides obtained from animal sources such as porcine myofibrillar proteins have demonstrated DPPH free radical scavenging activity [43–45]. Data from each treatment (L_{100}, F_{100}, L/F_{100} and L/F_{300}) were adjusted for the meat control to estimate the antioxidant activity due to the seaweed polysaccharides post digestion (Figure 4).

The DPPH free radical scavenging activity of digested L_{100} and L/F_{100} were similar (Figure 4). Laminarin is resistant to digestion in the upper GIT including acidic and enzymatic hydrolysis [46]. Salyers *et al.* [47] established two different types of enzymes (laminarases and β-glucosidases) were essential to fully degrade laminarin and were only synthesised after 4–6 h of incubation in the presence of the inducer. In the present study, the lack of suitable enzymes to break down laminarin in the *in vitro* digestion model used may explain the lack of enhanced antioxidant activity post digestion.

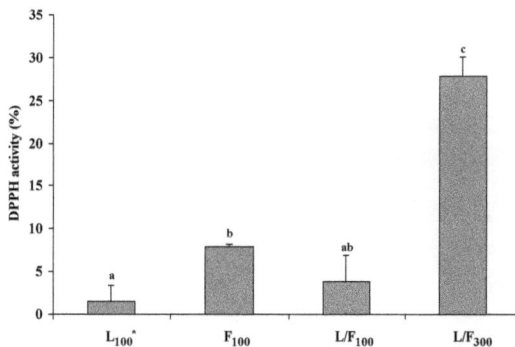

Figure 4. Free radical scavenging activity (DPPH) of L, F or L/F in digested cooked minced *longissimus thoracis et lumborum* (LTL) pork muscle stored for 20 h at ~20 °C. * Subscripts 100 and 300 denote concentrations in mg/g. [abc] Mean values (± standard deviation error bars) bearing different superscripts are significantly different, $p < 0.05$.

F_{100} and L/F_{300} significantly ($p < 0.05$) enhanced the DPPH free radical scavenging activity of cooked minced LTL post digestion. A few fucan-degrading enzymes have been obtained from marine bacteria and molluscs, however complete enzymatic breakdown has not been reported. The presence of sulphate groups attached to fucoidan has been postulated as a reason for resistance to enzymatic breakdown during digestion. The retention of the sulphate groups during digestion results in high ionic exchange capacities such as the binding of bile salts and scavenging of free radicals throughout the GIT before potential absorption [48]. The enhanced DPPH radical scavenging activity of F_{100} and L/F_{300} in cooked minced LTL, in the present study, may be due to the retention of the sulphate groups throughout the *in vitro* digestion procedure.

The DPPH free radical scavenging activity of digested L/F_{300} was significantly ($p < 0.05$) greater than F_{100}. Fucoidan may be partially responsible for the scavenging activity of the extract. The synergistic effect between components in the L/F extract, such as protein and mannitol, could have contributed to the observed enhanced free radical scavenging activity in cooked minced LTL post digestion. Antioxidant activity, post-digestion, of bioactive peptides extracted from seaweeds has been reported previously [49]. Mannitol is frequently considered as a reference for carbohydrate-type antioxidants due to its established scavenging abilities [24]. Additionally, MRPs formed during cooking may have enhanced the DPPH free radical scavenging activity of L/F_{300} post digestion.

2.6. Bioaccessibility of Seaweed Polysaccharides in Pork Meat after Incubation with Caco-2 Cells

The aqueous fraction of the control and L/F_{300} digestates was incubated with Caco-2 cells for 4 and 20 h to determine the bioaccessibility of L/F post digestion. The DPPH free radical scavenging activity of L/F_{300}, post digestion, was 56.49% higher than the meat control. Following incubation of the control and L/F_{300} digestates with Caco-2 cells for 4 and 20 h, the DPPH free radical scavenging activity of L/F_{300} was 12.34% and 19.85% higher than the meat control, respectively. The reduction in the DPPH free radical scavenging activity indicated theoretical uptake of some compounds with antioxidant activity. Therefore theoretical cellular uptake of seaweed polysaccharides was 44.15% and 36.63% (DPPH free radical scavenging activity) after incubation with Caco-2 cells at 4 and 20 h, respectively. Similarly, Soler-Rivas *et al.* [50] reported a decrease in ABTS free radical activity after digested grilled mushrooms were incubated with Caco-2 cells. Previously reported studies indicated that seaweed polysaccharides can be, to some extent, absorbed into the blood stream post digestion; however metabolism of these components after absorption has not been established [1]. Antioxidant compounds from L/F_{300} not absorbed through the intestinal wall would potentially be available to scavenge free radicals or be fermented by colonic bacteria and contribute to the overall antioxidant defence system of the GIT [1,51]. Further research is necessary to determine the fate of antioxidant compounds after absorption.

3. Experimental Section

3.1. Reagents

All chemicals used were "AnalaR" grade obtained from Sigma-Aldrich Ireland Ltd., Arklow, Co. Wicklow, Ireland and Merck KGaA, Darmstadt, Germany. Tissue culture plastics were supplied by Sarstedt, Wexford, Ireland and the Caco-2 cell line (Human Caucasian colon adenocarcinoma) were from the European Collection of Animal Cell Cultures, Wiltshire, UK. Fresh pork meat (*longissimus thoracis et lumborum* (LTL)) was supplied by Ballyburden Meat Processors, Ballincollig, Co. Cork, Ireland. Laminarin (L) (MW = 13 kDa) and fucoidan (F) (MW = 57 kDa) standards from Sigma-Aldrich were isolated from *Laminaria digitata* and *Fucus vesiculosus*, respectively. A spray-dried seaweed extract (L/F), containing laminarin and fucoidan was manufactured by Bioatlantis, Tralee, Co. Kerry, Ireland. The extract isolated from brown seaweed (*Laminaria digitata*) was prepared using an acid extraction technique, details of which are industrially-confidential. The extract contained 0.64% protein, 9.3% laminarin, 7.8% fucoidan, and 8.3% mannitol and further details are reported in Moroney *et al.* [15].

3.2. Measurement of the DPPH Free Radical Scavenging Activities of Seaweed Polysaccharides (L, F and L/F)

The 1,1-diphenyl-2-picrylhydrazyl (DPPH) free radical scavenging activity of L, F and L/F was measured using the method of Qwele *et al.* [52] with slight modifications. DPPH (0.2 mM, 3 mL) in methanol was added to 3 mL of L (1 and 10 mg/mL; L_1 and L_{10}), F (1 mg/mL; F_1) and L/F (1 and 3 mg/mL; L/F_1 and L/F_3). Trolox C (1 mg/mL; Trolox), was used as a positive control. Tubes were mixed and incubated for up to 20 h at room temperature (~20 °C) in the dark. The assay control contained 3 mL distilled water and 3 mL of DPPH solution. Absorbance measurements were recorded spectrophotometrically (Cary 300 Bio, UV-Vis spectrophotometer, Varian Instruments, Palo Alto, CA,

USA) against a distilled water blank after 1, 4 and 20 h at 517 nm. The DPPH free radical scavenging activity, expressed as a percentage of the assay control was calculated as follows:

$$\% \text{ inhibition of DPPH} = [1 - (\text{absorbance of sample}/\text{absorbance of assay control})] \times 100 \quad (1)$$

3.3. The Effect of Seaweed Polysaccharides on Lipid Oxidation in Pork Muscle Homogenates

Pork homogenates (25% w/v) were prepared by homogenising LTL (70 g) in buffer (210 mL) (0.12 M KCL 5 mM histidine, pH 5.5) on ice using an Ultra-turrax T25 homogeniser. L, F and L/F were solubilised in distilled water and added to LTL homogenates at final concentrations of 3 and 6 mg/mL (L_3, L_6, F_3, F_6, L/F_3 and L/F_6) homogenate. Lipid oxidation in muscle homogenate samples (20 g) held at 4 °C was initiated by the addition of 45 μM $FeCl_3$/sodium ascorbate (1:1). Muscle homogenates with and without $FeCl_3$/sodium ascorbate and without antioxidants (L, F and L/F) were run simultaneously as controls with each experiment. Lipid oxidation measurements were measured after 4 h in samples held at 4 °C.

Measurement of Lipid Oxidation in Pork Muscle Homogenates

A modification of the 2-thiobarbituric acid (TBA) assay of Siu & Draper [53] was used to measure lipid oxidation in pork muscle (LTL) homogenates. Homogenate samples (4 mL) were added to 4 mL 10% trichloroacetic acid (TCA) and centrifuged (Beckman J2-21, Beckman Instruments Inc., Brea, CA, USA) at 6160× *g* for 15 min at 4 °C. Following centrifugation, the supernatant was filtered through Whatman No. 1 filter paper. In a screw cap test tube, the clear filtrate (4 mL) was added to 0.06 M TBA reagent (1 mL) and incubated at 80 °C for 90 min. The absorbance of the resulting coloured complex was measured using a spectrophotometer (Cary 300 Bio) at 532 nm against a blank containing buffer (2 mL, 0.12 M KCL 5 mM histidine, pH 5.5), 10% TCA (2 mL) and 0.06 M TBA reagent (1 mL). Results were expressed directly as absorbance values at 532 nm.

3.4. The Effect of Seaweed Polysaccharides on Oxymyoglobin Oxidation

3.4.1. Preparation of Commercial Oxymyoglobin

Commercial horse heart oxymyoglobin (OxyMb) was prepared according to a modification of the method of Brown & Mebine [54]. Metmyoglobin (MetMb) (0.06 g) was dissolved in ice-cold distilled water (2 mL) to a concentration of 30 mg/mL and reduced to OxyMb by the addition of sodium dithionite at 1 mg/mL. To remove excess dithionite, OxyMb solution (2 mL) was applied to a glass column (2 cm i.d. × 25 cm) containing 10 g of mixed bed ion exchange resin (Amberlite MB-1A) and eluted from the column with approximately 20 mL cold distilled water. The OxyMb solution was passed through the column three times to reduce the conductivity to that of distilled water and was adjusted to a final volume of 50 mL with double strength buffer (300 mM KH_2PO_4-KOH, pH 5.5). The concentration of OxyMb in the final solution was calculated from its absorbance value at 525 nm divided by a millimolar extinction coefficient of 7.6 $mM^{-1} \cdot cm^{-1}$ [55].

3.4.2. Effect of Seaweed Polysaccharides on Oxymyoglobin Oxidation

Incubates (7 mL) containing OxyMb (~1 mg/mL) and L, F and L/F at two levels (0.1 and 1 mg/mL; $L_{0.1}$, L_1, $F_{0.1}$, F_1, $L/F_{0.1}$ and L/F_1) in 150 mM KH_2PO_4-KOH, pH 5.5, were prepared. Distilled water was used to prepare seaweed polysaccharide solutions (20 mg/mL). Additions to each OxyMb incubate were at a final concentration of 5% (v/v). Incubates were held at 4 °C and OxyMb oxidation was measured on days 0, 4 and 8 of storage.

Following centrifugation at 6160× *g* for 10 min at 4 °C, the absorbance spectra of the incubates (2 mL) containing commercial OxyMb were measured on a spectrophotometer (Cary 300 Bio) and spectral scans were recorded from 750 to 500 nm. The relative proportion of OxyMb (% of total myoglobin) was calculated using absorbance measurements at selected wavelengths (572, 565, 545 and 525 nm) as described by Krzywicki [55].

3.5. Effect of Cooking on DPPH Free Radical Scavenging Activity of Seaweed Polysaccharides in Pork Meat

Fresh minced LTL was assigned to one of five treatments: untreated pork (Control), L (100 mg/g pork; L_{100}), F (100 mg/g; F_{100}), L/F (100 mg/g; L/F_{100}) and L/F (300 mg/g; L/F_{300}). The levels of L, F and L/F added to fresh minced LTL were based on the DPPH free radical scavenging activities of the seaweed polysaccharides determined in Section 2.2. L, F and L/F were dissolved in water, immediately added to fresh minced LTL (5% v/w) and mixed vigorously. Minced LTL (1 g portion) from each treatment was retained for measurement of DPPH free radical scavenging activity of fresh minced LTL prior to cooking. The remaining fresh LTL (5 g portions) of each treatment were placed on aluminium foil lined trays and cooked at 180 °C for 5 min 30 s in a fan-assisted convection oven (Zanussi Professional, Model 10 GN1/1, Conegliano, Italy) until an internal temperature of 72 °C was reached.

Fresh and cooked minced LTL (1 g) were homogenised in 0.05 M phosphate buffer (9 mL), pH 7, using an Ultra Turrax T25 homogeniser and homogenates were centrifuged (Beckman J2-21) at 7800× g for 10 min at 4 °C. The supernatant fraction obtained (fresh/cooked minced LTL) was used for the measurement of the DPPH free radical scavenging activity [52]. DPPH (0.2 mM, 3 mL) prepared in methanol was added to 0.3 mL supernatant and 2.7 mL distilled water. The mixture was vortexed and left to stand at room temperature (~20 °C) in the dark. The assay control contained 0.3 mL phosphate buffer and 2.7 mL distilled water and 3 mL of DPPH solution. The absorbance of the solution was measured against a distilled water blank after 1, 4 and 20 h at 517 nm. The scavenging activity of the pork meat against the DPPH radical before and after cooking was expressed as a percentage of the assay control and calculated as:

$$\% \text{ inhibition of DPPH} = [1 - (\text{absorbance of sample/absorbance of assay control})] \times 100 \quad (2)$$

3.6. Effect of in Vitro Digestion on the DPPH Free Radical Scavenging Activity of Seaweed Polysaccharides in Cooked Pork Meat

The *in vitro* digestion procedure was adapted from that previously described by Daly *et al.* [56]. All experimental work was carried out in UV-light free conditions to reduce the possible photo-decomposition of L, F and L/F present in the cooked minced LTL. Briefly, cooked minced LTL (1 g) from each treatment were weighed into 100 mL plastic tubes and homogenized using an Ultra Turrax T25 homogeniser at 24,000 rpm for 10 s in 8 mL Hanks Balance Salts Solution (HBSS) containing BHT. HBSS (5 mL) was slowly pipetted down the homogeniser to rinse remaining residue into the plastic tubes. The homogenates were transferred into amber bottles (rinsed twice using 5 mL HBSS). In order to mimic the gastric phase of digestion, pepsin (1 mL) (0.04 g/mL in 0.1 N HCl) and HBSS (2 mL) was added and the pH was adjusted to 2 using 1 M HCl. Oxygen was displaced by blowing nitrogen over the samples for 5 s. Samples were then incubated at 37 °C for 1 h in an orbital shaking (95 rpm) water bath (Grant OLS200, Keison Products; Essex, UK).

After gastric digestion, the pH was increased to 5.3 using sodium carbonate (0.9 M NaHCO$_3$) followed by the addition of 200 µL bile salts (1.2 mg/mL glycodeoxycholate, 0.8 mg/mL taurocholate and 1.2 mg/mL taurodeoxycholate) and 100 µL pancreatin (0.08 g/mL HBSS). Subsequently, the pH was increased to 7.4 using NaOH, oxygen was displaced by nitrogen and samples were incubated at 37 °C in the orbital shaking water bath for a further 2 h. Following intestinal digestion, the digested minced LTL (digestates) from each treatment were centrifuged (Beckman J2-21) at 7800× g for 10 min at 4 °C. Undigested minced LTL samples were diluted using HBSS to the same final volume as the digestates and subsequently centrifuged at 7800× g for 10 min at 4 °C.

The supernatant (aqueous fractions) of the undigested minced LTL and digestate samples were frozen at −80 °C until required for measurement of DPPH free radical scavenging activity (described in Section 3.5). The assay control contained 0.3 mL HBSS buffer and 2.7 mL distilled water and 3 mL of DPPH solution. The absorbance of the solution was measured against a distilled water blank after 1, 4 and 20 h at 517 nm. The scavenging activity of the pork meat against DPPH radical post digestion was corrected for the meat control and expressed as:

$$\% \text{ inhibition of DPPH} = [(1 - (Ab_{sample}/Ab_{ac})) \times 100] - [(1 - (Ab_{meatcontrol}/Ab_{ac})) \times 100] \quad (3)$$

where Ab_{sample} = absorbance of sample; Ab_{ac} = absorbance of assay control; $Ab_{meatcontrol}$ = absorbance of meat control.

3.7. Bioaccessibility and Theoretical Cellular Uptake of the Aqueous Fraction of Digested Minced LTL

Caco-2 cells were maintained in Dulbecco's modified Eagle's medium (DMEM), containing 10% (v/v) foetal bovine serum (FBS) and 1% (v/v) non-essential amino acids. Cells were grown at 37 °C /5% CO_2 in a humidified incubator and were cultured with 0.5% Penicillin-Streptomycin (5000 U/mL). Cultures of Caco-2 cells were used between passages 46–51. To establish the Caco-2 intestinal model, the cells were seeded at a density of 6×10^4 cells cm^{-2} on a transwell plate (12-well plate, 22 mm diameter, 0.4 µm pore size membrane). Media was changed every 2–3 days and experiments were performed when monolayers were 17–20 days post-confluency. The aqueous fraction of the digestates (control and L/F$_{300}$) (125 µL) were diluted to a final volume of 500 µL with serum free media and added to the top chamber of the transwell plate. Serum free media (1 mL) was added to the basolateral chamber and the cells were incubated for 4 and 20 h. Preliminary work showed that the aqueous fraction of the digestates was not toxic to the cells (data not shown). The transepithelial electrical resistance (Millicell-ERS, Millipore, Cork, Ireland) was measured before and after the addition of the aqueous fraction of the digestates to ensure the monolayer remained intact. The media from the basolateral chamber was then harvested for the measurement of the DPPH free radical scavenging activity (see Section 3.5).

The assay control contained 0.3 mL serum free media and 2.7 mL distilled water and 3 mL of DPPH solution. The absorbance of the solution was measured against a distilled water blank after 4 h at 517 nm. The difference between the DPPH free radical scavenging activities of L/F$_{300}$ and the control, expressed as a percentage of the control, was calculated for the aqueous fraction of the digestate (AF) and the transwell basolateral chamber media (TW) as follows:

$$\% \text{ theoretical cellular uptake of antioxidant compounds} = [(AF_{L/F300} - AF_{meatcontrol})/AF_{meatcontrol}) \times 100] \quad (4)$$
$$- [(TW_{L/F300} - TW_{meatcontrol})/TW_{meatcontrol}) \times 100]$$

where $AF_{L/F300}$ = absorbance of aqueous fraction of the digestate L/F$_{300}$; $AF_{meatcontrol}$ = absorbance of aqueous fraction of the digestate meat control; $TW_{L/F300}$ = absorbance of transwell basolateral chamber media following incubation of L/F$_{300}$ with Caco-2 cells; $TW_{meatcontrol}$ = absorbance of transwell basolateral chamber media following incubation of the meat control with Caco-2 cells. The difference in activity between AF and TW was attributed to theoretical uptake of antioxidant compounds by the Caco-2 cells.

3.8. Statistical Analysis

Each experiment was carried out three individual times. All analyses were performed in duplicate. The DPPH free radical scavenging activities of L, F and L/F, fresh and cooked LTL pork muscle, cooked LTL digestates and lipid oxidation mean values were analysed by one-way ANOVA. Means were considered significantly different at ($p < 0.05$) using Tukey's post hoc test. A full repeated measures ANOVA was conducted to investigate the effects of L, F and L/F concentration and time on oxymyoglobin oxidation. L, F and L/F represented the "between-subjects" factor and the effect of time was measured using the "within-subjects" factor. Tukey's test was used to adjust for multiple comparisons between treatment means ($p < 0.05$). All analysis was carried out using the SPSS 18.0 for Windows (SPSS, Chicago, IL, USA) software package.

4. Conclusions

Due to the presence of sulphate groups and anionic charge, fucoidan is a more potent free radical scavenging antioxidant than laminarin. Furthermore fucoidan is at least, in part, responsible for the antioxidant activity observed by the L/F extract in previous studies. Fucoidan may be a potential natural antioxidant to enhance lipid stability in meat products. The antioxidant potential of fucoidan and the L/F extract is strongly influenced by the cooking and digestion processes. The L/F extract demonstrated superior antioxidant activity compared to fucoidan in minced LTL, after cooking and post digestion. The antioxidant compounds of the L/F extract were partially absorbed by Caco-2 cells confirming their bioaccessibility post digestion. Results demonstrate the potential for extracts containing fucoidan to enhance antioxidant activity of functional cooked meat products as well as contribute to human antioxidant defence systems.

Acknowledgments: This project (Grant-Aid Agreement No. MFFRI/07/01) is carried out under the Sea Change Strategy with the support of the Marine Institute and the Department of Agriculture, Food and the Marine, funded under the National Development Plan 2007–2013.

Author Contributions: Experiments were designed by N.M., M.O'G., S.L., C.S. and J.K., and conducted by N.M. and S.L. (cell culture work). All authors contributed to the analysis and interpretation of experimental data and the writing and review of the manuscript.

Conflicts of Interest: The authors declare no conflict of interest.

References

1. Holdt, S.L.; Kraan, S. Bioactive compounds in seaweed: Functional food applications and legislation. *J. Appl. Phycol.* **2011**, *23*, 543–597. [CrossRef]
2. Ngo, D.H.; Wijesekara, I.; Vo, T.S.; van Ta, Q.; Kim, S.K. Marine food-derived functional ingredients as potential antioxidants in the food industry: An overview. *Food Res. Int.* **2011**, *44*, 523–529. [CrossRef]
3. Devillé, C.; Damas, J.; Forget, P.; Dandrifosse, G.; Peulen, O. Laminarin in the dietary fibre concept. *J. Sci. Food Agric.* **2004**, *84*, 1030–1038. [CrossRef]
4. Choi, J.I.; Kim, H.J.; Lee, J.W. Structural feature and antioxidant activity of low molecular weight laminarin degraded by gamma irradiation. *Food Chem.* **2011**, *129*, 520–523. [CrossRef]
5. Anastyuk, S.D.; Shevchenko, N.M.; Dmitrenok, P.S.; Zvyagintseva, T.N. Structural similarities of fucoidans from brown algae *Silvetia babingtonii* and *Fucus evanescens*, determined by tandem MALDI-TOF mass spectrometry. *Carbohydr. Res.* **2012**, *358*, 78–81. [CrossRef] [PubMed]
6. Ustyuzhanina, N.E.; Bilan, M.I.; Ushakova, N.A.; Usov, A.I.; Kiselevskiy, M.V.; Nifantiev, N.E. Fucoidans: Pro- or antiangiogenic agents? *Glycobiology* **2014**, *24*, 1265–1274. [CrossRef] [PubMed]
7. Mak, W.; Hamid, N.; Liu, T.; Lu, J.; White, W.L. Fucoidan from New Zealand *Undaria pinnatifida*: Monthly variations and determination of antioxidant activities of fucoidan. *Carbohydr. Polym.* **2013**, *95*, 606–614. [CrossRef] [PubMed]
8. Kadam, S.U.; Tiwari, B.K.; O'Donnell, C.P. Extraction, structure and biofunctional activities of laminarin from brown algae. *Int. J. Food Sci. Technol.* **2014**. [CrossRef]
9. Gómez-Ordóñez, E.; Jiménez-Escrig, A.; Rupérez, P. Bioactivity of sulfated polysaccharides from the edible red seaweed *Mastocarpus stellatus*. *Bioact. Carbohydr. Diet. Fibre* **2014**, *3*, 29–40. [CrossRef]
10. Koleva, I.I.; van Beek, T.A.; Linssen, J.P.H.; de Groot, A.; Evstatieva, L.N. Screening of plant extracts for antioxidant activity: A comparative study on three testing methods. *Phytochem. Anal.* **2002**, *13*, 8–17. [CrossRef] [PubMed]
11. MacDonald-Wicks, L.K.; Wood, L.G.; Garg, M.L. Methodology for the determination of biological antioxidant capacity *in vitro*: A review. *J. Sci. Food Agric.* **2006**, *86*, 2046–2056. [CrossRef]
12. Machová, E.; Bystrický, S. Antioxidant capacities of mannans and glucans are related to their susceptibility of free radical degradation. *Int. J. Biol. Macromol.* **2013**, *61*, 308–311. [CrossRef] [PubMed]

13. O'Doherty, J.V.; Dillon, S.; Figat, S.; Callan, J.J.; Sweeney, T. The effects of lactose inclusion and seaweed extract derived from *Laminaria* spp. on performance, digestibility of diet components and microbial populations in newly weaned pigs. *Anim. Feed Sci. Technol.* **2010**, *157*, 173–180. [CrossRef]

14. Moroney, N.C.; O'Grady, M.N.; Robertson, R.C.; Stanton, C.; O'Doherty, J.V.; Kerry, J.P. Influence of level and duration of feeding polysaccharide (laminarin and fucoidan) extracts from brown seaweed (*Laminaria digitata*) on quality indices of fresh pork. *Meat Sci.* **2015**, *99*, 132–141. [CrossRef] [PubMed]

15. Moroney, N.C.; O'Grady, M.N.; O'Doherty, J.V.; Kerry, J.P. Addition of seaweed (*Laminaria digitata*) extracts containing laminarin and fucoidan to porcine diets: Influence on the quality and shelf-life of fresh pork. *Meat Sci.* **2012**, *92*, 423–429. [CrossRef] [PubMed]

16. Moroney, N.C.; O'Grady, M.N.; O'Doherty, J.V.; Kerry, J.P. Effect of a brown seaweed (*Laminaria digitata*) extract containing laminarin and fucoidan on the quality and shelf-life of fresh and cooked minced pork patties. *Meat Sci.* **2013**, *94*, 304–311. [CrossRef] [PubMed]

17. Elleuch, M.; Bedigian, D.; Roiseux, O.; Besbes, S.; Blecker, C.; Attia, H. Dietary fibre and fibre-rich by-products of food processing: Characterisation, technological functionality and commercial applications: A review. *Food Chem.* **2011**, *124*, 411–421. [CrossRef]

18. Rawson, A.; Patras, A.; Tiwari, B.K.; Noci, F.; Koutchma, T.; Brunton, N. Effect of thermal and non thermal processing technologies on the bioactive content of exotic fruits and their products: Review of recent advances. *Food Res. Int.* **2011**, *44*, 1875–1887. [CrossRef]

19. Gazzani, G.; Papetti, A.; Massolini, G.; Daglia, M. Anti- and prooxidant activity of water soluble components of some common diet vegetables and the effect of thermal treatment. *J. Agric. Food Chem.* **1998**, *46*, 4118–4122. [CrossRef]

20. Gawlik-Dziki, U.; Dziki, D.; Baraniak, B.; Lin, R. The effect of simulated digestion *in vitro* on bioactivity of wheat bread with Tartary buckwheat flavones addition. *LWT Food Sci. Technol.* **2009**, *42*, 137–143. [CrossRef]

21. Carbonell-Capella, J.M.; Buniowska, M.; Barba, F.J.; Esteve, M.J.; Frígola, A. Analytical methods for determining bioavailability and bioaccessibility of bioactive compounds from fruits and vegetables: A review. *Compr. Rev. Food Sci. Food Saf.* **2014**, *13*, 155–171. [CrossRef]

22. Hur, S.J.; Lim, B.O.; Decker, E.A.; McClements, D.J. *In vitro* human digestion models for food applications. *Food Chem.* **2011**, *125*, 1–12. [CrossRef]

23. Mirjana, M.; Jelena, A.; Aleksandra, U.; Svetlana, D.; Nevena, G.; Jelena, M.; Ibrahim, M.; Ana, Š.D.; Goran, P.; Melita, V. β-Glucan administration to diabetic rats reestablishes redox balance and stimulates cellular pro-survival mechanisms. *J. Funct. Foods* **2013**, *5*, 267–278. [CrossRef]

24. Tsiapali, E.; Whaley, S.; Kalbfleisch, J.; Ensley, H.E.; Browder, I.W.; Williams, D.L. Glucans exhibit weak antioxidant activity, but stimulate macrophage free radical activity. *Free Radic. Biol. Med.* **2001**, *30*, 393–402. [CrossRef] [PubMed]

25. Giese, E.C.; Gascon, J.; Anzelmo, G.; Barbosa, A.M.; da Cunha, M.A.A.; Dekker, R.F.H. Free-radical scavenging properties and antioxidant activities of botryosphaeran and some other β-D-glucans. *Int. J. Biol. Macromol.* **2014**, *72*, 125–130. [CrossRef]

26. Huang, D.; Ou, B.; Prior, R.L. The chemistry behind antioxidant capacity assays. *J. Agric. Food Chem.* **2005**, *53*, 1841–1856. [CrossRef] [PubMed]

27. Abu-Ghannam, N.; Cox, S. Seaweed-based functional foods. In *Bioactive Compounds from Marine Foods: Plant and Animal Sources*; Hernandez-Ledesma, B., Herrero, M., Eds.; Wiley & Sons Ltd.: Chichester, UK, 2014; pp. 313–327.

28. Yuan, Y.V.; Bone, D.E.; Carrington, M.F. Antioxidant activity of dulse (*Palmaria palmata*) extract evaluated *in vitro*. *Food Chem.* **2005**, *91*, 485–494. [CrossRef]

29. Zhou, G.; Ma, W.; Yuan, P. Chemical characterization and antioxidant activities of different sulfate content of λ-carrageenan fractions from edible red seaweed *Chrondrus ocellatus*. *Cell.Mol. Biol.* **2014**, *60*. [CrossRef]

30. Yan, J.K.; Wang, W.Q.; Ma, H.L.; Wu, J.Y. Sulfation and enhanced antioxidant capacity of an exopolysaccharide produced by the medicinal fungus *Cordyceps sinensis*. *Molecules* **2012**, *18*, 167–177. [CrossRef] [PubMed]

31. Schenkman, K.A.; Marble, D.R.; Burns, D.H.; Feigl, E.O. Myoglobin oxygen dissociation by multiwavelength spectroscopy. *J. Appl. Physiol.* **1997**, *82*, 86–92. [PubMed]

32. Kim, D.Y.; Shin, W.S. Characterisation of bovine serum albumin–fucoidan conjugates prepared via the Maillard reaction. *Food Chem.* **2015**, *173*, 1–6. [CrossRef] [PubMed]

33. Mulloy, B. The specificity of interactions between proteins and sulfated polysaccharides. *An. Acad. Brasil. Ciênc.* **2005**, *77*, 651–664. [CrossRef] [PubMed]

34. Varenne, A.; Gareil, P.; Colliec-Jouault, S.; Daniel, R. Capillary electrophoresis determination of the binding affinity of bioactive sulfated polysaccharides to proteins: study of the binding properties of fucoidan to antithrombin. *Anal. Biochem.* **2003**, *315*, 152–159. [CrossRef] [PubMed]

35. Imeson, A.P.; Ledward, D.A.; Mitchell, J.R. On the nature of the interaction between some anionic polysaccharides and proteins. *J. Sci. Food Agric.* **1977**, *28*, 661–668. [CrossRef]

36. Satoh, Y.; Shikama, K. Autoxidation of oxymyoglobin. A nucleophilic displacement mechanism. *J. Biol. Chem.* **1981**, *256*, 10272–10275. [PubMed]

37. Prabhasankar, P.; Ganesan, P.; Bhaskar, N.; Hirose, A.; Stephen, N.; Gowda, L.R.; Hosokawa, M.; Miyashita, K. Edible Japanese seaweed, wakame (*Undaria pinnatifida*) as an ingredient in pasta: Chemical, functional and structural evaluation. *Food Chem.* **2009**, *115*, 501–508. [CrossRef]

38. Kuda, T.; Hishi, T.; Maekawa, S. Antioxidant properties of dried product of "haba-nori", an edible brown alga, *Petalonia binghamiae* (J. Agaradh) vinogradova. *Food Chem.* **2006**, *98*, 545–550. [CrossRef]

39. Rajauria, G.; Jaiswal, A.K.; Abu-Ghannam, N.; Gupta, S. Effect of hydrothermal processing on colour, antioxidant and free radical scavenging capacities of edible Irish brown seaweeds. *Int. J. Food Sci. Technol.* **2010**, *45*, 2485–2493. [CrossRef]

40. Yoshiki, M.; Tsuge, K.; Tsuruta, Y.; Yoshimura, T.; Koganemaru, K.; Sumi, T.; Matsui, T.; Matsumoto, K. Production of new antioxidant compound from mycosporine-like amino acid, porphyra-334 by heat treatment. *Food Chem.* **2009**, *113*, 1127–1132. [CrossRef]

41. Bedinghaus, A.; Ockerman, H. Antioxidative Maillard reaction products from reducing sugars and free amino acids in cooked ground pork patties. *J. Food Sci.* **1995**, *60*, 992–995. [CrossRef]

42. Escudero, E.; Sentandreu, M.A.N.; Toldrá, F. Characterization of peptides released by *in vitro* digestion of pork meat. *J. Agric. Food Chem.* **2010**, *58*, 5160–5165. [CrossRef] [PubMed]

43. Chen, H.M.; Muramoto, K.; Yamauchi, F.; Fujimoto, K.; Nokihara, K. Antioxidative properties of histidine-containing peptides designed from peptide fragments found in the digests of a soybean protein. *J. Agric. Food Chem.* **1998**, *46*, 49–53. [CrossRef] [PubMed]

44. Saiga, A.; Tanabe, S.; Nishimura, T. Antioxidant activity of peptides obtained from porcine myofibrillar proteins by protease treatment. *J. Agric. Food Chem.* **2003**, *51*, 3661–3667. [CrossRef] [PubMed]

45. Sarmadi, B.H.; Ismail, A. Antioxidative peptides from food proteins: A review. *Peptides* **2010**, *31*, 1949–1956. [CrossRef] [PubMed]

46. O'Sullivan, L.; Murphy, B.; McLoughlin, P.; Duggan, P.; Lawlor, P.G.; Hughes, H.; Gardiner, G.E. Prebiotics from marine macroalgae for human and animal health applications. *Mar. Drugs* **2010**, *8*, 2038–2064. [CrossRef] [PubMed]

47. Salyers, A.; Palmer, J.; Wilkins, T. Laminarinase (beta-glucanase) activity in Bacteroides from the human colon. *Appl. Environ. Microbiol.* **1977**, *33*, 1118–1124. [PubMed]

48. Michel, C.; Macfarlane, G. Digestive fates of soluble polysaccharides from marine macroalgae: involvement of the colonic microflora and physiological consequences for the host. *J. Appl. Bacteriol.* **1996**, *80*, 349–369. [CrossRef] [PubMed]

49. Kim, S.Y.; Je, J.Y.; Kim, S.K. Purification and characterization of antioxidant peptide from hoki (*Johnius belengerii*) frame protein by gastrointestinal digestion. *J. Nutr. Biochem.* **2007**, *18*, 31–38. [CrossRef] [PubMed]

50. Soler-Rivas, C.; Ramírez-Anguiano, A.C.; Reglero, G.; Santoyo, S. Effect of cooking, *in vitro* digestion and Caco-2 cells absorption on the radical scavenging activities of edible mushrooms. *Int. J. Food Sci. Technol.* **2009**, *44*, 2189–2197. [CrossRef]

51. Palafox-Carlos, H.; Ayala-Zavala, J.F.; González-Aguilar, G.A. The role of dietary fiber in the bioaccessibility and bioavailability of fruit and vegetable antioxidants. *J. Food Sci.* **2011**, *76*, R6–R15. [CrossRef] [PubMed]

52. Qwele, K.; Hugo, A.; Oyedemi, S.O.; Moyo, B.; Masika, P.J.; Muchenje, V. Chemical composition, fatty acid content and antioxidant potential of meat from goats supplemented with Moringa (*Moringa oleifera*) leaves, sunflower cake and grass hay. *Meat Sci.* **2013**, *93*, 455–462. [CrossRef] [PubMed]

53. Siu, G.M.; Draper, H.H. A survey of the malonaldehyde content of retail meats and fish. *J. Food Sci.* **1978**, *43*, 1147–1149. [CrossRef]

54. Brown, W.D.; Mebine, L.D. Autooxidation of oxymyoglobin. *J. Biol. Chem.* **1969**, *244*, 6696–6701. [PubMed]

55. Krzywicki, K. The determination of haem pigments in meat. *Meat Sci.* **1982**, *7*, 29–36. [CrossRef] [PubMed]
56. Daly, T.; Ryan, E.; Aisling Aherne, S.; O'Grady, M.N.; Hayes, J.; Allen, P.; Kerry, J.P.; O'Brien, N.M. Bioactivity of ellagic acid-, lutein- or sesamol-enriched meat patties assessed using an *in vitro* digestion and Caco-2 cell model system. *Food Res. Int.* **2010**, *43*, 753–760. [CrossRef]

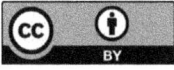

MDPI AG

St. Alban-Anlage 66

4052 Basel, Switzerland

Tel. +41 61 683 77 34

Fax +41 61 302 89 18

http://www.mdpi.com

Marine Drugs Editorial Office

E-mail: marinedrugs@mdpi.com

http://www.mdpi.com/journal/marinedrugs